Foundations for Integrative Musculoskeletal Medicine
An East-West Approach

Alon Marcus

D.O.M., L.Ac., D.A.A.P.M.

Foreword by

Michael L. Kuchera

D.O., F.A.A.O.

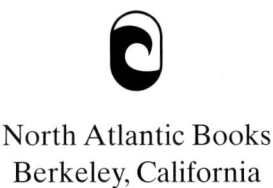

North Atlantic Books
Berkeley, California

Copyright © 2004 by Alon Marcus. All rights reserved. No portion of this book, except for brief review, may be reproduced, stored in a retrieval system, or transmitted in any form or by any means—electronic, mechanical, photocopying, recording, or otherwise—without the written permission of the publisher. For information contact North Atlantic Books.

Published by
North Atlantic Books   Book design by Alon Marcus
P.O. Box 12327   Cover design by Jan Camp
Berkeley, California 94712 Graphics by Joseph Marcus, Enrique Goldenberg, Puja Donak

Printed in the United States of America

Foundations for Integrative Musculoskeletal Medicine: An East-West Approach is sponsored by the Society for the Study of Native Arts and Sciences, a nonprofit educational corporation whose goals are to develop an educational and cross-cultural perspective linking various scientific, social, and artistic fields; to nurture a holistic view of arts, sciences, humanities, and healing; and to publish and distribute literature on the relationship of mind, body, and nature.

North Atlantic Books' publications are available through most bookstores. For further information, visit our website at www.northatlanticbooks.com or call 800-733-3000.

Note: Medical knowledge is constantly changing. As new information becomes available, changes in treatment, procedures, equipment, and the use of drugs become necessary. The editors/authors/contributors and the publisher have, as far as it is possible, taken care to ensure that the information given in this text is accurate and up to date. However, readers are strongly advised to confirm that information, especially with regard to medicine usage, complies with the latest legislation and standards of practice. Neither the publishers nor the author will be liable for loss or damage of any nature occasioned to or suffered by any person acting or refraining from acting as a result of reliance on the material contained in this publication.

ISBN-13: 978-1-55643-540-9

Library of Congress Cataloging-in-Publication Data

Marcus, Alon.
    Foundations for integrative musculoskeletal medicine : an east-west
approach / by Alon Marcus ; foreword by Michael L. Kuchera.
        p. ; cm.
    Summary: "An in-depth discussion of approaches to muskuloskeletal and physical medicine integrating Eastern and Western perspectives"—Provided by publisher.
    Includes bibliographical references and index.
    ISBN 1-55643-540-1 (hardcover)
    1. Musculoskeletal system—Diseases. 2. Medicine, Oriental.
    [DNLM: 1. Musculoskeletal Diseases—therapy. 2. Medicine, Chinese
Traditional—methods. WE 140 M322f 2004] I. Title.
    RC925.M33 2004
    616.7'06—dc22
                        2004023285

2 3 4 5 6 7 8 9   SHERIDAN   17 16 15 14 13 12

To my parents Joseph and Cila Marcus, my wife Ruth P Goldenberg, and my sons Sivan and Noam

Contents

Foreword xiii

Preface xv

Background and Acknowledgements xvii

1—FOUNDATIONS FOR INTEGRATIVE ORIENTAL MEDICINE 1
Essentials of Oriental Medicine 1

Basic Principles of Chinese Medicine: The Body Milieu 8

Qi 9

Blood (Xue) 14

Essence (Jing) 17

Fluids (Jin and Ye) 18

Yin and Yang 19

Disease Etiologies 22

Eight Principles (Ba Gang) 43

Five Phases (Wu Xing) 48

The Channels (Meridians/Vessels) (Jing-Luo) 51

Organs 81

Diagnosis 98

Typical TCM Intake Form 117

2—FOUNDATIONS FOR INTEGRATIVE PAIN AND PHYSICAL MEDICINE 123
Neural Mechanisms of Pain 125

Pain Mechanisms 136

Aspects of Pain 143

Pain Perception and Localization 150

Assessing Pain 155

Pain in TCM 159

TCM Treatments of Pain 161

3—FOUNDATIONS FOR TCM AND BIOMEDICAL ANATOMY, PHYSIOLOGY AND PATHOLOGY 165
TCM Classification of Soft Tissues 165

TCM Pathology and Etiology 167

Important Tissues: Biomedical Perspective 169
Joints 169
Muscles 172
Tendons 179
Fascia 180
Ligaments 180
Bone and Periosteum 180
The Spine 181
Normal Gait 196
A Systems Science Model For Biomechanical Construction 200

4—FOUNDATIONS FOR INTEGRATIVE ORTHOPAEDIC AND PHYSICAL MEDICINE ASSESSMENTS. 205
Reliability and Validity 205
The Diagnostic Process 207
Physical Examination 211
General Orthopedic Testing: Joints 222
Neurological Testing 232
Screening Examination 238
Laboratory and Technical Testing 243
Additional Tests 246
Imaging and Radiology 247
Imaging the Spine 252
Wrist Imaging 257
Ankle Imaging 257
Knee Imaging 258
Shoulder and Elbow Imaging 259

5—TREATMENT PRINCIPLES FOR INTEGRATIVE MUSCULOSKELETAL MEDICINE: ACUPUNCTURE AND DRY NEEDLING. 261
Acupuncture and Dry Needling 264
Acupuncture Mechanisms 267
Acupuncture Therapeutic Systems and Techniques 276
Main Channels 299

Connecting Channels/Network Vessels ... 299

Divergent Channels ... 300

The Sinew Channels ... 300

Extra Channels ... 303

Point Gateways and General Treatment Methods ... 304

6—ADDITIONAL ACUPUNCTURE SYSTEMS AND RELATED TECHNIQUES ... 333
Abdominal Assessment ... 333

Meridian Therapy (Keiraku Chiryo) ... 339

Auricular Therapy ... 343

Metacarpal Bone Systems ... 346

Wrist and Ankle Acupuncture ... 347

Korean Hand Acupuncture ... 350

Tong/Lee-style Acupuncture ... 350

Other OM and Related Western Therapies ... 368

7—FOUNDATIONS FOR INTEGRATIVE HERBAL MEDICINE ... 375
Chinese Herbal Therapy ... 375

Treatment of Blood Circulation ... 375

Commonly-Used Herbs In Painful Obstruction Syndromes ... 381

8—FOUNDATIONS FOR INTEGRATIVE ELECTROTHERAPUTICS ... 423
Bioenergetic Field Therapy ... 423

Introduction to Electromagnetic and Electrical Stimulation Therapy ... 430

Electroacupuncture ... 438

Static Magnetic Therapy ... 443

Laser and Photonic Therapy ... 447

9—INTEGRATIVE MANUAL THERAPIES, REHABILITATION, AND ORTHOSIS THERAPY ... 453
Massage/Manipulation ... 453

Western Manual Therapies ... 460

Osteopathic Medicine ... 460

Functionally Oriented Screen Tests ... 470

Osteopathic Treatment Methods ... 484

Manipulation with Impulse and Other Western Techniques 499
Additional Commonly Used Techniques 504
Rehabilitation and Exercise 513
The McKenzie System 526
Orthotics and Restraints 529

10—THE MANAGEMENT OF SPRAINS, STRAINS AND TRAUMA 537
Ligamentous Sprain 537
Muscle Strain 538
Treatment of Acute Sprain/Strain 539

11—MUSCULOSKELETAL DISORDERS: INTEGRATIVE PRACTICE 551
Inflammation 551
Three Phases of Degeneration 556
Joint Disorders 560
Ligamentous Disorders 579
Myofascial Disorders 584
Fibromyalgia and Myofascial Pain Syndrome 597
Nerve Disorders 632
Disc Disorders 638
Facet Disorders 646
Spondylolysis-Spondylolisthesis 647
Stenosis 648
Thoracic Outlet Syndrome 649
Whiplash 650
Mushroom Phenomenon 655
Iliocostal Friction Syndrome 655
Kissing Spine (Basstrap's Disease) 655
Periosteal Lesions 656
Scar Tissue and Interference Fields 656
Bursitis 657
Painful Obstruction (Bi) Syndromes 659
Perpetuating Factors 669
Medical Conditions. 681

REFERENCES ... 685
Works Cited ... 685
Works Consulted ... 710

INDEX ... 715

A NOTE ABOUT THE AUTHOR ... 751

Foreword

Through his text, *Foundations for Integrative Musculoskeletal Medicine: An East-West Approach*, Alon Marcus provides other healthcare practitioners (and the interested public) exactly what he seeks to provide for his patients -- **balance**. This is a balanced text. East meets west. Orthodox meets alternative. Somatic meets visceral. It manages to blend systems in a way that is useful to those who understand and value the concept of philosophic models.

The text provides a vehicle to transport understanding across professional degree boundaries and to introduce key concepts about the impact of the musculoskeletal system in diagnosis and treatment in a user-friendly fashion. Its even-handed overview of several healthcare systems welcomes readers with differing backgrounds to "come aboard" and comfortably absorb the new vistas presented without ever taking them too far from their respective homes.

Significantly more than a "how-to manual," this text offers insights built upon foundational concepts and promotes a deeper understanding of the many ways in which health may be encouraged. It interweaves practical advice with evidence-based data. It builds a foundation in one world while deftly bridging to another. It summarizes and encapsulates extensive specific data in tables that leave the reader free to grasp the concept being presented or the busy clinician to use as a time-effective resource.

In short, with this text Alon Marcus has made a major contribution to the healthcare field. He has deftly blended many of the best concepts and approaches offered by oriental, orthopaedic, and osteopathic medical practitioners into a vision of understanding the whole patient through the clues provided. The author doesn't promise nor force a single "integrative musculoskeletal medicine" approach upon us; instead, he delivers an excellent <u>foundation</u> to improve how we choose to practice. In this manner, I have become a better clinician and a better member of the healthcare community. What more can one ask for from a text?

Michael L. Kuchera, D.O., F.A.A.O.

Professor, Department of Osteopathic Manipulative Medicine Philadelphia College of Osteopathic Medicine
Director, Human Performance & Biomechanics Laboratory
Past President, American Academy of Osteopathy

Preface

Musculoskeletal complaints are very common and are often neglected by traditional Western medicine. As a result, many patients seek help from various "alternative and complementary" practitioners. Medical skills are best learned by apprenticeship, and no book can substitute for hands-on experience. Nonetheless, I have endeavored in this book to integrate several approaches that attempt to solve the many difficulties one encounters when treating pain patients. It is intended for clinicians interested in integrative medicine, that is, combining the best of both western and oriental medicine. It is all too easy to develop a myopic perception of health and disease when one is not exposed to a variety of models of medical perspective. Rather, I believe the ability to accurately diagnose and treat musculoskeletal and soft tissue disease is critically dependent on the ability to move fluently amongst medical paradigms, and doing so is the mark of a superior clinician. *Foundations for Integrative Musculoskeletal Medicine: An East-West Approach* covers basic principles of Traditional Chinese Musculoskeletal Medicine, Cyriax style Orthopaedic Medicine as well as traditional biomedical Orthopedics, Osteopathic Medicine, and "Bioenergetic" Medicine. These approaches are quite diverse, even antithetical in their view of pathophysiology, definition of health and disease, and strategy for diagnosis and treatment of those suffering from pain. Each of these methods has strengths as well as weaknesses – thus in my opinion integration often result in better outcomes. There have been many books written on these various models and approaches to musculoskeletal medicine. Few however attempt to integrate the body of information on the subject as well as discuss the possible limitations of each. In this text I have tried to do just that.

Traditional Chinese Medicine (TCM) is remarkable in that it is a complete system for medical diagnosis and treatment that has not only survived the millennia, but is as relevant today as ever. Treatment may consist of a wide variety of modalities from acupuncture to injection therapy, moxabustion, cupping, diet therapy, bloodletting, exercise regimens and physical rehabilitation methods, to a sophisticated scheme for the prescription of medicine in the form of herbal oral and topical formulae. Despite its lack of imprimatur from the Western medical mainstream and inadequate Western evidence base, the frequency of successful outcomes, the cumulative scientific evidence, and resulting popularity of TCM as a legitimate medical paradigm means it cannot be dismissed as only placebo. Its strength in modern times lies in its integrative view of the human body, and its low tech approach and lack of need for anatomical and/or physiological biomedical diagnosis. There is a great wealth of experience recorded over the past 2,000 years. However, even if one has the ability to read original texts, meanings can be misinterpreted due to the pictographic, multi-layered nature of the Chinese language. Compounding this is the difficulty of translation. Given the dilemma of language, the modern practitioner is further hamstrung by training via a model of education that was arbitrarily packaged as "TCM" during a time of political upheaval (which is slowly changing). While diagnostic and therapeutic tools available to the TCM practitioner are comparatively few, theoretical models abound. Numerous possible and all equally valid analyses of etiology are subject to the skill of the practitioner in applying them successfully. Therefore, there is high degree of inconsistency regarding diagnosis and treatment plans amongst practitioners, and outcomes are often diverse. Research is problematic in that the scientific model of randomized, double-blind, placebo controlled clinical trials compromises the basic tenet of TCM, that is, the individualization of treatment. Almost without exception, studies in the West have done a disservice to TCM by both compromising this basic tenet and by poor design. Insufficient frequency of acupuncture treatments and insufficient dosage of herbs are often problematic as well.

Cyriax style Orthopedic Medicine on the other hand is anatomically based and providers diagnose and treat specific anatomical lesions. The strengths of this system are the carefully thought out clinical assessments, the lack of reliance on imaging technologies which are often misleading, and the diverse treatment methods used. Cyriax used to say that all pain has a cause and therefore all treatments should be specific and appropriate to that specific lesion. Treatments used in Orthopaedic Medicine include massage, manipulation, injections, medications, minor surgery and exercise therapies. Lately many Orthopaedic Medicine specialists have expanded their use of "alternative" therapies. There have been many good clinical studies that verify the usefulness of Orthopaedic Medicine. The main weakness of Orthopaedic Medicine is the lack of organ systems integration within the diagnostic or treatment process. The lesion may have deeper, organ-based causes that may escape recognition.

Osteopathic Medicine may serve as a bridge between modern anatomically-based orthopedics and the more subtle, functionally oriented systems. Osteopathic methods integrate scientific principles, traditional medicine and manual medicine. While relying on modern anatomical and physiological principles, the practice of Osteopathic Manual Therapies is quite diverse and rely on individual skill and palpatory sensitivity. This has resulted in mixed clinical evidence with many positive and negative studies in the treatment of musculoskeletal disorders. As in Chinese medicine, Osteopathic methodologies are individualized, time dependent and tend to integrate the various systems of the body. There are many philosophical parallels between the two, some of which will be highlighted in the text.

"Bioenergetic" medicine is often used to describe therapies that rely on subtle and often scientifically controversial methods, and therefore may have little support in the literature. These include many of the bioelectrical systems for diagnosis and treatment, electromagnetic therapies, laser and photonic therapies and magnetic therapies. There is growing evidence for the clinical utility of some of these systems and they tend to be safe and not invasive.

Finally, as stated by Ken Wilber: "An integrally informed medical practice does not neglect the types of effective treatments that can or should be included in a comprehensive medical treatment. But all of that, truly, comes after the transformation of the practitioners themselves...An integrally informed medical practitioner is one who has let the most amount of the Cosmos into his or her mind, finds thereby the most potentials for health and healing and compassionate care, and brings the Big Mind to his or her practice in a way that inculcates both more confidence and more humility, all at once."

Alon Marcus D.O.M., L.Ac., D.A.A.P.M.

Background and Acknowledgements

When my schooling in Chinese medicine began in 1982, there were few schools in the US and acupuncture was not seen as a legitimate field of medicine. From the start of my training the emphasis was on herbal medicine while acupuncture was seen as secondary, especially when treating internal medical problems. This turned out to be quite fortunate as Chinese herbal medicine is much more difficult to learn. I would like to particularly thank C.S. Cheung M.D., L.Ac., and Yet Kai Lai L.Ac., for their teachings which gave me a good foundation in Traditional Chinese Medicine and herbology. I had the opportunity to increase my exposure to acupuncture by having been fortunate enough to study with Miriam Lee O.M.D., L.Ac. Dr. Lee was very generous with her teachings and exposed me to a totally different style of practice in her clinical setting. The majority of her acupuncture treatments were based on the Tong family style of acupuncture, and this greatly enhanced my appreciation of acupuncture. I would also like to thank Miki Shima O.M.D., L.Ac., for exposing me to and teaching me several Japanese style acupuncture systems. In 1985 I traveled to China where I did an internship at the Traditional Chinese Medicine Municipal Hospital in Guangzhou. During my internship I was able to visit many departments and was exposed to a wide variety of illnesses and their treatment using Chinese medicine. My interest at the time was in internal medicine and unfortunately I did not spend much time in the orthopedic department. However, I was very fortunate to be allowed to actually write herbal prescriptions under supervision, which greatly increased my confidence using Chinese herbs. This experience was greatly enhanced by the head of the internal medicine department, Dr. Zhang Jian Mei, who was my main teacher and to whom I am very grateful. Dr. Zhang increased my ability to understand Chinese pulse taking as well as to understand the Shang Han Lun. He was an adept practitioner of the Kidney and Purging schools and broadened my thinking to include these theories of practice. I would also like to thank Dr. Yang Gan Qian who exposed me to a family tradition of herbal medicine that uses mild formulas. Finally I would like to thank Fang Yao-hui, B.M., L.Ac., R.N., and Huang Guang chi B.M., for their indispensable translation and conversations throughout my stay.

The urge to improve my understanding of what can be offered to patients started early in my career when I realized that many of the methods I learned both in school and in China were palliative at best. While in China I had suffered an acute herniated disc and had first-hand experience being a patient; this only increased the desire to broaden my training. While my interest in varying approaches to medicine has evolved throughout the years, the seeds were planted on my first day of Chinese medical school by Dr. Cheung. Perhaps trying to support the use of Chinese medicine, Dr. Cheung reminded us that the reason there are so many pain pills on the market is that no one pill has been shown to work all the time. To me this message offered two deeper meanings, the first being not to oversimplify or blindly trust TCM as the ultimate and only way to practice medicine - to think critically; and second that there is a need for varying approaches to treat human suffering. While I have always been drawn to the specificity of Western medicine and studied it in tandem with what I was learning in Chinese medical school, my first few years of clinical exposure were exclusively to Chinese medicine. It was only my study in mainland China that truly impressed on me the importance of integrating modern biomedicine and Chinese medicine. As a matter of fact, every patient in the hospital was assessed by both TCM and Western methods and received a diagnosis from each. Treatment often integrated modern and traditional methods and I decided this to be the superior approach. When I returned to the U.S., I quickly realized that the majority of my patients were seeking treatment for musculoskeletal complaints. After several years of mainly having a Chinese medicine practice, in 1990 I had the good fortune of meeting Richard Gracer M.D., a Cyriax style Orthopaedic Medicine specialist. Dr. Gracer has been my mentor and friend for many years. He allowed me to take his courses as well as spend up to 3 days a week in his office for many years. This was my first exposure to Orthopaedic Medicine as well as prolotherapy, which also greatly helped my own low back pain. My Orthopaedic medical training has been greatly enhanced by the following individuals, to whom I owe a very great debt of gratitude: Thomas A. Dorman, M.D., Bjorn Eek M.D., Thomas H. Ravin, M.D., Stephen Levin, M.D., Robert Klein, M.D., Richard Derby, M.D., and my good friend Michael Brown, D.C., PA-C (M.D. student). Lenny Horwitz, D.P.M., has taught me the basics of foot biomechanics and orthotic therapy for which I am very grateful. I would also like to thank Len Saputo, M.D., for introducing me to the use of thermography and photonic therapy.

In 1991 I was introduced to Osteopathic Medicine via the American Association of Orthopaedic Medicine. My interest grew throughout the years and I was fortunate to study with Edward Styles D.O., F.A.A.O., Harriet Shaw D.O., F.A.A.O., Philip Greenman D.O., F.A.A.O., and Loren (Bear) Rex D.O. I would like to thank Fred L. Mitchell, Jr., D.O., F.A.A.O., for his helpful conversations and for allowing me to use illustrations from his texts. I would especially like to thank Michael Kuchera D.O., F.A.A.O., for his years of friendship and for supporting and encouraging my studies of Osteopathic medicine as well as his generous forward to this text. I would also like to thank William A. Kuchera D.O. F.A.A.O., for his generosity in allowing me to use so many of his illustrations in this text.

I owe a debt of gratitude to my father Joseph Marcus M.D., and my father-in-law Enrique Goldenberg M.S., M.B.A, both of whom created many of the drawings used in the book. Puja Donak improved many of my drawings. I would finally like to thank Richard Weissman L.Ac, Philip Cusick L.Ac., and Pamela Zilavy L.Ac., for their helpful reviews of the text.

1

FOUNDATIONS FOR INTEGRATIVE ORIENTAL MEDICINE

Essentials of Oriental Medicine

This text integrates several medical perspectives on musculoskeletal disorders. Many of the medical systems reviewed in this text, whether Western or Eastern, emphasize "holistic" approaches that take the patient's entire being into account. When the practitioner has attained a depth of understanding of these various systems, similarities among these approaches can be demonstrated even though each uses a different lexicon altogether. Integration of various approaches can increase the utility of each of these diverse systems.

This chapter covers *essential* principles of Oriental Medicine (OM) and is not intended to replace a basic text on the subject. Musculoskeletal disorders will be mainly described via OM principles, *biomedical* orthopedics (or Cyriax style Orthopaedic Medicine) and Osteopathy. In this text the term *Traditional Chinese Medicine* (TCM) is used to refer to modern *mainland-Chinese* style of Chinese Medicine, while OM refers to the diverse systems of medicine of the Far East that are based on Chinese Medicine.[1] The majority of ideas presented in this text are generally accepted *modern* Chinese Medicine/OM principles. However, some of the adaptations of these principles are novel. Most of information in this text combines: Chinese and Japanese materials; European perspectives on acupuncture; information this author has gathered throughout the years from lectures, teachers and a vast library of references (see "References" on page 685 and "Works Consulted" on page 710). It is important to understand that some of the westernized interpretations of OM are unique to the West and do not represent traditional Chinese writings or thinking. They do however exemplify the growth of ideas that have been influenced by both East and West, and may represent one possible future for "OM" practice. Table 1-1 lists a few of the thousands of important Chinese Medical texts and schools of thought, many of which are the bases of this text and of TCM in general.

Among OM methods, TCM may be the best documented. More standardized than historical Chinese medicine following China's Communist revolution, TCM is continuing a trend that started in the Song dynasty, or earlier,[2] to unify segments of existing methods. TCM is derived from the entire history of some twenty centuries of Chinese medicine and attempts to unify these segments by creating a *common theoretical framework* that can be used to categorize medical conditions into organized *diseases and their locations* (Bing Wei), *patterns* (Bian Zheng) *and pathomechanisms (*Bing Ji). The practice of Chinese Medicine has been summarized by the saying, "Bian Zheng Lun Zhi" which can be translated as: "The proposing of treatments based on the differentiation of patterns." It is important to understand that the modern version of Chinese Medicine (i.e., TCM) is strongly influenced by modern Western medicine, and much of the organization of the historic materiels is done to simulate biomedical thinking.[3] In TCM a "disease" is usually understood as manifesting with, and being caused by, diverse "patterns of dysfunction" and mechanisms that may be identical in different patients; more often, they are not.

---

1. There are many traditions of medicine in Asia, and some, such as Ayurveda from India, may have had a strong influence on Chinese Medicine.

2. It has been the general opinion that during the time of the "first emperor" (2698 BC), the theories of Yin-Yang, five-Phases, channels (for Blood and Qi), acupuncture points, Essence and Spirit were synthesized. This synthesis was first published around 221 BC in the *Yellow Emperor's Classic of Internal Medicine* (*Inner Classics*). However, the medical manuscripts found in 1973 at Mawangdui show that the early medical classics, especially the *The Classic of Internal Medicine*, which is revered as the "bible" of Chinese medicine, had not only been compiled much later than it has been commonly believed in the Chinese tradition, but also that the views represented in them (such as environmental factors effecting diseases, for example) could not have developed before the Han period (Galambos 1996, Unschuld 2003). The Mawangdui manuscripts, for example, do not mention acupuncture points. The *Classic of Internal Medicine* was probably compiled by many authors spanning many centuries. Galambos states that "regardless of their high esteem in Chinese tradition, almost everything about these classics is uncertain, especially their authorship and date." Unschuld states that we cannot be sure of what the classics meant in many cases, for example, even what they meant by the word "sinews" (Jin) is uncertain. According to Zhang and Rose (1995) significant standardization of Chinese medicine and education occurred during the Tang and Song dynasties. In the Tang dynasty, important texts appeared that integrated historical information such as the first comprehensive pharmacopoeia. During the Song dynasty, *standardized* editions of many of the Classics were printed, and consequently a more comprehensive and systematic theory on the causes and treatment of disease developed. At the same time, distinct schools of thought appeared, each with its own perspective on the diagnosis and treatment of disease. Finally, during the last of the Imperial dynasties (the Qing dynasty), many texts were written that updated and integrated much of the literature in Chinese medicine known at the time.

Conversely, two patients may have identical patterns (and visceral disorders) and yet suffer from different "diseases," both in biomedical and Chinese thinking. This essential difference between Western biomedicine and Chinese medicine must be understood. Perhaps the most striking difference is that modern (allopathic) biomedicine looks for "one disease-one cure," and treatment is often by searching for the "magic bullet" (i.e., lesion specific therapy). In OM/TCM no such emphasis is seen and treatment is often "systemic," rather then a disease specific magic bullet.[4]

Western medicine (biomedicine) and OM/TCM differ greatly in their approaches to, and understanding of, the human body. Western medicine for the most part is a reductionist, causal-analytic system that looks for the microscopic etiology of disease (Newtonian cause-and-effect). Even though the *World Health Organization* defines health as the physical, mental, and emotional well-being of a person, providing that person the ability to maintain a balance in life and participate in a fully active life to achieve the full potential of a human being, biomedicine often defines health as a "statistical norm."[5] Objectivity rather then "natural rationality" is emphasized.

Oriental medicine on the other hand takes a more qualitative approach, giving as much emphasis to historical and empirical experiences of physicians, to subjective feelings and thought, as it does to so-called quantitative objective data.[6] This may be compared to Aristotle's "natural philosophy," where all things and actions are considered to have a kind of inherent purpose and follow a simple "logic of observation."[7] In OM, emphasis is placed on the host (Zheng) and his/her reaction (behavior) to the disease (stresses and evils, or Xie), rather than on the so-called disease and its affected tissues; on human potential rather than the "norm." Disease is defined as an out-of-balance state between Yin and Yang (Ping or balance becoming Bing or disease).[8] Systems are viewed more as temporally complex relationships (including function, dysfunctions, and pathology) that change within time as compared to the anatomically and functionally fixed systems of modern medicine. This method allows for greater individual variation and flexibility. The *Classic of Internal Medicine* states:

Yellow Emperor asked: What constitutes a healthy person? Man has one exhalation to one pulse beat which is then repeated, and he has one inhalation to one pulse beat which is also repeated. Exhalation and inhalation determine the beat of the pulse. When there are five respiratory movements to one pulse beat, it means that there is one extra movement to one pulse beat, it means that there is one extra movement inserted, bringing about the deep breath of what is called a healthy and well-balanced person. A healthy and well-balanced person is not affected by disease...Those who are habitually without disease help to train and to adjust those who are sick, for those who treat should be free from illness. Therefore, they train the patient to adjust his breathing, and in order to train the patient, they act as an example.

The Systematic Classic of Acupuncture & Moxibustion states:

Those who are considered normal are without disease. Those who are without disease are characterized by a congruity of their *Mai Kou* (radial) and *Ren Ying* (carotid) pulses with the four seasons and by congruity [between pulses] in the upper

---

3. Much of what is called Chinese medicine is the Confucian (Han dynasty) version of historical medicine which by and large emphasized acupuncture as the main treatment modality. There are, however, other traditions within Chinese medicine and philosophy such as Daoism and their medical traditions. The Daoist tradition is not as well documented but has emphasized herbal medicine as the main therapeutic modality. In general, herbal medicine was and is the dominant modality in Chinese medicine.

    It must also be emphasized that Chinese medicine contains all the essentials of Kuhn's "standards" for what distinguishes "science" from "non-science," i.e., the existence of a basic theory and law, methodology, criteria, and instrumentation and techniques to apply and test the above. These however are often highly subjective.

4. In general, there are eight basic treatment methods (Fa) used in TCM: diaphoretics, dispersing, harmonizing, clearing, warming, tonifying, purging, and emetics.

5. Health in modern medicine is often defined as a bell shape curve. Many "discomforts" are considered normal because the majority of people report the same symptoms without observable pathology. In contrast, OM defines health as an ideal. However, the statement that Western medicine is reductionist and TCM "holistic/wholistic" is a great oversimplification. The consideration of statistical norms versus optimal health (and multiple causes and effects), is widely recognized by practitioners of *physiological medicine* (and many mainstream physicians) in the West as well. Many "nutritionally" oriented physicians use these ideas in their work and thus *individualized* therapies beyond the common allopathic biomedical model are prescribed. Osteopathic medicine is also systemic in its view where *optimizing* function is of major importance to both treat and prevent disease. Dr. A.T. Still, the founder of Osteopathy, says: "Basic principles must at all times precede each philosophical conclusion. Principles to an Osteopath means a perfect plan and specification to build, in form, a house, an engine, a man, a world, or anything for an object or purpose." Dr. Still saw the body as perfect (in the image of God), and therefore he thought that health can and should be optimized. In Osteopathy, life is believed to exist as a unification of *vital forces* and matter, and Osteopathy is said to rely on the law of mind, matter, and motion. Still was "keenly aware of the deleterious effects of environmentally induced trauma, or abrupt changes in the atmosphere, causing physical or emotional 'shock' or inertia, and therefore obstructing normal metabolic processes, body fluids, and nerve activity...His patient educational strategies highlighted *moderation* (as does OM)... He included advice for removing noxious or toxic substances from diet and environment, and behavioral adjustments such as adding exercises and stopping smoking...Each person is treated as a unique individual, not a disease entity." Normal function and practice is said to be dependent on the highly interdependent systems of body maintenance which are needed for optimal function. "These communication systems exchange substances via circulating blood and other body fluids and exchange of nerve impulses and neurotransmitters through the nervous system" (*OM: all of which are expressed as channels, vessels, Qi, Blood, Fluids, Nutrients, Essence, etc., in OM*). These show much philosophical overlap with Chinese medicine. Statements by Still such as, "look for health; anyone can find disease" sound quite similar to the writings of the ancient Chinese. Hulett and Downing trace the origins of various Osteopathic concepts to the philosophy and practice of medicine found in other ancient writings, such as those of the Prolemies, Brahmins, Chinese, and Hebrews (Ward 2003).

and lower parts of the body which are synchronous with one another.

As can be seen, the old classics advocated that the treating physician be healthy before treating a sick person. Health is monitored by *subtle* signs and not only by the absence of disease. When discussing the regulating effects of acupuncture, *Spiritual Axis* states:

> What are the symptoms [for which acupuncture is to be used]? The superior technique is to needle when the disease is not yet born. A secondary technique is to needle when it is not yet abundant. Following this is the technique of needling when the disease is already diminished. The lowest technique needles when the disease is in full attack, or when its appearance is abundant, or when the disease shows by the pulses being paradoxical.[9]

TCM/OM is *in part* a "holistic" method that evolved from the way body systems are *viewed* to affect one another and by the environment with great emphasis on *balance*. However, the concept of an innate healing capacity within humans and animals has not been part of historic Chinese medicine (Unschuld 2003). Healthy function (which may be attributed to automatic homeostasis in Western traditions) in Chinese medicine requires prompt intervention and proper behavior to prevent disharmony whenever imbalance is perceived. In discussing disease causes and treatments in the *Classic of Internal Medicine*, the Yellow emperor inquires as to why treatments that "seemed" to have worked during "antiquity"[10] do not work as well any longer, and Qi Bo answered:

> In high antiquity...people were strong...at the present time their shen (spirit) does not work...people's essence is ruined and their spirit is gone, the nutritive and Protective-Qi cannot circulate fully. And why is this? [Because] there is no limit to eating and drinking, and [people] worry ceaselessly. [Thus] essential Qi is ruined, Nutritive-Qi leaks out and Protective-Qi is lost, [and eventually] result in loss of spirit, and failure of the disease to be cured.[11]

This sense of perfection has prevailed in Chinese medicine and the *Yellow Emperor's Classic of Internal Medicine* as the *source* book has been referred to for virtually all of the important OM/TCM developments and commentaries in subsequent centuries. Therefore, TCM has been said to have "quasi-religious," mystical aspects (fundamentalist or revealed sources as opposed to information gained through research, Unschuld *ibid*). This *semi-fixed* nature of the various *canons* and *theories* that have characterized TCM from its beginning have had a defining role in how the medicine developed over the centuries. Paul Unschuld, in *Chinese Medicine: History of Ideas*, wrote:

> The common underlying conceptual basis of all these practitioners [those who were well-educated in the tradition] was exceedingly narrow, being limited to the acknowledgement of certain surviving works as classic texts and a belief in the fundamental truth of the central theories of the Five Phases and the all-encompassing dualism of Yin-Yang. But, even the interpretation of the universally revered classics, as well as the application of these theories to the concrete realities of daily life, gave rise to numerous contradictions, fragmenting the large community of private scholars and professional medical practitioners seeking solutions to health-related problems into countless individuals, groups, and traditions.

Consequently, developments and advances in Chinese medicine have not resulted in a basic *reinvestigation,* or in the *laboratory (research) style proof-or-disproof* of its principles (i.e., there has been no application of the core values of the modern scientific method). Rather, developments have emphasized further or novel applications within semi-fixed ideas. Therefore, when a traditional therapy has not worked (or does not), it is suggested that one consult the basic tenets (already written) to determine if an error has been made or a better approach is not available. Treatment failures are not attributed to any fundamental limitation in the traditional methodologies themselves, only to their incorrect application (Dharmananda 1999). The *Yellow Emperor's Classic of Internal Medicine* state:[12]

> The twelve Main channels and the 365 points (collateral vessels) are a [functional] feature that all humans possess. This is perfectly understood. Physicians use this knowledge for treatment. Therefore, the reason for an inaccurate diagnosis is that the physician's mind cannot concentrate. Their will and intention are not logical, causing the mutual interrelationship

---

6. On the other hand many scientific standards did exist in ancient China.

7. Aristotle's (384-322 BC.) natural philosophy can be described as a kind of "instinctive rational thought." For example, if an object is twice the size or weight of another, it should fall twice as fast when dropped (a belief that persisted in the West until Galileo's experiments around 1604). OM is very similar to Aristotle's philosophy in that "rational" observations are used to describe nature. Experimental testing has not been inherent in this medical system.

8. It's possible that, since automatic-healing (innate-healing) was not part of the Chinese construct, "successful" interventions were automatically credited for the healing. Thus, while TCM practice focuses on *process* (i.e., there is always a possible and appropriate intervention) Western medicine is "goal" oriented with an experimental emphasis. Chinese medicine pays more attention to process because a temporal (time and change related) emphasis is inherent in all Chinese medical theory.
   Homeostasis (Korr 2003) requires thousands of simultaneous dynamic equilibrations occurring throughout the body.

9. Obviously this is an approach that would not be acceptable in today's disease oriented environment. It does, however, show acupuncture to be a system used in preventative medicine.

10. The *Classic of Internal Medicine* (*Simple Questions*) is generally thought to have been written around 475-100 BC and is said to refer back to conversations between the "prehistoric" Yellow Emperor and his physicians. This and other sections suggest a process of mythication already occurring.

11. In the same text, the sages of high antiquity were said not to develop *abnormal diseases*. It is not clear, however, what an abnormal as compared to a normal disease is. Perhaps they still suffered from illnesses such as a common cold.

between the external and internal to be lost. This in turn causes the physician to experience dangerous disbelief and doubt.

Some newer developments were even viewed with disdain.[13] These views, however, were neither universal nor consistent, and there are many references to efforts by famous physicians to "correct or clarify" numerous mistakes or misunderstandings in the literature. There have even been official attempts to do so such as in the Song Dynasty by the "Imperial Bureau of Rectifying Medical Tests." Subhuti Dharmananda writes:

> ...the Chinese attempts at re-evaluation are usually philosophically based and argumentative: there is no well-established factual base for the opinion that has been rendered. Therefore, upon reading medical works, it becomes obvious that there is a lot of criticism, but not a conclusion to it: there is no evident consensus outside the basic tenet that practitioners must be humane and must pay attention to the performance of their craft. The continuing efforts to criticize and re-evaluate helps keep practitioners thinking about what they are doing, as opposed to allowing rote action on the basis of a past practice or allowing one's personal ambitions and problems get in the way of proper administration of medicine. The practitioner of Chinese medicine is expected to respect the past and turn to it for guidance, but not be blind to the current situation, which requires an attentive, and sometimes revised, application of the principles and methods of the past.

Oriental medical science views all life forms as being similar in "energetic essence" in sharing the vital forces of the universe.[14] The *Classic* of *Internal Medicine* states: "The principle of Yin and Yang is the way by which heaven and earth run, the rule to which everything subscribes, the parents of change, the source and start of life and death." Accordingly, all matter and life is affected similarly by natural forces such as windy, cold, and damp weather. Oriental sciences use these types of relationships to explain many activities in the universe, including human anatomy, physiology, and pathology. Many acupuncture points, for example, are named after astrological structures and phenomenon. Human anatomy and physiology, as well as the universe, are "centered" around pole stars, and have geographic meridians that have valleys, hills, seas, rivers, and function in relation to cycles of the stars and constellations. Therefore, to determine the cause of disease in OM, there is an attempt to integrate all natural processes and life's "movements" and their interactions with nature and social processes.[15] Irregular eating, irregular sleeping and waking, over taxation and mental pressure, unhealthy physical activities (including sexual), abnormal seasonal weather and cosmic influences, and even economic and political strife are said to lead to an unhealthy state and thus predispose one to disease. *(Biomedical: biomedical research concurs to some degree that environmental influences can effect pain. Cold and wet days make neuropathic pain [including complex regional pain, arthritic pain, myofascial syndrome pain, and pain from fibromyalgia] worse (Woessner 2003). Terms such as "frozen shoulder" and "catch a cold" are still used).*

As in Western medicine (and even more so), TCM recognizes that some bodily/Organ functions have both local and general/systemic effects. Many similarities can be demonstrated between biological/Western medicine and TCM, even though each is constructed from a distinct perspective and uses an altogether different language. Many of the systems that TCM describes are surprisingly similar to the current biomedical model (e.g., symptoms/signs related to an Organ/organ). Many of the relationships between Organ systems, bodily functions and Yin Yang relations (which sound ridiculous to the biomedicaly trained physician), can be demonstrated to have embryological bases (Lee 2002, Matsumoto and Birch 1988, Oshman 2000). As Unschuld points out in *Forgotten Traditions of Ancient Chinese Medicine*, there is no inherent conflict between the ideas of Chinese and biomedical medicine, and Kendall (2002) states: "As the story unfolds it becomes clear that the physiology of Chinese medicine is essentially the same as Western medicine."

Both Chinese medicine and modern Western medicine basically see two main reasons for the body's susceptibility to disease. The first is that the body, as the rest of the universe, is subject to natural laws. In modern medicine, these are the laws of physics, chemistry, and biology. In TCM the natural laws are the five Phases, (systems of correspondence), Yin Yang, etc. The second reason is the engagement

---

12. OM/TCM therefore can be described as a kind of traditionalist (or fundamentalist) system. "Truth" is said to have been mostly described in the past. Medical promise is placed in understanding the past rather then the future as seen in modern biomedicine. Because of the richness of treatment methods it is easy to do so, and to hope that a more skilled practitioner may do better ("secret" treatment methods abound as well). Therefore, there are an unlimited number of *potential* routes and methods within the larger matrix of Chinese medical tradition that can be pursued, vis-a-vis treatment.

13. As can be seen in Unschuld's translation of *Forgotten Traditions of Ancient Chinese Medicine*.

14. This view is also in agreement with the basic premise of *quantum theory* called the "superposition principle," which states that everything is related to, and connected with, everything else. However, in actual clinical practice, TCM/OM still groups symptoms and signs into syndromes (even though each pattern/syndrome is said to be individualized and thus treats the patient and not the "disease"). Treatment is said to change the specific values used to describe the syndrome. Therefore, the difference between modern medicine and TCM/OM is at times more conceptual than reflecting daily practice. The superposition of all phenomenon is also supported by DNA research as all life is constructed from similar base codes that may be affected by the environment. Another example of the interdependence of man and nature (and superposition) is the Kreb cycle: the sequence of enzymatic reactions involving the metabolism of carbon chains of sugars, fatty acids, and amino acids to yield carbon dioxide, water, and high-energy phosphate bonds. This energy producing cycle (ADP and ATP) is needed for plants, animals, and humans to function in a mutually interdependent ecosystem.

15. It is interesting to note, however, that most modern studies show that acute exposure to cold and wet environments do not increase the rates of flu or common cold infections in healthy medical students. At the same time, in TCM, environmental exposures are said to result in disease, mostly in patients with weakened immunity (antipathogenic-Qi).

Table 1-1: Chinese Medicine: Treatises and Medical Theories

TREATISE/MEDICAL BOOK	DATE
Book of Changes	7th Century BC
Yellow Emperor Classic of Internal Medicine (Simple Questions)	1-4rd Century BC
Spiritual Axis (part of Yellow Emperor Classic)	1st Century BC
Book of Difficulties	1st Century BC
Herbal Classic of Shen Nong (Divine Plowman)	2st Century BC
On Harm Caused by Cold	220 AD
Golden Chest Classic (originally part of same text as Harm Caused by Cold)	220 AD
Pulse Classic	285 AD
Miscellaneous Records of Famous Physicians	500 AD
Treatise On the Origins and Symptoms of Disease	610 AD
Nong's Newly Revised Materia Medica	659 AD
Prescriptions Worth Thousands in Gold	682 AD
Symptoms Arranged in Groups to Keep Man Alive	1108 AD
Cooling School	1200 AD
Purgative School	1228 AD
Discussion of the Spleen and Stomach	1249 AD
Clarifying Doubts about Injury from Internal and External Causes	1231 AD
Great Compendium of Acupuncture and Moxibustion	1601 AD
Teaching of Dan Xi	1481 AD
Compendium of Materia Medica	1593 AD
Yang Supplementation School	1640 AD
Pestilence School	1652 AD
On the Extraordinary Channels	1577 AD
Systematic Differentiation of Warm Diseases	1798 AD
Traditional Chinese Medicine (TCM)	Modern China

between the body's defenses and pathogens. In biomedicine this is the struggle between the immune system and pathogens. In Chinese medicine the engagement is between what is "correct" (Zheng, or Righteous) and evil (Xie).

Despite the similarities, it is important to note that the co-application or correlation of any OM/TCM with biomedical principle (or symptoms and signs) to each other must be viewed with great caution and skepticism. This includes many of the theoretical correlations discussed in this text. When and if combined clinically, they must be a beginning therapeutic consideration to be applied with great flexibility, always utilizing TCM logic.

Many modern TCM *pattern discriminations* (syndromes and diseases), especially as applied to biomedically defined diseases are hypothetical. In general, modern application of TCM pattern discriminations to a *biomedical disease* usually entails two main steps:

1. Identify TCM "disease" that seems to have symptomatic similarities to the biomedical disease in question (regardless of biological mechanisms).[16]

2. Analyze the possible clinical presentations of the biomedical disease (look at possible/common symptom sign patterns), and then apply TCM pattern differentiation and diagnosis from "recognized" TCM diseases.[17]

This process cannot differentiate between a symptom that occurs due to a functional disorder and one that is due to a specific tissue pathology; this is a strength of modern biomedicine.

The presumed overlap of symptoms, syndromes, and diseases can then be used to plan treatments. Although this may yield treatment strategies that have "logical" bases in TCM, treatment outcomes of biomedical diseases remain difficult to predict. Knowledge of biomedicine is important for safety as well as for prognostic assumptions. Nevertheless, this two step process can be helpful in assisting and leading the practitioner to a deeper understanding of the body systems and their relations to TCM logic.

TCM methodologies have been established as being useful (using modern research methods) for many maladies and diseases, including musculoskeletal conditions that affect humans and other animals as well. The *modern* TCM approach has both strengths and weaknesses. Examples of strengths are: texts are written more clearly and use less poetic language, euphemism and imagery; diagnosis and treatment are relatively standardized,[18] more consistent, often derived by consensus, *integrated* and flexible. However, the modern clinical relevance for many conditions has not been proven. Also, some "esoteric" systems that still may prove to be effective are said to have been purged from TCM. The integration of acupuncture practice and principles with the herbal traditions has been strongly criticized and has been referred to as "hebalized" Organ (Zhang Fu) TCM style acupuncture.[19]

The issue of the modern relevance of TCM is not new, for example in *On the Origin and Further Course of Medicine,* Hsu writes:

> Obviously, one particular illness can be treated not only with one particular prescription. Today, the name of an illness may still be quite similar to that [of an illness in ancient times], but the pathoconditions that appear in the course of this [illness today] may be very different [from those in ancient times], the drugs employed will not at all correspond to the [patient's] pathoconditions. Also, even though the names of [an ancient and a contemporary] illness may be identical, the manifestations of these illnesses may be in complete contrast. If the same prescription is used [today as in ancient times], all of its drugs will be contraindicated...past and present are on different tracks. Ancient formulas are not efficacious for new diseases.[20]

Despite these controversies and pseudo-weaknesses, within its own parameters TCM is comprehensive, logical, and inherently consistent.[21]

TCM sees the human body as a combination of vital *"energies"* (forces) and material substances that must stay in balance for health to be preserved. The bulk of TCM theory and practice is the description and manipulation of the functional relationships, *patterns of correspondences*, and quality of the body network of *channels, vessels, Organs, Fluids* and *energies*. This approach allows for a great amount of flexibility and treatment options.[22]

There has frequently been a tendency to assemble neatly woven and possibly linear connections in patterns of correspondences and other pattern discriminations ("root" causes of syndromes etc.), especially in the early days of Chinese medicine in the West, and usually with the promise that a single approach would cure all the symptoms. Many of this author's instructors have pointed out, however, that it is not always possible or correct to relate all symptoms and their development to a single "root." Patients often suffer from multiple and unrelated diseases that must be interpreted separately. These patterns, diseases, and symptoms may require "contradicting" treatment approaches for each to resolve.[23]

TCM Terminology

Chinese sciences use everyday language to describe the observable environment and to explain human physiology and pathology. Even though the same words are used in common language, however, their interpretation is a professional jargon, and untrained people, even if employing some of the same terms to describe symptoms and disease names, would not have any medical understanding of their meaning.

---

16. TCM diseases are often named after a symptom such as: abdominal pain, headache, fever, constipation, hemiplegia, jaundice, anger, etc. Others correlate to biomedical diseases such as: hemorrhoid, infertility, and worm infection. A TCM disease is then usually categorized by various possible *patterns* (syndromes) that are manifested as symptoms and signs, depending on the style of differential diagnosis used. However, TCM has also been aware of specific diseases (such as small pox for example) that affect all patients in the same way. In such cases the "disease" was often treated as compared to the patient "pattern" diagnosis (and many non-Confucian physicians have not used pattern diagnosis systems). There are many traditions within Chinese medicine that focus more on diseases and, according to Scheid (2002), from the period of the Han to Tang dynasties diseases rather than patterns functioned as the most important diagnostic classifications, as represented by the *Treatise Regarding the Origins and Symptoms of All Diseases*. Many modern TCM practitioners (especially in the West) insist that by treating the patient's pattern one treats the disease regardless of its biomedical name; a belief that abounds with problems. Also, while it is common to hear that "Chinese medicine differentiates patterns and Western medicine diseases; Chinese medicine treats the root while Western medicine only symptoms," these are great over simplifications as both TCM and Western medicines do both.

17. For example, headache, dizziness, numbness, tingling, and palpitations are often used to analyze possible *patterns* of hypertension, even though none are directly related to blood pressure. Atrophy, tremors, spasms, dysphagia, etc., are used for ALS. While for chronic renal failure, *diseases* such as lack of strength, anorexia, insomnia, and itching can be used. There would not be a mechanistic understanding which explains these symptoms, as they pertain, for example, to renal failure as apposed to another biomedical disease that causes similar *symptoms and signs*. For example, early Parkinson's disease and benign tremor may be viewed as the same disease even though treatment outcomes differ greatly.

18. In 1996 a Chinese national standard for clinical diagnosis and treatment terminologies was published.

19. Historically the tradition of acupuncture (a Confucian approach) and the herbal tradition (a more Daoist approach in part) have for the most part developed separately. At the same time, a report in 1992 stated that physicians of Chinese medicine currently employ more than one hundred different diagnostic systems with at least seven taught at state schools (Scheid 2002).

20. This paragraph also makes the point that proper differential diagnosis should be done on every and each patient. Thus, a thorough understanding of TCM/OM principles is essential.

A study of TCM vocabulary reveals an ordered system that describes complexes of symptoms and signs (syndromes) with terminology such as: *Vitality, Spirit, Affects, Soul, Essence, Qi, Blood, Fluids, Generating, Controlling, Excess/Fullness/Repletion, Deficiency/Emptiness/Vacuity, Stagnation/Depression, Obstruction, Veiling, Stasis, Wind, Wet, Heat, Fire, Warm, Cold, Phlegm, Water, Rheum, Pestilence, Worms, Food Stagnation and diseases, Poisons, and Toxins.*

Many terms in TCM have several meanings depending on context, and thus the argument has been made that one should read Chinese in order to understand Chinese medicine. The written Chinese language is such that words (images) are written in layered combinations of characters (radicals), often each with its own meaning. It is therefore possible to demonstrate, or conceive, of many layers of image-based interpretation. This, together with the fact that much of the classical literature was written in a somewhat cryptic and poetic format result in wide *interpretive* differences in meanings.[24]

TCM and Anatomical Terminology

The TCM anatomical model, which has been explained by reference to observable phenomena (including surgical dissection),[25] describes:

- A system of channels/meridians and vessels responsible for the circulation of "energy/air/forces/functions," Fluids, Blood, physical mobility, and other essential substances and nutrients.
- Organs that, when compared to the biomedical model, are somewhat different in function, shape, location and number. (However, the degree of similarity is surprising). The Organs' sizes, weights, lengths, connections with vessels, etc., are all described; however, these do not, for the most part, correlate with modern anatomy. At the same time, for example, the Heart is clearly described as being connected to Blood vessels. Classifications and locations, however, do not follow modern anatomical knowledge/classification; and the Spleen/pancreas, for example, is said to be on the right side and the Liver on the left side (although some have interpreted this to mean the practitioner side).
- Some structures are clearly described in anatomical terms, and different bones are given different names. For example, in the *Classic of Internal Medicine* (possibly being a later insertion) lower extremity bony anatomy is describe as follows (Unschuld 2003):

> Above the assisting bone, below the transverse [i.e., pubic] bone, this is the bolt bone. That which is on both sides of the hip bone is called the trigger (innominates?). The knee divide is the lower leg bone joint. The bone on both sides of the knee is the connection with the lower leg bone (lower femur?). Below the [connector] bone is the assistant [bone] (tibia?). Above the assistant [bone] is the knee bay (tibial fibular joint?). Above the knee bay is the joint. The transverse bone of the head is the pillow [bone] (patella?).[26]

Diagnosis (Zhen)

TCM uses differential diagnostic methods that involve grouping symptoms and signs in *patterns* (syndromes). These are often separate theories, or better, clinical tools, that apply to various clinical presentations and may not agree with one another all of the time.[27] Each theory is applicable for different clinical situations. For example, in an infectious disease of exogenous origin, one may use the Six-stages, Four-levels and Triple Warmer methods of diagnosis and treatment; in chronic insidious diseases, one may use the Organ/Bowel and/or the Qi, Blood, Fluid and Essence methods. The Channel and Connecting/Network-vessels (collaterals) differentiations may be used for localized disorders such as musculoskeletal disorders. In real life, of course, patients are complex, and disease mechanisms may overlap

---

21. There are many theories/methods in Chinese medicine, not all of which apply to all conditions or agree with one another at all times. Even the basic text that most of TCM/OM is based upon, *The Yellow Emperor Classic of Internal Medicine*, is full of contradictions (Unschuld 2003). The Chinese apparently never had the need for a "unifying theory," except for the absoluteness of Yin and Yang. It is the practitioner's job to know which theory applies to a patient at any particular moment. This is often difficult for Westerners to accept (for which Unschuld coined the phrase "cognitive aesthetics notion to contradictions.") Making the logic of TCM/OM even more diverse from Western "logic" is that these theories all have temporal (time dependent) aspects so that they are always relative as opposed to the fixed laws sought by most Western scientific pursuits.

22. It can also result in many varying systems and approaches as well as intertherapist disagreements and inconsistencies. It also makes the practice of TCM much more of an art than modern biomedical medicine, and, therefore, the practitioner's skill and style can lead to varying outcomes, a fact that needs to be considered when assessing modern research.

23. It is not uncommon to see orthopedic patients with Liver and Kidney Yin-deficiency (Organic dysfunctions that often relate to substance [actual tissues] and manifest with dryness, heat, degenerated tissues, etc.) and at the same time also have Spleen-deficiency (a condition of a hypofunctioning digestive system and often manifesting with symptoms related to coldness and Yang-deficiency), together with Stomach-Heat (often creating symptoms of mouth dryness, increased appetite [as apposed to decreased appetite seen with Spleen-deficiency], rapid digestion, etc.). Such a patient may not tolerate herbal treatment to his/her Kidney and Liver at the onset, which usually call for moistening and cloy (rich, greasy) herbs. One may need to treat the digestive system first so that the patient can tolerate as well as absorb the moistening herbs. This might be done by regulating Spleen and Stomach, harmonizing Spleen and Stomach, harmonizing Liver and Spleen/Stomach, tonifying Spleen, cooling Stomach, addressing Dampness or Dryness of the digestion system, food stagnation, etc., depending on each individual patient's symptoms and signs (which may constantly change and demand changing treatments). It is also important to understand that, for example, Stomach-Heat can easily affect the Kidneys because the Stomach moves downwards and may move too much Fluids to the Kidneys when hyperactive. This may cause excess urination that may be interpreted as Kidney-Yang/Qi weakness (a Cold condition) but which in fact is due to Stomach-Heat. Therefore, differential diagnosis in TCM is very complex and often subjective and open to disagreement. This also shows the difficulties one faces when designing a proper scientific study of TCM.

and mix. While both TCM and modern Western medicine use symptoms and signs to determine a diagnosis, in TCM the practitioner will ask questions and seek signs outside the patient's region or system of complaint. The integration of seemingly unrelated symptoms and signs makes TCM unique and holistic.[28] This text covers the orthopedic aspect of the pattern discriminations known as:

- Eight Principles.
  —Used to localize, stage, and characterize diseases. Can be used for most conditions.
- Five Phases.
  —Used mostly to describe balance, communication and control, environmental effects, and the transmission of disease within bodily systems as well as intervention effects via the body's servo systems.
- Organ/Bowel.
  —Used to describe the deepest structural and functional aspects of physiology and disease in the Organ systems. Often seen as describing the root causes of diseases.
- Channels, Connecting channels/Network-vessels.
  —Used mostly to describe localized or Exterior disorders (Wei) that have not affected the Organs (Zhang/Fu), and to describe vascular disease that can also have deep tissue and Organic effects.
- Qi, Blood, Fluids, Essence.
  —Used to describe disorders of the milieu (material basis of activities) of the body. Often used in combination with other methods such as Organ/Bowel.
- Disease Cause.
  —Used most often to describe endogenous (emotional), exogenous (environmental), and life-style causes of diseases.
- Six Stages/Levels.
  —Used to describe diseases caused by exogenous Cold, their location, depth, and progression. Also used to understand the effects of erroneous treatments.
- Four Stages/Levels.
  —Used to describe exogenous Warm-Heat (infectious) diseases, their location, depth and progression. Used also to describe the effects of hidden/lurking or retained pathogens.
- Triple Warmer.
  —Used most often to describe Warm-Heat, Summer-Heat, or Damp-Warm/Heat diseases. Can also be used to describe location of disease, communication functions and failure, and disorders of Fluid. Especially helpful in disorders with Yin-deficiency and Dampness.

The most difficult aspect of using the above theories/clinical tools is relating the classical (or modern Chinese) literature to what modern (Western) patients experience and communicate in a clinical setting. It is often necessary to interrogate the patient carefully and seek symptoms and signs Western patients are not sensitive to or aware of.

The following sections introduce the relationships among TCM principles, orthopedics, and modern biomedicine. (There is often an interplay between modern OM, TCM, and biomedical principles that this author believes only deepens one's understanding of the human body.) The integration of Chinese and Western medicine began in China in the 19th century by a group of physicians (Zhong Xi Yi Hui Tong Pai). In 1892, the text *Rudiments of Chinese and Western Medicine (Zhong Xi Yi Xue Ru Men)* was published.

Basic Principles of Chinese Medicine: The Body Milieu

In general, the body milieu is described as somatic structures, visceral Organs, channels, and vessels. There are substances that supply nutrients/functions (Ying/Jing) and Blood (Xue), defensive substances/functions (Wei), "vital energies/forces/substances," and "air" (Qi), many of which are dependent on constitution and which can *transform* and *change*. Constitution and the patient's condition relate

---

24. It has been argued that the linguistic divergence between European languages and Chinese results in radically different patterns of thought, especially as it has to do with causality and hierarchical organization; hence, words as they are related to TCM must be studied for their various meanings. At the same time, clinical presentation and disease outcome can transcend such interpretive divergence and allow for clear clinical evaluation.

25. Although it has been stated that in the past Chinese physicians rarely used dissection in the study of human anatomy and physiology (because a cadaver does not contain Qi), early writing suggested that physicians and "butchers" explored surgical anatomy on political prisoners. In *Spiritual Axis* it is said: "also when he dies, we can observe his internal anatomy." Thus post-mortems may have been used. The *Classic of Internal Medicine* also contains the measurement of the internal Organs, vessels, and membranes which implies the use of dissection.

26. As stated previously, according to Unschuld we cannot be sure what the classics meant by terms such as "muscles" and "sinews."

27. Unlike so-called deductive Western medical thinking, TCM logic (and historical writings) has less difficulty with what may be viewed as contradicting theories. TCM is an empirical as well as highly theoretical based system that is based on flexible clinical applications of many methods of correspondence and other pattern differentiations. Although difficult for the scientific "Western" mind, this should not lead to dismissal of TCM ideas. Of course, the questions of traditionalism as they pertain to accurate/effective medical theory should be addressed and tested.

28. This is an over simplification as many diseases in Western medicine affect multiple systems, organs, and tissues, and a complete history and physical is needed to make a diagnosis. In TCM it is not uncommon to only address and/or ask about symptoms and signs associated with the chief complaint especially in acute conditions and "non-holistic" treatments are used often. It is not uncommon for a Dr. in China to see as many as 150 patients in one morning. Obviously one cannot do a good holistic history and physical seeing this many patients.

closely to: prenatal or heavenly-Qi (Jing), and the Kidneys (Shen); postnatal functions of the Organs that digest and intake air (Spleen, Stomach, Lungs, Large Intestines, Small Intestines); the circularity and transport systems, the vessels (Mai/Luo), the channels (Jing), the hollow-Organs (Fu); and Organs and "seas" that store and distribute (Zhang). These are all reflected in the patient's "spirit" and vitality (Shen). The bodily functions are often compared to government officials, to irrigation systems (rivers, streams, seas, channels, ducts, flooding, containment, and blockage, etc.); struggles between armies and enemies; and healthy (Zheng) and Evil (Xie) factors. When the body functions correctly, health is maintained and disease is warded-off. Diseases occur when balance is disturbed in any of the above systems by external (Biao) environmental influences, by the internal (Li) environment (spirit, emotions), and by life style (diet, work, etc.). *Spiritual Axis* states:

> Concerning the hundred diseases, their beginning and birth, all are given birth by wind, rain, cold and heat, Yin and Yang, joy and anger, drink and food, swellings and position, great fright and sudden fear. They cause Blood and Qi to divide and to separate, Yin and Yang to break and to suffer, the main channels to labor under a perverse energy and to be cut off, the routes of the channels to be blocked, Yin and Yang to be mutually rebellious, the defensive-Qi to be delayed and detained, the collateral channels (vessels) to be hollow and vacant, Blood and Qi to be disordered, and constancy to be lost. These discussions cannot be found in the ancient classics but, if you please, this is the way (Dao) of their laws.[29]

Interestingly, while primitive societies must have had to recognize that people and animals can recover from injury and disease without any intervention, and therefore the concept of innate-healing was developed in the *West*, no parallel concept of innate or self-healing was developed in confucian Chinese medicine. Though the concept of Righteous (correct) Health (Zheng) has some similarities to internal order (health), it is dependent on proper behavior and prompt intervention (Unschuld *ibid*).

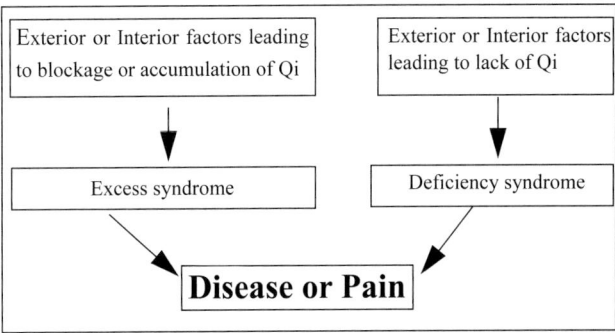

Figure 1-1: Qi and disease states.

function, when Qi gathers there is Yin and substance...*Qi can never be not moving*;" "Qi is that which cannot be seen while Form can be seen." Therefore, the concept of "universal energy/forces/organization/transformation of all substances and energies and primeval material" is central to OM and is used to describe both function and dysfunction. It is also clear that Qi is often used to describe reported symptoms and signs (or phenomena) which can not be "seen" and therefore has little objective findings.

The Chinese character that makes up the word Qi is composed of two characters that represent steam/gas/vapor and rice. When combined, the two characters signify the dynamic fluid quality of Qi: Qi can manifest, function, and transform itself to specific situations.[31] It can manifest as either form or so-called "energy." It is therefore a flexible term that can be used to describe disparate conditions that have many different meanings. Body-Qi originates in the Kidneys/Essence, is supported by Spleen/pancreas digestive functions,[32] is distributed by the Lung respiratory function, and is controlled by the Liver's function of governing movement. In general, it is said that "the Lungs govern Qi."

The movement of steam and by extension Qi, has a spiraling quality and therefore has been compared to the double

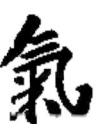 ## Qi

Qi (pronounced "chee") is a complex term describing many abstract concepts (like most terms in TCM) such as life force, functional aspects of the body, cell organizational forces, and some aspects of the material milieu and communication systems within all matter.[30] *The Classic of Internal Medicine* states: "Human beings are created by the Qi of heaven and earth;" "When Qi moves there is Yang and

---

29. Interestingly, the emphasis on *parasitic diseases* seen in older texts (pre-Han dynasty) is not included in the newer vision of health elaborated in the *Classic of Internal Medicine*. Parasitic diseases, however, continued to be part of Daoist medicine, and are included in modern TCM (Unschuld *ibid*).

30. It is important to understand that most TCM terms describe a kind of abstraction not commonly used in the English language. However, each term can still be defined and understood in languages other than Chinese. None of the functions or descriptions of Qi, or of any other term in TCM, is outside of the Western language of science, common experiences or common sense. Since these terms are often abstractions, no simple (one) word conveys their meaning fully. These terms are needed to organize information within the logic of TCM/OM.

31. The concept of transformation is important both as a physiologic process and as therapeutic method when treating musculoskeletal disorders. It is common to see Deficient patients with secondary Pathogenic Factors that result in accumulations in, and of, the bodily milieu. Such accumulations can result in continued worsening of Deficiency, as they consume normal healthy substances, while becoming painful as they block circulation. While some patients do well with dual attacking (resolving the accumulations and obstruction) and tonification (treating the root of Deficiency), many do not tolerate tonification. The concept of transformation can then be used to choose herbs that transform pathogenic accumulation (e.g., Phlegm, Blood) into healthy normal substances and in doing so both nourish health and eliminate pathogens.

helix of DNA. It is thought to be the shape of the forces that bind the universe, including both living and non-living things.[33]

In general, Qi serves six major functions in the body:

1. *Qi-transformation* is responsible for the conversion of nutrition (e.g., food, water, air, emotion, etc.) into Qi, Blood, and Fluids. Digestion and transformation of "food essence," and the separation of "clear" and "unclear substances," relay on the transforming ability of Qi. The concept of Qi transformation also pertains to growth (cell division) and reproduction. Therefore, most physiologic functions are dependent on the ability of Qi to transform, metabolize and gather to "form substances."

2. *Qi-transportation* moves all substances and is responsible for all movement in the body: Fluids, Blood, bowels, visceral motions, gait, etc. Qi-transportation is also responsible for directing movements in the "correct" directions. When disturbed, Qi accumulates (and may form insubstantial swellings, i.e., only felt by the patient) or can rebel, i.e., move in the wrong direction.

3. *Qi warms* the body in its entirety: channels, vessels, sinews, bones, viscera, and bowels. When Qi is weak or does not reach some of the body's tissues or areas/Organs, there will be coldness and hypofunction.

4. *Qi protects* the body from external and internal Pathogenic Factors.

5. *Qi holds* Fluids in place such as keeping Blood in the vessels, and controlling sweat, urine, and tears. When it fails the patient may suffer from nose bleeds, easy bruising, etc. Qi also holds the viscera in place preventing visceral prolapse.

6. *Qi maintains* balance and function by its ability to reach all parts of the body and by its ability to transform. It can function as a general (flexible) reservoir.

Table 1-2 summarizes several types of Qi that exist in the body. The Qi disorders are Deficiency (Emptiness/Vacuity) and Stagnation (Fullness/Repletion; Figure 1-1). There are general symptoms and signs of Deficient or Excess Qi, as well as symptoms and signs of Qi relative to each Organ. In general, each of these disorders consists of a group of conditions that can occur due to:

- *Qi-deficiency* that is characterized by general physical weakness; fatigue and inability to endure intensive mental and physical exertion; dizziness, shortness of breath, weak vocal strength, spontaneous (easy) sweating; poor Organ function due to: congenital causes or illness, dietary imbalances, excessive taxation from emotional or physical imbalances and aging; and from Yin or Blood-deficiency or hemorrhaging. Qi-deficiency is often related to Organ systems, especially the Spleen/pancreas controls the transformation/absorption of nutrients from foods; the state of the Lungs, with their intake of air and "ruling" of Qi; and the state of the Kidneys, which house Essence, the prenatal (genetic) materials needed for the healthy expression and ample supply of Qi.

  if Qi-deficiency is severe, this can lead to a sinking of Qi, causing prolapse of Organs, bleeding, "downward-dragging-distension" of the abdomen, loss of control over urine or bowels, and lumbar soreness.[34]

- *Qi-stagnation* is characterized by the loss of the *dynamic* character of Qi, can result from: emotional excess, external climatic influences or injury, weakness of Qi/Yang and/or Blood, accumulation of Fluids, and Organ dysfunction, especially of the Liver (or other Organs that can influence Liver function, particularly the Kidneys and Spleen). The Liver (a Yin Organ which is often associated with Yin and Blood) controls the moving/coursing of Qi. Qi *movement* is a Yang function and therefore the Liver is said to be dependent on receiving Yang from the Yang reservoir (Zheng), the Kidneys.

  Symptoms of Qi-stagnation are usually characterized by distension-ache of *unfixed* location and *character*. They are often described by patients as a feeling of bloatedness, fullness, swelling, achiness, and occasionally throbbing rather then frank pain (although frank pain may be related to Qi-stagnation as well). The patient may be suffering from frequent belching, sighing, or passing of flatus (all of which may result in temporary reduction of symptoms).[35] There may be subcostal or chest/trunk tension-distension, fullness and/or pain (or just difficultly taking a deep breath, often referred to as chest oppression).

  If severe, this can lead to *rebellious-Qi* (reverse flow of Qi), with symptoms such as: nausea, vomiting, hiccups (Stomach), cough, asthma (Lungs), urinary retention (Bladder), dizziness, irritability, hypochondrial pain distension (Liver), and non-substantial swelling (Channels).

---

32. TCM speaks of the Spleen (Pi, which may just be an erroneous translation as Spleen) as having functions more appropriately attributed to the pancreas and the rest of the digestive system. In a clinical study, a relation between Spleen Qi-deficiency syndrome and the pancreatic exocrine function was shown (Zhongguo Zhong 1996). Therefore, in this text, Spleen and pancreas are often combined.

33. The hexagrams of the *Book of Changes,* are composed of various combinations of broken and unbroken lines (codes) that are supposed to symbolize all phenomena. Together with the spiraling movement of Qi, they have provocative similarities to DNA codes and the spiraling shape of DNA strands.

34. There is a distinction made in TCM between "distension" and "fullness" of the abdomen. Distension usually pertains to a bloated hardness but with an elastic sensation on palpation. Fullness manifests with hardness but without distension (elasticity) on palpation.

35. It is not uncommon for patients to relate that passing gas or flatulence results in a temporary reduction of low back pain.

Pain and Qi

Pain can result from deficiency of Qi and/or stagnation of Qi as both may result in obstruction.[36]

Qi-deficiency Pain

Pain due to Qi-deficiency is intermittent,[37] chronic, dull, deep, achy and *is not* felt as distending or full. Associated with weakness, it becomes worse in the afternoon after activity, or at times, at night.[38] This type of pain responds favorably to palpation and massage.

If associated with excess-Cold (Yin-excess) or Phlegm (also a Yin-pathogen; i.e., mixed pain), the pain is aggravated by cold or wet weather and in some patients can respond poorly to deep palpation and massage.[39] Qi-deficiency pain is commonly seen in patients who have chronic myofascial pain and fibromyalgia. However, Stagnation/Excess is seen frequently in these patients as well, and both may be present in combination (Excess and Deficiency type pain and pathogens).

Qi-stagnation Pain

Pain due to Qi-stagnation is most often related to dysfunction of the Liver Organ/channel system and is felt as fullness, distension, bloating, and possibly throbbing or pulsating.[40] This type of pain changes in *location* or *character*, sometimes being sharp, then dull, then achy, and is usually poorly localized. It often affects large arias and becomes aggravated by lack of movement and alleviated with subsequent movement. This is typical of ligamentous and some myofascial pain syndromes (see chapter 3).[41] Distension, fullness, or swelling is said to precede the sensation of pain,[42] however, one of the most important characteristics of Q-stagnation pain is that it is "unseen," hence, it does not show externally. Qi-stagnation pain can be susceptible to emotional aggravation, because many emotional states affect the Liver, which further aggravates Qi-stagnation. Often it is associated with a numb-like sensation, usually from associated Wind and/or Blood-deficiency, which are often Liver related as well.

Although Qi-stagnation is usually classified as an *Excess* condition, pain that is caused by Qi-stagnation often responds, at least initially, to heat and deep invigorating massage, as this moves the Qi. However, this type of treatment may result in increased pain one or two days later in some patients, and the original pain often returns quickly.

Qi-stagnation can also result from other underlying mechanisms such as external Pathogenic Factors, congealed Fluids/Blood due to Qi-deficiency and/or Liver, Spleen and Lung dysfunctions. One must carefully analyze symptoms and signs to determine if this type of pain is primary or secondary. This precaution is critical because over-use of Qi-moving/regulating herbs, which are usually acrid, to treat Qi-stagnation pain is said to be capable of damaging the Qi, Yin, and Fluids, especially in a weak patient. While the Liver is usually associated with Qi-stagnation, it is the Lungs that are said to govern Qi, and therefor their role should always be kept in mind when designing or choosing a formula or acupoints.

Defensive-Qi (Wei Qi)

Defensive-Qi plays a particularly important role in musculoskeletal medicine. The classic *Simple Questions* states that Defensive-Qi is slippery and rough in nature and cannot enter the channels (vessels). It circulates under the skin and between the muscles and blood vessels, or between skin, subcutaneous tissues, and flesh. These areas are also called the *Cou Li*. (The Cou Li has been described as skin and pores, also called membranes/interstice and *may* relate in part to superficial and deep fascia. It is also referred to as a space between the Exterior and Interior, while membranes such as Mo Wai may also be related to fascia.) Defensive-Qi vaporizes between membranes, which gives it a material aspect. It disseminates over the chest and abdomen *(biomedicine: possibly relating to the diaphragmatic and abdominal pumps)*. When Defensive-Qi is harmonious, the Cou Li is firm, moist and supple.[43] *Spiritual Axis* says that Defensive-Qi warms the muscles. The least refined of the Qis and made from turbid-Qi,[44] Defensive-Qi is rooted in Mingmen, a Yang force. The production of Defensive-Qi depends greatly on the Kidneys, Mingmen,[45] and True-Qi[46] assisted by the

---

36. Most pain in Chinese medicine is caused by lack of free flow of Qi and Blood.

37. Many sources have associated Deficiency-pain also with *continual* pain when it is aggravated by physical strain.

38. Night pain is more often due to Blood-stasis, Heat, or any condition that causes turbidity and affects circulation.

39. The response to palpation is less informative in musculoskeletal disorders as compared to abdominal (organic) disorders. Patients with Deficiency type pain often do not report improvement with pressure. Patients with Excess type pain, on the other hand, are more likely to report increase pain with pressure.

40. Stagnation from any source can easily transform into Heat or Fire. Throbbing pain is primarily related to Liver-Fire (mostly head related pains). Clinically throbbing or pulsating pain is seen often with Blood-stasis sprains as well.

41. The hallmark of ligamentous pain in Orthopaedic Medicine is posain: meaning pain aggravated by lack of movement. This pain is worse in the morning because of lack of activity. Ligaments are also a common source of a numb-like sensation called nulliness.

42. For example, Qi-stagnation pain is common in the abdomen; the pain is relieved temporarily after passing gas.

43. Thus, palpation of surface tissue may give information related to Defensive-Qi.

44. *Spiritual Axis* states: "The Clear-Qi is the Nutritive-Qi, the turbid Qi is the Defensive-Qi...the Defensive-Qi comes out in the lower Warmer.

45. Mingmen has warming Yang functions associated with the Kidneys. "Life-Gate" is another name for Mingmen.

46. A combined Qi from digestive and endogenous factors.

Table 1-2: Types of QI

TRUE/SOURCE	• Formed by Ancestral and Original-Qi. • Assumes two forms: Defensive-Qi and Nutritive-Qi.
ORGAN	• The physiological activity and some material aspects of the Organ.
CHANNEL/VESSELS	• Transmitted and conveyed through a conduit system that is part of and inside the body.
DEFENSE	• Flows outside of vessels, between blood vessels, skin and in membranes. • In part circulates outside of the "body." • Coarse and slippery in nature. • Cannot enter the channels; however, enters the Organs at night. • Warms and moistens the muscles and skin. • Controls the skin pores, regulating sweat. • Main function: defense against exogenous pathological-Qi. • Closely related to Nutritive-Qi.
NUTRITIVE/NOURISHING/ CONSTRUCTION	• Flows within the vessels. • Derived from clear essence of food and Fluids. • Together with Fluids is precursor to Blood. • Moves with the Blood in the vessels. • Close relationship to Heart and with Defensive-Qi. • Helps the Blood in nourishing functions of Yin, Yang and Organs. • (Translated as "camp" Qi by Unschuld and is related to the military term of Defensive-Qi).
ORIGINAL	• Flows mostly in Eight Extra channels. • Most important and fundamental Qi (refers also to primeval cosmic creative stuff, even before the "Big Bang" or singularity that divided everything into Yin and Yang). • Circulates in all three burners and surfaces at the Source points. • Inherited vitality and constitution; closely related to Essence. • Precursor to all other Qi. • Non renewable.[a] • Resides in the Kidney and nourishes Kidneys, or dwells between the Kidneys at Gate of Life (Mingmen). • Has a historical aspect (memory of "old trauma" can be "stored" in Original-Qi). • Preservation of Original-Qi and True-Qi are said to be the secret of a long life.
ANCESTRAL/CHEST/ PECTORAL/GREAT	• Formulated from the interaction of Food-essence Qi and air. • The force and strength of respiration that circulates Qi and Blood by regulating the Heart and Lung functions. • The force that nourishes the Heart and Lungs. • Accumulates in chest and circulates throughout body. • Limb circulation and movement depends largely on Ancestral/Chest-Qi.
RIGHTEOUS/CORRECT/ RIGHT/ANTI- PATHOGENIC	• The sum of all of the body's Qis, Fluids, Blood, Essence and Organ functions. • All of the anti-pathogenic functions. • The patient's general condition. • Relates to "correct" behavior, both physical and emotional.

a. Treating source points, CV-4 through 7 and GV-4 (moxa) and the use of many herbs can support Original-Qi.

Lungs, Liver, Spleen/pancreas, and Large and Small Intestine.[47]

Defensive-Qi and Biomedical Analogies

Defensive-Qi is responsible for the elimination of or protection from exogenous factors.[48] It is an antipathogenic-Qi. It is also responsible for the body's reaction to the environment. Reflexive, inherent, instinctual (automatic) and the most Yang aspect of Qi, it performs its functions involuntarily.[49] Defensive-Qi is similar in many ways to the autonomic and immune systems in biomedicine.[50] The statement that Defensive-Qi flows outside the vessels *may* make the lymphatic system part of TCM's Defensive-Qi. The lymphatic system is dependent on the muscular and respiratory system (including the abdominal pump driven by the diaphragm and therefore corresponding to the respiratory function or Lungs in OM) for circulation.

TEMPERATURE REGULATION. Among the areas of influence of Defensive-Qi is temperature regulation—opening the skin pores to release heat or closing the pores in reaction to cold *(biomedicine: an autonomic nervous system function)*. The "battle" between Defensive-Qi and pathological influences is responsible for the development of fever and some types of inflammation *(biomedicine: immune system, which is closely related to autonomic system reaction)*. The Defensive-Qi function of warming the muscles is also related closely to the biomedical autonomic nervous system function that regulates circulation of blood to the muscles and skin.

DEFENSIVE-QI: SKIN AND FASCIA. Defensive and Triple Warmer Qi[51] protect the Organs and appear to have some functions that are ascribed to skin and fascia in biomedicine.

Both of these types of Qi are said to flow through the Cou Li *(possibly the ligamentous-fascial organ)*, where Fluid that is "white, moist, and wraps the periphery of the body" is said to circulate *(biomedical: possibly superficial and deep fascia)*. Skin and fascia are made of collagen and elastic fibers, ground substance and cellular elements that surround muscles and organs. They provide warmth, protection, the storage of elastic energy, and connect the *whole body (OM: possibly Triple Warmer)*. Defensive-Qi is in part the energy or the Sinew (tendinomuscular) channels and therefore provides potential (elastic) energy, as well. Skin and fascia are continuous throughout the body. Fascia is sometimes described as uniting in the abdomen, as is Defensive-Qi and the Triple Warmer. Fascia is moist, allowing movement and *communication* between tissues.

Skin and fascia contain small-caliber nerve fibers that play a role in the immune system (Ochoa and Mair 1969). In TCM, Defensive-Qi is the main immune force that circulates in skin and muscles.

Patients suffering from fibromyalgia, or any chronic generalized muscular aches, often suffer from disturbed sleep. Defensive-Qi circulates at the Exterior (skin, hair, muscles, and spaces between these and the Organs) during the day and in the Interior (Organs) during the night. When sleep is disturbed, the formation/supplementation of Defensive-Qi from True-Qi is disturbed, and the moistening and warming of muscles *may be* affected.[52] Myalgias may follow.[53] Treatment directed at Defensive-Qi (with Nutritive-Qi and Blood) is used often in these patients. *Spiritual Axis* states:

> ...The Defensive-Qi comes out, its fierce Qi is violent and quick. It moves first in the four limbs, in the divisions of the flesh and the gaps of the skin (Cou Li, skin, and pores), and is unceasing. During daytime it travels in the Yang. At night this Qi travels in the Yin; it follows the divisions and gaps of the Leg Shao-Yin as it moves in the five viscera and six bowels. When a perverse and deficient-Qi is a guest in the five viscera and six bowels, it causes the Defensive-Qi to protect only the outside, to move in the Yang, but not to gain entrance into the Yin. This movement in the Yang causes the Yang-Qi to be abundant. The Yang-Qi being abundant causes the Yang Motility channel to be dense. Not gaining entrance into the Yin causes the Yin to be hollow so the eyes cannot close.[54]

Defensive-Qi can become disharmonious with Nutritive-Qi,[55] resulting in excessive sweating *(biomedicine: sweating is associated with activation of the sympathetic nervous system. Autonomic nerve fibers provide innervation to sweat glands and fascia. Innervation to sweat glands comes from exclusively cholinergic innervation from the sympathetic cholinergic system which also affects muscular contractions)*. This results in lack of protection at the surface and allows the "penetration" of external pathogens. Lack of warmth provided to muscles as a result of the consumption of Defensive-Qi from sweating or from

---

47. The Transporting/Shu points (see chapter 5) for these Organs can be used to treat weakness of Defensive-Qi manifesting in patients who are weak, fatigued and susceptible to external influences.

48. Climatic factors that result in disease.

49. Daoist interpretations not found in modern TCM books.

50. Dr. John Shen has categorized the Tai Yang (the most superficial in the six level paradigm) depth as the nervous system. The nervous system and skin arise embryologically from the ectoderm all of which support some association between Defensive-Qi, the superficial aspects, and the nervous system.

51. Which Kendall translates as internal membrane [fascial] system.

52. Defensive-Qi is said to start circulation to the Exterior as soon as one opens his/her eyes.

53. Not a "classical," i.e., Chinese, conclusion. The Blood is also said to be replenished at night when it "enters" the Liver. Weakness of Blood is often associated with dysfunctions of sinews (the soft tissues), with tightness or weakness. Growth hormone is secreted by the anterior pituitary only when sleeping. It also stimulates the liver to secrete secondary growth hormones, or somatomedins which are the more active forms affecting bodily tissues and functions.

54. The suggested treatment is to tonify the Deficiency, disperse the Excess, harmonize the Hollow and Solid, penetrate and clear the routes, and remove Pathogenic Factors. Then a dose of medicine made from millet and Pinelliae (Ban Xia) is suggested to restore sleep.

55. Substances with trophic or nourishing properties.

battling exterior pathogens is said to be capable of causing muscle aches. Obstruction by pathogenic influences can also result in pain. Often it affects the joints, which may become inflamed and swollen as seen in Heat Obstruction (Bi) *(Biomedicine: inflammatory arthritis)*, or cold and painful, as seen in Wind-Cold-Damp Obstruction (Bi) *(Biomedicine: arthrosis)*. Disharmonious Defensive and Nutritive-Qi is a common finding in patients who have chronic fatigue syndrome, myofascial pain syndromes, and fibromyalgia.[56] The TCM possible origin of joint disease by exogenous pathogens is intriguing, as biomedicine has now shown that many rheumatologic disorders may be infectious.

Ancestral (Chest) Qi (Zhong Qi)

Ancestral (Chest) Qi provides another example of the similarities between TCM theory and biomedicine. Centered at the chest region, this Qi is derived from the interaction of Food-Qi and air: Food-Qi is transported to the Lungs, where it combines with air and becomes Ancestral (Chest) Qi.

Blood is closely related to Ancestral (Chest) Qi, postnatal-Qi and prenatal-Qi. The functions of Ancestral (Chest) Qi are said to control respiration and generation and the nourishment of Blood *(Biomedicine: oxygenation and transport of blood; heart/lungs)*; and to circulate Qi and Blood throughout the body. The close relationship between the Lungs and Heart is exemplified by the saying: "The Lung faces the hundred vessels."

The condition of Ancestral (Chest) Qi can be assessed by assessing the respiratory and circulatory systems. Ancestral (Chest) Qi clearly represents many of the biomedical functions of the respiration, blood oxygenation, and respiratory/cardiovascular systems in general.

Righteous-Qi (Zheng Qi)

The concepts of Righteous-(antipathogenic)-Qi, also called Right (Righteous) or Correct, is important in TCM, as it reflects the patient's general (total) healthy-influences. Righteous-Qi is the sum of all of the patient's Qi, Blood, Essence, Yin/Yang balance, and Organ functions. It represents the body's ability to fight disease, to maintain normal function and "correct" behavior. When Righteous-Qi is strong, the body can resist Pathogenic Factors, mount a battle and develop Heat (fever) to defend itself against invasion and stress. When Righteous-Qi is weak, pathogenic (evil) factors are not resisted and can infect the body and/or hide internally. Often symptoms are mild, enduring, and the patient is weak. While the classics often state that when one's Righteous-Qi is strong the body can resist diseases, the *Classic of Internal Medicine* also states: "The Yellow Emperor asked: In a given year, everyone may contract the same disease. What kind of Qi is responsible for this?" Shao Shi's answer, while considering the type of pathogens ("Eight Orientations, Eight Deficiencies, and Eight Winds"), clearly states that this occurs only when people are relaxed or fatigued, calling it deficiency-Wind. At the same time he states: "Even though people live an uneventful life, their interstices (skin and pores) open and shut and are slack and tense regularly...When the moon is waning to the close and, consequently, the eastern sea is at high tide, people experience a deficiency of Blood and Qi, their Defensive-Qi is gone, their interstices are open, their hair is thin, and the smoky grime as fallen off. At such a time, if a bandit Wind attacks, it will penetrate deeply and afflict people suddenly and acutely." He also states that deficiency-Wind can intrude upon the bone (i.e., interior of body; however, bone and sinews are also considered the Yin of Exterior, *Spiritual Axis*), without first affecting the exterior of the body (especially if the interstices or skin and pores are open). Righteous-Qi is therefore dependent on both Exterior and Interior factors.

Blood (Xue)

In TCM, the term Blood pertains to the same red fluid described in the biomedical model and is closely related to the circulatory system.[57] Blood flows throughout the collaterals, also called network-vessels (Jing/Luo which include the arterial and venous systems), to nourish the Organs and tissues of the whole body. Although it is not clear if the Chinese understood the concept of a closed circulatory system, and opinions differ (Kendall 2002; Unschuld 2003), statements in the classics such as: "The flow in the conduit vessels does not stop. It circulates without break" do suggest this possibility. On the other hand, the Blood is said to be stored in the Liver at night and leave the Liver during the day. When it does so people can see, walk, grasp and hold (although this can also mean that Blood/blood circulation is dependent on physiological use and therefore accurate). The *Classic of Internal Medicine,* in discussing the circulatory system, states:

> Food enters the Stomach; its Essence (refined nutrients) is then distributed into the Liver (possibly the portal system), and its vital force (Nutritive-Qi and Blood) flows over into the muscles (sinews). Food enters the stomach; its putrid gases (turbid Qi) are sent up to the Heart and its Essence (refined-Qi) overflows into the pulse (possibly circulation or Heart). The force of the pulse flows into the arteries and the force of the arteries (possibly veins) ascends into the Lung; the Lungs send it into all the pulses (possibly the right to left ventricle, venous to arterial), which then transport its essence to the skin and body hair. The entire vascular system unites with the secretions (possibly lymph) and pass the force of life (Qi) on to a storehouse (Chest Qi), which stores the energy, vitality and intelligence. These are then transmitted to the four [parts of body,

---

56. These conditions are commonly treated by harmonizing the Nutritive and Defensive-Qi, using variations of Cinnamon Twig Decoction (Gui Zhi Tang Jie Wei +/-). This is a formula with many uses including joint and soft tissue pain.

57. OM attributes other functions to this Fluid.

Table 1-3: Disorders of the Blood

DEFICIENCY	CHARACTERISTICS
Blood-deficiency	• Lusterless, pale, white, withered (emaciated), or yellow appearance. • Light headedness, especially when standing up (orthostatic hypotension). • Dizziness. • Flowery vision (floaters). • Numbness, itching. • Insomnia, excessive dreaming. • Fatigue. • Constipation. • Left sided paralysis and/or symptoms and signs.[a] • Dry Skin. • Pale tongue, lips, eyes and nails. • Thready, fine, or choppy pulse.
Blood-stasis	• see "Blood-stasis (Xue Yu)" on page 41.
Blood-Heat	Results from full-Heat, toxic-Heat [b] or empty-Heat in the Blood: • Often associated with infections. • Usually characterized by profuse bleeding of bright red or purple-black colored blood. • Bloody stools, nose or urine. • Red papules and/or macules or other red colored rashes. • Together with general signs of Heat: thirst, constipation or hot burning foul smelling. diarrhea, bitter taste in mouth, subjective/objective sensations of heat, etc. • Tongue red, yellow coating. • Pulse rapid.

a. Some practitioners use Blood-related herbs (both stasis and tonics) for left sided problems; for example, He Shou Wu for left-sided shoulder or elbow tendinosis.
b. Toxins usually pertain to infectious/high fever diseases, skin diseases or herbal/medicinal/food toxins. While toxins from environmental contamination have not been strongly related to disease in Chinese medicine, the understanding that foods, herbs, and floods have toxic effects have been described. Toxins from poor liver (biomedical) detoxification and from environmental heavy metals and chemicals can be an important factor in chronic pain patients.

limbs], and the vital forces (Qi) of the viscera, and are restored to their order...The viscera thoroughly expel into the Liver (possibly the portal system). Thus the Liver harbors the force of life of the muscles and the thin membranes...The viscera are in thorough communication and bound by circulation with the Heart and the Blood that is stored by the Heart, and thus the Blood fills the pulse (vessels) with the force of life (breath, Qi).

Spiritual Axis states:

The Blood vessels spread crosswise at the transport (Shu) points. They show clearly, and, when palpating them, they are firm.

As can be seen, while some of the portal systems, for instance, Liver, the respiratory system, and Heart, may have been understood, the "storing" of Blood and its refinements is not consistent with a closed circulatory system. There is also an understanding of the branching of large and small blood vessels.

The time estimated by the Chinese for the Blood to move through the body is said to be more accurate than the original estimate by Harvey, the first to describe a closed system in the West (Kendall *ibid*, *ibid*), however, states that the Chinese classics may be speaking of the circulation of Qi, Nutritive-Qi, and even seasonal influences, not necessarily of Blood/blood. Also, different vessels/channels are said to contain various proportions of Qi and Blood, a notion that would be difficult to understand if the Chinese were speaking of a closed circularity system, except perhaps, if this was one way of describing the difference between venous and arterial blood and the size of the vessels.

Circulation is achieved by the function of the Heart (although there is no mention of the heart as a pump), vitality of Qi (governed by the Lungs and Chest-Qi rhythmic movements), and a system of vessels (Jing) and collaterals (Luo). There is no clear description of the arterial verses the venous system; however, Blood is understood as moving up and down (Yin and Yang vessels). There is also no clear description of the lymphatic system except possibly in the section of the *Classic of Internal Medicine* that speaks of Fluids pouring into the vessels (from membranes and spaces that are outside the vessel and channel systems), and certain aspects of Defensive-Qi, which circulates outside the channels/vessels and can be understood, in part, as being the lymphatic system.[58]

Blood is governed/moved by the Heart (which also governs the vessels), produced by the Spleen/pancreas, regulated by the Liver with help from the Lungs (Chest-Qi), and supported by Kidney-Essence. In general, Blood is formed by Nutritive-Qi (also called Construction-Qi) and Fluids. This requires interactions of the Spleen/pancreas/Stomach, Liver, Lungs, Heart and Kidneys. Blood is derived from Food-Qi—the dense/Yin-flavored and Fluid part of food—and sent up to the Heart by the Spleen/pancreas *raising* function. The process of manufacturing Blood is achieved by interaction of the dense Food-Qi, Lung-Qi and Heart-Qi, all of which take root and interact with Original/True-Qi and Essence. The relationship between the Spleen/pancreas (Food-Qi), Lungs (Air), Heart and Essence (Kidney/bone marrow), and the creation and function of Blood was recognized in the Qing dynasty (Maciocia 1989).[59] Foods used to build the Blood tend to be of animal origin and/or red in color. Blood-deficiency is therefore common in vegetarians, especially females, as they loose Blood with menstruation.[60]

Functions

The main functions of Blood are the nourishing and moistening of the entire body. *The Classic of Internal Medicine* states:

> The eyes receive Blood and are capable of seeing. The feet receive Blood and are capable of walking. The palms receive Blood and are capable of grasping. The fingers receive Blood and are capable holding.

Qi is said to be the "commander of Blood" and retains Blood in its vessels, and Blood is said to be "the mother of Qi" and to "harmonize" Qi. Qi and Blood are therefore mutually generating and interdependent. The *left-side* of the body is said to relate more to Blood (Liver), and the *right-side* to Qi. Severe or chronic loss of Blood can result in Qi-abandonment/collapse (shock). *Spiritual Axis* states:

> If Blood and Qi are deficient, the vessels will not move freely. Thus, True/Righteous and pathogens will mutually attack each other. There will be chaos and this will lead to one's longevity being cut short.

Blood plays an important role in the nourishment and moistening of sinews, as was emphasized in the *Spiritual Axis*: "When the Blood is harmonized...the sinews are strong and the joints are supple." As Blood flows throughout the channels/network-vessels and Organs, it has multiple functions and can develop various dysfunctions. Blood-deficiency is said to "engender Wind and cause vascular (vessel) pain."

Dryness of Blood is said to cause "spasms." Table 1-3 lists disorders of the Blood with their principal characteristics and symptoms.

Blood Disorders

The two main disorders of the Blood are Deficiency and Stasis. While not the same as anemia, Blood-deficiency does share many of the symptoms and signs seen in anemic patients. It is associated with lack of Blood volume as well as weakness in activities associated with Blood. Blood-deficiency (Xu), is generally caused by weakness in the Spleen/Stomach (nutrition), Liver (storage), and/or bleeding. Kidney disease (by its affect on other systems) can also result in symptoms associated with deficiency of Blood (via the marrow). Blood-deficiency is also caused by taxation damage, consumption of Qi and Blood by chronic disease, and with stasis preventing the formation of new Blood. Blood-deficiency can result in symptoms associated with the Heart, sinews, and other tissues as well as other systems.

Blood-stasis is associated with the lack of movement of Blood, lack of vitality of Blood (sharing characteristics with Blood-deficiency), accumulation of Blood with or without transformation into a mass (Ji, Ju, Jia, etc.),[61] and with diseases of the vascular system. It is important to remember that Blood-stasis is also associated with the creating of abnormal Heat (as may be seen in inflammatory diseases with Heat signs). Blood-stasis is also associated with chronic and difficult-to-treat diseases. Modern research has shown Blood-stasis to relate to viscosity and cohesion of blood, vessel disease (arteriosclerosis, changes in the vessel endothelial linings, and reduction of cATP and cAMP), haematocyte alterations, haemoatoblast coagulation, increase in blood lipids, and thrombosis, among other effects (Xiao 2003).

Blood Disorders (Musculoskeletal Effects)

Lack of nourishment due to Blood-deficiency or stasis can result in stiffness and fragility of the tendons, ligaments, and other sinews. This is often described as "hardness" (hypertonicity) or "laxness." Blood-deficiency often results in the generation of internal-Wind (or allowing penetration of external-Wind), with symptoms such as: paresthesias (pins and needles), numbness (especially of the hands and feet), unfixed or radiating pain, and upper body symptoms. When Blood, a Yin substance, is deficient, it can also result in empty-Heat with burning pain *(Biomedicine: neuropathies, etc.)* and bleeding. Blood-stasis can result in fixed pain, hard fixed lumps, and may also result in Atrophy (Wei) disorders

---

58. The lymphatic channels (biomedical) drain the relatively cell-free extacellular fluid that accumulates outside the vascular system.

59. Many of the same systems are associated with biomedical blood, as well.

60. Blood-deficiency should not be confused with anemia.

61. Abdominal masses that are actual masses, fixed and immovable, are called Ji. "Masses" that come and go but are not fixed and movable are called Ju. Jia is equivalent to Ju (i.e., non-substantial masses usually from Qi-stagnation).

from trauma or chronic processes. Blood-deficiency is one etiology of vascular disease and pain. Blood-Painful-Obstruction-(Bi)-syndrome may cause numbness, painful limbs, and a pulse that is faint, choppy, and tight at the proximal position.

THE RELATIONSHIP OF BLOOD TO LIVER AND KIDNEY. The relation of the Blood to the Liver and Kidneys is especially important in musculoskeletal medicine. Athletic and physical activity demands increased Blood/blood circulation to muscles. Blood circulation is dependent on normal function of the Liver, because Liver stores and regulates (releases) Blood. Stagnation/congestion of the Liver can result in decreased Blood flow during physical activity, leading to a lack of nourishment of muscles and sinews. Patients who experience increased symptoms during or after physical activity often suffer from Liver-Blood and Kidney disorders *(biomedicine: often adrenal disorders)*. Patients with mainly Liver-Blood-deficiency often complain of increased pain following activity that easily improves with a short rest. Patients with primarily Kidney disorders often complain of increased pain following activity that may, or may not improve after a short rest. They may also complain of increased pain after sexual exertion. Increased physical activity must be balanced with rest, because Blood regenerates itself in the Liver when the person is lying down.[62]

Blood, Fluids, and Essence are interdependent. The Kidneys are the root of Essence and Fluids (which is made by refinement of Blood) and whole body Yin and Yang. The kidneys control the bone marrow and therefore the generation of Blood/blood.

THE RELATIONSHIP OF BLOOD TO LUNGS AND SPLEEN/PANCREAS. The Lungs and Spleen/pancreas (the root of postnatal-Qi) are important because Qi holds the Blood in the Blood vessels and Blood is formed by functions of Food/Construction-Qi and Lung-Qi. The Lungs also move the Blood to the Heart as it is said: "The Lungs connect to the hundred vessels." When Qi cannot hold the Blood, microbleeding may result in somatic fixed, sharp pain of unknown origin. (Although usually this mechanism is related to heavy menstrual and hemorrhoidal bleeding, bleeding is often caused by Blood-Heat as well.) Weakness of digestive energy or excessive bleeding can result in Blood-deficiency. Weakness of the Lungs can result in the pooling of Blood in the lower extremities and the formation of varicose veins. Lung function is important in venous circulation because rhythmic function circulates Qi (*Biomedicine: respiratory diaphragm which helps with both venous and lymphatic flow*).

RELATIONSHIP OF BLOOD WITH HEART. The Heart is the "monarch" and controls the Blood-vessels and therefore the Blood. Hence both the Heart and Blood are susceptible to emotional and physical stress. When Heart-Blood is weak, the patient may be restless, suffer from a poor memory, experience palpitations, and his/her sleep quality may be affected with excessive dreaming. Chronic pain is highly stressful, and emotional affects are common. Chronic poor sleep is a common factor in patients who suffer from myalgias and other chronic pain syndromes. The Heart is the monarch and is therefore affected by all emotional stresses (although, clinically, Liver-associated symptoms are seen often).

Essence (Jing)

Essence, which is said to reside in the Kidney system, is in part the material basis of life—potential material/energy, DNA, etc. Essence pertains to several *refined* or *potential* substances in the body from Essence-Qi to food-Essence. Essence, Fluids, and Blood are of the same source and share a similar nature, since they all are *Yin-substances*. Therefore, Essence, Fluids, and Blood are often affected simultaneously. Blood is stored in the Liver and Essence in the Kidneys. Essence has two main aspects:

- Inherited Essence (prenatal), which cannot be altered (but can be diminished or supported).
- Acquired Essence (postnatal), which can be supplemented and can then reinforce inherited Essence.

A Fluid-like (oily) substance, Essence relates to sperm and the egg and to "Tian Gui," the congenital substance that can promote human growth, development, and reproductive function. (It maintains a woman's regular menstruation and pregnancy.) It forms the basis of growth, sexuality, reproduction, and *aging*. According to *Simple Questions,* "Essence is the root of the body. If it is protected and stored, latent pathogenic-Heat will not appear in spring time," i.e., the immune system is strong.

Abnormal bone and mental growth is associated often with lack of Essence. Since Essence determines each person's *constitution*, Essence-deficiency is associated with many conditions that manifest by life-long disorders, such as: a weak immune system, lack of endurance, general fatigue, reproductive disorders, early aging, early degenerative diseases especially of bones, and brain disorders. The patient's history may include poor childhood health.

Thus, in many ways, acquired Essence resembles genetic material and the inborn constitutional condition of the individual. It is said, "Those who are endowed with sufficient Yin-Essence will reach longevity." Symptoms of patients with weak congenital Essence may begin in early childhood and last until death. Patients often present with changing symptoms and signs and have a sense of *instability*; they cannot trust their own health and bodies. They com-

---

62. As stated earlier, this may relate to growth hormones. Such patients can be given Bu Gan Tang Jia jie (Modified Tonify Liver Decoction): Shu Di (Rehmanniae) 12g, Dang Gui (Angelicae) 9g, Bai Shao (Paeoniae) 9g, Suan Zao Ren (Ziziphi) 9g, Chuan Xiong (Ligustici) 6g, Mu Gua (Chaenomelis) 6g, Zhi Gan Cao (Glycyrrhizae) 6g; Or: Kidney formulas such as Liu Wei Di Huang (Six Ingredient Radix Rehmanniae Pill).

plain of fatigue, a sense of living in a fog (foggy brains, *essence-spirit* weakness), dizziness, and blurred vision when fatigued. They often have vague pains that shift around and may also have multisystem complaints: gastrointestinal, gynecological, respiratory, multiple allergies, psychosomatic, psychiatric, hyperactive sympathetic nervous system (fibromyalgia and chronic fatigue syndrome), with shortness of breath and sweating easily. Their faces often show a bluish-green or dark color, especially around the chin and mouth and under the eyes (or are generally pale).[63] They tend to have a low tolerance of stress. Their pulses may be floating, changing and slightly rapid, and the left proximal position is often deep, thready, and weak (since Essence is associated with the Kidneys). Even though these patients are said to be Kidney-deficient, they often do not have symptoms and signs of cold or heat that are associated with Kidney-Yang or Kidney-Yin deficiency (or may not have any classic Kidney related symptoms). Also, because Essence is the most basic of the human building-block materials, it can affect any of the body systems and may do so, sometimes, without the typically associated symptoms/signs of the affected system, Organ, or tissue (and seen most often with degenerative diseases or congenital deformity).

Essence disorders often involve the nervous system and *may* be related in part to dysfunctions in the production and movement of *trophic* (growth) *factors* via the nerves. These are essential for the nourishment of many of the tissues/functions/organs that are related to Essence in TCM. When Essence is consumed, the patient may show signs of atrophy and catabolism, and trophic changes in affected tissues such as wilting of bones. *(Biomechanical: often caused by disturbance of exoplasmic flow of trophic factors via nerves)*. When the Blood-aspect is blocked or Deficient, sinews and muscles become "hard," hypertonic, and weak, as is often seen with lack of nourishment (*hypoxia*) and dysfunctional nerves with decreased trophic functions. These patients are also susceptible to many disorders characterized as dysfunction of the autonomic nervous systems in biomedicine: chronic fatigue syndrome and fibromyalgia, for example.[64]

Excessive sexual activity, overwork, drugs, and demanding life styles are said to deplete Essence, Fluids, and Yin (and may result in dystrophic disorders with pain). These types of patients must be differentiated clinically from patients in whom Essence is weak from birth (congenital). One cannot expect to see permanent therapeutic changes in patients who have genetic diseases. Weak Essence is a common factor in *early* degenerative joint disease, early degenerative disc disease, osteodystrophy, osteoporosis, and other degenerative spinal and bone disorders, which often have *genetic* influences.

Treatment of deficient-Essence often involves nourishing Liver-Blood and tonifying the Kidneys. The most important substance is said to be human placenta (Zi He Che). Other herbs and animal products that may be used are: Antler glue, (Lu Jiao), Tortosie Plastron (Gui Ban), Tortosie Plastron glue (Gui Ban Jiao), Fructus Lycii (Gou Qi Zi), Semen Cuscutae (Tu Si Zi), Radix Rehmanniae (Shu Di Huang), Fructus Corni (Shan Zhu Yu), Cortex Eucommiae (Du Zhong), Radix Morindae (Ba Ji Tian), Herba Cistanshes (Rou Cang Rong), Rhizoma Cibotii (Gou Ji), Rhizoma Drynari (Gu Sui Bu) and formulas such as Left-Restoring Pill (Zuo Gui Wan) and Right-Restoring Pill (You Gui Wan).[65]

Fluids (Jin and Ye)

Fluid pertains to all normal Fluids in the body and *interstitial fluids (biomed)* has been related to TCM Yin and Fluids.[66] Fluids such as urine, sweat, tears, and saliva moisten and nourish the skin, flesh, muscles, sensory Organs, and excretory Organs. Fluids are substantial and very sensitive to changes within the body systems (Qi, Blood, Organs, channels, tissues, etc.), as well as to the outside environment; for instance, they may be damaged in hot weather. The Kidney system is the Organ that governs Water and thus body Fluids, including being the "root" of Fluids. The Stomach, Spleen/pancreas, Lungs, Small Intestine, Large Intestine and Urinary Bladder are all important, as well.

Besides the above Organs, the *Triple Warmer* (an Organ system unique to TCM which has been compared to the fascial system) is "in charge of the waterways." The Stomach receives Fluids; the Spleen/pancreas absorbs, transforms, transports, and controls Fluids; the Lungs help in descending and moving Fluids to the Kidneys and are therefore called "the upper source of Fluids"; the Small and Large intestines separate the "clear and turbid" Fluids and absorb clear Fluids; and the Bladder receives all turbid Fluids, performing a final separation and excretion of the "turbid." The Triple Warmer provides a pathway for the Fluids. If the Triple Warmer (and/or any of the above described systems) fails to circulate Fluids, *pathogenic-Dampness* can arise (or Water which is a term always pertaining to pathogenic Fluid).

---

63. In Tong-style acupuncture, a dark (green/blackish) area around the chin and mouth reflect Kidney-deficiency. Needling Water Passing Through (1010.19) and Water Metal Gold (1010.20) is said to be useful (see page 350). The area around the mouth (Yi) is also related to the Kidney in the *Classic of Internal Medicine*, the color being black (soot).

64. Many of the above symptoms and signs are not "classical" (of Chinese origin) TCM associations with Essence. They are, however, commonly associated by modern practitioners, especially those that follow the Kidney school. Clinically, the wilting of sinews and bones seen in patients with complex regional pain (used to be called reflex sympathetic dystrophy) for example may be associated, in part, with weakening of Essence and treated with Essence tonics.

65. Unfortunately, it is not uncommon for these patients to have weak digestive systems that prevent them from taking strong and cloying tonics such as the above herbs. At times, the addition of Qi-moving, Heat-clearing, and digestion-aiding herbs can help the patient to better tolerate such herbs. It may be necessary to treat the Spleen and Stomach first.

66. This is interesting as modern research shows that all of the aging processes are related to dehydration of cells. In TCM aging is also related to decreasing Yin and Fluids.

Accumulated Fluids can result in Phlegm, especially if heated (i.e., becoming thick turbid Fluids). Accumulated Fluids can also block Qi-circulation, and therefore it is often necessary to add Qi-regulating herbs when treating Dampness, edema, or Damp/heavy-pain.

Fluids that arise from the Triple Warmer and are clear, light, and thin, circulate quickly with Defensive-Qi warming and moistening the muscles, flesh and skin, and are called *Jin* (Fluid). Controlled by the Lungs (and Triple Warmer), they fill extra-articular tissues (and possibly bursae) that may often be treated through the Sinew channels, Lungs, and Triple Warmer.[67] A thicker, denser/viscous, slow-circulating Fluid called *Ye* (Fluid) moves more deeply and is related to Nutritive-Qi, but does not "move" with the Qi and Blood. Ye is related to the Spleen/pancreas and Kidneys. Its function is to moisten, lubricate, and nourish the *joints*, brain, cerebral spinal Fluid and bone marrow, and to supplement Essence. Fluids help to "carry" Qi and at the same time are dependent on the Qi's physiologic functions of warming, transforming, and moving. That is why it is said that "Qi is the mother of Fluids."

In general, Fluids are harmed by excessive sweating, vomiting, diarrhea, or urination, Heat and Dry Pathogenic Factors, dry or hot environments, or spicy hot medications and foods, all of which can lead to dryness of mouth, lips and throat, causing thirst, constipation, and *concentrated* urine.

EDEMA. Most edema is thought to be caused by Yang-deficiency of the Lung, Spleen/pancreas, or Kidneys, or by retention of Dampness or Water. Edema in the legs is mostly associated with Spleen/pancreas-Yang-deficiency and/or Kidney Yang-deficiency. Edema of the upper body is associated with the Lungs as well. Edema and swellings (Zhong) are often discussed in TCM also in terms of water-swelling, skin-swelling, Qi-swelling, Cold-Swelling, Wind-water-swelling, and Drum-distension. Water-swelling is often used to describe collection at specific locations where water "spills" over, and if also associated with Cold, pitting edema may result (from either Interior or Exterior Cold). The skin may change in appearance, developing a shine. If, after pressure, the skin remains the same (i.e., no pitting or change in color), this is often referred to as skin-swelling. Qi-swelling is often associated with generalized body swelling (because Qi travels everywhere) and is not associated with any skin changes (i.e., in color or pitting). Wind-water-swelling usually refers to the onset of edema after exposure to wind. Drum-distension is usually associated with abdominal distension and generalized swelling.[68]

BIOMEDICINE AND YE. Ye may be closely correlative to biomedical synovial and spinal fluid. The Synovium (see

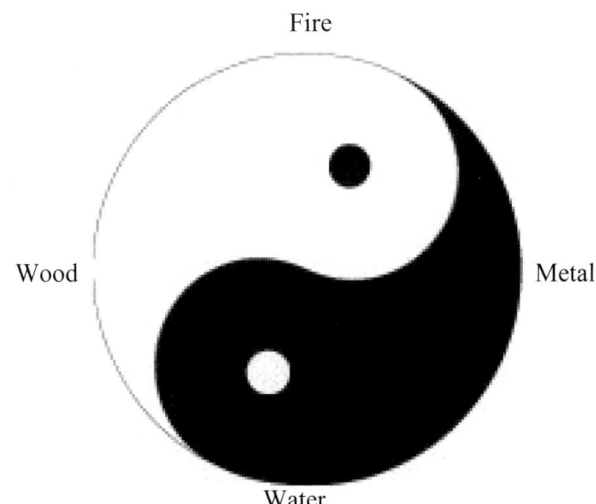
Figure 1-2: Yin and Yang Symbol.

chapter 2) is a colorless, viscid fluid that lubricates and nourishes the joint, including the avascular articular cartilage. The synovium plays a significant role in infection control (*OM: also Spleen, Kidney, Essence, and marrow functions*) and in production of hyaluronate, which gives synovial fluid its viscosity.

Yin and Yang

Yin and Yang are one of the earliest concepts described in Chinese sciences. First described around 700 B.C., Yin and Yang are *relative, interdependent* forces that both oppose and complement each other.[69] Yin and Yang are the two most primal manifestations of existence in the universe, after the division *(possibly the Big Bang)* of pretime "*singularity*."[70]

The Chinese character for Yin describes the shady side of a mountain, while the character for Yang describes the sunny side. One cannot exist without the other, and each transforms into the other. This concept is exemplified by the effects of morning and evening sun that result in opposite sides of the same mountain being more Yin or Yang at different times. A basic tenet of Yin Yang principles is that all subsystems (including the musculoskeletal system) are united, are part of a metasystem that is independent and interdependent at the same time. Although there may be local and specific variations, the underlying principles cannot be violated—disease begins when harmony and balance are disturbed. There is always Yin within Yang and Yang within Yin.

---

67. Not a classical association.
68. There are many other types of swellings associated with Fluids such as stone-water, mushroom-swelling, conglomerations and gatherings, Kidney-Wind-swelling, among others.
69. Although the mythical emperor Sheng Nung, about 2800 BC, is believed to be the source of the dual principles of the Yin and Yang.
70. These relate to Daoist ideas on the beginning of time.

Table 1-4: Basic Yin and Yang Aspects

Yin Aspects	Yang Aspects
Interior	Exterior
Lower	Upper
Anterior	Outer or Dorsal
Less active	More active
Cooler	Warmer
Slower	Faster
Substance	Function

According to Yin Yang theory, the seasonal cycle is the outcome of the mutually regulating, mutually generating, and mutually consuming activities of Yin and Yang. Either side of the two regulates and acts on the other, and one penetrates the other. This process of mutual regulation and interaction is at the heart of Yin Yang theory, without which change or harmony would not occur. Therefore, the two opposites of Yin and Yang do not exist as separate entities in a still or inactive state. They constantly interact with each other and allow for the alteration and development of objects and phenomena. At the same time, various phenomena are said to be always Yin or Yang; for example, the sun is always Yang and the moon always Yin, fire is always Yang while water always Yin.

The most basic tenets of the Yin and Yang concept are:

- Everything in the universe contains both Yin and Yang. The *Spiritual Axis* states: "Yin and Yang could amount to ten in number, be extended to one hundred, to one thousand, to ten thousand and even to the infinite....Man has physical shape, which is inseparable from Yin and Yang."
- The entire universe consists of dynamic, interdependent interactions between pairs of opposites (Yin and Yang). The *Spiritual Axis* states: "Yin is installed in the interior as the material foundation for Yang, while Yang remains on the exterior as the manifestation of the Yin function."
- Yin and Yang can transform into each other. The *Spiritual Axis* states: "Extreme Cold will bring about Heat, and extreme Heat will induce Cold...[furthermore], Excessive Yin may cause Yang syndromes or tend to transform into Yang and vice versa."
- Disease begins when balance is disturbed. The *Spiritual Axis* states: "When Yin keeps balance with Yang and both maintain a normal condition of Qi, health will be high-spirited. A separation of Yin and Yang will lead to the exhaustion of essential Qi."

Compared to Yin, Yang is more active, warmer, faster and lighter (less dense). Yin pertains more to dense material substance. Yang pertains more to function. Entities on the *Exterior*, upper, outer, or dorsal aspects of the body (such as skin, hair, skeletal muscles, head, limbs, trunk, vessels, and channels—body shell) are considered more Yang, as compared to the *Interior*, lower, and anterior aspects of the body (such as the viscera, although some aspects of the deep channels/vessels have functions that may be considered Interior as well). While Exterior, Excess, and Heat syndromes are considered Yang, Interior, Deficiency, and Cold syndromes are considered Yin. A boisterous voice indicates Yang, a low voice is Yin. Bright color is Yang, dim color is Yin. Coarse breathing is Yang, feeble and weak respiration is Yin. Superficial, rapid, and forceful pulses are Yang, slow, deep, feeble, and weak pulses are Yin (Table 1-4).

A few examples of Yin-Yang pairs are Qi and Blood, Exterior and Interior, Cold and Hot, Emptiness and Fullness.

QI - BLOOD. Qi, the vital force responsible for all life functions and all physiological activity, is more Yang than Blood. Blood, which is denser, is more Yin.

EXTERIOR - INTERIOR. Exterior (Yang, functional, muscular, hollow Organ) conditions are considered to be less serious than Interior (Yin, substance, bone, solid Organ) conditions.

COLD - HOT. Cold can be caused either by exogenous pathogens or by insufficiency of the body's Yang. When compared to Heat, it is considered to be Yin. Cold slows movement and contracts.

Heat is considered Yang in function or pathology. It can be caused by exuberant Yang (full-Heat) or by a relative weakness of Yin (empty-Heat), (Figure 1-4). Heat can also be caused by exogenous influences. Heat quickens movement and expands.

EMPTINESS - FULLNESS. Emptiness (also called "Deficiency" or "Vacuity") refers to a condition of insufficiency in any body substance or energy/forces (Yin, Yang, Qi, Blood, Essence, Fluids). It is Yin in nature.

Fullness (also called "Repletion" or "Excess") refers to any condition associated with exuberant pathogenic-Qi or the over accumulation/stagnation of a bodily substance. It is Yang in nature.

Yang and Exterior diseases are more easily treated, while Yin and Interior diseases are more difficult to treat. The *Classic of Internal Medicine* states:

> When the three Yang Channels and their collaterals are all affected by disease, but it has not yet entered the solid viscera (Zhang), it can be treated at this stage by inducing perspiration...When the three Yin and the Three Yang channels, and the five solid viscera and six hollow Organs (Fu) all suffer from the disease, Nutritive-Qi (nutrients) and Defensive-Qi cannot circulated freely. Hence the five solid Organs cannot perform their proper function, and death results.

Anatomical Orientation

Yin and Yang together with their channel attributions are used to describe anatomical orientation (Figure 1-3). In general, the ventral aspect of the body is Yin and dorsal aspect is Yang. The surface of the body is Yang while the interior is

Yin and Yang

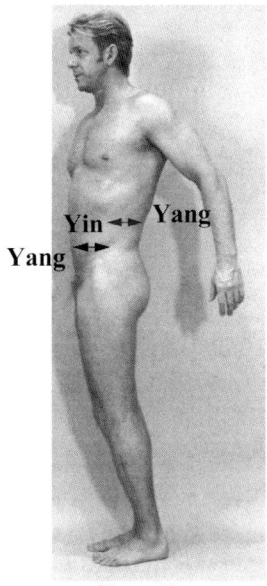
Shao-Yang

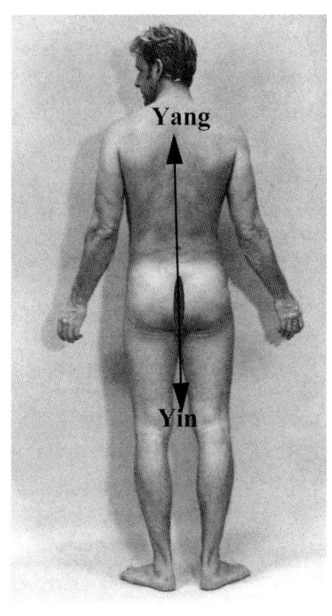
Yang

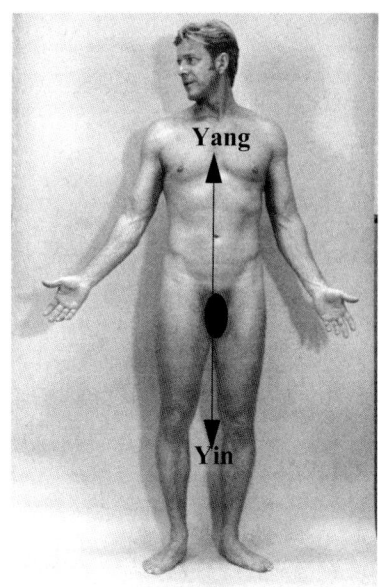
Yin

Figure 1-3: Anatomical orientations.

Yin. Superior areas such as the head and chest are Yang, while inferior areas such as the abdomen are Yin. The diaphragm separates the upper and lower. The little toe at UB-67 (even though on Yang/dorsal of Yin/inferior aspect) is named the most/reaching Yin (Zhi Yin). The lateral areas (sides) of the body are classified as Shao (lesser) Yang. Much of the medial and anterior areas are classified as Shao Yin or Jue (terminal) Yin. The perineum is considered to be the meeting of Yin and Yang (GV-1 and CV-1).

Biomedicine and Yin-Yang

Biomedical physiology describes balanced, interrelated, and interdependent servo-systems (i.e., regulating) as well. Many neural and endocrine functions are interdependent and interrelated, and are opposing in some situations and cumulative in others. Some are inhibitory; some are complementary. Goldenberg (1973) for example, compared the functions and relationships of cyclic adenosine monophosphate (cAMP) and cyclic guanosine monophosphate (cGMP) to Yin and Yang OM principals.[71] The density of cAMP and cGMP in cells are interrelated, at times oppose each other, and perform different functions in different cells. All servo-systems are, by their nature, Yin Yang balancing systems. The sympathetic nervous system may be thought of as being more Yang than the parasympathetic system when increased activity results in Yang-like activity, such as increased heart rate or increased sweating. This, however, is not consistent, since increased sympathetic activity can have inhibiting effects on digestive sections and motility (storage), and thus it is a Yin function (which may, however, be interpreted as Yang inhibiting Yin flow of Fluids, since it also results in dry mouth). While a nerve may be thought of as a Yin structure (and trophic factors transmitted via nerves function to nourish tissues), the transmission of information by action potential can be seen as the nerve's Yang function.

A study by Dong and Zuo (2002) showed the different effects needling Yang channel points (LI-4, 11, St-36, 37) and Yin channel points (P-6, Lu5, Sp-6, 9) had on different cerebral functional regions. They used positron emission tomography (PAT) to see if such effects could be documented. After needling the Yang channel points, the cerebral glucose metabolism was elevated in bilateral cross regions of the frontal lobe and temporal lobe, parietal lobe, thalamus, and basal ganglia, and in the contralateral cerebellum and hippocampus. After needling at Yin channel points, the cerebral glucose metabolism was lowered in the bilateral cross region of the frontal and temporal lobe, contralateral temporal lobe, cerebellum, and thalamus, and was elevated in the homolateral hippocampus and caudate nucleus.

Yin Yang and Musculoskeletal Medicine

In orthopedics, Yin and Yang can be expressed in various ways. For example, muscles that produce motion, acceleration, or concentric action can be considered Yang in nature. Muscles that stop motion, decelerate, and are eccentric in action may be considered more Yin in nature. Contractile aspects of muscles, myosin and actin (see chapter 2) may be

---

71. cAMP and cGMP mediate (second messenger) action of catecholamines, cholinergic receptors in parasympathetic nerve, vasopressin, adrenocorticotropic hormone, and other hormone functions.

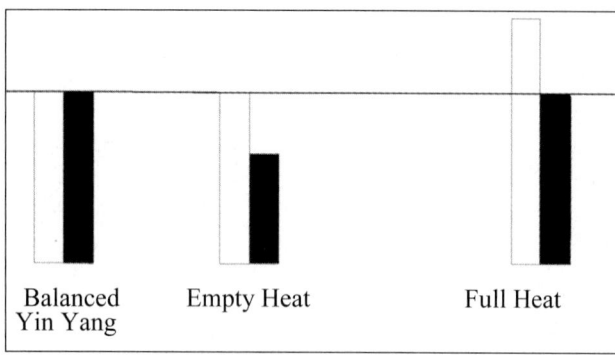

Figure 1-4: Yin and Yang balance. Empty-Heat presents with Heat symptoms due to lack of control by Water-Yin. Full-Heat presents with excess-Heat symptoms due to fullness of pathogenic-Qi.

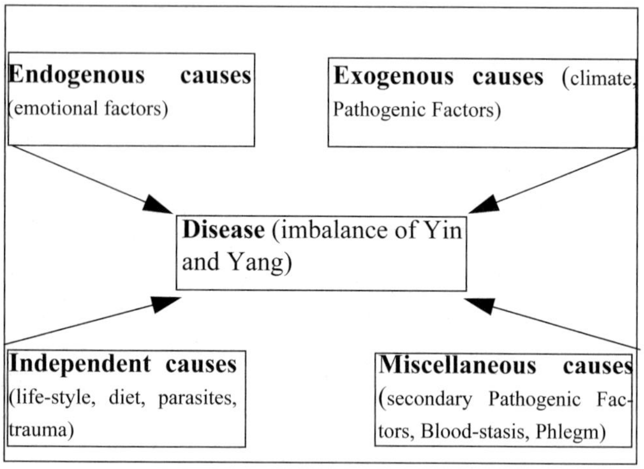

Figure 1-5: Causes of disease in TCM.

considered Yang. Tendons, which are noncontractile and denser, are more Yin. These functional aspects of muscles can transform and alternate (as can Yin and Yang).

To maintain normal gait and joint control, concentric Yang (*agonist*) muscles must interact constantly and sustain a working balance with eccentric Yin (*antagonist*) muscles. This fluid interdependence between agonist and antagonist muscles is a good example of Yin and Yang principles and interdependence.

Yin and Yang and Muscles

The biomedical model categorizes white muscles as having phasic functions and red muscles as having postural functions.

Phasic muscles are more Yang in nature because they tend to be located more superficially, can produce more force, and are faster acting.

Postural muscles may be classified as Yin because they tend to be deeper in the body, more vascular (they have increased density and are therefore red), and more resistant to fatigue than phasic muscles.

Postural Yin (red) muscles tend to develop Yang dysfunctions such as tightness. Phasic Yang (white) muscles tend to develop Yin dysfunctions such as weakness. It is said that "Yang produces Yin disorders and Yin produces Yang disorders" (see chapter 2).[72]

Disease Etiologies

TCM etiology classifies causes of disease (*factors*) as exogenous, endogenous, independent, and miscellaneous (Figure 1-5). In TCM, great attention is paid to Pathogenic Factors (both environmental and endogenous) and to the balance between antipathogenic forces and pathogenic forces (Zheng and Xie). It is said that whenever someone is a little uncomfortable (or is afflicted by external influences, such as a common cold), a balancing treatment should be initiated immediately. Even a single episode of becoming chilled is said to be capable of causing harm and of leading to serious and enduring disease. Thus minor illnesses (and dis-eases) should not be ignored, because once pathogenic influences ("evils" and dysfunctions) penetrate the Interior (deep aspects of the body), they may become very harmful and difficult to treat.[73] It is also stated that not all people will get sick due to environmental influences and therefore the condition of one's Righteous-Qi (total healthy influences, immune system) is important. The *Classic of Internal Medicine* states that if one conducts himself in "clarity and purity," he/she will not be affected by Wind, because his/her flesh and skin are tight and not open, the skin and pores being the door to Wind; however, if one sweats, the skin and pores open, and Wind can enter regardless of immunity.

Pathogenic Factors (Xie)

Pathogenic Factors are "Evil influences" that may arise internally or invade the Exterior from external environmental elements. In the *Classic of Internal Medicine* external pathogens are understood to invade the body via the skin and hair and to progress sequentially via the Minute (Sun) vessels (Mai) which meet all the Main channels at the acupuncture points (also called acupuncture holes). Pathogenic Factors may then settle in the skin, flesh, sinews, bones, channels, vessels, or Organs. When they only affect the Exterior and Channels, they are said to be easily treated. When settling in the Interior and Organs, they may be difficult to treat and even cause death. Therefore, it is essential to

---

72. Not classical associations.

73. At the same time some authors have stated that simple, self-limiting diseases should be left alone, and some advocated only treating 90% of an external illness and leaving the last 10% to the body's antipathogenic-Qi to overcome.

determine whether Pathogenic Factors are involved in the presenting complaint and to ascertain their depth of penetration, and if they are endogenously generated. The *Classic of Internal Medicine* elaborates on the progression of Exterior syndromes:

> The myriad of diseases always originate at the level of the skin and hair [Exterior]. When Pathogenic Factors attack the skin, the interstices and pores open. When they are open [the Pathogenic Factors] enter and reside in the network-vessels/collaterals (Minute vessels, Sun Mai). If they linger there and are not expelled, they will enter the Main channels. If they linger [in the Main channels] and are not expelled, they will enter the Yang Organs and gather in the Stomach and Large Intestine. When a pathogenic factor starts to enter the skin, chills and goose-flesh occur, and the interstices and pores open. When the Pathogenic Factors enter the network-vessels/collaterals, they are Excessive and the color changes. When they reside in the Main channels, the patient feels deficient and collapses. If The Pathogenic Factors linger between the sinews and bones and Cold predominates, the sinews spasm and the bones ache. If Heat predominates, the sinews become lax and the bones wilt, the flesh liquefies, the fleshy swellings disappear and the hair straightens and falls out.

Other alternative pathways are given in both the *Classic of Internal Medicine* (in "Simple Questions"/ "Su Wen") and in *Spiritual Axis* ("Ling Shu"), including the direct invasion of the Organs.

The Pathogenic Factors are: *Wind, Cold, Fire/Heat, Dampness, Dryness,* and *Summer-Heat* (Table 1-5). When they invade the body from the exterior, they are known as *exogenous Pathogenic Factors,* environmental influences that can cause disease. Wind, Cold, Fire/Warm, Dampness, Dryness, and Summer-Heat are known also as the *six environmental Excesses*. Unseasonal weather is said to be a major cause of disease. Early arrival of seasonal influences is said to cause Excess conditions and late arrival Deficiency. All of the Pathogenic Factors including Summer-Heat and Warm-diseases (Wen Bing) can arise from within as well.[74] However, external environmental pathogens are thought to be capable of damaging the body directly as compared to internal factors (emotions) that tend to affect physiological processes which then lead to disease or pathogenic processes. Warm-diseases are associated with hidden/lurking pathogens that can be activated by internal factors. The exogenous factors, which are associated with climatic influences, often manifest as acute disorders. They usually invade the Exterior (skin, hair, muscles, channels)[75] and obstruct the flow of Qi and Blood. This explains why a patient suffering from the flu (a respiratory virus) may also complain of muscle aches. The presence of muscle aches and aversion to cold and wind is said to be pathomnemonic with Pathogenic Factors at the Exterior. A patient with Exterior Pathogenic Factors often suffers from a runny or stuffy nose and may or may not have a fever. The pulse should be floating, but in clinical practice may not be.[76] Pain from Exterior syndromes, in a relatively healthy individual, should theoretically self-resolve in a few days.[77] All the Pathogenic Factors are mutually enforcing as it is said: "Dampness engenders Phlegm, Phlegm engenders Heat and Heat engenders Wind."

It must be emphasized that in TCM it is the manifestation of symptoms and signs that determines the patient's diagnosis, not the origin of the so-called pathogen (i.e., the patient does not have to be exposed to environmental wind to have external Wind.) The diagnosis of Exterior invasion of Wind-Heat or Wind-Cold may depend more on the individual response to the pathogenic factor than the pathogen, whether it is infectious and related to environmental exposure, or self-generating.[78] Thus the diagnosis of Exterior syndrome does not require exposure to climatic influence, although such exposure is certainly possible, and this diagnosis therefore does not contradict viral theories. Also, in modern times, the effects of weather and other environmental factors (except toxins) are moderated by clothing and shelter. Many Exterior syndromes may, in fact, be Internal/ miscellaneous diseases. In Zhu Dan Xi's *The Heart and Essence of Dan-Xi's Method of Treatment,* the discussion of Cold Damage states that internal damage is extremely common, while external contraction is only seen occasionally. This is in contrast with the classic *Damage By Cold* which relates many diseases to external Cold contraction, and possibly explains why some people contract viral diseases while others who have been exposed do not. It may also explain why Exterior symptoms, or signs are often lacking in patients with "cold and flu-like" complaints.[79]

Since symptoms of Wind, Cold, Fire/Heat, Dampness, and Dryness can originate from within or without, it is the pulse, tongue, and specific symptoms that determine if the condition is "*Exterior*" or "*Interior.*" In general, Exterior

---

74. The concept of Warm-diseases developed from the six environmental factors. Hidden Pathogenic Factors and Warm-diseases (pathogens) can linger in the body and be triggered spontaneously without a new exposure (although some stress is needed to activate the pathogens). This may suggest an incubation period or a period of dormancy. Much of the Warm-diseases literature, however, uses the phrase "hidden" (Fu) or "lurking Pathogenic Factors" to describe ongoing symptoms. Worm infections, insect bites, Phlegm, Blood-stasis, etc., are also types of pathogens.

75. Some texts consider the Exterior as being the endoskeletal frame, i.e., skin, flesh, sinews, and bones. Other texts, or sections within the same text, consider bones as being in the Interior, as they are under the control of the Kidneys.

76. Reading the radial pulse quality is an OM diagnostic method. If a patient does not have a floating pulse in the beginning of externally contracted Exterior syndrome, this is said, in part, to be due to a debilitated condition and to weak defenses not resisting the pathogen. In such cases the practitioner may need to decide whether to follow the pulse information or the pattern of symptoms and tongue. The floating quality probably occurs due to a widening of the capillaries, arterioles, and arteries, induced by the body dissipating heat.

77. Theoretically strong Defensive-Qi should prevent the invasion of most exogenous Pathogenic Factors.

78. Warm and Toxic (infectious) diseases, however, do tend to affect all people regardless of constitution and Defensive-Qi.

syndromes are said to have a floating/superficial pulse, and Interior syndromes have a deep pulse. The tongue coat is thin with Exterior and thick or peeled with Interior syndromes (see below).

In summary, it is important to assess every patient without preconceived ideas. While a patient may appear to have an Exterior condition such as a Cold or Painful Obstruction (Bi) (rheumatic and pain) syndrome, very similar symptoms can arise from Interior causes as well.

In TCM, most pain is caused by an obstruction of either Qi or Blood flow. Pathogenic Factors can result in obstruction and therefore pain, and are common factors in treating painful musculoskeletal disorders.

Wind (Feng)

Wind is said to be "the chief (or initiator) of hundreds of diseases" and is capable of carrying or guiding other Pathogenic Factors into the Exterior or Interior. (That is why it is called "the chief" of Pathogenic Factors.) Therefore, Wind is commonly associated with other Pathogenic Factors. The *Classic of Internal Medicine* states:

> When Wind harms a person, it may cause Cold and Heat; or it may cause a Heated center; or it may cause a Cold center; or it may cause Wind. These diseases are all different. Their names are not identical. In some cases [the Wind] internally reaches the Five solid Organs and Six hollow Organs...

Wind pathogenic factor invades the Exterior when the patient is constitutionally weak or when Defensive-Qi is temporarily depleted. The character of Wind is stirring, agitating, coming-on quickly, and intermittent. Therefore, Wind disorders come on or change quickly. Wind is considered a Yang pathogen that easily transforms to Fire that "strikes before noon." A Wind pathogen is light and therefore rises up and out. Often it results in symptoms of the upper/outer body such as dizziness, headaches, stiff neck, and itching, and has an affinity with the Lungs. When Wind is "widespread," it is said to cause tugging, convulsions, tremors, and shaking. Severe rigidity (spasm) is said to be caused by Wind, especially when Wind and Fire affect the channels and network-vessels. Exterior Wind is associated usually with a runny or stuffy nose and floating/superficial pulse. The tongue is usually normal when Wind is an external patogen but may be stiff and deviated when due to internal-Wind.

Head tremor is said to be generally associated with internal-Wind, which may arise from Liver disorders of Deficiency or Excess type.[80] In general, internal-Wind can arise from Liver disorders, Blood-deficiency, and extreme-Heat.

- The tongue in patients with Interior-Wind from Blood-deficiency is pale. The pulse is thready or choppy.
- The tongue in patients with Wind due to Liver-Yin-deficiency is red and the coat is peeled or very thin. The pulse is wiry, tight, and rapid or floating, quick, and empty.
- The tongue in patients with Wind due to Liver-transformative-Heat/Fire (which often arises from severe Qi-stagnation) is usually red. The tongue body is often slightly swollen (especially at the edges) or normal. The tongue coat can be yellow or off-white. The pulse may be wiry, tight, large, forceful, and quick.
- The tongue in a patient with Wind due to extreme-Heat is very red (especially tip and sides), and the coat is yellow. The pulse is rapid, often large and/or tidal, and may be tight.

Wind can also take advantage of traumatic injuries, open sores, bathing in hot or cold water or moxa and settle in the tissues. Wind, like most Pathogenic Factors, manifests differently in each Organ. The *Classic of Internal Medicine* states:

> The appearance of Lung Wind [is such that patients] sweat profusely and have an aversion to Wind. Their [facial] color is a pale white. They often cough and are short of Qi (breath). It is diagnosed above the eyebrows; the color is white.
>
> The appearance of Heart Wind [is such that patients] sweat profusely and have an aversion to wind. When the burning is extreme, they tend to be angry and to terrorize [others]. Their

---

79. There are many causes within TCM for the subjective feeling of heat (often with objective warmness but not necessarily with increased body temperature). These can include: externally contracted pathogens; congestion/depressive-Fire (often related to emotional effects); Qi/Yang-congestion/depression-transformation-Heat/Fire, Yin-deficiency-Empty-Heat/Fire; Yang-deficiency-Floating-Yang-*false*-Heat/Fire; Blood-deficiency-Heat; Blood-stasis-Heat (which can be related to Blood-deficiency or any other cause of Blood-stasis); Toxic-Heat (which can be related to severe-Heat, internal or external Toxins, etc.); Damage/taxation-Heat/Fire (usually Blood and Qi damage; or Yin and Yang damage; diet; general stress; excessive sexual activity; medical causes; etc.); Steaming-bone-Heat/Fire (often due to internal damage or Pathogenic Factors); and Water not controlling Fire (mostly Kidney Heart disharmony, or any Yin-deficiency-Empty-Fire), among others. Therefore, a sensation of "feverishness" is not necessarily due to infectious (external contraction, or internal penetration of exterior) pathogens, but can be due to many other causes that must be understood when treating musculoskeletal disorders. For example, an important herbal combination suggested by Li Dong for patients suffering from symptoms related to Heat, and that can be used often for musculoskeletal disorders, is Huang Qi 30g and Dang Gui 6g (Dang Gui Bu Xue Tang, Tangkuei Decoction to Tonify the Blood). This formula is used for a patient that feels heat (feverish, but without abnormal body temperature) within the muscle. This Heat is due to "floating-Yang" secondary to damage to Qi and Blood. This Heat is not due to external contraction but due to internal damage. It can be used to treat muscular atrophy and/or weakness. The patient's tongue is pale, the pulse is large and empty, and the patient prefers warm beverages.

80. Tremors, twitches, and tics of the head and face can also be caused by Liver-Qi-stagnation, Phlegm, and external-Wind. In general, spasticity, tremors, twitches, and tics are said to be caused by: Liver-Wind (most common) from Liver-Yang-rising; Liver-Fire (often transforming from Liver-congestion Qi-stagnation); Wind arising from deficiency of Blood or Yin (particularly Liver); exterior-Wind; Phlegm combined with Wind (external or internal); Heat in Blood division/level (four division theory); severe-Heat transforming into Fire-Wind (which may be due to Organic, pathogenic, or local effects. Pulling and "tenseness" of muscles can also be caused by Coldness of external or internal origins.

[facial] color is red. When the disease is severe, [the patient finds] it impossible to speak cheerfully. It is diagnosed at the mouth; the color there is red.

The appearance of Liver Wind [is such that patients] sweat profusely and have an aversion to wind. They tend to be sad. Their [facial] color is slightly greenish. When the throat is dry, they tend to be angry. At times they hate women. It is diagnosed below the eyes; the color there is green-blue.

The appearance of Spleen Wind [is such that patients] sweat profusely and have an aversion to wind. Their body is tired and [they are] lazy; their four limbs do not wish to move. Their [facial color] is slightly yellow. They do not wish to eat. It is diagnosed above the nose; the color there is yellow.

The appearance of Kidney Wind [is such that patients] sweat profusely and have an aversion to wind. Their face develops a surface swelling of the Yang-type. The spine aches, and they cannot stand upright. Their [facial] color is [that of] soot. The passage through the hidden bend is impeded. It is diagnosed above the jaws; the color there is black.

In musculoskeletal disorders Wind is usually associated with wandering or radiating pain, upper body (neck, shoulder, head) pain, or muscle twitches/spasms or with paresthesias.[81]

Cold (Han)

Cold pathogenic factor invades the Exterior when the patient is constitutionally weak, or when Defensive-Qi is temporarily depleted. An external Cold pathogen is often combined with Wind. Cold constricts and contracts so that muscles and movement are often affected. *Simple Questions* states: "When strong pathogenic Cold is in the muscles and the bones, it results in stiffness of the muscles and pain in the bones." Cold may also congeal Blood and affect the free flow of Qi, resulting in a Painful Obstruction (Bi) syndrome.[82] Congestion may also result in superficial edema. The stronger the pain and the tighter the muscles, the more exuberant the Cold pathogenic factor.[83] *Cold is said to govern pain.* In the time of the Han dynasty, Cold pathogenic factor was often viewed as the major cause of disease. The *Classic of Internal Medicine* states:

> The Yellow Emperor asks: Nowadays hot (febrile) diseases all belong to Cold. People may either recover from it or die. If they die, death always occurs between six or seven days. If they recover, it takes more than ten days. Why is that?

Qibo's answer to the Yellow Emperor's question is the basis for the later classic *On Harm Caused by Cold* (about 220 AD) which strongly infulenced OM practice for many centuries.

Because exogenous Wind-Cold usually penetrates the body through the Tai-Yang (UB) channel, the first associated symptom is often muscle ache and tension at the upper portion and/or back of the body (or UB sinew channel).

In modern times, heating and clothing are usually sufficient, so External Cold causing Painful Obstruction is likely not as prevalent as in older times. However, the use of air conditioning, walking barefoot or open sandals in cold weather, etc., can probably still result in overexposure to cold. Acute hypothermia and cold exposure are known factors causing both acute and chronic myofascial pain syndromes ("Fibromyalgia and Myofascial Pain Syndrome" on page 597).

Exterior Wind-Cold causes contraction of the blood vessels; therefore, the superficial pulses may tighten. The tongue is usually normal and the coat is thin white.

Weak or damaged True/Original/Righteous-Qi (constitution) can result in symptoms of Yang-deficiency and *internal-Cold*. Internal-Cold will usually manifest clinically as Yang-deficiency of the Kidneys or Spleen, or both. This results often in Cold accumulation which can become a *pathogenic factor* on its own. This condition is treated by warming the Interior with or without the addition of (Organ Yang) tonics. Here the patient may suffer from similar symptoms as seen in external-Cold, except that the onset is often insidious. The condition is chronic, and the patient is usually less sensitive to environmental wind and cold. The patient can be warmed by wearing extra clothing. The pulses may be deeper than normal and rise without force, and the tongue may be pale and swollen. Any prolonged External pathogenic infection can also lead to depletion of Yang, resulting in Interior-Cold.

Cold-obstruction is often combined with Dampness and/or Blood-stasis. Cold is said to be a common underlying cause of Blood-stasis. Cold is also said to "damage Form."[84] Deficiency of Yang (i.e., internal-Cold) is said to "engender external-Cold." Also, prolonged Qi-deficiency, especially if combined with retained Dampness or pathogenic water, can lead to the damage of Yang-Qi and result in internal-Cold. This is because Dampness is a Yin pathogen; by nature it is averse to Yang/Fire.

---

81. It is important to understand that Wind is not the only condition which is capable of causing movements and changeability. For example, Shao-Yang disorders, which are described as having Pathogenic Factors between the Exterior and Interior, a space that includes the Cou Li, can also result in changeability and large movements that not only pertains to depth (i.e., Exterior and Interior) but also pertains to regions. Qi-stagnation is also commonly associated with movement and changeability.

82. Most musculoskeletal pain disorders are described as Painful Obstruction disorder (Bi syndrome).

83. Acute traumatic arthritis, septic arthritis, and other acute frank inflammations (Heat disorders) usually result in more intense pain and restriction of movement. The restriction, however, is not due to tightness in muscles as is often seen with Cold-Damp pathogens, but rather to a reflexive protective action of muscle due to painful stimuli by joint capsules. At rest or in non-weight bearing the muscles are usually loose and only spring into protective spasm when the joint capsule is stressed. Cold-Bi (painful obstruction) is also called painful-Bi.

84. Form usually pertains to actual physical structure or substantial pathogen such as being fat related to excess-Phlegm. When Form is damaged there is actual physical change.

Painful symptoms associated with Cold are often worse in the morning (when Yin settles and Yang begins to increase) and improve with movement when circulation improves (Yang increases) and the tissues are warmed.

Heat/Fire (Re/Huo)

Heat Pathogenic Factors invade the Exterior when the patient is constitutionally weak or Defensive-Qi is temporarily depleted. But in contrast to Cold pathogens, which are said to enter the body through the skin and muscles, Heat/Warm-diseases enter the body through skin, nose or mouth. Therefore, Warm-diseases and Wind-Heat can often infect a patient regardless of the state of their Defensive (antipathogenic) Qi. External-Heat pathogens are usually combined with Wind. Warm-Heat/Fire or Summer-Heat are also common TCM etiologies of epidemic diseases.[85] External-Heat is usually associated with a fever. There is some thirst or dryness in the throat/lips and/or mouth, and the eyes are often red.

External invasion of Wind in a patient with exuberance of Yang is said to manifest often as Exterior-Wind-Heat. Heat/Fire is Yang; it expands, rises, and stirs (Wind and Blood), causing pain to radiate. The pulse may quicken, enlarge, and rise with force. The face and eyes are usually red. Heat consumes Yin/Blood and Fluids. Damage may also result in consumptive malnourishment of sinews and muscles, causing weakness and/or possible atrophy. As Heat is said to "stir Wind," the combination of "oppressive Wind-Heat" can result in severe muscle spasms and tetany. Hypertonicity may also be seen if Nutritive-Qi, Blood, and Yin are depleted.[86] In the *Spiritual Axis,* Tai-Yang tetany due to Heat is described as clonic in nature (alternating spasms with relaxation).[87] With severe Heat, the tissues and patient feel warm; the feet however, are often cold, as "extreme Heat can create Cold." The patient may still suffer from generalized chills if pathogens are at the Exterior. The tongue body may be red, and the tongue coat may be gray (off-white) or yellow. These descriptions, however, relate to internal medical condition.

Fire is usually used to describe Heat from endogenous origin, although it can be used to describe Exterior *severe-Heat*, or localized-Heat (binding/congested-Heat).[88] Endogenous-Heat/Fire is *usually* not (but can be) associated with a true fever (increased temperature). It is important to remember that any of the "six stagnations/depressions,"[89] especially Qi-stagnation and Damp-obstruction, can easily transform into Heat/Fire or Damp-Heat.[90] Also, Wind, Cold, Summer-Heat, Dampness, Dryness, poor Qi or Blood vitality, lack of regulation of the Organs, and emotional effects with Qi-stagnation can all transform into Fire/Heat. Symptoms associated with Heat/Fire often worsen at night, disturbing the patient's sleep, especially if associated with Blood-stasis or Yin-damage. When severe Heat-(inflammation) disturbs the patient's sleep, a serious disease is more likely. As Fire is said to be capable of "producing toxins," severe Heat/Fire or Damp-Heat, especially if in the Blood-division,[91] can result in skin eruptions, papular or macular, and bleeding. Damp-Heat can result in suppurative lesions. All of the above are sometimes used to describe *septic* joint and bone diseases with or without visible suppuration.

Heat may also arise from lack of Yin-Blood (Yin, Fluids, Blood) not controlling Yang (Fire), and is then called deficiency or Empty-Heat.[92] The Yin aspects of the body (chest, abdomen, palms and soles of feet) become warmer which is known as five-center-Heat. In Excess/Full pathogenic Heat/fever, the Yang aspects of the body (back, forehead, dorsal aspects of hands and feet) are warmer than the Yin/ventral aspects. To determine if Heat is Deficient or Excessive, the practitioner can palpate the patient's forehead and palms at the same time. If the palms are hotter than the forehead, this *may* indicate Deficiency/Empty-Heat; if the forehead is hotter, this *may* indicate Excess/Full-Heat. The pulse tends to be quick and weak in empty-Heat. It may also be tight or soft, floating or deep.

Dampness (Shi)

Damp pathogenic factor invades the Exterior when the patient is constitutionally weak, or when Defensive-Qi is temporarily depleted. It can also enter through the mouth (especially Damp-Heat) regardless of Defensive-Qi or constitutional strength. The nature of Dampness is heavy, sticky, viscous, substantial, and turbid. Therefore, it is said to linger, be difficult to cure, and thought to be "contracted first below." Consequently, Painful Obstruction due to Dampness is called *fixed-Bi*. External Damp pathogens are combined often with Wind, which, in contrast to Damp-pathogens, are erratic and moving. Patients with exuberant Yang are said to be susceptible to developing Wind-Damp-Heat disorders, whereas patients with weak Yang, True and Original-Qi or

---

85. Epidemic (Yi) is a category of diseases that have a definite infectious origin, are due to environmental factors, and infect entire communities regardless of the strength of their constitutional or Defensive-Antipathogenic-Qi. The cause of epidemic diseases is often said to be Warm-pestilential-Qi (Yi Li) and is similar to other seasonal diseases having to do with rhythmic, periodic processes of the universe (the Five Phases and the Six Pathogenic Factors). *Spiritual Axis* says: "... when the Five Epidemics occur, everyone becomes infected... Whether they be old or young, the symptoms of the disease are the same...In this epidemic (Yi), people are affected by the Pestilential-Qi from heaven and Earth...The severity of the epidemic varies in each year, and manifests differently in different localities and in different seasons... When this Qi has come, old and young, weak and strong who come in contact with it all get sick."

86. Spasm and tetany of the neck, for example, are also said to be caused by Dampness (a Yin pathogen). So, like so many symptoms in TCM, there may be many opposing etiologies.

87. In the *Systematic Classic of Acupuncture & Moxibustion*, Zhang Zhong-jing divided Tai-Yang spasms into "hard and soft" depending on the presence of aversion to cold. There are also Damp-tetany and Wind-tetany.

88. Fire is also used to describe *normal Yang* functions in the body such as Mingmen or Kidney-Fire.

constitution tend to be susceptible to developing Wind-Damp-Cold disorders. Dampness is associated with damp environments, climates, and even one's own sweat, especially if the patient does not change out of wet clothing after sweating from exercise, which leaves the skin-pores "open." Exterior-Dampness can result in swelling and thickening. If severe enough, Dampness can damage Yang. This could lead to pitting edema and even the formation of cysts (such as seen on tendons, i.e., ganglion cysts). When Yang is obstructed by turbid-Dampness, the skin and muscles may feel numb and the joints may feel stiff and painful. Dampness is said to be associated with the sensation of *fullness,* the sensation of being *boundup,* and the *cumbersome fatigue of limbs.* Dampness is a Yin pathogen that is capable of injuring Yang, especially Spleen Yang. However, since Dampness can result in accumulative-obstruction, Dampness can easily transform (Hua) into Heat and/or Damp-Heat. This may further transform into Fire/toxin.[93] Many skin disorders are therefore associated with Damp-Heat (toxin).[94]

Whether Exterior or Interior, Dampness is said to have a direct relationship with the Spleen's functions of transportation and transformation (digestive functions and movement of Qi and Fluid upwards). When external-Dampness enters the body (often through the mouth and Stomach/Earth), it tends to gravitate to Spleen/Earth related tissues, the flesh/muscles, and obstructs Spleen/pancreas functions. This results often in generalized symptoms of *heaviness/fatigue, fullness,* poor appetite, loose or sticky/pasty and difficult to move stools, a sensation of incomplete evacuation of stools, abdominal discomfort or distension, and swelling (especially after eating) in both Exterior and Interior Damp or Phlegm disorders. (For information on Phlegm see page 39).[95] While external Dampness is said to cause more "heaviness" and internal Dampness is said to result more in difficult urination, internal and external Dampness are mutually engendering. It is also important to understand that Dampness obstructing the Spleen/pancreas is an Excess/Full disorder (as disorders of the Spleen/pancreas are often thought of as Deficiency/Empty conditions). The *Classic of Internal Medicine* states: "In disease of Dampness the Head feels boundup. If Damp-Heat cannot be eliminated, the big muscles contract and there is spasms. The small muscles become flaccid and atrophied." *(Biomedical: interestingly this pattern of muscular reactions is also described by Janda. See chapter 3).*

With internal Damp disease, the disease process tends to be prolonged and may arise from failure to treat external-Dampness, constitutional weakness, or from other mechanisms that weaken the Spleen, Stomach, Lungs, or Kidneys. Since Spleen-Qi-deficiency, or any Qi-deficiency, and Dampness are associated with symptoms of fatigue, clinically one may need to differentiate between fatigue caused by *Deficiency* and *Excess* syndromes. Since Dampness is heavy and tends to settle with inactivity, fatigue that is due to Dampness is worse with inactivity and in the morning. Deficiency-fatigue is worse after activity and, therefore, is often worse in the afternoon. However, symptoms of Damp-Heat often increase during afternoon as well (mostly fever related), and therefore should be considered. Constitutionally strong patients with chronic or "constitutional-Dampness" tend to develop Damp-Heat and have strong and slippery pulses, especially at the right middle (Spleen) position. If Dampness leads to general Deficiency or is associated with constitutional-Deficiency, the pulse at the right middle (Spleen) position tends to be deep and weak. A deep, soft, and easily-dispersing-on-pressure pulse may be seen in patients with Dampness and Empty-Heat.[96]

Because the Spleen's transformation and transportation functions are dependent on Kidney-Yang, dual deficiency of Kidney and Spleen/pancreas are seen commonly in patients with chronic Dampness and Fluid/water disorders. When the Kidneys are involved, one may see additional Kidney symp-

---

89. Zhu Dan-xi's six depressions/congestions refer to Qi, Blood, Fire, Phlegm, Dampness, and food stagnation. Here, however, the six-stagnations refer to the six-Excesses (Pathogenic Factors). Stagnation/Depression describes flow stoppage associated with congestion or impairment of flow with so-called binding congestion. Zhu Dan-xi's *Qi-depression/congestion* mainly manifests as chest and hypochondrial pain/distension and a deep, rough pulse. *Blood-depression/congestion* refers mainly to weakness of the limbs, bloody stools, and a deep, hollow pulse. *Fire-depression/congestion* mainly manifests as clouded and distorted vision, concentrated (red) urine, and a deep, fast pulse. *Phlegm-depression/congestion* manifests mainly as asthma aggravated by physical exertion and a deep slippery pulse. *Damp-depression/congestion* manifests mainly as pain all over the body, or pain in the joints that starts after exposure to rainy, wet, and cold weather, with a deep, fine pulse. *Food-depression/stagnation* manifests mainly as acid reflux, belching with a sour taste, a full stomach with loss of appetite, and a leisurely pulse on the right with a tight and strong pulse on the left. The underlying cause of all the six-depression/congestions is Qi-stagnation and is often attributed to Excesses of the affects-mind causing Liver-congestion Qi-stagnation. All can easily transform into Heat and all are mutually engendering.

To treat the six-depressions use Six Depressions Decoction (Liu Yu Tang): Rhizoma Cypri (Xiang Fu), Rhizoma Atractylodis (Shen Qu), Fructus Gardeniae (San Zhi Zi), Fructus Forsythiae (Lian Qiao), Fructus Citri (Zhi Ke), Pericarpim Citri (Chen Pi), Radix Ligustici (Chuan Xiong), Radix Scutellariae (Huang Qin), Caulis Perillae (Su Geng), and Radix Glaycrrhizaie (Gan Cao).

90. Zhu Dan-xi also stated that Damp-Heat and Yin-deficiency cause most diseases.

91. Blood-division is part of Four-level diagnosis of Warm-Heat (Wen Bing) disease doctrine.

92. Empty-Heat (especially from Kidney and Liver) has been related to adrenal exhaustion in patients that feel a nervous-weariness (weakness-induced irritability and anxiety) and suffer from failure to regulate inflammatory and reaper pathways.

93. Toxic-Heat and Toxic-Qi are often used to describe epidemic, infectious, and skin diseases.

94. Exterior signs of toxins are often seen as skin lesions.

95. While the sensation of heaviness is often associated with Dampness, it can also be due to other causes. For example, heaviness is associated with external Cold pathogens blocking the Exterior and affecting the Nutritive-Qi in the classic *On Cold Damage* (Shang Han Lun).

96. Because Heat tends to rise, in Heat disorders the pulses tend to be more superficial. In this case, Dampness prevents the pulse from rising.

toms, especially increased and/or decreased urination (or night urination), tinnitus, shortness of breath, lightheadedness, cold extremities, and fatigue. All of these are *aggravated by exertion,* and all are chronic and "stubborn." Pitting edema of the lower extremity, especially around the ankles, may be seen. Lower abdominal pulsation may be palpated. (Often this is diagnostic of Kidney involvement; see "Abdominal Assessment" on page 333.) Because Dampness obstructs the flow of Qi, Qi-stagnation and Liver-Qi-stagnation (or congestion/depression) is seen often in Damp disorders. Humid weather (especially when hot and muggy) can result in symptoms of Dampness and Liver-Qi-stagnation.[97]

As Dampness is capable of damaging the sinews, bones, Blood, and blood vessels (and is frequently seen in Painful Obstruction Bi syndromes), it is often viewed as the central pathogenic factor in musculoskeletal pain. The pain tends to be achy, heavy, full, and fixed in location. The tissues are often damp, swollen, and possibly numb-like. The tongue may be swollen with teeth marks; the tongue coat may be greasy or thick. The pulse tends to be soft, slippery, or wiry. With Exterior-Dampness the pulse may be floating and soft. With Interior-Dampness the pulse is often deep and soft at the right middle (Spleen) position.

Damp-Heat is formed by the combination of two distinct pathogens: Dampness and Heat. Dampness and Heat are said to be *mutually transforming.* Damp-Heat is a hospitable environment for worms and thus is said to "engender-worms." In general, Damp-Heat can be caused by:

- An accumulation of endogenous-Dampness (Cold and Yin pathogens) which stagnates and transforms into Heat, and eventually combines with Dampness to form Damp-Heat. This, of course, can be a result of any dysfunction in which the strength or movement of Qi is affected.
- External-Dampness may accumulate and transform into Heat, resulting in Damp-Heat.
- Pathogenic Heat/Fire may congeal Fluids, causing pathogenic Damp-Heat.

A combination of the above three mechanisms is not uncommon. Because Damp-Heat is made up of a Yin (Damp) pathogen and a Yang (Heat) pathogen, the patient may present *contradictory or reduced* symptoms and signs. When Dampness dominates (in Damp-Heat), the Heat/feverishness symptoms are milder, because Water controls Fire. The skin may not be warm, the pulse may not be as fast, or tongue may not be as red, even though there is Heat or fever. The bowels may alternate from constipation and hard stools to loose and frequent stools. Other symptoms are *thirst or dry mouth without the desire to drink much*, possible increasing afternoon fevers, *scanty dark* or difficult urination, warm swelling, and yellow sticky tongue coat. Environmental Damp-Heat is said to be most common in "long summer," especially when the temperature is very hot and the earth is damp (muggy weather). Wu Ju Tong states: "Exclusively clearing Heat, the Dampness will not back off; restrictively draining Dampness, the Heat will blaze."

Dryness (Zao)

Dry pathogenic factor invades the Exterior when the patient is constitutionally weak, or if Defensive-Qi is temporarily depleted. The characteristics of pathogenic Dryness are dryness and astringency, which tend to injure Fluids and Yin. Exterior Dryness is associated with Pathogenic Factors contracted mostly in autumn or dry environments. Symptoms are said to include dry mouth and throat, dry lips, dry nostrils, nose bleeding, and dry cough. The tongue is dry and pulse is floating and often is quick.

Dryness can result also from Yin, Blood, or Fluid-deficiency and/or damage. The pulse in Blood-deficiency would be thready or choppy, and the tongue would be pale and dry. The pulse associated with Yin-deficiency would be quick, tight, wiry or thready, or floating and empty. The tongue would be red, dry, with little or no coat. There may be increased signs of tissue wrinkles, cracks, and "withering dryness." At times the only sign is a dry tongue coat or body.

In musculoskeletal disorders, Dryness is frequently associated with endogenous Yin/Fluids and Blood-deficiency (but not with exogenous Dryness), except that Exterior (i.e., at outer body skin and muscles) Dryness can damage Yin/Blood/Fluids. It is said that "when Dryness is located in the hands and feet, weakness may ensue."

Dryness of the mouth and lips (and tongue body or coat) may also be seen when the Spleen/pancreas fails to raise Fluids. In this condition usually symptoms and signs of Dampness and Dryness coexist. Dry lips, mouth, and tongue from Spleen/pancreas dysfunction should not be confused with Interior dryness, because treatment of the former is by warming and drying herbs which can aggravate Yin-deficiency or Dryness.

Summer-Heat (Shu Wen)

Summer-Heat Pathogenic Factors invade the Exterior when the patient is constitutionally weak or when Defensive-Qi is temporarily depleted. Summer-Heat is also associated with Warm-disease (infectious disease)[98] and may affect people regardless of their anti-pathogenic state. It is associated with

---

97. A dysfunction of Liver-Qi is often divided into two main types. The first is due to lack of flow and is often referred to in this book as congestion. Liver-Depression is also commonly used. The Second is abnormal movement of Liver-Qi and is often called Liver invasion of Spleen/Stomach/Center or Wood attack Earth in the five Phase paradigm.

98. The term "Warm Diseases" often implies *epidemic* febrile diseases. The theory by Wu Youxing (1582-1652) described *"transmissible"* causative agents and pestilential factors (Li Qi) before the germ theory in the West. In the Warm-Disease doctrine, diseases are categorized in 4-divisions/levels (Fen). The most superficial is the Defensive (Wei), then the Qi (often associated with Organs, especially Lung, Spleen or all the Yang Organs), Nutritive (Ying), and, the deepest, the Blood-division (Xue Fen).

the hot or damp weather of the summer months. Heat/sunstroke can affect the patient regardless of the condition of Defensive-Qi. Summer-Heat is associated also with latent/hidden/lurking Pathogenic Factors (Fu Shu) that, for the most part, are said to present clinically in the *fall* or *winter*. Summer-Heat can strongly damage the Qi and Yin/Fluids by excessive sweating and Heat burning Fluids. Summer-Heat-Dampness-*entrapment* can also result from drinking cold beverages in the summer months.

Triple Warmer pattern differentiation is often used in Summer-Heat and Warm-diseases diagnosis where Pathogenic Factors are seen as progressing from the upper-Warmer (Lungs) to the middle-Warmer (Spleen and Stomach), to the lower-Warmer (Liver and Kidneys); or where symptoms begin in the middle-Warmer.

Summer-Heat is not commonly associated with musculoskeletal disorders except that it can lead to Fluid damage with consequences of dryness, or result in hidden pathogens that also can damage Yin and Fluids.

INFLAMMATION. Inflammation (a biomedical concept) may be related to the reaction of the body's Defensive- and antipathogenic-Qis to insult.[99] Because *active* inflammation is usually associated with tissue warmth and swelling, it is often, but not always, classified as Damp-Heat or Wind-Heat.[100] Inflammation rids the body of foreign matter (exogenous or endogenous Pathogenic Factors), disposes of damaged cells, and initiates wound healing.

When inflammation affects a joint (Heat-Bi) as it does in rheumatoid arthritis, the cartilage can be damaged by Heat, which injures Fluids and joint nutrition *(biomedicine: by neutrophils and lysosomal enzymes that enter the area)*.

The body reacts to injury and infection similarly, since both activate Defensive and anti-pathogenic-Qi. The intensity of symptoms reflect the battle between the pathogenic and anti-pathogenic forces. Mild symptoms may be due to weak pathogens or weak anti-pathogenic forces. In general, symptoms reflect the states where Righteous-Qi (anti-pathogenic) is strong and the Pathogenic Factors are weak; the Righteous-Qi is strong but the Pathogenic Factors are even stronger; the Righteous-Qi is deficient and the Pathogenic Factors are Excessive; or the Pathogenic Factors are eliminated and the Righteous-Qi is recovering. In biomedicine, injury or infection also can result in many similar reactions. (see "Inflammation" on page 551.)

LATENT/LURKING AND RESIDUAL PATHOGENIC FACTORS (FU AND YI). The concept of an incubation period (or lurking pathogens) was described early in the history of Chinese medicine. The *Classic of Internal Medicine* states: "The cold of the winter causes a recurrence of illness in spring; the wind of spring makes peoples unable to retain food in the summer; the heat of summer causes intermittent fever in fall; humidity in the fall causes a cough in winter." Residual (Yi) pathogens are those that are left-over after an acute episode and that may not show symptoms unless they are activated (or combined) by other factors such as warming foods or stress and therefore may be latent. Residual factors, however, are most commonly associated with continued symptoms after a viral syndrome with chronic symptoms. Phlegm-Heat, Damp-Heat, or just Heat are the most common with symptoms such as a continued altered sense of dryness and/or thirst (which in Western patients needs to be carefully explored because it is unlikely to be reported or noticed), sleep difficulties, irritability, and concentrated urine (again not commonly reported).

Latent/lurking pathogens (especially Spring-Warm pathogens) are said most often to affect patients with weak Defensive-Qi, Yin-deficiency (Righteous) and/or Dampness (more in Wind-Warm/Feng Wen).[101] The *Classic of Internal Medicine* states: "If a person has sufficient essence, he will not suffer from a warm disease in spring, even though he has been attacked by cold in winter." Therefore, these patients (due to weakness) do not eliminate Pathogenic Factors, or the pathogens "stick" to Dampness and become hidden. Latent-Heat-Qi, or hidden/lurking Pathogenic Factors, are therefore a category of disease that *arises* from the Interior: Nutritive, Blood, and/or Qi divisions, or Organs,[102] and that usually progress to the Exterior (if improving). Thus patients

---

99. Acute inflammation has been related to a Yang-Ming reaction, which is one of the levels within the 6 level/division theory of penetration of pathogenic-Cold and which results in strong fever/Heat. Yang-Ming symptoms and signs are often similar to those of the Qi-division in the Warm Diseases (Wen Bing) doctrine. While the 6 level doctrine describes the abnormal penetration of "normal" Qi of "Heaven and Earth," the pathogens of Warm diseases are said to relate more to "Toxic Qi," which is said to be created by droughts, floods, and malarial affected areas (*Itemized Discrimination of Cold Damage and Warm Epidemics*). These concepts have been expend to include other clinical presentations were the pathogenic factor is thought to enter the Interior directly and to later move outwardly.

100. No single symptom is ever associated with one particular pattern in TCM. For example, a hot joint (which is usually due to inflammation or infection in biomedicine) can be due to: Yin or Fluid damage resulting in blazing Heat. This Heat can scorch the Blood or blood vessels (micro-injuries to vascular walls), causing bleeding, or leading to Blood-stasis and increased blockage; that again increases the Heat symptoms (each treated differently). Lack of Blood circulation due to injury or reduced vitality from Qi or Yang weakness, or Pathogenic Factors that block circulation, can also result in Stasis and transformative/congestion-Heat. Pathogenic Factors, especially Dampness (which can be external-Excess or internal secondary to Deficiency) can block Qi which congests and transmutes to congestion-transformative-Heat. Dampness can also transform into Damp-Heat via stagnation or when Dampness joins Heat from any other cause (lifestyle, external pathogens or internal processes). Prolonged Heat can damage the Kidneys and therefore the bones, which can lead to dryness of the joint and may lead to friction-Heat (if both Yin and Yang are affected then Heat symptoms are not pronounced as seen in arthrosis), etc. The last mechanism (friction-Heat) is not classically described, among other causes.

101. "Wind-Warm" and "Spring-Warm" are special terms used in the doctrine of "Warm-Diseases" (Wen Bing). Wind-Warm is associated more with new pathogens while Spring-Warm with latent or lurking pathogens. Other terms such as "Autumn-Dryness" (Qiu Zao), "Summer-Heat" (Shu Wen), "Damp-Warmth" (Shi Wen) as apposed to "Damp-Heat" (Shi Re) are used as well to describe other internal disorders or some external disorders. "Warm-toxin" (Wen Du) is often used in rapidly progressing severe Heat disorders.

Table 1-5: Exogenous Factors

Factor	Main Symptoms	Common In
Wind	Suddenness and changeability.	Paresthesia, neuralgia, arthritis, muscle contraction/twitching or spasms, ligamentous laxity.
	Symptoms with unfixed locations.	
	Upper body symptoms.	
	Convulsions, tremors, shaking, muscle twitching.	
	Labile emotions and symptoms.	
Cold	Pain combined with: contraction, constriction, tightening.	Pain, restricted movement from tight muscles, stiffness from joint arthrosis, morning pain, severe pain, self-reducing disc disorder.
	Slowness.	
	Subjective and Objective feeling of cold.	
	White or pale appearance.	
Heat / Heat/Toxin	Restlessness (less so than with Fire).	Inflammation, neuralgias, infections, autoimmune arthritis, septic arthritis, gout.
	Thirst.	
	Subjective sensation of heat.	
	Objective sensation of heat.	
	Red appearance.	
Fire (a degree of heat) / Fire/Toxin	Thirst.	Muscle atrophy, paralysis, neuritis, inflammation, infections, autoimmune arthritis, septic arthritis, gout.
	Restlessness, irritability, rage.	
	Subjective sensation of heat.	
	Objective sensation of heat; if with toxin may have ulcers or skin eruptions.	
	Red appearance.	
Dampness	Subjective sensation of heaviness, fullness, boundness and stickiness (symptoms of fixed location), persistent, difficult to cure.	Swelling, arthrosis, arthritis, edema, myalgia.
	Feeling of fatigue, sluggishness or apathy.	
Dryness	Dryness, such as of skin, lips.	Spasms, contracture, paresthesias.
	Thirst.	
	Constipation	
Summer Heat	High fever and profuse sweating.	Not related to orthopedic disorders.
	Seasonal in nature.	

… with latent pathogens may manifest severe or Interior symptoms and signs (Organ or Qi/Blood-division) at the onset of disease, that progress outwards in a positive direction. In more serious cases the pathogens do not exteriorize on their own. If the patient's anti-pathogenic forces are still somewhat strong, the first symptoms would probably manifest at the Qi-division first (classically with fever, irritability and thirst, or possibly *clear* inflammation). If anti-pathogenic forces are weak, the symptoms would probably first manifest at the Nutritive (or Blood)-division/depth. Spring-Warmth is said to be characterized by *acute/rapid*-onset, Interior-Heat, a *multitude of changes* and severe signs and symptoms. It often takes a new Exterior invasion or some kind of stress that weakness Righteous-Qi (antipathogenic forces) to trigger the hidden/lurking pathogens (such as: overwork, emotional stress, irregular eating, etc.). Lurking Pathogenic Factors are said to be capable of injuring the Yin and Blood and may include any of the Pathogenic Factors that remain in the body after unresolved external or internal pathogenesis (especially Phlegm and Blood-stasis, but also Wind, Heat, Cold, Dryness). It is important to understand that lurking/latent-Heat can present clinically as either Excess or Deficient syndrome. In Deficient syndromes (or more often combined Deficient-Excess syndrome) however, it is important to first address retained pathogens before tonifying the patient.[103] In general, Warm diseases from hidden pathogens are due to internal flaming of constrained/congested-Heat.

The etiology of painful disorders is said to relate often to external Pathogenic Factors (infectious). However, patients rarely relate a history of muculoskeletal pain that follows an infectious Exterior disease (except in fibromyalgia). Latent/lurking Pathogenic Factors *may be* one explanation, although classically, joint pains were not a part of the description of these patterns. They were mostly related to fever disorders arising in the middle Warmer and/or with Interior-Heat symptoms at the onset (e.g., irritability, rashes, concentrated urine, epistaxis, thirst, high fever, etc.), in which the pulse and tongue do not show Exterior signs (often with tidal, wiry-rapid, or soggy, *but not* a floating pulse).[104] However, Latent/hidden/lurking Pathogenic Factors are said to "reside in the bones and marrow, Cou Li *(membranes, space between Exterior and Interior)* and muscles." Therefore, one may *speculate* as to their role in musculoskeletal disorders. They would probably more appropriately be related to *inflammatory rheumatological disorders*. According to Liu (2001), Cold can lurk in the Kidney if the patient has Kidney-Yin-deficiency, and in the muscles if the patient does physical work and has a strong physical constitution. Another possible cause of hidden pathogens that may be considered in musculoskeletal medicine, is sweating excessively in patients, either through physical activity or from therapy. Excessive sweating is said to be capable of leading pathogens to the Interior, or to damage Yin, both of which can result in the patient's susceptibility to retain hidden pathogens. Latent Pathogenic Factors can also arise iatrogenically after an inappropriate use of cold herbs in the treatment of Exterior Wind-Cold (colds or flu).[105] The use of Yang-Ming cold herbs in cases of Tai-Yang disease (Exterior disease) are also said to draw heat into the muscles, and to result in deeper penetration (or suppression) of pathogens that then become latent and hidden. Symptoms resurface at a later date due to: a new Exterior syndrome, stress, overwork, emotional imbalance or spoiled and excessive food intake, with joint pains *possibly* being part of the syndrome. Some modern medication, such as antibiotics and NSAIDs, may also, at times, suppress or prevent complete healing (i.e., result in lurking pathogens) and may be considered as agents capable of creating lurking pathogens.[106] Finally, Hidden pathogens are also said to cause great Heat in the Exterior, Interior, and Triple Warmer where the patient cannot describe his/her symptoms.

In musculoskeletal practice, treatment strategies that use the concepts of lurking pathogens are probably most useful in patients that present with rapidly accelerating inflammatory processes, and that do not show any Exterior symptoms and signs. The patient may have a chronic condition that flares *suddenly* with symptoms of Heat and inflammation. These presentations can also be interpreted often as constrained or transformative/congested-Heat. The tongue is often dry especially in patients where Fluids are damaged. It is also common for the tongue and pulse to not coincide with

---

102. The terms "Nutritive" and "Blood" have special meaning in the Warm-disease four-division diagnostic scheme beyond their usual use in general TCM.

103. In musculoskeletal practice and when treating post viral syndromes (including fibromyalgia and chronic fatigue syndrome) the use of modification of Two-Cured Decoction (Er Chen Tang), Agastache, Magnolia Bark, Pinellia, and Poria (Huo Po Xia Ling Tang), Three-Nut Decoction (San Ren Tang), and Coptis and Magnolia Bark Decoction (Lian Po Tang) is often needed.

104. According to *The Itemized Discrimination of Cold Damage and Warm Epidemics*, Warm-diseases enter via the nose and mouth and directly move to the "middle pathways" to spread through the Triple Warmer until becoming depressed in the Blood. It must be remembered that if a new Exterior pathogen is the triggering condition, the patient may have Exterior symptoms at the same time as Interior symptoms, but the Interior symptoms should dominant. The patient may have a high fever without aversion to cold, have a dry mouth and be thirsty. The pulse may be flooding and slippery (at the middle or Blood-depth) or in some cases sinking and hidden (especially on the right side which is also more exuberant than the left pulses). Treatment is usually to clear Interior-Heat and eliminate Exterior pathogens. The Qi dynamic in the Triple Warmer must be freed and Heat-Toxin must be cleared from the Triple Warmer. This is not achieved by promoting sweating (the usual way of addressing Exterior symptoms, although herbs such as Cicadae [Chuan Tui]), and Menthae [Bo He] are still used) as these are often viewed as false Cold or false Exterior-Heat. If the triggering factor is not from an externally contracted pathogenic factor, the patient may present with a moist tongue without a coat. The pulse may be soggy, wiry, or slightly quick. The patient would complain of irritability, restlessness, aversion to heat, and *no* increase in thirst. The treatment for this patient would be to clear Heat from the Nutritive-division. As the patient improves, symptoms of Qi-division may arise, and the tongue may show an increase coat thickness which, in contrast to six-level diagnosis (of Cold-school), is an improvement.

105. Modern antibiotics are considered by many as cold in nature.

the presenting symptoms. Treatment is often achieved by working through layers (mostly the four-levels/divisions) during the course of treatment. This means that whatever else in done, some herbs or points are used to guide pathogens out of the body. This may include a combination of out-thrusting pathogens via the surface, and elimination via urine and bowels.[107] The Divergent channels which connect the Interior and the Exterior can be used as well.[108]

Endogenous Factors (Nei Yin)

The endogenous factors—influences that originate from within—consist of the *seven affects*: Joy, Anger, Sorrow, Anxiety, Preoccupation, Fear, and Fright/Shock (Table 1-6 on page 35).[109] These are normal emotional expressions of the Organs (Wu Zhi), and emotional expressions from evil-Qi (Wu Bing). While TCM clearly speaks of psychosomatic relationships, it does not separate the effects of the "mind" and body. According to (Kleirnman 1970), Chinese patients (at least in modern times) often express psychological problems by referring to somatic complaints. This may be due to the historic role of TCM and at times makes it difficult to correlate symptomatology expressed in the Chinese literature with clinical experience in the West. It is also interesting to note that in China, even though TCM has described complex relationships between bodily function and emotional states, psychological issues are most often viewed in relation to their social consideration (family, society, country) in contrast to the individual emphasis in the West.[110]

Unlike the external Pathogenic Factors, endogenous factors usually affect the Qi and then the Blood and Organs *directly*. When a person is angry, his/her face may become red, therefore it is said that anger raises Qi and Blood.[111] When frightened, he/she may need to urinate, so it is said that Qi and Fluids go down. Imbalance in one or more of these emotions can disturb homeostasis of Qi (and Organ functional balance) leading to endogenous-damage and dysfunction, and/or pathology of the Organs or channels and network-vessels. Endogenous-damage is caused by either a sudden violent emotional eruption (movement of "Spirit-Essence") or repeated emotional stress. These disharmonies can progress to Organ disease, Heat, Fire, Cold, Wind, Dampness, Qi, or Blood stagnation/stasis, channel obstruction, and tissue and/or Organ damage. Therefore, while external Pathogenic Factors (Wind, Cold, etc.) are said to be capable of damaging "form" directly, endogenous factors usually damage form secondarily. When the seven affects result in disease, it is frequently referred to as damage by *internal factors* and because their direct effects on the Organ systems they are often seen as the *"root" (Ben)* of disease,

including pain. *(biomed: Interestingly Sarno (1991) believes that the majority of musculoskeletal pain disorders, including acute and chronic pain, is due to repressed emotions. He believes repressed emotions cause muscle tension and lack of oxygen in muscular, tendinous, and nervous tissues which then leads to pain. He calls this kind of pain Tension Myositis Syndrome. In his view the subcontious mind is the "root" of most pain syndromes.)*

In TCM, the body and mind affect each other directly in an integrated system where the internal Organs play a *direct* role *(simultaneous occurrence)*. Emotional effects are not seen as secondary influences that only stress the human system, but rather as factors directly responsible for healthy Organ functions and for disease states. Emotions are a manifestation of Spirit-Essence-Qi *movement* related to each of the Organs and their associated functions (Table 1-6).[112]

TCM considers the "mind" to be part of the five solid Organ systems, especially the Heart.[113] The classic *Spiritual Axis* states:

> The Organ that is responsible for performance of mental activities is the Heart....The Heart is the monarch of the five solid and six hollow Organs... Therefore, grief and sorrow also disturb the Heart, and a disturbance of the Heart affects the five solid and six hollow Organs.[114]

The Heart controls the Blood vessels and therefore the Blood. Thus, Blood is said to be the foundation of mental activity. Lack of Blood circulation leads to pain; therefore, the association between pain and mind (Heart) is evident. "If there is plenty of Heart-Blood, the mind is clear, thinking is brisk, and one is full of spirit and vigor... If Phlegm is obstructing the Connecting-vessels of the Heart and Spleen, there will be stiff tongue and inability to speak." The Pericardium is closely related to the Heart. It is said that "Spirit

---

106. There has been much speculation, and some animal evidence, that NSAIDs may interfere with soft tissue healing and therefore be responsible for chronic, unresolved musculoskeletal pain. NSAIDs may also accelerate joint destruction, except the new COX-2 inhibitors which may actually protect the joints.

107. Common herbs used in *musculoskeletal disorders* to achieve a combination of up-bearing and down-bearing to eliminate lurking pathogens are: Bombyx Batricatus (Jiang Can), Rhizoma Rhei (Da Huang), Rhizoma Curcumae (Huang Jiang), Gypsum (Shi Gao), Fructus Gardenia (Zhi Zi), Herba Schizonepetae (Jing Jie), Radix Ledebouriellae (Fang Feng), Scorpio (Quan Xie), Uncariae Ramulus Cum Unicis (Gou Teng), Radix Trichonsanthis (Tian Hua Fen), Herba Lophatheri (Dan Zhu Ye), and Radix Puerariae (Ge Gen).

Depending on symptoms and signs *guiding* formulas modified for musculoskeletal use from Warm-diseases doctrine such as: Honeysuckle and Forsythia Powder (Yin Qiao San), White Tiger Decoction (Bai Hu Tang), Clear the Nutritive Decoction (Qing Yin Tang), Clear the Palace Decoction (Qing Gong Tang), Scallion and Platycody Decoction (Cang Chi Jie Geng Tang), Scutellaria Decoction plus Prepared Soybean and Scrophularia (Huang Qin Tang Jia Dan Dou Chi He Xuan Shen), Coptis and Magnolia Bark Decoction (Lian Po Tang), Three-Nut Decoction (San Ren Tang), Sweet Dew Special Pill to Eliminate Toxin (Gan Lu Xiao Du Dan), Artemisia Yinchenhao Decoction (Yin Chen Hao Tang), Newly Augmented Yellow Dragon Decoction (Xin Jia Huang Long Tang), Jade Woman Decoction (Yu Nu Jiang Tang), Universal Benefit Decoction to Eliminate Toxin (Pu Ji Xiao Du Yin), Cool the Nutritive and Clear the Qi Decoction (Liang Ying Qing Qi Tang), Wang's Decoction to Clear Summerheat and Augment the Qi (Wang Shi Qing Shu Yi Qi Tang), Immature Bitter Orange Decoction to Guide Out Stagnation (Zhi Shi Dao Zhi Tang), Rhinoceros Horn and Rehmanniae Decoction to Clear the Collaterals (Xi Di Qing Luo Yin), and Warm the Gall Bladder Decoction (Wen Dan Tang) can be used.

clouding and irrational speech is due to Heat entering the Pericardium."

Organ disorders are said to result in emotional and cognitive reactions. For example, it is said that, "if the Heart is weak there are palpitations and severe fright; if Heart-Yang is weak there are palpitations and forgetfulness; Heart-Qi-deficiency leads to sorrow, while an Excess leads to persistent laughter; weak memory (often associated in biomedicine with stress from chronic pain syndromes) is due mostly to Heart-Spleen-Kidney-weakness; if the Liver stagnates and does not spread, there will be anger and depression [and often pain]; Liver and Gall Bladder weakness leads to timidity."

Therefore, unbalanced emotions often affect the Liver and Heart, resulting in decreased Qi and Blood circulation, Blood-deficiency, and the generation of internal-Wind. Decreased Blood circulation and Blood-deficiency can lead to musculotendinous pain, tension, and rigidity. Intermingled they result in symptoms of numbness, paresthesias, muscle twitches, rashes, neck and wandering joint pains, and headaches. Liver (Wood) disorders, being the "child" of the Kidneys (Water),[115] can deplete the Kidneys, and may also deplete the Spleen/pancreas (Earth), which is under the control of the Liver, affecting the bones, muscles, sinews, and joints that depend on the Liver, Spleen, and Kidneys for normal function.[116]

Spiritual Axis states:

...When Liver-Qi is empty, the emotions are of fear. When Liver-Qi is full anger and irritability results...When Heart-Qi is empty, grief results. When Heart-Qi is full there is uncontrolled laughter...When Spleen-Qi is empty, the four limbs lose their normal motion and the five Yin Organs become insecure. When Spleen-Qi is full, the body is swollen, and urine and menses lose their smoothness...When Lung-Qi is empty, shortness of breath develops. When Lung-Qi is full, panting, fullness, chest discomfort and difficulty breathing will develop...When Kidney-Qi is empty, there is counterflow. When Kidney-Qi is full, there is swelling and the five Yin Organs are insecure.

Anger, depression, and *frustration* can all strongly affect the Liver, which controls the free flow of Qi, and therefore Blood. Liver-congestion-Qi-stagnation leads to symptoms of Qi-stagnation pain and often headaches, sighing, abdominal, chest, and subcostal/costal discomfort, as well as *distension/bloating* and a wiry pulse. Unhappiness in childhood or unfulfilled desires in adulthood may result in pent-up feelings of anger and frustration due to hopelessness and depression. They may also be the cause of disorders that affect the Liver and the tissues under its control, the sinews. Back pain that is strongly associated with stress and emotions may be seen, often with Gall Bladder channel, hip, and leg pain, i.e., L1-L3 or L4-L5 dermatomal distribution. When constrained/stagnated/congested/depressed Liver-Qi transforms into Fire, symptoms of anger, irritability, facial and eye redness, tinnitus and bitter/unpleasant taste in the mouth may be seen.[117] With time, transformative/congested-Fire will result in damage to the Yin and Blood with symptoms of insomnia, scant concentrated urine, thirst, constipation, night sweats, and palpitation.

LIVER QI-STAGNATION OR INHIBITION/CONGESTION/ CONSTRAINED WITHIN THE LIVER DUE TO EMOTIONAL FACTORS:[118]

1. Qi-stagnation of any kind can lead to Blood-stasis and the development of *substantial obstructions* with sharp, stabbing and fixed pains anywhere in the body, with or without palpable tissue hypertrophy.

---

108. For hidden-muscle-heat or for muscle pain from Spring-Warm and/or Summer-Heat the use of modified Ten Spirits Decoction (Shi Shen Tang) may be helpful: Notopterygii (Qiang Huo), Radix Puerariae (Ge Gen), Radix Ligustici (Chuan Xiong), Radix Angelica (Bai Zhi), Radix Paeoniae (Chi Shao), Folium Perillae (Zi Su), Pericarpium Citri (Chen Pi), Rhizoma Cimicifugae (Sheng Ma), Rhizoma Cypri (Xiang Fu), (Jiang Can), and Radix Glycyrrhizae (Gan Gao).

109. They have also been described as joy, anger, grief, fear, love, loathing, and desire. It must also be stated that while these are the modern translations of the so-called affects, in classical Chinese their meanings may have been quite different. For example, while the word Xi is translated as joy in modern Chinese, it may have been used to describe the kind of elation that comes from winning, and, as an internal-damaging- factor, may actually have been used to describe extreme elation and inappropriate giddiness or laughter and not simple joy (Bensky *ibid*).

110. Much of the psychological disorders were discussed in the traditional literature in terms of the mental derangements associated with quietness, activity/violence, hysteria, and epilepsy.

111. Although, at the same time, the Classics speak of anger cutting Qi and leaving the Blood to densely accumulate above, resulting in a red face.

112. Emotions can also arise as a direct result of Organic dysfunction.

113. The Chinese word Xin can be translated as either Heart or mind depending on context. In *Spiritual Axis*, the mind is often discussed in relation to the brain as well (e.g., discussion 80 on "Great delusions"). The Chinese word for brain is also used to describe mucus membranes in the head, especially when there is ceaseless discharge of a mucous that is seen as Fluid of the brain.

114. The heart and brain have similar embryonic origins. In early development, the heart tissues lie just above what later becomes the brain.

115. See "Five Phases (Wu Xing)" on page 48.

116. Liver dysfunction often results from Spleen dysfunction, as well.

117. Note that many of the symptoms are of the face and head as Fire tends to rise. Liver-Yang rising can also cause similar symptoms but as opposed to transformative/congested-Liver-Fire (sometimes called Qi-Fire), Liver-Yang rising is a Deficient (Yin or Blood) condition.

118. It is important to remember that, for example, Liver dysfunction can be caused or aggravated by Blood, Yin and/or Yang deficiencies. The Liver can perform its functions of moving Qi only if it obtains sufficient Blood to be nourished and lubricated, sufficient Yin to be enriched and moistened, and sufficient Yang to be warmed, motivated, and "steamed." Thus, all emotional-effects are inter-related to general systemic/Organic functions. Also, Liver dysfunction can be manifested as inhibited flow ("depression/congestion") or counter-flow (moving sideways or up from Qi-stagnation).

2. Transformative/congested-Fire can easily result from Qi-stagnation (Qi-Fire) and give rise to symptoms of pain in the upper body such as: red painful eyes, painful head and neck. Transformative/congested-Fire can also affect any local tissue such as the joints.

   If Fire lingers (chronic strong emotional states), Yin-Blood will be consumed and then the Liver may fail to nourish the sinews. This can result in tendinous and ligamentous weakness ("limp") as well as tightness ("hardness,")[119] fatigue, muscle cramps, and possibly spasms or twitching.

   If the Kidneys are affected, then Kidney-Yin-deficiency may develop with low back pain and possibly with deficient-Liver-Yang rising. Then dizziness, dry or sore throat, constipation, tinnitus, insomnia, a wiry thin and quick pulse and a *dry*, red tongue with thin coat are said to present.

3. Dysfunction of Spleen/pancreas is seen often with Liver-congestion Qi-stagnation, manifesting with symptoms of poor or other digestive symptoms that are affected by emotional states. The Spleen's transportation function is greatly dependent on the Liver's control of free flow. The rising and movement of Liver-Qi helps the Spleen/pancreas to transport and transform food-essence. Failure results in poor nourishment and accumulation. A combination of Deficiency and Excess type pains (or syndromes) can result.

4. The Gall Bladder, the paired-Organ of the Liver, can be affected by Liver-congestion with resulting stagnation and poor digestion and possibly symptoms of pain along the Gall Bladder channel, such as T11-L3 dermatomal/myotomal/sclerotomal symptoms. The state of emotional timidity, fear, and difficulty in making decisions is said to be related to Gall Bladder-deficiency

5. Blockage of channels can easily result from Liver-congestion Qi-stagnation with symptoms relating to secondary Pathogenic Factors, especially Blood-stasis. There is musculoskeletal pain, increased pain sensitivity, and possibly reduced skin and muscle sensitivity (Painful Obstruction (Bi) Syndromes).[120]

Anxiety and preoccupation can weaken the Spleen/pancreas and cause the accumulation of Dampness. Weakness of the Spleen/pancreas also affects muscle strength, especially of the four extremities. Dampness penetrates the muscles and joints, which become heavy, achy, and stiff. Pain along the Spleen channel can develop including hallux valgus and big toe bunions (described in Japanese traditions). Dysfunction of Spleen can also affect Liver function with all the above covered consequences of Liver-congestion Qi-stagnation.

Sorrow and grief are said to impact mostly the Lungs and possibly result in weakness of Qi-circulation, as the Lungs govern Qi. This may result in Lung channel dysfunction and Qi and Blood-stagnation, with chest, shoulder and upper arm pain. Pooling of Blood may occur with the development of varicose veins.

Fear and fright are said to mainly impact the Kidneys, which may then fail to distribute and conserve Essence needed to produce marrow and to nourish both the bones and nervous systems. This may result in symptoms such as weakness, bone and nervous system dysfunctions, low back pain, dizziness, tinnitus, and diminished bone strength.

The classic text, *Simple Questions*, in discussing the relationship of the mind, emotions, and spirit implies a psychosomatic relationship between pain and pain perception: "All kinds of pain, itching, and sores are due to Heart disorders...when the Heart is peaceful, any pain is negligible." Thus, general *pain sensitivity* in TCM is related mostly to Essence-spirit and Heart Organ functions and is not related to local tissue (nerve/channel) sensitization as is in some biomedical descriptions *(Biomedical: deafferentation)*. Patients with easy arousal of Essence-spirit from various causes are said to be over-sensitive to pain. When treating chronic and difficult to cure patients, it is wise to remember the role of emotional factors in obstructing Qi and Blood flow, and the balance and health of Organs and their possible general effects. This, however, can also be a double-edged sword, as emotional attributions to pain are made too commonly and often incorrectly. As can be seen in TCM, however, this does not simply mean the pain is in the patient's "head." ("Psychological Influences on Pain" on page 144; and "Pain in TCM" on page 159.)

BIOMEDICINE AND EMOTIONAL EFFECTS. The human brain has as many as 400,000 synaptic terminals in a single axon, and it contains one hundred billion neurons. These connections constantly form new connections, some of which can become permanent. Emotions may result in neuropsychological changes which can become "*hard wired*," resulting in permanent new synaptic connections. Biomedical sciences have shown physiological effects from emotions via the limbic, reticular, and autonomic systems (see chapter 2). These neural changes may explain some of the endogenous factor effects that TCM describes.

Although emotional effects may be viewed in a cultural framework (they may be expressed and experienced differently in various cultures), they do seem to have physiological effects that are more universal. For example, in TCM anger (both expressed and non-expressed) is considered a

---

119. As is often seen when hypoxia or atrophic changes occur in muscles and other soft tissues.

120. Skin and muscle numbness is said to be a common symptom in Bi syndromes (arthritic); however, it is not usually reported by Western patients except when there is neurological involvement. Numbness in Chinese medicine includes the characters for both numbness (Mu) and tingling (Ma). True numbness is often said to be caused by congested Pathogenic Factors (especially Phlegm and Blood) which block the Network-vessels. Righteous is blocked and "hidden" by pathogens, and the Defensive and Nutritive aspects are depleted and cannot flow (see page 633).

Disease Etiologies

Table 1-6: Endogenous Factors

Factor	Can Affect and Be Affected By	Effect
Excessive Joy	Mainly Heart.	Damages Heart. Over-relaxes Qi (relaxes functional activity). Disperses Qi and makes it circulate slowly (hypofunctioning).
		Symptoms that result from excessive lifestyles, burning the candle at both ends, over-eating.
		Disorders of thinking, exaggerated pain disorders, conversion pain disorders. Chest, arm pain.
Expressed Anger	Mainly Liver, Spleen, Stomach.	Causes Qi to rise. Damages Qi (mostly Blood). Damages Liver.
		Head, neck, chest, abdominal, subcostal, and/or trunk distension pain, vomiting, bleeding.
Repressed Anger	Mainly Liver or Spleen.	Knots Qi. Mental depression. Chest, abdominal, subcostal, and/or trunk distension pain.
Excessive Sorrow, Sadness, Grief	Mainly Lung.	Damages Lungs. Scatters Qi (mostly respiratory). Constricts (tightens), depletes and consumes Qi (vital substances).
		Mostly from loss or perception of loss.
		Fatigue, breathlessness/tightness of chest, venous congestion, edema, difficulty "letting go," Heat in chest. Upper back, shoulders, upper arm pain.
Anxiety, Preoccupation, Pensiveness	Mainly Spleen. Anxiety can also damage Heart.	Damages Spleen/pancreas. Causes Qi to slow and knot. Drains/disorganizes, and stagnates Qi (vital substances congest with poor distribution).
		Excessive thinking, worry, deception, confusion, excessive use of mind
		Dampness/Phlegm/Blood-stasis. Digestive symptoms; fatigue, heaviness. Muscle weakness pain, inability to raise limbs, joint swelling pain.
Fear	Mainly Kidney.	Damages Kidneys. Causes Qi (mostly Fluids) to descend.
		Mostly chronic fear.
		Increases urination, day/night urination w/fear, etc. Bone and spine disorders Spinelessness, lack of will. Low back and knees weak and painful.
Fright/Shock	Mainly Kidney/ Heart (Liver).	Qi drops, becomes chaotic, and flows in a disorderly fashion. Damages Gall Bladder.
		Related to actual fearful situations.
		Heart and Kidney symptoms. Insomnia, palpitations, pronounced fear, increased urination, day/night urination. Low back and knees weak and painful.

Table 1-7: Independent (Lifestyle) Factors

Factor	Affects (Mostly)
Diet	Spleen/pancreas, Blood, Damp/Phlegm, muscles.
Sexual Activity	Kidney, Essence, Yin, Qi, Blood, bone.
Excessive Consumption	Kidney, Spleen, Lung, Yin, Yang, Qi, Blood.
Trauma	Exterior (skin, muscles, etc.), Blood, blood vessels, channels, sinews.
Parasitic Infection and Poisons (smoking)	Spleen, Liver, Intestine, Lungs, Kidneys, Yin, Yang, Blood, Nutritive-Qi (Ying), Sinews.

primary factor in the etiology of high blood pressure and hypertension is a risk factor for developing brain attacks/strokes.[121]

Biomedical studies have shown a relationship between expressed anger and blood pressure (Laude, Girard, Consoli, Mounier-Vehier, and Elghozi 1997; Shapiro, Goldstein and Jamner 1996). The outward expression of anger has been linked to higher cardiovascular reactivity and risk of heart attacks (Siegman and Snow 1997; Verrier and Mittleman 1996). In a recent study a correlation between anger and platelet aggregation was shown (Wenneberg et al 1997). Shapiro et al (1997) have shown that high anger and sadness scores of healthy college students have significantly higher diastolic blood pressure at night (taken with automatic periodic recordings) than those with high happiness and pleasantness scores.

In TCM, anger can affect the Liver, is a manifestation of Liver disorders, and is said to engender Fire; all of which can impact Blood circulation. (Fire can thicken the Blood or possibly cause platelet aggregation. Fire can also result in pushing Blood out of the vessels and result in conditions such as brain attack/strokes). The effects of Liver Fullness/Excess (from acute anger or by anger being a result of Liver disorder) on the Heart can be explained by the Five Phases theory, Wood affecting Fire (mother child disorder).

INCREASED RISK OF DISEASE FROM DEPRESSION. More recently, biomedicine has shown that certain emotional states result in increased risk of developing various diseases. For example, depression is a risk factor in the development of osteoporosis (Schweiger et al 1994).[122] Researchers speculate that changes in appetite, decreased activity, and increased cortisol levels are responsible for this kind of effect

---

121. In the Framingham study, anger was not an independent predictor of hypertension in Western patients. However, anxiety was a predictor in middle-aged Western men.

122. Depression is associated with insomnia, changes in appetite, inactivity or agitation, and loss of libido.

In TCM, depression is related often to the Liver, Kidneys, Heart and Spleen with repressed anger (often Liver-related) and loss of will (often Kidney and Heart related) at the root (Ben). Congestion of Liver with Qi-stagnation results in poor Blood circulation, formation of pathogenic-Heat and, through Five Phases theory, in draining of Kidneys. Depression is also said to "transform Mingmen Fire into pathogenic Fire," which affects the Heart and Kidneys. Poor circulation, Heat, and Heart imbalances can result in disturbed sleep. Liver-congestion can also affect the Spleen/pancreas (Five Phases theory), influencing appetite. Kidney weakness, which has been shown to correlate to changes in steroid levels, also impacts libido. The Kidneys control the marrow and therefore the strength of the bones, which become osteoporotic.

SADNESS. Sadness has been shown to relate to lung function and asthma through cholinergically mediated airway constriction (Miller and Wood 1997).

EMOTIONS AND PAIN. Studies have shown a link between symptom-specific physiological reactivity and pain severity in reaction to stressful events. This occurs especially in depressed patients (Burns et al 1997). Anxiety, sensitivity, or the fear of anxiety-related bodily sensations (pain), arising from beliefs that the sensations have harmful consequences is associated with pain behavior and disability (Asmundson and Taylor 1996). Pain is often made worse by fear, by anger, or by a sense of isolation. The pain may be diminished if the patient understands the cause and loses his/her fear. Patients who keep busy find that sensory and other distractions relieve pain (Brand 1997).

Biomedical risk factors for development of pain chronicity are (CSAG 1994):

- Personal problems such as marital and financial.
- Psychological distress and depression.
- Adversarial medicolegal problems.
- Low job satisfaction.
- Disproportionate illness behavior.

In cases of pain chronicity, endogenous factors must be addressed medically and through education (physical exercise including breathing, meditation, *self-awareness*). This is important because dysfunctional behavior is a common factor in patients suffering from chronic pain, which may affect tissue and organ function. While many TCM practitioners attribute pain and other medical conditions to "spiritual" and existential problems, this can easily become an "excuse" for failed treatment and, in pain medicine, *primary* emotional causes of pain have been shown to occur only rarely (see page 144). At the same time Sarno (*ibid*) claims that as much as 80% of pain syndromes can be "cured" by understanding their underlying "emotional causes."[123]

Disease Etiologies

Independent, Not External or Internal Factors

Independent factors (Table 1-7) are related to disorders that are neither endogenous nor exogenous and therefore are numerous/limitless. They are often due to lifestyle, environment, or medical treatment. Diet, sexual activity, excessive consumption of physical resources, trauma, parasitic or other infection, poisons and iatrogenicity can all damage the Interior or Exterior and can lead to obstruction, tissue damage, and pain. "*Miscellaneous diseases*" is a term used to describe many diseases that are not External (febrile) in origin.

TCM stresses moderation as a way of maintaining health and longevity, and therefore dietary balance (between colors and flavours of food) was understood to be important for health maintenance. Failure of treatments is often explained as being due to the patient's lifestyle habits. Lack of moderation in any of the lifestyle factors is said to be capable of causing disease from taxation. The exploration of pathogenesis chapter in the *Classic of Internal Medicine* states:

> Excessive use of the eyes injures the Blood; excessive lying down or sleeping injures the Qi (gathering Dampness); excessive sitting injures the muscles; excessive standing injures the bones; excessive exercise and movement injures the sinews; and excessive sex injures the Kidneys.
>
> It happens that someone walks a long distance, and is exhausted to fatigue. He encounters massive Heat, and becomes thirsty. When he is thirsty, then the Yang Qi attacks internally. When it attacks internally, the Heat lodges in the Kidneys. Here now, the Water does not dominate the Fire. As a result the bones dry up, and the marrow is depleted. Hence, the feet cannot support the body. This develops into bone limpness.[124]

By and large, dietary imbalance weakens the Stomach and Spleen/pancreas; Spleen/pancreas weakness results in insufficiency of Nutritive-Qi and Blood, and the formation of Dampness and/or Phlegm; Dampness obstructs the channels; and lack of Nutritive-Qi and Blood result in insufficiency of raw materials needed for normal tissue renewal.

Simple Questions also states that excess of:

> Salty flavor hardens and congeals the pulse/vessels; bitter flavor withers the skin making hair fallout; pungent flavor knots the muscles and injures the skin and hair; sour flavor toughens/calluses flesh and sloughs the lips; sweet flavor causes aches in the bones and falling hair.

The treatise cites the importance of appropriately balanced flavors in keeping the Organs and tissues healthy, adding that:

> Sour flavor strengthens the Liver, the Liver nourishes the muscles, the muscles strengthen the Heart.

Different flavors are said to have different qualities. Sweet is relaxing and creates Fluids.[125] Sour flavor is astringent; bitter flavor is drying, clearing, and descending; salty flavor is softening and sinking, and it promotes defecation; spicy flavor is scattering, drying, and upbearing; and bland flavor can descend and drain Fluids. Foods are said to have hot, warm, cool, cold, and neutral qualities. The above qualities of foods can be used in treatment as well as to explain disease mechanisms such as indulgence in rich, fatty, and sweet foods, causing Dampness and Heat. Overeating is said to "damage the Spleen and Stomach"; having a "Cold" body and drinking cold drinks is said to "damage the Lungs;" starvation is said to "damage the Spleen;" over-eating sugar is said to "damage Stomach and create Phlegm;" addiction to alcohol is said to "damage Stomach and create Damp-Heat."[126] Alcohol can also vitalize Blood flow, and over-indulgence is a common factor in Damp/Phlegm-Heat diseases. Therefore, in general, it is thought that improper food consumption can result in Organ, channel, vessel, and pathogenic pains and/or dysfunctions. Intake of food and beverages should be regulated, as it is said in discussions on water illnesses: "At the moment [the patient] drinks, he should not eat; at the moment he eats, he should not drink." The *Classic of Internal Medicine* states: "Use medicinal herbs to eliminate illness and to then follow the formula with a diet that will nourish the patient."

FOOD DISEASES. Food diseases is a category in which diseases are mainly caused due to, or which relate to, indulgence in over eating, or consumption of contaminated food. These include diseases that result in damage to the digestive system, mainly the Spleen and Stomach, caused by food consumption; accumulation of food from various mechanisms; and disorders that result in temporary loss of consciousness. *The Heart Transmission of Medicine* says: "There is another theory saying that drink and food entering the Stomach are none other but Damp substances."

---

123. Studies also show that emotional factors are more predictive of pain and disability than any imaging information (MRI, x-rays, CT-scans, etc.).

124. These are known as damage by taxation. *Baopuz's Inner Treatise* lists thirteen: straining oneself beyond one's learning and wisdom, or beyond physical strength; being overcome with grief of joy; endless desires and endless talking with laughter; inadequate sleep, after drawing a bow; vomiting due to being drunk; lying down immediately after overeating; gasping while walking and jumping; being easily excited with tears; and Yin and Yang not interlocking. Ge Qian Xun adds: indifference to hunger, infinite desire for worldly things, driving oneself constantly without rest.

125. Sweet foods stimulate serotonin which explains the relaxing effects.

126. Wine is said to warm the Interior, resolve Blood-stasis, and sooth the channels and collaterals/network-vessels and is therefore also used to treat Cold-pain when mixed with herbs. Wine should not be given to patients with pain due to Yin-deficiency, Yang-excess, and Damp/Phlegm accumulation. Alcohol in general is said to flow outside the Main channels, flowing with Defensive-Qi, and to run into the skin to fill the Connecting vessels (channels/collaterals/network-vessels). It is therefore said to be capable of depleting the Main channels and Kidney-Qi (partly because of inappropriate behavior when one is drunk).

Food-Stagnation may occur due to over-eating in general; over-eating hard to digest heavy/rich foods in particular; and as a result of long term Spleen/Stomach insufficiency, impairing their ability to transform and transport food and liquid. Because Food-Stagnation is a Yin-accumulation, it tends to obstruct the Qi. Because the Qi moves the Blood and body Fluids, food stagnation can give rise to, or complicate, other associated pathologies. Also, since many of the above surpluses result in Dampness, and Dampness commonly combines with Heat, Damp-Heat is commonly seen.

The main manifestations of Food-Stagnation are abdominal distention, belching with food taste and smell, lingering food in stomach, a bad taste and a foul smell emitting from the mouth, nausea, vomiting, and restlessness. The pulse may be full and slippery and the tongue coat slimy/greasy and thick.

SEXUAL ACTIVITY. Excessive sexual activity depletes mainly the Essence and Kidney-Qi which may lead to joint and bone disorders, particularly of the spine and knees. It is said, "if Kidney Essence is lost, the bone marrow becomes empty and deficient." As sexual energy is rooted in Mingmen (Kidney-Yang/Gate of Fire), when depleted, Fire easily stirs upwards and harasses the Heart and spirit. This is often seen in patients with pain, restless spirit/emotions, and insomnia.[127]

CONSUMPTION/TAXATION. Regular physical exercise and balanced mental activity is paramount for optimum health. Appropriate exercise is extremely important for patients with myofascial pain syndromes and fibromyalgia. However, over-consumption of an individual's resources, whether mental or physical *may* tax the ability to self-heal (diminishes homeostasis) and "over-work" is said to be the most common cause of Yin-deficiency in industrialized nations. This overuse of Qi, Blood, Yin, Essence, and Nutritive-Qi may be seen in patients who have minor physical lesions (injury) and, nevertheless, suffer from chronic pain (*Biomedical: nervous exhaustion and facilitation*).[128] Excessive use of force, lifting, sitting, and living in difficult conditions (damp-earth, for example) can all damage the Kidneys and lead to bone disorders, lumbar/waist and knee pain. Pain may also be caused by too little activity, as is typically seen in patients that are bedridden and/or are sedentary. Liver-taxation due to over-emotional stimulation can damage Liver-Qi and result in slack and relaxed sinews and vessels, and difficulty in moving.

---

127. Treatment of insomnia, depression, anxiety, and fear, whether primary or secondary, in chronic pain patients is needed often.

128. Not classical associations. Overwork and taxation is often said to result in disease in TCM. This however must be questioned as some studies show that type-A personalities do not have any increase in mortality and some studies actually show these patients to have longer and healthier lives. Japanese tend to have long life-spans even though they may be one of the most overworked societies in the world.

WORMS, PARASITES AND INSECT BITES. In Chinese the word *chong/worm* generally refers to most earthly crawlers and some water invertebrates. However, when used in medicine, this term mainly describes infections by various types of worms, parasites, or insect bites. Worms are said to "arise" when there is Dampness and Damp-Heat. The etiology of diseases caused by bugs predates the ideas of atmospheric factors (Wind, Cold, etc., that are found in the *Classic of Internal Medicine*) as a major cause of disease. In terms of musculoskeletal disorders, Worm infections and especially insect bites can manifest as joint pains. They are seen in inflammatory type arthritis and in chronic myofascial pains with history of fatigue, immune responses, feverishness, digestive and biliary disorders, and respiratory disorders.[129] A history of a rash is often present. There may also be a history of travel in third-world countries, camping out, food poisoning and desire to eat abnormal foods. Examination may display bluish dots or lines in the sclera of the eyes. Modern blood titers and stool analysis may be useful in making the diagnosis.

EFFECTS OF SMOKING. Smoking, which is not traditionally included as an independent factor,[130] is a risk factor for many diseases. Smoke is a hot toxin that injures Yin substance, resulting in Phlegm-Heat, Yin-deficiency, Empty-Heat, Blood-stasis and reduced nutritional supply to tissues.

In biomedicine, smoking has been shown to decrease fibrinolytic activity and nutritional supply to tissues, including intervertebral discs. Decreased nutritional supply can lead to increased risk of poor healing and can cause disc pathologies, and surgical and fracture nonunion. Smoking lowers the interdiscal pH (Humbly and Moony 1992) and has been shown to increase the rate of disc degeneration (Battié et al. 1991; Holm et al. 1981). Smoking may double the risk of rheumatoid arthritis in men, but it does not seem to affect women's risk of the disease. This may explain why patients who smoke often develop chronic symptoms (Holm and Nachemson, 1988).

Secondary Factors

The *secondary* Pathogenic Factors that can lead to disease are *Phlegm* and *Static-Blood* (although many other mechanisms can result in "secondary" symptom/signs such as Qi-stagnation-transformative/congested-Fire, for example). These factors arise mostly due to dysfunctions in other systems, but can then cause disease by themselves. In-and-of themselves, both Phlegm and Blood-stasis are considered as Excesses. However, they are both commonly a result of Deficiencies in other systems, and *may* at times need to be

---

129. Although not described as such in TCM. Parasites may be important is some patients with chronic myofascial pain syndromes, fibromyalgia, multiple sclerosis, inflammatory arthritis and chronic fatigue.

130. As early as 1800, a TCM treatise described smoking as having hot, drying and toxic effects.

treated as a Deficiency syndrome. The *Heart Transmission of Medicine* says that Phlegm cannot engender itself, whenever there is Phlegm there must be a cause, possibly: Cold, Heat, Dampness, Summer-Heat, Dryness, Wine accumulation, food accumulation, Spleen-deficiency, and/or Kidney-deficiency. Both Phlegm and Blood-stasis share some of the same potential pathologic processes: arising from Deficiency or inadequate circulation, form firm coagulations/masses, and both can interact with Heat or Cold factors. Because Phlegm and Blood are of the same source (both are products of Yin-Fluids), Phlegm and Blood patterns are often seen together and can influence each other, resulting in a vicious cycle with dysfunctions resulting from one leading to the other, or which result in further weakening the Organs that have lead to their formation in the first place. Intractable diseases are often said to relate to Phlegm and Blood-stasis and clinical management can be very difficult. Table 1-8 summarizes symptoms and signs associated with Phlegm and Static Blood.

Phlegm (Tan, Yin)

Thick Phlegm (Tan), Thin Phlegm/Rheum (Yin) and Water/Fluid (Shui Shi) pathogens are all manifestations of pathological products of abnormal metabolism of Fluid and Grain. Thin-Yin-Phlegm (also called Rheum) is commonly found in the cavities of the chest, abdomen, and gastro-intestinal tract. Thick-Phlegm is a state where Dampness/Fluids congeal and become turbid (an abnormal metabolite of Water/Fluids), and usually is more confined than Damp or Yin-Phlegm Pathogenic Factors. Thick Phlegm can circulate with Qi to any part of the body. Because Phlegm is in part a product of Fluids, Phlegm may have both normal and pathogenic functions/effects in the body. Phlegm is required for normal lubrication of the mucous membrane lining, but it becomes a pathological substance when excess-Phlegm is derived from dietary factors; when normal Phlegm/Fluids (in mucus linings) is produced in excess; or when pathogenic Phlegm results from internal or external pathogenic/Evils (or pathological) factors. Phlegm is more often seen in overweight, middle-aged or elderly patients. It is also a common factor in children.

Phlegm may be diagnosed as visible or invisible Phlegm. *Visible Phlegm* is defined as the usual mucoid secretions (by mucus linings) seen in disorders of the Lungs, respiratory tract, Stomach, Large Intestines and in: palpable, localized, movable, and yielding masses. *Invisible Phlegm* is diagnosed in disorders of Interior Phlegm such as in arteriosclerosis, psychiatric disorders and diseases that impact consciousness (and possibly bone-spurs, loose bodies etc., that can only be seen on x-ray). Phlegm in the channels, network-vessels, sinews, or bones can result in Phlegm-nodes, Phlegm-swellings, scrofula, and numbness of the limbs and/or body. The five main Phlegm patterns are: Wind-Phlegm, Cold-Phlegm, Hot-Phlegm, Dry-Phlegm, and Damp-Phlegm. Phlegm can result from any of the Pathogenic Factors (six Excesses) and disorders of Yin, Yang, Qi, Blood, channels, Blood vessels, and any of the Organs. Phlegm can also result from diet, life-style factors, and medications. According to master Lin Pei Qin, "Eight out of ten people are plagued by Phlegm."

Because Phlegm follows Qi and Qi circulates' throughout the body, Phlegm can be associated with all clinical entities and at every stage of the disease process. By and large, disorders of the Spleen/pancreas ("Spleen is the source of Phlegm") and/or food stagnation, Lungs, Triple Warmer, and Kidneys are said to result in Dampness and/or Phlegm production. However, any disorder can result in Phlegm. The Liver controls free flow of Qi and Blood, and Phlegm follows Qi and is related to Blood. Therefore, Liver disorders are often associated with Phlegm. As Phlegm is moved by Qi, and Qi disorders are characterized by unpredictably/irregularity, symptoms and signs relating to Phlegm may come and go. Phlegm signs may show only during periods when Qi becomes significantly stagnant and/or rebels. It is therefore said, "strange sicknesses are usually Phlegm...Phlegm is the king of bizarre diseases."

In general, when disorders of Shen/spirit/emotions are said to result from Phlegm, it is the "substantial" aspect of Phlegm that is said to obstruct the flow of Yin and Yang. This may be expressed by *clear-Yang* not reaching the head, by loss of communication between the Kidneys and Heart, or by *veiling* the opening of Heart and Pericardium. Phlegm can also obstruct the channels resulting in Liver-congestion transformative/congested-Fire, with psychiatric symptoms of anger and irritability and/or agitation. Alternatively, Liver-Qi-stagnation can weaken the Spleen's transformation and transportation functions resulting in Phlegm. It is said, "Phlegm is produced by stagnation of Qi," and Qi-stagnation often involves the Liver; therefore, Liver disorders are a commonly the cause of Phlegm.

Phlegm is thought to have a similarity to grease or fat, and therefore, fatty foods are considered one potential source of Phlegm. Phlegm can also arise from dietary sensitivity, sugar, alcohol, or spoiled foods. In general, any food that is not completely digested (pure is not completely separated from impure) is said to give rise to pathological, turbid Phlegm. "Normal" thick Fluids are produced when pure substances are obtained from digested foods and then processed into a useful body lubricant/Fluids. Obese people are said to be displaying an excess of Phlegm in their extra body weight, which is seen as the equivalence of Phlegm. However, one should not automatically treat obese patients as having Phlegm disorders.

External Pathogenic Factors can obstruct circulation resulting in Fluid-accumulation transforming into Phlegm. Phlegm is therefore a pathogen that can be described as TCM's great imitator—it can be involved in any disorder, and is said to be "the cause of one hundred diseases." Phlegm is considered one of the most complex of the *secondary* Pathogenic Factors and may require *complex* treatment plans, since by definition it is often a secondary

Table 1-8: Secondary Factors

Factor	Symptoms, Signs
Phlegm	Complex presentations. Chronic diseases that come and go but which leave the patient physically strong or asymptomatic between attacks. Symptom aggravation during change of weather; foggy, muggy, rainy days. Symptoms that are worse in morning (after Dampness/Phlegm accumulate overnight) or after eating (due to Spleen Yang-weakness). Oppressive fullness in chest or stomach (shortness of breath, a sense as though one cannot get enough air, frequently taking deep breaths). Decreased appetite with preference for bland foods and drink, and dislike of oily foods. Nausea or Vomiting (Phlegm disturbing the Stomach descending functions). Absence of thirst or dry sticky mouth with strong desire to drink, but discomfort after drinking (especially with Phlegm-Heat). Difficultly swallowing or a sensation of a lump in throat (plum seed Qi). Dizziness, clouded spirit, hemiplegia. Lack of concentration, poor memory, "fogginess," "spaciness," all of which are usually worse in morning or on damp muggy days. Palpitation, fear, poor memory, mania, insomnia, depression, paranoia or other psychiatric symptoms. Soft lumps, scrofula, goiter. Elusive bizarre symptoms. Strong dislike of odors that may cause symptoms (can be a sign of easily aroused Yang as well). Achy distended extremities. Oily skin. Unpleasant bodily secretions (armpits, ears, palms, soles, eyes, etc.). Sticky/pasty, sluggish (difficult to pass) and incomplete bowel movements (but with soft stools), mucousy stools. Low grade fever or subjective feverishness. Localized heat, cold or numb patches that are fairly fixed. Reddish cheeks (especially if Phlegm-Fire) or complexion ashen and dull. Eyes and facial expressions are torpid (expressionless), puffy or oily shiny face, eye sockets dark, green circles around eyes Obesity with soft fleshy muscles or muscular nodules. Abdominal signs of Fluids with sloshing and gurgling sounds. Joint end-feels that are either soggy (in acute swellings) or hard; in acute Phlegm/Damp-Heat/Fire or in chronic arthritis with congealed Phlegm/Blood-stasis. Thick greasy tongue coat, that may be permanent or appear and disappear, may appear like accumulated powder, or at root only and even peeled in some patients (in which signs must be correlated with other symptoms. The patient may have combined Phlegm Yin-damage or Phlegm alone). Swollen tongue. Pulse: Slippery, variable, wiry, deep, or floating, soft/soggy, moderate (i.e., slightly slow).
Static Blood	Stabbing, Sharp, Fixed, Night pain. Pain that cannot be relieved quickly Excess pain, disliking pressure. Lumps that are hard and fixed. Obstruction (swelling, lumps) precede pain; however, mircobleeding or stasis may result in fixed pain without obvious signs of obstruction. Bleeding that is often chronic, difficult to stop. Blood dark or fresh red, and contains clots. Feverishness/heat usually low and can be localized (e.g., joint) or general (systemic). However, there may be persistent high fever. Or fevers may come and go, or may be tidal fevers. There may be bleeding or agitation. Dry mouth without desire to drink (like to only wet mouth). Numbness or feeling of electrical charges, shooting pains. Itching that is severe, or feeling of ants crawling between the skin and muscles. Blue-green-purple appearance/veins. Spider nevi/prominent veins that are dark. Dry rough skin, hair that easily breaks or falls out. Purple or red macules. Dark/soot color or blackish uneven facial complexion (or under eyes) and lips (or purple), static spots in iris or sclera (sclera may be tinged yellow), crab-claw lines (around eyes). Cheeks may be flushed or dark red (often with enlarged/congested blood vessels). Red scarred nose or facial rosacea. Abdominal drum bloating, bulging naval (umbilical hernia, also sign of Phlegm or Spleen damage), tender masses, lower abdominal tension (especially left); tenderness or hardness. Choppy, thready, wiry, inhibited (tight and submerged) pulse or normal when just associated with injury or channels. Static spots on tongue or normal when just associated with injury or channels. Enlarged, dark, crooked sublingual veins, or normal when just associated with injury or channels. Darkness of tongue, or normal when just associated with injury or channels.

disorder. Excess-Phlegm disorders often have an acute and rapid onset, while deficiency-Phlegm (Phlegm secondary to Deficiency) take time to develop and are difficult to treat. In all Phlegm disorders (especially Interior-deficient) treatment to the root (Gen) condition is imperative, otherwise Phlegm will regenerate. Careful Organ diagnosis is needed. Perpetuating life-style factors should be addressed. Zhu Dan Xi stated that when treating Phlegm one does not treat Phlegm directly; instead, taking care of Qi should be the priority. When Qi flows smoothly, Fluids will move freely; and resolution of Phlegm will take place easily.

An important cause of Phlegm that is often neglected is Yin-deficiency. Yin pertains to structure and form. Yin is stored, in part, in the channels, vessels, bone marrow, brain, spinal cord and muscles. When Yin becomes deficient (as commonly occurs in aging) an "empty space" is said to be created which becomes easily invaded with pathogenic Phlegm (or other Pathogenic Factors). Because Phlegm is in part a by-product of Fluids, the more generalized Phlegm becomes the more Fluid (and space) is used-up. Therefore, Damp/Phlegm can easily transform to Dryness/Yin-deficiency with Phlegm and Yin-deficiency presenting simultaneously. Yin-deficiency can also result in Empty-Fire that scorches the Fluids, resulting in Phlegm and Yin-deficiency. The key sign is often a dry tongue and lips. In all of these clinical presentations, one needs to both moisten and address Phlegm/Dampness. Moistening however is done using non-cloy herbs, or by transforming Phlegm with herbs such as Radix Trichosanthis (Tian Hua Fen).

Another important relationship is between Phlegm and Fire. It is said: Phlegm is simply Fire with From; Fire is simply Formless Phlegm." Any Pathogenic Fire, either endogenous or exogenous can therefore lead to Phlegm.

In musculoskeletal (and other) disorders, when Phlegm settles in the channels/vessels, tissues, and joints, numbness and/or pain of the limbs (due to blocked Qi and Blood), scrofula, subcutaneous swelling/nodes, hemiplegia, or fistulous infection of the tissues can develop. Phlegm is therefore a factor when swelling takes shape and is localized. By comparison, Dampness (or Rheum thin-phlegm) pertains usually to a more generalized edema or symptoms of heaviness/fullness (or, localized or general fatigue), with the appropriate signs. Swelling due to Phlegm feels harder and more confined (e.g., ganglion cyst) than swelling that is due to Dampness or thin-liquids-Rheum. Phlegm is often associated with the joints, tendons, and ligaments, while Dampness is associated more with muscular and skin disorders. The thickened Fluid that fills the bursae in patients with *bursitis* may be considered a Phlegm disorder; as it is usually manifested as local firm-swelling, which may or may not be palpable with the naked fingers, depending on location. Muscles afflicted by Phlegm develop nodules (as seen often in myalgic patients), whereas when afflicted by Dampness, they feel fatty (cotton-like) and lack tone only.[131] In arthritic and other chronic disorders, Phlegm and Blood may coalesce and result in stubborn disorders that are difficult to treat. This can be seen in arthritis with degenerative or proliferative changes.

Treatment in these cases is often a combined approach that integrates herbs that transform Phlegm, break Blood-stasis, warm the channels, and at times nourish weakness. (See "Treatment of Painful Obstruction According to TCM Pattern Diagnosis" on page 662).

Even though Phlegm is an Excess condition, patients often feel relief from massage/pressure, as it can move the Qi and thus move the Phlegm. Local accumulation such as ganglion-cysts and bursitis may need to be drained/bled, followed by other external and internal therapies (moxa, acupuncture, and application of herbs). To *penetrate* Phlegm-accumulation, highly aromatic herbs are often needed (see chapter 7)

Blood-stasis (Xue Yu)

Blood-stasis is a common and important etiology in musculoskeletal and Internal diseases, as it is a substantial pathogen that can block circulation and can also result in Heat or lack of nourishment of tissues. Blood-stasis refers to collection and stagnation of Blood-Fluids and to ecchymosis. Blood-stasis may result from injury that severs the channels and vessels, leading to bleeding. It also can be due to Qi-stagnation and/or Deficiency, either of which result in Qi failing to move Blood. Blood and Qi are interrelated, and simultaneous Qi and Blood patterns are commonly seen. Consequently congestion of microcirculation can lead to the symptom of pain that is associated with Blood-stasis. In recent times Blood-stasis has been receiving increased attention and biomedical research has shown that micro-injuries to vascular walls are quite common and can lead to reduced microcirculation and hypercoagulability. Vascular lesions and Blood-stasis can be mutually aggravating. Blood-circulation is often the key for resolving musculoskeletal disorders.

IMPORTANT CAUSES OF BLOOD-STASIS ARE:

- Phlegm and/or Dampness impeding the flow of Qi and therefore of Blood.
- Phlegm obstruction attracting Blood, which sticks to Phlegm and accumulates.
- Blood-deficiency failing to fill the vessels and therefore Blood does not flow properly.
- Organ disorders of the Liver, Lung and Heart.
   —The Liver stores, generates, and releases Blood and also controls free flow, especially of Qi.
   —The Lungs move Qi by their rhythmic movement (with Chest-Qi), which carries and moves the Blood.
   —The Heart commands the Blood vessels, and its Qi is the power that pushes Blood (by vessel contraction).

---

131. Not all are classical associations.

Table 1-9: Hot Cold Deficiency and Excess

Pattern	Deficiency-Cold	Deficiency-Heat	Excess-Cold	Excess-Heat
Primary Mechanism	Cold from Yang-Qi-deficiency.	Heat caused by Yin not controlling Yang (lack of Fluids to control fire).	Pathogenic Cold Factors, Yin-Excess.	Pathogenic Heat Factors. Yang-Excess-Heat.
Primary Symptoms/Signs	Pain responds to warmth and massage.[a] Feeling cold and bodily coldness. Liking of warmth and ability to warm up with extra clothing Fatigue and shortness of breath. Spontaneous perspiration. Paleness. Clear urine. Sticky stools or undigested food in stools.	Pain responds to cooling and massage.[b] Feeling warmth in Yin-parts of body. Irritability, restless, insomnia Night perspiration. Pale face, red cheeks. Yellow short urine. Dry stools. Dryness, thirst.	Pain responds to warmth but not massage.[c] Feeling chills without fever. Liking of warmth but difficult getting warm with extra clothing. No or little perspiration. Pain. Clear long urine. Diarrhea.	Pain responds to ice but not massage[d] Feeling and physical heat on Yang parts of body. Fever without chills. Liking of cold. Thirst. Profuse perspiration. Red face. Short, dark (concentrated) possibly painful urine. Constipation.
Tongue	Pale, tender, swollen, teethmarks. Coat moist and white.	Red, small, cracked, dry. Coat scanty or patchy.	Coat white and thick or white and moist.	Red, possibly swollen. Coat yellow and thick.
Pulse	Deep, slow, forceless.	Fine, rapid, wiry.	Slow, tight.	Tidal, rapid, floating.

a. Seen in many patients with chronic arthrosis.
b. Seen in many patients with chronic inflammatory conditions.
c. Seen in many patients with neuropathic pain.
d. Seen in many patients with active inflammatory conditions.

- Weakness of digestive functions from Spleen/pancreas-deficiency may result in deficient Qi/Blood and secondary stasis. Also, since Blood is supported by Kidney-Essence which is necessary for the production of Blood, and since Kidney-Yang is the source-Fire for Spleen digestion and Liver motion, Kidney disorders can result in weakness of Spleen-Yang, Liver-Yang (Qi) and Blood.
- Excessive-Heat (Interior or Exterior) can thicken Blood. Excessive-Cold (Interior or Exterior) congeals Blood. Therefore, either Heat or Cold can retard circulation and may lead to Blood-stasis.
- Excessive-Heat in the Blood-division (or Blood) can drive the Blood out of the vessels (as seen with infections) resulting in bleeding and stasis.
- Qi-deficiency (especially Spleen) can result in leaky vessels leading to Blood-stasis outside the vessels (ecchymosis). Qi-deficiency can also result in weakened propulsion of Blood, Blood-stasis forms. Stasis and ecchymosis then result in further consumption of Qi, resulting in decrease of tissue (or Organ) nourishment. This can result in a vicious cycle and is quite common.

Blood-stasis is thus a very common secondary complication of chronic illness. It is a common pathology seen in musculoskeletal disorders, especially after trauma, the elderly, and in chronic diseases, since it is a consequence of many chronic disorders. Blood-stasis is a substantial pathogen; therefore, swelling (obstruction) associated with it is said to *precede* the sensation of pain. When Phlegm, Dampness and Blood-stasis combine (seen commonly in severe arthritis, intra-articular body, spurs, some discogenic disorders, and stenosis), swelling and/or lumps develop that may be tender and especially difficult to treat. Blood-stasis from acute (or as a result of old) injury, is associated often with *little* or *no* other *generalized Blood-stasis signs*. The pulse and tongue may be normal.[132] This is often seen clinically. Zhu Dan Xi stated: "Painful swollen joints and a difficult pulse indicates the presence of Blood-stasis."

It is wise to remember that both Phlegm and Blood-stasis are a common consequence of chronic disorders and disease processes. Therefore, therapies such as blood letting and adding herbs that invigorate Blood flow (often with Qi tonics), and dispersing Phlegm are often used in chronic pain patients.[133]

---

132. Pulse taking is subjective and a very subtle art. Some people claim to be able to pick-up all obstructions (as well as other bio-medical disorders) via the pulse.

Eight Principles (Ba Gang)

"Eight Principles" is a diagnostic system that classifies disease according to Yin-Yang, Hot-Cold, Internal-External, and Deficiency-Excess. While the Eight Principles were only described as such in the Qing dynasty (fairly late in TCM history), their main ideas were described earlier in the *Classic of Internal Medicine*. The *Classic of Difficult Issues* (about 100 BC) states:

> Frequent movement in the vessels indicates an illness in the Organs [Internal]. Slow movement in the vessels indicates an illness in the Channels [External]. Frequency indicates Heat. Slowness indicates Cold...Yang symptoms are caused by Heat. Yin symptoms are caused by Cold. These principles can be employed to distinguish illnesses in the Channels and Organs [Exterior/Interior].

The Eight Principles comprise a method by which disease can be localized, the major characteristics and nature of pathogenic and healthy factors can be categorized, and the progression of symptoms can be understood. The Eight Principles can be applied to all other forms of diagnosis in Chinese Medicine.

The most basic aspect of the Eight Principles is the categorization of symptoms and signs into Yin and Yang. Deficiency, Cold, and Interior are Yin. Excess, Heat, and Exterior are Yang. Deficiency relates mainly to an insufficiency of the body's True-Righteous-Qi, the ability of the body to fight disease and to compensate for stress. Deficiency syndromes often relate to chronic diseases and old age. Excess relates mainly to the exuberance of Pathogenic Factors and/or retention, stasis, or congestion of any aspect of the body's milieu. In general, Excess syndromes relate more to the acute or middle stages of disease. However, the Eight Principles should never be seen as simple categorizations of "either-or," since mixed presentations are common and may involved all at the same time. Table 1-9 summarizes the most important aspects of Hot, Cold, Deficient, and Excess.

In general, Exterior syndromes are seen in patients in which Pathogenic Factors reside in the Exterior (skin and flesh/muscles), the pulse is floating, and the tongue coat is thin. They often relate to early or acute stages of disease. At the same time, gradual invasions of the *channels* by external Pathogenic Factors (Bi-syndromes by Wind, Cold and Dampness) are also considered to be Exterior syndromes. In general, Interior syndromes are found in patients in which Pathogenic Factors have entered the Interior (Organs or bones), the pulse is deep (or not floating), and the tongue coat is thick or lacking. They often relate to chronic diseases. At the same time, an acute disease in which external Pathogenic Factors enter the Organs or bones are considered Interior syndromes. External and Internal aspects of disease, their location and seriousness, have been interpreted differently throughout the years and even within the *Classic of Internal Medicine*. For example, while Interior serious diseases are usually interpreted as diseases of the *Yin Organs* by some authors, others have seen the *bones* and *marrow* as the most serious, deep and difficult to treat stage (e.g., Sima Qian 90 BC.).[134] The *Classic of Internal Medicine states*: "[the evil Qi] invades the bones and their marrow, and the disease cannot be cured." Elsewhere it relates end-stage disease as being related to the Jue (terminal)-Yin (Liver). Therefore, as with most concepts in TCM, every principle needs to be understood in the context of the patient and the disease. The Eight Principles can be used to categorize pain as summarized in Table 1-10.

PAIN FROM ACUTE MUSCLE STRAIN. Pain from acute muscle strain is a common occurrence. Accompanied by swelling and warmth, it is acute, sharp, burning, intense, and relatively superficial. The condition is classified as Yang, Hot, External, and Excessive because:

YANG	The condition is acute, and the pain is sharp and intense.
HOT	The tissue feels warm and responds to icing, and the pain can have a burning quality.
EXTERNAL	The lesion is located in the muscle.
EXCESSIVE	The area is sensitive to touch and acute.

Because the condition is Yang, Hot, External, and Excessive, treatment techniques that have Yin cooling and superficial effects, such as bleeding acupuncture points on Yang channels, would be appropriate.

---

133. It is a common mistake to overemphasize tonification in chronic pain patients. Even in older and so-called weak patients, Blood-stasis and Phlegm (often Phlegm-Heat) can be the central pathological mechanism responsible for pain and also aggravation of *secondary* or primary Deficiency (even though by definition both Blood-stasis and Phlegm are secondary mechanisms and the elderly are Deficient). Elderly patients often have full, tight and wiry pulses pointing to possible Excessive disorders (although according to some, wiry pulses are due to Empty-Heat). Even in patients with a weak pulse position (often distal or Kidney position) the possibility of obstruction of lower-Warmer or other area by Cold should be kept in mind. When the obstruction is removed or transformed, the patient's health (and pulse) improves. Obstruction is a common cause of (or can worsen), Deficiency, as it can hamper the formation of Blood and Qi. It is common also for Qi to be consumed by Blood-stasis (and/or severe pain). In some chronically Deficient patients, the dose of tonic herbs should be kept at a lower level (or not used at all) as compared to blockage removal. Harmonizing herbs are then added to the formula. Another strategy is to transform stasis, which both nourishes and eliminate stasis. The control of pain often results in increased Qi and reduces fatigue which may be confused with Deficiency or that can cause Qi-deficiency from poor sleep, etc.

134. Some texts refer to bones as being part of the body frame (especially when related to traumatic diseases) and place them in the Exterior. Also, many skin diseases are due to Interior causes even though manifesting at the Exterior (e.g., Blood-Heat).

CHRONIC MUSCULAR PAIN. An example of a condition that *may be* classified as Yin, Cold, Internal, and Deficient is *chronic* dull muscular ache. The patient may have pain that, for the most part, is constant, chronic, dull, deep, and achy (of moderate intensity), and is aggravated when the patient is tired, occurs usually in the afternoon, (and possibly in the morning when Yin-pathogens accumulate). The patient may feel cold and may find relief using heat and pressure (massage).

The practitioner uses treatments that are Yang in nature because the condition is Yin and Deficient. Energy from Yang channels is directed deeply to Yin channels (by selection of points and deep needling). Warming and tonifying techniques are used.

Clinical Use of Eight Principles

The Eight Principles is among the most commonly used diagnostic system for prescribing herbal medicines. It can be used for acupuncture as well. When using the Eight Principles, one prescribes treatments that result in balance; e.g., cold medicine for a hot condition and hot medicines for a cold condition.

In clinical practice, however, one often finds mixed syndromes (especially when Dampness and Phlegm are a component, or when there is both Yin and Yang deficiency), in which Hot and Cold, Deficiency and Excess, Internal and External, i.e., Yin and Yang, present at the same time. There may be Heat above and Cold below (e.g., irritability, bitter taste, thirst with profuse pale urine and cold extremities); Cold above and Heat below (e.g., Phlegm-Heat obstructing Clear-Yang, warm-swelling in extremities, scanty yellow urine, with clear runny nasal phlegm, stiff neck, and aversion to cold); Exterior Cold and Interior Heat (e.g., pre-existing Heat with invasion of Cold, body aches, stiff neck, lack of sweating, aversion to cold with irritability and thirst); and Exterior Heat and Interior Cold (e.g., pre-existing Yang-deficiency with fever, sore throat, thirst, sweating, with loose stools, cold extremities and profuse pale urine). One may also encounter false Heat (usually in very serious diseases when some symptoms of Heat are seen with signs, especially tongue signs, of Cold); false Cold (usual in very serious diseases when some symptoms of Cold are seen with signs, especially tongue signs, of Heat); false Deficiency (e.g., fatigue and shortness of breath caused by Pathogenic Factors); or false Excess (e.g., burning pain from Empty-Heat). Many disorders can be transmitted from one system to another (as seen with Five Phases—see page 48) and result in multiple system involvement. There may be one root disease mechanism responsible for multiple presentations (branch or presenting symptoms and signs), or there may be multiple roots (disease-mechanisms), each responsible for its own branch of symptoms and signs. Therefore, the practitioner must carefully assess symptoms and signs. In most cases the root condition of the patient (or of the pathocondition) determines which is "false," and the system that was affected *first* is often the root of the patient's complex presentation (therefore, a good history and analysis of risk factors is required).[135] In musculoskeletal practice the branch or presenting symptoms (i.e., pain) must always be addressed. If pain is not relieved, stress will result in emotional damage, which will further lead to Internal damage of the Organ systems and milieu of the body. *The Systematic Classic of Acupuncture & Moxibustion* states:

> If first there is a disease and then there is counterflow, then treat the root (if disease results in counterflow, the disease is the root and it should be treated first). If first there is counterflow and then disease, then treat the root as well (the counterflow is the root and should be treated first). If first there is Cold and this engenders a disease, then treat the root (Cold disease resulting in disease of another nature, Cold is the root and treated first). If first there is a disease and this engenders Cold, then treat the root as well (the disease is the root and treated first). If first there is Heat and this engenders a disease, then treat the root (Heat is the root and treated first). If first there is a disease and this engenders Heat, then treat the root as well (disease is the root and treated first). If first there is Heat and this engenders fullness in the center, then treat the branch (center is Stomach and is therefore the root and treated first)...If a disease arises with surplus (Excess), [it should be determined as] the branch as against the root, and one should first treat the branch and then treat the root. If a disease arises with insufficiency, [it should be determined as] the branch as against the root, and one should first treat the severity before regulation [of Deficiency and Excess]. Slight problems can be handled simultaneously, but severe problems must be dealt with separately. If inhibited urination and defecation precede and result in another disease, the root should be treated.

Mixed and Complex Presentations

Mixed presentations (mostly of internal origin) have been explored by the author Li Dong-yuan (among others) in his *Treatise on the Spleen and Stomach* and other writings. His concept of pathogenic Yin-Fire, which is centered around a deficiency of Original-Qi, mainly of the Spleen and Stomach, may be helpful when treating such patients. According to Li Dong-Yuan, a weak Spleen commonly results in a variety of syndromes accompanied by both Cold and Hot symptoms/signs, including a sinking of the Central-Qi. This is treated mainly by warming, tonifying, lifting and drying herbs. This strategy has led to vigorous criticism by other authors.

---

135. The "root" (Ben) of a disease is usually what is not easily seen (a root is under ground) and the branch (Ben) is the presenting symptoms. Therefore, to ascertain the root, a deeper analysis is needed. Root and branch may be also understood as primary and secondary disorders. Root is often viewed as Deficiency and branch as Excess. This, however, is not always correct, as root causes can be due to Excess as well. Sometimes "root" is used to refer to symptoms in the Interior (or Organs) and "branch" to symptoms in the Exterior. This, too, is not always correct.

Table 1-10: Pain and Eight Principles

Principle	Characteristic Pain	Changed by
YIN-YANG	**Yin**: Dull, continual achiness, deep, chronic.	*Helped* by pressure.[a]
	Yang: Severe, sharp, burning, acute, paroxysmal, superficial.	Usually made *worse* by pressure.
HOT-COLD	**Hot**: Severe, burning, hot, expending, pulsating, inflammation, swelling, worse at night.	*Alleviated* by cold, aggravated by heat (not always aggravated by heat as heat can move Qi and Blood).
	Cold: Cold, contracting (like in a vise), stiff, spastic, worse in morning.	*Alleviated* by heat, aggravated by cold (not always aggravated by cold as cold, especially local, has analgesic effects).
EXTERNAL-INTERNAL	**External**: Pain at muscles and skin.	*Worse* with exposure to wind and/or cold.
	Internal: Pain in Organs and deep channels and tissues.	Can be affected by many factors depending on other pathologies.
DEFICIENCY-EXCESS	**Deficiency**: Dull, achy.	*Improves* with pressure. Worsens with exertion.
	Excess: Sharp, severe.	*Worsens* with pressure and possibly with or lack of movement.
	If due to Excess/stagnation.	*Better* with activity.
	A Yang-deficiency pain: Would feel cold, achy, and dull. Worse in morning, and better after movement.	*Improves* with heat and pressure. Worsens with physical exertion.
	A Yin-deficiency pain: Would feel burning or hot. Worse at night and better after rest or in the morning.	*Improves* with cold and pressure. Worsens with heat and physical exertion.
	Deficiency of Blood: May be dull, hot or cold, tingling, and/or itching.	*Improves* with pressure, eating, cold or heat.

a. Not a reliable sign in musculoskeletal disorders, especially with Deficient type pain. A lack of response to pressure may be interpreted as improvement and thus as a sign of Deficiency. Excess syndromes (especially in abdominal region) reliably worsen under pressure.

Li believed that the causes of Spleen and Stomach damage are: improper food intake (over-consumption of cold, raw, fatty, or unclean foods); overstrain (exhaustion that leads one to need to rest in the middle of the day); and mental stress. The loss of regulation of the middle warmer results in disruption of the up and downbearing regulation of Qi (or Yang) and leads to the sinking of the Clear-Yang to the lower warmer. This may agitate Ministerial-Fire (Mingmen) and transform it into pathological Fire (Yin-Fire).[136] This pathological Fire is then displaced, impeding the Premier-Fire (healthy Heart-Fire) from descending to activate Kidney water. Yin-Fire then may result in disharmony of Kidney and Heart. Li Dong also used the term "Yin-Fire" to describe a pathogenic Fire (or Heart-Fire) that injures the Spleen (i.e., Spleen trouble is secondary to pathogenic Fire), so that Yin-Fire is not only the result of Spleen or Source-Qi weakness.

Another use of the term "Yin-Fire" is for external pathogenic Fire (Summer-Heat or Damp-Heat). Li writes:

> When Spleen/Stomach is deficient and degenerating, Original-Qi becomes weakened; Heart-Fire tends to be in excess. Heart-Fire is a Yin-Fire, which rises from the Lower Warmer and connects to the Heart. Heart loses command; Premier-Fire takes over. Premier-Fire of the lower Warmer relates to Pericardium-Lou [Ministerial-Fire]; it can ransack the Original-Qi. Excess-Fire (thief or evil) and Original-Qi are unable to comply with each other. One wins the other loses. When Spleen/Stomach-Qi is deficient, it will sink and drain into Liver and Kidney; at the same time Yin-Fire will take the opportunity to take over the position of Earth. Hence, the occurrence of the following pattern: Shortness of breath or dyspnea, fever with restlessness, flooding big pulse, headache, thirst without relief, inability of skin to resist Wind-Cold with appearance of chills and fever...Uncontrollable joy and rage, irregular life-style and consumptive damage invariably damages Qi. The Qi degenerates, Fire glows. Glowing Fire may counter-assault Spleen/Earth. Spleen governs limbs; when Heat is entrapped, Qi is unable to activate, which is manifested as disinclination to converse, exertional shortness of breath, superficial Heat with

---

136. Some authors contest the interpretation of Mingmen being the Fire of all the above Organs. Ministerial-Fire is usually used to describe the normal healthy Fire of the lower Warmer (Kidneys). Li Dong Yuan, however, also speaks of it as pathological Fire (Yin-Fire) that damages Source-Qi, an opinion that resulted in much debate.

resting perspiration...In order to nurture Qi, it is necessary to pacify Heart and tranquilize Spirit. Sweet-cold herbs are used to purge Heat-Fire; sour is used to astringe the dissipated Qi; sweet-warm is used to tonify central-Qi...The major cause of consumptive illnesses is due to dissipation of the Original-Qi of the Stomach, which can prevent moistening and nurturing of Channels and Vessels, and weakening the protective-Qi.

Master Wu Cheng has commented on the above approach stating that:

> It is important to note that this approach is definitely *not* for Deficiency damage in general. As a rule, Yin-deficiency of the inferior with raising of Qi should never be treated with this method; the same is true in elevation of Qi in Yang-deficiency...If diagnosis is inaccurate, using sweet warm herbs to treat an Excess-Heat case could end up with tragedy... Be extra cautious in making the diagnosis before using this strategy" (Cheung 2001).

While Li emphasized Yin-Fire and the rising of Ministerial-Fire as a result of Spleen/Stomach weakness, Zhu Danxi believed that Heat/Fire symptoms resulting from the flaring-up of Ministerial-Fire are caused more often by *Yin-deficiency*. Danxi also advised that Yin can be damaged by *excessive desires,* especially sexual, flavorful foods, alcoholic beverages, and the use of warm spicy herbs and foods. He treated these patients primarily by moistening, clearing, and lowering Fire. Zhu also considered the role of the Spleen/Stomach to be important as a key source of Yin-nourishing nutrients. Master Wu Cheng has commented on Danxi's ideas:

> The moistening and lowering Fire method is indicated for use in Yin-deficiency with floating deficient-Fire, where the *accompanying Yang is not yet significantly deficient.* However, if it is indiscreetly used in Yin-deficiency *associated with marked Yang insufficiency,* the cold bitter herbs will definitely annihilate the remaining Yang. Misfortune develops.

To solve this dilemma, Xue Ji introduced the method of warm tonifying, leading the "Dragon back to the Sea." This method is also known as the regimen of *leading the Fire back to the Source* (Cheung *ibid*).

In musculoskeletal disorders, mixed syndromes arise most commonly by pathogenic-Dampness, which is seen frequently in patients with weakened Spleen/pancreas and poor digestion. Dampness may transform into Damp-Heat and then a mixed Deficiency/Excess/Hot/Cold syndrome may arise. Another possible consequence of pathogenic Dampness, a "heavy" pathogen, is that it can "sink" to the lower-Warmer where the Kidneys and Liver are housed. This pathogen can stagnate and transform into pathogenic Damp-Heat. At the lower-Warmer, pathogenic Damp-Heat either consumes Kidney/Liver Yin and leads to Empty-Heat (with rising-Yang), or stirs Mingmen/Ministerial-Fire with symptoms of Fire *independent* of Kidney/Liver-Yin-deficiency. Both Empty-Heat and stirred Mingmen result in mixed syndromes and may affect the Heart with psychiatric symptoms because Mingmen is said to be the source-Fire of the Heart and Pericardium.

Dampness is a Yin pathogen and therefore can easily weaken healthy-Fire (Mingmen). Mingmen may then loose its root and result in floating-Yang (with Heat symptoms) in a Yang-deficient patient (leading to false-Heat).

Poor digestion, with or without Dampness, can also result in Yin/Blood-deficiency (Blood in part is a product of digestion) and the formation of Empty-Heat because Blood is a Yin substance.[137] Spleen dysfunction may counter-control (insult) the Liver and result in Liver-congestion-transformative-Heat, again having a mix of Spleen-Yang-deficiency (Coldness/deficiency) and Liver-Fire (Hot/Excess).[138]

Because Interior Dampness blocks Qi as well as the Organ and channel systems, the Blood often becomes obstructed, which can lead to complex symptoms of Stasis, Excess, Deficiency, Cold, and Heat.

Since any "stagnation/depression" can easily transform into Heat and/or localized-Fire (binding-Heat), Heat is often present regardless of other mechanisms, and often eventually leads to damaged-Yin and wiry pulses, as commonly seen clinically.

Blood-stasis, as well as most other Pathogenic Factors and/or Organic dysfunctions, can also result in a mixture of Deficient, Excess, Hot, and Cold symptoms, via common mechanistic interactions of the system of correspondences. The *Classic of Internal Medicine* states:

> Cold can settle inside the channels and confront its Heat; the channel in a state of Excess harbors a pain that cannot tolerate any pressure. If the Cold lingers, Heat rises, the vessel swells, and the Qi and Blood become disrupted...

Thus, when treating a patient with mixed, complex, and possibly confusing syndromes, one *may need* to combine several treatment principles or treat each at a different time. For example, In the *Classic of Internal Medicine* the Yellow Emperor asked:

> Suppose the Stomach desires cold drink while the Intestines desire hot liquids. These two desires are counter to each other. How are they treated? Qi Bo answered. In spring and summer, the branch should be treated prior to root, while in autumn and winter, the root should be treated prior to the branch...

In patients with Dampness/Phlegm or pathogenic-Fire, herbs that strengthen the Spleen (and possibly Kidneys), improve digestion (and Dampness), regulate the Liver, smooth the flow of Qi, and clear Heat may be needed. The above pathomechanisms may also complicate musculoskeletal disorders with Blood-stasis, Wind-Damp, Wind-Cold and Wind-Heat. However, *when possible*, it is always preferable

---

137. Empty-Heat is Heat that results from insufficient Yin/Fluids to balance the Yang/Fire/Heat of the body: Water not controlling Fire.

138. Any stagnation or blockage can result in transformation to Heat, similar to heat produced by friction.

to understand the *principal/pivotal* pathomechanisms of a particular patient and to emphasize treatment to that *pivotal* syndrome.[139, 140] Herbs and/or acupuncture points which deal with *secondary* pathologies that arise as a consequence of the pivotal mechanism, are added at a relatively *smaller* dosage, if needed. Combining too many treatment principles without a clear focus is said to result in poor outcomes.[141] Hsu writes in *On the Origin and Further Course of Medicine*:

> When, therefore, in later times the number of pharmaceutical substances [employed] increased significantly, this was not because [the people] loved to create confusion and chaos. It is just that the learning [of the people in later times] was inferior to that of the ancients, [and that the physicians] were unable to treat several pathoconditions with one single drug. Hence they changed to complexity what was simple before.[142]

Another important clinical musculoskeletal presentation to consider is that any *local (channel) obstruction* can result in simultaneous symptoms of Deficiency and Excess and/or Hot and Cold in the channels and vessels. Blockage of "circulation" can result in symptoms of Excess up-stream from the blockage-stasis (lesion) with accumulation of Qi and Blood (and symptoms and signs of Excess), and Deficiency down-stream (as the Qi and Blood is blocked due to the "blocked path"). This may be one explanation why somatic (musculoskeletal) lesions are often associated with Organic symptoms. For example, the obstruction of a Yang channel around a lower extremity or spinal joint may result in symptoms of stagnation (Excess) at the trunk or abdominal Organs (up-stream as Qi and Blood "backup") and symptoms of Deficiency distally to the affected joint; the wilting/atrophy of muscles in a disc disease, for example.[143, 144] The application of attacking herbal methods and bleeding techniques to remove obstruction should be considered. The French Barrier points system is said to be helpful.

In summary, in order to prioritize treatment strategies, one needs to carefully analyze the patient's symptoms and signs to ascertain if Deficiency or Excess, Hot or Cold, Interior or Exterior, Yin or Yang predominate. The "harmonizing" methods developed by Zhang Ji in *On Cold Damage* and *Golden Chest Classic* are particularly helpful for complex patients.[145]

---

139. The practice of herbal medicine is both a science and an art. According to several of *this* author's teachers, what often makes the difference between a "master" and student is the dosage of herbs used to address *secondary* symptoms, and knowing which symptom/signs are key for correct diagnosis and which should be disregarded. Complex presentations may also lead to the temptation to combine too many treatment principles (herbs) without emphasizing or understanding the *common pathomechanistic axis* that is said to be the cause of these secondary complications. Since Heat/Fire is so commonly seen, and since, for example, it can be secondary to Cold and Deficiency (i.e., transformation due to stagnation/congestion), using too many cold herbs can easily aggravate the "root" of such a patient. As TCM relies entirely on physical examination and history for diagnosis, "correct" diagnosis may be easier said than done. Some authors have stated that regardless of the amount or type of herbs combined, each herb would still function in its associated potential and nature, and therefore the practitioner may combine as many treatment principles as he/she feels necessary.

    The following clinical case illustrates these complex questions. Ms. N was seen by the author for chronic (several years) chest, thoracic spine, shoulder, and low back pains. She also complained of fatigue, PMS (with Liver S/S), night sweats, occasional abdominal and TMJ pain, difficulties with attention and concentration, sleep problems, palpitations, and weakness of knees. Her tongue and pulse could be interpreted as showing a variety of syndromes with a mix of Excess and Deficiency. Ms. N was seen previously by several practitioners including TCM doctors that gave her various herbs, and acupuncture therapies. This author treated her for AC joint sprain, rib and thoracic dysfunctions using manual therapies and herbal formulas to address a "*complex*" Painful Obstruction (Bi) syndrome, which also addressed the Kidney, Spleen, and Liver. Ms. N. improved significantly during her treatments; however, many of the symptoms came back several weeks after she stopped the therapy. Signs of AC joint sprain (painful adduction across the front) remained improved, and she did have much reduced shoulder pain. Her low back pain was somewhat improved, as well. All other symptoms remained, especially chest and thoracic pain. She was then referred to Dr. Zhu, a TCM doctor who trained as a barefoot doctor in his teenage years and then received his Masters in TCM from Shang Hai College of TCM. After giving her a Bi-syndrome type formula for two weeks, which did not help her, he decided that all her symptoms and signs were secondary to Spleen-deficiency. He then gave her a smaller variation of Shen Ling Bai Zhu San. In two weeks all her symptoms improved. At the time of writing this section, which is about one year after seeing him, she is still pain and symptom free. Dr. Zhu states (personal communication) that it is unwise to combine too many treatment principles in one herbal prescription. Although the author's prescribed formulas also contained all of the same Spleen tonic herbs, it was the elimination of many of the other herbs that may have led to success. At the same time, it is also possible that this approach would have not yielded good results if the patient had not been treated with the previous approaches first, which may have "pealed" some of the layers.

140. An herbal formula is chosen from the category that reflects this "main pivotal" diagnosis. If needed, other herbs are added.

141. Training and ideas vary widely in TCM. The above statement reflects this author's training and clinical experience and by no means conclusive.

142. In the experience of this author, people with very many different and diverse conditions that need addressing are often sensitive and prone to developing side-effects and are often non-compliant. This is commonly seen for example in patients with Dampness/Phlegm and Kidney/Liver Yin-deficiency. One may need to treat Dampness first as the patient may not tolerate *any* Kidney or Liver-Yin tonic herbs. It is this author's approach to use mild and *simple* herbal formulas in many "complex" patients—the more complex a condition gets, often, the simpler the herbal formula. The addition of harmonizing herbs (or formulas) is often helpful in resolving "conflicts." If it is difficult to ascertain which pathomechanism is pivotal, attention to central-Qi (Spleen and Stomach), which is said to relate to Earth (and center) may help clarify priorities. Gentle formulas that harmonize Spleen and Stomach and that support Righteous-Qi are given to the patient. As Righteous-Qi begins to recover, secondary issues *may* become clearer and are then addressed. Also, many complex and mixed syndromes are said to be caused by the Extra and Divergent channels which then should be the focus of treatment.

143. Since channel circulation differs depending on which channel theory one uses, the clinical application of these principles is best used based on *palpatory findings*, not theory.

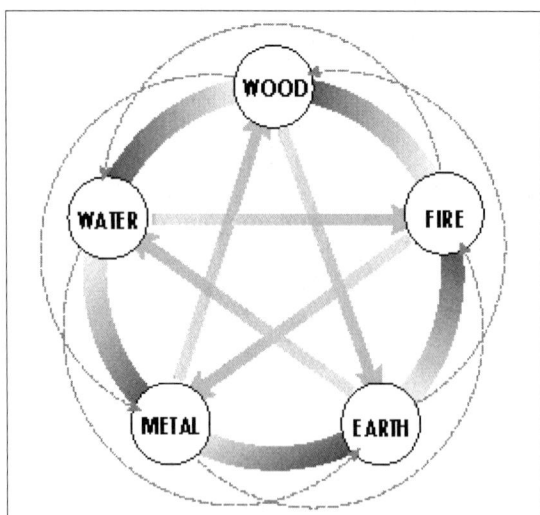

Figure 1-6: Generation cycle, inner thick circle; control cycle, thick inner arrows; over-regulation (insult) dysfunction, outer thin circle.

Five Phases (Wu Xing)

The Five Phases theory, one of the oldest in Chinese culture, was first developed to explain natural phenomena and normal cyclical movements in the universe including political structures. Later these principles were related to medical physiology. TCM suggests that all phenomena in the universe reflect five energetic/constructive phases (qualities) that are subject to positive and negative feedback mechanisms and have many interrelationships and intrarelationships. In Chinese the character for phases (Xing) denotes movement and therefore the Five Phases describe sequential (time-dependent) relationships that represent physiologic and pathologic processes. This theory describes a system of correspondence, that is, the relationships between specific categories such as the Organ systems, body tissues, climates, emotions, senses, vitalities, tastes/herbs/foods, etc. Table 1-11 summarizes the Five Phases characteristics.[146] The system was constructed to explain observable phenomena: water can extinguish fire; therefore, the Phase called Water can control the Phase called Fire. Rivers and man-made irri-

gation systems can control the flow of water; therefore, the Phase Earth can control the Phase Water; however, flooding can overcome irrigation systems and therefore, if the Phase Water is excessive, it can countercontrol (insult and overcome) the Earth Phase. When trees are burned, they turn into ashes and are incorporated into the soil; therefore, the Wood Phase can generate the Earth Phase, etc.

The Phases—five "elemental" configurations that are part of all material and natural order—are *Wood, Fire, Earth, Metal, and Water*. These describe complex categories/theories of quality and relationships, not simple physical elemental combinations. Physiologically, the Five Phases theory explains the unity of the mutual relationships between the Organs and body tissues, as well as between the human body and nature. Without the Five Phases there would be no Yin and Yang. In medicine, the Five Phases are patterns of associative relationships between different physiological and natural phenomena. For example, each of the seasons (late summer being a separate season) is related to one of the Phases and its associated Organ. Although the concept of a seasonal and environmental organ functional relationship seems obscure, a recent study of the affects of academic stress on the hypophyseal-pituitary-adrenal axis hormones has shown seasonal relationships (Malarky et al 1995). Also, seasonal affective disorder and the "flu season" are well recognized.

Each of the five-Phases is associated with one geographic direction. Recent studies show that brain function is affected by the direction one faces. There have been many studies showing a relation between human behavior and environmental phenomenon. Blair and Sharp (1995) have shown anticipatory head direction signals in anterior thalamus as evidence for a thalamocortical circuit that integrates angular head motion to compute head direction. A review and commentary on processing head direction cell signals was carried out by Taube et al (1996). Magnetic fields have been shown to influence human behavior and function. Friedman et al (1965) documented a relationship between increased geomagnetic activity and the rate of admission of patients to thirty-five psychiatric facilities. Perry et al (1981) showed a correlation between suicide locations with high magnetic field strengths due to 50 Hz power lines. Controlled studies have also shown a relationship between reaction time and magnetic fields (Wever 1974).

The physiological activities of the Organs can be classified according to the different characteristics of the Five Phases:

- Wood (Liver and Gall Bladder) is associated with germination, growth, extension, softness, bending, straighten-

---

144. This discussion is not a classical TCM interpretation of Channel flow. However, in this authors experience, this interpretation can be helpful in the clinical diagnosis and treatment of both sometovisceral and viscerosomatic disorders.

145. Minor Bupleurum Decoction (Xiao Chai Hu Tang) for example is often used in patients with conflicting and multi systemic symptoms and signs. The formula which was designed to treat Shao-Yang disease is particularly helpful in resolving conflict which is often related as Pathogenic Factors lingering between the Exterior and Interior. This formula has been used extensively in autoimmune disorders that almost by definition manifest symptoms of Excess and Deficiency and Hot and Cold.

146. The Five-Phases have been used to express many phenomena and objects such as: strains (Wu Lao), blockages (Wu Bi), types of stiffness (Wu Ying), movements (Wu Che and Wu Yun), materials (Wu Chu), serious conditions (Wu Si), exhaustions (Wu Duo), parts of body (Wu Xing), boils (Wu Ding), jaundice (Wu Dan), epilepsy (Wu Xian), confusions (Wu Luan), diets (Wu Yi), and so on.

Table 1-11: Categorization of Objects and Phenomena According To The Five Elements

PHASE CHARACTERISTICS	WOOD	FIRE	EARTH	METAL	WATER
TONE	Jiao	Zheng	Gong	Shang	Yu
FLAVOR	Sour	Bitter	Sweet	Pungent	Salty
COLOR	Green/Cyan	Red	Yellow	White	Black
CHANGE	Germination	Growth	Transformation	Harvest	Storage
CLIMATE	Windiness	Warmness	Dampness	Dryness	Coldness
DIRECTION	East	South	Center	West	North
SEASON	Spring	Summer	Late Summer	Autumn	Winter
ORGAN SOLID / ORGAN HOLLOW	Liver / Gallbladder	Heart / Small Intestine	Spleen / Stomach	Lung / Large Intestine	Kidney / Urinary Bladder
FLUID	Tears	Sweat	Saliva	Mucus	Urine
ORIFICE	Eye	Ear	Mouth	Nose	Anus and Urethra
SENSE ORGAN	Eye	Tongue	Mouth	Nose	Ear
TISSUE	Sinews	Vessels	Muscles	Skin and Hair	Bones
OFFENSIVE ODOR	Perspiration or odor of urine	Burnt	Sweet smelling	Fishy	Putrid
EMOTION	Anger	Joy	Rumination/ Excessive thinking	Melancholy/ Mourning	Fear
DIRECTION	East	South	Center	West	North
SOUND	Shouting	Laughing	Singing	Crying	Moaning
ENDOCRINE GLAND[a]	Pineal	Pituitary	Pancreas	Thyroid	Adrenal

a. Speculations by Kendall (*ibid*) based on the functional characteristics, vitalities, and emotions attributed to each organ system.

ing, orderliness, and harmony. Therefore, anything that has these characteristics can be categorized as having Wood Phase qualities.

- Fire (Heart and Small Intestines) is associated with Heat, upward movement, and the highest point of a hierarchy.
- Earth (Spleen and Stomach) is associated with growing, nourishment, generation of tens of thousands of things, center, and change. It likes warmth and dryness (Spleen).
- Metal (Lung and Large Intestines) is associated with separation, death, strength, and firmness.
- Water (Kidney and Bladder) is associated with cold, moisture, and downward flow.

The *Classic of Internal Medicine* states:

The heaven (sky) is the source of Qi (possibly air) for sustaining life. The earth is the source of the five flavors (food) for nourishing life. The five Qi (possibly air) is breathed through the nose and stored in the Lungs and Heart. The flavors and vital Qi are distributed above to reflect five colors [on the face] and to provide a bright complexion. The fact that Qi is responsible for producing the five sounds of the voice is evident.

The Five-Phases theory is used to describe regulatory systems (feedback/servo systems) and transmission pathways of both normal physiology and pathology. The positive feedback component of the Five Phases theory is called the generation cycle; the negative feedback component is called the control cycle. The *Simple Questions* states:

When the Qi of one of the Five Phases is excessive, it will overwhelm its subjugated [controlled] Phase (such as Wood overwhelming Earth) and counter-control its own subjugating Phase (such as Wood counter-regulating or insulting Metal).....The East generates wind, wind generates

Table 1-12: Physiologic Activity of the Channels

Channels (Meridians)	Physiologic Activity
Sinews	• Location of Defense-Qi circulation • Connection between Main channels and connective tissues and skin • With the muscles, provide a protective layer • Important in acute disorders such as sprain/strain and skin diseases • Important in musculoskeletal disorders
Connecting network-Vessels	• Link Main channels with surrounding tissues • Part of the Blood vessel system • Provide a functional connection between the ventral-dorsal and Yin-Yang aspects • Store Qi and Blood and release them to the Main channels when needed • Important in prevention of chronicity, emotional disorders, excess conditions
Main	• Connect Organs to rest of the system • The main channel system that has 360 acupoints
Divergent	• Reinforce Main channels • Provide functional connection between Yin-Yang Channels and Organs • Balance between the right and left • Important in Yin (substance) anatomical/pathological disorders • Complicated multisystemic diseases
Extra	• At a deep level, as all connect to the Kidneys • Store extra Qi and Blood • Release Qi and Blood when Main channels are vacuous • Balance between the left-right, superior-inferior, and diagonal aspects • Important in chronic disorders • Complicated multisystemic diseases

Wood, Wood generates sour, sour generates Liver, Liver generates Sinews.... The Five Phases theory is applied to the physiology and pathology of the human body by using the relationships of generation and control to guide clinical practice.

The generation cycle is an activating, generating, and nourishing sequence of phasic relationships (Sheng).

Wood⟶Fire⟶Earth⟶Metal⟶Water

The control cycle is a sequence of phasic relationships that restrict and inhibit (Key

Wood⟶Earth⟶Water⟶Fire⟶Metal

The *Classic of Categories* states:
If there is no generation, then there is no growth and development. If there is no restriction, then endless growth and development will become harmful.

Therefore, the movement and change of all things exists through their mutually generating and controlling relationships. These relationships are the basis of the never ending circulation of natural elements.

Five Phases Disorders

Five Phases theory is used also to demonstrate the transmission of pathological influences. In discussion on the transmission of diseases via the control cycle, the *Classic of Internal Medicine* states:

> When the Liver is diseased, the Liver will transmit [the disease] to the Spleen, and so one should replenish the Qi of the Spleen...When the Heart is diseased, first there is pain in the Heart, and in one day it results in coughing (transferred to the Lung), within three days there is pain in the ribs (transferred to the Liver), and in five days there is blockage causing pain and heaviness in the body (transferred to the Spleen). If the patient does not recover in three days, death will ensue. In winter the patient will die at midnight, and in the summer at noon.

Diseases of the Liver and Spleen/pancreas often interact with each other. For example, Liver disease may affect the Spleen/pancreas because Wood can over-control (Sheng) Earth, while Spleen/pancreas illness may affect the Liver because Earth can counter-control Wood (insult, Wu, and the disease can move contrary to its regular course, Ni and Fan). Liver disease may also influence the Heart by "mother affecting son" illness. If Liver disease is transmitted to the Lung, it can be categorized as Wood counter-controlling (insulting/invading) Metal. If it is transmitted to the Kidney, then it is considered a "son affecting mother" illness. The other Organs follow the same principles.

The control and generation relationships among Organs can be expressed as follows:

- The Lung's (Metal) function of clearing and descending can restrict the hyperactivity of Liver (Wood) Yang (via control cycle).
- The Liver's function of regulating the smooth flow of Qi is capable of reducing stagnation at the Spleen/pancreas (via control cycle).
- The Spleen's transportation and transformation function is able to subdue the overflow of Kidney Water (via control cycle). The rising of Spleen Qi helps the Liver and Kidney to move upward and bring Fluids up, as well as prevent Qi blockage (via control cycle).
- The Stomach's descending function helps descending functions of the Lung and Heart (via mother son cycle).
- The Kidney's nourishing and moistening function can prevent flare-ups of Heart-Fire (via control cycle) or Liver-Fire (via mother son [generation] cycle).
- The Heart's Yang (Fire-rising) can prevent hyperactivity of the Lung's (Metal) clearing and descending functions (via control cycle).
- Kidney-Yang warms Spleen-Yang, helping the Spleen's transformation function (via the Yang within Yin control cycle, or Fire generating Earth mother-son cycle [Kidney-Yang being Fire]).
- Sedating Liver can reduce over-activity of Heart-Fire (via son mother cycle).
- Strengthening Spleen/pancreas can strengthen the Lungs (via mother son cycle).
- Strengthening the Lungs descending function can bring Fluid to Kidneys and therefore strengthen Kidney-Water (via mother son cycle).

Therefore, the application of the Five Phases theory in explaining the complicated interaction between the Organs/channels and other phenomena can be summed up by these four relationships: over-regulation, counter-regulation, mother affecting son (depleting or nourishing), and son affecting mother (depleting or nourishing) (Figure 1-6).

The Five-Phase relationships can be used in emotional therapy as well, for example, if anger is excessive, melancholy can be stimulated in the patient to control anger, fear can be stimulated to control excessive joy, etc.

Some acupuncture systems rely almost entirely on the Five Phases theory for diagnosis and treatment. It is most useful for treatment of mental disorders; it is less effective for musculoskeletal disorders except when used as part of a larger treatment plan.[147]

The Channels (Meridians/Vessels) (Jing-Luo)

The body consists of matter and "energies" that "circulate" through a network of channels (Jing), network-vessels (Luo), and Organs.[148] The channels, also called "meridians," and the network-vessels (also called "collaterals") connect all the tissues of the body. Thus these intricate systems represent the body's "information" that "travel" via channels and vessels. In general, there are seventy-one channels in the body: twelve Main channels, twelve Sinew/cutaneous channels, twelve Divergent channels, fifteen longitudinal-Connecting channels, twelve transverse-Connecting channels, and eight Extra channels.

TCM uses the concept of *channels* and *vessels* to describe various systems: the muscular, circulatory, lymphatic, and nervous systems among them. Throughout TCM history, as the need to explain medical phenomena and prevailing philosophies have changed, channel theories have evolved and their sophistication has increased. The channels and vessels are described in part as circulatory systems akin to irrigation systems in agriculture. They contain Fluids and "energies" (Qi, Air, etc.) that circulates to every part of the body. Channels and vessels are arranged so that movement in a distal and proximal direction is possible. There are channels that function as the main throughways, others that are responsible for overflow (akin to systems that control flooding), some relate to flow and some to storage, others that connect various channels with each other or with the system they correspond to, and they can all become Empty or Full. Although the direction of circulation is different within each channel/vessel system (and historically different interpretations have occurred), undoubtedly the channel and vessel system was conceived to explain phenomena such as the distally flowing arterial and afferent systems, the proximally flowing venus and efferent systems, etc.

The information on channels in this text combines Chinese, Japanese, European, and information this author has gathered over the years from lectures and his teachers. It is therefore not strictly "classical" or Chinese. For sources please see works consulted in the references.

The Channels and Acupuncture

The channels are at the root of acupuncture theory; the belief is that acupuncture produces a physiological effect via the channel system. Researchers have attempted to verify the existence of acupuncture channels; however, data is contra-

---

147. The so called Worsley school of traditional acupuncture focuses almost exclusively on the relation of emotions to the internal Organs and on the inter-relationship of each of the "five elements" to emotions.

148. According to Unschuld (*ibid*), in early Chinese medical writings the channels (as well as points such as Transport points) are not strictly viewed as conduits of matter and "energies" (Qi and Blood, etc.) but where closely related to imperial controls and infrastructure systems and were even related to commerce. The theory therefore may have been developed out of, in part, general Confucian ideas on well-functioning societies and not strictly from medical thinking or experimentation.

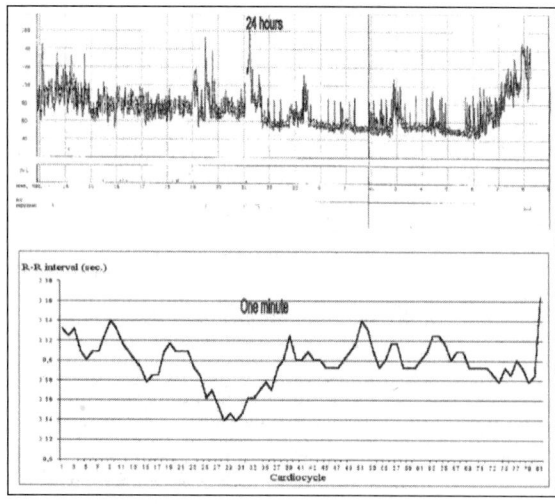

Figure 1-7: ECG patterns repeating at one minute and 24 hours. Note the self organization similarity between the one hour and 24 hours patterns (with permission Bouevitch 2001).

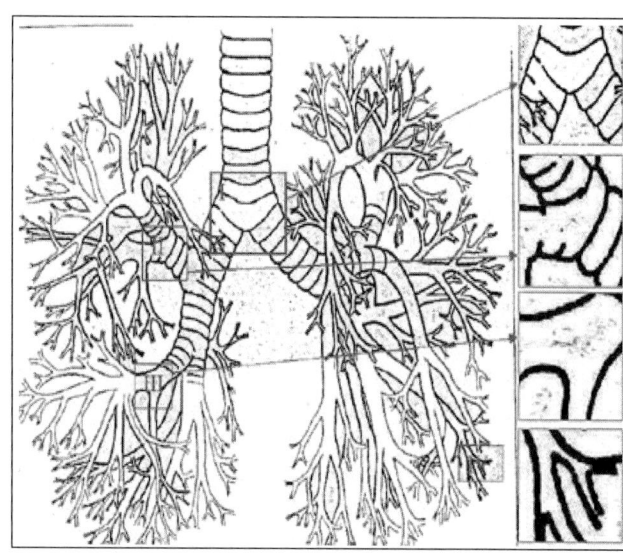

Figure 1-8: Fractal self-similarity of the respiratory tree. Note the similarities between the micro and macro tissue design (with permission Bouevitch 2001).

dictory and little linear relationship has been demonstrated between a given channel and any known anatomical or physiological entity or system (except for some embryological relations that may also include remnants of embryological organizing centers). Since all attempts at "finding" an "anatomical" substrate for channels have failed (even though bits of evidence such as possible electrical differentials and perivascular spaces along the channels have been described), it may be better to think of the channels as systems of communication similar to the immune system, at one extreme, and as mechanical relationships at the other extreme. The immune system does not contain a specific tissue or area; rather, it is a matrix of communication systems. On the other hand, the Sinew channels may correspond to myofascial structures and functional regional relationships as well as referred pain patterns can be demonstrated.

Many models have been proposed for such communication systems from bioelectrical, fractal (self-similarity, which may help explain the so-called microsystems of acupuncture), to wave theory (Bouevitch 2001). These may explain the channels as systems capable of transmitting information about the internal environment and facilitating the exchange of this information with the external environment via the acupuncture points. It is therefore possible that all information (or regional-system) can be found in particular surface areas such as an acupuncture point (i.e., a fractal). Bouevitch (*ibid*) states: "Microacupuncture systems are one of the manifestations of fractalizations, the universal principle of self-organization in nature. The number of possible microsystems is unlimited." Zhang Ying Qing described some 102 microsystems in the body that can be used for diagnosis and treatments (Maciocia 2004). The resolution of a microsystem and its influence on the organism depend on the size of its projection onto the surface of the skin, mucous membrane, and periosteum. *Self organization* can be shown within the all organ cells, organelles and systems (Figure 1-8), and even patterns of ECGs tend to self-organize (Figure 1-7). This influence may be most effective at the points of the classic acupuncture channels.

It is the so-called "propagated sensation of the channels" that is often cited as proof for the existence of the channel system. The "full" phenomenon of propagated sensation has been estimated to occur in about 1 out of 800-1000 patients. These people report feeling a propagated sensation through the entire channel when acupuncture points are stimulated. Some degree of propagation can be achieved in all patients, with about 10% of the population being capable of feeling the needling sensation propagated proximally. This in general is thought to be an inappropriate directionality for nervous painful transmission. The needle sensation (De Qi) is said to transmit sensation at approximately 10 cm per second, which is 10 times slower than the slow conducting C-fibers (Pomeranz (2001)). However, as discussed in the next chapter, referred pain (sensations) is a complex process that cannot be ruled out as the cause of De Qi, and the propagated sensation in these patients (which may or not follow the channels). Pain has been shown even to cross midline. (Again, this is thought to be inappropriate transmission of sensation.) Nerves are known to be capable of retrograde transmission, and some C-fibers have been shown to take as much as five seconds to conduct from the foot to the cord. In general, however, both pain and paresthesias propagate distally. Experimentally stimulated responses (i.e., acupuncture or other somatic stimulation) have been shown to not follow all the usual rules of orthodox neurology (Willard 1993, 2003).[149] De Qi can also be elicited in nonacupuncture points, although it may take more effort to do so.

Many attempts to document the existence of acupuncture channels has resulted in varied conclusions. For example, De Vernejoul et al (1985) injected radioactive technetium into a number of acupuncture and nonacupuncture points and showed scintigraphic evidence of specific radioactive paths which could be interpreted as acupuncture channels. Lazorthes et al (1990) attempted to reproduce this study but failed to show any such distribution. Recently Ma et al (2003) reported that perivascular space (PVS)—which has been demonstrated to be a body fluid pathway in addition to blood vessels and lymphatics in some mammalian tissues, such as brain, thymus, and lung—may relate to TCM channels. They studied characteristics of the tissues around the blood vessels along the Stomach and Gall Bladder channels with the goal of identifying anatomical structures corresponding to the channels. Through perivascular dye injection and frozen section histology, they found that there is PVS around the blood vessels along the channels that function as a fluid pathway. Subsequent physiologic studies revealed that the PVS shows significantly greater electrical conductivity and significantly higher partial oxygen pressure (pO(2)), compared to medial and lateral tissues. They concluded that PVS has properties offering a good explanation for the channel phenomenon.

There have been studies showing that channels and acupuncture points have a lesser degree of galvanic skin resistance than other sites, and thus many theories on electromagnetism and "information systems" have been proposed. An interesting experiment by Niboyet showed that when placing electrodes on points on a specific channel, the currents passed more preferentially within points in that channel than if the electrodes were placed on a non-related channel. None of the electromagnetic theories, however, yielded coherent, verifiable, and reproducible clinical procedures or evidence for the channels.[150]

There are possible embryological bases to the channel system. Lee (2002) proposes a mechanism by which the genetic information contained in the one-dimensional genome may be *converted into a three-dimensional body plan for development*. According to Lee and others, there are intimate relationships between the acupuncture channels and embryological development, evolution, the CNS, as well as the genome. Prior to mitosis of the fertilized egg, the chromatids, after being unpacked from the chromosomes, link up to form a giant circular loop which is then folded upon itself into a wired-frame structure that embodies the architectural embryological developmental scheme. This intranuclear spatial body design is then translated into a three-dimensional cellular plan surrounding the fertilized egg with the positional value of each surrounding daughter cell. This group of cells of the primitive embryo then leads to the formation of the Spemann Organizer, which directs the embryological development of the brain as well as the rest of the body. The Spemann Organizer thus retains control over the CNS which in turn controls the development and functions of the peripheral tissues. The chains of cells that compose the Spemann Organizer, forming a homunculus in the image of the wired frame formed by the chromatids are believed to be the equivalents of acupuncture channels. The high skin conductance of the channel system is supported by the finding of a high density of gap junctions at the sites of acupuncture points. Gap junctions are hexogonal protein complexes that form channels between adjacent cells. Gap junctions facilitate intercellular communication and increase electric conductivity. In early stages of embryogenesis, gap junction-mediated cell-to-cell communication is usually diffusely distributed, which results in the entire embryo becoming linked as a syncytium (a group of cells in which the protoplasm of one cell is continuous with that of adjoining cells). As development continues, gap junctions become restricted at discrete boundaries. This is consistent with the observation in the *Classic of Internal Medicine* that many channels and acupuncture points are distributed along the boundaries between different muscles (Shang 2001).[151] Mashansky et al (1983) have proposed that the channel system contains relatively under-differentiated epithelial cells connected by gap junctions which transmit signals and play a central role in mediating acupuncture effects (for more information see chapter 5).

Myofascial and sclerotomal triggers *(biomedicine: referred pain patterns)* often have distributions that are very similar to that of the Sinew channels. Because many of the Chinese words used in relation to the channels can also be translated as vessels, Kendall (2002) puts forth a speculative construction of channel systems being anatomical vascular structures ascertained by dissection.

Channel Distribution

Distributed from Exterior (Wei) to Interior (Zhang), the channels are arranged such that they cover the body in all directions and dimensions. Each channel corresponds to a functional and dysfunctional *level* within the body.

The Channels and Patterns of Discrimination

Use of pattern discriminations by channel systems (for diagnosis) is the oldest type of pattern discrimination in TCM. Responsible for communication between tissues in a closed/

---

149. For example, it is common for patients with de-Quervain's disease to report pain in the forearm and even upper arm. When the tendon is injected (at the wrist), the upper arm pain is reproduced, and, when local anesthesia is induced, the upper arm pain disappears.

150. "Electroenergetic" (or Bioenergetic) medicine is used extensively in Europe. There are many instruments for which claims are generous. These are said to be capable of diagnosing and treating a variety of diseases including allergies and organ diseases. There is however a lack of high quality scientific proof for any of the instruments.
Electromagnetic therapy is approved for bone nonunion and pain in the US. Even a clinical entity called "magnetic field deficiency syndrome" has been proposed (see chapter 5).

151. Protoplasm is the living substance of a cell, usually composed of a myriad molecules of water, minerals, and organic compounds.

Table 1-13: Channel Orientations

CHANNELS	DISTRIBUTION
Main	Longitudinal
Connecting/Vessels	Join the Main Yang channel to its paired Main Yin channel anteroposteriorly (superficial to deep). They also form the vascular tree and therefore connect all areas of the body.
Divergent	Cover the sagittal and axial plains and also have an anteroposterior (superficial deep connections).
Extra	Add a diagonal axis.

opened feedback system, each channel has its own physiologic activity and pathologic manifestations. TCM attribution of many distal symptoms to the Organs can be traced to the existence of the channels (*Biomedicine: visceratome, innervation and circulation*).

All channels, regardless of their location, are more superficial "energetically" than the Organ system. Often Painful Obstruction (*Bi*) syndromes (*Biomedicine: musculoskeletal disorders*) are obstructive channel disorders affecting the "body shell" only. When a patient has musculoskeletal pain without any Organ symptoms, the condition can be considered purely of channel/vessel and/or other bodily milieu origin (however not Organic). Because the channels and Organs are interrelated, and because channel Qi enters into the deeper Organ system at the Sea points,[152] Organic symptoms can be a part of the pattern discriminations of the internal course of the channels. *Spiritual Axis* states: "The twelve channels and vessels inside are ascribed to the Organs, the outside network to the limbs and joints."[153]

Importance in Musculoskeletal Medicine

Channel discrimination is especially important in musculoskeletal medicine and in acupuncture. The channels and network-vessels/collaterals can be invaded by exogenous pathogens, or they can develop dysfunctions due to endogenous disharmonies, both of which can result in symptoms and signs that appear along the course of the channel(s). Exogenous Pathogenic Factors, by and large, penetrate the body from the more superficial channels and travel through the channels and connecting network-vessels systems into deeper "energetic" or anatomical levels.

---

152. Acupuncture point at the level of knee and elbow.

153. Many practitioners tend to implicate TCM Organic malfunction in musculoskeletal disorders, and use Organ type diagnosis of the pulse and tongue to determine the patient pattern diagnosis. Musculoskeletal disorders often affect only the body shell or Exterior and are part of "Exterior-medicine." In Exterior-medicine, skin disorders for example, such diagnostic approaches are often secondary to direct examination of the skin (i.e. the pulse, tongue, and other Organic symptoms are often ignored, or considered less important). It is this author's opinion that the same applies often to musculoskeletal disorders. Tissue texture and feel should often be considered first.

The musculoskeletal system, including several aspects of the joints, is part of the Exterior system and of the external pathways of the Main channels. Other aspects of the musculoskeletal system that relate to structure and biochemistry may relate more to the deeper channel and vessel systems.

Table 1-12 on page 50 describes the physiologic activities of the channels and Table 1-13 their orientation.

The Sinew Channels

The most superficial of the channels, the Sinew (tendinomuscular) channels are the locus for circulation of Defense-Qi. With the muscles the Sinew channels:

- Provide a protective layer of the body.
- Govern movement and sustain the body in its erect posture.
- Connect the "100 bones."
- Serve as the connection between the Main and Divergent channels to the muscles, connective tissues, joints and skin.
- Serve to integrate the connections between the Yang channels and between the Yin channels.
- Closely related to the *twelve Cutaneous regions* which share Sinew channel functions of circulating Qi and Blood to the surface, nourishing the skin and pores, and protecting the body from external Pathogenic Factors. The cutaneous regions are the combinations of the territories of the leg and arm regions; i.e., hand Tai Yin and leg Tai Yin, etc. The close relationship between the skin areas of the twelve cutaneous regions with the channels and Organs is important in many aspects of diagnosis by observation and palpation. An affected region can reflect viscero-cutaneous (Organ/viscero-somatic) reflexes and pathologies. Signs such as pain, discoloration, dryness, or excessive moisture of skin, skin rashes, darkening or stasis of veins or venules, contraction of muscles, etc. are seen.

In *Spiritual Axis* the Sinew channels were mostly associated with muscular *spasm* and *weakness* and treated with Fire needle techniques. Defensive-Qi circulates through the Sinew channels. Patients who have myofascial pain syndromes and fibromyalgia often develop stagnation of Defensive-Qi (especially its Fluid quality). Fluid-stagnation transforms to Phlegm/Blood/Qi stasis that becomes nodular (*Biomedicine: fibrositic nodules*) called myofascial trigger points in biomedicine and Kori in Japanese OM. If only pressure sensitive they may be called "Ashi points." Treatment of local Ashi (painful or trigger) points mobilizes the Sinew channel Qi and disperses stagnation.[154]

---

154. Not classical descriptions.

The Channels (Meridians/Vessels) (Jing-Luo)

Table 1-14: Sinew Channels (Spiritual Axis)

CHANNEL	SYMPTOMS
LEG TAI-YANG BLADDER	Swelling and dragging pain between the little toe and the heel. Spasms at the popliteal crease of the knee. Backward bent spine, arched back rigidity. Spasms or tension in the neck muscles and sinews. Inability to raise the shoulder and cramping pain in the branch from the armpit to the center of the clavicle and inability to swing the arm. Bi syndrome of midspring.
LEG SHAO-YANG GALL BLADDER	Muscle spasms of the fourth toe, lateral side of the knee so that the knee cannot bend or stretch. Spasms or tension at the crease (popliteal area) of the knee and affecting the front of the thigh and back of buttocks (sacrum) (L3-L4). Pain in the depression under the bottom ribs, lateral abdomen, the chest, continuing up to the clavicle, breast, and cramped muscles in the neck. If muscle cramps go from the left to the right, the right eye will be unable to open because, as the channel goes up, it passes through the right corner of the forehead connected to right, and vice versa. Bi syndrome of early spring.
LEG YANG-MING STOMACH	Muscle spasms of the middle toe and leg, jumping/twitching hard/rigid feelings in the foot. Swelling of front part of the thigh, hernia, muscle spasms/tension of the abdomen which involve the clavicular area and cheek. If acute a sudden twisted mouth and eyes which will not shut. If Heat causes relaxed muscles/sinews, the eyes will not open. If the muscles/sinews of the cheek are cold, it causes spasms/tenseness and will induce twisting of cheek and mouth. If there is Heat, it will cause the muscles/sinews to relax deeply. This makes the muscles unable to contract and causes a distortion/deviation. Bi syndrome of late spring.
LEG TAI-YIN SPLEEN	Contracture in the big toe and pain in the medial ankle bone with spasms of muscles/sinews. Pain along the leg bone and medial side of knee and thigh which radiates to the hip. Knotting pain in sexual organs, which can lead up to the navel and both flanks and cause pain in the chest/costals and center of the spine. Bi syndrome of midautumn (or early spring).
LEG SHAO-YIN KIDNEY	Muscle spasms in the bottom of the foot and at the connection channel and/or entire channel and all its bindings. Epilepsy, spasms, and cramps if sinew proper is diseased. If back is affected, patient can not flex. When front is affected, (possibly deep muscles) patient cannot extend. If it is a Yang disease, (outer aspect) the waist opposes bending and one is unable to bow down (flex). There is an arched back. If it is a Yin (inner aspect) disease, the patient cannot extend or look up. Bi syndrome of midautumn (or early autumn).
LEG JUE-YIN LIVER	Spasms in big toe and along the channel up the front of medial ankle bone. Pain felt along medial side of leg and inner thigh. Malfunction or contraction of sexual organs. Bi syndrome of late autumn.
ARM TAI-YANG SMALL INTESTINE	Spasm and pain in the little finger, along the channel to the elbow on the medial side and behind the medial epicondyle. Pain along the Yin side of the upper arm, below the armpit, which runs around the shoulder blade (axila), and which then may include the neck. Ringing in ear with dragging pain in the chin and jaws. Delayed vision after prolonged closing of the eyes, and spasms in the neck muscles, which can cause ulcers and swelling in the neck and chills and heat at the neck. Bi syndrome of midsummer.
ARM SHAO-YANG TRIPLE WARMER	Cramps of the muscles/sinews at the points which pass through this channel, and rolled-up/retracted tongue. Bi syndrome of summer.
ARM YANG-MING LARGE INTESTINE	Pain and cramping/spasms of the muscles/sinews at the points through which this channel passes, and inability to raise the shoulder or to turn the neck either to the left or right. Bi syndrome of early summer.

Table 1-14: Sinew Channels (Spiritual Axis) (Continued)

CHANNEL	SYMPTOMS
ARM TAI-YIN LUNG	Cramping of the muscles/sinews at the points which this channel passes through. Extreme pain in the cardiac orifice with possible panting. Spasms in the ribs (diaphragm) may cause spitting Blood. Bi syndrome of midwinter.
ARM JUE-TIN PERICARDIUM	Cramping of the muscles/sinews on the points along the channel. Pain in sternum (diaphragm), chest, and throbbing of cardiac area. Bi syndrome of early winter.
ARM SHAO-YIN HEART	Pain and muscles cramping on the points along the channel. Spasm of the Heart which rise and fall like wooden beams, urgency in chest (possibly referring to heart attack) causing the elbow to feel as if it is in a net (wrapped). Bi syndrome of late winter.

The Sinew channels support and maintain skeletal integrity by connecting the "100 bones," thereby playing an important role in locomotion, the immune system, and the individual's sense of physical and emotional boundaries.

Although early Chinese writings do not describe the exact anatomical and functional delineations of *single muscles* (only the quadriceps, gastrocnemius [calf], sternocleidomastoid and diaphragm are mentioned by name in the early classical literature), the descriptions (and drawings) of general muscular chains-functions and distribution through the Sinew channels are fairly accurate and reflect both the function and dysfunction of muscle groups (*Biomedicine: pain distributions and functional groups of muscles*). Their distribution is similar to myofascial and sclerotomal referred pain patterns, which suggests that the Sinew channels were partly surmised to follow the distribution of needle sensations when muscles were stimulated. Distribution of the Sinew channels is supported by electromyography studies that have shown that during simple motions the frequency of muscle contraction potentials increases along the complete chain of fascia-muscle-tendon, even in muscles not involved in the motion.

The Sinew channels are made of muscle to joint connections (knots/Jie)[155] that include most of the soft tissues responsible for locomotion, as well as their "energetic" and functional aspects. They should therefore be viewed both as gross pulleys and as the mechanisms which make the pulleys work—i.e., the neurology and biochemistry of the muscular system. Because the Sinew channels are related to the more superficial aspects of locomotion, the entire channel/vessel system takes part in normal musculoskeletal function and shape.

ORIGIN AND POINTS. The Sinew channels originate at the extremities and do not have *specific* acupuncture points; however, their activating points are one fen proximal to the Well points (most distal points)[156] of the related Main channels. The channel then rises toward the Termination/reunion point on the trunk or head. Their broad muscle bends narrow to "knot/*Jie*" at the joints where a concentration of their Qi creates point-like focus. Other important areas are: *Ju,* or areas were two or more Sinew channels converge; *San,* the areas were the Qi disperses in the large muscles as they divide into smaller groups; and *Luo,* the areas were the Sinew channels connect to muscles, tendons, and ligaments. As Sinew channel Qi is said to accumulate around the joints, and joints are not smooth, stagnation of Qi as well as retention of Pathogenic Factors occurs often at the joints; therefore, pain is commonly felt at the joints. Ashi-sensitive/Kori-indurated-trigger points often manifest in the Sinew channel systems.[157] The Jue Yin (Liver) channel is said to be the gathering place of the sinews (as well as the ancestral sinew which is the penis or perineum).

Besides the activating, Ashi, joints, and termination points, there are some other points that are said to be important in Sinew channel function and *evaluation*. At GB-22, the Gall Bladder, Pericardium, Lung, and Heart Sinew channels meet. St-30 is said to be the meeting place of all the Yang and Yin sinews. The Sinew channels meet the Divergent channels at St-12. The Main channels Source/Yuan and Connecting/Luo points are said to affect the Sinew channels as well. Especially important in treatment and assessment of the Sinew channels are:

- Well points (or one fen proximal).
- Ashi-painful, Kori-indurated, or trigger points.
- GB-21, 22, 30, 13.
- St-3, 12, 30.
- SI-16, 18.
- CV-2, 3.

---

155. Same character used to describe the knots of a bamboo.

156. In some Japanese traditions. In French traditions, it is at the Well point. The Well points can be used to assess the Sinew channels by palpation or reaction to heat (Akabane testing).

157. As opposed to other channel points which often are said to be within depressions or "holes."

As the throughway of Defensive-Qi, the least refined and most reflexive Qi, the Sinew channels can amplify and externalize more endogenous and/or deeper dysfunctions. Since muscle tension can serve as a diagnostic-lens into the interior of the body, (visceral disorders often result in muscle tension and pain that can be used in diagnosis), interruption of muscle tension must be performed carefully.[158]

Sinew Channels and the Brain

The Sinews channels and the Main channels follow approximately the same external path. The Sinew channels are wider than the Main channels, and their forces always flow proximately and terminate in the trunk and head region ("brain" in some Daoist traditions).[159] This functional connection between the Sinew channels (*Biomedical: motor units*), trunk (spine) and brain (*Biomedical: upper motor neuron*) provides another example of the sophistication of the channel theory. It is through the Sinew channels that OM describes some aspects of motor activity and movement.

Symptoms and Signs

The Sinew channels provide an approach to the locomotive unit (*Biomedicine: muscles, joints, ligaments, tendons, bursae, and fasciae*). They are important in the treatment of acute conditions such as musculoskeletal sprains, strains, trauma, edema, and skin diseases including psoriasis, that can be associated with joint arthritis. They are often used in the initial stage of external pathogenic invasion. Acupuncture (by and large) functions through tapping the Defensive-Qi and directing it to tissues and deeper channels. The Sinew channels play an important role in this action. In general *Spiritual Axis* states:

> For the diseases of the sinew channels *Cold* [italic author emphasis] will cause violent contraction and spasms of the muscles, *Heat* will cause muscle relaxation, weakness and malfunction of the Yin Organs (Impotence). When *Yang* (superficial and posterior muscles) is in spasm, it will cause a bending backward. When the *Yin* (deep and anterior muscles) is in spasm, it will cause a bending forward and an inability to stretch. The fire needle may be used to needle Cold spasm. Do not use the heated needle when *Heat* causes muscles to relax and to be weak.

Fullness in the Sinew Channels

Acute injuries or invasion of Pathogenic Factors often result in Fullness of the Sinew channel and *relative* Emptiness of the related Main channel. This occurs as a result of release of Defensive-Qi from the Main Channel to the Sinew channel in order to help fight the Pathogenic Factors. Therefore, when the Sinew channel is Full, its corresponding Main channel may be Empty. Symptoms and signs of Fullness in the Sinew channels are related mainly to strong sensitivity to light pressure (hyperesthesia), pain, muscular spasms and contractions, edema, and signs of inflammation. Emptiness may also be seen proximal to the lesion (obstruction) while Fullness is seen distally (where Qi collects); because Sinew channel circulation is in a distal-to-proximal direction. Clinically however, Emptiness/Fullness of muscles may follow the other channel distribution more closely than Sinew channels. For example, with radiculopathy one often finds signs of Fullness above (at spine), on the Bladder and Governing channels, and weakness and atrophy below at the extremity Sinew channel.

Emptiness in the Sinew Channels

Chronic disorders can deplete the Sinew channels and result in movement of Pathogenic Factors to the Main channels, which may result in a relative Fullness of the Main channels. Therefore, when a Sinew channel is Empty, its corresponding Main channel can be Full. Symptoms and signs of Emptiness in the Sinew channels are related principally to dull and often deep ache, pain on deep pressure, lack of skin tone, hypoesthesia, muscular atonia and atrophy, numbness, coldness and pruritus.

Sinew Channel Functions: Yin Yang Pairs, Six Energetic Zones

Sinew, as well as Main channel functions can be classified in Yin Yang pairs and within the Six "Energy Zones" (stages) as well.[160]

The Six Energy Zones are layers of functional/pathological categories that describe the transformation or presentations of pathological influences from the External (Yang/energetic) to the Internal (Yin/substance) divisions/depth. They are:

- Tai (great) Yang.
- Yang (bright) Ming.[161]
- Shao (lesser) Yang.
- Tai-Yin.
- Shao-Yin.
- Jue (terminal) Yin.

The Six divisions were first described in the *Yellow Emperor's Classic of Internal Medicine* and *the Classic of Difficult Issues* and were expanded on in *Theses on Diseases*

---

158. Not a classical association.
159. Some sources describe the Yin leg channels as terminating at CV-3.
160. A Yin channel and its paired Yang channel. The following discussion is more a product of European thinking on acupuncture than TCM. The so called "energy zones" are discussed more in modern European literature.
161. In *Theses on Diseases caused by Cold*, Shao-Yang precedes Yang-Ming (Yang-Ming Organ is the first stage of Internal invasion). However, when considering common clinical presentations, especially in musculoskeletal disorders, Shao-Yang can be considered as the level between the External and the Internal.

caused By Cold, and *Theses on Exogenous Febrile (Warm) Diseases.* The latter book related these Divisions/levels mainly to the presentations and development of infectious diseases within the Four-Divisions. The first three Yang Divisions within the Six-Divisions were spoken of as a door, probably illustrating the entrance of Pathogenic Factors. There is an opening, a leaf (or door) and a pivot (hinge). The functions of the three Yang levels should therefore be thought of as an integrated system, each with its own perpose. In modern European and Japanese literature, the use of Six Divisions has been expanded beyond Exterior Cold and Heat damage and their traditional use.

Tai-Yang Level (Urinary Bladder, Small Intestine)

The most superficial layer of the channels, and anatomically the broadest of channels, the Tai-Yang level (Urinary Bladder and Small Intestine channels) is the first layer of defense against climatic and worldly influences. Said to open and move (gate) to the Exterior (outward), the Tai-Yang channels are strongly related to upright posture and movements that involve extension. Tai-Yang is said to be the first layer affected by external pathogenic Wind-Cold (or Wind-Heat). For disorders of Tai-Yang Wind-Cold, spicy-warm (or cool) herbs are used. Important points are UB-60, SI-5 or UB-67, SI-1, or UB-40 and SI-8 on opposite sides.

Tai-Yang Sinew channel disorders are said to apply mainly when movements away from the body are symptomatic. Tai-Yang disorders can also result in disorders of joint depression, rotation, adduction, and flexion. When the Tai-Yang external channels are affected, symptoms mostly are functional and have little or no affect on structure. Because the Tai-Yang (especially UB) sinew channel relates to the superficial back myofascial line, this channel is strongly related to changes in the primary and secondary curves of the body (from head to toe, convexities being primary curves and concavities secondary, viewed from behind).

Yang-Ming Level (Stomach, Large Intestines)

The Yang-Ming level (Stomach and Large Intestines channels) is the location where the immune system is strongly activated (by infection or injury) and inflammation (fever/heat, struggle between anti-pathogenic and pathologic-Qi) is most strongly induced. By and large this level is affected when Tai-Yang has failed in halting the progress of exterior pathogenic invasion. Yang-Ming is said to be affected when pathogenic Cold or Heat first affects the Organs (Interior) even when only affecting the *"Yangming aspect of the Lungs"* with severe cough and fever, and with or without symptoms of Stomach and Large Intestine-Heat. The Yang-Ming level is said to close on the Exterior, or being the inner door. When soft tissue or joint inflammation is apparent, the Yang-Ming level may be affected and herbs such as Gypsum (Shi Gao) and Anemarrhena (Zhi Mu) are used often. Important points are LI-1, St-44, or St-36, LI-11 on opposite sides.

Yang-Ming Sinew channel disorders are said to relate to pain on grasping and resistance. They are commonly involved in problems of joint elevation and depression and may also result in flexion, extension, and abduction disorders.[162] The Yang-Ming Sinew channel is related to the superficial front myofascial line, and, when tight, it shortens the front of the body and thrusts the head forward, compressing the cervical lordosis.

Shao-Yang Level (Gall Bladder and Triple Warmer)

The Shao-Yang level (the Gall Bladder and Triple Warmer channels) is an intermediate level between the External and the Internal.[163] Relating mostly to *rotational movements* the Shao-Yang is said to be a pivot and to open both inwards and outwards. Shao-Yang disorders are said to result often from weak antipathogenic-Qi and external pathogenic-Qi struggling. Both the pathogenic and Righteous-Qi (antipathogenic-Qi) are weak. Formulas that *harmonize* are often used for Shao-Yang disorders. Important points are GB-44, TW-1, GB-34, TW-10, or GB-40 and TW-4 on opposite sides.

Shao-Yang disorders may also result in symptoms related to sidebending, extension, abduction, and adduction. When affected, symptoms may have both functional and mild structural/cellular/inflammatory components: the immune system (acute/chronic inflammation) is still activated, but symptoms of weakness and possibly muscle atrophy are emerging. Both Cold and Heat are present and may alternate. Patients often complain of temperature disregulation that *started* after a common cold (feel like their internal temperature is not right).[164] The Shao-Yang Sinew channel is related to the superficial lateral myofascial line and strongly related to lateral movements and dysfunctions.

Spiritual Axis states:

> The Tai-Yang makes the gates. The Yang-Ming makes the inner door. The Shao-Yang makes the pivots. Breaking the gate will cause a flow of disease to the flesh and joints and a cruel disease will begin. Because of this cruel disease, one must treat the Tai-Yang and see if there is an excess or deficiency. This will weaken and emaciate the skin and flesh. Breaking the inner door will result in weakness because the Qi

---

162. Inflammation, the normal reaction to injury, should not be inhibited too quickly following an injury, as this may interfere with proper healing and chronicity may develop. For many inflammatory musculoskeletal disorders, especially for those that occur from injuries, only mildly cooling medications (or herbs that have anti-inflammatory effects) should be used with emphasis on vitalizing of Blood (see chapter 6). Modern anti-inflammatory agents may lead to chronicity. The use of plaster casts which are made from Gypsum (Shi Gao), a cold medicine, is said to "freeze" circulation and lead to chronic Cold-type pain. It is common in TCM to only use ice for the first twenty-four hours after injury, to be followed by heat and moxa.

163. The typical alternating hot and cold symptoms of Shao-Yang are considered as having both Tai-Yang and Yang-Ming (External/Internal) symptoms.

164. Often a sign of pathogenic factors and/or Yin and Yang weakness at the same time or by themselves. Again not classical associations.

The Channels (Meridians/Vessels) (Jing-Luo)

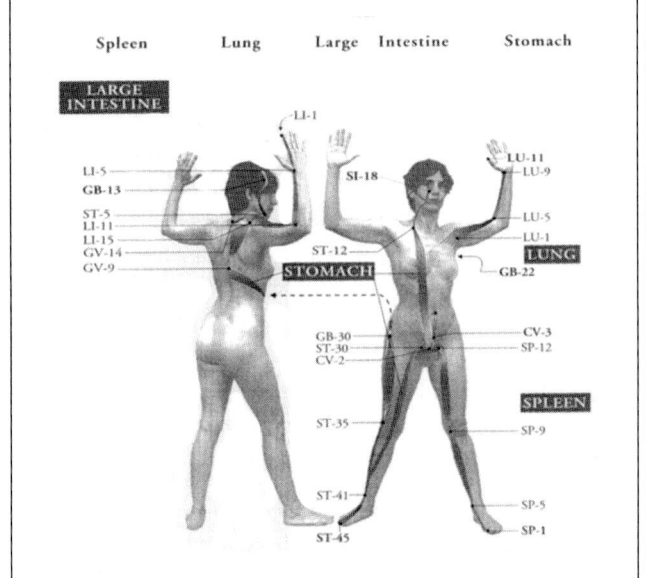
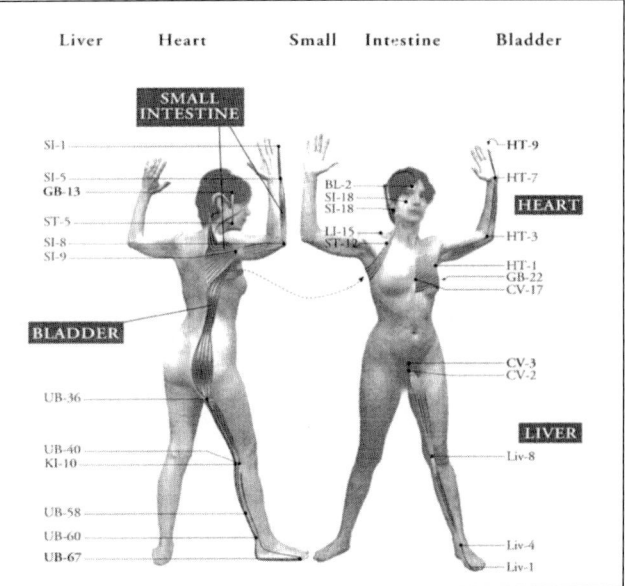
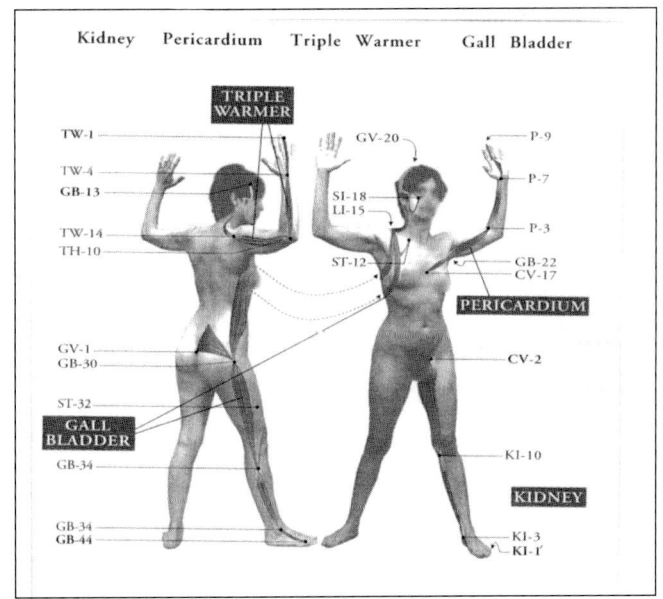

Figure 1-9: Sinew Channels.

is unable to stop and rest. Thus, for weakness, treat the Yang-Ming by seeing if there is an excess or deficiency. Without stop or rest, the Righteous-Qi is delayed and detained while the evil-Qi takes residence. When the pivot is broken, the bones are shaken, and it is not possible to be balanced on the ground. Thus, when the bones are shaken, treat the Shao-Yang by seeing if there is an excess or deficiency. Shaken bones cause the joints to be difficult to bend. Then discuss the bone shaking, the reasons for shaking, and thoroughly examine that point at its roots.

Yin Levels

When pathological influences enter the Interior, they begin to take form, and structural damage can be demonstrated. Soft tissue weakness or spasms are pronounced. Flexion dysfunctions are apparent and often involve the most superficial Tai-Yin channels—the Spleen/pancreas and Lung channels; and may be due to severe Warm-disease damage as seen in disorders such as acute dystonia (the Tai-Yin as well as deeper channels can be affected). Therefore, the Tai-Yin channels are said to be related to movement towards the body (adduction).

Once pathology enters the *Jue* (terminal) Yin channels (Liver and Pericardium), (or Shao-Yin), significant anatomical damage has occurred and paralysis/atrophy (Wei syndrome, Tan Huan) may set in.[165]

Shao-Yin Sinew channels disorders are related mainly to rotational movements with the limbs and are often related to spastic conditions.

Jue-Yin Sinew channels disorders are related to both spastic and wilting/atrophy with paralysis or flaccidity.

If the patient is able to flex but not extend, it is said that the "disease is in the sinews," and, if able to extend but not flex, the "disease is in the bones." The Sinews are related to both Liver and Spleen and the Bones more to Kidneys. In general, in TCM (not in six level diagnosis), Kidney disorders are considered to be at a deeper level than Liver or Spleen. Important points are:

- *Tai-Yin.* Lu-9, Sp-1 (or SP-3), or P-9 and Lu-5 on opposite sides.
- *Shao-Yin.* K-1, H-9 or K-10 and H-3 on opposite sides.
- *Jue-Yin.* Liv-1, P-9 or Liv-3, P-7, or Liv-8 and P-3 on opposite sides.

Disorders of Six Energetic Zones

One example of the affects and use of the "Six Energetic Zones" on muscles can be seen in the patient who has abnormal forward head posture. Along with Defensive-Qi, the Tai-Yang "energetic" level functions to maintain the defenses and psychological boundaries. Poor self-esteem,

---

165. Wei syndromes are conditions that involve wasting of muscular function such as myasthenia gravis.

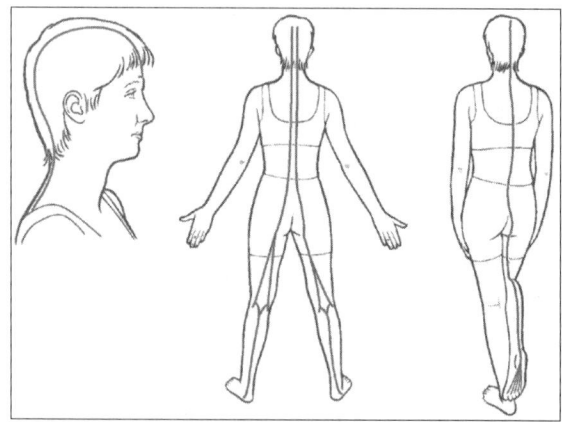

Figure 1-10: Superficial back line (with permission Chaitow 2001).

especially during the teen years, results often in slouched and forward head posture.

This posture stresses the Tai-Yang level and affects the Urinary Bladder and Small Intestines Sinews channels. The increased demand on these muscles to work eccentrically (as a strap) can result in fatigue of the suboccipital muscles, levator scapulae, and upper fibers of the trapezius, all of which can shorten as they work harder to maintain the head upright—due to excessive consumption of Qi and Blood from *maintained* eccentric anti-gravitational work. The upper flexor muscles (Yang-Ming/Tai-Yin) can become inhibited, stretched, and weak, a Yin Yang reaction. If this posture (and psychological state) remains, the upper flexor muscles, the sternocleidomastoid, and scalene muscles (Yang-Ming, Tai-Yin) become rigid and inflamed. Hyperactivity of Yang-Ming and Tai-Yin muscles can result in headaches and can, by a Yin Yang reaction, stretch and facilitate the suboccipital neck extensors and the levator scapulae, which often develops trigger (Kori-indurated or Ashi-sensitive) points at their attachments to the scapula—due to stagnation. Long-term dysfunction results in the involvement of the deeper Yin channels, and structural changes occur. When the deeper Yin channels are affected, it may be difficult to influence the patient's posture.

MYERS FIVE MAJOR FASCIAL CHAINS/MERIDIANS (Myers 1997, Chaitow 2002). Myers described five fascial chains that have many similarities to the Sinew channels:

The superficial back line starts with (UB):

- Plantar fascia, linking the plantar surface of the toes to the calcaneus.
- Gastrocnemius, linking calcaneus to the femoral condyles.
- Hamstrings, linking the femoral condyles to the ischial tuberosities.

The Channels (Meridians/Vessels) (Jing-Luo)

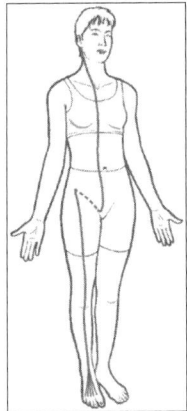

Figure 1-11: Superficial front line (with permission Chaitow 2001).

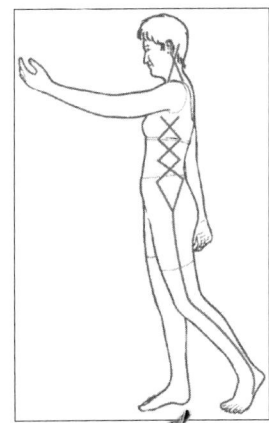

Figure 1-12: Lateral line (with permission Chaitow 2001).

- Sacrotuberous ligament, linking the ischial tuberosities to the sacrum.
- Lumbosacral fascia, erector spinae and nuchal ligament, linking the sacrum to the occiput.
- Scalp fascia, linking the occiput to the brow ridge (Figure 1-10).

The superficial front line starts with (St):
- The anterior compartment and the periosteum of the tibia, linking the dorsal surface of the toes to the tibial tuberosity.
- Rectus femoris, linking the tibial tuberosity to the anterior inferior iliac spine and pubic tubercle.
- Rectus abdominis as well as pectoralis and sternalis fascia, linking the pubic tubercle and the anterior inferior iliac spine with the manubrium.
- Sternocleidomastoid, linking the manubrium with the mastoid process of the temporal bone (Figure 1-11).

The lateral line starts with (GB):
- Peroneal muscles, linking the first and fifth metatarsal bases with the fibular head.
- Ilio tibial tract, tensor fascia latae and gluteus maximus, linking the fibular head with the iliac crest.
- External obliques, internal obliques, and (deeper) quadratus lumborum, linking the iliac crest with the lower ribs.
- External intercostals and internal intercostals, linking the lower ribs with the remaining ribs.
- Splenius cervicis, iliocostalis cervicis, sternocleidomastoid and (deeper) scalenes, linking the ribs with the mastoid process of the temporal bone (Figure 1-12).

The spiral line starts with (possibly the GB, UB, Liv, K, Sp and extra-channels):

- Splenius capitis, which wraps across from one side to the other, linking the occipital ridge (say, on the right) with the spinous processes of the lower cervical and upper thoracic spine on the left.
- Continuing in this direction, the rhomboids (on the left) link via the medial border of the scapula with serratus anterior and the ribs (still on the left) wrapping around the trunk via the external obliques and the abdominal aponeurosis on the left, to connect with the internal obliques on the right and then to a strong anchor point on the anterior superior iliac spine (right side).
- From the ASIS, the tensor fascia latae and the iliotibial tract link to the lateral tibial condyle.
- Tibialis anterior links the lateral tibial condyle with the first metatarsal and cuneiform.
- From this apparent end-point of the chain (first metatarsal and cuneiform), peroneus longus rises to link with the fibular head.
- Biceps femoris connects the fibular head to the ischial tuberosity.
- The sacrotuberous ligament links the ischial tuberosity to the sacrum.
- The sacral fascia and the erector spinae link the sacrum to the occipital ridge (Figure 1-13).

The deep front line describes several alternative chains involving the structures anterior to the spine (internally, for example) (possibly the K, St, H, P, Lu and extra channels):
- The anterior longitudinal ligament, diaphragm, pericardium, mediastinum, parietal pleura, fascia prevertebralis and the scalene fascia, which connect the lumbar spine (bodies and transverse processes) to the cervical transverse processes, and via longus capitis to the basilar portion of the occiput.
- Other links in this chain might involve a connection between the posterior manubrium and the hyoid bone via

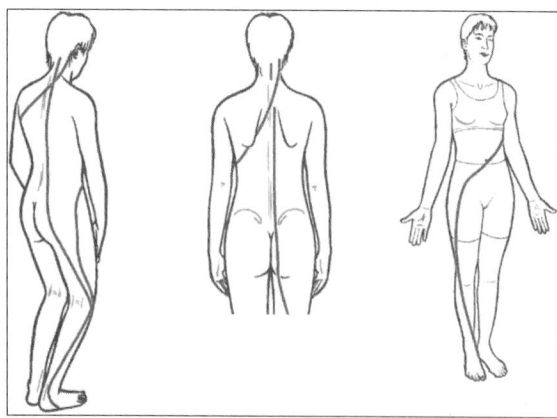

Figure 1-13: Spiral line (with permission Chaitow 2001).

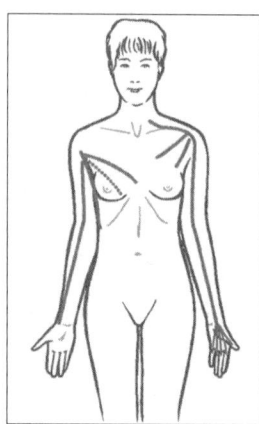

Figure 1-15: Front arm line (with permission Chaitow 2001).

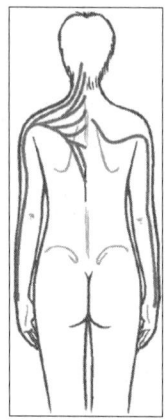

Figure 1-14: Back arm line (with permission Chaitow 2001).

the subhyoid muscles, and the fascia pretrachealis between the hyoid and the cranium/mandible, involving the suprahyoid muscles.
- The muscles of the jaw linking the mandible to the face and cranium.

Additional smaller chains involving the arms are described as follows. Back of the arm lines (possibly the SI, LI, TW and extra channels):
- The Broad sweep of trapezius links the occipital ridge and the cervical spinous processes to the spine of the scapula and the clavicle.
- The deltoid, together with the lateral intermuscular septum, connects the scapula and clavicle with the lateral epicondyle.
- The lateral epicondyle is joined to the hand and fingers by the common extensor tendon.
- Another track on the back of the arm can arise from the rhomboids, which link the thoracic transverse processes to the medial border of the scapula.
- The scapula in turn is linked to the olecranon of the ulna by infraspinatus and the triceps.
- The olecranon of the ulna connects to the small finger via the periosteum of the ulna.
- A stabilization feature in the back of the arm involves latissimus dorsi and the thoracolumbar fascia, which connects the arm with the spinous processes, the contralateral sacral fascia and gluteus maximus, which in turn attaches to the shaft of the femur.
- Vastus lateralis connects the femur shaft to the tibial tuberosity and (via this) to the periosteum of the tibia (Figure 1-14).

Front of the arm lines (possibly H, P, Lu and extra channels):
- Latissimus dorsi, teres major and pectoralis major attach to the humerus close to the medial intramuscular septum, connecting it to the back of the trunk.
- The medial intramuscular septum connects the humerus to the medial epicondyle which connects with the palmar hand and fingers by means of the common flexor tendon.
- An additional line on the front of the arm involves pectoralis minor, the costocoracoid ligament, the brachial neurovascular bundle and the fascia clavipectoralis, which attach to the coracoid process.
- The coracoid process also provides the attachment for biceps brachii (or brachialis) linking this to the radius and the thumb via the flexor compartment of the forearm.
- A stabilization line on the front of the arm involves pectoralis major attaching to the ribs, as do the external obliques, which then run to the pubic tubercle, where a connection is made to the contralateral adductor longus, gracilis, pes anserinus, and the tibial periosteum (Figure 1-15).

The Channels (Meridians/Vessels) (Jing-Luo)

Connecting Channels/Vessels and Collateral Branches (Luo Mai)

The Connecting channels and collaterals branches (Luo Mai, also called "network-vessels") (Figure 1-16), which run deeper than the Sinew channels, provide a defense system secondary to that of the Sinew channels. The word "Luo" has a sense of network, and, according to *Spiritual Axis*, the Connecting channels (and collateral branches or network-vessels) float to the surface of the body where they are visible; therefore, they are said to relate to vascular system. In the same text, the Connecting channels divide into smaller channels—*Minute* (Sun Mai, probably the arterioles, capillaries, and venules), *Superficial and collateral* (Luo Mai, probably the secondary branches of the main arteries and veins) *and main vessels* (Jing Mai, probably the main arteries and veins)—that branch throughout the entire body. They are said to constitute the Interior, but also fill the spaces between the muscles and skin (Cou Li). Branches that run transversely are the collaterals, and those that branch from the collateral are the minute. *Spiritual Axis* states: "The main channels/vessels make the foundation. The branches are horizontal and make the Luo channels. These channels divide and make the minute channels, which, when abundant with Blood, quickly train them." Thus the Connecting channels (network vessels) cover the entire body; the Interior, Exterior, Yin, Yang, Organs, Sinews, and skin. This makes the Connecting channels vulnerable to insult from both the Exterior and Interior, and most stagnation within the body is found in the Connecting channels. Therefore, many acute and chronic diseases may be treated by bleeding techniques, which act upon the Connecting channels/network-vessels.

The circulatory system is therefore described as a network of vessels that are ruled by the Heart. The condition of the Organs may be assessed by looking at superficial vessels. The *Spiritual Axis* states:

> When there is cold in the midst of the Stomach, the collaterals in the thenar-eminence are mostly a blue-green color. When there is heat in the midst of the Stomach the collaterals at the border of the thenar-eminence are mostly a dark red color.[166]

There are Connecting channels that link the twelve Main, Governing, and Conception channels with each other and with the surrounding tissues. In addition to these fourteen Connecting channels, a Great Connecting channel of the Spleen/pancreas links all of the Connecting channels. "Whole" body pain is said often to involve the Great Connecting channel of the Spleen/pancreas. Sp-21 is used to activate this channel and is found near the latissimus dorsi, a muscle (Vleeming, Stoeckart, Volkers 1990) that has direct fibrous connections from the upper arm to the opposite foot.[167]

Each Connecting channel separates from the Main channel at the connecting (Luo) point and connects with its paired channel at the source point. These channels, along with blood vessels, strengthen the Yin-Yang relationship between associated pairs of Main channels, and they connect the Main channel to its associated Organ and the skin (Sinew channels) and Organ. Connecting channels reinforce physiologically the ventral and dorsal somatic relationship of the Yin and Yang aspects. Surplus Qi can be stored in the Connecting channels and released to the Main channel when needed.

The Connecting channels/network-vessels relate mainly to movement of Nutritive-Qi and related Blood; however, the Connecting channels/network-vessels can also be affected by exogenous Pathogenic Factors before they penetrate to the deeper Main channels. According to the *Spiritual Axis*:

> The Connecting channels are unable to flow through the great joints. They must move by various routes to tissues and enter. Then they collect together on the skin, where their meeting points can be seen on the surface. Therefore, when needling the connecting channels, one must needle the places where they collect together on the surface, where there may be an accumulation of Blood. Even if there is no [local] concentration [of pathogens], one must needle quickly to disperse the pathogen and let out its Blood. If allowed to remain, it will cause a painful obstruction [*Bi* syndrome].

Symptoms of the Connecting channels are related to those of the Main channel and vascular systems. The condition of the Connecting channels/network-vessels can be assessed by looking at superficial vasculature and possibly the lymph system. The Connecting channels/network-vessels are affected often by strains, sprains, and contusions. They are used mainly in disorders of circulation, especially involving blood vessels, and for visible swelling. *Spiritual Axis states*: "The Nutritive-Qi follows the channels/vessels (travels with Blood). The Defensive-Qi, when rebellious and in conterflow (possibly inflammatory response), results in swelling of the vessles...causes skin swelling"

Pain of both the Yin and Yang aspect of a limb or joint, may be due to pathology in the Connecting channels and network-vessels. When the Connecting channels are involved, pain usually is local (stasis pain), although it may begin to expand as pathogenic influences move through the blood vessels and enter the Main channels. Chronic diseases are said to "enter the Connecting channels/vessels." The Connecting channels may be used to disperse external pathogens and may prevent the formation of painful obstruction (*Bi* syndrome).

---

166. A spotty red dotted palm is also called a "Liver-hand" and may be related to Liver disorders.

167. Texts position this point at the midaxillary line at the 7th or 6th intercostal space. The *Spiritual Axis* positions this point at 3 cun below the axillia.

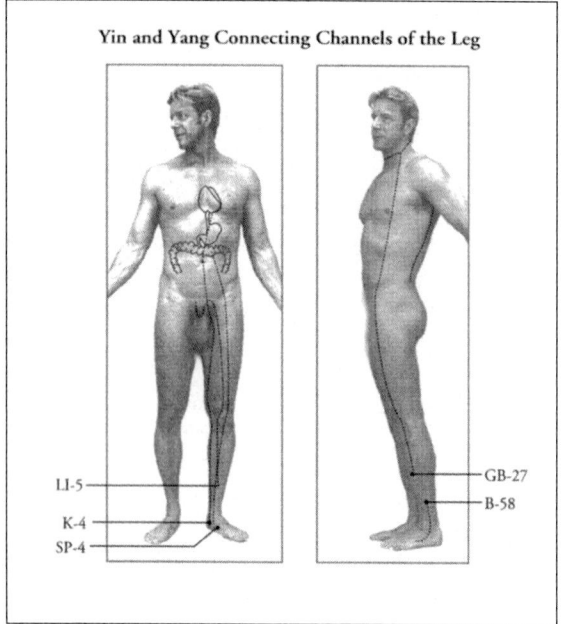
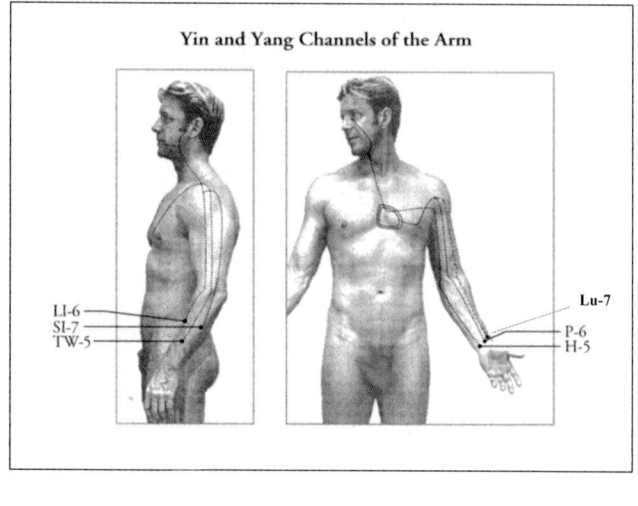
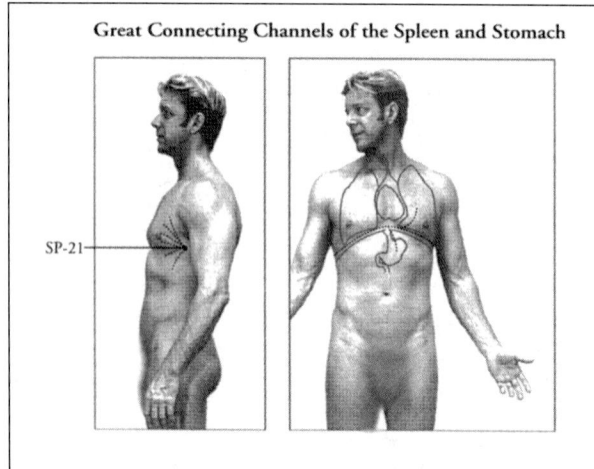
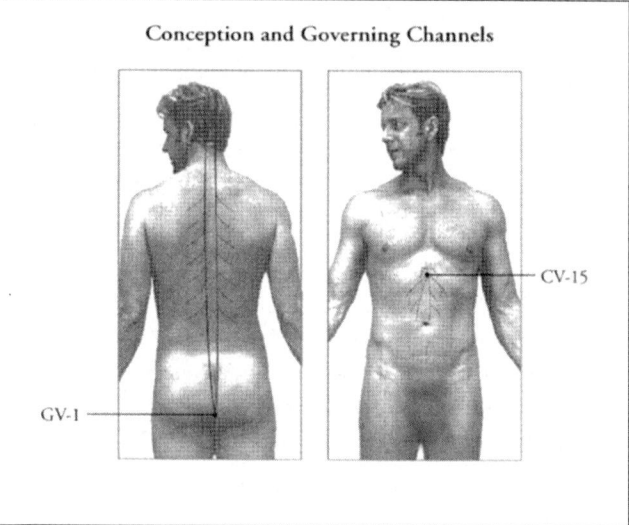

Figure 1-16: Connecting channels.

Table 1-15: The Main Channels

Main Channel/Associated Organ	Principal Symptoms and Signs
HAND TAI YIN Lung	**External.** Pain at the arm, supraclavicular fossa, shoulder, neck and upper back along the channel, usually associated with fever and/or chills; shoulder, elbow, wrist flexion disorders
	Internal. Organic symptoms such as cough, dyspnea, sore throat
HAND YANG MING Large Intestine	**External.** Swelling of the neck; locomotor dysfunction or pain of the fingers, wrist extensors, shoulder or upper arm elevators, SCM muscle; fever; dry mouth; sore throat; toothache; *dominates disorders of body (Jin and Ye) Fluids*[a]
	Internal. Lower abdominal pain; stool disorders
FOOT YANG MING Stomach	**External.** Swelling of the lower limbs and/or neck; pain along its path; SCM muscle, knee extensors, foot dorsiflexion and trunk stabilizer disorders; dry mouth; sore throat; fever; *dominates the disorders of Blood*
	Internal. Abdominal distention and pain; fever; thirst; loose stools; mania
FOOT TAI YIN Spleen/pancreas	**External.** Fatigue, weakness, atonia and flexion disorders of muscles of the limbs; lower limb adduction disorders; pain in the posterior mandibular area and lower cheek; cold along the inside of the thigh and knee; swelling of the leg and feet
	Internal. Diarrhea; reduced food intake; abdominal pain
HAND SHAO YIN Heart	**External.** Pain in the scapular region and/or medial aspect of the forearm; shoulder flexion disorders; coldness of extremities; general feverishness
	Internal. Chest pain; essence-spirit disorders
HAND TAI YANG Small Intestine	**External.** Stiffness of the neck; pain along the lateral aspect of the shoulder and upper arm; levator scapula disorders, numbness of tongue; pain in the cheek; *dominates disorders of body (Ye) Fluids*
	Internal. Pain in the lower abdomen radiating to the lower back or genitals; dry stools
FOOT TAI YANG Bladder	**External.** Stiff neck; headache; pain along channel, or intrinsic spine muscle disorders, of the cervical, thoracic, or lumbar spine; pain in the posterior aspect of the thigh, leg, and foot; eye disease; alternating chills and fevers; *dominates disorders of tendons and ligaments (sinews)*
	Internal. Various urinary disorders and mental disorders
FOOT SHAO YIN Kidney	**External.** Back pain; quadratus lumborum dysfunction; pain in the lateral gluteal region and in the posterior aspect of the thigh; pain in the soles of the feet; weakness of the legs and knees; dryness of the mouth
	Internal. Shortness of breath; urinary disorders; impotence; vertigo; blurred vision
FOOT JUE YIN Pericardium	**External.** Stiffness of the neck; spasm of the limbs; subaxillary swelling; hypertonicity of the elbow and arm
	Internal. Delirious speech; palpitations; restlessness; mental disorders
HAND SHAO YANG Triple Burner	**External.** Pain behind the ears, cheeks and jaw, or at the posterior aspect of the shoulder and the upper arm; disorders of shoulder and elbow extensors, suboccipital and intrinsic cervical muscles; rotation disorders and atonia; *dominates the disorders of Qi*
	Internal. May include abdominal distention and water metabolism disorders
FOOT SHAO YANG Gall Bladder	**External.** Pain under the chin, in the lateral aspect of the buttocks, thigh, knee, and leg; rotation disorders; fever alternating with chills; *dominates disorders of bone*
	Internal. Vomiting; bitter taste in the mouth; chest pain
FOOT JUE YIN Liver	**External.** Spasms of the limbs; upper motor (spastic) paralysis; headache; vertigo; tinnitus
	Internal. *(May include)* lower abdominal pain, oppressive feeling in chest

a. The Yin channels are said to dominate disorders of their own Organ.

The Twelve Main Channels

The Twelve Main channels which perform the most significant of the channel functions lie both in the deepest and the outer external layers of the body.[168] All other channels reinforce the Main channels, which connect the Organs to the rest of the system.

168. However, the Divergent and Extra channels often are more important for treating chronic and deep disorders.

Each Main channel reflects three aspects in its name:

1. External course (important in musculoskeletal medicine).
2. Location on the body, with Yin or Yang somatic aspects.
3. Associated Organ and internal course.

Each Main channel is associated with an Organ and has both internal and external pathways. The external aspects of the Main channels relate to the somatic components they influence. The internal aspects relate to the viscera. The accessory channels (Divergent, Connecting, and Extra) supplement and share points with the Main channels.

Of the Main channels, six are Yin and six are Yang, three each on the upper and lower extremities. Each Yin channel has a paired Yang counterpart, and vice versa. The balance of the Main channels determines health. Table 1-15 describe the principal symptoms and signs that indicate dysfunction of the Main channels (Figure 1-17).

The Channels (Meridians/Vessels) (Jing-Luo)

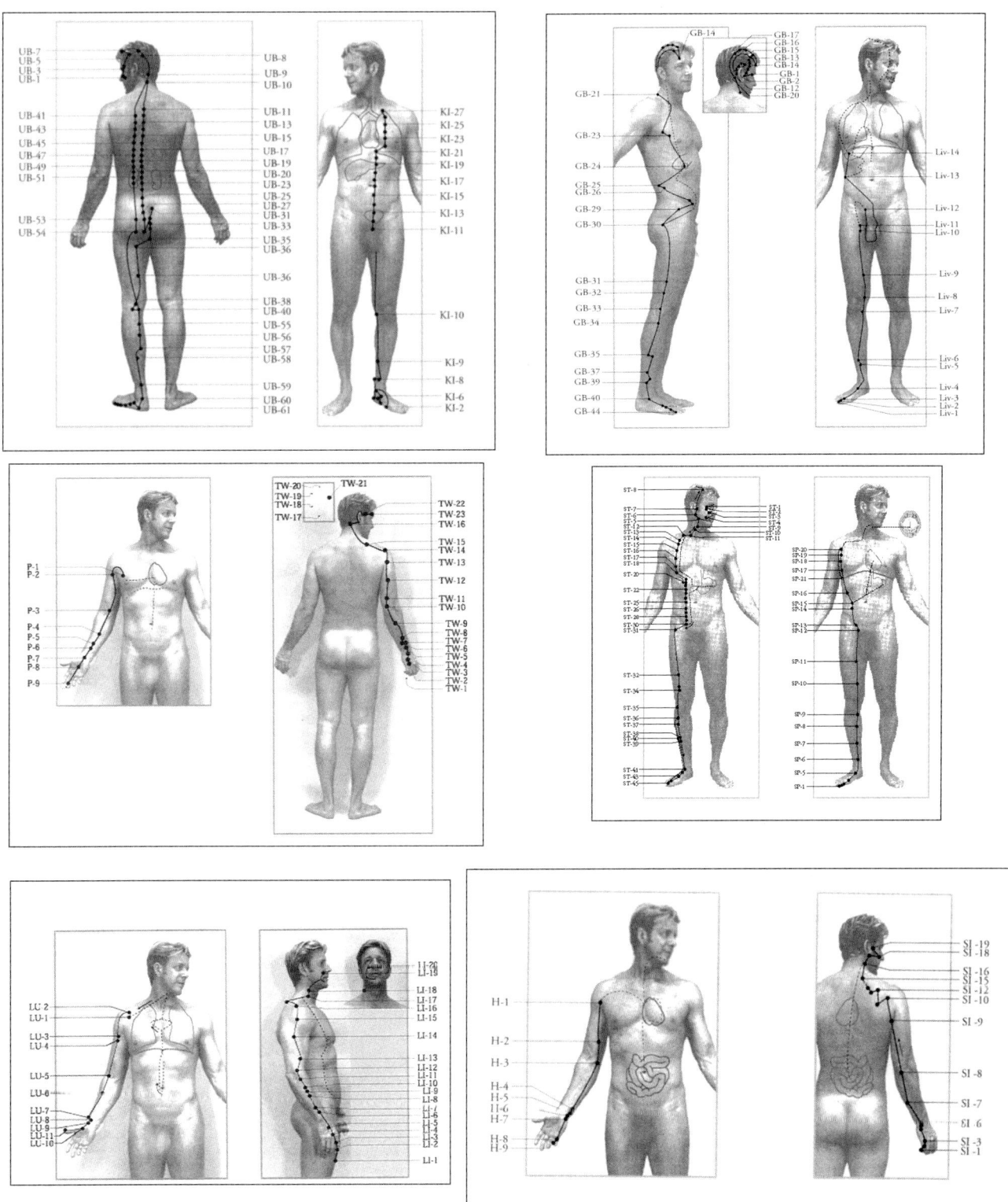

Figure 1-17: The Main channels.

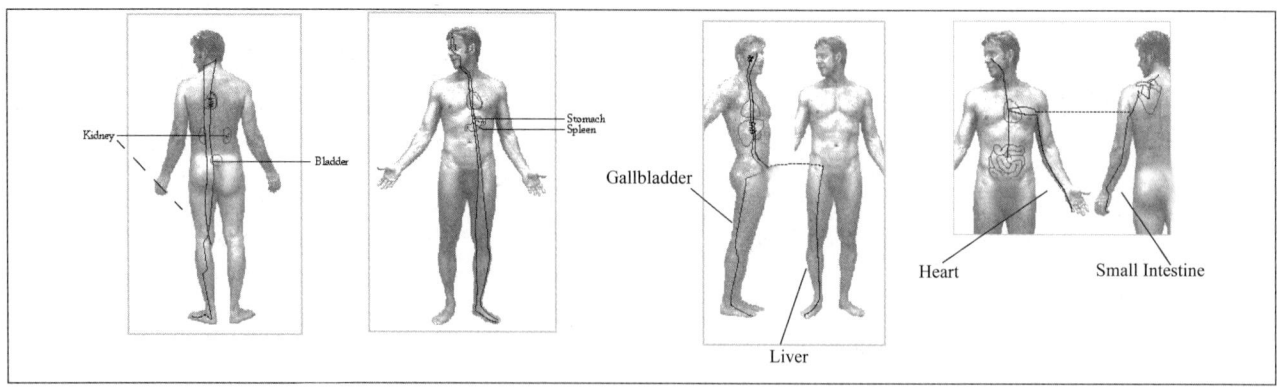
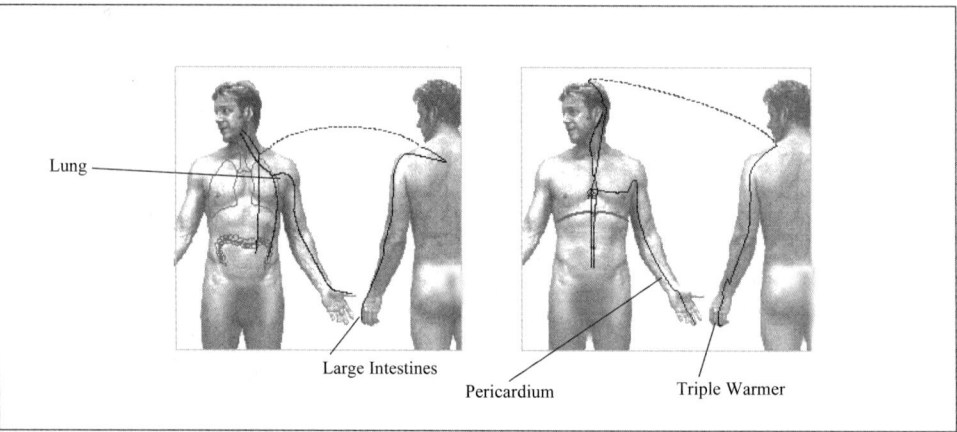

Figure 1-18: The Divergent channels.

Divergent Channels

Although not entirely clear, the Divergent channels are said to begin shallowly and then to flow deeply into the body. They diverge from the Main channels at origin points near articulations (hands, shoulders, pelvis, hips and knees) and are branches of the Main channels. They all connect or communicate with the Heart.[169] The Divergent channels reinforce the Main channels and may function as the functional/structural connection between the Yin-Yang channels and the Organs. According to Shima and Chace (2001), the Divergent channels lie at a level just between the Main channels and the Organs. Therefore, they may be considered as having a deeper function than that of the Main channels. One possible function is to internalize or materialize functional (Yang), autonomic instinctual experiences from Defensive-Qi (which is one type of their Qi) into Original and True-Qi (transform into Yin substance).[170] Except for the Triple Warmer Divergent channel, they are all said to run from the extremities to the trunk, face, and head. However, their type of Qi and direction of circulation is open to debate.

Yang Divergent Channels

From their points of divergence on the limbs, the Yang Divergent channels enter the Organs that are in the abdominal and chest cavities.[171] Moving through these cavities they enter the other Organs and then resurface at the neck, where they rejoin the Main channels at the return points. Because of their relation to Defensive-Qi (which is said to flow outside the vessels), of their origin at large articulations and resurfacing at the neck, and of their communication with the Heart (circulatory system), the Divergent channels may be associated with the lymphatic system.

Yin Divergent Channels

The Yin Divergent channels converge with the Yang Divergent channels (with which they are associated in a Yin-Yang relationship) and then join the Main Yang channel. A Yin

---

169. Although the Lung and Triple Warmer do not pass directly through the Heart.

170. Where postnatal-Qi influences and is integrated with prenatal-Qi (or Ancestral-Qi and Original-Qi i.e., True-Qi).

171. As Shima and Chase point out, however, these are open to debate and may originate at the Well/Jing points, as the Divergent channels also contain Defensive-Qi.

Divergent channel does not return to its own Yin Main channel (Figure 1-17).

Use of Divergent Channels

The Divergent channels are important for treating:
- Interior-Exterior coupled disorders.
- Pathologic (beyond functional) disease processes and deep Organ disorders.
- Deep or lurking Heat or other Pathogenic Factors.
- Chronic disorders including joints, muscles, and sinews.
- Left (Yang) right (Yin) imbalance.
- Disorders of Defensive-Qi.
- Disorders of the throat, face, sense organs, and head.
- Lymphatic, hormonal, and autonomic disorders, often via the Pericardium and Triple Warmer.
- Patients that suffer from extreme fatigue and intermittent symptoms, often via the Pericardium, Triple Warmer, Kidney, and Bladder.
- Disorders of their Main associated channels.

The Divergent channels are important in treatment of fibromyalgia and chronic fatigue syndrome. Defensive-Qi circulates outside the channels during the day and via the Divergent channels to the Organs at night, allowing Defensive-Qi and Blood to regenerate. Any sleep disturbance (common in pain patients and with fibromyalgia) interrupts this process and may result in Organic dysfunction and chronicity. Disruption of Defensive-Qi day/night circulation is said to result in intermittence of symptoms (also common in fibromyalgia patients). When treating fibromyalgia patient the Divergent channels are used with the Sinew channels.

According to Dr. Shima, the Divergent channels are used often with the Extra channels as follows:
- Kidney/Bladder with Chong/Ren and Du/ Yang Qiao.
- Liver/Gall Bladder with Dai/Yang Wei and Du/Yang Qiao.
- Spleen/Stomach with Ren/Chong.
- Heart/Small Intestine with Du and possibly Ren.
- Pericardium/Triple Warmer with Yin /Yang Wei.
- Lung/Large Intestine with Ren /Chong.

Eight Extra Channels (Curious Channels, Extra Vessels)

The eight Extra channels (Figure 1-19), (also called the Eight Curious channels or Eight Extra vessels), which also lie deep, are an important part of the channel system. The classic *Difficult Issues* says the eight Extra channels are separated from the circulation of the Main channels, even though the majority of these channels branch from the Main channels and share the Main channel function of circulating Qi (especially Original/Yuan-Qi) as well as share points with them. The Extra channels are said to have embryological origin, and the Governing and Conception channels are the first to divide and separate the left and right sides of the body (both of which have their own points). The eight Extra channels also store extra Qi and Blood (collecting overflowing or flooding), releasing them when the Main channels are Empty, and they provide additional connections among the twelve Main channels. *Difficult Issues* states: "The Yang-Wei and Yin-Wei channels tie the vessels together to handle overflow of Qi and Blood." Their association with Original-Qi and their ability to release Qi and Blood, explains their use in constitutional illnesses and general weakness. If the Liver and Kidneys are damaged, the Extra channels loose their nourishment, and thus it is said, "the Extra channels originate at the Liver and Kidneys." This is also why these channels are said to be particularly important when treating brain, marrow, bone, and mental diseases.

The Extra channels also absorb excess Pathogenic Factors that were not expelled by the Sinew, Connecting, and Main channels, a circumstance that may explain the use of TW-5 in disorders of external origin. Since the eight Extra channels are said to have little circulation, Pathogenic Factors can accumulate in them, and therefore conditions that involve swelling and Heat (especially chronic) are associated with the Extra channels. Tenderness will be found in *large regions* and scattered throughout the *territories of several* of Main channels. With time, disorders of the bones including hypertrophy (possibly spurs), are said to develop. Therefore, the Extra channels are used in *complex syndromes* (involving many systems and pathologies, and in wide spread pain and/or symptoms (as they integrate several channels and Organs).

Late in OM history, several Master points were created and the use of the Extra channels was expanded.[172] Use of these channels has been expanded greatly in modern times, especially in Japan.

A vascular *interpretation* by Kendall (*ibid*) speculates that the Chong is the aorta, carotid, posterior tibial artery, and veins of the kidney, spleen, and liver; the Ren is the vena cava, medial branches of the superior and inferior epigastric veins, internal and external jugular veins, and vertebral, retromandibular, middle occipital, and temporal veins; the Du is the azygos and hemiazygos, and the ascending lumbar veins; the Dai is the subcostal and ascending lumbar veins.

Extra Channel Use

The Extra channels are said to be especially effective for treating chronic, deep seated, or constitutional conditions. They are also used for treating other conditions that involve several channels (wide spread pain), and that involve left right or diagonal imbalance. They are particularly important in treating psychological disorders.

---

172. Said to control and activate the Extra channels.

Each Extra channel is associated with specific pathological signs. Of particular importance for *musculoskeletal* disorders are:

- The Governing (Du) channel is used often in disorders of the head, neck, and back, especially midline pain. Mental and cognitive symptoms, psychosomatic pains, and disorders of locomotion and articulation (mostly in men) are treated by combining the Governing (Du) and Yang Motility (Qiao) channels. The channel is used for foot disorders and pain, especially when associated with a *collapsed arch* or *heel pain*. A sense as though one cannot hold-up the head is often associated with the Governing (Du) channel. With the Girdle (Dai) channel, the Governing (Du) channel is also used for many neurological disorders, especially when manifested with weakness (neuritis with palsy, multiple sclerosis, etc.).

- Conception (Ren) channel is used in patients with poor abdominal muscle tone and tight lumbar muscles as well as pains that have an allergic component with periumbilical sensitivity.

- Girdle (Dai) and Yang Linking (Wei) channels support and keep the muscles and Sinews strong and tight. The Girdle (Dai) channel influences the low back and pelvis while the Yang Linking (Wei) has more generalized effects. Both of these channels are associated with pain elicited by rotation. In musculoskeletal disorders they are used to treat *weakness* and *instability*.

  The Girdle (Dai) channel is particularly used for lumbar/hip pains and low back pains that radiate to the abdomen/pelvis, genitals, and/or medial thigh (in the author's experience, disorders of T12 to L3 levels, often with psoas tension, and innominate dysfunctions). The Girdle (Dai) channel can be affected by life stresses and used as an adaptogenic or stress fighter. Disorders accompanied by motor deficit (paralysis) are treated often via this channel.

- The Yang Linking (Wei) channel is used in patients with arthritic pains that worsen on rainy days (Wind-Damp-Bi); headaches that radiate from the base of the neck to the eye, unilateral symptoms, lateral neck and shoulder pains, upper extremity pains and swelling.

- Yin Linking (Wei) channel is used to treat patients with poor coordination between the upper and lower body, especially with weakness of an upper extremity and contralateral lower extremity. The channel can be used in patients with back pain due to desiccated discs and circulatory problems, especially when seen with abdominal wall (fascial) symptoms ("oily membranes" symptoms). It is used also in patients with restlessness, general weakness, and shortness of breath on light exertion. This channel is said to closely relate to the parasympathetic nervous system, is thus used to treat Heart and digestive disorders and is often used in patients with musculoskeletal disorders.

- Yin and Yang (Qiao) Motility channels are associated often with imbalances between the medial and lateral sides of the legs and postero-lateral and antero-medial areas with difficulties in walking or standing (Yin and Yang aspects of body). Symptoms that are worse in the day or night are associated as well. Fullness in the Yin Motility (Qiao) is associated with limpness of the (Yang) postero-lateral aspects of the leg and back and with symptoms increasing during the *day*. Fullness in the Yang Motility (Qiao) is associated with limpness of the (Yin) antro-medial aspects of the leg and back and with symptoms increasing during the *night*. These two channels are often used to treat muscular hypertonicity (spasms), sedating the Yang (Qiao) Motility if Yang sinew channel(s) is hypertonic and tonifying the Yin (Qiao) Motility channel. For hypertonic Yin Sinew channel(s) the Yin (Qiao) Motility channel is sedated while the Yang (Qiao) Motility channel is tonified.

  Yang Motility (Qiao) is associated also with acute Wind, headaches, and muscular problems of a Yang nature (spasms).

  Patients with low back pain, a tight iliotibial tract, and weak abdominal muscles, may be treated via the Yang Motility (Qiao). This channel is said to release ACTH and may be used in most inflammatory disorders. In patients with occipital pain, the channel is combined with Governing (Du) points.

  The Yin Motility (Qiao) channel is related to tightness of the back muscles and weakness of the abdominal muscles as well. Here the quality of movement is affected and the muscles are stiff but not spastic. This channel is associated with unilateral headaches near the eye. Patients with weak thyroid, often associated with myofascial pain syndromes, may be treated via the Yin Motility (Qiao) channel.

- The Penetrating (Chong) channel, which controls the Blood and its ability to penetrate tissues, is associated with an inability to express a source for symptoms (vague symptoms), often due to internal-Wind arising from deficient-Blood and poor vascular supply (and possibly symptoms arising from connective tissues). Confusing, conflicting, and various combined pathogenetic processes, such as Heat above and Cold below and combined Deficiency and Excess, are often treated using the Penetrating (Chong) channel. The channel is used for moving-pains, autonomic and inflammatory joint disorders, and in patients over forty years of age. This channel is said to activate a deep Kidney pathway.

Table 1-17 through Table 1-23 on page 79 summarize the Extra channels/vessels, the principal symptoms and signs associated with them, and their Master (Meeting/Confluence), Activating, and Departure points. The tables integrate various ideas and sources, both modern and classic, with personal experience. Table 1-24 on page 80 summarizes the different approaches in pulse diagnosis as it pertains to the Extra channels.

The Channels (Meridians/Vessels) (Jing-Luo)

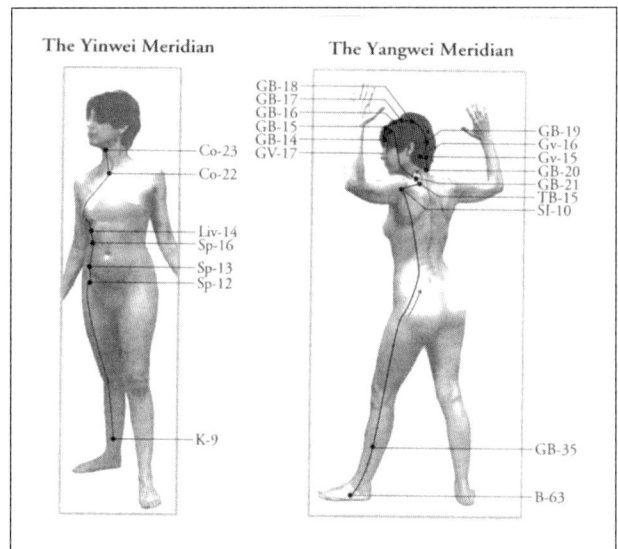
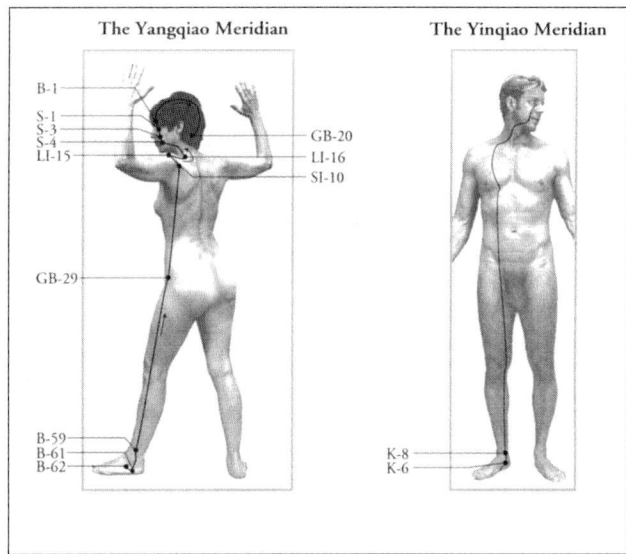
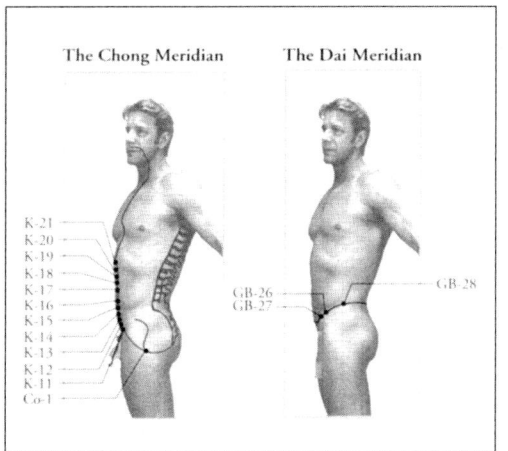
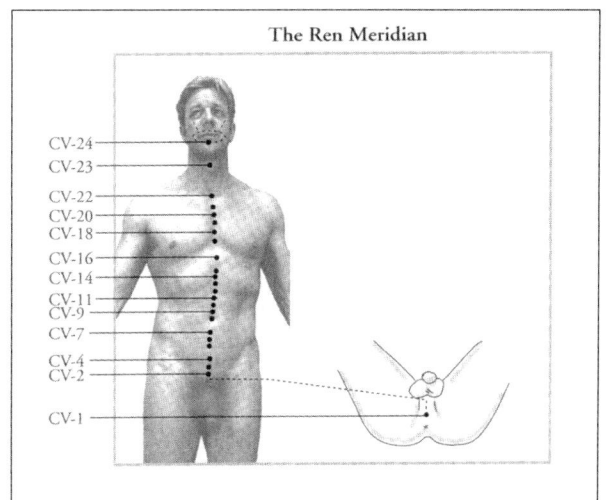
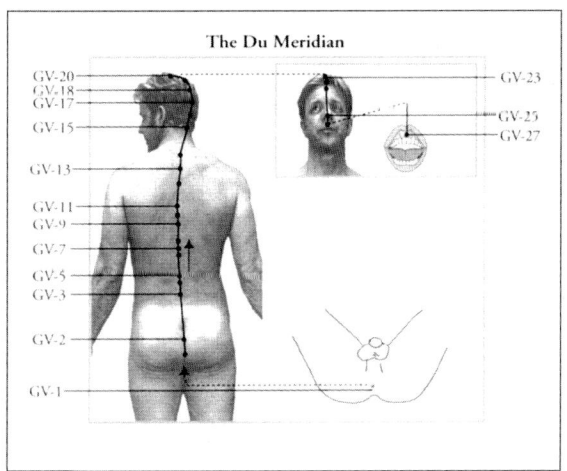

Figure 1-19: The Extra channels/vessels.

Table 1-16: Governing (Du) Channel

FUNCTION	Controls/governs Yang channel functions; absorbs Yang surplus (both healthy and pathologic), provides heat to Organs and channels. Home to Brain and Kidney (marrow). Affects mental and reproductive functions, spine, nerves, cerebrospinal fluid, and brain. Influences musculoskeletal and sensory activity; expels pathogens.
GENERAL SYMPTOMS	Lowered immunity, weakness of many Yang functions. Symptoms and/or pain of upper body. Spinal pain (especially midline), neck pain, and stiffness. Or abnormal curvature of spine. Heavy sensation in head. Vertigo. Urinary retention. Hemorrhoids. Mental/neurological disorders. Anterior-posterior Qi disharmony. Unregulated nervous system.
DEFICIENCY/EMPTINESS SYMPTOMS	Lack of strength. Stiffness of spine. Heavy head. Sterility. Impotence Hemorrhoids. Phlegm epilepsy. Weak character.
PHYSICAL FINDINGS	Pulse floating and uninterrupted in all three positions (proximal [*cubit*], middle [*bar*] and distal [*inch*]), wiry and long. Or floating excess wiry or tight. Or floating straight up and down. Or proximal (*cubit*) and distal (*inch*) both excess and strong in the superficial level. Or wiry, taut in Qi (superficial depth) level. Tenderness along medial-back/spine, neck, top of head, GV-20, and SI channel, especially SI-3.
MASTER/MEETING POINT	SI-3 (+) (or red ion) often unilaterally.
COUPLED POINT	UB-62 (-) (or black ion) often unilaterally.
ACTIVATING POINT	GV-1.

Table 1-17: Conception (Ren) Channel

FUNCTION	Called the Sea of Yin; circulates Yin-Qi, Blood, Essence, and Fluids to nourish and lubricate all Organs and channels. Controls lower abdomen and anterior chest and abdomen; regulates function of the internal Organs. Regulates menstruation. Nurtures the fetus. Nourishes the uterus, regulates reproduction. Controls body Fluids, especially in the abdomen.
GENERAL SYMPTOMS	Urogenital disorders. Lower abdominal symptoms; hernias. Pains in the genitalia or the umbilicus with radiation to the chest and tense abdomen. Reproductive disorders. Anterior/posterior Qi disharmony. Phlegm anywhere in the body.[a] Cough. Bronchitis. Asthma. Emphysema.
EXCESS/FULLNESS SYMPTOMS	Menstrual problems. Vaginal discharge. Male genitourinary disorders. Head and neck pain. Mouth sores. Hernia. Abdominal distention.
DEFICIENCY/EMPTINESS SYMPTOMS	Miscarriage. Uterine hemorrhaging. Sterility. Enuresis. Menstrual problems. Skin disorders.
PHYSICAL FINDINGS	Pulse tight at the distal (*inch*) position; thin, full, and long from distal (*inch*) to middle (*bar*) positions. Or all positions mildly deep, flat, deficient, and choppy. Or tight. Or tight, thready, full, from distal (*inch*) to proximal (*cubit*). Or wiry, taut at the Blood level (middle depth) and diminished at Qi (superficial depth) level. Abdominal tenderness and tightness along channel, mid-abdomen feels like a "chop stick." Tenderness along Lu channel, especially Lu-1, 2 and Lu-7.
MASTER/MEETING POINT	Lu-7 (+) (or red ion) usually bilateral.
COUPLED POINT	Ki-6 (−) (or black ion) usually bilateral.
ACTIVATING POINT	Ki-1.

a. Lu-7 is the commend point which may explain this function.

Table 1-18: Penetrating (Chong) Channel

FUNCTION	The Central reservoir (Sea) of Blood and Essence; treats all disorders of Blood. Called the Sea of the Twelve channels and therefore has been related to connective tissues and li (lining); regulate, and opens the 12 channels (important in treating all stasis and blockages, especially of Blood). Source of Qi for channels. Governs sexual characteristics. Regulates menstruation. Connects prenatal and postnatal Qi. Governs reproduction. Affects gastrointestinal system and Heart/heart.
GENERAL SYMPTOMS	Urogenital disorders. Sexual symptoms, both sexes. External/Internal Qi disharmony. Rebellious-Qi (rushing upwards) leading to a wide range of symptoms affecting the whole torso, including nervousness and "butterflies in the stomach." Complex syndromes and multiple pathologies. Inability to express a source for symptoms (vague symptoms), possibly arising from connective-tissues. Abdominal pain and distension, chest fullness and oppression, palpitations, mental symptoms, panic disorders with the feeling of suffocation and rushing upward feeling (so called "running piglet syndrome," cold below hot above).
EXCESS/FULLNESS SYMPTOMS	Sensation as though body is increasing in size (or is large and puffy), constant thinking and no awareness that there is disease. Deficient lactation. Impotence. Menstrual irregularities.
DEFICIENCY/EMPTINESS SYMPTOMS	Sensation as though body is decreasing in size (or is diminishing in size), constant thinking and no awareness that there is disease. Pain. Prostatitis. Urethritis. Orchitis. Seminal emission. Menorrhagia. Hematemesis.
PHYSICAL FINDINGS	Pulse tight and uninterrupted in all three (proximal [*cubit*], middle [*bar*], and distal [*inch*]) positions; wiry and full. Or very deep, close to bone, and tight. Or proximal [*cubit*] and distal [*inch*]) both strong and firm at the deep level. Or pounding and forceful in the Organ depth (deep level). Tenderness around the umbilicus, SP channel, in particular SP-6, 4, 13, 15, 16, 21, CV-17 and possibly suprapubic.
MASTER/MEETING POINT	SP-4 (+) (or red ion) often on right side (may be part of cross syndrome).
COUPLED POINT	P-6 (-) (or black ion) often on right side (may be part of cross syndrome).
ACTIVATING POINT	K-3.

Table 1-19: Girdle (Dai) Channel

FUNCTION	Connects, controls and binds all the longitudinal channels at the trunk. Regulates balance of Qi between upper and lower body. Supports the abdomen and low back. Regulates the Gall Bladder channel (disorders of sides of body).
GENERAL SYMPTOMS	Limpness of the lumbar region (instability). Menstrual disorders. Lumbar/hip dysfunction. Lumbar pain radiating to abdomen, pelvis, genitals, or medial thigh. External/Internal Qi-disharmony. Paralysis. Deficiency in lower body, Excess in upper body. Laxity of ligaments.
EXCESS/FULLNESS SYMPTOMS	Excess of the Yang channels. Weakness of upper extremities. Lumbar or loin pain. Unilateral weakness in eye, breast, or ovary.
DEFICIENCY/EMPTINESS SYMPTOMS	Weak loins or lumbar ("feels like sitting in water"). Hypermobility (laxity of ligaments). Pain in opposite shoulder, eye, breast, or ovary. Abdomen distention.
PHYSICAL FINDINGS	Pulse tight at middle (*bar*) position and beats that vibrate left and right. Or middle (*bar*) pulse floating and others deep, tight, or slippery. Or middle (*bar*) left to right pellet like (moving). Or full in both middle (*bar*) positions; diminished distal (*inch*) and proximal (*cubit*). Tenderness around umbilicus, along the channel, ASIS, St-25, GB-24, 41 and possibly UB-23 and 52.
MASTER/MEETING POINT	GB-41 (+) (or red ion cord) often on right (may be part of cross syndrome).
COUPLED POINT	TW-5 (-) (or black ion cord) often on right (may be part of cross syndrome).
ACTIVATING POINT	GB-26.

Table 1-20: Yang Motility (Qiao) Channel

FUNCTION	Rules the left side of the body (Yang). Regulates the movement of Yang-Qi and Fluids. Regulates muscular activity. Nourishes the muscles and joints of lower extremities. Controls opening and closing of eyes. Fullness condition of this channel implies an Emptiness condition of the Yin Qiao channel, and vice versa. Regulates Yin/Yang of lower extremity with Yin Qiao channel.
GENERAL SYMPTOMS	Pain in lumbar region and/or spasm along lateral lower extremity with corresponding weakness along the medial aspects Acute headaches and Wind problems (CVA), stiff neck, etc. Muscular problems of a Yang nature (tightness, spasm) on dorsal unilateral aspect of body. Toe-out gait and stance. Symptoms often bilateral, however worse on one side or show an opposite reaction on opposite side. When "diseased" Yin becomes slack and Yang cramped. Symptoms related to Urinary Bladder channel; back, spine, joint symptoms; aversion to wind, headache, numbness of feet and hands. Back pain, leg pain (sciatica) along lateral side (L4-5). Mania, epilepsy, (day seizures), insomina.
EXCESS/FULLNESS SYMPTOMS	Deficiency/Emptiness of Yin organs and Excess/Fullness of Yang organs. Upper body Excess. Symptoms worse at night. Restlessness. Anger. Epilepsy during the day. Eye diseases. Open eyes (will not close). Excess tearing. Throat pain. Male genitourinary conditions. Shoulder pain. Pain of the lateral leg.
DEFICIENCY/EMPTINESS SYMPTOMS	Deficiency/Emptiness of Yang with Excess/Fullness of the Yin organs. Upper body Empty. Complaints worse during day. Night epilepsy. Inability to keep eyes open. Hypersomnia. Migraines. Throat pain. Difficulty breathing. Lower Warmer Excess/Fullness. Gynecological problems. Waist pain. Tightness of medial leg. Bi syndromes of joints.
PHYSICAL FINDINGS	Pulse tight at distal (*inch*) position; beats vibrate to the right and left (moving). Or distal (*inch*) pulse high/superficial/floating and proximal (*cubit*) pulse is deep (may be normal for man). Or forcefully striking at the inner and outer (moving) aspect of the distal (*inch*) position. Or distal (*inch*) left to right pellet-like (moving). Or fills the whole distal (*inch*) position on both left and right and diminished elsewhere. Tenderness around ASIS, PSIS, around spine, especially around upper back and sides of cervical spine, posterior axilla (SI-9, 10) and possibly suprapubic.
MASTER/MEETING POINT	UB-62 (-) often bilateral.
COUPLED POINT	SI-3 (+) often bilateral.
ACTIVATING POINT	UB-59.

Table 1-21: Yin Motility (Qiao) Channel

FUNCTION	Rules the right side of the body (Yin). Regulates Yin aspect of movement of Qi and Fluids (quality and flexibility, essence, and free movement); opening and closing of eyes; muscular activity. Excess/Fullness condition of this channel implies Deficiency/Emptiness condition of Yang Qiao channel, and vice versa.
GENERAL SYMPTOMS	Tightness and spasms along medial lower limb with flaccidity along lateral aspect of limb. Back and hip pain radiating to the groin and/or genitals. Tremors of legs. Toe-in gait. Accumulation in the Yin channels (lumps, tumors, spurs). Unilateral headache near eye. Tightness of back muscles with weakness of rectus abdominus. Eye, circulatory, gynecological disorders. When "diseased," Yang becomes slack and Yin cramped.
EXCESS/FULLNESS SYMPTOMS	Deficiency/Emptiness of Yang Organs with Excess/Fullness of Yin Organs (worse during day). Night epilepsy. Inability to keep eyes open Hypersomnia. Difficulty breathing. Feeling cold. Migraine. Throat pain. Lower Warmer Excess/Fullness (gynecological problems, waist pain, tightness of the medial leg, Bi syndromes of joints).
DEFICIENCY/EMPTINESS SYMPTOMS	Excess/Fullness of Yang channels (fever; headache with heat). Symptoms worse during weather changes.
PHYSICAL FINDINGS	Pulse tight at proximal (*cubit*) position, beats vibrate to the right and left (moving). Or proximal (*cubit*) superficial/floating and distal (*inch*) deep (K-Yin Excess or Deficient). Or forcefully striking at the inner and outer aspects of the proximal (*cubit*) position. Or proximal (*cubit*) left to right pellet-like (moving). Fills the whole proximal position on both sides and diminished elsewhere. Tenderness/tightness along CV channel, especially above umbilicus, and soft superficial/deep tight below umbilicus. Findings also at: suprapubic (K-11,12), periumbilical, mid-clavicle (ST-12) and SCM (ST-9), K channel along abdomen and K-8, K-6 and Ki-3.
MASTER/MEETING POINT	K-6 (-) (or black ion cord) usually bilateral.
COUPLED POINT	Lu-7 (+) (or red ion cord) usually bilateral.
ACTIVATING POINT	K-8.

Table 1-22: Yin Linking (Wei) Channel

Function	Carries Ancestral-Qi and functions on deepest level of Yin. Ruling Interior; especially Heart, Lung, Stomach, and Spleen Organs; balances the emotions. Links the Yin of the body. Together with Yang Wei connects and regulates all Yin-Yang channels of body.
General Symptoms	General weakness. Lumbar or genital pain. Vague thoracic heaviness (chest oppression) and pain dyspnea. Circulatory problems. Distension in subcostal region, pain in Hear/heart region, fullness of chest. Ache in waist. Insomnia and other emotional symptoms; low self-esteem, weak will power. Nightmares. Restlessness, anxiety, fear; timidity, lack of will power, depression. Easily angered. Palpitations. Delirium. Weakness of homolateral upper extremity and contralateral lower extremity.
Excess/Fullness Symptoms	Delirium. Nightmares. Weakness of homolateral upper extremity and contralateral lower extremity. Dyspnea. Chest oppression.
Deficiency/Emptiness Symptoms	Pain in homolateral upper extremity and contralateral lower extremity. Hypotension. Hypothyroidism. Impotence. Rectal prolapse. Depression. Timidity. Fear. Nervous laughter.
Physical Findings	Pulse at the proximal (*cubit*) position seems to roll toward the thumb (radially) or up toward the distal (*inch*) with beats that are sinking; big and full. Or floating at proximal (*cubit*) and sunken at distal (*inch*) position. With excess, deep pulses stronger than superficial ones. With deficiency, deep pulses weaker than superficial ones. Or beating from radial portion of the proximal (*cubit*) to the ulnar portion of the distal (*inch*) position. Or proximal (*cubit*) inner slanting upward, arriving at the distal (*inch*). Subcostal tenderness or tightness, especially on right (Liv-14, GB-24), CV-17 (female), P-1 (male). Possibly tenderness of medial clavicle, suprapubic, periumbilical and SP-6.
Master/Meeting Point	P-6 (-) (or black ion cord) usually on right (may be part of cross syndrome).
Coupled Point	Sp-4 (+) (or black ion cord) usually on right (may be part of cross syndrome).
Activating Point	K-9.

Table 1-23: Yang Linking (Wei) Channel

FUNCTION	Unites and regulates Yang channel activity. Impacts Defensive-Qi. Rules Exterior; superficial and acute pathologies; pathologies having to do with rotations and extension; Tai-Yang and Shao-Yang channels. Connects to brain and balances emotions.
GENERAL SYMPTOMS	Unilateral symptoms, unilateral (or lateral) leg pain. Neck-shoulder pain, especially with headache radiating from base of head to forehead or ipsilateral eye. Pain in lateral aspect of body. Headaches, especially unilateral. Muscular fatigue and/or stiffness, weakness of limbs. Arthritis with sensitivity to weather changes. Vertigo (with quick head or eye movements), dizziness. Fevers, chills, alternating chills and fevers.
EXCESS/FULLNESS SYMPTOMS	Excess of Yang channels. Fever. Headache with heat. Symptoms worse during weather changes. Mumps. Manic-depression, anger.
DEFICIENCY/EMPTINESS SYMPTOMS	Deficiency of Yang channels. Lack of body heat. Loss of strength, especially during rainy or cold weather. Obsessive compulsive behavior.
PHYSICAL FINDINGS	Pulse at proximal (*cubit*) position seem to roll toward little finger (as though flowing in opposite direction or ulnerally) or up to the distal (*inch*) position with beats that are floating; big and full. Or distal (*inch*) position is floating (normal) and sunken in proximal (*cubit*) position. Or beating from the ulnar portion of proximal (*cubit*) to radial portion of distal (*inch*) position. Or distal (*inch*) position inner slanting upward, arrive at distal (*inch*) position. Or running diagonally from ulnar proximal (*cubit*) position to radial distal (*inch*) position. Tenderness/ tightness around ASIS, especially left side. Tenderness and positive findings at TW-5, along GB channel — especially GB-21 to GB-29 and GB-35, GB-34.
MASTER/MEETING POINT	TW-5 (-) (or black ion cord) usually right or (may be part of cross syndrome).
COUPLED POINT	GB-41(+) (or red ion cord) usually right or (may be part of cross syndrome).
ACTIVATING POINT	UB-63.

Table 1-24: Eight Extra Channels Pulses (Morris 2002)

Channel	Li Shi-zhen (Huyn)	Wang Su-he (Yang)	Wang Shu-he Lakeside Master (Flaws)	Miki Shima	Will Morris
Governing (Du)	Wiry and Long Floating and Uninterrupted in all Three positions	Proximal and distal both Excessive and Exuberant in the Superficial depth	Straight Up and Down Floating	Floating Wiry and Excessive and Tight	Strong-taut in the Qi depth
Conception (Ren)	Tight at Distal position Thin Full and Long	Tight, Fine, Excess, from Distal to Proximal positions	Straight Up and Down Floating	Mildly Sunken almost to Bone	String-taut in the Blood depth Qi depth diminished
Penetrating (Chong)	Firm and Uninterrupted Wiry and Full	Proximal and Distal both Exuberant in Deep depth Firm	Confined	More Sunken Deficient and Choppy	Pounding and Forceful in the Organ depth
Girdle (Dai)	Tight at the Middle position. Pulses Vibrating Left and Right	Forcefully Striking at the Outer and Inner Sides of the Middle position.	Middle Left to Right Pellet-like movement.	Floating in the Middle. Sunken at Distal and Proximal positions.	Running Diagonally from the Radial portion of the Proximal position to the Ulnar portion of the Distal position.
Yin Linking (Wei)	Beats are Sinking Big and Full. They Roll from the Distal toward the Proximal position.	Beating from the Radial position of Proximal position to the Ulnar portion of the Distal position.	Proximal Outer Slanting Upward. Arrives at the Distal position.	Sunken Distal. Normal Middle. Floating Proximal.	Running Diagonally from the Radial portion of the Proximal position to the Ulnar portion of the Distal position.
Yang Liking (Wei)	Beats are Sinking, Big and Full. Roll from the Distal toward the Proximal positions radially.	Beating from the Radial portion of the Proximal position the Ulnar portion of the Distal position.	Proximal Inner Slanting Upward. Arrives at the Distal position.	Floating Distal. Normal Middle. Sunken Proximal.	Running Diagonally from the Ulnar portion of the Proximal position to the Radial portion of the Distal position.
Yin Motility (Qiao)	Tight at the Proximal position. Vibrate Left and Right.	Forcefully Striking at the Inner and Outer aspect of the Proximal position.	Proximal Left to Right Pellet-like movement.	Sunken Distal. Normal Middle. Floating Proximal.	Fills the Whole Distal position on Both Sides. Diminished elsewhere.
Yang Motility (Qiao)	Tight at the Distal position and Vibrate Left to Right.	Forcefully Striking at the Inner and Outer aspects of the Distal position.	Distal Left to Right Pellet-like movement.	Floating in the Distal position. Normal Middle. Sunken Proximal.	Fills the Whole Distal position on Both Sides. Diminished elsewhere.

Organs

The Organ system in TCM describes Solid (Zhang) Organs that are said to be Yin, and Hollow (Fu) Organs that are said to be Yang. Each Yin Organ is paired with a Yang Organ. The Hollow Organs are associated with the digestive system and mostly have connection with the Exterior body (via orifices). The paired Organs are, therefore, said to have Interior Exterior relationships. An interesting discussion speculating as to why the Chinese chose to associate each Yin Organ with a paired Yang Organs can be found in the *Dao of Chinese Medicine* (Kendall *ibid*).

The following review of Organ functions and dysfunctions, that are commonly dealt with in patients with musculoskeletal disorders is only a partial survey of TCM/OM patterns. The information on Organs in this text combines Chinese, Japanese, European, and information this author has gathered over the years from lectures and his teachers. Some of the information is novel. For sources please see works consulted in the references.

The anatomy, physiology, and pathology of TCM Organs are quite different from those of the scientific medical model.[173] TCM emphasis is often on the relationships of the Organs to related systems. The *Spiritual Axis* states:

> The five solid Organs store up essential-Qi and regulate its outflow. The six Hollow Organs transform and transport substances without storing them and for this reason they may be over-filled but cannot be filled to capacity.

The Organs influence distal tissues through the systems' channels and vessels. The Liver, for example, controls nourishment to the eyes; it is in charge of communication (by being in charge of free-circulation), distribution, and the dredging of channels and vessels (Gan Zhu Shu Xie). The Kidney influences hearing. Each of the solid Organs controls a tissue system: the Lung rules the body's skin and hair; the Heart rules the body's Blood and vessels; the Liver rules the sinews and membranes; the Spleen rules the body's muscles and flesh; the Kidneys rule the bones and marrow. Each Organ is also responsible for a particular form of emotional and mental expression and health. These types of physiologic attributions, their relationships and their balance are at the root of TCM Organ pattern discrimination.[174] Nonetheless, many similarities between biomedicine and TCM Organs/organs can be demonstrated. One example is the TCM Kidney system, which controls growth, the bones, Fluids, reproduction and hearing. It houses the prenatal-Qi and stores Essence and Original-Qi, thereby governing the body's energy reserves and ability to cope with stress. Kidneys are the root of Qi and respiration. The taste related to the Kidneys is saltiness.[175] Most chronic disease processes eventually affect the Kidneys. The Heart and left-(Yin)-Kidney are related.

Embryological relationships can be demonstrated between the left kidney and heart, and both kidneys are connected via the perirenal fascia to the aorta stemming from the heart. The kidneys, adrenals, and sexual organ develops from the same embryological tissue, and therefore it is not surprising that the Kidneys in TCM are associated with many of the hormone and reproduction systems in biomedicine. The three midline lines: pronephros, mesonephros, and metanephros, lie in lines on the sides of the midline of the embryo and extend upward as far as the somites that are the precursors of the developing cervical vertebrae. These lines also extend downward as far as the somites of the developing lumbar vertebrae. The mesonephric tubules' tissues extend up to the sixth cervical and down to the third lumbar somites. Thus, kidney functions may be related to tissues that transverse nearly the whole length of the embryo, from head to toe (Matsumto and Birch *ibid*). Kidney-Yang is said to denote the hypothalamic-pituitary-adrenal, thyroid and gonadal axes, secretion of the corresponding hormones, sodium pump activity of red blood cells, caloric energy production, and immunomodulating functions. The Kidney-Yin involves cAMP/cGMP activity (Wu 1998).

Gate-of-Fire/Mingmen/Ministerial-Fire

The Yang of the Kidneys (Fire within Water), also called the "Gate-of-Fire" (*Mingmen*) contains the Ministerial-Fire (which is also the source of Fire of the Liver, Gall Bladder, and Triple Warmer), and is *located* between the Kidneys, or at the seventh vertebra (*Classic of Difficult Issues*). In other texts, Mingmen is said to be in the right-Kidney, or to be an "oily membrane." The Gall Bladder is said to be the "storehouse" of Ministerial Fire.[176] This separate location may reflect the adrenal system, as adrenal insufficiency has been shown to correlate closely with the TCM Kidneys (mostly Yang-deficiency). Mingmen is said to be the "sea of Essence and Blood, mansion of Water and Fire, house of Yin and Yang, root of Original/Source-Qi and lair of life and death." Mingmen-Fire (also called small-Fire, true-Fire, small-

---

173. The word "Organ" is not what Unschuld uses to translate "Zhang" and "Fu," since these words were also used to describe ideas of storage, administrative centers, palaces, commerce, army camps, etc. He uses the word "depots" for the solid Organs and "palaces" for the hollow Organs. The solid Zhang are said to store items for extended periods, while the hollow Fu may only store items temporarily. The "Organs" were also associated with governmental institutions, and, again, their functions may have, in part, come about from general Confucian ideas and not strictly medical thinking or experimentation.

174. TCM is a system in flux, and ideas have changed with time. For example, most mental and cognitive functions are attributed to the Heart and Kidneys. In the Yuan and Ming dynasties however, some physicians attributed these functions to the brain. Also, the sea of marrow (brain) has always been thought to be under the influence of the Kidneys, showing some understanding of the role of the brain in early writing as well. The *Spiritual Axis* says the original spirit-Qi is housed in the brain.

175. Although in *Simple Questions* it is also said that saltiness is associated with Heat.

176. In the Ming dynasty theories were advanced linking the Triple Warmer to the fatty tissues around the Kidneys, or possibly adrenal.

Table 1-25: Biomedical and OM Kidney Systems

Condition	Biomedical Renal and Adrenal	OM Kidneys and Gate of Fire (Mingmen)
Anabolic Functions	Responsible for production of many anabolic steroids.	Producing and sustaining body milieu.
Multiple Causes	Causes of renal failure and disease are numerous and multisystemic. They can be from intrinsic or extrinsic causes. Acute adrenal insufficiency can result from many severely stressful circumstances. Vast embryological distribution and development.	Causes of K disorders are numerous as most disorders eventually affect K energy.
Urinary Symptoms	Often result in urinary symptoms of anuria, polyuria, retention, and nocturia.	Often results in urinary symptoms of anuria, polyuria, retention, and nocturia.
Pregnancy	Disorders often related to pregnancy and both systems have similar embryological origins.	Ks control reproduction and are affected by pregnancy.

Table 1-25: Biomedical and OM Kidney Systems (Continued)

CONDITION	BIOMEDICAL RENAL AND ADRENAL	OM KIDNEYS AND GATE OF FIRE (MINGMEN)
BACK AND FLANK PAIN	Renal colic and flank pain are associated with K and urinary tract disease.	Back and flank pain is often related to Ks.
GROWTH FAILURE	Preadolescent adrenal insufficiency is related to growth failure and delayed puberty.	K Essence-deficiency is related to growth failure and delayed puberty as well.
IMPOTENCE AND AMENORRHEA	Disorders are associated with development of impotence and amenorrhea.	Ks regulate reproduction and are associated with impotence and amenorrhea.
GYN ANOMALIES	GYN congenital anomalies are highly associated with renal system anomalies as both have similar embryological origins.	Ks house the prenatal-Qi, thus GYN disorders and congenital anomalies are related to the Ks.
PULMONARY CONGESTION AND CONGESTIVE HEART FAILURE	Disorders of renal and adrenal system are associated with pulmonary congestion and congestive heart failure, both of which result in shortness of breath and edema.	Disorders of Ks are related to pulmonary congestion and shortness of breath as the Ks are the root of breath and control Fluid. Edema, and pulmonary congestion is often related to K-Yang.
BONES	Kidneys have a role in calcium regulation. Chronic renal disease can result in osteodystrophy and osteomalacia. Cushing's disease (adrenal excess) is related to osteoporosis. Vertebrae and Ks have similar embryonic origins.	K disorders are related to osteoporosis, osteomalacia and osteodystrophy as the Ks control the growth and strength of bones.
PROTEINURIA PYURIA	Proteinuria and pyuria seen in renal disease, (protein or pus in urine) can result in cloudy urine.	Loss of Essence and Damp-Heat from K disorders can manifest as cloudy urine as well/
MENTAL SYMPTOMS	Encephalopathy can be seen with renal disease. Insomnia is commonly seen with chronic K disease.	Symptoms of cognition and brain function often are related to K disorders as the Ks control the Essence and sea of Marrow (brain). Sleep disorders are often related to K-Yin.
SKIN PIGMENTATION	Hyperpigmentation is a common sign of renal or adrenal disease.	Darkening of skin is associated with K disorders as well.
DIGESTIVE SYMPTOMS ANEMIA	Anorexia, nausea, vomiting, and diarrhea are associated with renal failure. Anemia is often seen in chronic K disease.	K and Sp interrelation (dysfunctions through Five Phases theory) are associated with same symptoms. Blood-deficiency (and anemia) often result from K-Sp-deficiency.
SALT	Salt overload can result from renal disease.	Saltiness is the taste associated with the Ks.
STRESS TOLERANCE AND WEAKNESS	Adrenal cortex glucocorticoid hormone insufficiency results in weakness, dizziness, and reduced stress tolerance.	Dizziness is a symptom associated with K and Essence-deficiency. The Body's ability to cope with stress (energy reserves) is controlled by the Ks.
TEMPERATURE	Heat and cold intolerance is seen with renal and adrenal disorders.	Heat and cold intolerance are commonly related to K disorders as all of the body's Yin-Yang is rooted in the Ks.
FATIGABILITY	Fatigability, especially in the afternoon, is commonly seen in renal and adrenal disorders.	Afternoon fatigue is a K associated symptom, as the Ks circadian time is in afternoon.
HAIR LOSS	Hair loss seen with adrenal disorders.	Hair loss is a symptom of K disorders.
APATHY	Apathy is commonly seen with both renal and adrenal disorders.	Apathy is a common manifestation of K disorders as the emotion associated with the Ks is the will.
LIBIDO	Loss of libido can be seen with adrenal and renal disorders.	Libido is a cardinal function of K.
HEART AND KIDNEYS	Heart disease can cause Kidney disease. Kidney disease can cause Heart disease. Both organs have common embryonic origins. Left kidney and heart and both kidneys are connected via the perirenal fascia to the aorta stemming from the heart.	There is a clear relationship between the Heart and Ks; the left K being Yin is said to control Fire (Heart).

Heart) is the main anabolic force in the body and is said to be capable of "producing and sustaining body milieu (things)...basis of the production of life."

Therefore Mingmen Fire is said to be needed for: supporting digestion allowing the Stomach to except food and Spleen/pancreas to transport and distribute Fluids; allow the Heart to rule consciousness and move the Blood; steam the Liver allowing it to govern the movement of Qi and control reflection; move bile (with Liver and Gall Bladder) and allow the Gall Bladder to rule decision making; support the Lungs so that they can rule rhythmic regulation over Qi and movement of Fluids to the Kidneys; allow the Large Intestines to move the bowel; allow the Small Intestines to separate pure and impure Fluids; allow the Urinary Bladder to receive and hold the urine/Fluids; and finally to allow the Triple Warmer to regulate Fluid pathways. Kidney-Yang (Mingmen) should therefore be suspected as being the root in all conditions involving Yin Pathogens, especially Phlegm associated with chronic diseases.

The main formulas that treat Mingmen are Restore Right Beverage or Pill (You Gui Yin or You Gui Wan), Kidney Qi Pill from the Golden Cabinet (Jin Gui Shen Qi Wan) and Construction-Nourishing Essence-Invigorating Powder (Qiang Yang Zhong Jing Dan).

Suprarenal (Adrenal) Glands

The adrenal glands, which are located at the upper end of each kidney, are important in the regulation of many bodily functions, including the nervous system. Each adrenal gland has an external layer of cortex and an internal layer of myelonic material. The adrenal cortex and myelonic material secrete hormones that have direct effects in the regulation of various nutritional and defense activities. Their action is important also in the process of acupuncture analgesia and anesthesia. Many adrenal steroids have anabolic (building-up) functions (*OM: many of which are related to Kidney-Mingmen function*).

SUPRARENAL MYELONIC MATERIAL. The suprarenal myelonic material is controlled by fibers of the anterior lowest splanchnic nerve that contains the sympathetic fibers for the renal plexus. It secretes adrenaline and demethyladrenaline (noradrenaline/norepinephrine), and in action is similar to sympathetic nerves.[177]

SUPRARENAL CORTEX. The suprarenal cortex secretes many adrenocortical hormones (corticosteroids and sex hormones) that are necessary for maintaining many of the basic activities of life. Adrenocortical hormones can strengthen the body's capacity to resist harmful factors such as injuries, diseases, infections, and painful stimulation.

Glucocorticoids (hormones) are produced from cholesterol in the zona fasciculata of the adrenal cortex under negative feedback control of both the hypothalamus and pituitary glands. The hypothalamus produces corticotropin-releasing hormone (CRH), which stimulates the pituitary gland to synthesize adrenocorticotropic hormone which, in turn produces *cortisol*. Glucocorticoids are needed for cell *homeostasis* and to maintain normal carbohydrate, lipid, and protein metabolism. Cortisol facilitates catecholamine (norepinephrine, epinephrine) production and modulates beta-adrenergic receptor synthesis, regulation, coupling, and responsiveness. Glucocorticoids can enhance normal immune activity and wound healing, and maintain cardiovascular integrity and cardiac contractility. Mineralcorticoid synthesis occurs in the adrenal zona glomerulosa when stimulated by the renin-angiotensin-aldosterone system or hyperkalemia. Aldosterone is the main endogenous mineralocorticoid, which enhances sodium and potassium homeostasis and *maintains intravascular volume*. Autoimmune disease is the most common etiology of *primary* adrenal insufficiency. Pituitary dysfunction or failure with insufficient adrenocorticotrophic hormone (ACTH) production causes *secondary* adrenal insufficiency and is uncommon. *Tertiary* adrenal insufficiency develops from hypothalamic or the hypothalamic-pituitary-adrenal (HPA) axis dysfunction or failure. The most common cause of adrenal insufficiency is therapeutic glucocorticoids administration (steroid therapy). Recovery of the HPA axis after the discontinuation of exogenous glucocorticoids may take up to a year (Coursin and Wood 2002).

Excessive hormonal secretion, as seen in high stress states, may be deleterious to soft tissues. Increased cortisol levels is known to *decrease* the pain threshold.

Glucocorticoid insufficiency (Eddison's disease) occurs when 90% or more of the adrenal tissue is destroyed. Symptoms usually include fatigability, weakness, anorexia, nausea and vomiting, cutaneous and mucosal pigmentation, hypotension, and occasionally, hypoglycemia. So-called *adrenal fatigue* (Wright 2001) may be seen in patients suffering with fatigue, weakness, and *exercise intolerance*. They often suffer from low blood pressure (and hypoglycemia), dizziness upon standing (orthostatic hypotension due to loss of sodium and increase in intercellular potassium), heart palpitations, and a tendency towards low weight. They often also suffer from allergies, other hormonal dysfunctions, learning difficulties, and ulcers of the duodenum.[178]

Glucocorticoid excess (Cushing's disease) is mostly due to iatrogenic steroid therapy or bilateral hyperplasia due to various tumors. Glucocorticoid excess causes muscle weakness, cutaneous striae (streaks), easy bruisability, and promotes fat deposition in face (moon face), the interscapular (buffalo) hump, and the mesenteric bed (truncal obesity).

---

177. It is interesting to note that German acupuncturists have related the functions of the Triple Warmer to the adrenal system. According to Teitelbaum (2000), both the back-Shu-Transport and Alarm-Mu points are located in the range of sympathetic output to the adrenal medulla. These points are used in acupuncture to coordinate the activity of the Organs found in the upper, middle, and lower Warmers. This may be similar to the biomedical understanding of a coordinated sympathetic control of these same organs (possibly Organs), effected through release of epinephrine by the adrenal gland.

Hypertension and emotional changes are common, and diabetes mellitus occurs in more than 10% of patients.

There are numerous similarities between the known pathologies of biomedicine and the theorematic basis of TCM/OM theory. Some example have a distinct relationship, while other are more tenuous. Table 1-25 highlights some similarities between *biomedical renal and adrenal diseases and the TCM Kidney system.* (Again, clinical parallels should be viewed with caution as the two systems have completely different clinical interpretations of symptoms and signs.)

A recent study supports TCM's relationships between hearing and bone mass by showing that in women 65-85 years old, hearing loss and bone mass are related (Clark 1995). Another clear association in TCM is cognitive function and bone health, as the Kidneys and the "sea of Marrow" (brain) are of the same source. In TCM, memory is also closely related to the Heart, and the Kidneys and Heart have clearly defined functional relations. Embryological relationships (Birch *ibid*) can be demonstrated between the heart and brain and between kidneys and vertebral bones. Thus cognitive functions, hearing and bone mass are related to Kidney functions (in TCM) and may have close embryological origins and thus functional relationships. The association of memory and bone mass was studied by Zhang, Seshadri, Ellison, et al (2001). In evaluating 4,304 elderly subjects who were sixty years of age or older in the Third National Health and Nutrition Examination Survey between 1988-1994, bone mineral density and the prevalence of verbal memory impairment were evaluated by a 3-item word list and a 6-item story and bone mass studies. After adjusting for variables, the prevalence ratios of verbal memory impairment for each increased bone mineral density quintile were 1.00, 0.64, 0.65, 0.55 and 0.44, respectively. The data suggests that bone mineral density in the elderly is associated with verbal memory impairment. The prevalence of verbal memory impairment decreased with increasing bone mineral density.

A look at osteoporosis as it relates to Kidney-deficiency syndromes in TCM, and at where bone density examination was performed by DEXA technique and the diagnosis of osteoporosis was made by finding 2.5 standard deviations below the bone density of healthy youths was undertaken by Chen, Hsue, Chang, and Gee (1999). The study showed a marked association between Kidney-deficiency syndrome and postmenopausal osteoporosis. Patients with Kidney-Qi-and-Yin-deficiency syndrome were more likely to get osteoporosis than those with Kidney-Qi-deficiency syndrome or Kidney-Yin-deficiency syndrome alone. Other common associations are Kidney and Spleen deficiency and Qi and Blood deficiency.[179]

A few of the *many* examples of similarities between TCM and Biomedical organ and other physiological dysfunctions are: bleeding, Liver disorders, and Spleen/pancreas disorders.

SPLEEN DISORDERS. As in biomedicine, in TCM the Spleen is associated with the immune system. Dysfunction of the TCM Spleen can result in Phlegm production and lymph node enlargement (seen also with biomedical spleen disorders). The biomedical spleen is part of the extramedullary hematopoiesis system and therefore is associated with blood formation in both TCM and biomedicine. The Spleen in TCM is associated with digestive functions more appropriately attributed to the pancreas in biomedicine. This apparent difference may be in name only. One section in the *classic Difficult Issues* may include the pancreas as part of the Spleen: "The Spleen weighs 2 pounds and 3 ounces. It is 3 inches wide, 5 inches long and has ½ pound of fatty tissue surrounding it." This description generally and the mention of "fatty tissue" in particular sounds more like the pancreas than the spleen. As noted before, a clinical association between Spleen-Qi-deficiency syndrome and the pancreatic exocrine function was shown. Also the word "Pi" is used to describe this organ, and the translation of it as "Spleen" may be erroneous. At the same time, other functions of the Organ Pi, especially as relating to Phlegm, Dampness, and Blood do fit the biomedical spleen. The Spleen is said to control the flesh and muscles. Muscle and flesh emaciation is therefore related to the Spleen.

In a comprehensive review article Wu (*ibid*) has documented many functional and structural (biomedical) alterations in patients and animals with TCM Spleen-deficiency. *Changes in secretory and absorption functions* have been shown. These include reduced gastrointestinal (GI) tract salivary flow, reduced salivary amylase activity, changes in gastrin and acid secretion, and decrease in xylose excretion in chronic atrophic gastritis patients. Differences in serum motilin level with motility disturbances that led to loss of appetite and epigastric fullness after a meal have also been shown (all symptoms associated with TCM Spleen).

Structural and biochemical changes in gastric mucosa (Stomach is the paired Organ of the Spleen) have been

---

178. Adrenal function can be tested by 24 hour urine collection, blood tests, and by saliva testing. Measuring blood pressure supine and standing normally result in increased pressure standing of about 8 mm Hg. In patients with significant adrenal insufficiency, the pupalery reaction to light may be reduced, reversed, or delayed. Chapmen's reflexes (page 498) may be positive, and in Applied Kinesiology, weakness of the sartorius muscle has been related to the adrenals. Treatment may include low glycemic index diet, salt, multiple vitamins, 1 gm of pantothenic acid BID, vitamin C, DHEA, licorice (Gan Cao), ginseng (Ren Shen), astragalus (Huang Qi), and possibly low dose natural cortisol. When using licorice, one must watch for signs such as: headaches, lethargy, sodium and water retention, excessive loss of potassium and high blood pressure. Relora, a proprietary blend of patented extracts from cortex magnolia officinalis and cortex phellodendron amurense is said to promote healthy cortisol and DHEA production.

179. Commonly prescribed herbs for osteoporosis are: Eucommiae (Du Zhong), Epimedii (Yin Yang Huo), Dipsaci (Xu Duan), Psoraleae (Bu Gu Zhi), Cervi (Lu Rong), Beef Marrow (Niu Gu Sui), Salviae (Dan Shen), and Astragali (Huang Qi) which are added to herbs that address the pattern diagnosis.

shown in patients with superficial gastritis and Spleen disorders. The turnover rate of epithelial cells has a short life span, and differences in the mucosal lamina propria have been shown. In Spleen-deficiency patients, glandular atrophy was more severe, intestinal metaplasia more frequent, whereas in patients with disharmonic Liver and Stomach type the metaplasia was modest. Ultrastructural studies revealed reduced microvilli of epithelial cells, increased junctional width, membrane damage, swollen mitochondria with disrupted cristae and dilated endoplasm in parietal cells, decreased pepsinogen granules within chief cells, and increased plasma cell infiltration in lammia propria. These changes were not seen in disharmonic Liver and Stomach type patients. Substance P and VIP were found increased in sigmoid colon, correlated with loose bowel movement (a symptom of Spleen-deficiency). Elevated cAMP levels in gastric mucosa and plasma of Spleen-deficiency patients were found, and plasma cAMP/cGMP ratio was decreased markedly in those patients with intestinal metaplasia. Likewise, gastric mucosal SOD content and plasma LPO also decreased significantly and may have correlated with metaplasia.

Studies have also shown varying *dysfunctions of the vegetative (autonomic) nervous system* of the gastrointestinal tract in relation to Spleen-deficiency. Cerebral cortical function was extensively suppressed and presented with unstable somatic evoked potential, diminished amplitude, and poor reproducibility. The hypofunction of sympathetic nervous activity manifested a decrease in skin electric potential activity, reactivity of peripheral vessels to cold, urine VMA content as well as plasma dopamine hydroxylase; all of which increased after adequate treatment. In these patients, blood acetylcholine level was elevated, usually accompanied by bradycardia and lower systolic and diastolic blood pressure; these indicated the presence of relative hyperfunction of parasympathetic nervous activity.

Studies of *immunologic functional changes* in Spleen-deficient patients showed the peripheral blood lymphocyte count to be lower than normal. Patients with chronic hepatitis B, Liver-congestion (depression), and Spleen-deficiency pattern diagnosis have lower lymphocyte count than normal. This can be restored to near normal by Spleen-fortifying therapy. A T-cell subset study revealed significantly decreased total T-cells and TH-lymphocytes. Among cancer patients with Spleen-deficiency, CD4 was shown to be lower than normal, whereas CD8 had no change. Herpes-infected patients have weaker lymphocyte and plasma cell infiltration and local SIgA response. Recently, it was found that Spleen-deficient patients had a high frequency of HLA-B12 whereas patients with pattern diagnosis of disharmony of Liver and Stomach had a high frequency of HLA-B15. These showed that immune response is closely related to vulnerability to disease.[180]

Endocrine changes in patients with Spleen-deficiency patterns showed urine 17-ketosteroid to be significantly lower than normal, but there was no significant change in 17-hydroxysteroids as compared with normal. The level of catecholamine was also low. There was thyroid hypofunction with total T3 and fT3 significantly lower than normal, whereas rT3 was significantly higher; low metabolic rate, low skin temperature, poor tolerance to cold and lack of adaptation to environmental changes were also present. This poor tolerance to cold is a special feature of Spleen-Yang-deficiency pattern diagnosis. Asthenia and loss of weight might also be due to hypofunction of thyroid and are common symptoms and signs seen in Spleen-deficiency patients.

Changes of trace elements in the blood of chronic hepatic disease patients with Spleen-deficiency pattern diagnosis showed the blood Zn to be significantly lower than normal, but Cu was the reverse. Zn is important in enzymatic action, nucleic acid synthesis, membranous function of red blood cells, hemopoiesis, and cell respiration. In Spleen-Yang-deficiency patients serum Mg was increased, whereas in Spleen-Yin-deficiency it was extremely low. Fe was elevated in Spleen-Qi-deficiency and in Spleen-Yang-deficiency patients at the ages of fifty to sixty years, and ten years after it was first found to be elevated. In Spleen-Qi-deficiency Mn and Cr were both increased significantly.

Muscle metabolism is affected as well in patients with Spleen-deficiency patterns. Muscle glycogen and CPK activity in the quadriceps and plasma all decrease significantly. The resulting asthenia and muscular weakness were primarily due to energy depletion from lowered hepatic and muscle glycogen content. Besides, ATP, ADP and AMP contents were also much lowered, and LDH and succinyl dehydrogenase activities significantly elevated because of anaerobic glycolysis; those ions relevant to muscle contraction were decreased. Serum total free amino acids and essential amino acids including branch chained amino acids were all decreased; lysine, valine, glycine, theonine, tryptophan, isoleucine, serine, alanine, and histone were all lower than normal. These may all contribute to muscle emaciation.

Changes of fecal bacteria flora and Helicobacter in Spleen-deficiency mice was shown. Lactobacillus bifidus and other lactobacilli were decreased but could be restored to normal after the Si Jun Zi decoction treatment. The enterobacteria pathogens were increased but could be reduced after

---

180. Studies on Spleen-fortifying herbal formulas have shown that these formulas restore NK activity and TK activity in cancer patients. Astragalus (Huang Qi) and Atractylodis (Bai Zhu) can elevate CD4 significantly in patients with lowered CD4. Treatment with Four Gentlemen Decoction (Si Jun Zi Teng) of patients with GI diseases and Spleen-deficiency pattern diagnosis showed very little change in immunoglobulin G, but the content of secretory IgA decreased significantly. Some Spleen-fortifying prescriptions can enhance proliferation of mice splenic cells and increase significantly the mice specific antibody secretory cell number, antigen-induced delayed allergic reaction, and mixed lymphocytic reaction. They also enhance the cytotoxic action of lymphocytes and promote ConA-stimulated mice splenic cells to secrete IL-2. Phagocytic function of monocyte-macrophages also increases as seen by the clearance of carbon particles. Astragalus (Huang Qi) and Four Gentleman decoction (Si Jun Zi Teng) can restore the immunologic function of red blood cells, probably through their promoting effect on C-3b receptor expression and the activity on the red cells surface (Wu *ibid*).

treatment. and Helicobacter pylori was also decreased in amount.

LIVER DISORDERS. In biomedicine, liver disease results often in anorexia, nausea, vomiting, diarrhea, fatigue, weakness, fever, jaundice, amenorrhea, impotence, and infertility. Signs such as spider telangiectasis, palmar erythema, nail changes, Dupuytren's contracture, testicular atrophy, and gastrointestinal bleeding are recognized.

In TCM, via the Five-Phases theory, Liver disorders affect the Spleen/Stomach and also lead to anorexia, nausea, vomiting, diarrhea, fatigue, and weakness. Heat and Dampness in the Liver or Gall Bladder result in fever and jaundice. Interruption of the Liver's function of regulating the Blood can result in amenorrhea, infertility, and bleeding disorders. The Liver channel passes through the penis and testicles; hence, disorders of the Liver channel and Organ are associated with impotence and testicular atrophy. The Liver controls the sinews; the nails reflect the condition of the sinews. When Liver-Blood fails to nourish the sinews, soft tissue contracture (including Dupuytren's) can result. Nail changes, including Muehrcke lines, Terry's nails, and finger clubbing are manifestations in part of Liver disorders.

BLEEDING. Bleeding and thrombotic disorders are related to the Liver and Spleen in both TCM and biomedicine. Liver disease results in deficiencies of all clotting factors except factor VIII. The TCM Liver controls the storage of Blood. In TCM, Spleen-Qi holds the blood in the vessels and is dependent on proper digestive function. Vitamin K deficiency impairs production of clotting factors II, VII, IX and X. The major source of vitamin K is dietary and therefore is dependent on good digestive function and food. The spleen also contributes to plasma proteins involved in controlling blood coagulation. Infections are related to bleeding in both models.

Extraordinary Organs

There is another category of Organs called "the extraordinary hollow Organs," which include the Brain, Marrow, Bone, Vessels, Uterus, and Gall Bladder. They are named hollow but their functions are considered to be similar to that of the five solid Organs as they "store."

YIN ORGANS. Table 1-27 on page 89 through Table 1-30 on page 93 together constitute a brief summary of the most common Yin Organ functions and dysfunctions that may be attended to in musculoskeletal patients. There are many more combinations and dysfunctions not covered in these tables; however, they are less significant in musculoskeletal patient population.

YANG ORGANS. The Yang organs, which also have patterns of symptoms and signs, are located more superficially than the Yin organs and therefore are often considered by many to be less important. Table 1-31 on page 94 through Table 1-36 on page 97 summarize the general characteristics of the Yang organs.

Table 1-26: Yin Organs: Liver/Wood (LIV)

FUNCTIONS	Control free flowing Qi and Blood, both storage and discharge (Yin in structure but Yang in function). Control the Interior of body. Upbearing functions of the right side of body. Nourishing of the sinews. Healthy vision. Orderliness of functions.
GOVERNS	Storage and movement of Blood and nourishment of sinews (seen in nails), muscle tone, and strength.
OPENS	At the eyes and "makes" the pupils.
HOUSES	The ethereal soul.
EXPRESSES	Decisiveness, control of emotions, principle of emergence (spring and the power of action).
HEALTHY EXPRESSIONS	Kindness, spontaneity, and ease of movement.
UNHEALTHY PSYCHOLOGICAL EXPRESSIONS	Anger, erratic behavior, tension, depression (repressed anger), frustration and resentments, feeling stuck, dysthymia ("the blahs"), lack of direction in life, fear. Said to be the "Bandit of the 10, 000 diseases."
PERSONIFIES	Pioneer.

Table 1-26: Yin Organs: Liver/Wood (LIV) (Continued)

PAIR EXTERNAL ORGAN	Gall Bladder.
DISEASE PATTERNS	**LIVER DISEASE PATTERNS AND THEIR CHARACTERISTIC SYMPTOMS INCLUDE:**
LIVER-BLOOD-DEFICIENCY (LIVBD)	Mostly due to Spleen/pancreas weakness or blood loss, diet, constitutional weakness of Kidney-Yin or Essence. **Dizziness**, insomnia, **flowery vision** (floaters), restriction of movement, tightness of sinew-muscular components and/or tingling and numbness of the limbs, headache (especially on left side),[a] muscle twitching, **increase of pain with physical labor, eased by half hour rest.** Pale or shallow (emaciated) yellow complexion, or lips and nails. Pulse: thready, wiry, choppy, possibly rapid. Tongue: pale especially on sides, with thin white coat.
LIVER-YIN/BLOOD-DEFICIENCY	Mostly due to constitutional weakness, Kidney-Yin-deficiency, or blood loss. Can be due to lifestyle or chronic diseases, or iatrogenicity. This is a pattern of Kidney-Yin and Liver Blood-deficiency. Symptoms seen with LivBD and Kidney-Yin-deficiency **with Heat**, **dryness**, thirst, night sweats. Pulse: thready, wiry, **quick.** Tongue: red or pale, red especially on edges.
STAGNATION/OF LIVER-QI (SLIVQ) **AKA.** **LIVER-DEPRESSION QI-STAGNATION, LIVER-QI-STAGNATION**	Liver-Qi either fails to flow (congestion/depression) or overflows sideways (Qi-stagnation).[b] Mostly due to emotional factors and stress, or Spleen/pancreas weakness, or Kidneys and Blood failing to moisten (sooth) the Liver. **Irritability**, **depression**, frustration, frequent sighing. **Painful distention/bloating** of: chest, breast, subcostal, lateral costal regions, abdomen (may indicate sideways movement of Liver-Qi, i.e., Liver invading Spleen/Stomach). There may be distention/bloating without pain, but never pain without distension/bloating. Irregular menstruation. Pulse: **wiry.** Tongue: normal or slightly dark.
UPFLAMING OF LIVER-FIRE (UFLIVF)	Mostly due to SLivQ (or more accurately Liver-congestion) with transformative/congested-Fire (an Excess disorder). Strong or long-term stress, anger, frustration, or depression results in Liver-Qi-stagnation that transforms into Heat/Fire; or from iatrogenicity, or spicy foods. Symptom seen with SLivQ and **short temper**, severe anger, impetuosity, **headache**, dizziness, sudden tinnitus, **bitter (unpleasant) taste** in mouth, **red** eyes and complexion, acne. Pulse: **wiry, rapid**, weak or strong. Tongue: **dark red**, thin or swollen, swollen edges, yellow coat.
HYPERACTIVE LIVER-YANG	Mostly due to chronic or strong Liver-Qi-stagnation and transformative-Heat that then damages Yin/Blood. Or secondary to Kidney and Liver-Yin-deficiency failing to control Liver-Yang (a Deficiency disorder). Possibly symptoms of UfLivF with headache, **dizziness**, vertigo, and **low back pain.** Pulse: wiry, **rapid**, and **weak.** Tongue: red, **thin body, fissures especially on edges, no or little coat.**
LIVER-WIND	Can be due to Blood-deficiency or progression of SLivQ and UfLivF, or iatrogenicity, or recreational drugs, or high fever (Warm-disease), or animal bites. Symptoms more in the head region are often do to SLivQ and UfLivF. If symptoms are mostly at the extremities Wind symptoms often are due to Blood-deficiency. **Rigidity** of the neck, dizziness, **tremors** or jerking, muscle twitches, headaches, **convulsions**, tidal red facial color. Pulse: **wiry**, quick or slow, tight, floating. Tongue: red, or pale if Blood-deficiency, thin or swollen, often yellow coat.
INVASION OF STOMACH BY LIVER	Symptoms/signs seen in SLivQ, **nausea**, *vomiting, acid reflux, sour taste* exacerbated by emotional factors.
LIVER AND SPLEEN DISHARMONY	Symptoms/signs seen in SLivQ; **abdominal pain** *and diarrhea or loose stools*, both of which are exacerbated by emotional factors.
LIVER/WOOD FAILING TO MOVE SPLEEN/STOMACH/ EARTH	Similar symptoms as Invasion of Stomach and Liver and Spleen Disharmony (with primarily Liver affecting Stomach symptoms), except that treatment is focused on Stomach/Spleen and Dampness as this is a Deficient condition. (It is related to Liver-congestion without Qi-stagnation.)

Table 1-26: Yin Organs: Liver/Wood (LIV) (Continued)

Liver-Yang (Qi) Deficiency **Liver-Cold**	General Liver related symptoms and signs, with disorders of movement (often a combined pattern of **Kidney-Yang/Qi-deficiency** and **Liver-Blood-deficiency**). Movement disorders, as pertain to gait as well as Qi, as Liver controls free-flowing Qi and Blood. (It is important to realize that Yang-Qi is needed for Liver function of moving Qi. If Kidney-Yang/Qi is weak, this easily results in Liver failure to move Qi and thus Liver-congestion Qi-stagnation, which must be treated with Kidney-Yang/Qi herbs). **Withering** or **tenseness** (hardness) of sinews, weakness and movement disorder of the extremities (mostly feet). Feeling cold and cold extremities. **Fear.** Liver-Cold is an acute condition due to external Cold pathogenic factor. Paleness, bright-white facial complexion. Pulse: deep, **wiry**, fine and **slow** or tight. Tongue: pale with white coat.

a. If Blood is deficient with Wind the headache will be on the left side. If Qi is deficient with Wind the headache is on the right side.
b. While often difficult to differentiate in the clinic, Liver-congestion pertains more to lack of flow with symptoms attributed primarily to the Liver such as chest oppression, impaired digestion, subcostal fullness, etc. The lack of movement of bodily Qi (which is mainly controlled by the Liver) can result in inhibited Qi flow anywhere and other symptoms in other systems, most commonly slow digestion and bloating. Liver-congestion Qi-stagnation often refers to an Excess of Qi within the Liver (due to congestion) which then moves sideways to attack the middle Warmer. While Liver-congestion can transform to Qi-stagnation (sideway moving), it does not go the other way from Qi-stagnation into Liver-congestion. Liver-congestion is also said to produce Heat, while some authors state that so-called Liver-Qi does not (others disagree). Liver-congestion usually requires treatments that move and open the Liver, while, when advancing to Liver-Qi-stagnation, harmonizing therapies are often called for.

Table 1-27: Yin Organs: Kidney/Water (K)

Functions	Growth, reproduction, regeneration, generation; stores Essence and essential forces of body (fullest at birth, depreciates throughout life), metabolizes Fluid, and roots Qi.
Governs	The bones, Essence, brain, Fluids, Yin (left K) and Yang (right K) of the entire body, low back and legs, knees (although the knees are also said to be the dwelling place of the sinews and therefore Liver as well).
Opens	Into the ears, the spine is the K pathway, Essence "makes" pupils and its vigor is seen in the hair and teeth.
Houses	The will, fear, desire, mind.
Expresses	Ambition, creativity, vigor, focus.
Healthy Expressions	Gentleness, endurance and groundedness.
Unhealthy Psychological Expressions	Fear, indecisiveness, apathy, discouragement, negativity, lack of will, impatience, frequent spitting.
Personifies	Philosopher.
Mingmen Life-gate	Mingmen/lifegate is the sum of the two Kidneys. Origin of Triple-Warmer. An oily membrane (possibly adrenals).

Table 1-27: Yin Organs: Kidney/Water (K) (Continued)

PAIR EXTERNAL ORGAN	The Urinary Bladder.
DISEASE PATTERNS	**KIDNEY DISEASE PATTERNS AND THEIR CHARACTERISTIC SYMPTOMS INCLUDE:**
KIDNEY-QI-DEFICIENCY (KQD)	Mostly constitutionally or due to chronic disease. May be due to K-Yin or Yang deficiency. **Low back and knee soreness and weakness**, pain often aggravated by physical activity or sexual exertion; and may or not get better with a short rest; frequent urination, **nocturia**, tinnitus, dizziness, hearing loss, **low libido**, impotence. Pulse: deep, **weak.** Tongue: pale red.
KIDNEY-YANG-DEFICIENCY (KYAD)	Mostly due to aging, chronic disease, excessive life styles; drugs, sexual activity, iatrogenicity. Symptoms seen in KQD plus symptoms and signs of **coldness** (especially low extremity), lower abdominal tension/pain, early morning diarrhea, **nocturia**. Pulse: **deep** fine, or floating at the proximal (*chi*) position and deep distal (*inch*) position, or generally slow and **weak**, or may be slippery due to dampness. Tongue: pale, swollen, moist, and white coat possibly thick.
SPLEEN AND KYAD	Mostly seen with aging, chronic disease, or damage from cold and unclean food, or cold medicines. Symptoms and signs seen in KQI and/or KYaD, with *persistent* or **early morning diarrhea.**
KIDNEY FAILURE TO HOLD THE QI	Mostly constitutionally or due to chronic disease. Symptoms and signs seen in KQD and/or KYaD, **asthma**, rapid and short breath, **difficult inhalation**, short breath when laying down.
HEART AND KYAD	Mostly seen with aging, chronic disease, drugs, early life shock Symptoms and signs seen in KQD and/or KYaD, **palpitation**, dyspnea, **edema** (heart failure)
INSUFFICIENCY OF KIDNEY-ESSENCE	Mostly constitutionally, or life style abuses: drugs, sexual activity, chronic disease, strong shock especially early in life. **Premature aging**; graying of hair and degenerative disorders, constant dull back and heel pain, soft bones, lack of muscle strength, intellectual deficiency, **slow growth** (standing, walking, hair growth, development of teeth, closure of fontanel), **physical abnormalities** (scoliosis, etc.) hair loss, **low energy reserves.** Pulse: deep, weak, choppy or constantly changeable, or floating soft and weak especially at the distal (*inch*) positions (or on right side). Tongue: variable.
INSECURITY OF KIDNEY-QI	Mostly seen with aging, chronic or acute disease, iatrogenic. Symptoms and signs seen in KQI and/or KYaD, **polyuria** more severe, and/or incontinence, cloudy urine.
KIDNEY-YIN-DEFICIENCY (KYID)	Mostly seen with aging, chronic disease, or damage due to Heat burning Essence, Fluids or Yin, life style abuses: drugs, sexual activity, iatrogenicity, prolonged stress. **Dry throat and lips**, dizziness, tinnitus, back pain, night sweats, **feeling of warmth**; especially in the Yin aspects of body (palms, soles, and chest, also called five center heat), symptoms **aggravated by heat** or exertion, concentrated **scanty urine**. Pulse: deep fine and rapid, or: deep rapid at proximal (*chi*) or floating at distal (*inch*) position, or generally rapid and weak or generally tight-wiry, or possibly slippery weak, or floating quick and weak, or surging at distal (*inch*). Tongue: Red, **thin**, **dry**, fissures, little or no coat, or thin dry yellow coat, mostly in rear of tongue.
HEART AND KYID	Symptoms signs seen in KYiD; palpitation; **insomnia**; cognitive symptoms. Tongue: may be cracked, or show changes at tongue tip.
LIVER AND KYID	Symptoms seen in KYiD; headache; **flowery vision** (floaters); severe **dizziness.** Tongue: May show changes at edges (Liver areas), may be less red if Liver-Blood is also deficient.
LUNG AND KYID	Symptoms seen in KYiD; dry **cough**; severe night sweats.

Table 1-28: Yin Organs: Spleen/Pancreas/Earth (SP)

Functions	Controls digestion, helps in production of Blood, maintains the Blood in the vessels, stirs and therefore transports substances, raises Fluids.
Governs	Flesh (muscle bulk, mass), four limbs, mind, intelligence, center, Nutritive-Qi, eye lids, paranasal area, Qi of five viscera.
Opens	Into the mouth and its vigor seen at the lips.
Houses	Thought.
Expresses	Centeredness, persistence, care, reflection.
Healthy Expressions	Fairness, openness, deep thinking, recollection.
Unhealthy Psychological Expressions	Excessive use of the mind (obsessiveness), melancholia, agitated sleep and nightmares, stubbornness and rigidity, excessive ruminating on the past.
Personifies	Care giver, farmer.
Pair External Organ	Stomach.
Disease Patterns	**Spleen disease patterns and their characteristic symptoms include:**
Spleen (SP) Qi-deficiency (SpQD)	Usually due to over or under eating, eating cold or poor quality foods, excess sweets, over-thinking, over-taxation, cold medicines (iatrogenicity). Fatigue, **sleepy/fatigue after large meals**, lack of strength, thin, loose, or sticky stools, abdominal discomfort or distension, **poor appetite**, dusky or white-yellow complexion. Pulse: Leisurely/relaxed, weak, soft, deep, especially in middle (bar) position; may be slow or fast. Tongue: **Swollen**, moist, thin sticky or thick white coat.
Spleen-Yang-deficiency	Often due to iatrogenicity, chronic disease, cold foods, prolonged SpQD. Symptoms seen in SpQD, **abdominal pain** relieved by warmth and pressure, **cold** body and extremities (especially upper extremities and nose), sensitivity to cold, edema, drained white complexion. Pulse: Deep and weak, leisurely/relaxed, often slow or rapid large and empty. Tongue: Pale, **swollen, moist.**
Central-Qi-Sagging (Spleen Stomach, frequently referred to as Central-Qi)	May be due to weak Original-Qi from a difficult birth, prolonged disease, or most frequently due to aging. Symptoms seen in SPQD, **dizziness on standing** (orthostatic hypotension), bloating after meals, **sagging distention** feeling in abdomen, **prolapse** of viscera or rectum. Pulse: **Large empty**, rootless especially in right middle (bar), short. Tongue: Pale, **swollen** with **teeth marks**, thin white coat.
Spleen Failure to Hold the Blood	May be due to all the above factors as well as hemorrhage injuring Spleen-Qi. **Bleeding** (mainly menorrhagia, hemafecia occurring with Spleen-deficiency symptoms), early periods, blood that is pale, thin, or dripping. Pulse: Thready, weak, faint, choppy; or floating, large, empty, and rootless. Tongue: Pale, swollen with teeth marks, thin white coat.
Spleen and Heart-Qi and Blood-deficiency	Often due to chronic stress, or post viral infection, or other diseases. Symptoms of SpQD, poor sleep, **dream disturbed sleep**, palpitation, forgetfulness. Pulse: Thready and weak. Tongue: Pale, tip of tongue may show changes; swollen or thin, thin white coat.
Central Qi-deficiency-Cold	Often due to vegetarian and cold diet, constitutional, or chronic disease. **Abdominal dull pain** relieved by pressure, warmth or food, fatigue, cold limbs. Pulse: Deep and slow. Tongue: Pale, often swollen.
Spleen-Yin-deficiency	Usually due to chronic disease with some Heat, consumption of alcohol or spicy foods. Symptoms of SpQD, **dry often red lips** and mouth, **epigastric discomfort or burning** (if with Stomach-Heat), indigestion, **alternating** constipation and loose sticky stools. Chronic diseases with lack of nourishment of muscles (also sinews, bones, skin, vessels). Hunger but dislike eating or no thought of food. Dryness but no desire to drink. Pulse: Thready, weak, soft or slightly tight, rapid. Tongue: Red, thin or swollen, **peeled center coat**, or scanty coat.

Table 1-29: Yin Organs: Lung/Metal (LU)

FUNCTIONS	Governs respiration, downbearing of Qi (left side), regulates the flow of waterways and are the upper source of water.
GOVERNS	Surface skin and hair (Exterior), Qi of the whole body, parting.
OPENS	At the nose, the throat is Lungs' gate.
HOUSES	Corporeal soul, Qi
EXPRESSES	Expression, clarity of speech.
HEALTHY EXPRESSIONS	Appropriate sadness and cheerfulness.
UNHEALTHY PSYCHOLOGICAL EXPRESSIONS	Grief, worry, sadness, difficulty letting go.
PERSONIFIES	Sensitive type.
PAIR EXTERNAL ORGAN	Large Intestine.
DISEASE PATTERNS	**LUNG DISEASE PATTERNS AND THEIR CHARACTERISTIC SYMPTOMS INCLUDE:**
LUNG-QI-DEFICIENCY	Usually due to chronic illness or Spleen/pancreas weakness. Cough, **shortness of breath**, panting worsened by exertion or speaking, low voice, weak enunciation, spontaneous sweating. Pulse: Weak, floating, big and weak, or deep and faint, slow or fast. Tongue: Pale, normal or swollen, thin white coat.
LUNG-YIN-DEFICIENCY	Usually due to chronic illness with Heat, or acute-Heat, Dryness, or Heat-toxin. **Dry cough**, cough with sticky/scant/bloody phlegm, **night/sleep sweating**, flushed cheeks, afternoon or low grade fevers, dryness. Pulse: Weak fine, floating or deep, especially in distal (inch) position, often rapid. Tongue: Red, thin, fissures, little dry or no coat.
NONDIFFUSION OF LUNG-QI	Usually due to exterior Pathogenic Factors resulting in counterflow of Lung-Qi. **Paroxysmal cough** and/or dyspnea with rapid breathing, itchy throat, phlegm. Pulse: depends on if Heat or Cold predominate, tight if Cold, rapid slippery or wiry rapid with Heat. Tongue: depends on whether Heat or Cold predominate, white coat if Cold, yellow if Heat.
IMPAIRED DEPURATIVE DOWNBEARING OF LU QI/FLUID	Usually due to Heat from Pathogenic Factors. Persistent cough and/or **water metabolism disorders.** Pulse: depends on if Heat, Cold, Dryness or Dampness predominate. Tongue: depends on if Heat, Cold, Dryness or Dampness predominate.

Table 1-30: Yin Organs: Heart/Fire (H) (Pericardium/Fire) {P}

FUNCTION	Supplies Blood to the entire body.
GOVERNS	The vessels, Fire, speech and its vigor can be seen in the face.
OPENS	Into the tongue.
HOUSES	The spirit and the Heart's Fluid is sweat.
EXPRESSES	Clarity of thought.
HEALTHY EXPRESSIONS	Rosy complexion, clarity, ordered thinking and expression, joyfulness.
UNHEALTHY PSYCHOLOGICAL EXPRESSIONS	Disturbances of mental function, irrational behavior, hysteria, delirium, bipolar mood disorders, coma.
PERSONIFIES	Intellectual.
PAIR EXTERNAL ORGAN	Small Intestine.
PERICARDIUM	Closely related to Heart function. Protects the Heart. Associated with sympathetic nervous system, coma, psychiatric symptoms, and Warm-diseases.
DISEASE PATTERNS	**HEART DISEASE PATTERNS AND THEIR CHARACTERISTIC SYMPTOMS INCLUDE:**
HEART-QI-DEFICIENCY (HQD)	May be due to constitution, chronic illness, overtaxation, emotional stress (early life shock), aging, or blood loss. Dizziness, **palpitations**, **shortness of breath** especially with exertion, tendency to perspire, fatigue, poor sleep, anxiety. Pulse: **Weak**, fine, irregular, especially at left distal (inch) position. Tongue: Normal or swollen pale, thin white coat.
HEART-YANG-DEFICIENCY	Usually due to aging, overtaxation, long-term HQD, chronic disease, or iatrogenicity. HQD symptoms, **cold** limbs, cold sweat, **cyanosis** of nails and lips, **edema**, dull white complexion. Pulse: **Irregular**, **weak**, deep, slow, may be slippery, or fast, large and empty. Tongue: Pale or dusky, purple, swollen, thin or thick white coat.
HEART-BLOOD-DEFICIENCY (HBD)	Usually due to weak Spleen/pancreas or constitutional, aging, blood loss, chronic illness. Dizziness especially on standing (orthostatic hypotension), palpitation, fright, **insomnia**, **excessive dreams, poor memory,** lusterless complexion. Pulse: Weak, **thready**, choppy, may be rapid. Tongue: **Pale**, thin whit coat.
HEART-YIN-DEFICIENCY (HYID)	May be due to aging, constitution, chronic emotional stress or illness, chronic HBD. HBD symptoms with **night sweating**, tidal fever, **restlessness**/agitation and flushing red complexion. Pulse: Weak, fine, floating, rapid, especially at left distal (inch) position. Tongue: Thin, **red**, dry, no or little coat.
UPFLAMING OF HEART-FIRE	May be due to excess syndrome from Pathogenic Factors, overeating: spicy rich/greasy, hot, alcohol or sweet foods, or mixed syndrome from upflaming of Mingmen/Ministerial fire (pathogenic Yin-Fire), or from Kidney-Yin-deficiency. Restlessness/agitation, palpitations, **anxiety**, erosion of oral mucosa, **sores in mouth or tongue**, insomnia, red complexion, and/or associated Kidney-Yin-deficient symptoms. Pulse: **Rapid**, slippery, weak or strong, deep or floating, often tight and surging. Tongue: **Red tip.**
HEART-OBSTRUCTION	Often due to aging, chronic Qi-stagnation, chronic debility or illness, poor diet or Bi-syndrome **Angina, chest pain**, sharp pains, choking sensation when drinking water, other Heat-related symptoms, **purple complexion,** dark lips or circles around eyes. Pulse: Weak or strong, **choppy**, tight, or wiry. Tongue: **Purple**, dark red, static patches, enlarged sublingual veins.

Table 1-31: Yang Organs: Urinary Bladder/Water

FUNCTIONS	Receives the "impure/dirty" part of Fluids after the Small Intestine separates the Fluid from the "pure/clean" Fluids. • In charge of Qi-transformation (transforming and excreting Fluids by the power of Qi—Fluid disorders due to Qi-dysfunction). • Controls storing of Fluid.
HEALTHY INDICATIONS	Balanced mental state.
EMPTINESS/DEFICIENCY	• Fright affects the Bladder adversely (loss of urine). • Paranoia/suspicion and jealousy. • Back and neck pain. • Neurological disorders. • Lack of confidence. • Lethargy. • Low sexual energy; frequent, excessive or cloudy urination; incontinence. • Epistaxis. • Fear.
EXCESS/FULLNESS	• Agitation. —Excessive erections. —Headaches. —Olfactory problems. • Pain along spine or waist.
MENTAL SYMPTOMS	• Changeable moods. • Over-enthusiasm. • Suspicion, jealousy. • Lack of confidence.
PRINCIPAL SYMPTOMS	• Stiff neck. • Pain along cervical, thoracic, or lumbar spine. —Headache. —Pain in posterior aspect of thigh, leg and foot. —Eye disease. —Alternating chills and fevers.

Table 1-32: Yang Organs: Small Intestine/Fire

FUNCTIONS	• Separates the "pure" from the "impure." • Controls Fluid reabsorption. • Responsible for quality (pureness) of Blood. • Proclaims Qi. • Protects spirit by filtering out negative input (pure/impure).
HEALTHY INDICATIONS	• Confidence. • Appropriateness and sharp mindedness.
MENTAL SIGNS	Poor mental assimilation. • Feeling of mental deficiency due to inability to assimilate ideas. • Insecurity.
EXCESS/FULLNESS	• Small Intestine Organ disorders. • Pain, discomfort or abnormal sensations in lower abdomen ("mounting Qi pain.") • Tenderness in hypogastric area. • Pain at temples and sides of neck. • Flaccidity of arm muscles and joints, especially elbows. • Cystitis, urethritis, painful urination. • Over-confidence, delusions, restlessness.
EMPTINESS/ DEFICIENCY	• Swelling and nodules (may be from Excess), testicular pain. • Hemicrania/Migraine (sides and back of head). • Tinnitus; pain around ear. • Cystitis, urethritis. • Mental deficiency.
PRINCIPAL SYMPTOMS	• Neck stiffness. • Pain, sores, or heat sensation along the channel or related to Heart. • Tongue numbness, ulcers. • Urethritis, cystitis and small intestine organs disorders (abdominal pain).

Table 1-33: Yang Organs: Triple Warmer/Fire

Functions	• Has no "form", i.e, encompasses the whole body, and has been associated with the fascial-organ. May correspond to the three cavities of the trunk (pleural, pericadial, and peritoneal) integrating respiration, digestion and elimination. • Regulates metabolism (water) and has been related to the lymphatic system. • Distributes and is the origin of Original-Qi. • Responsible for the differentiation of Original-Qi into various functions. • Governs the flow of Ancestral, Nutritive, and Defensive-Qi. • Comes out of the right-Kidney (Mingmen) connecting the Heart and Kidneys. • Regulates basal temperature. • Helps communication among lower, middle, and upper parts of body and the Organs. —Upper Warmer mist/fog (water vapor). —Middle Warmer foam (gruel). —Lower Warmer swamp/dregs (waste water). —(It is said, "if the upper and lower are diseased treat the middle.") • Associated with the parasympathetic nervous system. • Affected by Warm-diseases.
Healthy Indications	Balanced mental state.
Mental Signs	• Poor elimination of harmful thoughts. • Emotional upsets caused by breaking of friendships or family relations. • Suspicion. • Anxiety.
Principal Symptoms	• Abdominal distension; hardness and fullness of lower abdomen. • Urinary difficulty or frequency. • Edema. • Pain behind ears, cheeks, neck, and jaw or at posterior aspect of shoulder and upper arm. • Warm febrile disease.

Table 1-34: Yang Organs: Large Intestine/Metal

Functions	• Elimination. • Absorbs water. • Drains turbid, retains clear.
Healthy Indications	• Appropriate sadness. • Cheerfulness.
Mental Signs Weakness, Dysfunction, Illness	• Sadness. • Grief. • Worry.
Excess/Fullness	Heat and swelling along channel. • Dryness, thirst, dark urine. • Abdominal distension, dizziness, constipation.
Emptiness/deficiency	• Coldness • Borborygmus • Diarrhea.
Principal Symptoms	Stagnation of Qi in the Large Intestine produces: • Spastic abdominal pain. • Constipation. • Alternating small stools and diarrhea.

Organs

Table 1-35: Yang Organs: Gall Bladder/Wood

FUNCTIONS	• Stores and secretes bile. • Provides expression through the sinews (ligaments, tendons and other soft tissues). • Serves as the source of courage and initiative. • Responsible for proper judgment, clarity of vision, decision-making. • Controls circulation of the nourishing and protecting "energies"/functions.
HEALTHY INDICATIONS	Good judgment and confidence.
MENTAL SIGNS WEAKNESS, DYSFUNCTION, ILLNESS	• Impulsive behavior. • Rashness of judgment. • Indecisiveness. • Fear.
FULLNESS/EXCESS	• Abdominal, head, shoulder discomfort or pain, lateral headache (especially right side). • Muscular spasms. • Tinnitus. • Agitation, impulsiveness.
EMPTINESS/ DEFICIENCY	• Wandering pains; pains and dysfunctions on sides of body, neck or head. • Weakness in muscles and tendons of legs. • Difficulty standing. • Chest pain. • Vertigo chills. • Insomnia. • Timidity, indecisiveness, excessive sighing.

Table 1-36: Yang Organs: Stomach/Earth

FUNCTIONS	• Receives and ripens food. • Serves the sense of taste. • Moves food and Qi downwards. • Regulates body flesh.
HEALTHY INDICATIONS	• Balanced mental state.
MENTAL SIGNS WEAKNESS, DYSFUNCTION, ILLNESS	• Bipolar mood disorder. • Erratic behavior. • Delusions.
FULLNESS/EXCESS	• Painful, burning sensation in stomach. • Hunger, halitosis, mouth ulcers and bleeding of gums. • Vomiting and constipation. • Pains and cramps in legs. • Loud psychotic behavior; manic phase of bipolar mood disorder.
EMPTINESS/DEFICIENCY	• Nausea. • Hiccough. • Loss of appetite. • Leg weakness. • Worry, obsessiveness; depressive phase of bipolar mood disorder.

Diagnosis

TCM diagnosis is accomplished through the Four Examinations: visual, audio-olfactory, inquiry, and palpation.

Visual Examination

Table 1-37 on page 107 and Table 1-38 on page 108 describe the basics of the visual examination. One of the most useful sources of visual signs in TCM diagnosis is the tongue. In comparison to other diagnostic procedures, tongue diagnosis is fairly clear and objective. Each area of the tongue represents various Organs and/or regions of the body. Figure 1-20 depicts the areas of correspondence on the tongue. The tongue is often reliable when other signs may be less so, especially as compared to pulse diagnosis: the pulse is affected frequently by drugs/medications, changes rapidly, and is affected by many factors, while the tongue is less affected. Tongue diagnosis can often help to shed light on complex patterns when contradicting and mixed symptoms and signs are seen. Table 1-38 on page 108 summarizes the most important aspects of tongue diagnosis. While Tongue (and Pulse) diagnoses are usually used within the context of all the Four Examinations, they can be used as the sole bases for diagnosis and treatment and may, at times, trump information from the other examinations.

Audio-Olfactory Examination

Auscultation (listening) is part of the basic examination. The practitioner observes quality of voice and enunciation, verbal expression, respiration, cough, and breath.

- Loud, pressured speech often indicates Heat and/or Liver and Heart disorders.
- Unclear thinking/expression may indicate Heart and Pericardium disorders, especially with Phlegm.
- Weak enunciation and a disinclination to talk may indicate Deficiency, especially of Lung-Qi.
- Muttering to oneself may indicate Heart-Qi-deficiency.
- Stuttering suggests upward disturbance of Wind and Phlegm.
- A fast respiratory rate can indicate Heat or Deficiency.
- A dry cough may indicate Dryness and Deficiency of Yin.
- A rattling cough may indicate Phlegm and Dampness.
- Foul breath suggests pathogenic-Heat in Stomach, indigestion (food stagnation), tooth decay, or unclean mouth.
- Foul offensive secretion or excretion usually indicates Heat.
- A stinking (rotten fish) smell may indicate Cold.

Examination by Inquiry

The practitioner poses questions to the patient about his chief complaint and about temperature, perspiration, the head, the body, stools, digestion and micturation, diet, chest, hearing, thirst, sleep and emotions, and history of present and past illnesses. Past treatments are reviewed. Table 1-40 on page 113 summarizes examination by inquiry.

Inquiry About Pain

In TCM, as is also the case in biomedical orthopedics, it is important to ask the patient about their pain, because the character, timing, location, and response to pressure and temperature are important for the clarification of the etiology of the pain. The information can inform us as to a diagnosis of Deficient or Excess and also help differentiate the various involved pathomechanisms. Information about the location of pain can tell us about the channels involved and should be as detailed as possible. Localized pain is often due to Blood-stasis, Phlegm, obstruction by Cold, Dampness or Damp-Cold blocking the sinews and network-vessels. Moving pain is often due to Wind or Qi-stagnation affecting the channels.

While some information can be gathered by questioning, response to pressure is better assessed clinically. When treating Western patients, there is always some difficulty in translating traditional TCM terminology (and descriptions of pain, which are difficult to begin with) to what Western patients describe (see page 155). A discussion and suggested vocabulary about the qualities of the pain are therefore often needed. This, however, must be done carefully so as not to influence the patient's responses. When asking the patient about the pain's reaction to temperature, it is often necessary to clearly ascertain if the patient likes to use heat or ice to alleviate the pain. Here again, however, there is often difficulties encountered when treating Western patients. Many have ideas acquired from other health care providers that may influence their experience (which can be said about Asian patients and literature as well).

Examination by Palpation

During palpation, the practitioner examines the radial pulse, skin, limbs, chest, abdomen, channels, Back-Shu, Alarm (Mu), and Command points. For more information on TCM orthopedic palpations see page 220.

Palpation: Radial Pulse

Palpation of the radial pulse is one of the most difficult and important aspects of TCM diagnosis. Each of six positions has three depths and at least twenty-eight qualities that reflect different Organs or pathologies. Different areas around the radial pulse represent different regions and Organs in the body (Figure 1-21). Pulse diagnosis is therefore a skill that takes great effort to learn. The reliable measurement of radial pulse characteristics has been studied by

Diagnosis

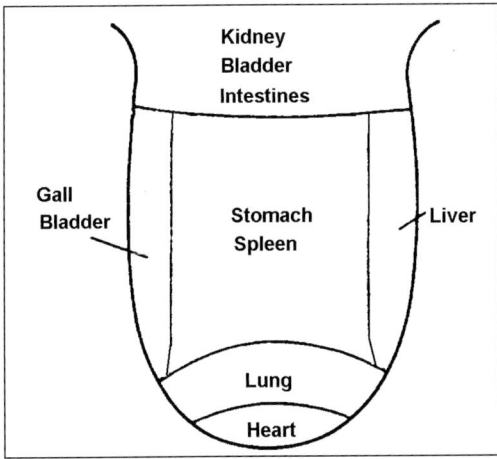

Figure 1-20: Areas of correspondence on the tongue.

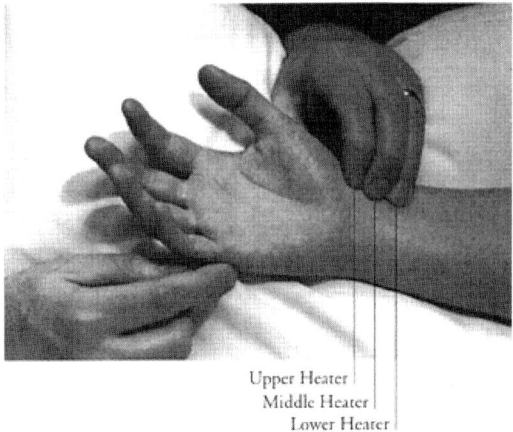

Figure 1-21: OM radial pulse taking.

King, Cobbin, Walsh, and Ryan (2002). They report on the physical sensations that are detected under the fingertips when the radial pulse is palpated, rather than attempting to translate these into the complex and typically ambiguously defined TCM pulse qualities. The inter-rater reliability of the pulse-taking procedure and operational definitions was assessed by determining agreement levels between two independent pulse assessors for each characteristic. Inter-rater agreement averaged 80% between the two assessors in both the initial data collection (sixty-six subjects) and in a replication collection (thirty subjects) completed two months later. Considering other studies of inter-rater reliability in physical examinations in general, these results are quite high.[181] Modern pulse-measuring devices have been advocated as a diagnostic and educational instrument (Broffman and McCullock 1986). At the same time, it must be emphasized (at least in this author's experience) that clinically it is difficult to predict which pulse a patient may manifest and that, nevertheless, the pulse would always convey the patient's *true* or most important condition/pathocondition. Also, there is much disagreement on how pulses should be taken regarding depths, positions, and what pulse images mean.

Hsu states:

> A physician may recognize the nature of the [patient's] illness by observing his complexion or by feeling the [movement of his] vessels [pulse]. But this is not as truthful as the words spoken by the [patient] himself...if the physician does not accept the truth [reported] by the patient [as his guideline] for designing a therapy that focuses on specific pathoconditions, and if he, on the contrary, clings to his own biased views and forces them onto his patient, then harm will be unavoidable...Those experts who discussed the [movement in the] vessels through the ages have all contradicted one another, and they all differed in what they considered right and wrong. They all cling to their specific doctrine, and their advantages and errors balance each other. All this results from their ignorance of the essential meanings of changing relationships [among movements in the vessels, pathoconditions, and illnesses]. and, the more detailed [their discourses become], the further away [they move from perfection].

Subhuti Dharmananda writes:

> The utility of pulse diagnosis may be more properly viewed as belonging to the realm of confirming a diagnosis attained by other means, including modern medical testing, or implying that something is missing from the diagnosis when the pulse does not agree, setting off a series of questions or investigations for additional information. This application of pulse as confirmation is one that Bob Flaws has argued against having modern practitioners rely on, even though he observed it as a common situation in China. He wrote in the introduction to his book on pulse: This Western ambivalence toward and pervasive lack of mastery of the pulse examination is, I believe, exacerbated by a somewhat similar attitude towards pulse examination current in the People's Republic of China at least in the 1980's.[182] When I was a student in China during that time, the importance of pulse examination was deliberately played down by many of my teachers and clinical preceptors....I never had a teacher tell me a pulse was anything other than wiry, slippery, fast, slow, floating, deep, or fine...it seems that many modern Chinese TCM practitioners relegate pulse examination to a minor, confirmatory role....I believe that mastery of pulse examination is vitally important to making a correct TCM pattern discrimination. And, I believe the pulse examination is, perhaps, even more important to Western practitioners than for our Chinese counterparts...In his book, Flaws goes on to argue that the importance of the pulse in modern practice lies with the complexity of chronic conditions suffered by many patients who turn to acupuncture in the West.

---

181. For discussion of physical assessment reliability see page 205.

182. In the text *The Treatment of Modern Western Diseases with Chinese Medicine,* however, when discussing reliable signs and symptoms in Western patients, Flows and Sionneau state: "In particular, the tongue and pulse are not good indicators of cold in the body...In particular, when there is a dual kidney yin and yang vacuity the tongue and pulse typically show the signs of the vacuity heat rather than the vacuity cold."

The idea is that these patients typically present a picture that is difficult to sort out, and that the pulse can provide information that resolves the dilemma. I would argue, contrarily, that this complexity of the patients makes pulse diagnosis more difficult to rely on, rather than more valuable. One can come to this view by reading the indications of the pulses in the Mai Jing, in which the interpretations are very succinct and focused: this pulse is common in the spring, this pulse means taiyin disease, this pulse means a fever, etc. By contrast, the complexity of modern patients, especially those who are older and suffer from numerous diseases, means that within one individual there is a complex of deficiencies and excesses, of internal and surface disorders, of stagnation and looseness, and influences of drugs, surgery, and daily habits that don't fit any traditional pattern. The resulting pulse is more difficult to analyze and less informative.

On the other hand in Unschuld's *Medical Ethics in Imperial China* Chang Chan states:

> Nowadays we have diseases which take a similar course with different patients, yet from the outside they appear to be different; and there are others, which take a different course with different persons, yet from the outside, they appear to be similar. For this reason, it will never suffice to examine exclusively with the eyes and ears the symptoms of excess and deficiency in the five granaries and six palaces as well as the flow or blocking of the blood and the pulses and the constructive and the protective influences. In the first place, one has to examine the symptoms of an illness which can be felt in the pulses to determine the specific illness. Only someone who gives his undivided mental attention can begin to elaborate on these symptoms. This undivided attention must be given even to the last details which are related to the irregularities in the depth and the marking of various kinds of pulsations, which conditions the variations in the acupuncture points, and which are responsible for the deviations in the thickness and strength of flesh and bones. Today, however, the prevailing effort is to grasp the most subtle details with the crudest and most superficial thought. This is truly dangerous!

THE MOST IMPORTANT QUALITIES ARE PULSE RATE, DEPTH, STRENGTH, AND STABILITY.

- A pulse that is quick, superficial, and strong may indicate a Yang condition and acute disease, but not always.
- A pulse that is slow, deep, and weak may indicate a Yin condition and a chronic disease, but not always.
- A pulse that is not congruent with the patient's disease is said to be a sign of poor prognosis and a disease that is difficult to treat. Therefore, a patient with a chronic disease should have a Yin-type pulse while a patient with an acute and short-lived disease a Yang-type pulse.
- An unstable, rootless, and "spiritless" pulse (i.e., lacking Stomach-Qi)[183] may indicate severe Deficiency ("separation of Yin and Yang") or Heart and Kidney (or *biomed: sympathetic/parasympathetic*) disorders. The normal Earth (Stomach/Spleen) pulse is said to be moderate/leisurely and thus to contain a moderate amount of the characteristic of all the Organ pulses, and therefore reflect the body whole (Righteous) Qi. This quality is also referred to as having spirit and root. The moderate pulse is often used to describe a leisurely rate as well.

IN MUSCULOSKELETAL PRACTICE THE MOST FREQUENTLY ENCOUNTERED PULSES ARE:

- *Tight* or *wiry,* seen most commonly in patients with pain due to Cold, Empty-Heat, stagnation in general, or Liver disorders. Sometimes one can feel a double wiry pulse which may be interpreted as Phlegm and Qi-stagnation. If a small, thin wiry pulse is felt within the larger vessel (pulse within a pulse) this may be interpreted as Excess-Cold and Deficient Organ systems.
- *Slippery* pulse, seen in patients with pain due to Dampness, Phlegm and Heat disorders, or other obstructions causing Blood turbulence including strong anxiety.
- *Difficult/Choppy* pulse, seen most often in patients with pain from Blood-stasis, and/or Deficiency of Qi and Blood.
- *Floating* pulse, seen most often in patients with pain from an Exterior pathogen, and/or a Deficiency of Yin or Yang.
- *Deep* pulse, seen most often in patients with pain from severe or chronic disorders, deep obstructions, and/or Cold and Interior conditions.

In the classic of *Difficult Issues,* different depths within the radial artery are said to represent various tissues and Organs. The fifth difficult issue states:

> The [movement in the] vessels may be light or heavy. What does that mean? It is like this. First one touches the vessel [at the inch-opening[184] by exerting a pressure] as heavy as three beans and one will reach the Lung section on the [level of the] skin [and its] hair. If [one exerts a pressure] as heavy as six beans, one will reach the Heart section on the [level of the] Blood vessels. If [one exerts a pressure] as heavy as nine beans, one will reach the Spleen section on the level of the flesh. If [one exerts a pressure] as heavy as twelve beans, one will reach the Liver section on the level of the muscles. If one presses down to the bones and then lifts the fingers until a swift [movement of influences] arrives, [the level reached] is the Kidneys [section]. Hence, one speaks of light and heavy.

Spiritual Axis states:

---

183. The "root" of the pulse most commonly refers to the proximal positions (Kidneys). Having root means that the position is deep, even, moderate, and forceful. A lack of pulse at the proximal position, however, can also result from obstruction in the lower burner and does not necessarily mean weakness and Deficiency. A spiritless pulse is scattered, chaotic, sometimes present and sometimes not, and may change its characteristics often. It is called "Qi-wild pulse" in the Shen-Hammer system.

184. A location on the radial artery. See Meridian Therapy in chapter 5 for details.

The left pulse at the inch [distal] position superficially reflects the Heart. Deeper it reflects CV-17 [chest qi]. At the left bar [middle] position, the surface reflects the Liver, the deeper pulse the diaphragm. At the left foot [proximal] position, the superficial pulse is the Kidney, the deeper pulse is inside the abdomen. In the right pulse, at the inch position, the Lungs are reflected at the surface, the deeper pulse reflects the chest. At the right bar position, the superficial pulse is the Stomach, the deeper pulse is the Spleen. Both bar positions reflect the rib cage. In the right foot position, the Kidneys are reflected at the surface, the deeper pulse is the abdomen.

Table 1-39 summarizes the pulses and indications and integrates various schools of thought, both modern and clasical. The general qualities of the pulse can be assessed at the carotid artery as well. In *Spiritual Axis,* the relative sizes of the carotid (Ren ying)[185] and radial pulses are said to show which channel is involved. For example, when the carotid pulse is twice as large as the radial pulse, the disease is said to be located in the leg Shao-Yang; when twice as large and rough, the disease is said to be located in the arm Shao-Yang. The Ren ying pulse is also said to govern the Exterior while the wrist pulses the Interior. The classic of *Difficult Issues* and *Spiritual Axis* also state that the skin of the ventral forearm may be used, with the same principles as pulse diagnosis. *Spiritual Axis* states:

> A hurried pulse means the skin at the elbow is also hurried. A slow pulse means the skin at the elbow is also small. A large pulse means the skin at the elbow is also thick and slow. A slippery pulse means the skin at the elbow is also slippery. A rough pulse means the skin at the elbow is also rough.

Pulses that relate to conditions of the Organs, channels, and regions can be palpated at arteries in the vicinity of specific acupuncture points summarized in Table 1-3 on page 219. For more information on pulse diagnosis, see Meridian Therapy in chapter 6

Diagnostic and Treatment Priorities

Since TCM diagnosis is established by the history and physical alone (with no "objective" lab work),[186] the practitioner must rely upon data collected through the five senses. Often patients present with conflicting information that must be prioritized. While at times necessary, it is unwise to overly theorize and combine elaborate mechanisms that may sound rational but ignore one of nature's basic principles: simplicity. Nature's problem solving is more often simple—as is so commonly demonstrated by biological sciences. If possible, a simple and historically substantiated solution/treatment should be used.[187] Complex and multisystem disorders are often said to involve the Eight-Extra channels, Divergent channels and/or to be of Essence-Qi.[188] On the other hand, in discussing Deficiency Damage, the master physician Wu Cheng of the Qing Dynasty (1644-1908) stated that "multiple pattern manifestations are the rule. The determination of primary and secondary patterns is not an easy matter, but it is an absolute requirement in order to form an effective formula."

THE FOLLOWING ARE GENERAL RULES THAT CAN AID IN THE DIAGNOSTIC AND TREATMENT PROCESS THAT THE AUTHOR HAS FOUND TO BE HELPFUL:

- Physical signs take precedence over symptoms *often*.
- Information concerning the entire body takes precedence over data concerning any one part of the body, except when treating acute and severe disorders.

For example, a patient with low tolerance of *physical activity* (becoming fatigued and developing symptoms after physical activity, especially Spirit-fatigue with a weak pulse) is often of a weak confirmation even though his/her body (or affected area/joint) may look muscular and strong. They may however, have Interior or Exterior Pathogenic Factors accounting for their fatigue, and then often should be treated as Excess or mixed confirmation. A strong patient that, as a result of his/her disease, is now fatigued and weak can still be characterized as strong but depleted. (This often occurs in musculoskeletal disorders due to severe pain, such as disc herniation resulting from lifting in a constitutionally strong patient.) Such a patient can usually still tolerate strong and possibly sedating techniques. If, however, the pulse has become very deficient, the patient should be tonified first and then sedating and strong methods used.

---

185. "Ren ying" (man prognosis) is the name of an acupuncture point on the front of the neck and therefore may be interpreted as the carotid artery. However, some interpretations claim Ren ying to be the pulse of the left distal (cun) position (reflecting Exterior or Stomach-Qi), with the right distal (cun) position (Kou cun) being the position that reflects the Interior. In discussing the condition of Stomach-Qi in patients with chronic diseases, Zhu Dan-Xi states that, if in females the left cun position is stronger than the right, the patient's Stomach-Qi is still strong and the disease curable. In males, if the right cun position is stronger than the left, the Stomach-Qi is strong and the disease is curable. These are consistent with men having more Qi and women more Blood. The *Pulse Classic,* however, states the opposite; and Zhu Dan-xi claimed that in that text the sides referred to the physicians' hands.

186. In modern times, laboratory work is being incorporated increasingly into the OM paradigm.

187. This may sound like a contradiction in a text that emphasizes the development of ideas, however, it is consistent with much of the history of OM. Using pathomechanistic principles in OM is not just the stacking up of patterns, but understanding the interaction between systems. As master Wu Cheng stated, when seeing evidence for "multiple patterns" it is always important to ascertain what is central and what is secondary and tertiary. TCM is a *logic-system-medicine* in which treatment is often a logical (theoretical) continuation of the diagnostic process. Therefore, while "logical" conclusions may be made from symptoms and signs, every treatment is still an experiment (since there are no truly objective criteria) that should be always followed by re-examination and evaluation. It is therefore important to not get trapped in process and keep clinical outcome and reassessment foremost.

188. At the same time complex formulas and treatment approaches may be necessary and appropriate.

Patient with pulses, tongue, abdomen (see abdominal diagnosis chapter 6), nails, and general body that suggest a weakness, Cold and Deficiency, is often treated as such even though he/she may have an inflamed and warm joint (unless acute or severe). Zhang Jie Bing (Warm Yang school) approaches are often useful. At the same time a mild-neutral approach to herbal therapy may be needed. Individual consideration as to the degree of attention to localized (or secondary) symptoms is always applicable and depending on severity may take precedence.

- The patient's *general constitution* and body type (or the *primary disease mechanism*) is often more important than any information concerning excretion and secretion (or other "branch" symptoms/signs), except when treating acute-infective, Exterior, or *severe* disorders in which attention to localized (acute) secretion or excretion (or area) may be more important. This is known as treating the root first and branch second. In general, it is said that one should first clear any Pathogenic Factors, external or internal, before using tonifying or astringent herbs or acupuncture techniques. However, if pathogenic accumulations are caused by Deficiency (secondary to Deficiency), it may be impossible to remove the Pathogenic Factors without the addition of, or sometimes emphasizing, tonifying herbs (especially in deficiency-Phlegm, i.e., Phlegm [an Excess pathogen] in an underlying Deficient patient). Sometimes it is necessary to tonify first and only when the patient is stronger to use sedating methods. Tonification is often (but not always) emphasized in protracted chronic cases as Pathogenic Factors are said to eventually damage the Organs. According to the *Classic of Internal Medicine*, the Five Tissue Bi (painful obstructions) are caused by Yin and Blood deficiency and the use of strong sedating methods that cause excessive sweating, urination, or purging is discouraged.

Therefore, treatment of a chronic musculoskeletal disorder in a weak patient with a weak pulse that also has some yellow phlegm, constipation/hard stools, and strong local point tenderness (possible signs of Excess and Heat) is often mostly by strengthening (usually done in Interior conditions, i.e., not acute or traumatic). Herbs that deal with Excesses or Heat may be added (i.e., treating both root and branch). Thus it is said, "Different diseases same pattern, same pattern different diseases." Again, a mild-neutral approach to herbal prescription may be best, especially if side-effects develop or the patient does not tolerate stronger formulas. If, however, for example, an acute warm joint with a capsular pattern and with signs of Excess (severe tenderness to pressure and limitation of ROM) is seen in a weak patient, one may need to strongly resolve local Excess before attending to the patient's general constitution or condition. This is known as "attending to the branch first and root second." Also, one always needs to keep in mind that Pathogenic Factors may be responsible for or lead to Deficiency, and tonifying a patient with retained Pathogenic Factors may result in an aggravation of the Deficiency (even if symptoms are not severe or particularly acute). It may be difficult to ascertain if Internal Damage mimics External contraction or External contraction simulates Internal Damage. A good history is often the key to resolving such a question. In protracted and chronic diseases, the tonification of Qi, using high dosage (up to 60g) of Astragali (Huang Qi,) is needed often, as this herb is indicated for "strong-Wind" and can assists Defensive-Qi and Yang in eliminating pathogens. In such situations, this herb is often combined with *variations* of Cinnamon Twig Decoction (Gui Zhi Tang+-) that can treat Pathogenic Factors while at the same time treating Yin, Yang, Defensive, and Nutritive-Qi and can easily be altered to clear Heat or Warm and expel Cold and Dampness.

The balance of treating root and branch symptoms is one of the more difficult issues one must resolve clinically (especially when using herbs). There are no hard rules, and opinions defer greatly. For example, the famous physician Zhu Dan-xi (Nourishing Yin School) often emphasized the supplementation of Righteous-Qi-Yin (over elimination of pathogenic influences) while others such as Liu Wansu (Cold/Cooling School)[189] and Zhang Cong-zhen (Purge and Attack School) emphasized the direct elimination of Pathogenic Factors first (and/or clear Fire) which may then result in automatic recovery of Righteous-Qi.[190]

The questions of root and branch (primary and secondary) are not always clear and should *not* be viewed as two separate entities, but, rather, as two aspects of the same condition. Diseases that *arise* from the Interior often have Organ (or Blood and Nutritive-Qi) related symptoms at the onset while diseases that arise from the outside may not. Careful history is therefore necessary to understand which is primary and which is secondary. Pure tonification is usually used only in Interior conditions where Righteous-Qi is weak. Since most musculoskeletal disorders are not purely Interior or Deficient (particularly where Deficiency, Excess and possibly Interior/Exterior are mixed), it is this author's general (but flexible) rule to treat *clearly* identified obstructions (or Excesses/Exterior and Pathogenic Factors) first, and only secondly to treat underlying root-Deficiency. As the saying goes, "First treat the Exterior, then the Interior,"[191] especially if there is Dampness. If the patient is, however, *severely* or *clearly* Deficient (showing *clear* patterns with symptoms *and* signs of

---

189. Although Liu Wansu designed treatments with regard to time and place, the patient's health condition (e.g., constitutional factors), and the characteristics of the disease, he stated that at the same time pathogenic-Fire/Heat was an underlying force that often had to be dealt with using cool and cold herbs. He often tonified Yin as well.

190. Together with the school of Spleen and Stomach, these are the four schools of the Jin-Yuan period.

191. In *Spiritual Axis*, however, it is also said: "One should first treat the root, then later treat the symptoms."

Diagnosis

Deficiency), it is this author's approach to use mild-neutral herbal tonic formulas with the addition of secondary herbs, and, at lower dosages, to treat Excesses and obstructions. This is done in order to minimize unwanted side-effects and maximize patient compliance. This is important when treating protracted diseases, because the patient may need to take herbs for extended periods. Manual therapies and acupuncture (with which the above rules are less important) are aimed at obstructions, restrictions of flow, restricted movements/motions and Pathogenic Factors (i.e., Excesses and Exterior). At the same time, for example, when treating back pain due to "malalignment" (vertebral dysfunctions) one may use massage to treat the muscle spasm which is the branch and manipulation to treat malalignment which is the root. As the channels are more superficial than the Organ systems and therefor more Yang, and Yang tends towards Excess, it is not a mistake to sedate Excesses in somatic areas (channels) using acupuncture in a generally weak and Deficient patient.

To ascertain if symptoms are so-called "false," or to discern if Excess or Deficiency is predominant, both general information such as pulse, tongue, nails, abdomen, spirit, chronicity, age, and localized tissue-feel and function should be considered carefully. Again, a good history is often the key to successful treatment.

- Almost all chronic disorders are Internal conditions, often with Blood-stasis, Phlegm, involvement of network-vessels and Kidneys. If degenerative in nature, they often involve Essence-Qi as well. The patient's digestive system must first be restored in many such cases, as normal digestion is needed to absorb and *tolerate* many of the herbs that treat the Interior, especially tonics. The use of modern digestive enzymes and addressing abnormal intestinal flora is often helpful. The stressful effects caused by chronic disease or pain almost always result in Qi-stagnation and Liver disorders which need to be addressed; and also help with digestive functions.
- Almost all acute disorders are External conditions. However, many diseases such as nuclear disc herniations for example, are Internal or mixed.
- When both Yang and Yin are deficient, the patient may show symptoms and signs of both Heat and Cold, which should not be confused with Shao-Yang (external pathogenic) disease. The key is a more regular appearance (timing) of Heat symptoms (e.g., nightly fever) as opposed to the erratic character of Exterior conditions (although Shao-Yang is often characterized by *cyclical* manifestations as well. The cyclical nature is, however, said to be not as regular, except that, for example, malaria, often a Shao-Yang disease, can manifest regularity).
- Prolonged stress (pain) can exhaust Righteous and Defensive Qi. An external pathogen can then be concealed in the Connecting channels (Network-vessels), membranes, and muscles without any manifestation of Exterior syndrome, and is said capable of injuring Yin and Essence. Later, often with additional weakness or a new exposure to pathogens, symptoms arise and simulate Internal Damage. In Warm-diseases, this type of manifestation is considered to manifest in the Interior, and appropriate Interior therapies are given. In musculoskeletal disorders, however, attention to Pathogenic Factors first or in combination may be more appropriate. The pathogens are usually guided outwards (a layered approach).
- Signs and symptoms of Heat are common, as all stagnations/congestions (depressions) and Deficiency (Qi, Yang, Blood, Yin, or Essence) can result in: transformative/congested-Heat, Exterior or Interior pathogenic-Heat, Empty-Heat or un-rooted Yang syndromes (false-Heat).

Most musculoskeletal disorders of Excess-Heat are acute, come on quickly, and usually have a clear precipitating factor that can be identified. This may be due to internal or external origin, except in lurking/hidden Warm-diseases. Most musculoskeletal disorders caused by Empty-Heat come-on slowly and arise from chronic physiological or disease processes which are due to Deficiencies and insidious processes (except when they are a result of acute Heat/fever damaging Fluids).

- True Excess results often in persistent (constant) symptoms. Deficiencies often result in symptoms that come and go. Thus, symptoms such as distension, fullness, and strong point tenderness, that may be interpreted as Excess but that come and go, may still be due to (or rooted in) Deficiency.
- The conditions of uppermost areas (trunk, head, upper back) often take precedence over the conditions of the lower parts, *when using acupuncture.*

For example, a patient with red complexion, a feeling of warmth in the head, tight subcostal areas, and with cold feet (a possible Cold-Deficient sign), often has a primary Heat or Qi-stagnation (Excess) disorder that accounts for the cold extremities. One, for example, should not conclude that a patient is Kidney Yang-deficient just because he/she has cold lower extremities. Cold extremities are often due to Damp-Heat or any other factor that obstructs or affects circulation.[192]

When using *herbs* and in *chronic illness,* however, following information from the lower body may takes precedence. This is because acupuncture is by and large a sedating external therapy, while oral herbs may be more useful as tonics and are an internal therapy.

The *Classic of Internal Medicine* states: "When the patient's body is in poor condition, his or her vitality can be improved with warm herbs. If the patient has a deficiency of Nutrient-Qi (vital essences), this can be

---

192. Although, as with all information, all symptoms and signs have meaning only within the context of the whole picture of symptoms and signs.

strengthened by using the five flavors (nutrition and herbs)...If [disease] results in an Excess condition, it should be dispersed and drained off (by using acupuncture and bleeding)."[193]

- Patients with chronic musculoskeletal disorders but who show a *vacuity* of systemic symptoms and signs (except for their musculoskeletal pain), often suffer from Phlegm and Qi-stagnation disorders. They often have pain that comes and goes and appear generally healthy (and they may have little of the usual symptoms and signs related to Phlegm and Qi-stagnation), especially between attacks. They tend to be in the postural/dysfunction stage of the degenerative cascade (see "TCM and the Degenerative Cascade" on page 556), even though they have been suffering from occasional pain for a long time.

PRIORITIES IN TREATMENT MUST BE SET OFTEN. Prioritizing and choosing treatment principles is often complex and may differ widely between different practitioners and schools of Chinese medical thought. The following are some general ideas this author finds helpful when treating *musculoskeletal* disorders:

- In the presence of both Dampness and Dryness (or Yin-deficiency), Dampness is often treated first, although treating Organ Yin-deficiency can resolve pathogenic Dampness, especially when Dampness/Phlegm is due to Empty-Fire congealing the Fluids. The use of drying herbs in patients with Yin-deficiency must be done with care, even though they may have a combined secondary Phlegm/Dampness or Damp-Heat.[194] The correct balance between Yin tonifying, Blood nourishing and Dampness expelling/transforming herbs must be used. Treatment must be adjusted often to reflect frequent changes. Neutral (mild) quality herbs (not too hot, spicy, cold, or cloying/greasy) may be preferable. This is especially true in patients with *secondary* symptoms/signs of Damp-Heat due to *Deficiency-accumulation-transformative-Heat,* and in patients with Dampness and Yin-deficiency. The formulas should *gradually* improve Spleen health (which is often the source of Damp/Phlegm) by using mildly sweet herbs which are not too warm, and that tonify Yin and clear-Heat with herbs that are not greasy (cloy) or very cold. Cold herbs are added with caution as they can easily damage Yin-Yang and Spleen/pancreas. Formulas that treat Spleen-Yin can often be used.[195]

On the other hand, Phlegm or Dampness can also result from Yin-deficiency which thickens Fluids/Yin, and then moistening-Yin may be used as the principal treatment. When treating a patient with Phlegm or Dampness by using warming Yang and draining Fluids herbs results in dryness (often seen only on tongue), increased thirst, or constipation, the diagnosis of Yin-deficiency and Phlegm must be considered. The main treatment principle may need to be shifted to moistening Yin.

If moistening Yin results in trapped Dampness, Phlegm, or digestive symptoms arise, herbs such as: Fructus Hordei Germinatus (Ma Ya), Fructus Oryzae Germinatus (Gu Ya), Endothelium Coreum Gigerae Galli (Ji Nei Jin),

---

193. Dr. Miriam Lee used to say that all acupuncture techniques have draining effects, even though acupuncture can be used in Deficient patients and conditions. Moxibustion is said to have tonifying effects especially on Blood.

194. The use of spicy herbs that "open" the surface and cause "sweating" are to be used with caution in patients with Yin/Fluid/Blood deficiency. Sweating can further damage Yin, Fluids and/or Blood. According to the classic, *On Cold Damage*, spicy herbs to open the surface should not be used (or used with caution) even in a patient with an acute Exterior-Cold syndrome, if the patient is significantly deficient in Yin, Blood, Fluids, or Yang. Such an approach is said to be capable of causing a collapse of Yang with chills, shivering, shaking, spasms, and disturbed spirit. It is therefore important to remember that excessive sweating can injure not only Fluids, but also Yang. Therefore, the promotion of sweating is also said to be contraindicated in patients that are Yang-deficient and sweat spontaneously or too easily. At the same time, some cases of trapped-Heat, excess-Heat, and Yang-stasis (all Excesses) can be treated using Ma Huang Teng (a spicy warm formula) which is said to push the Heat out via the surface or even by causing a nose bleed.

195. The following herbs are said not to be excessively cloying (greasy and sticky): Radix Glehniae (Sha Shen), Rhizoma Polygonati (Yu Zhu), Rhizoma Phragmitis (Lu Gen), Herba Pyrolae (Lu Xian Cao), Ramulus Loranthi (Sang Ji Sheng), Fructus Ligustri (Nu Zhen Zhi), Herba Ecliptae (Han Lian Cao) and Bulbus Lilii (Bai He). The following herbs can treat Dampness without being overly harsh and damaging to Yin/Fluids: Semen Coicis (Yi Yi Ren), Poria (Fu Ling), Radix Dioscoreae (Shan Yao), Talc (Hua Shi), Semen Lablab (Bai Bian Dao), Flos Lablab (Bai Bian Hua), Herba Agastaches (Huo Xiang), Herba Eupatorii (Pei Lan) and Semen Nelumbinis (Lian Zi). These are commonly used in neutral and mild herbal formulations.

Examples of mild formulas used by the Yang-Gao family style are:

Nourish Joint Clear Heat (inflammation) Tea: Qin Jiao 6g, Fang Feng 6g, Gao Teng 6g, Bai Shao 6g, Cao Ju Ming 12g, Suan Zao Ren 12g, Ju Hua 6g, Mai Ya 12g, Bai Zhi Ren 9g, Wei Ling Xian 6g.

Nourish Spleen Tea: Can Cao 3g, Fu Shen 9g, Mai Ya 12g, Bai Zi Ren 5g, Lian Zi 12g, Da Zao 4g, San Yao 9g, Wu Dou Hua 9g.

Harmonize Center Tea: Su Gen 5g, Gu Ya 12g, Fu Ling 12g, Bai Shao 5g, Ju Hua 3g, Gan Cao 5g, Nan Dou Hua 5g, Da Fu Pi 9g, Shen Qu 5g, Mian Yin Chen 9g.

Stomach-Heat food stagnation Tea: Bu Ja Ye 12g, Chun Tui 4.5g, Bian Dou Hua 6g, Gan Cao 3g, Gu Ya 12g, Bai Shao 4.5g, Shi Hu 6g, Cao Jue Ming 12g, Mai Ya 12g, Lian Zi 12g, Fu Shen 12g, Mian Yin Chen 9g, Suan Zao Ren 12g.

Food stagnation Spleen-deficiency Tea: San Yao 12g, Fu Ling 12g, Bian Dou Hua 6g, Suan Zao Ren 12g, Gan Cao 1g, Gu Ya 12g, Sang Ji Sheng 6g.

Common Cold Tea: Su Gen 3g, Bian Dou Hua 5g, Ju Hua 5g, Ge Hua 5g, Gu Ya 9g, Gan Cao 3g, Gou Teng 3g, Mian Yin Chen 9g, Wei Jing 9g, Bai Wei 3g.

Nourish Liver Tea: Suan Zao Ren 12g, Fu Ling 12g, Mai Ya 12g, Zhi Mu 5g, Rui Ren Yo 9g, Tu Si Zi 12g, Lian Xu 5g, Gan Cao 5g, Gou Qi Zi 9g, Su Xin Hua 5g.

Tonify Blood Tea: Fu Ling 10g, Bai Zi Ren 10g, Shang Ji Sheng 10g, San Yao 10g, Tu Si Zi 10g, Lin Su 3g, Nu Zhen Zhi 10g, Huang Jing 10g, Sha Ren 5g.

Tonify Qi and Blood Tea: Chuang Xiong 5g, Fu Ling 10g, Tu Si Zhi 10g, Bai Shao 6g, Dang Gui 4g, Bai Zi Ren 10g, Dang Shen 15g, Huang Jing 15g, Huang Qi 15g, Sha Ren 4g.

Radix Curcumae (Yu Jin), Pericarpium Trichosanthis (Gua Lou Pi), and Semen Armeniacae Amarum (Xing Ren), are used to restore proper digestive function and free trapped Dampness or Phlegm.

- Dampness often takes precedence over other pathogens as it can attract and bind to other Pathogenic Factors making them worse. Also, since Dampness is often a result of Spleen/Stomach's failing to transform and transport, care must be taken so as not to injure the Spleen/Stomach further by using too harsh, spicy, fragrant or cold formulas.

  With Damp-Heat, attention to Dampness often takes precedence since with the expulsion of Dampness the Heat often resolves. However, if Heat far exceeds Dampness, more emphasis is put on clearing Heat first, as this may help resolve and prevent Fluid-stagnation-accumulation and thus the formation of *pathogenic*-Dampness or Phlegm. Dampness can easily obstruct Qi and result in symptoms of fatigue, cold extremities, and paleness, all of which can easily be mistaken for a Yang-deficient condition. This should not be confused with deficiency-Fatigue.

  Slightly warming and fragrant herbs are therefore needed often even in patients with Damp-Heat, and Qi moving herbs are essential for treating Damp-accumulations as Dampness always obstructs Qi.

- In the presence of both Heat and Cold, Heat is often treated first or emphasized, unless the Fire (often local) is the result of accumulation from Cold/deficiency-stagnation-transformative/congested-Heat. In that case, it is better to use both cold and hot medicines, or warming herbs alone. In such cases, often the body of the tongue shows Coldness/deficiency, and the coat (or local tissue) shows Heat (or vice versa).

  Transformative/congested-Heat, in patients with a root disease mechanism of Yang-deficiency-Cold, and who show a *large moist* tongue with teethmarks, a deep weak pulse (weak or limited rising of pulse wave) and no *moons* under their finger nails,[196] (even if for example, they suffer from herpatic neuralgia with burning pain which may suggest Heat), may best be treated with formulas containing Radix Aconiti praeparata (Fu Zi). Heat signs and symptoms then often resolve on their own. A small dose of Heat clearing herbs can be added if needed.

It is not uncommon to see a yellow tongue coat change to a normal thin white coat in patients treated with hot formulas when the root disease mechanism is Yang-deficiency-Cold.

If however the tongue is dry, red, or small, and the patient does *not* have *moons* under the finger nails, a neutral or often Spleen-Yin tonification may be appropriate. If both Yin and Yang are deficient and the patient easily develops symptoms of Heat (Empty, transformative or Mingmen rising), a large dose of Radix Reumanniae (Sheng Di Huang) and Rhizoma Alismatis (Ze Xie) can be used together with warm Yang tonics.

Also, it is important to remember that Heat signs from hidden-Heat are often said to be secondary to being trapped by the use of cold natures medicinals or foods. In such cases it is important to use warming herbs combined with colder herbs. For example, for hidden-muscle-Heat or for muscle pain from Spring-Warm and/or Summer-Heat the use of modified Ten Spirit Decoction (Shi Shen Tang) is said to be helpful: Notopteryggi (Qiang Huo), Radix Puerariae (Ge Gen), Radix Ligustici (Chuan Xiong), Radix Angelica (Bai Zhi), Radix Paeoniae (Chi Shao), Folium Perillae (Zi Su), Pericarpium Citri (Chen Pi), Rhizoma (Cimicifugae (Sheng Ma), Rhizoma Cypri (Xiang Fu), Bombycis (Jiang Can), and Radix Glycyrrhizae (Gan Gao).

- The balance between addressing Excess/Fullness, Deficiency/Emptiness, Interior, Exterior, Hot and Cold demands skill and experience. Pathogenic Factors can be trapped (or hidden) and can result in extreme fatigue that can simulate Interior (Deficiency) syndromes. Prolonged and hidden pathogens may produce transformative/congested-Heat that can sometimes simulate Yin-deficiency-Empty-Heat. Tonifying and moistening can sometimes aggravate the condition. Therefore, deeply seated Pathogenic Factors (or when they enter the network-vessels) are often treated first (by sedating techniques often using animal and insect medicines, and/or blood-letting), even though the patient may appear Deficient and weak. Moistening and tonifying herbs erroneously administered in a chronic and enduring disease, in which Pathogens are deep and account for Deficiency symptoms and signs, can sometimes help retain and aggravate the condition further. For example, in many acute abdominal disorders (such as appendicitis), unless the Pathogenic Factors are purged, the patient's Righteous-Qi will not recover, particularly if the patient is weak or elderly. (A combined approach may be needed.) Weak patients with Excess-Damp/Phlegm often do worse if one tonifies the Spleen before, or without, eliminating the pathogenic Damp/Phlegm and regulating Qi. This is often true in weak patients with Blood-stasis and other retained Pathogenic Factors as well.

  If the patient's disease is a result of external (climatic) influences, and the patient is seen some (or even fairly long) time after the onset, and then shows some symp-

---

196. The presence or absence of moons under the finger nails are helpful signs that may indicate the condition of the patient's Yang-Qi. Many patients with unclear symptoms/signs and with no moons, swollen thick tongue, and no other obvious tongue Heat signs, do very well on formulas such as Fu Zi Li Zhong. Often, even when there are some signs or symptoms of Heat, these patients still do well on Aconite formulas. Herbs such as Shi Gao, Sheng Di, Huang Bai and Zhi Mu may be added to address *secondary-stagnant-Heat* or possible side-effects. Large dosage of Fu Zi (upto 60g/day) is often the key for successful herbal therapy in musculoskeletal disorders. If the patient develops thirst, dry mouth or tongue, however, this approach must be reconsidered or the dosage of Shi Gao and Di Hunag can be increased.

toms/signs of Interior depletion, treatment often should still first focus mainly on eliminating external influences. Tonifying too early is said to be capable of "strengthening" the pathogens and further depleting Righteous-Qi. Again, a neutral-mild tonification and dispersion at the same time may be the best approach in some patients. When using combined tonification and elimination (purging, out-thrusting/opening surface, etc.), close attention to dosage of herbs is paramount. Another helpful approach is to use herbs and formulas that mainly "transform" (Hua). This treatment approach usually focuses on movement (of the bodily milieu and pathogens) rather than strongly affecting either Righteous-Qi or pathogens. Harmonizing (He Fa) which also *adjusts* function rather than attacking or tonifying is often a useful approach as well.

On the other hand, because in chronic and prolonged diseases the pathogens may attack and lodge in the channels, network-vessels, and Organs, and because chronic disease affects the Kidneys, the pathogens may enter the bones becoming "glued" and difficult to remove. Phlegm and Blood-stasis coalesce, obstructing flow, congealing, stagnating, and accumulating. Pathogens and Righteous-Qi may mix, and swelling, degeneration, and pain become chronic and difficult to separate or treat. In such patients, primary attention to Deficiency may be required in order to increase the body's ability to eliminate Pathogenic Factors; as Sun Zi says: "Open a corner for the thief to escape." Primary attention to Deficiency then may prevent unnecessary injury to the patient. Although treatment may involve many Organs, symptoms of Kidney-Yang-deficiency are quite common, and tonifying the Kidneys and strengthening the Governing (Du) and Girdle (Dai) channels may be required.

Frequent external contractions can also occur easily in Deficient patients. Nutritive and Defensive Qis are disharmonious and weak. Symptoms such as chills, fatigue, fever, headache, Phlegm, and bleeding may simulate Internal syndromes. Care must be given not to overly tonify, as this easily results in the exhaustion of Righteous-Qi and the retention of Pathogenic Factors.[197] However, if Central-Qi is insufficient and Nutritive and Defensive Qi are weakened (or the patient's constitution is weak), he/she can easily be infected by external Pathogenic Factors. Just using surface expelling herbs may not work and may even result in a deeper penetration of pathogens. Simultaneous tonification and surface expelling/resolving herbs are combined. In patients that do not tolerate tonification (which may lead to congestion, stagnation, and increased symptoms) the Harmonizing or Transforming methods may be used. For example, a variation on Cinnamon Twig Decoction (Gui Zhi Teng) can be used to both Transform and Harmonize and is commonly used in musculoskeletal disorders.

- Two or more *unrelated* disease *processes* may be seen in the same patient, and may even manifest in the same joint (area/system). This occurs if one, for example, has a meniscal tear (acute or repeated *derangements*) at the knee, and at the same time the patient suffers from, lets say, Qi and Blood-deficiency with Cold-Damp Painful Obstruction (Bi) syndrome of the same knee, or some other joint problem (arthrosis). Symptoms arising from meniscal derangement (often acute and come-and-go) may manifest as local excess-Damp-Heat and Blood-stasis, thus manifesting two disparate pathomechanisms at different times within the same joint.

A patient that suffers from back and leg pain caused by Kidney-deficiency, Blood-stasis, and Wind, who then suddenly develops acute shoulder capsulitis, may show contradictory symptom/signs in the low back and shoulder with one being predominately Cold and the other predominately Hot. The shoulder symptoms may be due to a normal progression of Kidney-deficiency-Cold which then transforms into Heat (at the shoulder), or the two conditions may be unrelated and represent two distinct processes. One then needs to carefully ascertain which disease process is predominant (again considering local and general signs) and emphasize herbs that treat the dominant condition. Even if one decides to treat both at the same time (which in some patients can aggravate more than help) still, the relative portions of herbs need to be considered carefully. At times, one can use an external formula for one and oral herbs for the other. At other times, more than one formula is given at different times (i.e. one can treat each pathocondition or pattern separately; for example, taking a formula before a meal to treat the lower body, and a second formula after the meal to treat the upper body). Formulas from the Harmonizing category are often appropriate in dealing with conflicting clinical presentations because of their balanced design. Manual and acupuncture therapies can be used locally while at the same time treating the patient's general condition with herbs. Again, dosage must be considered carefully. It may even be necessary to ignore one condition until the other improves. Different areas on the same or different channels may feel different. In *Spiritual Axis*, when discussing the minute needle, it states:

> When it is said that Emptiness should be tonified, it means the opening of Qi is empty, and should be tonified at that point. Overflowing should be drained, which means the Qi opening is full and should be drained at that point. When it is stagnant and spoiled, it should be removed, which means to drain from the Blood channels. Evil to be overcome must be drained, which means when the channels are full, they should be drained and dispersed of evil.

---

197. Zhu Dan Xi states: "Try to astringe sweat, but the sweat increases. Try to calm spirit, but restlessness augments. Try to moisten Yin, but the congested Heat worsens. Try to tonify Qi, but bloating intensifies. Failure is due to inability to recognize the presence of external evil [pathogens], and to note that this is not a genuine Deficiency."

Table 1-37: Visual Examination General

OBSERVATION OF SPIRIT	Spirit/Shen is the external manifestation of the individual's life and health. Brightness of eyes, facial expression, clarity of speech and thought, coordination, alertness are all evaluated and provide information as to the condition of the Spirit/Shen. *Lack of Spirit*: dullness and slowness of eyes, weakness of breath and speech, confusion, emaciation, swellings, listlessness, pale dull complexion. A patient who has Spirit is fundamentally healthy; the prognosis is good. If form is damaged it can affect Spirit.
OBSERVATION OF BODY	Complexion, skin color, sheen, texture. Lack of sheen (moisture and luster) means disease is serious and difficult to cure. Rough, coarse, and scaly skin often indicates Blood-stasis. Dry, emaciated (withered) often indicate Fluid/Blood/Yin-deficiency. Papular eruptions are generally Tai-Yin Wind-Heat. Macular eruptions are generally Yang-Ming Heat-Toxin or Blood-Heat and more serious than papular eruptions. Can also be caused by strong-Cold condition (Yin-macule), the color would be pale or dusky. • Red— Heat (Deficient or Excess). —Malar flush with bright red color especially in the afternoon or with otherwise pale face—empty-Heat. —Entire face, interior signs of excess; constipation, irritability, thirst, tidal or constant redness—excess-Heat. —Exterior symptoms and red eyes—Wind-Heat, if with Interior Liver symptoms/signs and red eyes—empty or excess Liver-Heat. —Infections, autoimmune diseases. • White—mostly Cold and/or Deficiency. —Pale with swelling—Qi-deficiency. —Lusterless (emaciated) face—Blood-deficiency. —Cold from Exterior or Interior. —Anemia, cardiovascular, respiratory disease. • Cyan/Bluish/Purple/Green—mostly stagnation/stasis. —If under eyes often Liver related. —Cold mostly from Wind-Cold. —Constitutional weakness; often around chin and mouth as well as eyes. —Pain. —Convulsion/spasm, blood vessel constriction. —Cardiovascular or respiratory stasis. —Fright. • Yellow—mostly Dampness, Spleen-deficiency. —Flabby—Damp accumulation due to Spleen failure of transportation and transformation. —Weakness, pale yellow, dry and puffy skin—post illness from deficiency of Qi, Blood and Spleen/pancreas. —Jaundice, orange yellow or bright—Damp-Heat. —Jaundice, dark—Cold-Damp or Damp-Heat with predominance of Dampness. —Liver, Spleen, Pancreas and Gall Bladder diseases. • Black, Gray—mostly Kidney-deficiency, Essence-depletion, Blood-stasis, Phlegm-accumulation, Cold. —Deep in color and withered (emaciated)—serious disease with damage to Qi and Essence. —Dark gray around eyes and swollen—Phlegm due to Kidney-deficiency, or Phlegm and Blood-stasis. —Renal, or end-stage Kidney, Liver or other serious diseases. Weight. • Excessive weight may result in dampness/Phlegm and more Blood less Qi. • Excessive leanness is often due to Yin-deficiency, Heat or Spleen and Stomach weakness and more Qi less Blood. General condition. • Muscular indicates a strong (Yang) constitution. • Weak muscles indicate a weak (Yin) constitution. Limbs. • Swelling is usually ascribed to Excess/Full patterns. • Atrophy, lack of strength, softness, often due to Deficiency, Wei-syndromes, and malnourishment. • Extension restriction usually due to Sinew diseases, more superficial disease. • Flexion restriction often due to bony diseases, deep disease.

Table 1-38: Visual Examination Tongue

TONGUE	Reflects the state of Qi and Blood, progression and location of disease, degree of Cold and Heat (for example in deficiency of both Yin and Yang shows which is predominant), depth of penetration of exogenous pathogens, condition of the Organs. Tongue spirit is observed mainly on the root of the tongue because of the relations to the Kidneys.
GENERAL CONSIDERATIONS	**Tongue body** may reflect the patient's general constitution or if there is false Cold/Heat. Useful more in chronic conditions. Reflects primarily conditions of Deficiency or Excess. Cracks, depressions, localized swelling or drawn-in-areas reflect disharmony of the specific Organ or related body area, but must be correlated to symptoms and signs. The degree of tongue body swelling is often inversely correlated to strength of Yang or True-Qi. The patient is often suffering from hypofunctioning systems and/or Phlegm/Damp accumulation. Blood-stasis from trauma often does not show on the tongue. Localized somatic tissues-Fire may or may not show on tongue. In Liver, skin (and musculoskeletal) disorders the tongue may not show the condition, especially in Liver Qi-stagnation/Wind (or may see false impressions). Rough, coarse, hard, tough tongue often relate to Excess/Fullness conditions. Tender, fine, swollen, with teeth marks, or shrunken often relate to Deficiency/Emptiness conditions. **Tongue coat** is an important indicator in acute febrile/infectious disorders, showing disease depth (level of penetration of pathogens). In general the quality of coat is more reliable than the body in Damp disorders; the body color more reliable in Hot disorders. The coat reflect more the condition of the Yang (Fu) Organs and is easily influenced by short-term factors. Rootless, or no coat at root of tongue, may be due to Stomach-Qi-weakness, Yin or Kidney-Yin-deficiency, and therefore, seen in a weak patient that must be treated with more care. Illness due to pathogenic-Heat almost always affects the coating (*reduced* in deficient-Yin-Heat, or Warm pathogens in the Nutritive or Blood depth/divisions). Smoking, hot spices, many foods may dry the tongue coat. May affect color.
TONGUE FORM (BODY)	**Enlargement.** A swollen enlarged tongue indicates Deficiency of: Qi, True-Qi, Yang. Or Excess: Phlegm, Damp or Phlegm-Fire. Phlegm may affect more the tongue body while Dampness more the tongue coat. Seen in edema, digestive (Sp/St) disorders, kidney disorders, chronic illness or severe infections. (Swollen enlarged tongue is often due to hyperplasia of connective tissue, tissue edema, or blood and lymphatic drainage disturbances). If *body and edges* are swollen this often indicates Spleen/pancreas weakness. If swollen *at edges only*, often indicates Liver-Qi-stagnation. Pale and narrow (center of tongue body not swollen) and *rolled-up slightly/swollen edges*, often seen with deficiency of Blood and Liver-Qi-stagnation or Qi and Blood-deficiency resulting in impaired circulation (Qi/Blood-stagnation). Upper 1/3 wider-shaped and *pale* is seen in severe exhaustion of Central-Qi. Upper 1/3 wider-shaped and *red* is seen in severe exhaustion of Yin. May also look contracted at rear. Swollen at the *tip* seen often in Heart or Lung disorders. **Shrinkage.** A thin, shrunken or contracted tongue usually indicates Yin/Fluids or Blood-deficiency or damage. If pale with depression/shrinkage *at root* often indicates weakening of Essence and/or Kidney-Yin-deficiency. Short and red may be seen in severe exhaustion of Kidneys and/or Liver-Yin-deficiency with Heat. **Fissures.** Fissures/Cracks may indicate Fluid depletion and conditions that affect the Spleen and Stomach; however, this condition may also be normal. Small *horizontal cracks* are seen with Heat and dryness, or Yin-deficiency, especially if tongue body is red or slightly red. Small cracks and *pale* tongue body seen in Blood-deficiency. If *only superficial* cracks may be Spleen/pancreas Qi and Blood-deficiency. If cracks are *deep* there is Fluid injury. Small *irregular horizontal* cracks at *center* of tongue, together with *pale body*, often indicate Stomach-Yin-deficiency. If tongue body also *red* indicates Heat.
PAPILLAE AND SPOTS	**Speckles and Prickles** (elevated papillae, or flakes of coat on papillae) indicate excess-Heat. Occurs in patients suffering from constipation, insomnia (especially if at tip of tongue) or Lung (upper 1/3) and other infections/Fire/Heat/Phlegm-Fire. Flaring upwards of Ministerial-Fire. Red spots are sometimes seen at the root of the tongue which are larger than red papllae and reflect Heat with Blood-stasis. Purple spots are usually related to Blood-stasis or extreme Heat. A single relatively large purple spot may relate to trauma with the location reflected on the tongue; the tip reflecting the head and root the lower extremities.
BODY COLORS	Reflects mainly the state of the Yin Organs and Blood and shows conditions of Heat or Cold, Yin or Yang deficiency. Pale red Normal. Pale Deficiency, hypofunction, Cold. Red Heat. Purple Stagnation, stasis, severe-Heat, possibly Cold. Dusky/dark Cold, stagnation, stasis or severe-Heat. Blue-green Yin Cold and Blood-stasis.

Table 1-38: Visual Examination Tongue (Continued)

MOISTURE/YIN	**Condition of Body Fluids/Yin/Blood and Heat.** **Mirror or Shiny** with a light-reflection on tongue seen in Yin/Fluid-depletion. Mirror tongue is caused by the papillae disappearing, making it look like a mirror and indicating Qi and Yin-deficiency. A *pale* mirror tongue is seen with deficiency of Blood due to Spleen and Stomach deficiency and is seen often at the tongue's edges. A shiny tongue is *always red* or dark red, and always indicates severe Kidney-deficiency. In Kidney-Yin-deficiency the tongue is red and its coat is peeled. May also see a pale red tongue and no coat at root *or discolored reddish root, or increased roughness at root.* The dryness of Yin can create an *old looking* coat (often looks thick, layered and yellow). Seen often as sequelae of severe-Heat. In Stomach-Yin-deficiency, first the center of tongue dries; if also red it indicates Heat. Typically Stomach-Yin-deficiency if red and peeled; if *no coat,* then Kidney and Stomach-Yin-deficiency. If *also swollen pale* or pale red, then complicated with Spleen/pancreas deficiency and Dampness. Dry pale can also indicate Hot condition. Dry or dry/pale or pale *on edges only,* often indicates Liver-Blood-deficiency. *Tip dry red* and possibly cracked indicate Heart-Yin-deficiency or flaming Fire. If affects the *front 1/3* indicates Lung is affected.
MOVEMENT	**Trembling.** Often seen in diseases such as Wind, Hyperactivity of Liver-Yang, excess-Heat, and Qi-deficiency (tongue quivering). **Stiffness (Wry).** Seen in serious diseases such as Wind-Strike (stroke), Heat in the Pericardium, diseases of the sea of marrow (brain), depleted Essence.
COAT	Generally indicates the depth of pathogenic factor penetration, Stomach condition, level of Dampness/Phlegm, Food stagnation, Yin/Fluid condition. Dampness tends to reflect as slippery and smooth coat, while Phlegm in slightly rough and sticky coat. Dry — Dry pathogenic factor, Heat, Qi-damage—even if white and thick. Greasy, sticky, glossy (with strong reflection) — Dampness, Phlegm, food stagnation. Peeling, patchy — Yin-insufficiency or deficiency and damage of Stomach-Qi Rootless (floating, easily scrapped off) — True-Qi weakness. White — Cold. Yellow — Heat. Black — Abundant pathogen.

Table 1-39: Pulses

PULSE	PULSE DESCRIPTION	INDICATION
FLOATING PULSES	Floating, surging/tidal, deficient/empty, scallion, scattered, soft/soggy, drum skin/leathery.	Various deficiencies, Heat, Exterior syndromes.
FLOATING/ SUPERFICIAL	*Floating,* felt at superficial level as soon as touching skin (above Qi-depth) but less perceptible with slight pressure. (Some consider the Qi-depth as being at the surface of the blood *vessel* when first feeling the pulse; others as at a fixed depth with pre-determined pressure). Must not be confused with the Deficient pulses.	Superficial, Exterior disorder or Deficient patient. If deeper levels strong, then Superficial syndrome. If deeper levels weak, then Deficient patient.
TIDAL/SURGING	*Floating,* (but not all the way to surface) forceful, large, coming-on with force/speed, departing with less force/speed. or Departing deeply at proximal position (*chi*) with less force but emerging with force at distal position (*inch*) (with severe deficiency often more pounding than tidal).	excess-Heat at Qi-division. Heat with Yin-Blood-Essence deficiency (often more pounding than tidal). Kidney-deficient-Fire, Heart and Kidney not communicating.
DEFICIENT/VACUOUS/ EMPTY	*Floating,* (but not all the way to surface) large, slow, empty, soft, forceless.	Blood/Yin-deficiency. Qi/Blood-deficiency. Yin-deficiency-Heat (often has a wiry quality). Essence-deficiency. Summer-Heat damaging Qi and Yin.
SCALLION	*Floating,* (but not all the way to surface) soft, large body, empty center (Blood [middle] depth disappears) but usually with some presence deeply.	Blood severely deficient (often due to bleeding).
SCATTERED	*Floating,* (occasionally above Qi-level at skin level) large, no root, with light pressure irregular, disappears quickly with strong pressure (edges of pulse not clear).	Desertion: Blood/Yin/Essence and Qi. Separation of Yin and Yang.

Table 1-39: Pulses (Continued)

Soft/Soggy	*Floating*, (but possibly not all the way to surface)[a] *fine*, soft and flexible (forceless with soft vessel). It gradually disappears with pressure but not as quickly as the scattered pulse.	Deficiency taxation. Qi/Blood-deficiency. Central (Sp/St) Yang-deficiency may also have concave vessel. Yin-deficiency if also fast. Dampness.
Leathery/Drum Skin	Floating (but not all the way to surface) hard vessel/surface, empty on pressure (yielding).	Sudden loss or severe deficiency of Yin/Blood/Essence. Separation of Yin and Yang. Deficiency-Cold (rarely). Extreme exterior-Cold (rarely).
Deep Pulses	Deep, weak, hidden, confined.	Various deficient or Interior conditions or deep obstructions.
Deep/Sinking	*Deep*, felt only on deep pressure at Organ/bone depth (some consider the Organ depth to be just above the level at which pressure obliterates the pulse near the bone; others at fixed depth/pressure).	Interior disorder, depletion of true-Qi, K Qi/Yang-deficiency. Rarely, form Exterior pathogens with obstructed Yang-Qi (severe infections and/or Qi-stagnation from cold). Obesity. Deep and tight/wiry—Qi and Yin-deficiency. Deep and slippery often due to stagnation or deficiency with stagnation (food, Phlegm, Blood).
Weak	*Deep*, fine, soft, thready, weak rising pulse force.	Deficient-Qi, Clear-Yang not rising, Yang-deficiency.
Hidden/Deep Feeble	*Very Deep* fine, not obvious, and forceless.	Qi/ Yang-deficiency. Blood-stasis. Qi-stagnation.
Confined/Hidden Excess	*Deep*, hard, firm, not changeable, large, wiry.	Cold-Damp congealed obstruction (may be transformed to Heat), severe pain. Or confined stagnant-Blood, Phlegm, food, Interior-Wind.
Pulse Rates	Slow, rapid, bound/irregular, regularly irregular, skipping/rapid irregular.	Cold, Heat, blockage, stasis and deficiencies.
Slow	*Below* 60 per min.	Cold, Deficient Qi/Yang, healthy athlete.
Rapid	*Above* 90 per min.	Heat (Yin-Heat or Yang-Heat). Fine soft, or tight/wiry→deficiency-Heat. or: Large forceless→deficient-Yang floating. Stress, anxiety, etc.
Bound/ Irregular	*Slow*, relaxed, stops at irregular intervals.	1)Forceful→ blockage. 2) Forceless→ Yang-deficiency. 3)Relaxed→ Heart-Qi-deficiency with stasis.
Regularly Irregular	*Slow*, relaxed, weak stops at regular intervals.	Visceral Qi-deficiency.
Rapid/Irregular (Skipping)	*Rapid*, irregularly interrupted.	1) If Forceful-→Yang-Heat hyperactive, Internal congestion (Qi, Blood, Phlegm, food). 2)If Forceless→Desertion (Qi, Blood).
Excess	*Long, wiry, **large, forceful**, hard, slippery, tight.*	Excess disorders.

Table 1-39: Pulses (Continued)

WIRY	Fine, thin, long, strong, clear edges, taut, has a cutting edge, may be felt on letting go. Found very often (with a range from a taught/pipe-like pulse to the very thin, hard unyielding string wiry-like quality).	*Liver Qi-stagnation, Yin-deficiency from the following causes*: 1) Emotion→Liver-congestion→Yin-deficiency, 2) Blood/Yin-deficiency→ Liver-congestion, 3) Spleen deficiency→Liver-congestion→Yin/Blood-deficiency, 4) Kidney-Yang or Yin-deficiency→Liver stagnation. If pulse *wiry and*: 1) Tight Fine=Yin-obstruction, or very deficient with Heat (Damp, Phlegm, food, Blood, or pain, with tansformative or deficiency-Heat). 2) Deep=Yin/Essence-deficiency with Qi-deficiency. 3) Large Slippery=Yang condition (pulse often more tight than wiry) if fast often due to infections. 4) Large Pounding=deficiency damage, mostly deficiency-Heat (hard artery) (usually more tight than wiry) or infection. 5) Both hands=Yin-deficiency with Heat, pain, chronic Cold. 6) Hard=Serious disease, arterial sclerosis, (often more tight/ropy than wiry). 7) One side double wiry pulse (as though two parallel arteries)=Phlegm with Qi-stagnation or mass. If felt more at Blood-depth, then usually pertains to Blood-Heat. The thinner and harder the more the Yin-deficiency with Heat.
TIGHT/ROPY	Tight, cord/pipe-like and easily separated from surrounding tissues, wider than wiry, strong, twisted like rope, pulse hits the finger moving from side to side.	Pain or Cold. Tight and Yielding (leathery-long) severe deficiency. Heat causing arterial sclerosis.
SLIPPERY	Smooth, uninhibited, rolling, tickling—independent from pressure.	Blood swirling (abundance or obstruction), Stagnation; Heat, Phlegm, Damp, food diseases. Fine= Damp with Spleen-deficiency, Phlegm from various Deficiencies. At Blood-depth (middle depth) seen with high lipids and Blood-Heat.
LARGE	Forceful, fills blood vessel.	Robust health.
VARIOUS WEAKNESSES	Short, Stirring/Bean, Choppy, Fine/thready, faint.	Various deficient conditions.
SHORT	Felt only in middle (*bar*).	Great Chest-Qi or Spleen-deficiency, (Heart and/or chest symptoms and signs). Yang-Qi-stagnation in middle warmer.
BEAN/SPINNING/STIRRING	Hard, short, or slippery, rapid and felt in middle position (*bar*) only. Moving back and forth.	Yin/Yang fighting, pain, fright.
CHOPPY/DIFFICULT/ROUGH	Stagnant, rough, uneven, variable, fine, hesitant. Pulse wave changes in amplitude, strength or timing. Pulse wave does not continue from position to position. Felt by rolling finger across positions mostly at Blood and Organ depths.	Qi Blood Yin-Yang deficient (often Essence-deficiency, serious condition). Mix Deficiency/Excess. Qi-stagnation or Cold-Dampness. Blood-stasis.
FINE/THREADY	Soft, thready, weak, but not scattered by pressure.	Qi/Blood-deficiency, (Yin/Blood-deficiency) Dampness.
FAINT	Very fine, soft, barely palpable, variable by adaptation of vessel to pressure (changes)	Extreme Qi and Blood-deficiency.
NON-CONGRUENCE	Pulse not congruent with condition (weak in a new acute disease, strong in a chronic weak disease etc.)	Denotes a serious and difficult to treat disorder.
ADDITIONAL INFORMATION[B]		
SPECIAL LUNG LOCATION **OTHER SPECIAL LOCATIONS**	Should have no special quality, should be the same as normal location. If different quality.	Lung disorder.
SLIPPERY LEFT DISTAL	Felt as the wave coming from under scaphoid. In general: rate normal or slow. Rapid. One small lateral area just over the tendon.	Phlegm in orifices. Phlegm-Fire. Mitral valve problem.

Table 1-39: Pulses (Continued)

Hollow/Full	When with pressure one feels diminished substance at Organ and/or Blood and Organ-depths (but still some present), but on release Blood-depth fills up, feels tense and/or slippery.	Blood-Heat, Blood-toxicity, Blood-stasis. When Blood-depth more tense → "Blood Unclear/Heat." When even more substantial at Qi-depth then "Blood thick."
Tense Hollow Full-Overflowing	Here the pulse rises from the Blood-depth to above the Qi-depth and feels swollen in a sine wave pattern.	Severe Heat from excess in Blood especially if rapid.
Taut → Tense → Tight Wiry	No-fluid qualities ranging in thickness and flexibility from about the D to A string of a violin. The taut pulse is like D string and wiry more like A string.	Degree of tightness of pulse as it has to do with the progression of Qi-stagnation excess-Heat, to deficient-Heat and their effects on the Yin/Blood and blood vessels. The harder and thinner the pulse the more Yin-deficiency and deficiency-Heat present.[c] The wider the pulse the more Qi-stagnation excess-Heat. The tense pulse roughly fits the traditional tight pulse.

a. According to Dr. Hammer. Others however disagree and say it is floating to surface.
b. These and other terms are special areas and qualities described by Dr. Hammer after Dr. Shen. Dr. Hammer teaches that the Qi, Blood, and Organ-depths are at fixed depths with little to no variability due to the patient's shape/weight.
c. Many other sources, however, emphasize the loss of tension in the vessel and soft-soggy qualities of the pulse as indicating a Yin-deficiency Empty-Heat.

Table 1-40: History and Inquiry

Topic	Indication
Aversion to cold with fever	At beginning or middle stage of infectious disease usually indicates Exterior syndrome. If with thirst and perspiration is due to Heat. Warm disease/Fire toxin i.e. epidemic disease. Localized infection/ Fire-toxin entering Blood/Nutritive-Qi, e.g. from sores, ulcers, etc.
High fever without chills	May be due to exogenous pathogenic chill penetrating the Interior and turning into Heat. Interior-Heat, Damp-Heat, Heat in Blood, Heat/Fire-toxin, Warm diseases.
Low fever without chills	Pathogenic Factors at Exterior or retained. Qi-deficiency. Yin/Blood-deficiency. Vigorous Dampness subdues Fire (may have chills or may even have slight fear of heat if from Damp-Heat).
Night fever	Yin, Nutritive division/depth illness, or Blood damage by Warm diseases. Yin-deficiency (Heat). Damp-Heat (more often in afternoon). Blood loss. Reactivation of hidden/latent pathogens in Nutritive division/depth.
Tidal fever	Yin/Blood-deficiency: Usually in afternoon or night. Yang-Ming-Heat or Qi division/depth Heat: Usually starts at dusk with constipation and abdominal distension, (often with cold extremities due to Warm-Heat Pathogenic Factors blocking Qi-circulation). Damp-Heat: Usually starts in afternoon. If Dampness dominates, fever will be low. Blood-stasis: Usually starts in afternoon or evening. Deficiency or damage of Qi: Usually starts in morning.
Alternating chills and fever	May indicate Pathogenic Factors are between Interior and Exterior, (Shao Yang division/depth, GB/TW).
Perspiration	Exterior syndrome without sweat may indicate Cold-Excess, with sweat indicates Heat or disharmony of Defensive and Nutritive-Qi. Night/sleep sweat usually indicates Yin or Blood-deficiency, but can also be any other Heat, Phlegm/Damp-Heat or food stagnation. Spontaneous sweating (or with extremely mild exertion) usually indicates Qi or Yang-deficiency, or disharmony of Defensive and Nutritive-Qi. May be seen also in retained Heat or Damp-Heat (pathogenic factor) i.e. after a history of illness. Profuse sweating with night fever usually indicates internal-Heat. Dripping with severe weakness can be from total collapse of Yang (shock). In head only may be from Heat in upper Warmer or Damp-Heat in middle-Warmer (often while eating). In head and face, with cold limbs, weak Qi/shortness of breath, and deep pulse, may be due to Yang-deficiency. Excessive when nervous usually indicates Heart disharmony (especially in palms and armpits as they are associated with Heart).
Appetite	No appetite usually indicates Spleen/pancreas dysfunction or Dampness; Exterior or Interior. No appetite with chest fullness/discomfort (short breath) often indicates Phlegm. Repulsion to food usually indicates food stagnation. Excessive appetite usually indicates Stomach-Heat. Hunger, but unable to eat, may indicate Stomach-Yin-deficiency. Craving for dirt may indicate pestilence disease.
Thirst	Generally indicates the condition of the body Fluid. *Excessive* thirst may indicate: • Consumption of Yin or stagnation of the body Fluids which fail to rise. • Heat syndromes. • Extreme thirst with preference for hot drinks can indicate a Phlegm-Cold-obstruction. • High fever with thirst but patient cannot drink, can indicate Pathogenic Factors in the Nutritive division and Blood. *Lack* of thirst can indicate Dampness/Phlegm, Spleen, Kidney, Qi or Yang-deficiency.
Taste	Bitter (bad) taste in mouth usually indicates Heat, especially in Liver and Gall Bladder (often in morning only). Sweet taste in mouth usually indicates Damp-Heat in the Spleen and Stomach. Sour taste in mouth usually indicates accumulation of Heat in Liver and Stomach. Tastelessness in the mouth usually indicates dysfunction in Spleen/pancreas or Damp pathogens.
Ears	In general related to Kidney health. • *Acute* tinnitus or hearing loss often due to Heat/Fire in Gall Bladder, Triple Warmer, or Liver, or to external Pathogenic Factors such as Wind-Heat or Damp-Heat. • Chronic tinnitus or hearing loss often related to Kidney weakness, Liver Yin/Blood-deficiency, Qi and Blood-stasis or Phlegm.

Table 1-40: History and Inquiry (Continued)

Topic	Indication
Eyes	Poor or clouded vision is often due to deficiency: of Blood, Kidneys, Liver or Spleen. Or obstruction: by phlegm and/or Qi/Blood. Poor night vision usually indicates Liver-Blood-weakness or Blood-stasis. Other deficiencies such as Spleen, Kidney, Heart can affect clear-Yang and Blood and also result in poor night vision. Spotty vision (floaters) usually indicates Liver-Blood-deficiency or phlegm/Blood stasis (often acute onset). Photosensitivity usually indicates poor nourishment of eyes due to Liver-Blood-deficiency with/without Heat, Pathogenic Factors obstructing nourishment to eyes, or general Qi and Blood deficiency. Dry eyes mostly due to Yin/Blood-deficiency or Exterior pathogenic Heat, or Spleen not raising Fluids. Itchy eyes usually indicates Wind due to internal (Blood-deficiency, Yin-deficiency, transformative-Heat) or external source (Wind-Heat, Heat-toxin, Wind-Cold). Damp-Heat often results in sensation of sand in eye. Red eyes usually indicate Exterior Heat (Wind-Heat, Fire-toxin) or Interior Heat (transformative-Heat, deficient-Heat, toxic-Heat). Sleeping with eyes open: Deficiency of Spleen/Stomach-Qi and Blood.
Stool	Dry stool shaped like sheep-dung usually indicates stagnation-Heat or Fluid exhaustion or Qi-stagnation with transformative-Heat. Dry stool followed by loose stool usually indicates dysfunction of the Spleen and Stomach with imbalance of Dryness and Dampness, Damp-Heat or Liver-Spleen imbalance.. Alternating dry and loose stool (or constipation and loose stool) often indicates Liver-Qi-stagnation and Spleen-weakness. Watery stool with undigested food usually indicates Yang-deficiency of Kidney and Spleen. Diarrhea with yellow burning anus usually indicates Damp-Heat. Formed or loose stool with undigested food and foul smell usually indicates food stagnation. Tarry (black) stool usually indicates hemorrhaging in the Spleen and Stomach (Intestines). Mild prolapse of anus during bowel movements may be due to chronic diarrhea and Spleen-Qi-deficiency, central-Qi sinking. Tenesmus usually is a sign of Qi-stagnation or Damp-Heat. Irregular habit often is caused by Liver failing to regulate the Spleen and Stomach. Diarrhea soon after abdominal distension and pain, which then relieves the pain, usually indicates food or Qi-stagnation. Abdominal pain not relieved (or only relieved for a short time) by bowel movements can be due to Spleen-deficiency and Liver over-controlling Spleen (Wood attacks Earth). Thin and sticky stools often seen with deficiency-Cold patterns.
Urine	Deep yellow (or tea color) urine usually indicates Heat. Clear and profuse urine usually indicates Cold. Turbid or a mixture of urine and sperm may indicate Damp-Heat, or Kidney not restraining Essence. Brownish urine may indicate Heat damage to blood vessels. Increased urine volume usually indicates Kidney Qi-deficiency (from Yin or Yang deficiency). Decreased urine volume is caused mostly by consumption of body Fluid or by dysfunction of Qi. Dribbling or retention of urine can indicate exhaustion of Kidney-Qi with Damp-Heat, or Phlegm/Blood-stasis. Stabbing pain accompanied by urgency and burning usually indicates Damp-Heat. Pain following (not during) urination usually indicates Kidney-weakness. Nocturnal urination is usually caused by Kidney-Qi or Yang-deficiency.
Sleep	Insomnia: • Palpitations, dreams and easily awakened, nervousness, poor memory, mostly due to Heart-Blood-deficiency. • Sores in mouth, thirst, red face often due to Heart-Fire. • Restlessness of mind, and difficulty falling asleep often because of Yin-deficiency. With profuse dreaming often with Essence-deficiency. • Back pain, tinnitus, dizziness, night sweats, and Heart symptoms mostly due to Kidney and Heart not communicating (K and H Yin-deficiency). • Bitter taste, vomiting/nausea, chest fullness, irritability/agitation and difficulty falling asleep often caused by Phlegm-Fire. • Restless mind during sleep, possibly night sweats, abdominal discomfort, often due to Stomach dysfunction food stagnation. • Fear of sleeping alone, fear/fright, frequent sighing, dizziness, phlegm signs, can be due to Gall Bladder-Qi-deficiency. • Headache, irritability, dizziness when going to sleep (or when lying down with closed eyes), bitter taste, often due to Liver Fire/Wind. • History of infectious disease, sweating, fatigue, often due to retained/lingering Pathogenic Factors. Hypersomnia: • Mostly Qi, Yang, Essence, Kidney, Spleen, Heart deficiency caused by chronic disease. • Dampness, failure of Spleen or clear-Yang to rise. • Retained/lingering exogenous Pathogenic Factors.

Table 1-40: History and Inquiry (Continued)

Topic	Indication
Menstruation and Leukorrhea	Early menses with red colored blood may indicate Heat. Early menses with light-colored blood may indicate Qi and Blood deficiency. Late menses with dark purple blood and pain mostly indicates Cold. Late menses with scanty light-colored blood mostly indicates Blood-deficiency, Irregular menses mostly indicates Liver-Qi-stagnation. Amenorrhea may be caused by pregnancy, Blood-stasis, Blood-exhaustion, consumptive diseases, and Liver-Qi-stagnation. Heavy flow is mostly due to Heat. With dark purple blood, clots and pain, it may indicate deficiency of Penetrating (Chong) and Conception (Ren) channels or sinking of Central-Qi (Spleen Qi).

Table 1-40: History and Inquiry (Continued)

Topic	Indication
Pain or Numbness	Wandering pain: Mostly from Wind. Changing characteristics of pain: Mostly from Qi-stagnation. Pain with sensation of heaviness, tightness, being boundup or fatigue: Mostly from Dampness. Pain with numbness: Mostly associated with Phlegm and/or Blood-deficiency. Severe pain: Often from Cold or Heat or Blood-stasis. Pressure pain, severe, clenching, like squeezed in a vise: Often from Cold, Cold may be due to Qi and Blood-blocked not warming tissues. Burning, hot pain: Mostly Heat/Fire, but can also be due to Qi and Blood-blocked not warming tissues with injury to vessels/nerves. Pulsating, throbbing pain: Mostly from Blood-stasis Qi-stagnation in acute injury, often with Heat, Liver-Fire, Liver-Yang-rising, Liver-Wind. Pain with redness and swelling: Mostly from Damp/Phlegm-Heat. May be with Blood-stasis. Pain and/or discomfort and feeling of distension/bloating: Mostly Qi-stagnation. Pain aggravated by pressure/massage: Mostly Excess condition. Pain alleviated by pressure/massage: Mostly Deficiency condition. Pain aggravated by lack of movement: Mostly due to stagnation of Qi or Blood-stasis or Cold. Lower body pain: Often with Dampness. Cramps of calves: Mostly Liver-Blood-deficiency, retention of Cold, Phlegm or Wind (may also cause tingling). If also painful-cramps often also Blood-stasis. Upper body pain: Often with Wind or Heat. Vague pain: Often Blood-deficiency and Chong/Penetrating channel/vessel disorder, or Qi-stagnation. Sharp, cutting, lacerating, boring pain: Mostly Blood-stasis or Heat/Fire or Stone. Dull, achy, intermittent pain (or very dull continuos pain): Mostly deficiency, Qi and/or Blood. Night pain: Mostly Blood-stasis. May be with Heat; Deficient or Excess, or any turbidity that effects circulation (or serious condition). Morning pain that improves quickly after movement: Often due to Phlegm, Cold, Blood stagnation/stasis-reduced sinew nourishment. Pain aggravated by activity or in afternoon: Often due to Deficiency. Pain and stiffness or inability to move the joint (or severely restricted movement): Often due to retention of Cold, Pathogenic Factors, especially Dampness or Phlegm obstructing the sinews, Bleeding and Blood-stasis within the joint space, Heat-Toxin affecting the joint. Headache: • Occipital referring to the nape and upper back—Tai-Yang channel. • Frontal referring to supraorbital ridge—Yang-Ming channel. • Temporal—Shao-Yang channel. • Vertex—Jue-Yin channel. • With teeth pain—Shao-Yin channel invaded by Cold. Chest pain: Mostly obstruction of Phlegm and Blood with Qi-stagnation (Liver and Gall Bladder). Lateral trunk, chest, chest wall, subcostal pain: Mostly by Qi/Phlegm obstruction or dysfunction of the Liver and Gall Bladder. Epigastric pain: Mostly by disorders of the Stomach or invasion by Liver-Qi. Abdominal pain:[a] • Lower lateral pain mostly by Liver-Qi-stagnation, intestinal abscess (appendicitis) or hernia. • Umbilical pain mostly by food stagnation, constipation, parasites, and Spleen or Large intestine disorders or hernia. • Lower abdominal pain and distension mostly by Urinary/Kidney disorders. If without urinary symptoms mostly by food stagnation. Low back pain: Mostly by Kidney-deficiency, Cold-Damp painful Obstruction, Blood-stasis, or Liver-Qi-stagnation. Limb pains: Mostly by Painful Obstruction syndromes (Bi), or Deficiency or Excess in channels and collaterals/Network-vessels, Kidney-deficiency. Numbness in limbs: Mostly associated with Phlegm, Wind, or Blood-deficiency (more tingling). Numbness or tingling improving with activity: Mostly associated with Qi-stagnation and obstruction of Qi and Blood.
Cold limb(s)	Yang-deficiency: Often affects the entire limb. Kidney-Yang-deficiency mostly lower limbs (important sign of Kidney-Yang). Upper or all four limbs: Heart-Yang-deficiency associated with palpitations and dizziness. Qi-stagnation: Mostly affects the hands and feet only, particularly the fingers and toes. Improves with movement and relaxation. Severe Heat: Mostly in severe infectious diseases with Interior Heat signs (reversal syndrome). Qi and Blood deficiency or retention of Pathogenic Factors: Mostly affects feet, or feet and hands, or one limb.
Edema	Lower limb: Mostly Kidney-Yang-deficiency, Spleen/pancreas-Yang-deficiency, Water over flowing, Heart and Kidney Yang-deficiency. Upper limb: Mostly Lung or Spleen Yang-deficiency. None pitting: May be due to Qi-stagnation.

a. For further information see the author's book *Acute Abdominal Disorders,* Blue Poppy Press.

Typical TCM Intake Form

My Pain or Symptoms are:
__Relieved with heat
__Intense, spastic
__Achy, dull, continuous
__Worse in morning, better mid-day
__Local, not radiating
__Tissues feel shortened/tight, pulling, or cold
__Relieved with ice
__Tissue and hands and feet feel warm
__Tissue feels loose, lax, not contracted
__Burning
__Radiating
__Pain area, or body, feels heavy or fatigued
__I need to lie down a lot
__Area of pain is swollen or feels damp
__Worse on rainy days or when weather changes
__Comes on suddenly
__Changes location often
__Constant (same all of the time)
__Feels sharp, cutting, like a knife, like pins and needles
__Usually worse at night
__Feels inflated, swollen, pushing outward, pulsating, or throbbing
__Difficult to describe
__Difficult to localize
__Affected by my emotions, stress
__Worse with pressure or massage
__Better with pressure or massage
__Worse after activity
__Better after activity
__I feel totally normal between attacks
__Feel oppressive fullness in chest, difficulty taking full breath etc.
__Feel worse after drinking fluids
__Lack of concentration, poor memory, "fogginess," "spaciness," all of which are usually worse in morning or on rainy or muggy days
__Feel severe itching, or feeling of ants crawling between the skin and muscles
__Numbness or feeling of electrical charges, or shooting pains

Water/Kidney/Bladder
__Hearing loss
__Ringing, low humming in ears
__Dizziness often, especially when fatigued or in afternoon
__Low back pain often, especially when fatigued
__Weak or unsteady feeling in knees or legs
__Knee soreness, pain
__Swelling of legs
__Feel cold in lower body
__Feel cold easily
__Cold feet all of the time
__Darkness under eyes
__Thinning hair, hair loss, early gray hair
__Frequent urination
__Difficult urination, or small amount frequently
__Night urination, # times_____
__Urinary incontinence
__Long clear/water/color urine
__Difficult getting a full breath in
__Feeling like not enough air
__Asthma
__Difficulty breathing in when lying down
__Chronic cough
__Loose teeth
__Uterine prolapse
__Bone problems
__Early morning diarrhea
__Chronic diarrhea with undigested food in stools
__Fatigued spirit
__Frequent sexual activity for a long time
__Any longstanding chronic disease
__Prolonged overly-physical stress
__Prolonged emotional stress
__History of blood loss
__History of very high fever
__Night sweats
__Dry or sore throat only <u>when</u> fatigued or overtired
__Afternoon fever, or feeling feverish, or sweats
__Low grade fever
__Increased sex drive
__Reduced sex drive
__Impotence
__Seminal leaking
__Lack of sexual secretion
__Flushing of face
__Chronic dry or sore throat
__Urine is dark yellow/tea color or very smelly
__During childhood, slow development in standing, walking, hair growth, teeth, closure of fontanel (head)
__Lack of muscle strength, especially in lower extremities
__Great exhaustion, life-long weakness, lack of willpower
__Poor memory
__Frequent terror, fear, fright

Earth/Spleen/Stomach
__Indigestion
__Stomach distension or pain

__Acid regurgitation, heartburn
__Nausea
__Nausea before eating, or after eating
__Nausea better after eating
__Loss of appetite
__Loss of taste
__Loose, pasty, soft, sticky stools
__Constipation often
__Hard stools followed by loose stools
__Frequent over-thinking, worry allot, obsessive, you are a student
__Pale white complexion
__Yellow complexion
__Weak voice
__Weakness of four extremities
__Excessive drooling
__Chronic hemorrhoids
__Blood in stools, Fresh__ Not Fresh__
__Organ prolapse
__Bloating after eating
__Feel sleepy, fatigue after eating, or after a large meal
__A sagging feeling in abdomen or distension feeling
__Difficulty gaining, losing or regulating weight
__Much phlegm in body, nose, lungs, ears (wax)
__A lot of thin, clear phlegm
__Yellow or green phlegm
__Watery discharges
__Frequent gurgling sounds in abdomen
__Cough on exertion or talking
__Spontaneous sweating, sweating easily
__Undigested food in stools
__Dull abdominal pain
__Full feeling in chest, epigastric area
__Alternating constipation and loose stools or diarrhea
__Feel full after eating a small amount of food
__Often eat fast
__Problems digesting foods
__Sweet taste in mouth
__Crave sweets
__Dry, cracked lips
__Mouth sores
__Painful or bleeding gums
__Toothaches
__Bad breath
__Headaches at forehead
__Constantly hungry, lingering hunger after meals
__Dry heaves
__Hiccups
__Stabbing, piercing stomach pain

Fire/Heart/Small Intestines

__Palpitations (can feel the heart beating in my chest)
__Insomnia
__Difficulty falling asleep
__Frequent waking up at night
__Forgetfulness
__Allot of dreams at night
__Often feel suspicious
__Dizziness/vertigo with exertion
__Perspiration, or palpitations with excitement
__Dry mouth and throat
__Tongue sores
__Chest pain
__Purple lips or nails
__Circulation troubles
__Shortness of breath *especially during exertion*
__*During physical exertion,* nausea, pain or tingles in: chest, teeth, face, shoulder, or arm
__A choking sensation when drinking water, desire but unable to vomit
__Emotional problems or withdrawal
__Laugh inappropriately
__Can't stop talking
__Skin rashes that are red, burning or itching
__Burning urination
__Increased urination or defecation when nervous
__Incessant hiccups

Wood/Liver Gall Bladder

__Irritability, moodiness often
__Impetuosity
__Depression
__Mental restlessness
__Distension or tight feeling in chest or side of trunk, breasts, or abdomen
__Sighing or needing to take a deep breath often
__Feet cold when nervous but warm when not
__Burping, belching, hiccups often
__Stools hard like little balls or very stringy (long and thin)
__Redness, pain or distension of eyes
__Headaches frequent, one-sided, temples, top of head, come on suddenly, with eye pain
__Dizziness or vertigo that comes on suddenly
__Strong ringing in ears or ringing that comes on suddenly
__Any symptom that comes on suddenly
__Blurred or poor vision
__Poor night vision (difficulty driving at night)
__Eye floaters (moving spots in vision)
__Dizziness when getting up from sitting or lying

Typical TCM Intake Form

__Dizziness after physical exercise
__Brittle nails, dry skin
__Twitching of muscles
__Numbness of limbs
__Tremors
__Convulsions
__Sudden loss of hearing
__Ear pain
__A feeling of swelling anywhere
__Genital itching
__Genital sweating
__Turbid, unclear urine
__Bloody urine
__Bloody nose and cough
__Proneness to fear and depression
__Body feels cold/hot/normal
__Impotence
__Flushed cheeks in afternoon
__Sharp lower abdominal or testicular pain
__Awaken in middle of sleep with fright or palpitations
__Easily startled
__Alternating fever and chills, or difficulty regulating temperature
__Cramping pain in testes or scrotum
__Bitter/bad taste in mouth, especially in morning
__Very sensitive to smells
__Feeling a lump or phlegm in throat often, or difficulty swallowing
__ "Liver" spots, skin discolorations, Liver hands-red spotty palms
__Broken veins, varicosities

Metal/Lung Large Intestine

__Respiratory problems
__Fevers
__Flu or cold w/itchy throat, cough w/thin watery phlegm, runny or stuffy nose, headache, body aches, sweating, no sweating
__Cold or flu with sore, painful throat, dry throat, sticky thick phlegm; occasional sweating, thirst
__Cold or flu with dry cough, itchy dry painful throat, dry lips and nose, no or scanty phlegm that is stringy thick, little sensitivity to cold
__Flu or cold with high fever, thirst, blurred vision, dizziness, nose bleed, cough with blood, rapid breathing
__Cough worse after meals, with allot of phlegm
__Chronic cough and difficult breathing worsened by exertion or speaking
__Spontaneous sweating
__Chronic asthma, coughing w/ thick yellow phlegm or pus and/or blood in sputum, facial swelling
__Dry cough with some phlegm that is thick and difficult to expectorate
__Cough and constipation

__Chronic low grade fevers, low-grade sore throat, dry throat and lips, night sweats
__Fatigue and dislike to talk, weak voice strength
__Bowel incontinence, chronic diarrhea
__Diarrhea with foul smelling stool, burning anus during or after passing stool
__Facial edema or swelling

Women

__Have children? How many___
__Yeast or other infections
__Clear watery vaginal discharge
__Thick or yellow vaginal discharge
__Irregular menses
__Heavy bleeding
__Dark blood with clots
__Bright red blood
__Pale color blood
__Spotting or dribbling for many days
__Menstrual pain
__Menstrual low back pain
__Short/early cycle
__Long/delayed cycle
__PMS (headaches, tender swollen breasts, bloating, emotional or irritable, sugar craving)
__Painful swollen breasts often
Last mammogram___
__Cysts, lumps, tumors
__Use or used birth control pills
__ Hot flashes
__Sexually transmitted disease
Age began menses___
Menopausal age ___

Men

__Prostate trouble
__Dribbling urination
__Weak or slow urine stream
__Burning urination
__Urethral trouble or discharge
__Testicular swelling or pain
Last testicular exam___
__Low sperm count
__Impotence
__Premature ejaculation
__Sexually transmitted disease

Do you or a Blood Relative (indicate who) have (or

had in the past):

__Alcoholism/drug abuse
__Arthritis or joint pains
__Bleeding problems
__Blood in stools
__Swollen glands (painful/not painful)
__Black stools
__Cancer
__Diabetes
__Digestive trouble
__Change in bowel habits
__Epilepsy
__Glaucoma or eye trouble
__Heart trouble
__Kidney trouble
__Liver trouble
__Lung trouble
__Spleen trouble
__Immune disorder
__High blood pressure
__Mental disorder
__Stroke or TIA
__Thyroid trouble
__Tuberculosis or positive PPD
__Diabetes
__Strong body odors
__HIV, AIDS
__Ulcers
__Lumps or swelling anywhere

Other   (specify)
_____
_____
_____

Lifestyle

Coffee/Tea cups per day_____
__I eat a lot of salads, fruits and *raw* vegetables
__I am a vegetarian
__I drink mostly cold drinks
__I drink mostly hot drinks
__I eat a lot of spicy foods
__I eat a lot of sugar, sweet foods
__I eat a lot of fatty or fried foods
Cigarettes per day_____
Beer/Wine per day_____
Distilled liquor per day_____
__I get plenty of exercise
__I do not exercise

__I am under significant emotional stress

__I am under significant physical stress

2

FOUNDATIONS FOR INTEGRATIVE PAIN AND PHYSICAL MEDICINE

The word pain is derived from the Latin poena and the Greek poine, which mean penalty or punishment. Pain is the most frequently presenting symptom in medical practice in the industrialized world and is almost always a symptom, not a disease or disturbance itself. It is pain as a result of problems within the human body that this text is addressing. The complementary approach to musculoskeletal medicine combines the benefits of Western science with principles and techniques developed throughout the world. Integrated methods have significant benefit to patients, some of whom have not responded to "traditional" approaches. This section summarizes the biomedical and TCM principles that are important for the application of this approach. The chapter presents a brief review of basic concepts and builds on information gradually, so that both practitioners with limited biomedical science training and scientifically trained practitioners can follow and benefit. This section is not intended to be a state of the art review; only basic information pertinent to the pain practitioner is covered.

Pain

Pain—a sensation in which a person experiences discomfort, distress, or suffering—is the most common complaint that patients present to the doctor. For the family physician, the incidence of patients who request treatment for back pain is second only to that of patients whose complaint is a common cold. Some 40% of the American population (and of the populations of other industrialized countries) is afflicted with acute or chronic pain that requires medical management. Inadequate management and out-and-out mismanagement of these patients is common (Bonica 1990). Unfortunately, even today some clinicians and scientist continue to promulgate the concept of nonorganic pain. At the present time, however, our knowledge of the pathophysiology of chronic pain is incomplete, and the few tools available for diagnosis are neither sensitive nor specific. It is important to note that only recently did the medical profession accept that migraine headache, post herpetic neuralgia, and phantom pain are neurologic disorders. Not very long ago, many patients with these disorders were referred to psychiatrists or psychonanalysts and then admitted to psychiatric hospitals for treatment (Galer and Dworkin 2000). Pain is now recognized by the Joint Commission for the Study of Pain as the "fifth vital sign."

In general, pain may be divided into nociceptive, neuropathic, idiopathic, and psychogenic pain. *Nociceptive* pain pertains to pain within normal functioning neural sensor-wire-perception systems. *Neuropathic* (which includes *Central pain* from spinal cord and brain) pain pertains to dysfunctional sensor-wire-perception systems. *Idiopathic* pain pertains to pain that does not relate to known neural anatomy or pathology, and if present, does not account for its distribution or intensity. *Psychogenic* pain pertains mainly to pain associated with a major psychiatric illness (Williams and Spitzer 1982) or resulting from neurosis and stress. Sleep disturbance, depression, and heightened risk of suicide are among the most clinically significant sequelae of chronic pain (Smith, Perlis and Haythrornthwaite 2004).

MUSCULOSKELETAL PAIN MAY OCCUR DUE TO:
- Injury.
- Unsound posture and uncoordinated movements.
- Mechanical stresses to soft tissue from dislocation of bony structures or other restrictions of tissue motions.
- Muscular imbalances.
- Inflammatory processes from acute trauma, immune dysfunctions, metabolic and repetitive injuries such as tendinitis, and degenerative conditions and neurogenic inflammation.
- Abnormal neurological self-regulation (such as facilitated segment, neuropathic, psychological, and neuropsychological).
- (Possibly) environmental factors such as Wind-Wet.

In addition to the above, Chaitow (2002) lists:
- Congenital factors such as short or long leg, small hemipelvis, fascial influences (e.g. cranial distortions involving the reciprocal tension membranes due to birthing difficulties such as forceps delivery).
- Overuse, misuse, and abuse factors such as injury or inappropriate or repetitive patterns of use involved in work, sport, or regular activities.
- Immobilization–disuse. (Irreversible changes can occur after just 8 weeks.)
- Postural stress patterns that are often related to emotional states.
- Inappropriate breathing patterns.

- Chronic negative emotional states such as depression, anxiety, etc.
- Reflexive influences (trigger points, facilitated spinal regions).

Musculoskeletal pain may also occur due to the Biomechanical stress sequence:
- Something occurs leading to increased muscular tone.
  If this is anything but short-term, retention of metabolic waste commences.
- Increased tone then simultaneously results in a degree of localized oxygen deficit resulting in relative ischemia.
  Ischemia does not produce pain but an ischemic muscle which contracts rapidly does.
- Increased tone may lead to a degree of edema.
  Retention of wastes/ischemia/edema all contribute to discomfort or pain, which, in turn, reinforces hypertonicity.
- Inflammation or at least chronic irritation may evolve.
- Neurological reporting stations in the distressed tissues will bombard the CNS with information regarding their status, resulting in neural sensitization and the evolution of facilitation – a tendency toward hyper-reactivity.
- Macrophages are activated as are increased vascularity and fibroblastic activity.
- Connective tissue production increases with cross-linkage leading to shortened fascia.
- Chronic muscular stress (a combination of the load involved and the number of repetitions, or the degree of sustained influence) results in the gradual development of hysteresis in which collagen fibres and proteoglycans are rearranged to produce an altered structural pattern.
- This results in tissues that are more easily fatigued than normal and more prone to damage if strained.
- Since all fascia/connective tissue is continuous throughout the body, any distortions or contractions developing in one region can create fascial deformations elsewhere, thereby negatively influencing structures supported by or attached to the fascia, e.g. nerves, muscles, lymph structures, blood vessels.
- Hypertonicity in muscles leads to inhibition of antagonist(s) and aberrant behavior in synergist(s).
- Chain reactions evolve in which some muscles (postural muscles) shorten while others (phasic muscles) weaken.
- Sustained increased muscle tension ischemia in tendinous structures leads to the development of periosteal reactions and pain. Tension and ischemia in localized areas of muscles can also lead to myofascial trigger point evolution. (Ischemic influences and trigger points are discussed in chapter 3 of this text).
- Compensatory adaptations evolve leading to habitual, 'built-in', patterns of use emerging as the CNS learns to compensate for modifications in muscle strength, length, and functional behaviour.
- Abnormal biomechanics result, involving malcoordination of movement. (For example, erector spinae tightens while rectus abdominis is inhibited).
- The normal firing sequence of muscles involved in particular movements alters, resulting in additional strain.
- Joint biomechanics are directly influenced by the accumulated influences of such soft-tissue changes and can themselves become significant sources of referred and local pain, reinforcing soft-tissue dysfunctional patterns.

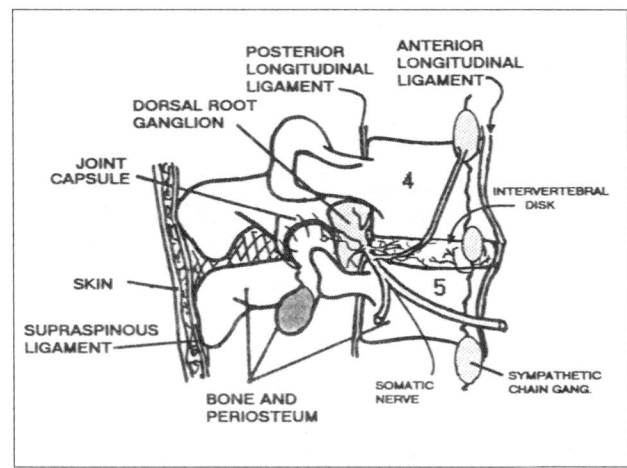

Figure 2-1: Structures capable of producing pain around the vertebra (From Kuchera WA and Kuchera ML, Osteopathic Principles in Practice, KCOM press 1993, with permission).

- Deconditioning of the soft tissues becomes progressive as a result of the combination of simultaneous events involved in soft-tissue pain: 'spasm' (guarding), joint stiffness, antagonist weakness, overactive synergists, etc.
- Progressive evolution of localized areas of neural hyper-reactivity occurs (facilitated areas) paraspinally, or within muscles (myofascial trigger points).
- Within these trigger points increased neurological activity occurs (for which there is EMG evidence) which is capable of influencing distant tissues adversely (Hubbard 1993, Simons 1993)
- Energy wastage due to unnecessarily sustained hypertonicity and excessively active musculature leads to generalized fatigue.
- More widespread functional changes develop; for example, changes affecting respiratory function and body posture, with repercussions on the total body economy.
- In the presence of constant neurological feedback of impulses to the CNS/brain from neural reporting stations indicating heightened arousal (a hypertonic muscle status is the alarm reaction of the flight/fight alarm response) there will be increased levels of psychological arousal and a reduction in the ability to relax, with consequent reinforcement of hypertonicity.
- Functional patterns of use of a biologically unsustainable nature emerge.

One can thus see that musculoskeletal disorders are usually accompanied by some degree of mechanical dysfunction, degenerative conditions, such as ligament and tendon insufficiency, fibrosis and myotendinosis. Injury can cause sensory, motor, and/or autonomic dysfunctions in the corresponding dermatome, myotome, sclerotome, or viscerotome. Neoplastic and other medical diseases must be kept in mind, since they can result in pain that seems to have musculoskeletal origin.

Understanding and diagnosing the origin of musculoskeletal pain is complex, as pain can arise from so many near by structures, all of which can interact to complicate matters even more. For example, Figure 2-1 illustrates some of the structures capable of producing pain in one motion segment in the spine.

Neural Mechanisms of Pain

The nervous system is usually divided into components such as central, peripheral, and autonomic systems, all of which actually function as one continuous functional system. Pain therefore involves the whole neural communication system. A complex experience in which psychological factors play a critical role, pain can even influence the sensory transmission processes, i.e., pain can change the circuitry in the nervous system.

Basic Elements of the Nervous System

Nerves provide neural control of skeletal, smooth muscle and glandular tissue. They also deliver trophic factors (the exoplasmic transport of growth promoting chemicals, both antegrade and retrograde or regulatory factors to the muscles or organs that they innervate). For these nourishing factors to travel up and down the nerves, they must be relatively free from structural pressure.

In order to consider the neural mechanisms of pain, the practitioner must have a fundamental understanding of the nervous system. The basic functional and structural component is the *neuron*, which receives information, processes it, and sends it to other neurons. Nerves and neurons are long tubes of protoplasm which may, or may not, be surrounded by insulating myelin. A neuron is composed of a cell body (like all normal cells) and its processes, a single *axon*, and one or more—often several more—*dendrites* (Figure 2-2). There are primarily two main types of neurons: *motor (efferent)* neurons which mostly carry signals from the CNS to muscles and organs, and *sensory (afferent)* neurons which mostly carry signals from the periphery to the CNS.

An axon is the process of a neuron by which impulses travel away from the cell body. A dendrite is a tree-like, branched process of a neuron. Dendrites conduct impulses to the cell body from the axons of other neurons. Dendrites are believed to produce graded electrical responses, in contrast to the all-or-nothing responses produced by the axon and cell body. At the other end of the axon (away from the cell body) are terminals called *synaptic bulbs*. These are buttons or knobs that form a functional connection to other nerve cells (to the cell body or to the dendrites of the next neuron) through *synaptic transmission*. Information travels down an axon by a *nerve impulse* (also called *action potential*), an all-or-nothing response. A nerve impulse is created by depolarization of the axon, which is caused by the inflow of sodium ions across the cell membrane from the outside to the inside, giving the inside of the membrane a positive charge. When triggered at the origin of the axon, the information travels all of the way down the axon (although more recent studies show bidirectional transmission). The amount of stimulation needed to initiate a nerve impulse reaction in the axon is called the *threshold* (Waxman and deGroot 1985).

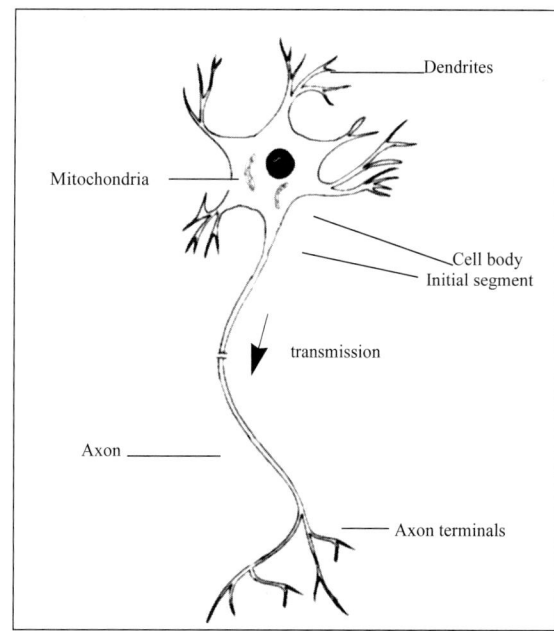

Figure 2-2: Axon and processes.

Many characteristics give a neuron its identity or phenotype. These include its shape, location, the type(s) of transmitters and neuropeptides it produces and uses to communicate with other neurons, the cell with which it forms connections (both presynaptic and postsynaptic), and the types of receptors it bears on its cell surface to "hear" what other neurons have to say (Koslow et al 1995).

Abnormalities in or loss of communication between neurons result in neurological disorders such as Alzheimer's disease, Parkinson's disease, amyotropic lateral sclerosis (ALS), and congenital epilepsy. Newer information shows many neurological diseases, such as multiple sclerosis, Parkinsonism, and diabetic neuropathy to be caused by problems that develop in the surrounding support cells, which are more numerous than the neurons, about 9:1 ratio. These are the astrocytes, Schwann cells, oligodendrites and other neuroglia (Koslow et al *ibid*).

According to Oschman (2000), the "neuron doctrine" is incomplete and holds that all functions of the nervous system are the result of activities of the neurons. It is incomplete because it ignores an evolutionarily more ancient informational system residing in the perineural connective tissue cells that constitute more than half of the cells in the brain. Perineural cells encase every nerve fiber, down to their finest terminations throughout the body. This ancient system is a direct current (DC) communications system that is related to the "current of injury" that controls injury repair. Becker and Nordenström theorized that a naturally occurring current of injury is measurable.[1]

Newer information, however, has shown that while glia contain the same voltage-sensitive ion channels that generate electrical signals in axons, in glia these channels only allow the indirect sensing of the level of activity of adjacent neurons. Glial cells lack the membrane properties required to actually propagate their own action potentiations. Glia rely on chemical signals instead of electrical ones to communicate information, using mostly calcium and ATP (Fields 2004).

The Synapses

Synapses (or gap junctions) are functional connections between nerve cells. They are located between the synaptic bulbs and the adjacent target nerve fibers, often a dendrite of the next cell. The bulb of the source nerve is covered by a membrane called the *presynaptic membrane*. The membrane of the adjacent neuron at the synapse, called the *postsynaptic membrane*, contains receptor sites for chemicals released from vesicles in the bulb (Figure 2-3). Synapses are among the most abundant structures in the brain; estimates suggest that a mammalian brain may contain 10^{15} (Koslow et al 1995). Synaptic transmission occurs across the thin synaptic space between the two neurons via the release of chemicals called *neurotransmitters*. The neurotransmitter diffuses within the synapse and binds to its receptor, a large protein embedded in the membrane of the receiving neuron. Some examples of neurotransmitters are epinephrine, norepinephrine, serotonin, acetylcholine, histamine, dopamine, and even some amino acids such as gamma-aminobutyric acid (GABA) and glycine. Nitric oxide (NO) is a gaseous neurotrasmitter. This chemical release is initiated by the nerve impulse (action potential) travelling down the axon to the bulb. Neurotransmitter substances may be inhibitory or excitatory, and therefore may either promote or inhibit nerve impulses. When enough synaptic excitation occurs to reach the threshold, the *sodium gate* opens. (A sodium gate is a gate in the membrane of the nerve that keeps the sodium outside until the threshold is reached). The opening of this gate causes the interior of the membrane to be charged more positively than the outside of the membrane, and it initiates a nerve impulse in the axon. However, if synaptic inhibition occurs, the cell membrane becomes more negatively charged, often by opening some chloride channels in the cell membrane. This prevents the membrane from reaching the threshold (Waxman and deGroot 1985). Recently, neurotransmitters have been shown capable of triggering gene expression providing a means by which neuronal activity can produce long-term changes in the activity at a synapse (Koslow et al *ibid*)

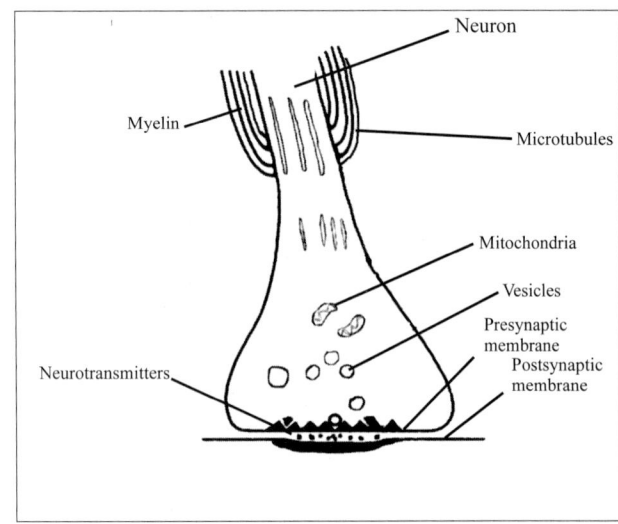

Figure 2-3: Axon and synapse.

Other modes of chemical-mediated communication between cells include dendrite release of chemical transmitters and the recently discovered systems involving small, soluble gases such as nitric oxide whose mode of action is still unclear (Koslow et al *ibid*).

The synapses are probably the most important part of the system that regulates transmission across neurons. Their regulatory effect is achieved by (Ornstein and Thompson 1984):.

•Controlling the direction of transmission;

•Allowing for facilitation and inhibition;

•Creating summation by allowing weak and repetitive stimuli (subthreshold) to produce an accumulation of chemical transmitters, which eventually leads to a level equal to the threshold;

•Creating a synaptic delay due to the time it takes to release neurotransmitters;

•Causing fatigue due to neurotransmitter depletion;

•Allowing for the action of drugs [or acupuncture] on the secretion, and for the removal and blocking of neurotransmitters.

Recent information has shown that neuronal and synaptic transmission do not follow linear models. It is not unusual for a neuron to receive thousands of synaptic inputs arising from diverse sources in the central nervous system. These effects will not be the same from moment to moment. Such non-linearity gives neurons integrative and computational capabilities previously unimaginable. Retrograde[2] transmission has been documented as well (Koslow et al *ibid*).

---

1. Becker hypothesized that this current was conducted via the Schwann and glial cell sheaths (perineural tissues) that surround neurons. The current is said to be in the microcurrent range within 10-30 µA (microamp). Becker found that the human body is positively polarized along the central spinal axis and negatively peripherally. The normal voltage reading is said to be -10 µV (microvolt), however when a fracture occurs, the voltage is decreased toward zero. For more detailed information about the "body electric" see "Bioenergetic Field Therapy" on page 423.

2. Transmission going in the other direction.

Neural Mechanisms of Pain

Table 2-1: Types of Nociceptors (Pain Receptors)

MECHANICAL	Mechanoreceptors, activated by mechanical stimulation.
THERMAL	Activated by injuries induced by thermal input of approximately 45°Celsius and higher.
POLYMODAL	C fiber nociceptors, a catch-all for all other nociceptive signals. Also can respond to mechanical and thermal stimulation.

PRESYNAPTIC INHIBITION. The binding of neurotransmitters to axo-axonic synapses (the receptors that mediate presynaptic inhibition) leads to a reduction in the amount of neurotransmitter liberated by the postsynaptic axon. Presynaptic inhibition provides a mechanism by which the "gain" at a particular synaptic input to a neuron can be lowered without reducing the efficacy of other synapses that might impinge on that neuron (Waxman and deGroot 1995). Presynaptic inhibition probably works, in part, by reducing calcium current inflow during the action potential in the terminals of cells (Koslow et al *ibid*).

Types of Nerve Fibers

Nerve fibers can be *myelinated* (laminated) or *unmyelinated* (unlaminated). Myelinated nerve fibers are surrounded by *Schwann cells* (a type of fatty glial cell), which wrap the nerve tightly in a multilayered structure, called a myelin sheath, that serves as an electrical insulator. Unmyelinated nerves do not have this sheath. Myelinated nerves—one of the nerve types in the peripheral nervous system—are fast conductors of information.

Nerve fibers are divided by their fiber diameters, conduction velocities, and physiologic characteristics. The three categories of nerve fibers (A, B, and C fibers) each have several subtypes.

The term nociception refers to the body's response to and perception of pain. Nociceptors (pain receptors) belong the smaller fibers the A-δ (A-delta, a subtype of A fibers) and C afferents (sensory nerves) that are equipped in the periphery with receptors that are sensitive to noxious or potentially-noxious mechanical and chemical stimuli. Pain receptors are divided into three categories, each of which is activated by different mechanisms and is made of different fiber types (mostly A and C fibers; Table 2-1). Activation of these primary afferents (sensory) neurons by noxious stimuli renders the nociceptor membrane permeable to sodium ions, leading to the generation of an impulse. These impulses (action potentials) are propagated to the central nervous system (CNS) by the A-δ and C-fibers that synapse in the dorsal cord of the spinal cord.

A-fibers

A-fibers, which are large, somatic, and myelinated, are fast conductors. They:
- Act as proprioceptors (see below);
- Provide motor supply to muscle spindles (see muscle spindle in this chapter);
- Receive pain, temperature, touch, and pressure sensations.

A-Alpha Fibers

A-α (A-Alpha) fibers (a subset of A-fibers) are large (12-20 μm in diameter) and conduct at a rate of 70-120 meters per second. They function as proprioceptors, and they innervate the muscle spindles, annulospiral endings, and golgi tendon organs (see "Muscles" this chapter). In muscles these fibers are known as *type I receptors*.

A-Beta Fibers

A-β (A-Beta) fibers (a subset of A-fibers) are low-threshold mechanoreceptors found in skin, muscle, tendons, and joints. They connect to the dorsal horns of the spinal cord. A-β myelinated fibers are large-diameter in being 5-15 μm in diameter. Relatively fast conductors, they conduct at a velocity of 30-120 meters per second. In muscles they are known *type II receptors*.

A-Delta Fibers

A-δ (A-Delta) fibers (a subset of A-fibers), also called *high-threshold mechanoreceptors* (see below), are medium-diameter fibers (1-5 μm in diameter) that connect A-fiber nociceptors (pain sensors) to the dorsal horns (sensory horn) of the spinal cord. Pain from A-δ fibers is felt as a local, sharp, and relatively brief pain. Found mostly just under the skin, these fibers transmit messages principally from the skin and mucous membrane. They are important for superficial acupuncture stimulation. A-δ fibers are pressure and pain fibers. They are divided into large A-δ (IIIa) and small A-δ (IIIb). The small A-δ (IIIb) fibers are responsible for the first/immediate pain. In muscles they are know as *type III receptors*.

B-Fibers

B-fibers are smaller, autonomic, myelinated fibers that are fast conductors yet slower than A-fibers, and function as preganglionic sympathetic fibers (see "Sympathetic System" this chapter).

C-Fibers

C-fibers, also known as "C-polymodal nociceptors," are found everywhere in the body except the brain. They carry pain signals from peripheral cells, transmitting messages from deep tissues and from the skin and mucous membranes. These unmyelinated fibers measure 0.25-1.5 μm in diameter, the smallest of the nerve fibers. C-fibers are the slowest conductors, with conduction velocity rates of 0.5-2 meters per second. (However, some C-fibers are thought to be very slow, taking up to five seconds to conduct from the foot to the cord). They:

- Function as pain fibers;
- Function in reflex responses;
- Are also postganglionic sympathetic fibers (always end at the sympathetics);
- Are known in muscles as *type IV fibers;*
- Are activated by mechanical, thermal, or chemical stimuli.

When stimulated electrically, C-fibers can produce pain. Pain in deep tissues, felt as a deep-seated, ill-defined and widespread ache (such as seen in sclerotomal and myotomal pain), is produced by stimulation of C-fibers. Gunn (1977) has demonstrated that painful stimuli from muscles have implicated muscle fiber types III and IV.

Researchers have shown that cutaneous nerves have more than four times the number of small-diameter A-delta and C-fibers, than larger myelinated A-β fibers (Ochoa and Mair 1969). Kruger, McMahon, and Kolzenbug posit that this occurs because, apart from their function of pain transmission. Nociceptors serve other regulatory and trophic functions, such as regulating:

- Blood flow and vascular permeability in both visceral and somatic tissues;
- Trophic functions such as maintenance and repair of skin integrity;
- Immunological processes, such as emigration of leukocytes at sites of tissue injury (OM: *Defensive-Qi circulates largely in the skin areas*);
- Activity of autonomic ganglia and visceral smooth muscle.

The very slow-conducting C-fibers may explain, in part, the "De-Qi Phenomenon" (propagated needling sensation) of acupuncture, which is also slow conducting—said to be about one cm per second, and thought to be related to slow excitatory postsynaptic potentials (Katayama and Nishi 1986). In general, type II (muscle) afferents are thought to signal the "numbness" of De-Qi, and type III, the fullness (heaviness and mild aching) sensation. Soreness (deep achiness) is probably due to unmyelinated type IV afferents. In more superficial stimulation the A-δ (type III) afferents are probably responsible of the sharp sensation and De-Qi.

Mechanical and Proprioceptive Receptors

Mechanoreceptors (mechanical receptors) gather information about the *outside* mechanical forces acting upon the body and transmit this information to the central nervous system (spinal cord and brain). These receptors may be stimulated by pressure, touch, movement, gravity, and even sound and vibration.

Proprioceptors are a large group of nerve receptors that respond to stimuli produced *within* the body. A-fibers, for example, supply proprioceptors that function as sensors of posture and equilibrium. There are three main groups of proprioceptors: joints, ligaments, and skin (Ruffini's end organs, Pacinian corpuscles, and free nerve endings); in the neck and in the labyrinthine (often associated with balance), and muscle proprioceptors (monitoring length and tension, see this chapter) (Willard 1993; 1997).

Brain

The brain (Figure 2-4) is composed of neurons and glia[3] and their specific interactions with one another. The brain has three main divisions: starting at the base of the skull (where the brain meets the spinal cord) we have the hindbrain (rhombencephalon), then midbrain (mesencephalon) and forebrain (prosencephalon). The hindbrain contains the medulla oblongata, the pons, and the cerebellum, *collectively known as the brainstem.* In humans the forebrain is the most massive part of the brain. It consists of two parts: the interbrain (diencephalon) and the cerebrum (telencephalone). The interbrain (also called "midbrain") includes the thalamus, hypothalamus, and pineal gland. It also contains the nerves connecting these to the cerebrum.

Unlike other organs which are composed of a relatively homogenous population of cells, the brain is diverse. In general, neural pathways controlling information and action are linked from the bottom to the top.

Brain Stem

The brain stem (medulla oblongata, pons, and the cerebellum), thought to be the oldest part of the brain ontogenically (500 million years old), resembles the entire brain of a reptile. The *medulla oblongata* connects the rest of the brain with the spinal cord. The *pons* is the signal bridge between the medulla and the middle brain. The *cerebellum* is wrapped around the brainstem and fills the back bottom of the cranium. It is the largest part of the hindbrain (brain stem), and the second largest in the brain. The cerebellum is mainly involved with the motor system and with maintaining posture, balance, and skeletal muscle function. It maintains, adjusts, and directs the coordination of muscular movement,

---

3. Glia is the non-nervous or supporting tissue of the brain and spinal cord. While glia has been thought to only provide support (carry nutrients, etc.) to the "main" communication systems of the brain and peripheral nervous system, the neurons. Newer information now show that glia engage in a two-way dialogue from embryonic development through old age. Glia influence the formation of synapses and help to determine which neural connections get stronger or weaker over time; such changes are essential for learning and for storing long-term memories. The most recent work shows that glia also communicate among themselves, in a separate but parallel network to the neural network, influencing how well the brain performs. Glial communication is achieved mainly by chemical release using calcium and ATP (Fields 2004).

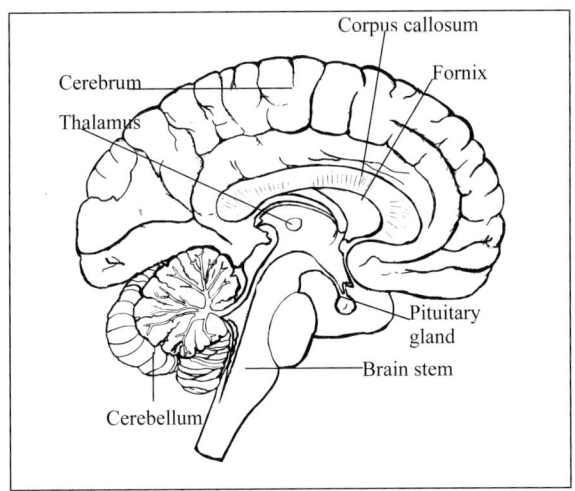

Figure 2-4: Brain.

and it stores memories for simple learned responses (Ornstein and Thompson 1984).

The brain stem giving rise to ten of the twelve pairs of cranial nerves, determines the general level of alertness, and warns the organism of important incoming information. It directs attention to specific events and handles basic bodily functions such as respiratory and heart rates (Ornstein and Thompson *ibid*). It contains a spatial map of the body and its relationship to its surrounding and has been described as an imageless space of will, direction, intuition, subconsciousness, intention, and life-saving defensive reactions (Oschman 2000). Often involved in post-traumatic injuries, the brain stem is also implicated in chronic pain syndromes that involve the cranial nerves, which in part innervate shoulder and neck muscles. Osteopathic functional techniques may be effective in treating such injuries (Ward 1995).

RETICULAR SYSTEM. The reticular system is a diffusely-organized neural apparatus that extends through the central region of the brainstem into the subthalamus and the intralaminar nuclei of the thalamus. A complex system that occupies a large portion of the brainstem, the reticular structure has major ascending sensory tracts to the cerebrum and cerebellum, and descending (reticulospinal) motor tracts to the spinal cord and to the central nuclei related to the cranial nerves (Waxman and deGroot *ibid*). The descending fibers can activate the spinal cord non-specifically, determining the excitability of skeletal muscles and their susceptibility to tightness and *trigger point formation*. It acts as a selective filter for information on touch, pain, and temperature, as well as visceral information. It can modulate ascending information from A-δ and C-fibers (Bekkering and van Bussel 1998).

CLINICAL DEFICIT OF BRAINSTEM. Lesions in the brainstem result primarily in sensory loss (proprioception, discriminative touch and vibratory sense) from the body and face; loss of motor control (spastic paralysis, also called ataxia) of the limbs; loss of pain and temperature sensations from the body and face; loss of hearing or balance; loss of speech (dysphagia) and swallowing (dysarthria); paralysis of the tongue; heart arrhythmias; dyspnea; and/or coma and death (Willard 1993).

CLINICAL DEFICIT OF CEREBELLUM. Lesions in the cerebellum can result in coma and death; loss of primary sensory modalities (vibratory sense, discriminative touch, and proprioception) and loss of pain and temperature sensations from the body and face; abnormal motor control (ataxia and paralysis); eye movement dysfunction; and decerebrate posturing, with the upper and lower limbs going into extreme, extensor-dominated positions (Willard *ibid*).

The Midbrain

Located in the midbrain/interbrain (the diencephalon, which is the division of the brain between the cerebrum and mesencephalon, consisting of the hypothalamus, thalamus, metathalamus, and epithalamus) are the most important control centers for unconscious body functions (in the thalamus and hypothalamus). The *thalamus* is a pair of oval shaped organs forming most of the lateral walls of the third ventricle of the brain. The thalamus receives and transmits incoming nerve signals from the body and between most parts of the brain. The information from the cerebellum is processed in the thalamus, where it is prepared for becoming conscious. The *hypothalamus* is the main director of the autonomic nervous system which directs all the functions like digestion, secretion, metabolism, etc., that are not normally under conscious control. The hypothalamus controls the *pituitary gland* which is called the "master gland" of the body, that in turn controls all of the endocrine system (Ornstein and Thompson *ibid*).

Cerebrum

The *cerebrum*, the largest part of the human brain, is divided into hemispheres that each control a side of the body. The two hemispheres are connected by the *corpus callosum*, a band of some three hundred million nerve cell fibers. A cross section of the cerebrum reveals the thick grey cerebral cortex of nerve cells surrounding a white core of nerve fibers.

The cerebral cortex, which is thought to have evolved some 200 million years ago, has several lobes: frontal, temporal, parietal, and occipital. The cortex allows humans to organize, remember, communicate, understand, appreciate, and create (Ornstein and Thompson *ibid*). All patterns of movement and mental pictures are stored within the cerebrum. It gathers and processes the reports of sensory impressions from sight, sound, touch, etc.

LONG TERM POTENTIATION (LTP). LTP is a mechanism by which short-term memory is converted to long-term memory, as a result of frequent stimulation which may be

Table 2-2: Thalamocortical Projections and Related Aspects of Pain

Projection	Termination	Aspect of Pain
1	Superior paracentral of cortex.	Perception (localization).
2	Frontal lobe.	Emotion.
3	Ipsilateral temporal lobe.	Recent and long-term memory.

encoded and stored at the synaptic level. It was observed first at synapses in the hippocampus,[4] which may play a role in associative learning. In early stages of development and in primitive mammals, the hippocampus is located anteriorly and constitutes part of the outer mantle of the brain. The hippocampus is involved in converting short-term memory of up to sixty minutes to long-term memory of several days or more. The anatomic substrates for long-term memory probably include the temporal lobes as well hippocampus (Waxman and deGroot 1985). Studies on LTP suggest that postsynaptic neuron may release one or more diffusible substances (including nitric oxide; [NO]), and retrograde transmitters that affect the presynaptic neuron. In other words, LTP is initiated by events that occur in the postsynaptic neuron. The presynaptic neuron then undergoes some change that perpetuates the phenomenon. Opioid peptides may serve as retrograde inhibitory transmitters. LTP currently is the most compelling model in the mammalian brain for a neural mechanism related to learning and memory (Koslow et al *ibid*). Therefore, the connections the hippocampus has with the hypothalamus and other structures dealing with somatovisceral, emotional, and endocrine functions (among others) that combine parts of the brain to form a "cognitive map," may explain the actual changes in all these areas seen with associative pain memories.

A speculative possibility as to why acupuncture reports from China are more positive than reports from the West is that in China treatment is often given daily and therefore may provoke *LTP like* mechanisms, including the "windup-winddown" phenomenon. (Acupuncture has been shown to modulates the expressions of NO and c-Fos in the gerbil hippocampus post transient global ischemia (Kim et al 2003)).[5]

CLINICAL DEFICIT OF CEREBRUM. Clinical deficit ranges from specific sensory and motor losses to alterations of cognitive functions such as language, speech, writing, reading; and to changes in awareness, social mores, memory, or consciousness. Damage to the subcortical structures can result in memory loss, aberrant emotional behavior, personality changes, and movement disorders such as hyperkinesia or hypokinesia (Willard *ibid*).

Limbic System

The limbic system, a group of cellular structures rather than a single brain region, is located between the brain stem and the cortex. It interconnects structures within the cerebrum, frontal lobe, temporal lobe, thalamus, hypothalamus, and circuitous neuron pathways that connect all parts. The limbic system, which contains the hypothalamus and the pituitary gland, is involved in many of the body's self-regulating systems and is strongly involved in the emotional reactions that have to do with survival (Ornstein and Thompson *ibid*). After the brain stem, the limbic system can be said to be a "viewer-centered" space of image, dream, or hallucination, in which "objects" are selected on the basis of memory (Oschman *ibid*). The limbic system can also relay information to the spinal cord and can cause inhibition at the spinal cord "gate," making it more difficult for the pain signal from the peripheral nervous system (PNS) to reach the brain (this is called *stress analgesia*). However, if the limbic system is activated for prolonged periods, such as in chronic pain, the limbic activity results in opening of the gate, more pain impulses reach the brain, and increased pain intensity is felt (Galer and Dworkin *ibid*).

The Brain and Pain

Although researchers have identified several spinal-supraspinal (spinal-brain) tracts that are involved in the transmission of pain, current data suggests that nociception is not related solely to a unique or exclusive system of pathways. Several neurons within a number of reticular, cortical, and diencephalic structures are responsive to noxious stimulation and are not associated with these pain related tracts (Wall *ibid*). Axons from the thalamic nuclei, which ascend to the cerebral cortex, have been defined as three thalamocortical projections, each of which relates to a different aspect of pain (Table 2-2; Melzack and Casey *ibid*; Hand and Morrison 1970; Desijaru and Purpura 1970; Newcombe 1972).

Studies using positron emission tomography (PAT) and functional magnetic resonance imaging (MRI) provide the bases for a conceptual model of the brain regions and mechanisms involved in the following pain functions and behaviors (Galer and Dworkin *ibid*):

- Sensation;
- Emotion;
- Autonomic nervous system;
- Motor system;
- Attention and orientation;

---

4. The hippocampus is an elevation of the floor of the lateral ventricle of the brain. It is an important component of the limbic system and its efferent projections form the fornix of the cerebrum. The fornix is nerve fibers that lie beneath the corpus callosum (band of fibers that connect the two cerebrum hemispheres).

5. Windup is an abnormal temporal summation of peripheral nervous system input into wide-dynamic-range neurons. Acupuncture as also been shown to modulates nitric oxide activity in the brainstem somatic sensory paths (nucleus gracilis), basal ganglia striatum, and the cerebral cortex.

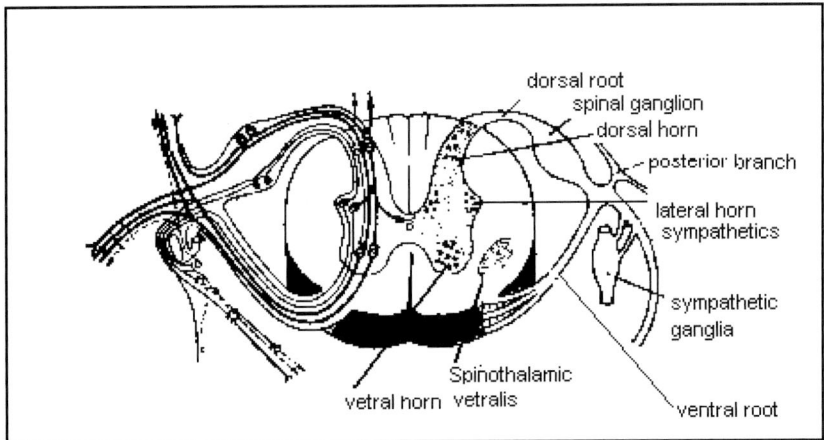

Figure 2-6: Spinal cord and nerve roots.

- Pain modulation;
- Past experience;
- Labeling pain.

Recent studies using PET and magnetoencephalography scanning have revealed changes in the activity, size, and location of brain cortical structures relevant to the sensation of the body parts after amputation. Interestingly, these neuroplastic cortical changes revert to normal state when the phantom pain is relieved (Galer and Dworkin *ibid*).

Spinal Cord

The spinal cord (Figure 2-6) is an intricate core with complex circuitry and biochemistry that receives sensation and routes motor signals and reflexes. This system is important in pain perception and modulation, and in integration of sensory, motor, central, and sympathetic signals. The spinal cord has two horns, with laminae that have specialized functions.

Spinal Cord Core

Each segment of the spinal cord has an inner column of gray matter that contains nerve cell bodies, and an outer sheath of white matter. A cross-section of the spinal cord reveals a central, H-shaped area. Table 2-3 and Figure 2-6 lists sections of the H-shaped area and the areas and/or functions they affect.

THE CORE SPINAL LAMINAE. Bror Rexed discusses the core spinal segments in terms of laminae of the neural tube (Figure 2-5). This tube gives rise to neurons that compose the sensory nuclei of the spinal cord and the brainstem. Each lamina organizes connections. Some neurons, such as at laminae I and V (which contribute significantly to perception of pain), cross to the contralateral side and ascend to the brain. At lamina V, somatic and visceral input converge with fibers that descend from the brain. Other laminae— II to III —integrate multiple segments without exiting the spine. Since

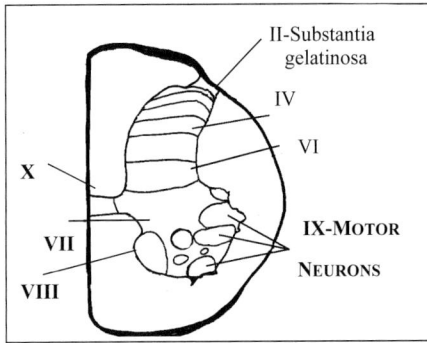

Figure 2-5: Spinal cord laminae (After Willard).

incoming information converges, cells in these laminae contribute to referred pain (Willard *ibid*). Table 1-4 on page 133 summarizes functions of the laminae.

$A\text{-}\delta$ nociceptive fibers terminate in laminae I and V. *C-nociceptive* fibers terminate mainly in laminae I and II, and also in lamina III, where their axon terminals secrete substance P (Thompson 1988). Nociceptor sensory *C*-fibers enter the spinal cord, where they divide into short, descending and ascending branches. Some of the sensory nociceptor fibers cross the cord to the contralateral side and form the anterolateral spinal tract. This anterolateral tract, called the *spinothalamic tract*, connects the basal spinal nucleus with the thalamic nuclei (Willard *ibid*).

One group of cells that receives input from both low threshold and nociceptive afferents is called *multiconvergent* or *wide dynamic range* (WDR) cells. These cells may be activated by noxious stimuli in a large peripheral area and by tactile stimuli in part of that area. They also seem to be involved when pain inhibitory modulation is disturbed, when a patient is experiencing non-noxious stimuli as painful (Andersson 1997). These cells are associate with N-methyl-D-Aspartate (NMDA) receptors and windup of neuropathic pain. WDR cells have been implicated in acupuncture analgesia.

Table 2-3: Spinal Cord Core

Section	Location	Affected System
Dorsal Horn	Posterior.	Processing of sensory information from. • somata. • viscera (internal organs).
Ventral Horn	Anterior.	Motor system.
Intermediary Region	Between the dorsal and ventral horns.	Formed by interneurons linking the: • sensory system (from dorsal horn). • suprasegmental system (brain). • motor system (from ventral horn).

SPINAL NERVES. The spinal cord receives thirty-one pairs of spinal nerves. Each pair of nerves has a ventral and a dorsal root, made up of one to eight rootlets. A spinal segment is defined by the level at which an associated nerve enters the cord. With development, the segmental posterior and anterior branches from each anterior primary ramus unite to form large posterior and anterior nerves. The union of the original segmental posterior and anterior branches from each anterior primary ramus is the basis for the formation of the brachial and lumbosacral plexuses. A segmental spinal nerve provides both sensory and motor innervation of the limbs. One segmental level can innervate more than one type of tissue. For example, dermatome, myotome, and sclerotome receive their innervation from the same segmental level, the nerve root. However, conscious perceptions of sensation from these tissues do not overlap and may be separated by considerable distance; see Figure 2-10 and Figure 2-11 (Willard *ibid*).

The Dorsal Horn

The dorsal roots (except C1) contain afferent (sensory) fibers from the nerve cells in their ganglia. The roots also contain a variety of fibers from cutaneous and deep structures. Most of the axons in the dorsal nerve roots are small C-unmyelinated fibers and A-δ myelinated fibers that carry information about noxious and thermal stimuli. The dorsal roots also contain large A-α fibers that come from muscle spindles, and medium-size A-δ fibers that come from mechanoreceptors in skin and joints (Waxman and deGroot *ibid*).

Once thought to be a simple relay station, the dorsal horn is a complex, medullary core. The intricate circuitry of the dorsal horn includes diverse types of neurons and synaptic connections that have prolific biochemistry. These aspects of the dorsal horn make possible not only reception and transmission of nociceptive (pain) input, but also sensory processing such as the integration of several signals, the selection of signals from numerous signals, the abstraction (removal) of particular signals, and the appropriate dispersion of sensory impulses. This complex local processing is activated by (Bonica 1990):

- Central convergence: The coming together of several sensory receptors on one or a few motor neurons;
- Central summation: The cumulative action of stimuli;
- Excitatory and inhibitory influences that come from the periphery, local interneurons, and the brain.

The functional state of the dorsal horn varies according to the circumstances of somatosensory involvement. The dorsal horn can function in a:

- Normal control state;
- Suppressed state.
  A higher threshold of pain is achieved by descending inhibition (commonly seen in acute athletic injuries);
- Sensitized state;
  A low threshold to pain.

Sensitization of the dorsal horn can occur following peripheral tissue injury or inflammation, and as a result of damage to the peripheral and central nervous systems. In some instances, a pathological response can form a reorganized state in which abnormal synaptic circuitry is established. This reorganization, which can be irreversible, is thought to be secondary to the degeneration of various elements of the system and to the formation of new inputs. Following injury, such reactions have been documented in both the PNS and the CNS (Woolf 1979). Prolonged pain and release of glutamate by pain fibers may act on N-methyl-D-Aspartate (NMDA) receptors in the spinal cord. These receptors become more responsive to all of their inputs, resulting in *central sensitization*. NMDA-receptor activation not only increases the cell's response to pain stimuli, but it also decreases neuronal sensitivity to opioid receptor agonists. (Bennett 2000). NMDA-receptors have been implicated in acupuncture analgesia.

Documented changes in the dorsal horn from ongoing pain have been shown to have bilateral effect even when pain is coming from a unilateral area. These changes include (Galer and Dworkin *ibid*):

- Reorganization.
- Enlargement of the second-order neurons receptive field.
- Modulation of sensory input.
- Alteration in opioid receptors.
- Abnormal ingrowth of sympathetic nerves.
- Windup.

The Ventral Horn

The ventral horn roots carry the axons of large-diameter *alpha* motor neuron axons to extrafusal skeletal muscle fibers (contractile muscle fibers); smaller axons of *gamma* motor neuron to intrafusal (spindles) muscle fibers, preganglionic autonomic fibers, and a few afferent, small-diameter axons that arise from cells in the dorsal root ganglia and convey sensory information from the thoracic and abdominal viscera (Waxman and de Groot *ibid*).

Table 2-4: Spinal Cord Lamina (Waxman and deGroot 1995)

LAMINA I	A thin marginal layer. • Contains neurons that respond to noxious stimuli.
LAMINA II	Also called *substantia gelatinosa*. • Made up of small neurons, some of which respond to noxious stimuli.
LAMINAE III-IV	Known together as *nucleus proprius*. • Main input from fibers that convey position and light-touch senses.
LAMINA V	Contains cells that respond to noxious and visceral afferent stimuli.
LAMINA VI	Deepest layer of dorsal horn. • Contains neurons that respond to mechanical signals from joints and skin.
LAMINA VII	Large zone that contains. • cells of dorsal nucleus medially. • large portion of the ventral gray column. • intermediolateral nucleus in thoracic and upper lumbar regions. • preganglionic sympathetic fibers that project to sympathetic ganglia. Dorsal nucleus contains cells that give rise to posterior spinocerebellar tract.
LAMINAE VIII AND IX	Motor neuron groups in medial and lateral portions of ventral gray column. • Medial portion contains lower motor neurons that innervate axial musculature. • Lateral motor neuron column contains lower motor neurons that innervate distal muscles of arm and leg. Flexor muscles are innervated by motor neurons located centrally in the ventral horn, close to the central canal. Extensor muscles are innervated by motor neurons located more peripherally.
LAMINA X	Represents small neurons around central canal or its remnants.

Table 2-5: Core Brain Segments and Neural Tube Laminae

CORE SEGMENT	LAMINA(E)	ARRANGEMENT
Dorsal Horn	I to VI.	Posterior to anterior.
Ventral Horn	VIII to IX.	Posterior to anterior.
Intermediary	VII.	Between ventral and dorsal.
Auxiliary Column of Cells	X.	Concentrated around central canal.

The Peripheral Nervous System

The peripheral nervous system (PNS) is composed of forty-three pairs of nerves.

- The cranial nerves (twelve pairs) connect with the brain.
- The spinal nerves (thirty-one pairs) connect with the spinal cord.
- Estimated to extend 93,000 miles within the body.

Each peripheral nerve is comprised of smaller functional units—nerve fiber and its axon and sheath. A nerve trunk is composed of different fasciculi (bands of fibers), bound together by the epineurium. The epineurium consists of longitudinal collagen and fibers, fat cells, fibroblasts, blood and lymph vessels (Figure 2-7; Waxman and deGroot *ibid*).

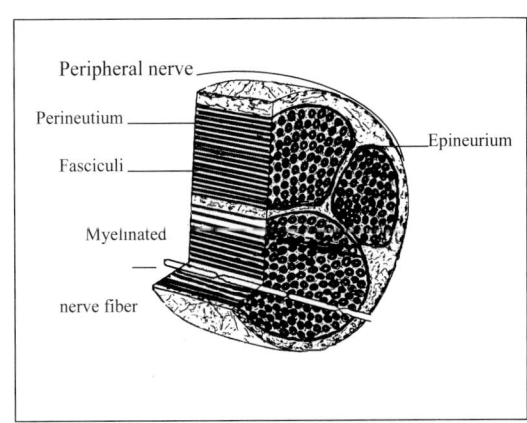

Figure 2-7: Peripheral nerve.

Afferent and Efferent Nerves

The PNS has both *afferent* (sensory) and *efferent* (motor) nerves.

- Afferent nerves (sensory nerves) convey information from receptors in the periphery to the CNS. The cell bodies of afferent neurons are located in structures called "ganglia," which are close to the spinal cord and brain.
- The efferent system (motor system) projects from the CNS to the periphery. It has an autonomic nervous system and a somatic nervous system.
    — The autonomic nervous system innervates smooth muscles, cardiac muscles, glands, and skeletal muscles. The somatic nervous system innervates the musculoskeletal system.

The peripheral somatic neurons are made up of large-diameter, myelinated axons, often called *motor neurons* (Waxman and deGroot *ibid*).

The Autonomic Nervous System

The autonomic nervous system (ANS), (Figure 2-8), involving elements of both the CNS and PNS, is controlled by the hypothalamus gland (and the limbic structures), and pertains to the automatic regulation of all body processes, such as breathing, digestion, heart rate, vascular tone, etc. The hypothalamus itself is closely integrated into a complex network involving the endocrine and immune systems. The autonomic nervous system is highly integrated, in both structure and functionality, with the rest of the nervous system and with the body structures (through numerous somatovisceral and viscerosomatic reflexes). Many of these systems are also associated directly with pain and emotion. In fact, a number of these structures are part of the limbic system, including the anterior cingulate cortex, amygdala, periaqueductal gray (PAG), and hypothalamus (Galer and Dworkin *ibid;* Willard *ibid*).

The autonomic system is an efferent system, that is, it sends information out to the structures away from the cord. All nerves containing autonomic efferent axons also carry primary afferent (sensory) fibers. The primary targets of these primary afferent fibers are the dorsal horn of the spinal cord from approximately T1-L2 and S2-4, and the solitary nucleus of the vagal complex in the medulla. A system called the "visceral afferent nerves" carries afferent impulses from the viscera to the cord. The autonomic system provides input to: the vasculature and fascia throughout the body; the visceral organs of the head and neck; the visceral organs of the thoracoabdominopelvic cavity; thymus, bone marrow, and lymph nodes (Willard *ibid*). The ends of the autonomic motor nerves project out from their insulating myelin sheaths into the ground substance of cells. Their signals are carried up to 2000 nm through the ground substance along fine collagen fibers to the basal membrane of the connective tissue or organ cells. Thus the nervous control of cells does not occur through synapses but through the chemical medium of the ground substance (Frost 2002).

The autonomic nervous system is organized within the central and peripheral nervous systems. The major autonomic components of the central nervous system (CNS) include: limbic forebrain, hypothalamus, several brainstem nuclei and intermediolateral cell columns of the spinal cord. The autonomic components of the peripheral nervous system (PNS) include numerous ganglia (collections of neuron cell bodies located outside of the CNS) and a network of fibers distributed to all tissues of the body with the exception of the hyaline cartilages, the centers of the intervertebral discs, and the parenchymal tissues of the CNS. The axons from neurons located in the CNS enter the periphery through spinal and cranial nerves. Input and output for the peripheral autonomic nervous system occurs via spinal, cranial, and splanchnic (visceral) nerves. Ganglionic neurons of the autonomic system are found primarily in three locations:

1. The paravertebral ganglia or sympathetic trunk lying along the sides of the spinal cord;
2. The prevertebral ganglia or collateral ganglia scattered in several clusters associated with the large organs of the pelvis;
3. In isolated ganglia or hypogastric ganglia embedded in the tissue of specific visceral organs of the pelvis (Willard 2003).

Although the autonomic nervous system has been thought to perform almost entirely involuntarily, this system responds to conscious stimulation. For example, it is well-documented that by vasodilation, blood pressure can be lowered with meditation or biofeedback training.

The Sympathetic and Parasympathetic Nervous Systems

The autonomic system is one of the most important systems as it can integrate many functions. It is, however, one of the least understood systems. According to Korr the sympathetic and parasympathetic systems have usually been thought of as two antagonistic regulatory systems (negative feedback systems). However, they have different origins and functional organization, and their distributions work on different areas. This separation is easy to see by looking at the somatic structures that receive only sympathetic innervation (although the cholinergic [which controls muscle contraction] system is associated with the parasympathetic system).

Sympathetic fibers exit the spinal cord from the thoracic and lumbar regions (thoracolumbar division) that arises from cholinergic preganglionic neurons. The parasympathetic fibers originate from the brain and the sacral portion of the spinal cord (craniosacral division). After exiting, the CNS autonomic fibers synapse in cell clusters called *sympathetic ganglia* and *parasympathetic ganglia*. Many sympathetic ganglia are close to the cord. All others are between the spinal cord and the organs they innervate. Parasympathetic gan-

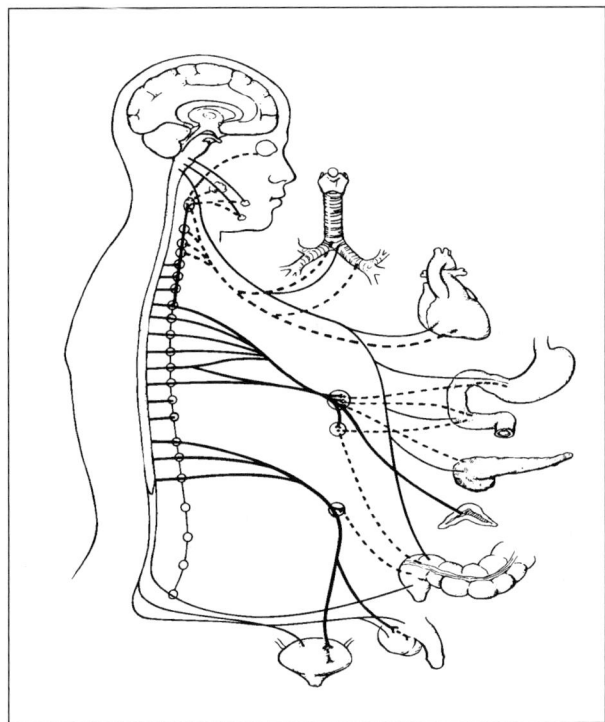

Figure 2-8: The autonomic nervous system.

glia are found within the walls of the effector organs. Preganglionic fibers are found between the CNS and the sympathetic and parasympathetic ganglia. All preganglionic cell bodies are located in the lateral horn of spinal cord segments primarily between T1 and L2; however, they can extend as high as C7 and as low as L3. Their axons leave the spinal cord through ventral roots. Postganglionic fibers are between the ganglia and the effector organs. In general, the postganglionic fibers of the sympathetic system are adrenergic and secrete norepinephrine. However, there are important exceptions. For example, some cholinergic ganglionic neurons contribute to the innervation of the hair follicles and sweat glands as well as possibly innervating the vasculature in skeletal muscles (Willard *ibid*).

The sympathetic (thoracolumbar) division is rapid to respond and produces wide-reaching and varied effects, even as a result of a single afferent impulse. It tends to become very active when a person is stressed, needs to react quickly, and needs to change the physiologic state of the entire body in a matter of seconds (fight-flight, or fright response). Recent information shows that the sympathetic segments of the autonomic nervous system play an important role in sensory processing. Investigations have also demonstrated autonomic innervation of skeletal muscle (Baker and Banks 1986). Axons that stain positive for tyrosine hydroxylase and neuropeptide Y (which suggests sympathetic efferent function) also have been found in the posterior longitudinal ligament, the ventral dura, the periosteum of the vertebral body, the intervertebral disc, and the vertebral body that reaches into the marrow cavities (Ahmed et al 1993). Thus, the sympathetic nervous system innervates all viscera, glands, and all blood vessels. It also affects somatic tissues such as bone, muscles, connective tissue, and even the CNS, peripheral nerves, and the lymph vessels. According to Korr "in all disease processes, there is hypersympathetic activity." Sympathetic hyperactivity strongly inhibits the rate at which injured tissues are regenerated and reduces the body's ability to establish collateral circulation after injury. Reduced circulation from the vasoconstriction that results from sympathetic hyperactivity can increase the risk of infection and increase the rate at which arteriosclerosis is formed (Kuchera and Kuchera 1993).

The *parasympathetic* (craniosacral) division is slower to react and cares for the body when it is resting, relaxing, digesting, recovering, and secreting. Its innervation is strictly to the visceral organs, glands, and smooth muscles. Typical responses include salivation, lacrimation, urination, defecation, and erection (Kuchera and Kuchera 1993). The vagus nerve (cranial nerve X) is the largest of the parasympathetic nerves and is a significant source of parasympathetic innervation to the thoracic and upper abdominal viscera. It enters the thoracic cavity along the upper portion of the mediastinal wall and passes posterior to the root of the lung to gain a position on the walls of the esophagus. Vagal branches are given off to the cardiac and pulmonary plexuses and to the esophageal plexus. Efferent vagal axons arise in the dorsal motornucleus and nucleus ambiguous of the medulla. The vagus is largely a sensory nerve; afferent fibers out number efferent fibers in about 10:1 (Willard *ibid*).

ERGOTROPIC FUNCTION. When postural and musculoskeletal demands change, changes also occur in physiologic demands on circulatory *(OM: Liver)*, metabolic, and visceral activity. Hess (1954) labeled this regulatory sympathetic nervous system (SNS) task an *ergotropic function*. For the SNS to perform this task, it must receive sensory input from the musculoskeletal system, directly through segmental afferent pathways and indirectly through the higher centers, (Korr 1987). Segmental (vertebral) dysfunction can disturb this activity and therefore may have systemic affects (see "Facilitated Segment" this chapter). Respiration and circulation are seen as crucial functions in the Osteopathic model of disease. When discussing respiration, Osteopathic practitioners often speak of respiration at a cellular level, and fluid circulation is seen as essential to this process. Nerves are said to control blood circulation. The arteries supply a route and means for fluids to reach the tissues and the veins and lymphatics allow for the return and purification of blood and extracellular fluids (Patterson 2003).

PERIPHERAL VASCULATURE. The vascular tree is divided into four different types of vessels based on their distinct functions: Conduit vessels comprise the arterial system prior to arterioles; Resistance vessels represent arterioles; Exchange vessels are capillaries; Capacitance vessels consist of veins. Most aspects of the vascular tree receive autonomic innervation that controls the resistance of these vessels to

Table 2-6: Sympathetic Innervation

REGION	LEVEL	COMMENTS
Body in General	T1-12.	Originates in thoracic spine, except for those innervated by sympathetic cell bodies originating at L1 and L2.
Mucous Membranes Vessels of Head Vessels of Neck and Eyes	T1-T3.	
Esophagus	T1-8.	
Upper Limbs	T3-7.	
Heart	T1-5.	Also C3, 4.
Lungs and Pericardium	T1-8	Also C3,4.
GI Tract in General	T5-L5.	Large Intestine also S2-4.
Stomach/Liver/Gallbladder	T5-10.	
Spleen/Pancreas	T5-11.	
Appendix	T10-L5.	Also S2-4.
50% of Legs (upper)	T10-T12.	
50% of Legs (lower)	L1, L2.	
Kidneys	T10-L2.	
Adrenals	T8-L2.	
Gonads/testicle/ovary	T9-L1.	
Bladder	T11-L2.	Also S2-4.
Uterus/Ureter	T11-L2.	Also S2-4. Ureter also S1-4.

blood flow. The vasomotor fibers to the head and neck come from spinal segments T1-4. The vasomotor fibers to the upper extremity come from spinal segments T5-7. The vasomotor fibers to the lower extremity come from spinal segments T10 through L2-3 (Willard *ibid*).

In summary, most structures of the body receive their sympathetic innervation from the thoracic nerves, from which the preganglionic sympathetic cell bodies emanate. The exceptions are structures that are innervated by sympathetic cell bodies that originate at L1 and L2. (Table 2-6 summarizes the innervation levels.) The sympathetic nervous system is commonly involved in chronic pain and in the facilitated segment phenomenon.

Pain Mechanisms

Control of nociception (pain) requires a multi-leveled mechanism that involves not only the brain, but peripheral and spinal controls. Among the many hypotheses proposed to explain the origin, mechanisms, and regulation of pain are the Gate Control Theory, Neuromatrix theory, chemical effect theories, central biasing, hypersensitivity, loss of inhibitory function leading to recruitment of other relay stations, and ectopic (extra) impulses, among others (Bonica 1990; Melzack 1999). The most important theories are covered below. For information on neuropathic pain see page 634.

Gate Control Theory

Melzack and Wall's Gate Control Theory (Melzack and Wall 1965) has probably been the most comprehensive hypothesis on the nature of pain, encompassing even emotional and cognitive facets (Bonica *ibid*). It basically states that impulses in large diameter afferent (sensory) fibers, conducting information about pressure, touch, and vibration, inhibit the central excitation of cells in the dorsal region of the spinal cord. Melzack and Wall have modified their theory several times as information has become available, and many components of it have been confirmed by new evidence. Several elements of the gate theory are applicable broadly (Baldry *ibid*). Wall uses it mostly to explain what he refers to as the "immediate" phase of acute pain. In 1999, Melzack proposed a new theory which he calls the "neuromatrix" theory.

Normally, noxious and non-noxious stimuli transmit from small-diameter (nociceptive pain) nerve fibers to second-order neurons in the spinal cord (the spinothalamic tract; Willard *ibid*). According to Melzack and Wall, before transmission continues up to the brain, a sensory input "gate"—speculated to be located in the dorsal horn of the spinal cord (substantia gelatinosa on lamina II)—is opened by the activity of small-diameter nociceptive nerve fibers and is "closed" by the activity in large-diameter afferent nerve fibers, inhibiting painful stimuli transmission temporarily. They suggest that this gate regulates transmission by integrating information that is coming from the periphery, from the brain, and from within the dorsal horn itself.

The "opening" part of the gate theory has been challenged, however, the conceptual closed gate that inhibits transmission has been verified satisfactorily (Schmidt *ibid*). The information that Melzack and Wall have incorporated recently includes:
- The existence of both excitatory and inhibitory interneurons in the substantia gelatinosa;
- The existence of postsynaptic inhibition in addition to the originally-posited presynaptic inhibition.

Although Wall and Melzack believed at first that large fibers always inhibit small fibers, they now say that, at times, large and small fibers may summate (an additive action) (Baldry *ibid*). Also, stimulation of A-α and A-β (large) fibers of the tibial nerve results in only slight inhibition of the C-fiber, evoking cell activities of the spinothalamic tract. However, when the stimulus intensity that activates A-δ (smaller) fibers is increased, a more powerful inhibition is observed (Chung, Lee, Hori, Endo, and Willis 1984).

Signals from peripheral sensory C-nociceptor fibers (pain fibers) travel at a relatively slow rate of 0.5 to 2 meters per second. Faster A-δ (pain fibers) fiber signals travel at 5-15 meters per second. The A-δ fibers transmit signals from the skin and mucous membrane. C-fibers transmit both from deep tissues and from skin. Nonpainful impulses for pressure and temperature transmit via A-β mechanoreceptors at a faster rate of 30-70 meters per second, and by A-γ fibers that transmit touch and pressure at velocities of 15-40 meters/sec. All these various signals are routed together with painful signals toward the spinal cord. Painful signals and nonpainful signals converge in the dorsal horn and terminate primarily in the upper two lamina (Waxman and deGroot *ibid*; Willard *ibid*).

The gate control theory suggests that an increased activity of large-diameter mechanoreceptive fibers, and other afferent (sensory) fibers that are in competition with or inhibit the slower painful messages, may "close or crowd the gate" to pain signals. Since information travels faster via large-diameter fibers, their stimulation causes them to arrive faster at the spinal cord, thereby inhibiting the pain messages from small-diameter fibers.

There is also a brain component to inhibition of pain that results from stimulation of low-threshold mechanoreceptive fibers located in the skin, tendons, and joints. This stimulation may be able to activate an opioid peptide-mediated serotinergic inhibitory descending system and inhibit pain transmission to the brain (descending from the brain to the spinal cord). A-β fibers from mechanoreceptors travel up the cord to the medulla oblongata's gracile and cuneate nuclei.[6] Axons from these nuclei, and those from the medial lemniscus after it dessicates[7] in the medulla, terminate principally in the ventrobasal thalamus. The medial lemniscus is connected to the periaqueductal grey area in the midbrain, at the upper end of the opioid-peptide mediated serotinergic descending inhibitory system (Baldry *ibid*). Descending tract analgesia involves both serotonin (5HT) and norepinephrine, and analgesia is completely abolished if both sets of neurons are cut (Hammond 1986; Figure 2-9).

It is known now that many of the gate theory mechanisms are regulated chemically. For example, stimulation of certain neurons by acupuncture needles can lead to action potentials of the neuron, which then releases its neurotransmitter and neuropeptide substances. In turn, the neuropeptide

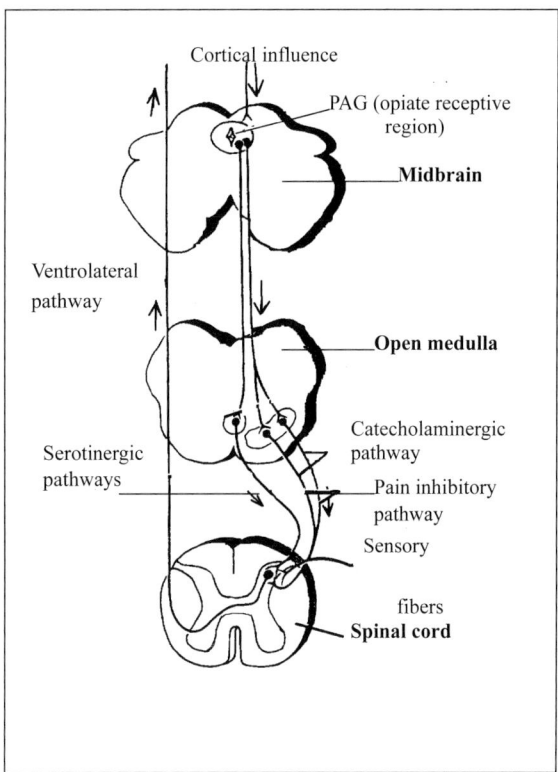

Figure 2-9: Schematic of pain suppression by periaqueductal gray (PAG) matter (the opiate system) and serotinergic systems. The PAG is a primary reception center for ascending nociceptive information, and it also receives descending inhibition from the somatosensory cortex via circuits that distribute to the nucleus dorsal raphe (After Waxman and deGroot 1995). Microinjection of morphine or electrical stimulation of the PAG in the midbrain suppresses behavioral nociceptive reaction in animals and gives a profound inhibition in the spinal cord of neuronal responses to noxious stimuli (Andersson 1997). There are also norepinephrine and GABA systems that influence interneurons and are often involved in neuropathic pain.

substances are thought to be responsible for pain inhibition, or in Wall and Melzack's terminology, the closing of a gate. To stop pain, the practitioner can stimulate these fast-conducting nerves by using shallow subcutaneous acupuncture to stimulate the local A-δ and larger fibers. The gate theory is often used, in part, to explain the action of treatments such as counter-irritation therapies (TENS; topical application of tingling, cooling, or warming ointments; manual therapy; and acupuncture).

The Neuromatrix Theory

The neuromatrix theory has been developed to address the complexity involved in the experience of pain, beyond the simple psychophysical concepts that seek a simple one-to-one relationship between injury and pain (Melzack *ibid*). It is a theory in which a genetically determined template for the body-self is modulated by the powerful *stress system* and the *cognitive functions* of the brain, in addition to the traditional

---

6. The medulla oblongata is the most vital part of the brain continuing as the bulbous portion and the spinal cord.

7. Cross in the form of an "X".

sensory inputs. It proposes that the brain possesses a neural network—the body-self neuromatrix—which integrates multiple inputs to produce the output pattern that evokes pain. The body-self neuromatrix comprises a widely distributed neural network that includes parallel somatosensory, limbic, and thalamocortical components that subserve the *sensory-discriminative, affective-motivational* and *evaluative-cognitive dimensions* of the pain experience. The synaptic architecture of the neuromatrix is determined by genetic and sensory influences. The "neurosignature" output of the neuromatrix—patterns of nerve impulses of varying temporal and spatial dimensions—is produced by neural programs genetically built into the neuromatrix and determines the particular qualities and other properties of the pain experience and behavior. Multiple inputs that act on the neuromatrix programs and contribute to the output and experience of pain (neurosignature) include:

1. Sensory inputs (cutaneous, visceral, and other somatic receptors).

2. Visual and other sensory inputs that influence the cognitive interpretation of the situation.

3. Phasic and tonic cognitive and emotional inputs from other areas of the brain.

4. Intrinsic neural inhibitory modulation inherent in all brain function.

5. The activity of the body's stress-regulating systems, including cytokines as well as the endocrine, autonomic, immune, and opioid systems.

Chemical Theories and Implications

The discovery of endogenous opiates such as endorphins and enkephalins (Snyder 1977) contribute significantly to the understanding of pain perception.

Opioid Peptides/Endorphins are any of the opioid-like endogenous opiates that are composed of many amino acids (peptides) that are secreted by the pituitary gland and that act on the central and peripheral nervous systems. They can effect several systems in the body including the hypothalamus and a neuronal network that projects to midbrain and brainstem (Andersson 1987). Generally, opioid peptides are divided into three distinct peptide families: enkephalins, endorphins, and dynorphins.[8] These peptides are known to have a direct effect on pain awareness and emotional behavior (Thompson 1984). There are also antiopioid substances, the most widely studied and probably the most potent of which is cholecystokinin octapeptide (CCK-8), (Han 2001).

Endorphins exert their effects by binding to opioid receptors and function as synaptic neurotransmitters, possibly modifying the movement of sodium and potassium across nerve membranes and affecting action potentials. Researchers have isolated several endorphins, classified as *alpha, beta,* and *gamma* endorphins. Endorphins not only effect pain but also regulate blood pressure and body temperature (Wall *ibid*).

Enkephalins are two closely related polypeptides found in the brain called *met*-enkephalin and *leu*-enkephalin. Frequently enkephalinergic interneurons are localized in the same areas as opiate receptors that produce pharmacological effects similar to morphine. The amino acid sequence of met-enkephalin has been found in alpha-endorphin and beta-endorphin. The amino acid sequence of beta-endorphin has been found in *beta-lipotropin*, a polypeptide secreted by the anterior pituitary gland (Snyder 1977). Plasma met-enkephalin levels have no relation to other endorphins during circadian studies and corticosteroid suppression tests. Unlike other endorphins, which are produced in the pituitary, met-enkephalins seem to be produced in the adrenal gland, gut, sympathetic ganglia, and peripheral autonomic neurons (Baldry *ibid*).

The inhibition of pain that occurs in the substantia gelatinosa (lamina II) of the spinal cord—as proposed in the gate theory—is achieved in part by chemical mechanisms through the production of enkephalins and dynorphins that interrupt nociceptive transmissions.

Substance P, one of the first polypeptides to be discovered,[9] is a neurotransmitter messenger formed by eleven amino acids found in the hypothalamus, substantia nigra, and dorsal roots of the spinal nerves. It acts to stimulate the vasodilation and contraction of intestinal and other smooth muscles. Substance P also serves as a transmitter for signals carried by alpha and delta nerve axons traveling to and from the periphery, into the dorsal horn of the spinal cord (Marx 1979), where it can mediate long-lasting excitation. Substance P, in particular, appears to transmit and mediate pain signals up the spinal cord segments (Henry 1976). In the brain, it may have an analgesic effect (Stewart et al 1976). Research has suggested that the "gate" in the substantia gelatinosa is partly mediated through release of Substance P (Marx 1977). High levels of Substance P are found in the spinal cord in fibromyalgia patients. Substance P can also be proinflammatory and is involved in neurogenic inflammation (Willard *ibid*).

Peripheral electrical stimulation and acupuncture have been demonstrated to be capable of releasing Substance P (Jin Wenquan et al 1985) as well as other endorphins and antiopioid substances (Han *ibid*).

Other Chemical Theories

Other important chemicals involved in pain are inflammatory mediators such as bradykinin, histamines, and prostaglandins; neurotransmitters such as serotonin, norepinephrine,

---

8. Recently, two novel opioid peptides were reported, Orphanin and endomorphin.

9. Discovered by Von Eurler in 1931. It was not recognized as an endorphin.

dopamine, gamma-aminobutyric acid (GABA), acetylcholine, nitric oxide, glutamate and histamine; gut brain peptides such as neurotensin and Substance P; simple ions such as calcium and magnesium ions, and even adenosine triphosphate (ATP) the energy source of all cells.

INFLAMMATORY MEDIATORS. The nociceptors (pain receptors) belong predominantly to the small and medium size neurons in which algogens such as weak acids,[10] bradykinin,[11] and serotonin produce inward currents that can generate impulse activity (Vyklicky and Knotkova-Urbancova 1996). Nociceptive receptors can be sensitized by chemicals that are secreted by injured tissues. Prostaglandins,[12] for example, make nociceptors fire more easily. As a result, the nociceptor endings become even more sensitive and reactive to chemicals such as bradykinin and histamines, which are capable of firing these pain nerves. The analgesic activity of NSAIDs such as aspirin may be the result of prostaglandins inhibition, which may desensitize nociceptors (Wall *ibid*).

NEUROTRANSMITTERS. Serotonin, norepinephrine, and GABA have been implicated in pain perception by acting as synaptic inhibitors and by influencing the release of Substance P. Medications that affect serotonin and norepinephrine, such as anti-depressants, are often used to treat pain, and decreased levels of blood serotonin have been shown to occur in chronic pain patients (Barson and Solomon 1998). Sensitivity to norepinephrine is often seen in sympathetic nerve fibers post-traumatically. This sensitivity is thought to be one of the causes of sympathetically-maintained pain (Wall *ibid*).

- Serotonin is a neurotransmitter synthesized by the enzymes that act on tryptophan and/or 5-HTP. It is stored in presynaptic vesicles and released to transmit electrochemical signals across the synapse. Serotonin acts, in most cases, as an inhibitory neurotransmitter and like GABA modulates neuron voltage potentials to inhibit glutamate activity and neurotransmitter firing. Serotonin ascending fibers have been demonstrated to run from the midline raphe nuclei in the midbrain, and from the ventromedial reticular formation, with axons projecting through the ventral tegmentum and medial forebrain bundle, to innervate forebrain structures. Descending serotonin fibers have been demonstrated to run from the raphe magnus nucleus, with axons projecting through the anterior and lateral funiculi, to innervate the spinal cord dorsal horn, and sympathetic lateral column cells (Kho and Robertson 1997). Increasing serotonin levels raise the pain threshold. Drugs such as clomipramine and pargyline that raise serotonin levels, can potentiate acupuncture analgesia (Zao, Meng, Yu, Ma, Dong and Han 1987). The gut is the largest organ in which serotonin is found.

- Norepinephrine is synthesized from dopamine by means of the enzyme dopamine beta-hydroxylase, with oxygen, copper, and vitamin C as co-factors. Cells that use norepinephrine for formation of epinephrine use SAMe as a methyl group (the radical CH_3) donor. Norepinephrine acts as an excitatory neurotransmitter and modulates neuron voltage potentials to favor glutamate activity and neurotransmitter firing. Norepinephrine has complex effects, being different in the brain and spinal cord and in different animals. In the brain, norepinephrine seems to have an antagonistic effect on analgesia produced by acupuncture and morphine, whereas in the spinal cord it potentiates acupuncture analgesia (Han et al *ibid*; Xie, Tong, and Han 1981). Studies of norepinephrine networks in the primary somatosensory cortex have shown that the net effect of norepinephrine release is to raise the signal-to-noise ratio of neural signals (Koslow *ibid*). Animal models of neuropathic pain, as well as studies performed in patients with neuromas and complex regional pain have demonstrated that the damaged peripheral nerves become sensitized to norepinephrine (Wall *ibid*).

- GABA is a true neurotransmitter and is the major inhibitory neurotransmitter of the brain, occurring in 30-40% of all synapses. GABA is second only to glutamate the brain's major excitatory neurotransmitter. Its concentration in the brain is 200-1000 times greater than that of the monoamines or acetylcholine. GABA has two different effects on morphine and acupuncture analgesia, and probably on pain perception. In the brain, GABA seems to be antagonistic, whereas in the spinal cord it may have agonistic effects (Fan, Qu, Zhe and Han 1982; Pomeranz and Nguyen 1987).[13]

- Dopamine is an amine neurotransmitter derived from the amino acid tyrosine. It serves as a precursor to norepinephrine and epinephrine. Dopamine acts, in most cases, as an excitatory neurotransmitter and modulates neuron voltage potentials to favor glutamate activity and neurotransmitter firing. Dopamine seems to have antagonistic effects in the brain, and acupuncture analgesia results in decreased concentration in the caudate nucleus in rats (Sun, Boney and Lee 1984).

- Acetylcholine is an ester (combination of an organic acid with an alcohol) of choline occurring in various organs and tissues of the body. It is the major transmitter across the myoneuroal junctions. Acetylcholine reduction, by administration of hemicholine (HC-3) to the intracerebroventricular, does not alter the pain threshold but does

---

10. Pain producers.
11. Bradykinin is a peptide of nonprotein origin containing nine amino acid residues. It is a potent vasodilator.
12. Prostaglandins are eicosanoids formed by fatty acids which are part of the arachidonic acid inflammatory cascade.

13. The drug Valium, which increases central GABA levels, has antagonistic effects on acupuncture analgesia. When using amino acid therapy to augment neural functions it is often important to first increase GABA by supplementing with L-theanine and 5HTP. This may help prevent over stimulation by excitatory amino acids such as tyrosine and phenylalanine.

reduce the analgesic effects of acupuncture (Ren, Tu and Han 1987).

- Nitric oxide (NO) is a gaseous neurotransmitter that has important effects in the CNS, peripheral nervous system, vascular system, and endocrine system. NO may be involved in central sensory and memory areas related to pain. Acupuncture seems to modulate NO activity in the hippocampus, brainstem (nucleus gracilis), basal ganglia striatum, and the cerebral cortex, all of which are important in pain perception and behavior (Koslow et al *ibid;* Kim et al *ibid*; West et al 2000; Ma *ibid*).

Acupuncture and electroacupuncture have been shown to stimulate the release of all of the above neurotransmitter mediators with different electrical frequencies stimulating different neurotransmitters.

ATP (ADENOSINE TRIPHOSPHATE). ATP has been shown to function as a messenger in the glial communication system. ATP has many features that makes it an excellent messenger molecule between cells. It is highly abundant inside cells but rare outside of them. It is small and therefore diffuses rapidly, and it breaks down quickly. All these traits ensure that new messages conveyed by ATP molecules are not confused with old messages. Moreover, ATP is neatly packaged inside the tips of axons, where neurotransmitter molecules are stored; it is released together with neurotransmitters at synapses and can travel outside synapses, too. Astrocytes (a type of glial cells) have been shown to release ATP when excited. The ATP binds to receptors on nearby astrocytes, prompting ion channels to open and allow an influx of calcium. The rise triggers ATP release from those cells, setting off a chain reaction of ATP-mediated calcium responses across the population of ostrocyes. ATP release has also been shown to trigger calcium influx into Schwann cells. This influx can cause signals to travel from the cells' membrane to the nucleus, where the genes are stored, causing various genes to switch on. Amazingly, by firing to communicate with other neurons, an axon could instruct the readout of genes in a glial cell and thus influence its behavior (Fields *ibid*).[14]

ATP has been shown recently to bind to P2X-3 protein. P2X-3 is a gene that encodes a protein found to exist only in sensory C-fibers. This creates a protein that floats on the surface of nociceptors and helps mediate specific biochemical properties of the pain-mediating neurons, giving the neuron its uniquely defined function. When ATP binds to this protein the nerve fires. Since ATP is found in all cells (giving cells energy), when the cells are destroyed, ATP is released into the extracellular space, where it can come in contact with this protein, on nociceptor nerves, and initiate pain sensation. The initial pain, from tissue damage, may result from the release of cytoplasmic components that act upon nociceptors.[15] ATP was proposed to fill this role, because it elicits pain when applied intradermally and may be the active compound in cytoplasmic fractions that cause pain. Additionally, ATP opens ligand-gated ion channels (P2X receptors) in sensory neurons, and only sensory neurons express messenger RNA for the P2X3 receptor (Cook, Vulchanova, Retrieves, Elde, and McCleskey 1997).[16] Administration of ATP results in a delayed time-course affect and suggests that it may occur in concert with other mediators that are recruited by the inflammatory process, rather than reflecting a direct depolarization of sensory nerves (Sawynok and Reid 1997). Localized acidosis, associated with tissue injury, may enhance pain perception via an action on ATP-gated ion channels on mammalian sensory neurons (Li, Peoples, Weight and Li 1996).

Ancillary Pain Mechanisms

Researchers have posited several ancillary pain mechanisms.

Peripheral Mechanisms

Most types of musculoskeletal pain probably occur due to peripheral (non-central nervous system) mechanisms, especially when the pain involves nerve endings (Bonica *ibid*).

In such cases, the causes of pain are probably secondary to the direct irritation of the peripheral nervous system (Asbury and Fields 1984). This assertion is supported by the fact that treatment of the peripheral joint often relieves pain. Involvement of the peripheral nervous system can be due to noxious stimulation such as inflammation, hypersensitivity of nerves due to nerve injury (Cannon and Rosenblueth's law of supersensitivity in denervation), joint dysfunctions (lack of normal motion) (Iggo 1984), and various reflexes and other mechanical dysfunctions that probably stimulate one of the above conditions. The newly discovered NMDA receptor cells in peripheral joints may explain the windup like phenomenon seen often in patients with chronic joint disease (Brown personal communication).

Peripheral-Central Mechanisms

Peripheral-central mechanisms, or the interaction of peripheral and central pathways, are seen in the vicious cycle of reflex pain. Livingston has described a vicious cycle of reflexes in which nociception increases in the primary afferent and then activates preganglionic sympathetic neurons (between the ganglia and the CNS). This leads to activation of postganglionic neurons that sensitize and activate primary afferent nociceptors, which feed back to the spinal cord, maintaining the pain cycle. Although this cycle is said to be also set up by painful input (within a muscle) that leads to

---

14. Laser, photonic and microcurrent therapy are said to stimulate ATP production and may initiate genes to be "turned on."

15. Cytoplasm is all of the substance of a cell other than the nucleus.

16. Ligand is an organic molecule attached to a specific site on a surface or to a tracer element, like vitamin B12.

muscle spasm, which activates more motor neurons, sustaining the spasm. And that the spasm activates nociceptors, which feed back to the spinal cord, creating a vicious cycle, newer information has shown that pain originating within a muscle lead to inhibition rather than facilitation (spasm) of the same muscle. In severe manifestations of peripheral central mechanisms (such as reflex sympathetic dystrophy), the peripheral-central reflex is commonly due to a more serious lesion in the peripheral, dorsal root, and ganglion. These are often due to deafferentation (Bonica *ibid*).[17]

In phantom limb pain it has been shown that any input to the hyperactive central cells (which can also come from any nearby injured tissue, from visceral sensory nerves, from small afferents in the sympathetic chain, and from higher psychoneuronal processes), can trigger abnormal, prolonged firing and produce severe, persistent pains in discrete areas of the denervated limb or other body parts (Melzack *ibid*).

The *facilitated cord segment* is an important concept in the osteopathic evaluation and treatment of both musculoskeletal and organ dysfunctions. A facilitated segment is an abnormal or exaggerated response within a spinal segment created by peripheral-central mechanisms. Sherington and Korr have proposed that a low threshold exists in this syndrome, and that any sensory excitation via somatovisceral (the body structure influencing the organs) or viscerosomatic (the viscera influencing the body structure) mechanism can cause a reflex and a vicious cycle of dysfunction and pain.

The segment is said to be in a hypersensitive state, and it is said to produce exaggerated responses to any stimulation, physical or emotional. Work by the Sato demonstrated the affect of somatic stimulation on various visceral functions, to range from heart rate to adrenal output. Sensitization can occur within the spinal cord or from afferent activity from the somatic stimulation which travels up the spinal cord to the brainstem, resulting in a cascade of activity from the brainstem back down to the spinal autonomic motoneurons (Kuchera and Kuchera 1993; Patterson and Wurster 2003). The multiconvergent or wide dynamic range (WDR) cells that may be activated by noxious stimuli in a large peripheral area and by tactile stimuli in part of that area, are probably involved when pain inhibitory modulation is disturbed, and when a patient is experiencing non-noxious stimuli as painful (Andersson *ibid*). This facilitation of the peripheral-central pathways have been associate with N-methyl-D-Aspartate (NMDA) receptors resulting in the so-called "windup" of neuropathic pain. (*OM: Peripheral-central reflex mechanisms fit very well with OM's internal-external channel Organ relationship, Bladder channel Shu/back points, and coactivation theories*).

Nerve Sprouting

It has been shown that injury can induce a sprouting of nerves in the injured area, and that it can lead to the creation of connections between motor (including sympathetic) and sensory (afferent) nerves. Also, the repeated stimulation of a nerve causes it to grow in diameter and to invade more receptor sites than before. Repeated stimulation at the dorsal horn can lead to changes at the receptor site. These pathological neural circuits, along with a decrease of synaptic thresholds—probably due to neuropeptides such as substance P, inflammatory mediators, and other neuromuscular and atrophic changes—lead to increased pain activation by other normal motor nerves and in a wider distribution of pain. This may explain why mild activity aggravates pain in chronic pain sufferers (Willard 1995). A stated before, lately NMDA receptors, which are associated with windup, neuropathic pain, and WDR cells, have been found in peripheral joints and may be increased in numbers by chronic pain states.

Sympathetic Nervous System Involvement

The sympathetic nervous system is often involved in chronic pain. Many of the primary afferent fibers in autonomic nerves are of the small-caliber variety (the B-afferent system); a few larger myelinated fibers are also present (the A-afferent system). In general, the input over visceral afferent to the medullary brainstem involves the non noxious regulation of organ function. Conversely, many of the primary afferent fibers targeting the spinal cord have characteristics of nociceptive fibers. They produce neuropeptides such as substance-P and calcitonin gene-related polypeptide and respond to nociceptive stimuli. In addition, some are capable of eliciting a neurogenic inflammatory response in surrounding tissue (Willard *ibid*). This system has been shown to innervate muscles, ligaments, and discs (Raja *ibid*). Currently the term *sympathetically maintained pain* is used to describe conditions that respond to medical intervention to the sympathetic system.

When chronic pain patients experience pain adrenaline levels rise and can cause a significant increase in abnormal ectopic discharges in damaged, and therefore sensitized, nociceptors, culminating in the perception of worsening pain. Sympathetic ectopic foci (windup or extra-firing of nerves, with an expression of novel sodium channel receptor subtype) may be responsible for Travell's trigger point activity. In patients with myofascial dysfunction affected muscles can be very sensitive to norepinephrine—by increasing norepinephrine levels, stress can cause muscle spasm which results in increased pain (see page 584; Galer and Dworkin *ibid*). In sympathetically maintained pain one may finds trophic changes such as:

- Skin becomes pale, cold, clammy, showing goose flesh and increased red response or dermographia.
- Trophic edema with subcutaneous thickening and reduced pliability.
- Muscle tension, reduced stretchability, and increased motor point tenderness.
- Joint restrictions and hypertrophy.

---

17. Interruption in the afferent nerve system.

Table 2-7: International Association for the Study of Pain (IASP) Definition of Pain Terms (Galer and Dworkin *ibid*).

PAIN TERM	DEFINITION
ALLODYNIA	Pain due to a stimulus that does not normally provoke pain
ANALGESIA	Absence of pain in response to stimulation that would normally be painful
HYPERALGESIA	An increased response to a stimulus that is normally painful
HYPERESTHESIA	Increased sensitivity to stimulation excluding the special senses
HYPERPATHIA	Abnormally painful reaction to a stimulus, especially a repetitive stimulus, as well as an increased threshold
HYPOALGESIS	Diminished pain in response to normally painful stimulation
HYPOESTHESIA	Decreased sensitivity to stimulation, excluding the special senses

Sensitization/Deafferenation

Chronic pain research is increasingly showing involvement of the nervous system in chronic pain, due to sensitization. Nervous system plasticity (re-wiring) may also be responsible for the maintenance of some types of chronic pain (Miller 1997). The exact changes and causes in peripheral or central nervous sensitization that occur in the presence of chronic pain and dysfunction are unknown. Perl et al (1976) eliminated acetylcholine, histamine, 5-HT, bradykinin, pH, potassium, and prostaglandins as candidates for being the cause of sensitization in unmyelinated afferents. More recent studies show that sensitization by prostaglandins and norepinephrine is implicated with pain that is maintained sympathetically. Tasker (1991) proposed that the use of "deafferenation pain" is appropriate for all conditions that commonly are called neuropathic pain (Bonica *ibid;* Wall *ibid*). NMDA receptors may be associated with peripheral sensitization as they have now been found in pathologic joints.

Sensitization can also occur in the central nervous system. For example, magnetoencephalographic and evoked potential studies in patients who have chronic back pain have demonstrated central nervous system hyper-responsiveness in the primary somatosensory cortex (Flor, Birbaumer, Fust 1993). Migration of substance P from the tip of the dorsal horn to deeper areas was found following protracted stimulation of pain (Loeser 2000). Multiconvergent or wide dynamic range (WDR) cells have been implicated as well.

Unlike physiologic pain which has an adaptive role, pathologic pain is a pathogenic factor causing disturbances in the activity of the organism and its systems. Current views on the nature of pathologic pain are mainly concerned with neurochemical and plastic processes occurring in nociceptive neurons but not with systemic mechanisms of pathological pain. This limitation has been overcome with the elaboration of the pathophysiologic theory of generatory and systemic mechanisms of algesic syndromes. According to this theory, a pathogenetic basis for a pathologic pain is the formation and functioning of new pathologic integrations within the algesthesia system—an aggregate of changed nociceptive neurons acting as a generator of pathologically enhanced excitation and a new pathodynamic organization from changed parts of the algesthesia system which represents a pathological algic system. This theory can explain many peculiarities of pain syndromes without contradicting cell-mediated and neurochemical mechanisms of pathological pain (Korsakova 1999).

ALLODYNIA AND HYPERALGESIS. An injury to the skin or to an internal organ evokes a discharge in the nociceptive afferents (pain sensory fibers) that innervate the damaged area and, as a consequence of the ensuing inflammatory process, sensitizes these nociceptive endings. The activity of sensitized nociceptors evokes two different alterations of pain sensation:

- A change in the modality of the sensation evoked by low threshold mechanoreceptors, from touch to pain (allodynia).
- An increase in the magnitude of the pain sensations evoked by mechanically sensitive nociceptors (hyperalgesia).

Allodynia and hyperalgesia show that pain sensation is a dynamic process whose presence and intensity depend on the past history of an affected area and not only on the magnitude of the stimulus. During the initial injury and for the duration of the repair process, there will be increased nociceptive activity from the injured region. These afferent barrages cause, in turn, central changes in excitability mediated circuits by positive feedback loops between spinal and supraspinal neurons and by the enhanced synaptic actions of certain neurotransmitters. Among these transmitters, attention has currently focused on the actions of NMDA receptors and neurokinins as putative mediators of the increases in central excitability induced by noxious stimuli. The overall mechanism combines the features of the classical "pain pathway" with the dynamic plastic changes mediated by non-conventional neurotransmitters (Cervero 2000).

Many other hypotheses have been proposed to explain the mechanisms of pain (and causalgia/complex regional pain II), such as central biasing, hypersensitivity, loss of inhibitory function leading to recruitment of other relay stations, and ectopic (extra) impulses (Bonica *ibid*). More details on some of these can be found in the "Referred Pain" section of this chapter.

Gunn (*ibid*) states that myofascial pain syndromes as well as many organic disorders (allergies for example) are manifestations of denervation supersensitivity. Acupuncture needling is believed to result in the stimulation and healing of these nerves.

Table 2-7 summarizes the International Association of the Study of Pain definition of pain terms.

Aspects of Pain

An understanding of phase, perception, localization, source and severity of pain is helpful in determining an approach to treatment. The phases of pain can be described as acute or chronic.

Acute Pain

Bonica has defined acute pain as:

> ...a complex or constellation of unpleasant sensory, perceptual, and emotional experiences and certain associated autonomic, psychologic, emotional and behavioral responses.

Acute pain results from noxious stimulation produced by injury or disease. Its function is to warn the individual that something is disordered. It may limit the patient's activity, thereby preventing further injury, or it may cause the patient to seek attention and/or to pay attention. Associated physiological responses from the stress reaction are increased: respiration, blood pressure, heart rate, blood flow to muscles, and enhanced attention. The resulting inflammation also aids in healing.

In the case of acute trauma, a painless period (known as stress analgesia) following the injury is common and serves to allow the "fight or flight" option. Injury elicits impulses in all types of fibers. Some are inhibitory impulses that may deter further excitation of the neuron, such as large, myelinated A-β fibers, and some are excitatory impulses, such as unmyelinated C-fibers and myelinated A-δ fibers which can increase excitation of the neuron (Bonica *ibid*).

Wall divides acute pain into two stages that he calls *immediate* and *acute*.

Wall's Immediate Pain Stage

Wall's *immediate* (nociceptive) pain signals tissue distress and/or immediate damage. This happens, for example, when one is slapped on the face. The quick signal occurs by way of injury-sensitive A-δ and C-fibers.

Immediate pain is associated with an activation of the nervous system, not with injured tissues. However, it can change the subsequent excitability/threshold of these nerve terminals. As a response to the initial excitation, some terminals become more sensitive, and others become less sensitive. Therefore, even brief pain is dynamic rather than static, and it can cause changes within the nervous system. A short, quick trauma may change the circuitry and the perception of pain for a longer duration. Immediate pain is not considered a significant cause of chronic pain (Wall *ibid*).

Wall's acute pain stage

The second of Wall's acute-pain stages is usually caused by tissue damage such as occurs in trauma. This kind of tissue damage fires nerve endings by mechanical, thermal, or chemical effects. Inflammatory processes that occur in this phase are due to the production of substances such as vasoactive amines,[18] acidic lipids, lysosomal components, and lymphocyte products. Some of these inflammatory mediators can activate nociceptors as well. Various chemicals such as bradykinin, histamine, prostaglandins, and potassium ions are capable of sensitizing C (type IV) and A-δ (type III) sensory nerves. These chemicals, especially bradykinin, also can sensitize sympathetic nerve fibers (Bonica *ibid;* Wall *ibid*).

Acute pain sets in motion:
- Diminishment of inhibition;
- Change in the environment of nerve endings;
- Change in the cord reaction to some types of peripheral stimulation.

This results in an increase in all remaining sensory input, which usually consists of painful stimuli (Wall 1984). In Wall's acute phase, the pain is thought to be mostly due to C-afferent fibers, and possibly to various chemical mediators that act intraspinally. An *acute* nociceptive input can induce prolonged functional and physical changes in the nervous system. *Prolonged acute nociception* may result in neuroplastic changes that may not be reversible. There is growing data suggesting that the control of acute pain with narcotics or local anesthetics if necessary, can prevent the development of chronic pain.

Chronic Pain

Chronic pain is not simply a repetition of acute pain. The patient's anxious, emotional response to acute pain is often replaced by a depressed, obsessed, and irritable mood. Bonica defines chronic pain as:

> ...pain that persists a month beyond the usual course of an acute disease or a reasonable time of an injury to heal, or that is associated with a chronic pathologic process that causes continuous pain, or pain that recurs at intervals for months or years.

Others define chronic pain as being of more than six-months in duration. Chronic pain is different from and less understood than acute pain. Often this type of pain does not produce the obvious autonomic nervous system reactions

---

18. Amine is a type of organic compound that contains nitogen.

that result from acute pain. Usually such reactions are present, but tend to be less obvious.

Chronic pain is caused by pathogenic processes in the soma (non-internal organ parts of the body) and viscera (internal organs); by inflammation; changes within the nervous system; and psychological factors. Often acute pain is followed by functional and structural changes within the central or peripheral nervous system (Gunn *ibid*). These include alterations of cell phenotype; changes in the expression of proteins such as receptors, transmitters and ion channels; and modifications of neural structure (Dray, Urban, Dickenson 1994). These changes often result in sensitization of nociceptors that may acquire ongoing (spontaneous) discharge, a lowered activation threshold, and an increased response to subthreshold stimuli and stimulation from other, possibly normal, tissues (Bonica *ibid*; Wall *ibid*; Willard *ibid*). Chronic pain most likely, but not necessarily, involves all three types of pain: *nociceptive, neuropathic*, and *central* (Woessner 2003).

Chronic pain can develop when pain is due to tissue damage. If the pain results from mechanical forces such as subluxation, ligament, and tendon overstress and/or weakening, trigger point activation, or inflammation (from repeated irritating injuries as in tendinitis), stimulation of pain receptors can be ongoing and continuous. Chronic inflammation that appears as redness, increased local temperature, and swelling (such as rheumatoid arthritis and lupus) is most often caused by abnormal immunologic responses. Chronic inflammation (Ryan and Majno 1983) can be present without these obvious signs as well.

Most patients with chronic pain use the same words to describe their pain as do patients with acute pain, including aching, throbbing, burning, shooting, stinging, and sensitivity or tenderness of the skin. However, most patients with chronic pain report that their pain is worse than any acute pain they have experienced, especially if they have neuropathic pain. This may be a result of secondary emotional reactions due to the uncertainly of an unknown prognosis (Galer and Dworkin 2000).

As with acute pain, chronic pain is frequently associated with a stress reaction, including increases in blood pressure, heart rate, and respiration rate. Guarding and protection of the painful body part may also continue. Unlike in acute pain, the stress reaction and guarding of the painful area are maladaptive and may actually become part of the problem. In most people with chronic neuropathic pain, the stress reaction and protection of the painful region occur involuntarily (Galer and Dworkin *ibid*).

In summary, most chronic musculoskeletal pain is probably due to mechanical dysfunctions that lead to, or are caused by, disturbances of tissue structure and function. Often these result from degenerative processes and the reactions to them (i.e., secondary effects). Subtle changes affect the mechanically-linked systems of the musculoskeletal body, causing stresses on tissues, injuring them and leading to activation of the nervous pain perception systems. The nervous mechanisms can become facilitated and cause pain on their own. The health effects of chronic pain are vast and include: increased risk of heart disease, lowered immunity and increased risk of illness, as well as psychological sequelae such as depression, fatigue, anxiety and suicide. Secondary guarding and physical deconditioning can become an additional source of pain with:

- Muscle atrophy causing pain;
- Muscle tightness and spasm causing pain (myofascial reaction);
- Shorting and loss of elasticity of tendons and ligaments, causing loss of range-of-motion and pain;
- Brittle bones, increasing the risk of fracture.

Psychological Influences on Pain

Psychological causes of chronic pain are complex and may represent a psychiatric disorder or a complex dynamic reorganization among converging neurons. Considering that it has been estimated that the brain has as many as 400,000 synaptic terminals in a single axon, and that it has 100 billion neurons (Melzack 1984), it is not surprising that many neuropsychological changes occur with chronic pain (Bonica *ibid*). Secondary psychosocial illness behavior, including depression, anxiety, inactivity, and pain avoidance, are the consequent rule in chronic pain sufferers (Naliboff et al 1985). Inflammation has also been shown to influence serotonin level by inducing indolamine 2, 3 dioxygenase (IDO), which is a rate-limiting enzyme in the degradation of tryptophan needed for the production of serotonin (Wichers and Maes 2004).

Emotional influences can have strong modulation effect on the perception of pain. The result of research provide support for the importance of the individual's interpretation of his or her pain. The meaning attributed to pain not only has a direct effect on the behavioral response to it, but also influences the intensity of the pain experienced. Humans have the innate ability to modulate the pain sensation as well as the emotional, autonomic, and motor responses to pain. If the meaning of pain involves threat or harm, the pain will be perceived with more intensity. If a pain is labeled as potentially damaging, the limbic system is activated. A headache that is considered a result of stress and muscle tension is perceived as less painful than one that is thought to be symptomatic of a brain tumor. Modulating pain by altering its meaning (for example, by providing understanding and reassurance) is an important, but often neglected, therapeutic tool in pain management. If the patient focuses on pain, the brain actually perceives more pain, but when an individual is distracted, the brain perceives less pain. Distraction elicits a true neurophysiological response within the brain that results in alleviation of pain. (Galer and Dworkin *ibid*). Dr. Sarno (1991) reports the compleat resolution of pain and disability in 79% of his patients, regardless of medical diagnosis, by having the patient acknowledge that his/her pain is due to emotional repression (because it is so-called "caused" by the brain attempt to further hide emotional anger or pain).

As Korr (1976, 1986) points out, the musculoskeletal system involves a complex functional interaction between the nervous system and the somatic systems which include input from the limbic system and emotional effects:

> It is no semantic accident that posture and attitude apply to both the physical and psychological domains. Given the unity of the body and mind, posture reflects the history and status of both and helps in determining where and how the body framework is vulnerable.

Studies have shown a link between symptom-specific physiological reactivity and pain severity in reaction to stressful events, especially in depressed patients (Burns et al 1997). Anxiety, sensitivity, or the fear of anxiety-related bodily sensations, arising from beliefs that the physical sensations have harmful consequences, is associated with pain behavior and disability (Asmundson and Taylor 1996). Pain is often made worse by fear, anger, or a sense of isolation. The pain may be diminished if the patient understands the cause and loses his/her fear. Patients who keep busy find that sensory and other distractions relieve pain (Brand 1997). Depression, hypochondriasis, anxiety, and hysteria are related to poor clinical outcomes (Cats-Baril and Frymoyer 1991). The pain associated with depression is commonly represented by headache, back pain, or nonspecific musculoskeletal complaints. In fact, in one study of 1146 patients with major depression, physical symptoms were the *chief* or *exclusive* complaint for 69% of those identified. Anxiety is often comorbid with depressed mood and, in terms of patients affected, is roughly as common as physical symptoms. Physical symptoms may have predictive value in depression screening, with one investigation finding back pain and nonspecific musculoskeletal pain significantly predictive (43% and 39%, respectively). Both patients and physicians may so emphasize these physical presentations that the diagnosis of depression can be delayed or missed altogether. Kirmayer and colleagues documented that highly somatic presentations of depression were missed more often than those with significant psychosocial contexts. This may be due to interference from symptoms attributable to previously diagnosed comorbid illness (e.g., diabetes, asthma, arthritis) or to new somatic diagnoses created to account for individual presentations of depression. Regardless, it is important to realize that depression may "amplify" the intensity or distress attributable to an existing complaint or serve as the basis for any one of a number of pseudonymous diagnoses—aliases for depression that may be specialty specific. Therefore, any patient with symptoms out of proportion to objective findings, chronic or "functional" pain, irritable bowel syndrome, disequilibrium, "hypoglycemic" episodes of undetermined cause, "hormone imbalances," fibromyalgia, and the like should be considered fertile ground for the diagnosis of depression (Medscape 2003).

Many individuals with chronic pain also have clinical depression. The depression should not be ignored, since depression, when present, influences the pain and, in turn, depression can be influenced by the level of pain. Those who treat pain should screen for depression with tools such as the *Beck Depression Inventory*, and should work with mental health professionals to treat the more distressed individuals. To have an optimal outcome, both the pain and the depression need to be treated (Rush, Polatin and Gatchel 2000). Case histories of patients who later developed low back pain show that often the patient was under stress before experiencing pain, and that the episode of trauma that resulted in pain was minor (Kirkaldy-Willis 1990). Dual action antidepressant medications (acting on both serotonin and norepinephrine such as Effexor) seem to work best in patients suffering from depression accompanied by somatic symptomes. However, physical symptoms often improve only in the beginning of treatment and then plateau even when depression continuously improves.

To determine whether a loss of function and the pain behavior is primarily psychological or chiefly neurophysiological, Simons, Travell and Simons (*ibid*) suggest asking three questions:

1. How effective were the patient's skills in coping with the problems of life prior to the onset of pain?

2. Does the patient concentrate on finding ways to do things that circumvent the pain, or focus on reasons why not to?

3. Is function something the patient tries to do, or only talk about?

Chaitow (2001) writes:

> A patient with major social, economic, and emotional stressors current in her life and who presents with muscular pain and backache is unlikely to respond—other than in the short term— to manual approaches which ignore the enormous and multiple coping strains she is handling. In many instances, the provision of a job, a new home, a new spouse (or removal of the present one) would be the most appropriate treatment in terms of addressing the real causes of such pain or backache. However, the practitioner must utilize those skills available so that suitable treatment will, if nothing else, minimize the patient's mechanical and functional strains—even if they do not always deal with what is really wrong!.......Suitable treatment for pain and dysfunction which has evolved out of the somatization by the patient of emotional distress might well be helped more through application of deep relaxation methods, non-specific "wellness" bodywork methods, and/or counselling and enhancement of stress-coping abilities, rather than specific musculoskeletal interventions which impose yet another adaptation demand on an already overextended system. The art of successfully applying manual approaches to healing lies, at least in part, in recognizing when intervention should be specific and when it needs to be more general.

Psychological Diagnosis

Primary gain is defined as when neurotic patients unconsciously develop (physically expressed) psychological symptoms that tend to relieve their high level of anxiety and tension. Secondary gain occurs when some patients discover that there are privileges for being sick in regard to exemption from the normal responsibilities of work and/or mature social interactions; the patients become accustomed to the benefits of having pain (Simons, Travell and Simons *ibid*). In the DSM-IV pain disorders are divided into: pain disorder associated with psychological factors (307.80) and pain disorder associated with both psychological factors and a general pain condition (307.89).

FUNCTIONAL OVERLAY SYNDROME. This syndrome may be defined as whatever else the patient brings along with their organic (physical) disease to the clinical setting. These may include psychological, emotional, coping, and interactional styles. Lechnyr and Holes (2002) divide functional overlay syndrome into eleven types:

1. The *"frightened"* patient either directly or indirectly conveys his or her fear. This may be conveyed in language noting a high physiologic arousal (fear), or in protective posturing (an attempt to avoid any further damage). The patient's internal images of what their symptoms mean are perceived in catastrophic terms. As a result, the patient may talk too much, ask too many questions, be overly-dramatic, emotional, and have a sense of on-going panic and reactivity that makes exposure to this patient somewhat overwhelming.

   These patients need in-depth education, that may need repetition several times.

2. The *"please me"* patient complains either verbally or non-verbally that no one cares or takes the time to listen and understand them. This patient values relationship above technical information, and before developing confidence in any treatment (or practitioner), this patient needs to feel that they are seen as an "individual" that is being heard and cared for.

   A close relationship needs to develop before any treatment commences. A patient who seems depressed, may in actuality just be a patient wanting to be heard.

3. The *"I hurt everywhere you touch"* patient may have a low pain tolerance and is often difficult to perform a physical examination on. The patient exhibits a poor ability to discriminate the severity of his/her felt sensations. An exact "diagnosis" is often difficult to make. Usually the patient is suffering from symptoms of endogenous depression with exhaustion, sleep disorder, mood and concentration difficulties. The patient expects a great deal of him/her-self and may exhibit embarrassment, a fear of having psychological problems, or a sense of inadequacy. He/she may be *genetically* programed to feel things more intensely. This does not reduce the reality of their "physical" disease and only makes them feel more sensitive and helpless.

   The practitioner may need to explain that his/her pain condition can "deplete" their brain and pain sensing "chemistry," which makes them more sensitive. Medication is often needed to "boost" brain chemicals, so that sleep improves and pain threshold increases. The patient needs to understand that he/she may have a low tolerance to stress and that they may need to back-off a little. Cognitive therapy and physical exercise are very helpful.

4. The *"overwhelmed"* patient may present similarly to the low pain tolerance patient. The difference is that their stresses are more external—marital, financial, family, behavioral, or health problems, death in family, etc.—that have become overwhelming. The emotional energy behind their complaints is a "cry for help."

   The practitioner should explain that treatment of their medical or painful disorder has to be performed at the same time that their life stresses are addressed. The crisis intervention model may be appropriate. The patient should be connected with resources for support and problem-solving, to regain control and stability in their situation. The medical problem should not be the sole source of attention, or else the underlying causal factor or "dis-ease" will remain unresolved.

5. The *"angry/blaming"* patient expresses anger either directly or indirectly which, in turn, interferes with establishing or maintaining adequate doctor-patient or other relationships. Anger is an emotion/communication that needs a deeper understanding—it's often a "smoke screen," and may function to alert the patient that something is going on, which otherwise, he/she may or may not be aware of.

   It is important to let the patient express his/her anger, but, if the anger is persistent, the practitioner should comment on and validate the anger (making sure not to take it personally), and make certain that a good relationship is maintained. Understanding the anger may allow the practitioner to change strategy and better serve the patient. Giving a sense of control to the angry patient may be helpful.

6. The *"somatizer"* patient describes a condition that is emotional (dis-ease) but which he/she express physically or somatically. The intensity of the focus on symptoms reflects the intensity of the emotional disturbance. These patients tend to search for help everywhere except in their emotional being. They often have a history of poor childhood emotional training, and may even have a history of abuse. There is a spectrum of somatization from simple to complex conversion disorders somatization disorders such as hysterical paralysis or amnesia.

   When taking a history, the practitioner should inquire about physical and emotional symptoms equally. Listening carefully to the imagery of the patient's symptom description for clues (most somatizers are not difficult to spot) and emanating acceptance and a non-judgemental attitude towards the patient and their condition is very helpful. Attention to physical symptoms may be needed, but the focus should be shifted towards their emotional causes.

7. The *"passive"* patient does little to actively participate in their own care. He/she often fails to follow through with treatments, appears helpless, overwhelmed, incapable of acting on his/her own behalf, or offers numerous excuses, usually based on being controlled by others or by circumstances. The patient may be asking for validation and often compliments the practitioner, which may become a trap.

    The practitioner may need to draw "contracts" with the patient, demanding that in return for intervention and time, the patient participate in clearly defined activities that will eventually empower him/her.

8. The *"secondary gain/malingering"* patient may learn that continued illness has benefits. These may be emotional or physical. The patient may be trying to receive emotional support, relief from responsibilities at home or work, and even securing access to drugs in dependency states. True malingering is rare, while secondary gain factors are common and will remain so as long as the patient lacks viable options or the confidence to successfully make changes in his/her life. It is important to understand that *secondary gain factors* are ones the patient is *not aware* of on a conscious level, yet may strongly motivate a patient toward specific goals of an unconscious psychological nature. On the other hand, *primary gain factors* are those the patient is *very aware* of and is trying to obtain, such as increased or continuing compensation. The latter behavior is not as common as one might think, even in cases where compensation is involved.

    Focusing on objective findings and goals as well as referring the patient to a pain psychologist or pain center program can be helpful for secondary gain patients. It is not helpful to push the patient beyond his/her current psychological or physical abilities.

9. The *"hysterical personality/over-dramatic"* patient simply expresses themselves with greater vigor, color, and flamboyance. This is often a learned behavior and it may be cultural. This style of communication often gets such a patient in trouble with doctors, who may think the patient is just seeking attention and/or exaggerating their symptoms. It may be helpful to explain this to the patient; however, this style of communication may be difficult to change. It is very important to remember that a true physical problem can exist even with dramatic presentation of symptoms.

    Examination and treatment should focus on objective signs and goals.

10. The *"major psychiatric disorder"* patient may develop "real" medical illness and complaints more frequently than the population at large. It may be difficult to understand such a patient, because he/she may express emotional symptoms in terms of physical symptoms and employ medical terms in describing them.

    Treatment must combine psychiatric or psychological with appropriate medical care.

11. The *"normal"* patient can easily develop "psychological" reactions to disease and pain. Severe stress can bring-out the worst in all of us. The patient may react with fear, anger, immature behavior, and become "difficult." These are often normal reactions to stressful events.

    While the patient's physical complaints are being taken care of, he/she should be taught coping and self-care management skills.

As can be seen in a chronic pain patient, emotional responses to pain *can* become the major component of his/her suffering. It must be stressed, however, that physicians often shift blame to the patient when the pain is poorly understood—and commonly incorrectly. Slater and Glithero (1965), for example, showed that 60% of patients diagnosed by neurologists as having hysteria did not have hysteria, and that eventually they developed symptoms that related to a physical disease that could account for their symptoms. Hendler and Kolodny (1992) have estimated that the true incidence of "psychological pain" is about one in 3,000 patients. Bugdok (1997) has shown that in patients with neck pain related to whiplash injury, successful treatment can resolve all psychological distresses as well as pains that were previously considered to be of non-physiological origin. Bugdok also states that he can identify the cause of low back pain (by anesthetic techniques) in 60-70% of patients, in spite of the literature which states that 80% of low back pain is idiopathic (of unknown origin and often thought to be non-physiologic). In one study, using discography, among subjects with "somatization disorder," ¾ had at least one disc that had an outer annular rupture (6/13 discs), with ¾ having at least one positive disc. Of the six discs with significant structural abnormalities, two were positive and four were negative for post injection pain flare. The more disrupted the annulus, the greater the chance of a positive response (Derby 2004).

At the same time, it should be understood that patients suffering chronic pain tend to *resist* the diagnosis of depression, even when clearly present. It may be necessary for the practitioner to educate the patient about chronic pain syndromes and about the relationships among pain, neurotransmitters, pain thresh-holds, and depression. Pain behaviors/suffering, whether primary or secondary, must be addressed. Often, changing this kind of pain behavior (mostly depression, anger and despair) takes some time and a multidisciplinary approach is best. Treatment should *focus on function, not pain reduction*. Early return to activity and work may help prevent the emergence of chronic pain syndromes and reduce the costs of back care (Deyo et al 1986). Herbal and nutritional therapies, pharmaceuticals anti-depressants, trans-cranial electro stimulation (LISS or Alpha-Stim, page 435), physical activity, and cognitive therapy can be very useful.

Acupuncture and relaxation exercises have been shown to be helpful in treating anxiety and can decrease the experience of pain. The anxiolytic effects of ear acupuncture for patients receiving TCM style ear acupuncture versus "relaxation" (tranquilizer and master cerebral) ear points and controls showed that anxiolytic effects or TCM style ear acupuncture was not as significant as those in the group who received ear acupuncture with French "relaxation points," (see chapter 5). Ear acupuncture decreases preoperative anxiety in patients undergoing elective, ambulatory surgeries. The acupuncture can be administered in less than one minute, is relatively inexpensive, and has minimal adverse side effects (Wang, Peloquin, Kain 2001). Ear acupuncture, or at least the use of stimulatory techniques (seeds, electricity, or pressure) to ear points, can be easily taught to the patient or a family member. In this author's experience, *frequent* acupuncture treatments can be beneficial in patients with secondary psychosocial (abnormal) illness behavior, including anxiety and depression. Ear and other forms of acupuncture can be used successfully to treat the patient's primary complaints, affective symptoms; they can also serve as an aid in facilitating manual and rehabilitation therapies. Acupuncture should, therefore, be part of the primary approach to such patients.

There are several approaches to the treatment of depression and anxiety within TCM. Some herbs commonly used to nourish the Heart and calm the Spirit, and often prescribed for both depression and anxiety, can also open the collaterals/network-vessels and treat musculoskeletal pain. Cortex Albiziae (He Huan Pi) beside nourishing the Heart, calming the Spirit, and opening the channels and collaterals, is often used to treat swelling, invigorate the Blood, and to facilitate the healing of soft tissues and bone. Caulis Polygoni Multiofolori (Ye Jiao Teng) is used to treat soreness and pain in the limbs from Blood-deficiency. Radix Polygalae (Yuan Zhi) can eliminate Phlegm from the channels and collaterals (mostly from orifices associated with the Heart and Pericadium) but can be used also to treat Phlegm associated with pain. Radix et Rhizoma Valerianae (Xie Cao) can be used to relieve cramps, spasms, and pain due to Liver-congestion-Qi-stagnation (seen often with depression and anxiety). For more information on herbs see chapters 7 and 11.

The practice of Tai Chi Chuan, or other exercises that promote relaxation such as yoga and Qi Gong, are particularly useful in patients in pain and for so-called secondary or primary psychological symptoms. Studies have shown a 34% higher oxygen consumption peak, higher skin blood flow, higher cutaneous vascular conductance and skin temperature, and higher levels of plasma nitric oxide metabolite than in a sedentary group at rest and after other types of exercise (Wang, Lan and Wong 2001). The practice of Tai Chi Chuan has also been shown to positively affect patients with brain injuries (Shapira and Chelouche et al 2001). These and other studies suggest a strong relaxation response and the integration of the somatic and nervous systems. Clinical experience shows great benefit to chronic pain sufferers with these types of exercises.

DIFFERENTIATING NONORGANIC PAIN. It is important to understand that a finding that all "tests" are normal does not prove that the patient's pain is nonorganic or "psychological." The absence of evidence is not evidence of its absence. While some patients may have a psychiatric "factitious disorder," in which patients produce symptoms in order to assume a sick role. And some patients malinger; that is, they intentionally report pain they do not have, these are very uncommon. Unfortunately, even today some clinicians and scientist continue to promote the concept of nonorganic pain. At the present time, however, our understanding of chronic pain is incomplete, and the few tools available for diagnosis are neither sensitive nor specific (Galer and Dworkin *ibid*).

To differentiate so-called nonorganic back pain from other types of back pain,[19] Waddell devised the "Waddell signs"—seven signs elicited by the practitioner while observing patient responses (Waddell et al 1980):[20]

1. Superficial or nonphysiologic tenderness that is widespread to light touch.

2. Pain provoked by axial loading when light pressure is applied to the top of head.

3. Pain when rotating the trunk fully (rotating from the pelvis, to avoid twisting the spine).

4. A contradiction in sitting and supine straight-leg raising, one being painful while the other is not.

5. Nonphysiologic weakness.

6. Nonphysiologic sensory disturbance (uncoordinated motor and sensory signs).

7. Patient exaggeration response to all provocative testing.

Nonorganic "psychiatric" pain may be caused by somatoform disorders such as somatization and pain disorders. In somatization disorder, the patient's symptoms start before age thirty, and there are at least four pain symptoms, two gastrointestinal symptoms, one pseudoneurological symptom, and one sexual symptom. In pain disorder, there is one or more pain symptoms that cause significant social or occupational impairment, and there is an apparent link between the pain symptom or symptoms and psychological factors. *(OM: It is interesting to note, however, that in* Spiritual Axis, *the ability to tolerate pain (including needling, moxa, and fire-needles) is associated more with the patient's body-type [ten-*

---

19. These principles can be used with other pain as well.

20. Waddell has recently expressed regret over publishing these signs.

dons, bones, skin, and muscle thickness] than their emotional-courage).

In *Chinese Medical Psychiatry* (2001), somatoform disorders (which include somatization, conversion, undifferentiated somatization, pain, hypochrondriasis, and body dysmorphic disorders) are divided into twelve TCM syndromes:

1. Liver-Qi-stagnation (depression) & binding, Heart Spirit delusional pattern.
   Treated with Bupleurum Course the Liver Decoction plus Licorice (Chai Hu Shu Gan Tang) and Wheat & Red Date Decoction (He Gan Mai Da Zao Tong).

2. Liver-congestion (depression) Transformative/congested-Fire with Qi-counterflowing upwards.
   Treated with Running Piglet Decoction (Ren Tun Tang).

3. Liver-congestion (depression) Phlegm-obstruction.
   Treated with Pinellia & Magnolia Decoction (Ban Xia Hou Po Tang).

4. Phlegm-Heat harassing above.
   Treated with Coptis Warm the Gall Bladder Decoction (Huang Lian Wen Dan Tang).

5. Qi-stagnation & Blood-stasis.
   Treated with Persica & Carthamus Four Materials Decoction with Added Flavors (Tao Hong Si Wu Tang Jia Wei).

6. Heart Spirit deprived of nourishment.
   Treated with Licorice, Wheat & Red Date Decoction with Added Flavors (Gan Mai Da Zao Tang Jia Wei).

7. Heart Liver Qi-counterflow with malnourishment of the network-vessels.
   Treated with Licorice, Wheat & Red Date Decoction (Gan Mai Da Zao Tang) plus Rambling Powder with Additions & Subtractions (Xiao Yao San Jia Jian).

8. Heart Spleen dual deficiency (vacuity) Qi & Blood insufficiency.
   Treated with Restore the Spleen Decoction (Gui Pi Tang).

9. Liver Kidney insufficiency with malnourishment of the sinews & bones.
   Treated with Hidden Tiger Pills with Additions & Subtractions (Hu Qian Wan Jia Jian).

10. Yin-deficiency (vacuity) Heat.
    Treated with Nourish Yin & Clear the Lungs Decoction (Yang Yin Qing Fei Tang).

11. Cold Water-counterflowing upward, Heart-Yang-insufficiency.
    Treated with Cinnamon Twig Plus Cinnamon Decoction (Gui Zhi Jia Gui Tang).

12. Phlegm-turbidity blocking the orifices, Liver-Wind internally stirring.
    Treated with Abduct Phlegm Decoction with Added Flavors (Dao Tan Tang Jia Wei).

Gender Variations

A critical review of research examining gender variations in clinical pain experience demonstrates that women are more likely than men to experience a variety of recurrent pains. In most studies, women report more severe levels of pain, more frequent pain, and pain of longer duration than do men. Women may be at greater risk for pain-related disability than men, but women also respond more aggressively to pain through health related activities. Women may be more vulnerable than men to unwarranted psychogenic attributions to their pain by health care providers (Unruh 1996). It is possible that since estrogen increases the release of peripheral cytokines, such as gamma-interferon, which in turn produces increased cortisol, that women are more susceptible to the distractive effects of chronic high levels of cortisol in the blood. This may explain why more females than males suffer from most kinds of chronic pain as well as painful autoimmune diseases such as multiple sclerosis and lupus (Melzack *ibid*).

Female soldiers are more likely to sustain an injury than their male counterparts. Specific injuries account for the majority of this difference. Military training, work, and recreation are more likely to be the cause of injury in the female soldier. Conditions existing prior to military service were also more common (Strowbridge 2002).

Stress

Stress has been defined by Selye (1974) as "the nonspecific response of the body to any demand." It is therefore the bodies reaction to psychological and physical burdens. Stress is a normal response of the adaptation systems, and was divided by Selye into *distress* and *eustress*. Distress is caused by activities that the individual does not like to do, but must do. Eustress is produced by performing an activity the individual likes and which is good for him or her. Selye divided stress into three basic phases: the *alarm reaction, state of resistance,* and *state of exhaustion*. The alarm reaction is the initial shock to stressful events. It is followed by the state of resistance which is a "fight or flight" reaction. If this phase of stress continues, it can result in a state of exhaustion. Selye notes that chronic stress results in muscular tension, which is known to decrease the *pain threshold* (by both tension and stress), especially in patients with neuropathic pain as their nerves and muscles are over sensitive to adrenaline. According to Selye, stress is associated with:

- Infections and allergies.
- Organic dysfunctions, especially digestive symptoms such as: diarrhea, constipation, changes in appetite, etc.
- Mental symptoms such as: insomnia, difficulties in concentration, confusing thoughts, depressive tendencies, etc.

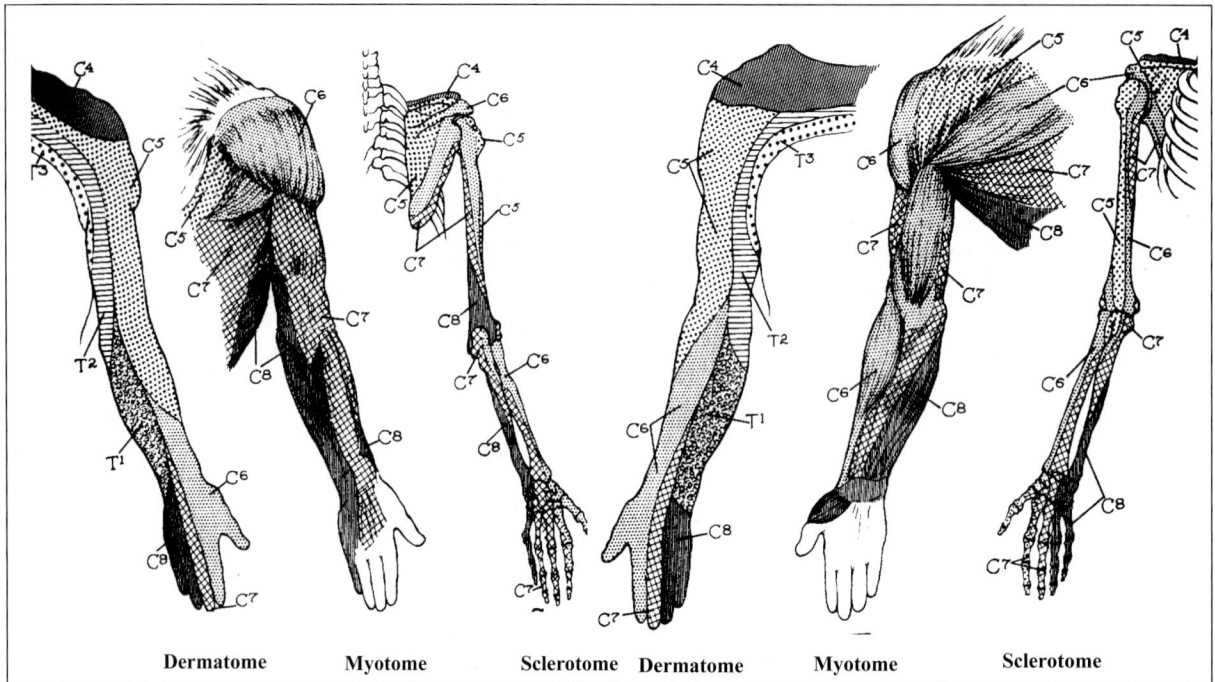

Figure 2-10: Segmental innervation (Reproduced with permission, Inman VT. Referred pain from skeletal structures J Nerv Ment Dis 99:660, 1944).

- Pains such as: low back and neck pains, migraines, recurring injuries or aches that in spite of good treatment are enduring.
- Use of drugs such as: nicotine, alcohol, coffee, or other stimulants.
- Chronic fatigue.[21]

Therefore stress appears to relate most commonly with the stomach, thymus, and adrenal systems. Frost (2002) related the three phases of stress to Applied Kinesiology testing. The causes of stress should therefore be identified and treated in patients with chronic musculoskeletal disorders.

Pain can disrupt the brain's homeostatic regulation systems, thereby producing "stress" and initiating complex programs to reinstate homeostasis. While the stress reaction may be a healthy bodily reaction in acute pain, the stress reaction and guarding of the painful body part in chronic pain are maladaptive (Galer and Dworkin *ibid*). These "inappropriate" responses to chronic pain may actually become part of the problem. By recognizing the role of the stress system in pain processes, we discover that the scope of the puzzle of pain is vastly expanded and new pieces of the puzzle provide valuable clues in our quest to understand chronic pain. Stress is a biological system that is activated by physical injury, infection, or any threat to biological homeostasis as well as by psychological threat and insult to the body-self.

---

21. It is interesting to note that these are the most common disorders for which patients seek "alternative" health care.

Stress and injury can activate the hypothalamic-pituitary-adrenal (APA) system, in which corticotropin-releasing hormone (CRH) produced in the hypothalamus enters the local blood stream which carries the hormone to the pituitary, causing the release of adrenocorticotropic hormone (ACTH) and other substances. ACTH activates the adrenal cortex to release cortisol. If the output of *cortisol* is prolonged, excessive, or of abnormal patterning, it *may destroy* muscle, bone, and neural tissue and produce the conditions for many kinds of chronic pain. Cortisol dysregulation has been documented to affect muscles (myopathy) and bones (decalcification), and to be implicated in fibromyalgia, rheumatoid arthritis, chronic fatigue syndrome, and accelerated neural degeneration during aging (Melzack 1999).

Individuals with chronic pain often experience a worsening of their pain with stress, and this is sometimes considered evidence that the pain is psychological in origin. However, although stress often accompanies pain, it is usually a consequence of the pain itself or of the disruption that pain, distress, and disability have caused in the patient's life. Much of the natural stress responses results from the body's neurochemical response to stress, in which norepinephrine (and adrenaline, epinephrine) play a large role (Galer and Dworkin *ibid*).

Pain Perception and Localization

For the patient, the most compelling aspect of pain is perception, which is subjective and should be accepted accordingly.

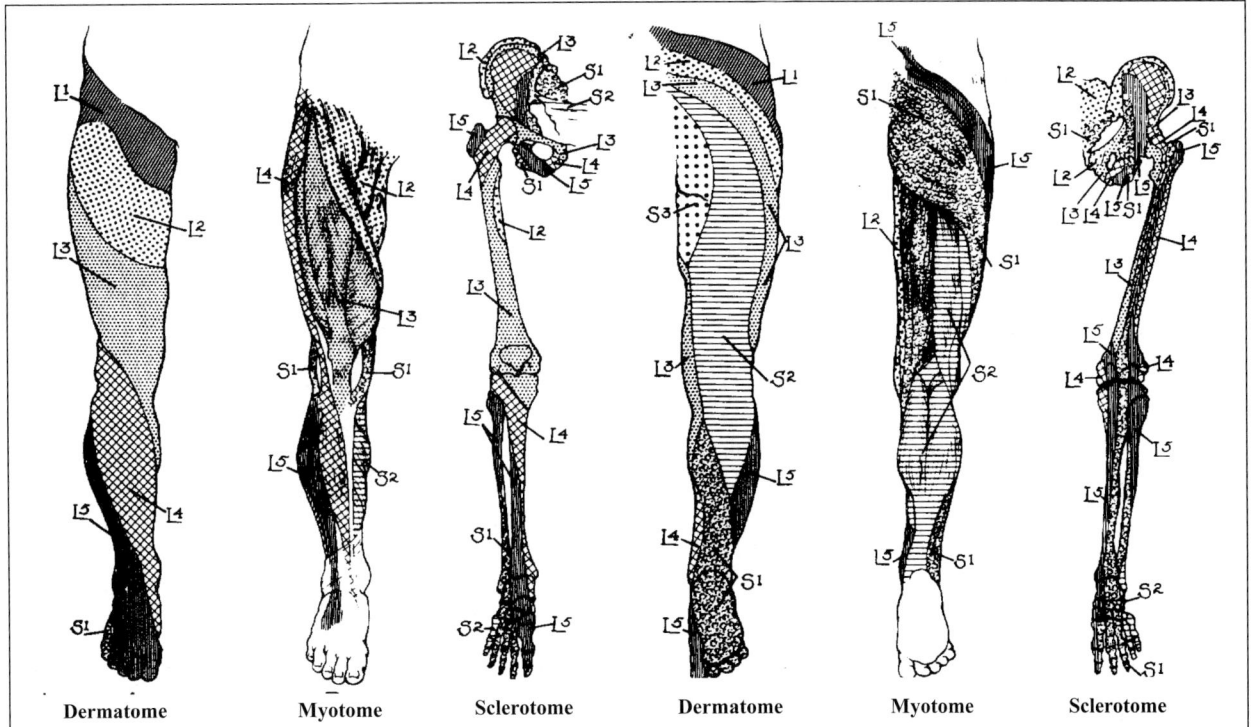

Figure 2-11: Segmental innervation: A—Dermatome, B—Myotome, C—Sclerotome (Reproduced with permission, Inman VT. Referred pain from skeletal structures J Nerv Ment Dis 99:660, 1944).

The patient's impression of the pain is often the first clue the practitioner has for diagnosing and localizing the source. Table 2-10 summarizes some typical descriptions of pain.

The patient's perception and localization take place through complex mechanisms within the nervous system. Pain signals travel mainly via A-δ and C-fibers to the limbic system in the brain, where pain is perceived first. The faster A-δ signals travel in the anterolateral spinothalamic tract to the limbic system, and then continue to the cortex. These signals, which require only three relays on the way to the cortex, travel very quickly (Gunn ibid). Therefore, the combination of painful stimuli from A-δ fibers and the reacting motor system allow the patient to localize pain quickly and to act appropriately, such as pulling the hand away from a hot fire.

C-afferent nociceptive messages travel up to the spinal cord and then to the brain more slowly than A-δ nociceptive messages, via fibers called the pleospino-reticulothalamic tract. On the way up, these signals, which enter at lamina I and II and travel to lamina V, VII, and VIII, must pass several relays. At lamina I and V the fibers cross to the contralateral side and integrate with other levels (Willard ibid; Gunn ibid). The complexity of the C-fiber nociceptive signals probably leads to the phenomenon of referred pain.

By contrast, most of the information from the mechanoreceptors (A-β fibers) is transmitted directly and quickly to the brain stem via posterior fibers (Gunn ibid). All of these messages are modified and are managed by the brain through the descending fiber systems. Some of the responses are voluntary, some are not.

Types of Localization

Cyriax divides pain localization into three types:
- Shifting pain.
  — Results from a shifting of a lesion, such as the shifting of a disc fragment, as may be seen in back pain that changes from one side to the other.
- Expanding pain.
  — Increases the reference area as the local pain intensifies. When this pattern develops, one must consider serious conditions such as cancer.
- Referred pain.
  — Originates in a fixed location. As it intensifies, its area of reference (but not its local pain) increases.

Referred Pain

Referred pain is often difficult to localize and may move and change as the disease progresses. Initially, the pain may be vague or gnawing and felt close to the origin of symptoms (close to midline or other lesion). Later, or if inflammation is

Table 2-8: Embryonic Segmental Derivations

Organ	Derivation	Organ	Derivation
Heart	C8-T4 (left). (possibly C-3).	Small Intestine.	T9-10.
Lungs	T2-T5.	Appendix and ascending colon.	T10-L1.
Esophagus	T4-T6.	Epididymis.	T10.
Diaphragm	C3-C4.	Kidney.	T10-L1.
Stomach & Duodenum	T6-T10.	Ovary, testis, & suprarenals.	T11-L1.
Liver and Gallbladder	T7-T9 (right).	Bladder fundus, colonic flexure, uterine fundus.	L1-L3.
Spleen	T7-T10 (left).	Sigmoid colon.	S3-S5.
Pancreas	T8 (left).	Rectum, cervix, neck of bladder, prostate, and urethra.	S2-S5.

increased, the pain may refer distally and follow a segmental or dermatomal distribution (the innervation of tissues by the same spinal nerve level and/or the development of tissues from similar embryonic tissue). Segmentation begins during embryological development. The formation of somites in the developing embryo, composed of embryonic mesoderm (mesenchyme), is specifically related to the segmentation of the neural tube. The ventral somite eventually differentiates into *dermatomes*, *myotomes*, and *sclerotomes*. The segmentally organized nervous system provides the connection between somatic and visceral tissues, which develop internally in a similar segmental manner. The projection of these segments is one factor that determines the extent of pain reference. Since individual differences occur (probably due to developmental differences, post-traumatic rootlet anastomosis, and other causes), it is impossible to draw comprehensive maps of these distributions and therefore impossible to draw absolutely accurate referred pain maps. Kellgren (1938), Whitty (1967) and Hackett (1958) have demonstrated that when ligaments, musculature, and zygapophyseal joints are stimulated by chemicals, both local and referred pain occur, in both segmental and nonmanagement patterns. The embryonic segmental derivations of the viscera are summarized on Table 2-8. It should also be understood that any pressure on a nerve can refer pain (Figure 2-12).

The deeper the origin of pain, the more difficulty the patient has localizing it, hence, patients have difficulty localizing soft tissue pain that is deeper than skin level. Often such pain is referred from structures the patient does not recognize. This referred phenomenon is thought to be due to the organization of the nervous system. Therefore, for accurate and tissue-specific diagnosis the practitioner must have a clear understanding of the concepts of referred pain and the conditions that stimulate it.

Fundamental to the concept of referred pain is an understanding that the human body's interrelated parts influence each other mechanically and neurally. The tensegritous interdependency (or mechanical chain) of the body's parts can make diagnosis difficult, because an injured tissue can

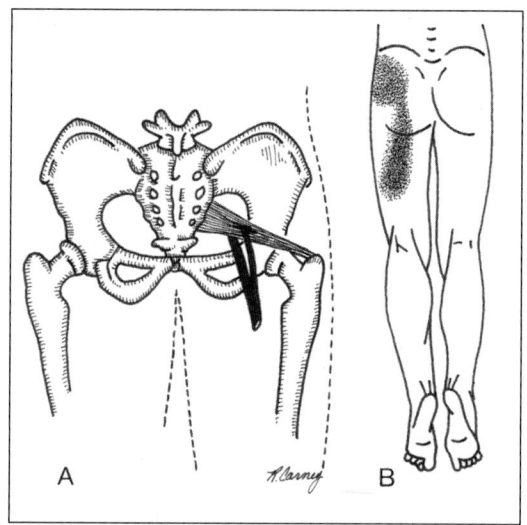

Figure 2-12: Possible compression on the sciatic nerve by the piriformis muscle can cause referred pain down the leg.

cause a cascade of dysfunctions or reactions in other tissues. For example, an upslip innominate on the sacrum (at the SI joint) can result in mechanical tension on the sacrotuberous ligament, which can refer pain to the heel. When the shoulder joint is inflamed, the practitioner commonly finds secondary myofascial trigger points, muscle spasms, and other compensatory misreactions, all of which can cause their own symptoms and signs. If the practitioner does not understand the possible pain patterns and does not recognize the primary tissues at fault, he is likely to focus on the secondary manifestations and undoubtedly will chase the pain's tail.

The presentation of referred pain patterns is summarized in table Table 2-9. Figure 2-10 and Figure 2-11 on page 151 show the myotomes, sclerotomes, and dermatomes. Referred pain often follows these distributions.

Table 2-9: Pain presentation

PATTERN	PRESENTATION PATTERN	ORIGIN OF PATTERN
MYOTOMAL	Muscle Pain, Ache. Tightness. Tenderness.	Muscles innervated by a spinal root. • The area of reference of those muscles.
SCLEROTOMAL	Deep, Dull Ache. or Piercing pain, numb-like sensation that is difficult to localize.	Connective tissue structures and bone innervated by a spinal root. • The area of reference from connective tissue.
DERMATOMAL	Sharp Pain, Ache. Paresthesia. —prickling. —tingling. —numbness. —heightened sensitivity.	Superficial sensation innervated by a spinal root. • The area of reference from nerves felt on the skin.

Theories of Referred Pain

Referred pain has been explained as errors occurring in the spinal cord or perceptual errors in the sensory cortex. The most coherent hypothesis postulates that individual pain transmission neurons in the spinal cord receive afferents from both somatic pain fibers in the body wall and visceral pain fibers in deep organs and that this results in perceptual errors in the sensory cortex (Ombregt, Bisschop, ter Veer and de Velde 1995). In general, there are four physiological theories that can assist in understanding musculoskeletal referred pain: convergence-projection; convergence-facilitation; peripheral branching and sympathetic mediation.

SPINAL CORD COMPONENTS. Melzack and Wall (*ibid*) and Bonica (*ibid*) attribute the false sense of pain localization to the organization of nociceptive afferent (pain sensory nerves) systems in the spinal cord. For example, spinal cord neuron input from cats knees have been shown to converge with input from muscles in the thigh and skin in the lower leg, and, therefore, can activate pain in the knee and in the thigh. Electrophysiological studies in animals have demonstrated convergence of nociceptor input from deep and cutaneous tissues into the same somatosensory spinal neurons (Cervero et al 1992). Viscerosomatic convergence may be involved in RSD of an upper limb following an episode of cardiac pain (Bonica *ibid*).

Mackenzie (1989) has described an "irritable focus" created by visceral afferents in the spinal cord so that other segmentally somatic inputs could produce referred pain.

Sinclair et al (1948) suggested that the bifurcation (division) of the axons of some primary sensory neurons that innervate both somatic and visceral targets leads to confusion about the source of the afferent activity and explains the segmental nature of referred sensations. Sympathetic nerves can release substances that sensitize primary afferent nerve endings resulting in referred pain.

SENSORY CORTEX ERRORS. The peripheral branching of a single sensory nerve to separate parts of the body may cause difficulty in the brain's ability to interpret the parts and the source of an incoming sensory impulse. The *convergence-projection* theory states that, since nociceptive sensory afferent fibers innervating both the visceral and somatic structures enter the spine at the same level and converge on the same dorsal horn transmission cells, pain from either one can be perceived as originating from the same level. Furthermore, since the brain is more used to receiving stimulation from somatic structures, it tends to "dislocate" pain of visceral origin to somatic structures (Ruch and Patton 1965), as seen in cardiac infarct with radiating arm pain.

Hackett, Hemwall, and Montgomery (1991) posit that ligament and tendon relaxation produces a hypersensitive state in these tissues. Subsequently, normal tension causes a barrage of afferent, somatic, proprioceptive, and sensory impulses to the posterior spinal root ganglion. From the ganglia, some impulses are conducted to the brain and are perceived as local pain. Others create exteroceptive impulses,[22] which also enter consciousness as superficial pain in a pattern associated with the sensory distribution from the same spinal segment. Hackett's proposed mechanism is similar to the *convergence-facilitation hypothesis* (Ruch 1965) which states that when a noxious (injured tissue) stimulus exceeds the resting background activity level of the sensory nerves, the effect of the background signal from the reference zone on the ascending spinal cord neuron is facilitated. Thereafter, nociceptors that normally do not initiate pain will do so when "facilitated" by sensory impulses from deep structures.

Lewis (1942) proposed that interactions at supraspinal levels lead to the referred pain and phenomenon..

---

22. Sensory receptors that get activated from stimuli that originate from outside the body.

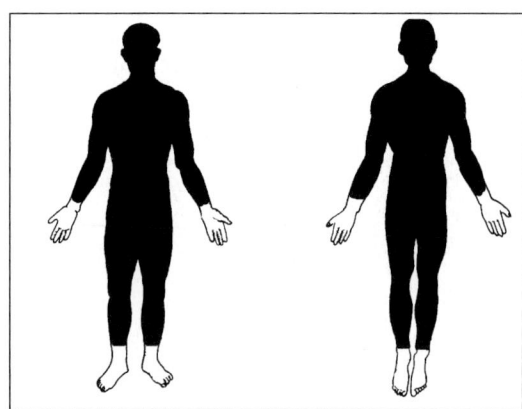

Figure 2-13: Extrasegmental dural pain.

EXTRASEGMENTAL REFERENCE. Cyriax believed that the dura mater[23] does not follow the "rules" of segmental reference and posited that pressure from the spinal disc is responsible for most pains that show these nonsegmental pain patterns. Input to the dura has been shown to impact as much as four segments above and four below the level in which stimulation enters the spinal cord (for a total of eight segments which explains the possible wide-spread pain felt from dural irritation). The dura is a centrally located structure so that pain can be bilateral or felt at the midline. Dural reference may be very difficult to understand and diagnose. For instance, dural pain originating in the low back may affect the whole back, buttocks, and both legs, or just, for example, one groin. Dural stimulation *also provokes referred tenderness* (Ombregt et al *ibid*).

Extrasegmental pain may also represent some sclerotomal reference (referred pain down the sclerotome or connective tissue innervated by a spinal nerve) and not necessarily only dural reference. Orthopaedic Medicine specialist Thomas Dorman has suggested that these spinal pain references have a ligamentous origin (Dorman 1991). Nervous supply to many spinal structures, such as the facets for example, are multisegmental as well. New information shows that this type of referred pain may be due to the chemical irritation of the dura, nerve roots, facets, and ligaments and not just physical pressure. Moreover, many painful disc pathologies are due only to internal disc tears and the chemical stimulation of the disc annulus nerves (the annulus is also a ligament). These only show on special MRI studies and discography (Brown *ibid*)

According to Cyriax, extrasegmental (dural) pain reference (Figure 2-13):

- Of *cervical origin* may be perceived all the way from the head to the mid-thorax;

- From *mid and low-thoracic* lesions may radiate to the base of the neck;
- From the *low lumbar levels* may reach the lower thorax (posteriorly), the lower abdomen, groin, the upper buttocks, the sacrum, and the coccyx. It does not extend to the upper limbs or hands, although it often reaches down to the lower limbs and ankles, but not the feet.

Cyriax believed that, as a rule, pain is referred only distally and never crosses the midline. Theoretically, only centrally localized structures such as the vertebral body, discs, longitudinal ligaments, intra-and-supraspinal ligaments, and dura mater are capable of causing bilateral or midline pain. Midline pain cannot result from a unilateral structure such as a facet joint (unless affected bilaterally).

This concept however cannot be used as an absolute rule, because at times, for example, when tissue is stimulated with a needle, the patient perceives pain proximally, or even contralaterally. More recent anatomical research supports these observations. This is especially true if deep scars are present, and is probably due to extra nerve development. It is known now that the ventral and dorsal horns and the sympathetic system communicate with each other, and that the function of one may transform into the function of the other in chronic dysfunction (Willard 1994). Unilateral neuropathic pain has also been shown to influence the spinal cord bilaterally (Galer and Dworkin *ibid*). In these cases, messages may cross midline. Clinically, however, the above guideline is still useful.

REFERRED TENDERNESS. Cyriax considers these disc pressures to be the cause of referred tenderness (and myofascial trigger points) within these regions. He posits that, when these trigger points are pressed forcefully, the patient identifies the pressure as the source of his/hers pain. Cyriax regards this type of referred tenderness as a major obstacle to the diagnosis of the true nature of these conditions, and adds that these spots can be either moved around or eliminated by manipulation and by joint or epidural injections. Scmorl and Junghanns (1968) and Dvorák (1990) also find that secondary muscle pain is often caused by vertebral dysfunction—not just by disc dysfunction—and that it will improve when the vertebral dysfunction is treated. Thus, while most Orthopaedic Medicine physicians consider myofascial pain syndrome (MPS) as an inappropriate primary diagnosis, secondarily it still need treatment.[24]

Referred tenderness and hyperalgesia (tissue sensitivity) has been shown to involve both peripheral and central mechanisms (Meyer, Campbell and Raja 1994). Referred tenderness and hyperalgesia may result from the sensitization of the secondary dorsal horn neurons or from a decreased threshold of primary peripheral afferents—with pain result-

---

23. The dura mater is the outermost and most fibrous of the three membranes surrounding the brain and spinal cord.

24. The most recent Simons, Travell and Simons text integrates more information to the affect that joint dysfunctions are a likely cause of "trigger points."

Table 2-10: Typical Pain Quality Descriptions

TYPE	DESCRIPTION AND EXAMPLES
DULL (ACHY) PAIN	Often poorly localized. Arising from deep-seated structures, organs, abdominal wall, or may be referred.
DULL (PIERCING) BORING PAIN	Often from deep-seated lesion, organs, chronic/subacute derangements.
DULL PAROXYSMAL PAIN	Comes on in waves of spasm-like pain. Usually from sudden irritation of a chronically irritated tissue. Seen in mild derangements, chronic disc irritations.
DULL DIFFUSE PAIN	Felt over large areas of body, several quadrants of body, or over a whole limb. Seen in inflammation, infection, fibromyalgia, referred.
SHARP PAIN	Often felt locally, often searing (burning) in quality. Seen in superficial lesions, neuralgias, referred.
SHARP (PIERCING) BORING PAIN	Felt as sharp penetrating pain (often acute paroxysmal). Seen in some neuralgias, severe discogenic pains, abdominal diseases, GYN diseases, urological diseases.
THROBBING PAIN	Felt as pulsations. Usually due to vascular congestion. May be seen in visceral or somatic problems, inflammation, trauma.
TWINGES (ACUTE PAROXYSMAL) PAIN	Felt as sudden severe local or referred pain. Usually due to derangements, disc lesions, neuralgias, tabes dorsalis, visceral obstruction, and shifting/movement of lesion (stone).
EXPANDING PAIN	Felt as rapidly increasing in extent and intensity. Usually seen in serious lesions, cancers.
SHIFTING PAIN	Felt in different areas at different times. Seen in midline lesion (disc), inflammatory disorder, fibromyalgia, psychosomatic.
GIRDLE PAIN	Felt as a constricting sensation around waist. Can be seen with some cord disorders.
AGONIZING PAIN	Felt with a strong emotional component (fear). Usually due to visceral pain.
IMPERATIVE PAIN	Felt persistent with urgency. Usually indicates an overlying or underlying psychological factors.

ing from normal input of mechanoreceptor afferents (Cohen at el 1993; 1992).

Factors that Influence Referred Pain

Factors significant in the patient's perception of referred pain are:
- The more tenacious the incitation/stimulation (inflammation and/or painful lesion), the *less* likely the patient will be able to localize it, and the more likely the patient will be able to feel it distally.
- The more superficially the lesion lies, the more precisely the patient will be able to localize it, and the less reference of pain there will be.
- The deeper the lesion (excluding bone), the less accurately the patient will be able to localize it, and the more referral of pain there will be.
- The more central the lesion, the more reference of pain. Lesions that involve the shoulder, the hip,[25] the SI joint, and spine can refer pain extensively.
- The more distal the lesion, the more accurate the patient's perception regarding its origin and the less the reference of pain. Pain that arises in the elbows, wrists, hands, knees, ankles, and feet commonly refers an ache to the forearm or leg, but rarely enough to mislead the patient as to its source.
- Pain is likely to be referred from muscles, tendons, bursas, ligaments, and joint capsules in a way that the patient cannot identify the origin.
  Muscles can refer pain. And joint capsules, ligaments, tendons, bursa, dural sleeve, and perineurium can refer even more.
- Pain from bone hardly ever radiates. However, pain from the periosteum may radiate a little.
  Thus, serious localized pain may point to a bone.

The practitioner should always suspect that pain is referred, especially if local function is not disturbed, or if pain affects large areas and is felt with great intensity. The closer referred pain is felt to midline, the better the patient is becoming.

Local anesthesia is the most effective way to confirm the location of the suspected lesion. Local acupuncture can be of some use in trying to reproduce the symptoms. However, it does not reproduce or eliminate the pain as reliably as local anesthesia does.

Assessing Pain

Since pain perception is subjective, relative intensity of pain is difficult to measure. There is a growing trend to try to measure and quantify the results of the physical examina-

---

25. It is not uncommon for a hip facture to be missed as the patient may complain of knee pain only.

tion, during which patients tend to report more subjective findings than objective ones. Several methods are available to help the practitioner assess the patient's pain—none of which are flawless.

Patient Drawing

The practitioner can begin the patient interview by reviewing a pain drawing done by the patient. Such drawings contain a great deal of general information that can assist the practitioner in the diagnosis of the patient's complaint (Figure 2-14). The drawing should include various symbols to designate the type of pain and may include symbols for tingling/pins and needles, numbness, burning, ache, boring, tension, shooting/radiating, sharp, etc. A numbering system can be used to prioritize each area. Symbols for durations such as for occasional, constant, almost constant can be used as well. The practitioner may want to evaluate the drawing using the Wiltse's point evaluation method.

Wiltse's Point Evaluation Method

A patient's pain drawing can be helpful in differentiating between organic and nonorganic pain. The practitioner can assign a "score" using a point method from seven categories, as described by Wiltse (Kirkaldy-Willis and Burton 1992). For each category, a score of one point (one irregularity) indicates a "normal" score; a score of five points or more indicates a strong psychological component to the patient's pain. The scoring categories are:

- Writing (anywhere) on the drawing.
- Nonphysiological pain pattern.
- More than one type of pain.
- Involvement of both upper and lower areas of the body.
- Markings outside of body contours.
- Unspecified symbols.

CORRELATION WITH OTHER PAIN ASSESSMENT METHODS. Nonorganic drawings have been shown to correlate with elevated hypochondriasis and hysteria scores on the MMPI; higher hospitalization rate and chronicity; and high scores on the McGill Pain Questionnaire (Tait et al 1990).

Dolorimeter

One means of quantifying a subjective examination is a dolorimeter (pressure meter), which measures in units called *dols*. Examples of dolorimeter readings are (Bonica *ibid*):

- Childbirth: 10.5 dols.
- Migraine: 5 dols.
- Toothache: 2 dols.

    Aspirin may help pain under 2 dols.

Visual Analog Scale (VAS)

The Visual Analog Scale (VAS), also called the Pain Visual Analog Scale (PVAS), is a common method of pain measurement. A subjective estimate of pain intensity, the VAS consists of an unmarked, 10cm line labeled at one end as "no pain" and at the other as "unbearable pain" (Merskey 1973). The patient conveys the intensity of his/hers pain by marking a line between the two extremes (Figure 2-14).

Verbal Scale

The patient is asked to rate his pain on a scale of zero to ten or zero to one hundred, zero being no pain and ten/one hundred being the worse pain he can imagine (a medical emergency). The practitioner should define the scale every time it is used. The author has found it useful to define the worst pain as being run over by a car at a rate of one inch/hour Patients that still rate their pain as high on this scale usually have a high psychological aspect to their pain and are unlikely to benefit from treatment.

West Haven-Yale Multidimensional Pain Inventory (MPI)

The West Haven-Yale Multidimensional Pain Inventory (MPI or MHYMPI), a multidimensional pain inventory developed by Kerns, Turk, and Rudy, is intended to supplement behavioral and psychophysiological observations and was specifically developed for the evaluation of chronic pain patients (Kerns, Turk and Rudy 1985). It classifies patients as dysfunctional, interpersonally distressed, or adaptive-copper. The MPI provides information in nine clinical scales including:

- Pain dimensions and severity, including:
  — interference by pain on various functions
  — role of significant others
  — pain severity, and mood
- Specific responses of significant others
- Functional activities

This test was compared with the Minnesota Multiphasic Personality Inventory (MMPI) and was shown to be much more useful for chronic pain patients (Berstein, Jaremoko, and Hinkley 1995).

McGill Pain Questionnaire

The McGill Pain Questionnaire (MPQ), developed by Melzack, uses classes of words that have been determined to represent the affective, sensory, and cognitive components of pain experience. The MPQ is able to separate sensory, affective, and evaluative dimensions providing an assessment of different qualities of pain. The questionnaire provides three kinds of pain detail:

- Intensity of pain.

Assessing Pain

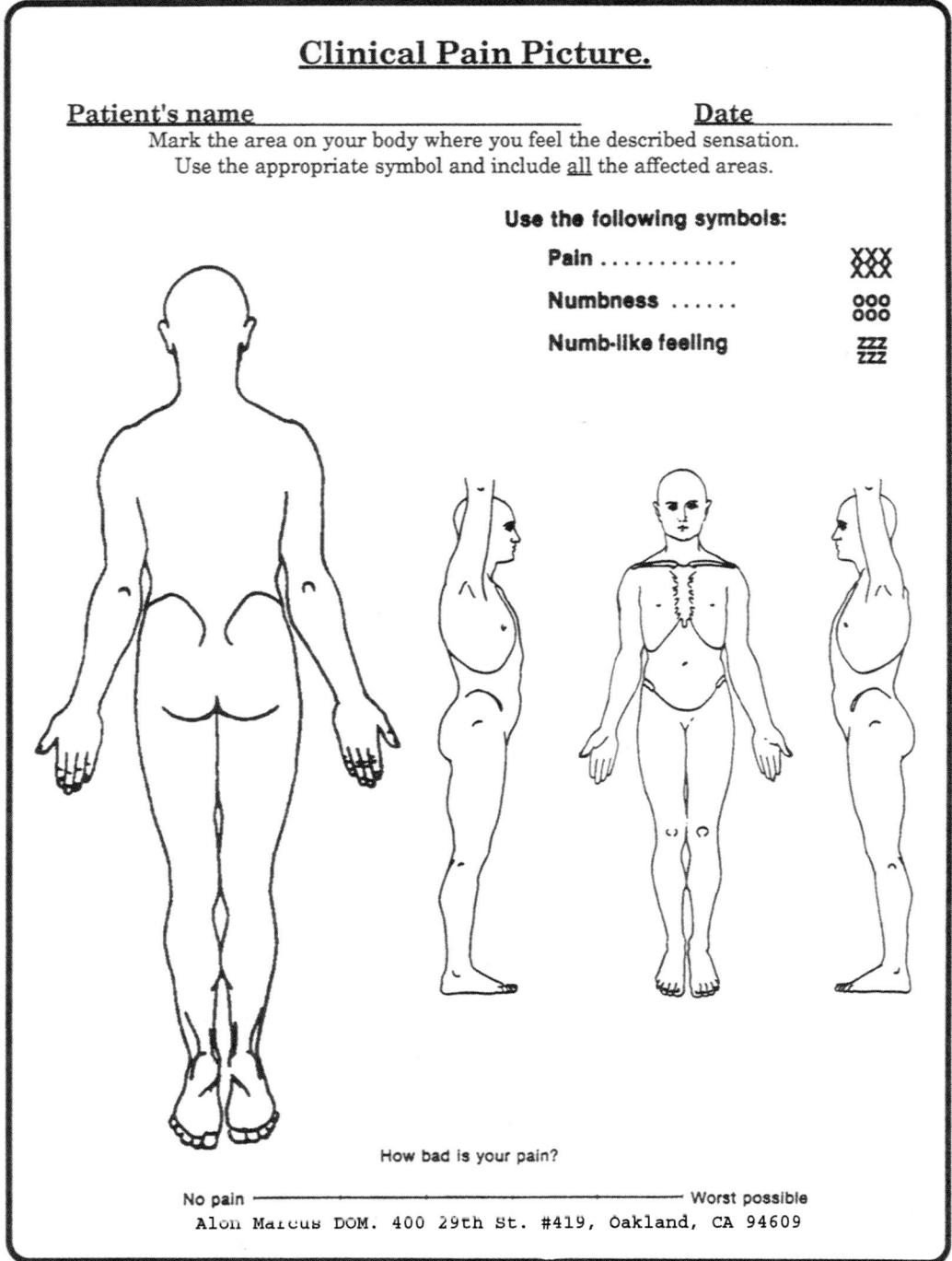

Figure 2-14: Pain drawing and visual analog scale (VAS).

- Number of words chosen in each category.
- Pain rating index.

This questionnaire has been the subject of many studies that have confirmed its validity and reliability (Bradley, Prokop and Gentry et al 1981).

Minnesota Multiphasic Personality Inventory (MMPI)

The Minnesota Multiphasic Personality Inventory (MMPI) is the most thoroughly researched of the personality inventories in both psychopathology and pain management. Studies by Bradley et al showed that MMPI profiles of pain patients consistently clustered into categories:

- Depression
- Somatization
- Hypochondriasis
- Manipulative reactions

They found that chronic pain patients are not homogenous in personality makeup. These patients bring to the pain situation their own unique, pre-illness personalities that can either contribute to or inhibit the clinical pain picture (Bradley, Prokop and Margolis et al 1978). The utility of the MMPI, the most commonly used inventory scale, has been questioned (Main and Spanswick 1995).

Oswestry Low Back Questionnaire

The Oswestry Low Back Index (Fairbank et al 1980) is commonly used to assess the pain and functional capacity of patients suffering from low back pain. It is given here as an example of pain and functional capacity questionnaires and can be modified for other painful areas. After asking the patient how long they have had back pain and how long they have had leg pain, the questionnaire is divided into ten sections:

SECTION 1- PAIN INTENSITY

1. I can tolerate the pain I have without having to use pain killers.
2. The pain is bad but I manage without taking pain killers.
3. Pain killers give complete relief from pain.
4. Pain killers give moderate relief from pain.
5. Pain killers give very little relief from pain.
6. Pain killers have no effect on the pain and I do not use them.

SECTION 2- PERSONAL CARE (Washing, Dressing, etc.).

1. I can look after myself normally without causing extra pain.
2. I can look after myself normally but it causes extra pain.
3. It is painful to look after myself and I am slow and careful.
4. I need some help but manage most of my personal care.
5. I need help everyday in most aspects of self care.
6. I do not get dressed, wash with difficulty, and stay in bed.

SECTION 3- LIFTING.

1. I can lift heavy weights without extra pain.
2. I can lift heavy weights but it gives extra pain.
3. Pain prevents me from lifting heavy weights off the floor, but I can manage if they are conveniently positioned, e.g., on a table.
4. Pain prevents me from lifting heavy weights but I can manage light to medium weights if they are conveniently positioned.
5. I can lift only very light weights.
6. I cannot lift or carry anything at all.

SECTION 4- WALKING.

1. Pain does not prevent me from walking any distance.
2. Pain prevents me from walking more than 1 mile.
3. Pain prevents me from walking more than 1/2 mile.
4. Pain prevents me from walking more than 1/4 mile.
5. I can only walk using a stick or crutches.
6. I am in bed most of the time and have to crawl to the toilet.

SECTION 5- SITTING.

1. I can sit in any chair as long as I like.
2. I can only sit in my favorite chair as long as I like.
3. Pain prevents me from sitting for more than 1 hour.
4. Pain prevents me from sitting for more than 1/2 hour.
5. Pain prevents me from sitting for more than 10 minutes.
6. Pain prevents me from sitting at all.

SECTION 6- STANDING.

1. I can stand as long as I want without extra pain.
2. I can stand as long as I want but it gives me extra pain.
3. Pain prevents me from standing for more than 1 hour.
4. Pain prevents me from standing for more than 30 minutes.
5. Pain prevents me from standing for more than 10 minutes.
6. Pain prevents me from standing at all.

SECTION 7- SLEEPING.

1. Pain does not prevent me from sleeping well.
2. I can sleep well only by using tablets.
3. Even when I take tablets I have less than six hours sleep.
4. Even when I take tablets I have less than four hours sleep.
5. Even when I take tablets I have less than two hours sleep.
6. Pain prevents me from sleeping at all.

SECTION 8- SEX LIFE.

1. My sex life is normal and causes no extra pain.
2. My sex life is normal and causes some extra pain.
3. My sex life is nearly normal but is very painful.

4. My sex life is severely restricted by pain.

5. My sex life is nearly absent because of pain.

6. Pain prevents any sex life at all.

SECTION 9- SOCIAL LIFE.

1. My social life is normal and gives me no extra pain.

2. My social life is normal but increases the degree of pain.

3. Pain has no significant affect on my social life apart from limiting my more energetic interests, e.g., dancing, etc.

4. Pain has restricted my social life and I do not go out as often.

5. Pain has restricted my social life to my home.

6. I have no social life because of pain.

SECTION 10- TRAVELING.

1. I can travel anywhere without extra pain.

2. I can travel anywhere but it gives me extra pain.

3. Pain is bad but I can manage journeys over two hours.

4. Pain restricts me to journeys of less than one hour.

5. Pain restricts me to short necessary journeys under 30 minutes.

6. Pain prevents me from traveling except to the doctor or the hospital.

Other indexes that are often used in the assessment of pain include: Millon Behavioral Health Inventory (Gatchel RJ, et al. 1986), the Neck Disability Index (Vernon and Mior 1991), and the Roland Morris Scale and Illness Behavior Questionnaire (Roland and Morris 1983).

Pain in TCM

As stated before, most pain theories in TCM are predicated on the saying from the *Yellow Emperor's Classic of Internal Medicine;* "If there is free flow there is no pain,"[26] in which pain is associated with the disruption of the flow of Qi and Blood. In that text, pain is classified by thirteen types, most of which are related to exogenous-Cold. Pain is also understood as it relates to Deficiency (with Deficiency-type pain), as well as other causes (e.g. food disorders) that may lead to obstruction of Qi/Blood and *Excess-type-pain*. Even Deficiency-pain due to lack of Qi or Blood is considered to be a form of inhibited flow. Excess pain is almost always suggestive of Pathogenic Factors. It is important to remember that Qi-stagnation, in general, is what is not "seen" while Blood-stasis often manifests in the body Form, and therefore may be seen, e.g., swelling and hematoma. Clinically pain almost always presents with complicated and multi-pattern presentations. There is always individual variations and often one sees multiple pathologies associated with various Root causes.

In general, pain in TCM may be caused by:

- External penetration of Pathogenic Factors (six Excesses) usually resulting in Excess-type pain.
- Internal damage by emotional factors, usually affecting Organ functions and Qi and Blood circulation, usually with Excess or mixed Excess-Deficient type pains.
- Secondary Pathogenic Factors: Blood-stasis and Phlegm, usually with Excess-type pain, but also with mixed pains.
- Excessive consumption of bodily resources (mental or physical), or an over-leisurely life style. This is usually seen with Deficient-type pains, but also in mixed pains. Leisurely life styles can result in mainly Excess-type pains.
- Dietary irregularities or food contamination, seen with both Deficient and Excess type pains.
- Parasitic diseases. Often with Excess or mixed type pains.

The idea of "lack of flow and congestion" causing pain certainly agrees with biomedical ideas of stasis and congestion-chemotactic "inflammatory soup" factors that activate and sensitize pain receptors—as seen mostly in acute pain states. Chronic pain in biomedicine is often said to result from deficient nourishment (e.g., disruption of trophic factors flow) from blocked or dysfunctional nerves and/or vessels with hypoxia, and with deafferention (often with neuropathic type pains) which results from failure in nervous communication and/or regulation. Also, in the field of "electro-energetic" medicine, studies by Ionescu-Tirgoviste and Pruna suggest that blockage in the "normal" flow of bodily currents leads to a high concentration of positive or negative electrical charges (i.e., lack of flow and congestion) which may cause pain and other symptoms of disease. While these chronic pain states may manifest as either Excess or Deficient type pains in TCM, their causes are often related to a decrease in the endogenous milieu influencing the nervous system (which then can lead to the hyper- or hypoactivity of the system, or Excess and Deficient pains as they often manifest in TCM). The channels in TCM function as information and communication systems (described in terms of the nervous and other systems in biomedicine), and "lack of flow" therefore disrupts communication and nutrition. Hence, many conceptual similarities can be demonstrated between the biomedical and the TCM understanding of pain.

While localized pain in TCM is by and large caused by Pathogenic Factors such as Blood-stasis, obstruction by Cold or Dampness, or both, and at times by Phlegm, generalized or specific pains can also be caused by TCM Organic dysfunctions (which are often seen as root causes) such as: Liver-congestion Qi-stagnation, Yin-deficiency of Liver and Kidneys, deficiency of Kidney-Yang, Heart-Blood-stasis, Urinary Bladder-Heat or stone, etc. Dysfunctions within the Spleen/pancreas and Lung systems can affect Blood/Qi production and lead to deficiency of Qi/Blood and Deficiency-type pain (and then may be associated also with numbness

---

26. It has been pointed out that in Chinese this saying can be translated as "loss of communication," an interpretation which would be closer to many modern understandings of chronic pain mechanisms.

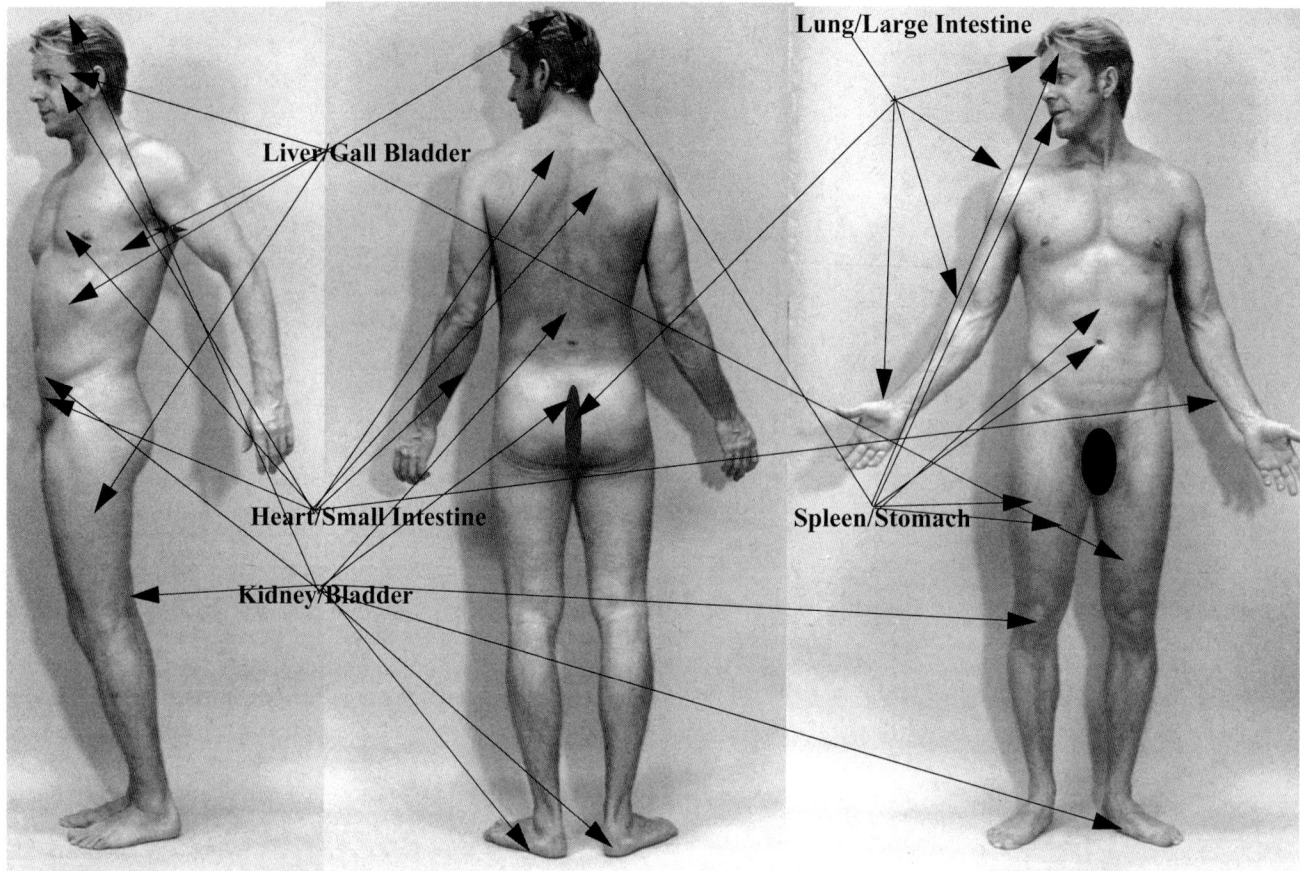

Figure 2-15: Referred Organ pains.

and/or insensitivity). They can also result in a lack of vitality (or movement) of the Qi and thus of the Blood, which can then lead to Excess or *mixed* (Excess and Deficiency) type pains. Deficiency-pain is related more to *lack* of nourishment and/or consumption of the body Fluids (Yin/Blood). It tends to be chronic and is said to be *always dull* in character.[27] *Mixed* pain etiologies often lead to *changing* pain characteristics and conflicting symptoms and signs.

Regional pains often relate to Organs or channels. For example, left-sided pain is often said to relate to the Liver, Blood, Wind, and/or Dampness. Right-sided pain is said to relate often to the Lungs, Qi, Phlegm and/or Dampness. It is said, if Blood is deficient with Wind the headache will be on the left side. If Qi is deficient with Wind the headache is will be on the right side.

In general, pain from (Figure 2-15):

- Lung and Large Intestine is felt in the face (nose, throat, or lower teeth and jaw), shoulder, upper back, arm, elbow, hand, chest, anus.
- Spleen and Stomach is felt in the face (frontal, vertex, or forehead, upper teeth, tongue), epigastric region, general abdomen, outside of anterior leg and thigh.
- Heart and Small Intestine is felt in face (corners of eye), chest, upper back, periscapular region, inside arms, Bladder.
- Kidney and Urinary Bladder is felt in vertex of head, spine in general, lumbar spine and coccyx in particular, lower abdomen, knees, feet.
- Liver and Gall Bladder is felt in vertex or sides of head, ear, lateral trunk and chest, lower abdomen, inner medial aspects of thigh and leg.

Although referred pain is not clearly described in TCM, pain is understood to *transmit* through, or relate to, the channels. Also, Liver-Fire, for example, is said to be capable of invading the Lungs and of causing chest pain and Lung symptoms that are due to *it,* and not just to the Lungs or chest. When Liver-Qi-stagnation occurs, its Qi is said to move sideways and attack the Stomach where it may cause Stomach, hypochondriac, and trunk pain. Thus, most *radiating* pains are thought to be caused by the stagnation of Qi (and thus of the Blood, although Blood-stasis is character-

---

27. It is important to understand that dull pain can be severe. "Dullness" pertains to not being sharp or having a well defined edge.

ized by fixed pain), by Wind, or by the accumulation of stone and sand in the Organs. The Shao-Yang, since it is related to the three Warmers and the spaces between the muscles (Cou Li, and other membranes), may also result in changing and moving pains.

Pain in TCM is often classified by its nature (pathocondition: Damp, Wind, Heat, Cold, etc.), location (area, channel, network-vessel, Organ, tissue), severity (Excess, Deficient) and character (sharp/dull, fixed/moving, constant/intermittent, expanding/contracting, hot/cold, local/generalized, one-sided/bilateral, upper/lower, flaccid/contracted, hard/soft).

The experience of pain is almost always an interplay between the Righteous and the Pathogenic (evil) which would dictate the location (Interior/Exterior), severity (Excess/Deficient), and character (Hot/Cold). The *magnitude* and *resolution* of pain reflects often the relative strength and struggle between Pathogenic Factors and Righteous-Qi (anti-pathogenic forces).

Daytime pain is often associated with dysfunction of Qi or Blood and with external Pathogenic Factors. *Night* pain is associated more with Blood-stasis, Empty-Fire, and Yin-deficiency. *Constant* pain is associated mostly with Excesses, especially Blood-stasis. *Intermittent* pain is associated with Deficiencies, mostly Qi and Blood, but also with Qi-stagnation, which is an Excess.

TCM Treatments of Pain

Even though all the above-discussed pains are generally due to some degree of inhibited flow of Qi and Blood, therapy that only moves Qi and Blood is not necessarily appropriate or effective. For example, if inhibited flow is mostly due to Cold, any successful treatment must include techniques or herbs that dispel the Cold. In general, the patient is said to have symptoms/signs that correspond to one or more "pattern" of pain, Organ, channel, pathogen, Fluids/Yin, Blood, and/or Qi/Yang dysfunctions. These patterns are repeated and often sound the same for almost all types of pains, regions, tissues and diseases. However, treatment is always specific to the patient, with disease diagnosis combined with pattern identification determining the approach and specific interventions. Herbs and acupoints that treat Blood-stasis in the head and Blood-stasis in the foot would have some commonalities but significant differences as well.

Herbs that direct a formula to a particular Organ, channel, or tissue would be used. For example, for a patient with Blood-stasis pain in the bones, in addition to Blood-stasis herbs, Rhizoma Drynariae (Gu Sui Bu) may be added to direct the formula to the bones. Radix Dipsaci (Xu Duan) may be added to direct the formula to the sinews and bones. If pain is in the low back or lower part of the body, Radix Cyathulae (Chuan Niu Xi), Radix Angelicae Pubescentis (Du Huo), Cortex Acanthopanachis (Wu Jia Pi), Caulis Trachelospermi (Luo Shi Teng), and/or Ramulus Loranthi (Sang Ji Sheng) may be added; while, if in the neck, Radix Pueraria (Ge Gen), Rhizoma et Radix Notopterygii (Qiang Huo), and/or Ramulus Cinnamomi (Gui Zhi) may be added. Rhizoma Atractylodis (Cang Zhu) may be added for 1st metatarsophalangeal joint (Spleen channel) swelling and pain (bunions). Rhizoma et Radix Notopterygii (Qiang Huo), Ramulus Cinnamomi (Gui Zhi) and Rhizoma Curcumae (Jiang Huang) may be added to treat the shoulder. For left-sided shoulder pain, Radix Polygoni (He Shou Wu), and for right-sided shoulder pain, Radix Astragali (Huang Qi) may be added. Radix Pueraria (Ge Gen) may be added to formulas to guide the herbs to the Stomach channel and therefore may be used to treat temporomandibular joint (TMJ) or temporomaxillary pain. Radix Bupleuri (Chai Hu) is said to free the flow of Qi on the left side of the body. Rhizoma Cimicifugae (Sheng Ma) is said to free the flow of Qi on the right side of the body. To guide herbs to the channels, collaterals/network-vessels, muscles and sinews Lumbricus (Di Long), Squama Manitis Pentadactylis (Chuan Shan Jia) and Caulis Trachelospermi (Luo Shi Teng) can be added. Herbs that conduct formulas to a particular channel are listed in Table 1-3 on page 402.

The *Practical Dictionary of Chinese Medicine* (1998) lists twelve types of pain. Table 2-11 summarizes some of the more common types of pain. Table 2-12 summarizes the most fundamental aspects of pathoconditions as they relate to pain. For information on pain and the Eight Principles, see Table 1-10 on page 45; for pain and Qi see "Qi-deficiency Pain" on page 11; for pain and Blood-stasis and Phlegm, see Table 1-8 on page 40; for pain and Pathogenic Factors, see "Pathogenic Factors (Xie)" on page 22; for pain and emotions, see "Endogenous Factors (Nei Yin)" on page 32.

Table 2-11: Types of Pain in Traditional Chinese Medicine

Pain	Characteristics	Mostly Felt At
ACHING PAIN (SUAN TONG)	Mostly felt as continuous pain. Usually attributed to deficiency factors and/or weak Pathogenic Factors (mostly Dampness and Cold). *Continuous* pain is usually attributed to Excess conditions in which the antipathogenic-Qi and pathogens are struggling. *Intermittent* pain is more often associated with Deficiency of Qi, Blood, Yin or Yang, and implies that the antipathogenic-Qi is weak.[a] It is often accompanied by a feeling of weakness on the affected body part.	Mostly felt in musculoskeletal tissues commonly in thick and soft muscles or joints. Can be in extremities or trunk.
DISTENDING PAIN (ZHANG TONG)	Felt as expansion and inflation,[b] bloated, or throbbing. Associated mostly with Qi-stagnation; however, it can also be seen with uprising Liver-Yang, Wind-Heat, Phlegm, and food diseases. Can also be caused by the Stomach, Spleen/pancreas, and Lungs, depending on location. Fluctuates in intensity and location and is strongly affected by emotions.	Mostly felt in the chest, subcostals, trunk, and abdominal areas. Can also be felt in the head (as migraines), eyes, and, much less frequently, in the limbs and musculoskeletal tissues, except in acute sprains and strains when throbbing and pulsating pains are common.
DULL PAIN/SORENESS (YIN TONG)	Muted, persistent and generally bearable. Associated with Deficiency of Qi, Blood, and Yang.	Felt anywhere, but most often in limbs or head.
EMPTY PAIN (KONG TONG)	Felt as emptiness, lightness. Likes warmth and pressure. Associated with Deficient-Essence, or Deficiency of Yang, Yin, Blood, or dual Yin Yang (failure to nourish the channels). Associated with the Kidneys.	Usually felt in head, low back, or abdomen.
COLD PAIN (LENG TONG)	Felt with a sensation of chill. Relieved by warmth. May be sharp, stabbing, achy, or spastic. Associated with external pathogenic Cold. Or internal Yang-deficient/Cold.	Usually felt at the Exterior (musculoskeletal and skin) Organs, abdomen.
GRIPPING (COLIC) PAIN (JIAO TONG) SPASTIC PAIN	Felt as excruciating acute pain that feels as if the painful area were being wrung and twisted, or stabbed. A sudden sharp pain with spasms. Associated with tangible pathogens obstructing an Organ (Intestines, Gall Bladder, Urinary Bladder, Kidney and Heart) or channels and network-vessels. Caused by accumulation of Cold (internal or external), Qi-stagnation, stones, sand, Blood-stasis or Phlegm.	Organ colic (acute abdomen, gallbladder or kidney stones etc.) Usually *not* associated with musculoskeletal pain, except possibly with strong twinged of discogenic pain, and with some internal derangements.
HEAVY PAIN (ZHONG TONG)	Usually felt as achy and not severe with a feeling of heaviness, a tendency to remain lying down, and a feeling of being boundup. Associated with Dampness from exogenous or endogenous source. There may be a feeling of suffocation.	Often occurs in the limbs, head, chest, and/or abdomen.

Table 2-11: Types of Pain in Traditional Chinese Medicine (Continued)

Pain	Characteristics	Mostly Felt At
PULLING PAIN (CHE TONG) SPASMODIC PAIN	Felt as tension or pulling or pain that stretches into another area. Associated with malnourishment of the sinews, vessels and with hypertonicity. Often associated with Liver-Heat or Wind which damages Yin/Blood leading to malnourishment of sinews. *Spasm* (pulling) pain can also result from Cold that causes tissue contraction from exogenous or endogenous sources. Spasm can also result from Deficiency of Blood (Liver), especially with Cold (exogenous or endogenous).	Felt with chest Painful Obstruction (Bi) and pain that stretches through to the back. Musculoskeletal in general, especially if following physical exertion such as sports, associated with Qi-stagnation. Exogenous Cold often results in cervical or fascial spasms. Also associated with Liver-Yang-rising, felt in head Deficiency of Blood can cause spastic pains in the limbs, often at night or when cold (such as nocturnal calf spasms).
SCORCHING (BURNING) PAIN (ZHUO TONG)	Felt as hot burning pain. Tissue hot and often swollen. Associated with Fire-Heat, Damp-Heat, Toxic-Heat, Dry-Heat (external or internal) in the channels, Or deficiency-Heat scorching the channels and network-vessels. Relieved by cold. Also associated with transformative-Heat/Fire from Cold (area may not be hot), Qi or Blood-stagnation.	Mostly surface pain caused by burns, sores, infections, etc. Some types of neuralgias. Organ-Heat such as chest pain from Liver-Heat. Can affect any area or tissue.
SCURRYING (WANDERING) PAIN (CUAN TONG)	Felt as moving and changing pain that comes and goes and is difficult to pinpoint. Associated with Wind of external or internal source. Associated also with the Liver (Qi-stagnation) and then with changes in emotional states.	In musculoskeletal tissues and related channels. Abdominal, chest, trunk, head.
STABBING PAIN (CI TONG)	Felt as pins and needles, as though being stabbed or cut. Associated with Blood-stasis from: Qi-deficiency or Qi-stagnation, Blood-deficiency or anything that obstructs Blood circulation. Associated also with chronic disease states. Can worsen at night, when lying down, or being still. Improves with movement.	Always felt in a fixed location. Can be felt in channels, vessels, Organs, and musculoskeletal tissues; however, may also be generalized and then pain may not be fixed but the patient has many signs of Blood-stasis.
SORENESS (TONG)	Pain that is associated with open wound or with redness and swelling.	Surface pain.
LURKING PAIN (YIN TONG)	Pain associated with hidden pathogens, mild but chronic. Associated with Qi and Blood deficiency, Yang-deficiency Cold with malnourishment.	Abdomen or low back.

a. At the same time some sources associate Deficiency type pains with continuos pain that is aggravated by activity.
b. There is a distinction in TCM between the sensation of fullness and distension.

Table 2-12: Fundamental Pathogenesis of Pain in Traditional Chinese Medicine

		Temperature	Skin/Tongue Color	Aggravated by	Other Symptoms
Cold Pain	Usually local. May be intense, may be worse at night, better during the day after activity.	Tissue/patient feel cold.	White/pale/pale purple.	Cold.	Tissues cold, contracted, muscles tight or spasmed.
Hot Pain	Often radiates. Feel burning, hot. Often intense. May be worse at night. May be throbbing.	Tissue/patient warm.	Red.	Heat.	Tissues hot; muscles may be flaccid or atrophied; or very tight/severe spasms, but only when loaded.
Damp/Phlegm Pain	Local, usually not radiating. Often lower body. Patient/affected area usually feels heavy/fatigued/boundup.	Patient/affected area may feel heavy, damp, and numb (Phlegm).		Weather change.	Tissues feel damp, swollen.
Wind Pain	Movement, radiation. Often upper body. Often sudden onset and changes.	Hot or cold.	Cyan/green Normal.	Exposure to wind.	Muscle may twitch.
Blood-stasis	Fixed location. Often stabbing or paresthesia. May be throbbing.	Hot/cold.	Dark/dry lusterless/purple	Immobility, Sleep.	Often worse at night; Common with injury; Common in women and elderly or chronic diseases.
Qi-stagnation	Often at disease onset; distention/pulsating, nonfixed, poorly localized.	Normal.	Normal	Wind and Emotions. Immobility.	Frequently related to emotional factors; often subcostal tenderness and pain.
Qi/Blood-deficiency	Usually in chronic stage, intermittent, dull achy, area weak, often poorly localized.	Normal or cold.	Normal or pale.	Fatigue.	Pain worse in afternoon after activity. Possibly at night.

3
FOUNDATIONS FOR TCM AND BIOMEDICAL ANATOMY, PHYSIOLOGY AND PATHOLOGY

The musculoskeletal system is the largest system in the body, composing about 75% of the body mass. It is the largest consumer of energy and the bodily resources. These requirements demand functioning cardiovascular, respiratory, digestive, renal, visceral, endocrine, and nervous systems to provide fuel and nutrients, remove the products of metabolism, and control the composition and physical properties of the internal environment. Musculoskeletal medicine therefore must not be reduced to a mechanical reductionist method. This system deserves spacial attention as it is highly affected by gravitational forces on the vertical human framework. This in turn can lead to both musculoskeletal problems as well as visceral and neurogenic dysfunctions. As stated earlier, pain is the most frequent presenting symptom in medical practice in the industrialized world and is almost always a symptom, not a disease or disturbance itself. Well over half the older adults in the US. report chronic joint symptoms, and 80% of the adult population will suffer disabling low back pain in their life time.

TCM Classification of Soft Tissues

The *Classic of Internal Medicine* states:

> The bone is the mainstay, the vessels are the battlements, the sinews are the superstructure, and the flesh is the [exterior] wall... The gathering of the vessels binds the bones and promotes flexibility of the joints.

Joints (Jie)

Joints are formed by sinews and bones. They are classified often as being part of the channels, vessels, Liver, Spleen, and Kidney systems and therefore part of the Exterior and Interior levels. It is said that "the twelve channels and vessels reside internally in the five viscera, and they network externally with the joints of the limbs." Joints are important for the circulation and storage of Qi and Blood. The knees and elbows are the places where Qi enters and exits the Interior (at the Sea points). Joints rely on nourishment from Blood, Fluids, and Essence and are therefore influenced by these and their related Organs. "When Nutritive-Qi and Blood lose their moistening and nourishing, Liver-Wind may enter the sinews and Connecting vessels." Because the Spleen is said to govern the extremities, all peripheral joint pains can affect the Spleen.

Blockage of circulation often occurs at the joints due to excess or lack of physical movement, or to the invasion of external Pathogenic Factors. Because joints are movable and bend, (they are "crooked"), it is easy for Pathogenic Factors to become "trapped" in them, resulting in a Painful Obstruction syndrome. The *Classic of Internal Medicine* says that if joints are pierced and the Fluid leaves the body, the patient will not be able to bend and stretch the joint (possibly referring to traumatic capsulitis). It also states that *all diseases of the joints* result from transmission via the Main channels.[1]

Sinews (Jin)

The Chinese charcter for Sinews (Jin) is made of radicals that denote flesh, tendons, bamboo (joints), and the costal region. The term "sinews" therefore covers a wide range of tissues that are stringy, tough, and elastic, and that overlap with many tissues that are categorized as flesh (Rou). Sinews are also described as "the strength of flesh." The anatomical areas encompassed by the TCM definition of Sinews are: Fascia, tendons, ligaments, subcutaneous tissue, aspects of muscles, joint capsules, cartilage, some blood vessels, and the penis (i.e, sinew gathering).

The sinews are often related to the connective parts of contractile units and joints, and to the tendons and ligaments which are controlled by the Liver and Blood. According to the *Spiritual Axis*:

> When there is an abundance of Blood, the sinews are solid and strong; when there is a deficiency of Blood, the sinews are weak and hard.

In the *Classic of Internal Medicine* the Liver is said to govern the sinews. "If the Blood is deficient the sinews may atrophy." The knees are the "palaces/Organs" (Fu) of the sinews. Therefore, sinews are related to the *Liver-Wood* characteristics of flexibility and strength. The *Spiritual Axis* says: "The color of the eyes, whether green, yellow, red, white, or black tells of disease in the Sinews (because the

---

1. The Chinese term for joint subluxation (partial dislocation) is "Guan Jie Ban Tuo Wei" (or "Tuo Jiao"), complete dislocation is called "Guan Jie Chuan Tuo Wei," and the term for joint dysfunction is "Gong Neng Zhang Ai."

eyes relate to the Liver)." In general, if the Liver (especially Liver-Blood) is deficient, the sinews become vulnerable to invasion of Wind, Cold, and Dampness. Lack of nourishment from Liver-Blood-deficiency may also cause contraction of the sinews. Liver-Blood-stasis or stagnation of Liver-Qi can also cause stiffness of the sinews and joint. Liver-Wind can cause tremors and spasms.

Sinew disorders were classified during the Qing dynasty as Sinew *Rigidity, Flaccidity, Deviation, Laceration, Contusion, Slippage, Enlargement, Twitching, Fatigue, Turned Over, Coldness,* and *Heat*.[2]

In *Spiritual Axis* there are discussions of various oily and greasy (pasty) tissues and membranes that can possibly be interpreted as fascia and connective tissue. In *Spring and Autumn Annals* it is said:

> Above the huang (which has been translated as connective tissues) and below the gao (the region below the heart and above the diaphragm),[3] [is a place that] can not be attacked.[4] It is not possible to reach and to touch this. Even herbs cannot reach it.

This is notable because many fascial, ligamentous and tendinous structures have a poor blood supply and are therefore difficult to treat once damaged. *Difficult Issues* state:

> The strands of oily membrane passing through the spinal bones...[are] called the Kidney connector. It passes down to the net-like membrane...[and] spreads to the dantian, the source of the lower warmer.

Spiritual Axis states:

> ...The sinew [lie along] neither the Yin or Yang [channels], nor to the left or right [side]. They are treated only insofar as they are locally diseased.

Flesh (Rou) and Muscles (Ji)

Muscles in TCM are mainly related to the Sinew channels. Only the quadriceps, gastrocnemius, sternocleidomastoid, and diaphragm are mentioned by name (Kendall *ibid*). Muscle mass is related mostly to flesh (Rou) and, according to *Simple Questions*, is under the control of the Spleen as well as the Liver.

> The Liver controls the muscles; the Liver stores the Qi of the muscular membranes; the Spleen controls flesh...

Spiritual Axis states:

> A pathogenic factor in the Spleen and Stomach will lead to pain in the muscles and flesh...The color of the lips, whether green, yellow, red, white, or black tells of disease located in the muscles and flash (the lips are related to the Spleen)...The fleshy columns (masses of flesh that support) are located between the partings of the flesh of the arms and the lower legs on the routes of various Yang [channels] and between the partings of the flesh on the route of the foot Shao-Yin.

The Spleen/Stomach, by their function of transportation and transformation, provide for the shape/mass, form, and possibly the tone of the muscles, subcutaneous tissue, and fascial mass.[5] The Liver, being Wood, is in charge of flexibility, including that of the muscles and tendons. Therefore, good muscle tone, strength, shape, and flexibility are dependent on the health of both the Liver and the Spleen/Stomach. Since Spleen-Yang and Blood are dependent in part on healthy Kidney-Yang and Essence, Kidney health is important as well. The Stomach is said to govern and moisten the gathering of sinews (penis or possibly also the perineum), to tie the bones and to inhibit joints.

When the Spleen's transformation and transportation functions are weak, "Dampness may pour down to Kidneys (earth disease transferred to water), the bones may atrophy, the marrow may become deficient and empty, and the person may be unable to walk." Severe overuse of muscles can damage Spleen-Qi. With disease, flesh often becomes numb or has a feeling of moving insects; it can wither or harden. The muscles may weaken, may be numb, or tighten and spasm (twitch).

Bones (Gu)

Bones are said to be mostly under the control of the Kidneys and are the surplus of Kidney-Essence. It is said, "Kidneys engender bone and marrow." "When Kidneys are full, the marrow is replete." Essence damage "leads to bone marrow atrophy." (Kidney atrophy is sometimes understood as a synonym of bone atrophy [*Simple Questions*]). Kidney-Heat (Yin-deficiency) can result in low back pain, spine and knee weakness, fragile bones, and decreased marrow; it may lead to bone atrophy/wilting. Healthy and strong bones are also dependent on Nutritive-Qi and Fluid-Ye and their functions of moistening and lubricating. This nourishes the bone marrow, and supplements the Essence. It is said, "If Yin-Qi does not flow freely, the bones will ache." Kidney-Qi is responsible for the nourishment and support of the Sinews and bones, especially the low back and knees. *Spiritual Axis* states:

---

2. Such as: Jin Qiang (*Golden Mirror of Medicine*), Jin Wei (*Simple Questions*), Jin Zhuan (*Golden Mirror of Medicine*), Jin Fan (*Golden Mirror of Medicine*), Jin Ji (*Treatise on the Causes of Diseases*), Jin Duan (*Golden Mirror of Medicine*), Jin Zao (*Essentials of General Collection for Holy Relief*), Jin Chi (*Monograph on Etiology and Pathogenesis of Miscellaneous Diseases*), etc.

3. The same character is used for paste.

4. Although this is usually interpreted to mean early stages of fetal development, umbilicus or disease of the region below the Heart (where the Heart alarm point is located, (and therefore may relate to Heart disease), in *Difficult Issues* Huang is said to be "the space between the Organs, bones and flesh." It may be treated by stimulation of UB-46 (Huang or Triple Warmer back-Shu point, which has been related to fascia by several authors). In the same section, UB-46 was associated with the Yang character of Huang and therefore may also pertain to Defensive-Qi (again however, this section mainly refers to pain below the sternum).

5. Flesh pertains to all soft tissues except viscera and skin.

"The ears, when hot and dry and suffering from dust and dirt, tell of disease of the bones (ears are associated with Kidneys)." The strength of the bones is dependent on normal weight bearing exercises. The *Classic of Internal Medicine* states: "The bones are the home of the marrow. When for a long time one has not been able to stand up and to walk, then one flaps and shakes and the bones will deteriorate (possibly referring to osteoporosis which occurs more often in sedentary patients)." The bones are the palaces (Fu) of the marrow. It is also notable that, when discussing febrile diseases caused by Cold, the *Classic of Internal Medicine* associates the bones with the foot Shao-Yang channel or the Gall Bladder channel.

Injury to the sinews and bones is also said to be capable of injuring the Organs: "Sinew and bone damage leads to damage of the Liver and Kidneys." Thus, the overexertion and lack of rest so common in modern times, especially in athletes, may result in damage to the Spleen, Liver, and Kidney spheres of influence on their related tissues.[6]

As we can see, mixed etiologies, complex patho-mechanisms and involvement of multiple Organs are common when dealing with musculoskeletal disorders.

TCM Pathology and Etiology

In their simplest form most musculoskeletal disorders can be described as follows. Mechanical (Independent) factors such as sprains, falls, and collisions can cause acute tissue damage. Trauma damages the channels and network-vessels/collaterals, blocks Qi and Blood circulation, and induces hematomas/stasis, all of which result in Excess-type pain, and localized dysfunction or pathology (including Phlegm nodes). The formation of Blood-stasis and Phlegm as independent pathologies (i.e., not from an external origin or secondary to internal Organ dysfunction) has been described by some authors.

Alternatively, Deficiency allows for the invasion of environmental Pathogenic Factors which also block Qi and Blood circulation giving rise to pain and/or dysfunction. If Pathogenic Factors are not treated effectively or soon enough, further damage can occur due to increasing blockage and malnourishment that leads to chronic soft tissue dysfunction and/or *pathology,* with Blood-stasis, Phlegm, adhesions, tissue hyperplasia, or atrophy.

The continual overuse of any musculoskeletal structure, especially weight-bearing joints, ligaments, and tendons, can cause break down due to increased metabolic need for Qi and Blood (nutrients).[7] Alternatively, the weakness of Organs, Qi, Blood, Fluids, and Nutritive-Qi result in poor nourishment and failure of tissues. Chronic disorders are characterized by pain of the affected structures, stagnation/stasis of Qi/Blood and/or Fluids/Phlegm; manifesting with diminishing strength, fatigability, inactivity, and hypertrophy or wasting of tissues.

Organic and Interior Influences—TCM

An important consideration in soft tissue damage and Painful Obstruction (Bi) disorders is whether Organic (Interior) causes are affecting the musculoskeletal structure. As it is said in *Spiritual Axis:* "For external factors to invade, there must be Deficiency." *Precise Explanation of Pulse in Familiar Conversations* states: "Inability to turn or bend is due to Kidneys....Lumbar region is the Fu (Palace/Organ) of the Kidney." *General Treatise on the Causes of Symptoms of Disease* states: "The Kidneys dominate the lower back and feet.... Lower back pain is caused by overtaxing of Kidneys [this allows] overexertion [strain] to damage the channels and collaterals...When the Yang aspect is damaged, the patient has difficulty flexing... When Yin is damaged, the patient has difficulty extending... If both Yin and Yang are damaged, the patient has difficulty in both flexion and extension." The *Golden Mirror of Original Medicine* states, "Frequent attacks of Wind, Cold and Damp accompanied by traumatic impairment causes Blood-stasis, hard mass, damage to sinews...In addition, disharmony of Qi and Blood allows for invasion of Wind, Cold and Dampness." *Spiritual Axis* states:

> When evil-Qi is located in the Liver, it causes pains in the middle and on the sides of the ribs. There is cold in the center. Evil-Blood is located on the inside. When walking, frequently there are spasms of the joints, and at that time a swelling of the feet...When evil-Qi is located in the Spleen and Stomach it results in disease. The muscles and flesh are painful...When evil-Qi is located in the Kidneys, it will cause disease. The bones will be painful, and there will be Bi (obstruction) of the Yin. *For Bi of the Yin, pressing with the hand may not localize the pain* [italics emphasis by author], for the abdomen swells, the loins are painful, bowel movements are difficult, the shoulder, back, and neck are painful, and there is occasional dizziness.

When discussing hypertonicity it states:

> The Yellow Emperor asked: People have eight hollows. What is the indicators of them? Qi Bo answered: If there is evil in the Lung and Heart, their Qi will be retained in the elbows. If there is evil in the Liver, its Qi will be retained in the armpits. If there is evil in the Spleen, its Qi will be retained in the hip joint. If there is evil in the Kidney, its Qi will be retained in the back of the knee. The eight hollow parts are all cavities of joints. The True-Qi passes through them and the Blood con-

---

6. And should not be confused by the commonly associated symptoms and signs for these Organs.

7. *Overuse* bone pain is often treated with Psoralea (Bu Gu Zhi), Beef Marrow (Niu Gu Sui), Deer Horn (Lu Rong), Drynaria (Gu Sui Bu) and Tiger [Cat] Bone (Hu Gu). These may be soaked in wine. If the ligaments and tendons are affected, Liver and Blood tonics are added. As Tiger is an endangered species, Cat (or any other) bones are substituted.

necting/network-vessels flow across them. Hence, evil-Qi and bad Blood find it easy to become lodged, and then, they damage the sinews and bones, inhibiting movement. This results in hypertonicity.

Examples by Unschuld (*ibid*) from translations of the *Classic of Internal Medicine* discussing "deeper" causes of musculoskeletal pain are:

> Hence, the shoulder and the shoulder blades may have pain or may be hot in the case of an Excess of Fire Qi. When the shins are swollen, this may be a sign of Kidney disease; when they are painful, this may be attributed to Lung disease; and when they are sore, this may indicate a Liver disease. Similarly, the thigh bones as well as the shins may experience lameness, the feet may be unable to support the body, and limbs in general may be sluggish.

In general, *acute* musculoskeletal disorders are due to Excess/Full patterns. At the acute/severe stage, attention to the Organ (or root) systems is secondary to channels, vessels, soft tissues, or bones, and is limited often to the Exterior. The Lungs, which together with Defensive-Qi and Sinews channels control the Exterior (skin, muscles/body shell) are often treated when external factors (Wind, Heat, Cold, or Damp) are involved. However, many *acute* disorders lack clear Exterior symptoms/signs (except pain and soreness of muscles) and can present without floating pulses and other Exterior symptom/signs, and therefore may actually be manifestations of Interior or Deficiency-Excess patterns.

During *chronic* stages, attention to Deficiency/Emptiness is often needed. The Liver and its connections to Blood, sinews and muscular strength, the Spleen/Stomach and their connections to muscular texture, mass (flesh), Blood formation, and Dampness; and the Kidneys and their connections to Essence (marrow) and bones are often addressed. The Defensive and Nutritive levels are often treated in cases of chronic muscular pain and chronic Painful Obstruction Bi syndrome problems especially in patients that sweat inappropriately. Attention to Blood, Yin and Yang is also commonly needed beyond addressing the related Organs.

Differential Diagnosis

When diagnosing a patient with acute or chronic pain, the practitioner must palpate carefully for maximum tenderness. Often in TCM, these painful sites are said to be the location of *blockage* and therefore the *source* of pain. This is particularly important in chronic diseases,[8] because often the areas have abnormal lumps, scarred tissues, and acupuncture points that can be treated. In addition, the practitioner should evaluate how well the involved structures are functioning.[9] New diseases are often said to be in the channels, and chronic diseases in the Connecting vessels and/or Organs. With chronic disorders, if there is no change in appetite or Organic symptoms, often the condition is said to be due to a "cutting of Channels and Vessels."

Acute Pain

When the patient presents with an acute injury, the practitioner should first exclude other medical conditions that might appear to be traumatic in nature or that allow damage such as latent-toxin/cancer resulting in bone weakness or erosion (Gu Shi) and fracture (Gu Zhe). For example, Heat-Bi *(Biomedical: inflammatory arthritis)*, Damp-Heat/toxic-abscess *(Biomedical: gonococcal arthritis)*, Bone-clinging flat-abscess *(Biomedical: osteomylitis)* may present similarly to acute traumatic disorders; however, ordinarily Heat-Bi and Damp-Heat-abscesses do not have a history of trauma, and hematomas are not usually present. With fractures that are due to cancer or infection, a history of mild trauma is common. Organic diseases must be excluded as, for example, it is said, that "hollow Organ disease makes the upper back painfully-distended," Liver-congestion "results in chest wall (rib-side) and trunk pain;" "all pain pertains to Liver, and if there is Liver disease there is pain." Kidney disease results in back pain as the "lumbar region is the Fu (organ) of the Kidneys." Kidney-deficiency leads to "bone marrow emptiness and therefore atrophy, weakness, and inability to walk." Pain and aching of the foot and heel are said to be due to "Liver and Kidney weakness." Thus Organic disease must be considered in acute and chronic illness.

General symptoms such as a fever that is not allayed by perspiration; malaise, and poor appetite are common both in acute trauma and in internal medical conditions. These should be evaluated carefully, using modern lab work, if needed.

Chronic Pain

When the patient presents with a suspected chronic condition, the practitioner should exclude the possibility of Latent/hidden-toxins *(Biomedical: such as cancer)* and Latent-Fire-toxin infections *(Biomedical: such as tuberculosis)* that, in early stages can easily be mistaken for musculoskeletal conditions. The practitioner should watch the general condition of the patient carefully and may use both modern and traditional diagnostic techniques. As many low-grade tumors and infections are elusive, the best clues come from observation of the patient and from biomedical studies.

---

8. This contrasts with Orthopaedic Medicine, in which local tenderness is considered less important during the chronic stage because often both pain and tenderness are referred.

9. Channels, Collaterals/vessels and Organs are responsible for neurological and motor function.

Important Tissues: Biomedical Perspective

The following are *basic* descriptions of the makeup and function of several important tissues and structures. The understanding of basic biomedical concepts helps explain many of the treatments proposed in this text and can deepen one's use of TCM/OM principles.[10] All tissues are basically built of three basic structures: the capillary, the ground substance or matrix, and the cell. The functional units of the musculoskeletal system are the synovial joints, musculotendinous complexes, and fascial/ligamentous elements, which support the muscles and bones, and their neurovascular supply. For disorders related to these tissues see "MUSCULOSKELETAL DISORDERS: INTEGRATIVE PRACTICE," page 551.

Joints

Joints, the structural foundation of locomotion, are complex structures that can function only by an intricate integration of compression, tension, locomotive, and proprioceptive elements.

Connective Tissue

It is now known that all cells are filled with filaments, tubes, fibers, and trabeculae collectively called the "cytoplasmic matrix" or "cytoskeleton." The entire interconnected system has been called the "connective tissue/cytoskeleton" (Oschman 1994). All elements in a joint complex contain connective tissue. Connective tissue, which includes cartilage and bone, develops from the mesenchyme,[11] which arises largely from the mesodermal somites and the somatic and splanchnic mesoderm.[12] There are three basic types of fibers: collagen, elastin, and reticulin. Ordinarily, connective tissue consists mostly of fibroblast cells;[13] the rest are mast cells,[14] macrophages,[15] plasma cells, pigment cells, lymphocytes, and leukocytes.[16] *Fibroblasts* are involved in the production of fibrous elements and nonfibrous ground substance of connective tissue. The fibrous components are collagen and elastin (Ombregt et al *ibid*).

Collagen is the most abundant protein in the body and is a component of all types of connective tissue. It tends to have great tensile strength (approaching that of steel) because of its triple helix configuration, but it is relatively nonelastic. Collagen can be stretched only 4% or so before it ruptures, or is subjected to irreversible hysteresis (loss of elasticity, although this has been challenged). Its basic building blocks are amino acids: proline, glycine, and lysine, and the biochemical configuration is highly dependent on the incorporation of proline which is the most abundant amino acid in collagen. It requires vitamin C for normal production (Bates and Levene 1969). *Elastin* which is often incorporated with collagen in the makings of connective tissues can stretch to 150% of its original length.

There are eleven types of collagen found in connective tissue. Each type is genetically determined and differs in the chemical nature of the polypeptide chains that form the tropocollagen molecules found in the collagen fiber. Type 1 is the primary component of tendons and ligaments. Type 3 collagen is smaller in diameter and is weaker. In degenerated tendons and ligaments type 3 collagen is often abundant. During repair (the maturation phase), type 3 collagen is replaced by the stronger type 1 (see "Wound Healing" on page 553; Bogduk and Twomey *ibid*). Reticulin is a very fine fiber, a kind of immature collagen which predominates in the embryo but is largely replaced by collagen in the adult (Myers 2001).[17]

The *extracellular matrix* (the sum total of exracellular substances within connective tissue) consists of nonfibrous *ground substance* and is composed of proteoglycans. Proteoglycans are polysaccharide molecules of six to sixty glycoaminoglycans (GAGs). GAGs are also referred to as mucopolysaccharides that are bound to protein chains in covalent complexes (sugar amine bound together by a polymer; Figure 3-2). These long-chain molecules, when linked to the collagen fibers, help form connective tissues. Ground substance is thus a complex connective tissue that lies between all the cells of the body and facilitates tissue metabolism and provides support, shock absorption, and resiliency. Within cartilage there are two main types of GAGs: chondroitin-4-sulfate and chondroitin-6-sulfate. All GAGs (Hascall and Hascall 1981) contain sulfate ester moieties which are required for normal GAG synthesis.[18] GAGs do

---

10. This is a controversial statement; however, this author believes strongly that it is true.
11. Embryonic tissues.
12. Frozen mesenchyme tissues, orally or by injection, can be used in treatment of musculoskeletal disorders.
13. Fibroblast is an undifferentiated cell in the connective tissue that gives rise to various precursor cells, such as the chondroblast, collagenoblast, and osteoblast, that form the fibrous, binding, and supporting tissue of the body.
14. Mast cells are constituents of connective tissue containing large batholithic granules that in turn contain heparin, serotonin, bradykinin, and histamine. When injured, they release heparin that acts as an anticoagulant, histamine that acts as a vascular dilator, and bradykinin that acts as an inflammatory regulator.
15. A macrophage is any phagocytic cell of the reticuloendothelial system, including histocyte in loose connective tissue.
16. A leukocyte is a white blood cell. Five types of leukocytes are classified by the presence or absence of granules in the cytoplasm of the cell. The agranulocytes are lymphocytes and monocytes. The granulocytes are neutrophils, basophils, and eosinophils.
17. A polypeptide is a chain of amino acids joined by a peptide bond. It is heavier than a single molecule peptide but lighter than a molecule of protein.
18. That is why sulfur-containing compounds such as methylsulfonylmethane (MSM) and glucosamine sulfate are often used to treat soft tissues.

not bend around into a circles like most other proteins but rather lie flat and take up lots more room than other molecules of the same molecular weight. On their flat sides they bind large amounts of water and positively charged ions (especially sodium), which assists the amorphous ground substance to become viscous and gives the structural ground substance turgor (fluid pressure) or even hardness (Frost *ibid*). In cartilage, they are bound to hyaluronic acid chains to form a proteoglycans aggregate (Bogduk and Twomey *ibid*). GAGs also form the microfilaments, microtubles, and the microtrabeculae of the *intracellular matrix* and thus help determine what chemicals enter and exit the cells. The primary function of GAGs is to provide flexibility and serve as a lubricant between adjacent collagen fibers, and maintain interfiber distance by their negative electric charge (Bogduk and Twomey *ibid*). The "ground substance system" has been theorized to form a communication system that uses chemical, electrical, and electromagnetic signaling to "oversee" much of the body systems, including the acupuncture channel systems.

Connective tissue *ground substance* can vary from a *watery sol-state* to a *viscous gel-state*. With a higher metabolic rate, motion, electrical stimulation, and warmth, the "energy level" of the tissue is raised, and the ground substance is more fluid and ductile. With a lower energy level from reduced metabolism, lower temperature, and/or inactivity, the ground substance is more of a gel, and the tissue is less able to soften and stretch (Juhan 1987) and may lead to an accumulation of "toxins" (Oschman *ibid*). This may be why rubbing an acupuncture point before inserting the needle is said to facilitate its Qi. Ground substance facilities tissue metabolism and provides support, resiliency, and shock absorption.

At a microscopic level, connective tissue fibers extend into every cell in the body and can be thought of as the living matrix of the continuous and dynamic web that is responsible, in part, for the regulatory effects of "informational" systems of medicine such as acupuncture. When bone or any connective tissue is compressed, or stretched, a minute electric charge is set-up. These oscillations and their harmonics are precisely representative of the forces acting on the tissues involved. In other words, they contain information of the precise nature of the movements taking palace. This information is electrically and electronically (tissues have been characterized as semi-conductors) conducted through the surrounding living matrix.[19] One of the roles of this information is in the control of form (Oshman *ibid*). Connective tissues are therefore capable of enabling communication and connections, and are capable of energy/information storage and conduction. Oshman (*ibid*) states:

- All of the great systems of the body—the circulation, the nervous system, the musculoskeletal system, the digestive tract, the various organs and glands—are everywhere covered with material that is but a part of a continuos connective tissue fabric.

- The connective tissues form a mechanical continuum, extending throughout the animal body, even into the innermost parts of each cell.
- The connective tissues determine the overall shape of the organism as well as the detailed architecture of its parts.
- All movement, of the body as a whole or of its smallest parts, is created by tension carried through the connective tissue fabric.
- Each tension, each compression, each movement causes the crystalline lattice of the connective tissues to generate bioelectronic signals that are precisely characteristic of those tensions, compressions, and movements.
- The connective tissue fabric is a semiconducting communication network that can carry the bioelectronic signals between every part of the body and every other part.

STRESSES AND LOADS. The terminology used to describe stresses on the somatic frame is often that of mechanical systems and taken from the behavior of *nonbiologic* materials. While this approach has many drawbacks (see page 200) and may not take in account the placticity, complexity, and remodeling of biologic systems, it is commonly found in the literature. The magnitude of force applied to somatic structures is usually described as pounds per square inch (psi) or as pascals (N per square meter). *Tension* is defined as the force applied perpendicularly outward from the surface of an object (pull) so that the object is elongated or stretched. *Compression* is a stress force applied perpendicularly inward (push) to the surface of an object, so that the object is shortened or compressed. *Shear stresses* are forces applied parallel to the surface of an object. *Torsion stresses* are rotation-like forces, which, on a constrained object, act to twist it about a neutral axis (an axis that would not be translated or moved by the force). The sum of all stresses on an object is termed *load* (Wells 2003).

The ability of connective tissue to return to its former shape (without loosing its shape) once a loading stress is reduced is called *elastic* behavior. Tissue elasticity is related to its viscoelastic properties and due to the spaces between molecules of collagen containing large amounts of water with salts and other small, relatively mobile molecules. When an applied stress is greater than the elasticity which the tissue can tolerate, it is termed material *failure*. Stress to connective tissues including fascia and ligaments can result in a kind of damage known as hysteresis or "*creep.*" This

---

19. Electrical conduction is usually described as one of three types: metallic conduction, ionic conduction and semi-conduction. Metallic conduction is said to occur only in metal wires (although when non-metallic materials are formed to make tensegrity tubes they can become conductive as well). Ionic conduction occurs through cell membranes and travels minute distances. Semi-conduction is possible within the body (via crystalline-like protein structures, such as perineural glial cells), or other crystalline structures (e.g., transistors), and is capable of conducting small currents (information) over long distances. Piezo-electricity describes the tendency of a crystalline structure to release electrical charges when deformed or struck. Movements within the body are said to constantly release and trigger piezo-electric activity.

Table 3-1: Types of Cartilage

GENERAL	Description	Non-vascular tissue made of a variety of fibrous connective tissues. Three types, depending on structure.
ELASTIC CARTILAGE	Location	Ligamenta flava, ear, and larynx
	Elasticity	More pliant than other cartilage.
	Color	Yellow.
HYALINE CARTILAGE	Location	Comprises the costal, nasal, and articular cartilages on ends of bones.
	Elasticity	Considerable
	Color	Often bluish
	Notes	The most abundant cartilage in the adult body • Contains 80% H2O, which is bound by the negatively-charged proteoglycans • High H2O content results in swelling of cartilage, allowing it to absorb mechanical forces • Sustained pressure can result in plastic deformation • Avascular • Does not have a nerve supply
FIBROCARTILAGE	Location	Intervertebral discs of vertebral column Symphysis pubis A few other joints
	Elasticity	More elastic than hyaline but less than elastic cartilage
	Color	Whitish
	Notes	Appears as a transition between tendons, ligaments, bones Subject to hysteresis

often occurs when the tissues are fatigued. *Fatigue* is a multifaceted term that is used to describe material failure after repeated application of stresses that, if applied individually, would not produce failure. *Creep* is a term that accurately describes the slow, delayed, yet continuous stretch that occurs in response to a continuously applied load. This stretch occurs as long as it is gentle enough not to provoke the resistance of colloidal *drag*. It therefore describes a slow phase after an initial stretch in which a viscoelastic material undergoes an even slower deformation as fluid in the matrix reaches a new equilibrium. *Hysteresis*, or the loss of elastic energy after prolonged or repetitive loading, can become permanent and result in an increase of tissue length known as *set* (i.e., loss of elastic behavior, Bogduk and Twomey *ibid;* Wells *ibid*). Most somatic tissues, when under stress (including bone and soft tissues), are capable of producing a change in their shape called a *deformation*. Wolf's Law states that collagen places or displaces itself in the direction of functional pressure and movement, and that it increases or decreases its mass (and the structures it makes), to reflect the amount of functional pressure and tension (stress). The stress/strain, deformation, and biologic design relationships for most materials (regions) have a linear correspondence; for example, the vertebral bodies and discs become larger at the bottom of the spine in response to increased load (Brown *ibid*). Therefore, all connective tissue is subject to Wolf's Law.

Cartilage

Cartilage, a non-vascular tissue, is comprised of a variety of fibrous connective tissues in which the matrix (intracellular substance of a tissue) is abundant and firm. Table 3-1 lists the types of cartilage, based on their structure. Due to complex processes within the chondrocytes (cartilage cells), articular cartilage undergoes constant degeneration and regeneration. As articular cartilage lacks blood vessels, lymph vessels, and nerves, the joint's environment is greatly dependent on synovial fluid for nourishment and regeneration. Cartilage has some similarity to bone in that it consists of chondrocytes surrounded by an extensive extracellular matrix that they secrete, except that the matrix is not calcified as in bone (Wells *ibid*).

Articular cartilage guarantees coherent distribution of stress on the osseous surfaces, participates in articular sliding movements with a low friction coefficient, and helps dampen impact during daily activities and trauma (Barral and Croibier 1999). Under conditions of rapidly repeated fight-impact loading, the fluid forced from the matrix that would normally provide a cushioning effect cannot be reabsorbed in time to cushion subsequent impacts. This may also produce a plastic deformation of cartilage surfaces that does not sufficiently recover for smooth surface contact upon subsequent loading and can lead to degenerative joint disease. This may explain why some professionals such as football

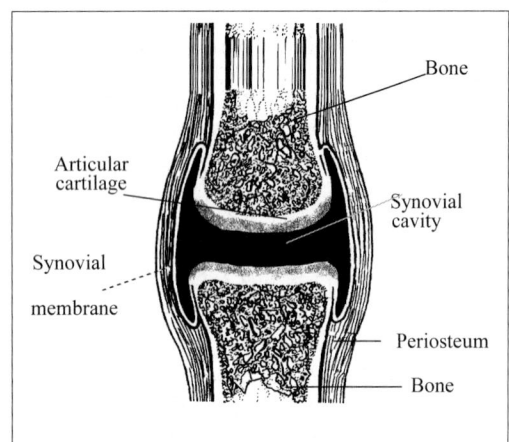

Figure 3-1: Synovial Joint.

players and dancers commonly suffer from arthrosis (Wells *ibid*). *(OM: Tai Chi exercises, which are designed to open and close the joints, are believed by some to aid in the regenerative process).*

Synovium

The synovium is a colorless, viscous fluid that lubricates and nourishes the joint, including the avascular articular cartilage. The inner surface of the joint capsule is lined with several synovial layers. Innervated by sympathetic nerve fibers, these layers are abundant in capillaries, venules, and lymphatic supply. The synovium plays a significant role in infection control and in the production of hyaluronate, which gives synovial fluid its viscosity. While the synovium is derived from the mesenchyme (Jacobs and Falls 2003), mircoscopically and functionally it is similar to epithelial tissue, which is an ectodermal derivative. Trauma and disease can change the viscosity of the synovium so that it no longer circulates properly (Brown *ibid*).

Categories of Joints

Joints can be categorized as freely-movable (diarthrodial) hinges, such as the shoulder and the zygoapophyseal (facet) joints, or semi-movable (amphiarthrodial), such as the intervertebral joints and the symphysis pubis. The sacroiliac joint has characteristics of both.

FREELY-MOVABLE JOINTS. Freely-movable joints are synovial in structure, held together by a capsule of dense, fibrous tissue and ligaments. Additional support is provided by muscles, tendons, and atmospheric pressure (the inner joint space has negative pressure). One example of this structure is the hip joint: the two surfaces can stay together even if the soft tissues around them are severed. However, if a small hole in the synovial sac develops, and air penetrates, the hip joint loses this adherence (Bonica *ibid*). All synovial joints are similar in structure. The two articular surfaces of a synovial joint are separated by a monolayer of synovial fluid in the joint cavity. The capsule is formed by two layers: the fibrous outer layer is in continuity with the periosteum of the proximal and distal bones and can be described as the free periosteum which envelops the joint. The inner layer is the synovial membrane that lines the fibrous outer layer. This layer secrets the synovial fluid that lubricates and protects the joint (Jacobs and Falls *ibid*).

Movable joints are kept stable and mechanical forces are distributed by a system that combines elements of tension and compression from the capsule, ligaments, muscles, fascia, and bone. This system allows joints to survive great mechanical stresses. Ligaments may be classified as capsular or accessory. A capsular ligament is a part of the fibrous outer layer of the joint capsule, while accessory ligaments are either located within the joint cavity (intracapsular) or outside the joint capsule, separated from the fibrous outer layer (extracapsular) (Brown *ibid*).

SEMI-MOVABLE JOINTS such as the vertebral bodies are separated by a disc. The bony surface of the joint is covered by articular cartilage of type 2 collagen, which has significant tensile strength.

Many semi-movable joints such as the acromioclavicular, sacroiliac, etc., are dependent almost entirely on ligaments for stability and do not have any primary muscle movers.

Joint Neurophysiology

Synovial joints are supplied by mechanoreceptors and nociceptive receptors (pain-receiving nerve endings). The joint capsule has four types of receptors: the Raffini, Pacinian, Meissner's, and Merkel's. They also contain free nerve endings (C-fibers). Joint receptors have myelinated and unmyelinated fibers that have several functions, some of which are inter-regulating. Joint (and ligament) receptors are capable of reporting position throughout the range of the joint. The characteristics of joint receptors are summarized in Table 3-2 on page 173 (Wyke 1979, 1977; Mitchell 1993).

Muscles

Skeletal muscles make up about 40% of body weight. They are comprised of 75% water, 20% protein and 5% inorganic material, organic "extractives," and carbohydrates. Skeletal muscle tissue is derived from mesenchyme and is modified for specific junction of contraction. Muscles are well-vascularized, allowing them to recover from injuries relatively faster than tissues that have a smaller blood supply.

Muscle Fibers

Muscles are composed of muscle fibers bound by connective tissue and are arranged in a regular, systemic manner to facilitate contraction when stimulated by a nerve impulse. A single skeletal muscle cell is a thin cylinder, 10-100 microns in diameter, that can extend up to 4cm in length. Skeletal

Table 3-2: Joint Capsule Receptors

TYPE I	Functions	Proprioception, pain suppression, tonic reflexogenic effect on muscles, report tension of joint capsule outer layer
	Size	Small (6-9 μm)
	Myelinated	Yes
	Location	Joint capsule outer layer
	Most Active	At initiation and at end of range of motion
	Notes	Static and dynamic mechanoreceptors, low threshold, slow adapting
TYPE II	Functions	Phasic reflexogenic effect on muscle, pain suppression
	Size	Medium (9-12 μm)
	Myelinated	Yes
	Location	At deeper layers of capsule and articular fat pads
	Most Active	Mid-range of motion
	Notes	Dynamic mechanoreceptors, low threshold, very slow adapting
TYPE III	Function	Probably proprioception
	Size	Large (13-17 μm)
	Myelinated	Yes
	Location	Typical receptors of ligaments and tendons that insert close to, but not in, joint capsule
	Most Active	Probably in extremes of motion
	Notes	High-threshold mechanoreceptor, very slow adapting, more receptive to load than to degree of stretch
TYPE IV	Functions	Nociception, tonic reflexogenic effect on muscles, respiratory, and cardiovascular reflexogenic effect
	Size	Very small (2-5 μm)
	Myelinated	Myelinated and unmyelinated
	Location	Throughout joint capsule, walls of articular blood vessels, and articular fat pads
	Notes	High threshold, nonadaptive

muscle fibers may extend the entire length of the muscle and join with tendons at their ends. An electrically-polarized membrane surrounds each fiber. If the membrane becomes temporarily depolarized, the muscle fiber contracts.

Muscle fibers are composed of a huge number of slender, tiny contractile threads of *myofibril,* each of which has two fine, longitudinal fibrils lying side by side. The myofibrils composed of many regularly-overlapping, ultramicroscopic, thick and thin *myosin* and *actin* myofilaments that may extend the entire length of the muscle. A muscle fiber has about 1500 myosin filaments and 300 actin filaments. These two types of filaments together form large protein molecules responsible for muscle contraction. Myofibrils are embedded in connective tissue that transmits the pull of the muscle cells during contraction. Myosin is the thicker of the filaments and is twice the size of the thin filament, actin. (There are also other fiber types such as titan fibers.) Muscle contraction is achieved by nervous stimulation by the motor (alpha motor nerves) system which results in attractive forces between these filaments that cause them to slide together (Chusid 1982; Figure 3-3).

Muscle Contraction

Three mechanisms that induce action potentials (electrical depolarization of muscles) lead to the initiation of muscle contraction: stimulation by nerve fibers, stimulation by hormones and local chemical agents, and spontaneous electrical activity within the membrane (found in the heart).

Smooth muscles and heart muscles are stimulated by all three mechanisms; normally, skeletal (striated) muscles are stimulated only by nerve fibers (Chusid *ibid*). The skeletal muscle fibers contract in response to *acetylcholine* release by the motor nerves.

Muscle Functions

Muscles *produce motion*: acceleration and concentric action, and *stop motion*: deceleration, isometric and eccentric action. These are both types of contraction. With the first the muscle fibers shorten, and with the second they lengthen. The resting contraction of muscles has been called *muscle tone*. Muscles also contribute to functions such as respiration, defecation, and the generation of body heat. Muscle

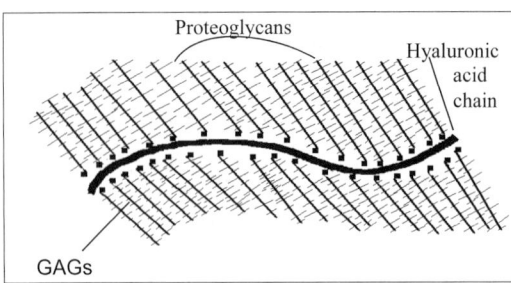

Figure 3-2: Ground substance.

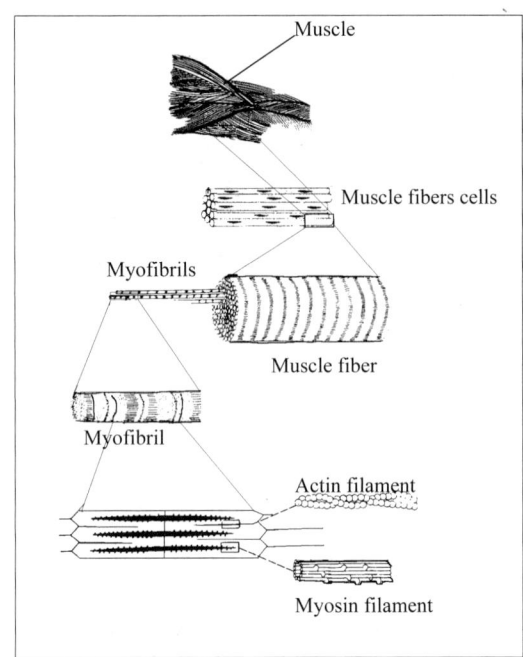

Figure 3-3: Fibrillar organization within skeletal muscle (after Bloom and Fawcett). There are also other types of fibers in muscles such as titan fibers.

health and function depend on the nervous, digestive, respiratory, and circulatory systems to provide food (trophic factors) and oxygen, on the skin for protection and to help dissipate heat produced during muscle contraction, and on the kidneys to excrete metabolic waste. Muscle contraction that does not involve muscle shortening (i.e., no movement) is called *isometric* (constant length) contraction. Muscle contraction that involves movement of an object is known as *isotonic* (constant tension) contraction. The muscle that acts isotonically (concentrically, is shortened by activity) to move the joint is called the *agonist*. The muscle being lengthened is called the *antagonist* (it controls and slows down the primary motion). For example, when the elbow is flexed the biceps shorten, functioning as the agonist, while the triceps lengthen, functioning as the antagonist.

Postural and Phasic Muscles.

Skeletal muscles are composed mainly of two fiber types: slow twitch (type I) and fast twitch (type II) (summarized in Table 3-3.) Table 3-4 on page 178 lists postural and phasic muscles. Muscle fiber types are distinguished by the rate at which adenosine triphosphate (ATP) can be made available to the sarcomeres for contraction and by the metabolic pathways through which ATP is generated. The rate of availability of ATP directly affects the rate of contraction or twitch time of a muscle fiber. Many muscles, called intermediate muscles (Wells *ibid*), are complex and composed of both fiber types.

POSTURAL MUSCLES: Postural muscles, also called *Tonic* or *red* muscles, have a significantly larger number of type I (slow) fibers than phasic muscles have. Type I fibers are more vascular (containing more myoglobin) and resistant to fatigue than type II fibers. Their metabolism is oxidative (due to myoglobin). Myoglobin has a six times greater affinity for oxygen than the hemoglobin which carries the oxygen in the blood. Slow fibers utilize sugar (glucose) for fuel and can completely oxidize the glucose to carbon dioxide and water. Twenty times more ATP can be produced by the oxidation of glucose in the slow fibers than by the splitting of glucose in fast (tonic) fibers. Slow fibers can also use fatty acids for their fuel (Chusid *ibid*; Wells *ibid*). Tonic muscles can withstand several hundred contractions before becoming fatigued. Often they are relatively deeper than phasic muscles. They tend to be monoarticular (span only one joint), richly innervated (spindle-rich), and have many mitochondria. They have relatively small motor units (Mitchell 1993).

Tonic muscles are often the first muscles recruited during an involuntary reflex such as maintaining posture. Since tonic muscles often span one joint and are prone to tightness, they can perpetuate type II (non-neutral) somatic dysfunction in the spine (see page 461; Mitchell *ibid*). These muscles are thought to have primary responsibility for countering the effects of gravity, e.g., for maintaining posture, and therefore are required to withstand work of long durations.

The small, deep, monoarticular vertebral muscles are thought to have important proprioceptive functions, to make fine adjustments of the relative positions of the two bones, and to stabilize that relationship in preparation for the more powerful leverage forces exerted by the polyarticular muscles. These muscles may also prevent nociceptive information from passing the "spinal cord gate" (Mitchell *ibid*).

According to Janda (*ibid*), these muscle are prone to tightness.

PHASIC MUSCLES: Phasic muscles (*white* muscles), which consist predominantly of fast twitch (type II) fibers, are used for short periods when extra strength or quick response is needed. Their metabolism is anaerobic (glycolysis) and they have fewer mitochondria (i.e., they get their energy by splitting glucose in the absence of oxygen). Fast fibers contain little or no myoglobin and are therefore white in color. They are thicker than slow (red) fibers. The end product of the

Table 3-3: Muscle Fiber Types

MUSCLE FIBER TYPES	
TYPE I SLOW TWITCH	Strength training and interval training transform Type I into Type II
TYPE II FAST TWITCH	Endurance training converts Type II to Type I
MUSCLE TYPES	
TONIC (POSTURAL)	Have significantly larger number of Type I Fibers than phasic muscles. More vascular than Type II. More resistant to fatigue than the phasic muscle. Can withstand several hundred contractions.
PHASIC	Predominantly type II muscle fiber. Used for short periods when extra strength or quick response is needed.

anaerobic splitting of glucose is lactic acid, which may be responsible in part for the soreness felt after strong exercise (by becoming acidic).

Phasic muscles are often relatively more superficial than tonic muscles and tend to be polyarticular (span several joints). Innervated by relatively large motor units, they are under voluntary reflex control. Because they are polyarticular they can perpetuate rotoscolioses.[20]

According to Janda (*ibid*), these muscles are prone to weakness. Tight muscle often result in inhibition of other related muscle which then function as though they are weak. The relationship between a tightness-prone muscle and its weakness-prone (inhibited) *partner* muscle is *one-way*. As the tightness-prone muscle becomes tighter and stronger, its inhibition of the weakness-prone muscle also becomes stronger. The weaker muscle does not provide reciprocal feedback (Mitchell *ibid*). When phasic muscles are contracted continuously, such as in reflex guarding, they become congested and sore.[21]

Although there is a distinction between phasic and tonic muscles, many muscles display both characteristics of both, and contain a mixture of Type I and Type II fibers. The hamstring muscles, for example, have a tonic stabilizing function yet are polyarticular and are notoriously prone to shortening. Phasic and tonic muscle functions are always integrated with each other, with the CNS activity, and other tissue. It is advisable not to consider muscle function in purely mechanical and reductionist manner.

Table 3-5 provides summaries of some of the patterns which can be associated with imbalances between stabilizers and mobilizers. Possible observational evidence of dysfunction is reviewed on Table 3-6 (Chaitow *ibid*).

TRANSFORMING MUSCLE FIBERS. With training or electrical stimulation, muscle fibers can be transformed from one type to the other.

• Strength training and interval training transform type I-tonic to type II-phasic.

• Endurance training converts type II to type I (Dvorák 1990).

• Lack of use due to injury or inactivity can also result in a transformation of fiber types, which in turn may result in imbalance and stress on other structures (joints, discs, ligaments, etc.).

In the lumbar spine, both hypomobility and nerve root compression result in the transformation of muscle fibers. These factors have been demonstrated histochemically to increase the proportion of slow twitch fibers, resulting in decreased dexterity (Jowett and Fidler 1975). Fatigue of muscles with prolonged contraction activity results from the depletion of the nutrients and oxygen required to produce adenosine triphosphate (ATP) as an energy supply from either aerobic or anaerobic glycolysis.

Muscle Innervation

Skeletal muscle fiber is innervated both by efferent (motor, from the CNS) and afferent (sensory, towards the CNS) nerves. Efferent axons arise from nerve cells located either in the brainstem or the spinal cord. These nerve cells are called *motor neurons* or *somatic efferents*. Motor neuron axons are myelinated. They are the largest-diameter axons in the body and are therefore fast-conducting. A large number of muscle nerve fibers are sensory in function (Sherrington has estimated at least 40%). Many muscles have considerable individual variation in their innervation, from both spinal and peripheral nerves. Rarely do anatomists agree completely on the segmental innervation of muscles (Simons, Travell, Simons 1999).

A motor neuron and the muscle fibers it innervates is called a *motor unit* (Figure 3-4). The region of the muscle membrane together with the terminal portion of the axon (nerve) is the *motor endplate*. The junction that includes the axon terminal and the motor endplate is called the *neuromuscular junction*. The location and size of endplate zones are related to muscle functions. The relative length of individual fibers to total muscle length has important functional consequences (Simons, Travell, Simons *ibid*). Muscles like the *quadriceps, scalenes,* and *gastrocnemius,* with relatively low fiber length/muscle length ratios (short fibers), are designed for force production.

---

20. Rotoscolioses can occur from osteopathic type I neutral spinal dysfunction. Phasic muscles seem to be affected by problems in spinal joints and the deep postural muscles may have some regulatory effects on phasic muscles. Phasic muscle therefore often develop trigger points as a result of vertebral dysfunction and the monoarticular tonic muscles, on their convex side. The pain and spasm are not confined to the precise site of the primary dysfunction (Mitchell *ibid*).

21. It is also possible, however, for a muscle to have too little tone (from being weak) resulting in its antagonists reacting with increased tightening and shortening. The tightening of the antagonists may then further inhibit agonist which then may in turn result in further tightening of the antagonists, creating a vicious cycle. In this scenario, the strengthening of the primarily weak muscle takes precedence.

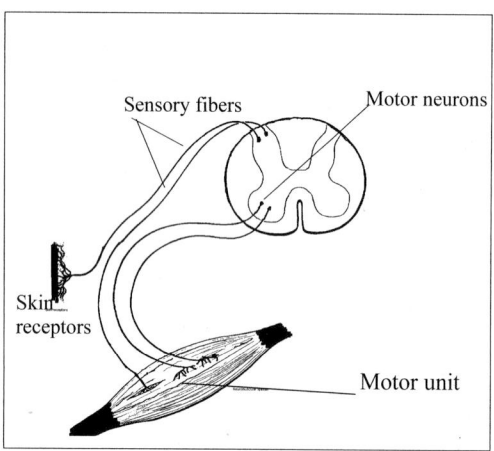

Figure 3-4: A motor unit (After Crouch).

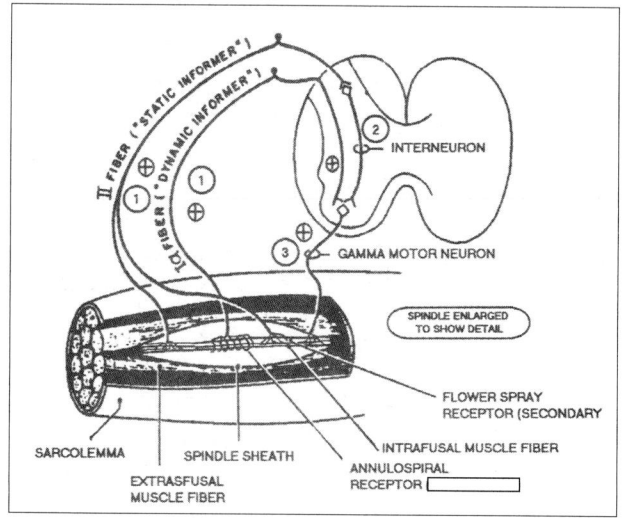

Figure 3-5: The spindle mechanism (From Kuchera WA and Kuchera ML, Osteopathic Principles in Practice, KCOM press 1993, with permission).

- *Biceps, hamstrings,* and *tibialis anterior* have a high fiber length/muscle length ratio and are designed to produce high-velocity movements.
- Muscles designed to produce force have endplate zones that run the length of the muscle.
- Muscles designed for rapid movements have endplate zones that run relatively transverse to the muscle (depending on structure), but are always near the midpoint of the muscle fibers.

Muscles have three major types of receptors (Chusid *ibid*): Muscle spindles (annulospiral ending, nuclear bag region and flower-spray endings), golgi tendon organs, and free nerve endings.

Muscle Spindles

Muscle spindles are specialized mechanoreceptive (proprioceptive) contractile fiber units that contain *intrafusal fibers* surrounded by connective tissue.

The spindles are bundles of about three to ten intrafusal fibers that are several milliliters long (2-4 mm) and are therefore shorter and thinner than the contractile fibers. Muscle spindles are arranged parallel to *extrafusal fibers*, which are the regular contractile fibers that provide the muscle's contractile force. The ends of muscle spindle capsules are attached to tendons at either end of the muscle, or to the sides of adjacent, extrafusal fibers. These fusiform (spindle-shaped) structures are found throughout the muscle, with a high concentration around the slow twitch fibers (Richmond and Abrahams 1979), and concentrated in the muscle "belly." Muscles responsible for fine and precise motor movements, such as tonic (postural) and hand muscles, have a considerably higher concentration of spindles than phasic muscles (Mitchell *ibid*).

NUCLEAR BAG REGION. The two ends of each muscle spindle are contractile. The middle portion or receptor portion of a muscle spindle, the *nuclear bag region* (Figure 3-5), is noncontractile. Wrapped around the muscle spindle fibers in a complex manner are two types of sensory endings that are found in the muscle spindle. These sensory endings are the nuclear bag that contains *annulospiral endings* (primary endings), which are continuous with rapidly-conducting afferent (sensory) nerves; and *Flower-Spray Endings* (secondary endings) found on either side of the annulospiral endings, which are receptors for the smaller myelinated fibers (Waxman and deGroot *ibid*).

MUSCLE SPINDLE FUNCTION. The primary function of intrafusal fibers (spindles, nuclear bag and flower-spray endings)—which serve as the sensory organ of muscles—is to register changes in muscle length (the static response) and rate of change in muscle length (the dynamic response), both of which regulate muscle tone and help to protect the muscle. These stretch-sensing receptors send their messages along the "primary" type Ia afferent nerves to the CNS. Muscle spindles are responsible for the stretch reflex and for muscle tone, which is essential for maintaining posture. In general therefore, the spindles can evaluate, report, and initiate re-setting of muscle length and tone (Waxman and deGroot *ibid*). They may be involved in myofascial pain syndromes, and, according to Korr (*ibid*), may be the primary cause of joint restrictions and somatic dysfunction.[22]

The receptors in the nuclear bag region, which adapt rapidly to changes in muscle length, velocity, and acceleration of contraction, serve the stretch reflex. Flower-spray endings produce increased flexor and decreased extensor motor neuron activity (Waxman and deGroot *ibid*).

---

22. However, others disagree (Simons, Travell and Simons *ibid*).

Muscles

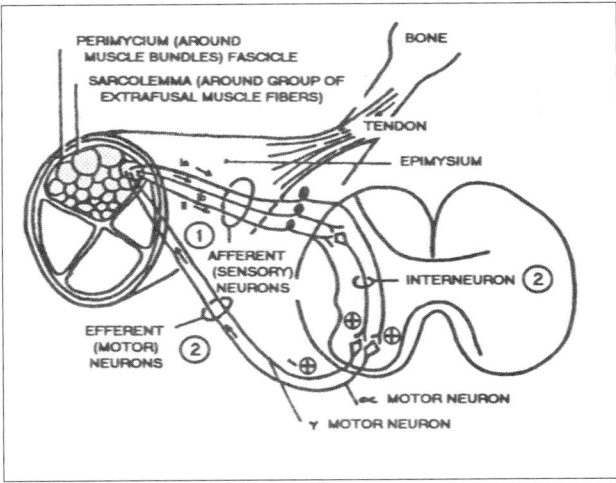

Figure 3-6: Muscle mass innervation (From Kuchera WA and Kuchera ML, Osteopathic Principles in Practice, KCOM press 1993, with permission).

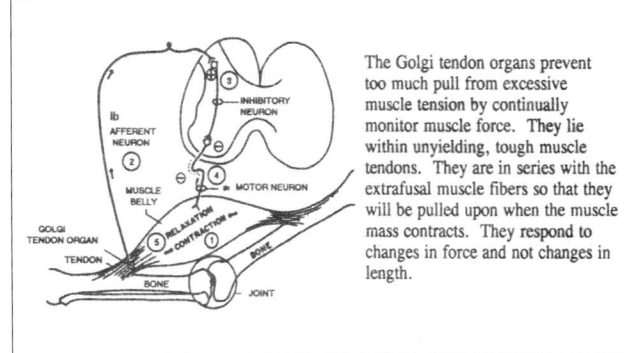

Figure 3-7: Golgi tendon organs (From Kuchera WA and Kuchera ML, Osteopathic Principles in Practice, KCOM press 1993, with permission).

The arrangement and number of spindles (for example, the fact that a muscle with the tendency to tightness has many spindles), helps explain Janda's clinical observation that postural muscles tend to become short, whereas phasic muscles tend to become weak (Dvorák and Dvorák *ibid*).

Muscle spindle and end-plate stimulation by acupuncture is probably one of the most important aspects of this treatment technique in myofascial pain.

GAMMA AND ALPHA MOTOR (EFFERENT) NERVES. The efferent (motor) nerves send responses and commands from the CNS to the muscles and are divided into the *Gamma* and *Alpha* systems. Gamma nerves supply the motor innervation to the muscle spindles and comprise the small motor neuron system, whose cell bodies are located in the ventral horn (spinal cord). These nerves are distributed to the motor end-plate on the contractile ends of the intrafusal fibers (muscle spindles).

Gamma motor nerves set the gain or resting tone of muscle spindles which increase the muscle's sensitivity to overall stretch. The gamma motor system is regulated by descending activity from a number of areas in the brain. The gamma "loop" is a length-regulating reflex mechanism for each muscle and is protective against excessive stretch. It is important for coordinated movement and postural control. (Waxman and deGroot *ibid*).

Alpha motor nerves supply the regular contractile, extrafusal, muscle fibers (not the spindle). Alpha motor nerves arise from large anterior horn neurons (of the spinal cord), called alpha motor neurons. When alpha motor neurons fire, the action potential in their axons propagate via the ventral roots and peripheral nerves to the motor end-plate where they excite the muscle. There are two types of alpha motor nerves: the "tonic" system innervates the postural muscles, and the "phasic" system innervates the phasic or fast muscle fibers (Waxman and deGroot *ibid*), (Figure 3-6).

A muscle receives about 70% of its motor innervation from the alpha system and 30% from the gamma system.

Golgi Tendon Organs

The Golgi tendon organs, which lie in series with the muscle fibers, serve as inhibitors of muscle spindles and contractile forces in the muscle. The Golgi tendon organ therefore functions in opposition to the spindles. About ten to fifteen muscle fibers attach to each Golgi tendon organ. They are found at the musculotendinous junctions. When tension at the muscle tendon fiber approaches a dangerous level (when the length of the muscle is shortened causing it to pull on the tendons), the Golgi tendon organs limit muscle contraction automatically, by reacting to tension in the (extrafusal) muscle fibers that mass-activate Golgi receptors. The Golgi receptors then send impulses to the spinal cord, which in turn excites inhibitory interneurons that relax the muscle (turning off the alpha system that stimulates muscle contraction). In contrast to the muscle spindles, which are said to be always active, the Golgi tendon organs become active only when the muscle is forcefully shortened (contracts), which then pulls on Golgi receptors (*ibid*).

Golgi tendon organs have a much higher threshold than muscle spindles do, and, therefore, they do not over-control the muscle but still can allow for forceful contractions. (They can be overridden by the CNS to the extent that, at times, muscles can be torn by forceful contraction, as is seen in athletes.) The nerve fibers of Golgi tendon organs, which are myelinated, are believed to synapse in the ventral horn of the spinal cord with inhibitory interneurons (Renshaw cells) that terminate directly on alpha motor neurons of the same muscle. Therefore, Renshaw cells appear to be part of local feedback circuits that prevent overactivity in alpha motor neurons (Waxman and deGroot *ibid*). This inhibitory reflex which differs from the muscle spindle stretch reflex is discussed by Sandler (1983):

Table 3-4: Postural and Phasic Muscle Pairs

Postural Muscles		Phasic Muscles
Suboccipital	Inhibits	Digastrics
Cervical erector spinae	Inhibits	Short cervical flexors
Masticatoris	Inhibits	Deltoids
Sternocleidomastoid (scm)	Inhibits	Scaleni[a]/longus colli (short cervical flexors)
Temporalis	Inhibits	Digastric, Short cervical flexors
Short, deep extensor muscles	Inhibits	Deep cervical flexors[b]
Upper trapezius	Inhibits	Lower/middle trapezius
Levetor scapulae, (Scalenes)	Inhibits	Lower trapezius, short cervical flexors
Pectoralis major	Inhibits	Lower stabilizers of scapula, Rhomboids
Latissimus dorsi	Inhibits	Serratus anterior, deltoid
Subscapularis	Inhibits	Spinatti and middle trapezius
Upper extremity flexors	Inhibits	Upper extremity extensors
Quadratus lumborum	Inhibits	Thoracoabdominal diaphragm, gluteus medius/minimus, abdominal int/ext obliques
Lumbar paraspinals (erector spinae)	Inhibits	Rectus abdominus[c], thoracic erectors
Piriformis	Inhibits	Gluteus maximus, medius and minimus
Iliopsoas	Inhibits	Rectus abdominus, glutei (gluteus maximus)
Tensor fascia latae (TFL)	Inhibits	Gluteus maximus, medius and minimus
Rectus femoris	Inhibits	Vastus medialis and lateralis (gluteus maximus?)
Lower extremity adductors	Inhibits	Gluteus minimus/medius, abdominals int/ext obliques
Hamstring	Inhibits	Glutei, tibialis anterior
Tibialis posterior	Inhibits	Tibialis anterior
Triceps surae	Inhibits	Vasti (quadriceps)

a. The subject of whether the scalenes are phasic is controversial
b. Jull, Janda 1987, Janda 1996.
c. The subject of whether the rectus abdominus obliques are phasic is controversial.

Table 3-5: Patterns of Imbalance as Some Muscles Weaken and Lengthen, and Synergists Become Overworked, While Antagonists Shorten (Chaitow *ibid*)

Lengthened or underactive stabilizer	Overactive synergist	Shortened antagonist
Gluteus medius	TFL, quadratus lumborum, piriformis	Thigh adductors
Gluteus maximus	Iliocostalis lumborum and hamstrings	Iliopsoas, rectus femoris
Transverse abdominis	Rectus abdominis	Iliocostalis lumborum
Lower trapezius	Levator scapulae/upper trapezius	Pectoralis major
Deep neck flexors	SCM	Suboccipitals
Serratus anterior	Pectoralis major/minor	Rhomboids
Diaphragm		Scalenes, pectoralis major

Table 3-6: OBSERVATIONAL EVIDENCE OF IMBALANCE INVOLVING CROSS-PATTERNS OF WEAKNESS/LENGTHENING AND SHORTNESS (CHAITOW *IBID*)

MUSCLE INHIBITION/WEAKNESS/LENGTHENING	OBSERVABLE SIGN
Transverse abdominis	Protruding umbilicus
Serratus anterior	Winged scapula
Lower trapezius	Elevated shoulder girdle (gothic shoulders)
Deep neck flexors	Chin poking
Gluteus medius	Unlevel pelvis on one-legged standing
Gluteus maximus	Sagging buttock(s)

When the tension on the muscles, and hence the tendon, becomes extreme, the inhibitory effect from the tendon organ can be so great that there is sudden relaxation of the entire muscle under stretch. This effect is called the lengthening reaction and is probably a protective reaction to the force which, if unprotected, would tear the tendon from its bony attachments. Since the Golgi tendon organs, unlike the spindles, are in series with the muscle fibres, they are stimulated by both passive and active contractions of the muscles.

Free Nerve Endings

The third group of muscle-nerve structures is the free nerve endings, which are associated mostly with blood vessels and pain receptors. Deep palpation and stimulation of free nerve endings can produce muscle pain.

Sympathetic Innervation

Earlier researchers thought that skeletal muscles did not have sympathetic innervation (except for the blood vessels). Now direct sympathetic innervation to the intrafusal fibers of muscle spindles is known, and the fact that sympathetic stimulation causes muscle tension is recognized (Baker and Banks 1986). Muscle paralysis of animals that have been injected with curare (a plant alkaloid that induces the paralysis of muscle by selective action on the myoneural junction) can be blocked by alpha-adrenergic antagonists, which act on sympathetic neurons. This sympathetic innervation has been demonstrated physiologically and anatomically (Passatrore, Filppi, and Grassi 1985; Bridgman and Eldred 1981; Santini and Ibata, 1971; Baker and Daito 1981).

Tendons

Tendons are fibrous connective tissues that attach muscles to bones and other structures. Their collagenous fibers are arranged fairly regularly running parallel and partly interweaving. Tendons appear to be white because they are *relatively* avascular. The vascular supply is found in three areas, each suppling one third of the tendon: small vessels at the musculotendinous junction, vessels in the paratendon, and at the tendon-periosteum junction with direct anastomoses between tendon vessels and those in the periosteum. There is often a reduced circulation in areas of increased friction and compression, referred to as the "critical zone" (Brown *ibid*).

Collagen represents about 60-80% of the total dry weight of a tendon. Tendons are slightly stretchable although they have little or no elastin fibers. The slight, rope-like interweaving pattern of collagen fibers allows for some elongation, which can mitigate pull at the tendon insertion. Tendons are highly resistant to extension. In a normal state, tendons consist of 30% collagen and a maximum of 2% elastin, embedded in an extracellular matrix containing 68% water. Some evidence suggests that they are capable of inert motion as they contain a small amount of actine and myocine. Tendons are also visco-elastic, which allows them to store energy and to recoil back after being stretched.

Tendons are constructed by groups of fibers, each of which is composed of several fibrils, which form fascicles surrounded by the endotendon. The endotendon is an areolar connective tissue sheath (or small space) that houses the nerves and blood vessels. The endotendon is enclosed by the epitendon, and the outermost layer is the paratendon. Tendons appear to receive only afferent (sensory) nerve supply. The strength and size of young growing tendons can be increased by exercise. In adults only minimal effect on size is seen, but exercise is needed to maintain structural integrity (Brown 1995).

In most cases tendons attach to the skeleton. The tendon of the muscle that attaches to the less movable or proximal structure is called the *tendon of origin*. The tendon that attaches to the more movable or distal part is called the *tendon of insertion*. Frequently the origin of a muscle is attached directly to the periosteum of a bone without an intervening tendon, but usually the insertion is tendinous. The dense fibrous connective tissue is anchored to the compact cortical substance of bone by microscopic connective tissue penetrating fibers (*Shrapes fibers*). The connective tissue here forms the mass of the tendon, becoming feathered to interdigitate with the skeletal muscle fibers, which will form the substance of a given muscle. The same architecture is duplicated at the proximal and distal muscle attachments to bone (Jacobs and Falls 2003).

Tendons can vary in shape from short and stocky to long and slender. Some tendons are broad sheets of connective tissues called *aponeuroses (*Bugdok *ibid).*

Fascia

Fascia as a structure literally ties everything together, from the soles of the feet to the meninges that surround the brain. Soft tissue dissection shows that fascia is anatomically inseparable from muscles, although some authors suggested that fasciae move independently. Work done at Michigan State University suggests that fasciae probably move in response to complex muscle activities acting on not only bones and joints but also ligaments, muscles, tendons, and other fascia. After joint and muscle spindle activity is accounted for, 75% of remaining proprioception occurs in fascial sheaths (Ward 2003).

Fascia is made of collagen and elastin fibers, ground substance (which follows the laws of fluid mechanics), and cellular elements. The fascial system has been divided into two parts: the subcutaneous and the subserous. The subcutaneous system has two distinct layers, the superficial and the deep. Together they form a continuous sheet over the body. The superficial fascial system connects the skin, muscles, and skeletal structures. The deep layer (deep fascia) invests and separates muscles of the limbs and trunk. The spaces that form between muscles are known as the intermuscular septa and contain the nerves, the blood, and the lymph vessels.[23] The subserous system lines the body cavities (e.g., peritoneum, pleura, mesenterium). A third system is the intracranial-dural system. Fascia define the individual muscle and muscle groups. Groups of muscle of similar location and function are further ensheathed in an enveloping fascia forming compartments. Fascial compartments typically enclose arterial, nervous, lymphatic, and venous supply to the muscles that compose the compartment. The fascia defines the extent of a compartment and enhances the extensor functions of the muscles, while at the same time it protects and supports the muscles. Fascia also constrain injuries, preventing the spread of bleeding, infection, and even tumor growth into adjacent compartments (Ombregt et al *ibid*, Brown *ibid*, Ward *ibid*.). The deep fascia, which contains longitudinally arranged compartments accommodating nerves, blood vessels, and lymphatics has been compared to the channel system in OM.

Fascial structures are slightly elastic membranes that allow organs and muscles to slide smoothly against each another. Since fascia is subject to Wolf's law, it may be said that fascial structure follows function. Therefore, when posture or gate patterns result in a chronic shorting of muscles, the fascia, which ideally should be the same length as the muscle, can become structurally shortened and further restrict normal movement and inhibits blood and fluid circulation. The nerves and stretch receptors found within fascial tissues become adhesed and therefore painful when stretched (Ward *ibid*). (Nerves need to be freely moveable).

Ligaments

Ligaments are bands or sheets of strong, fibrous, connective tissue. Their main function is to connect the articular ends of bones, forming support for the joints. They often brace cartilages and organs, and they provide support for the connecting muscles and fasciae of other structures.

Hinge joints such as the elbow or finger joints need collateral ligaments to support the relatively lax joint capsule (Bonica *ibid*). Ligaments can facilitate the release of stored elastic energy and both assist in and limit motion.

Ligaments get their tensile strength from collagen, which comprises 70-80% of the structure's dry weight. The ligament's elastin fibers, about 4% of its dry weight, give the ligament its elastic quality (Ombregt et al *ibid*).

Structurally, ligaments are similar to tendons; however, the collagenous fibers of ligaments are not arranged as regularly as those of tendons. Because ligaments are innervated richly by both mechanoreceptors and sensory receptors, they are a frequent source of pain. This is seen (and recognized) regularly in acute sprains. However, ligaments are also a common source of chronic pain in patients who may or may not have a history of acute trauma (Dorman *ibid*). The richness of innervation to and from ligaments should not be underestimated and probably contribute significantly to regulatory mechanisms of posture and muscular tone. Ligaments and joint receptors have considerable affects on the gamma loop which regulate muscle tone. This explains why muscles become painful and shortened when ligaments are damaged (Brown *ibid*).

Bone and Periosteum

The skeletal organ is a living tissue with multiple functions. Bones are dense, hard, and slightly elastic. There are 206 bones in the human skeleton. Bony tissue is composed of a frame of collagen and mineral salts, in which the osteocytes (bone cells) are distributed. The osteocytes of bone are maintained in a rigid matrix, which is calcified and reinforced by connective tissue fibers. There are two types of osteocytes: the osteoblasts and osteoclasts. Osteoblasts lay down new bone (calcified, reinforced connective tissue); osteoclasts cleanup old bone and may be directed by piezo-electric factors.[24] The spongy, cancellous tissue is surrounded by compact osseous tissue. This spongy tissue is permeated by many blood vessels and nerves and is enclosed in membranous periosteum. The composition of the osseous substance changes from birth to old age, and the ratio of collagen to

---

23. It is interesting to note that most Tong-style (as well as other) points and lines are located within intermucular septa and therefore in close relationship to all the above structures.

24. An electric charge is often used to heal a non-union fracture by reproducing the normal piezo-electric charge of the bone which guides the collagen to fill the bridging gap. Calcium salts follow (Ressett, Mitchell, Norton et al 1978).

mineral salts also varies, with the mineral salts tending to predominate over time. In a child, the proportion of collagen is higher, so that bones do not break as frequently as in the adult. Bones are a viscoelastic material that is more resistant to rapid than slow deformation. Bones are also more resistant to compression than to traction (Bogduk and Twomey *ibid*, Ombregt et al *ibid*, Barral and Croibier 1999).

Bone grows well only when subjected to normal mechanical stress. When these stresses occur outside their normal axis and are repeatedly poorly damped, the spans and osteons are deformed, leading to deformation. Increasing the force of compression on a bone leads to hypertrophy while, when normal stress is decreased (such as when one is confined to bed), osteoporosis and fragile tissue develops. Fractures may be caused by compression, traction, torsion, flexion, and fatigue (Barral and Croibier *ibid*).

PERIOSTEUM. The periosteum is a fibrous vascular membrane covering the bones, except at their extremities. It consists of an outer layer of collagenous tissue containing a few fat cells and an inner layer of fine elastic fibers. The periosteum is permeated with the nerves and blood vessels that innervate and nourish the underlying bone. The membrane is thick and markedly vascular over young bones, but thinner and less vascular in later life. Bones that lose periosteum through injury or disease usually scale or die. Its external fibrous layer joins the fibers of inserting tendons, muscles, fasciae, and ligaments (Bogduk and Twomey *ibid*, Ombregt et al *ibid*, Barral and Croibier *ibid*).

The Spine

Normally the spine is composed of seven cervical, twelve thoracic, five lumbar and five fused sacral vertebrae. The spinal column has four anatomical curves: the lumbar and cervical lordosis, which have a forward convexity, and the structures adjoining either one, the thoracic and sacrococcygeal areas, which are kyphotic with a backward convexity. Normal spinal curvatures develop through embryology and into adulthood. In the uterus, in order to conform to the uterine walls, the spine is convex posteriorly in its entirety. Hence, all posterior convexities are called primary curves. When a baby turns onto his abdomen and begins to look up, the cervical lordotic curve develops. Lumbar lordosis develops into adulthood, probably beginning when the baby begins to crawl on all four limbs. The lordotic lumbar and cervical curves with their posterior concavity are called secondary curves (Mitchell *ibid*).

Stability, as well as posture, is maintained mainly by ligamentous structures, muscles, and their fasciae. In humans, the forces of weightbearing at the spinal vertebrae increase progressively from the cervical to the lumbar spine, therefore the size of the vertebrae and discs increases. The curvatures of the spine provided by the discs and other structures allow for regional weightbearing capabilities by preloading tension components of the spine.

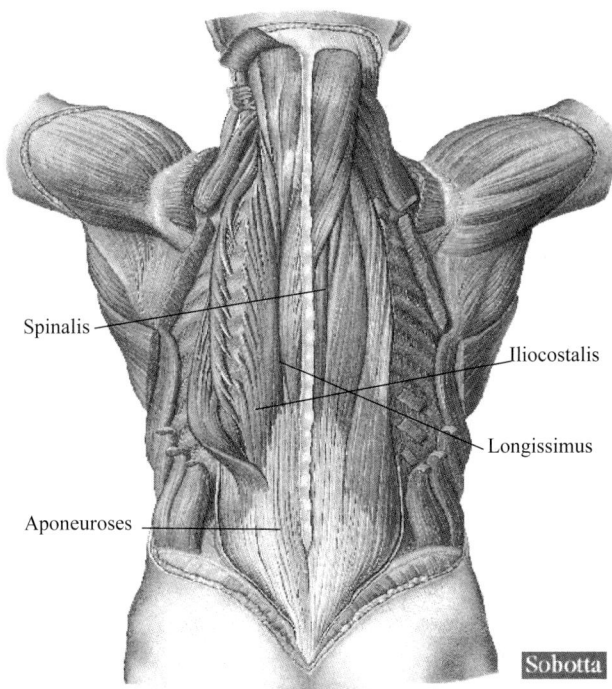

Figure 3-8: Posterior muscles.

Pain in the spine may arise from all structures containing free nerve endings, such as muscles, fasciae, ligaments (including the posterior longitudinal ligament and the anterior longintudinal ligament), annulus fibrosus, the periosteum of vertebral bodies, posterior arches, facets, dura mater, blood vessels, and spinal cord (Hrisch et al 1964). Pain often arises from sacroiliac structures, as well.

Ligaments of the Spine

Ligaments provide stability to the entire spine and are important in proprioception.

The Anterior and Posterior Longitudinal Ligaments

The anterior and posterior longitudinal ligaments secure the vertebral bodies to one another and provide protection for the disc and cord. They are both *extrinsically* and *intrinsically* innervated (Willard *ibid*).

ANTERIOR LONGITUDINAL LIGAMENT (ALL). The anterior longitudinal ligament is a broad, strong band of fibers that runs from the axis of the cervical vertebra to the sacrum. The ligament is narrower in the cervical region and widens inferiorly, the greatest dimension and strength being in the lumbar spine. The ligament is made up of dense longitudinal fibers that are tightly adherent to the discs and to the margins of the vertebral bodies (Bogduk and Twomey *ibid*).

POSTERIOR LONGITUDINAL LIGAMENT (PLL). The posterior longitudinal ligament also runs along the posterior surfaces of the vertebral bodies, from the axis of the neck to the sacrum. Unlike the ALL, the PLL is relatively narrower in the lumbar spine than in the rest of the spine. This unfortunate arrangement is one possible reason that disc lesions in the lumbar spine are more common than in any other region (Cyriax *ibid*). The longitudinal fibers of the PLL are denser and more compact than those of the ALL (Bogduk and Twomey *ibid*).

Ligaments of the Posterior Arch

The ligaments of the posterior vertebral arches are important for stability and provide elastic energy during movements.

INTERSPINOUS AND INTERTRANSVERSE LIGAMENTS. The interspinous ligaments are thin and membranous in composition, binding adjacent spinous processes. The intertransverse ligaments connect adjacent transverse processes. They are contiguous with the deep muscles of the back, especially in the thoracic spine (Bogduk and Twomey *ibid*). Tenderness of the interspinous ligaments is a good indicator of a dysfunctional vertebral level.

SUPRASPINOUS LIGAMENTS. The supraspinous ligaments connect the apices of the vertebral spinous processes, providing stability and acting as a counterforce to flexion of the spine, as well as assisting in the restoration of posture from the flexed to the erect posture (by releasing elastic energy/ springing). The supraspinous ligament becomes progressively less organized and, in some individuals, may not extend inferiorly to L4 (Bogduk and Twomey *ibid*).

The interspinous and supraspinous ligaments act as force transducers, translating the tension of the thoracolumbar fascia to the lumbar vertebra (Willard *ibid*).

LIGAMENTA FLAVA. The ligamenta flava (or yellow ligament) is more elastic than other ligaments in the spine, allowing separation of the lamina during flexion. They connect adjacent laminae of the vertebral bodies, and they function to restore the spinal column to a neutral position. The ligamenta flava are thickest and strongest in the lumbar spine (Bogduk and Twomey *ibid*).

Muscles of the Spine

Muscle actions are always coupled with those of other muscles and fascia to distribute loads, increase stability, perform concentric and eccentric functions (as well as agonist/antagonist functions), and for the storage of energy.

Flexor and Extensor Muscles of the Spine

Functionally, muscles affecting the spine can be divided into two major groups, the flexors and the extensors. However, flexion extension and stability of the spine and pelvis are dependent also on other associated muscles and their fascia,

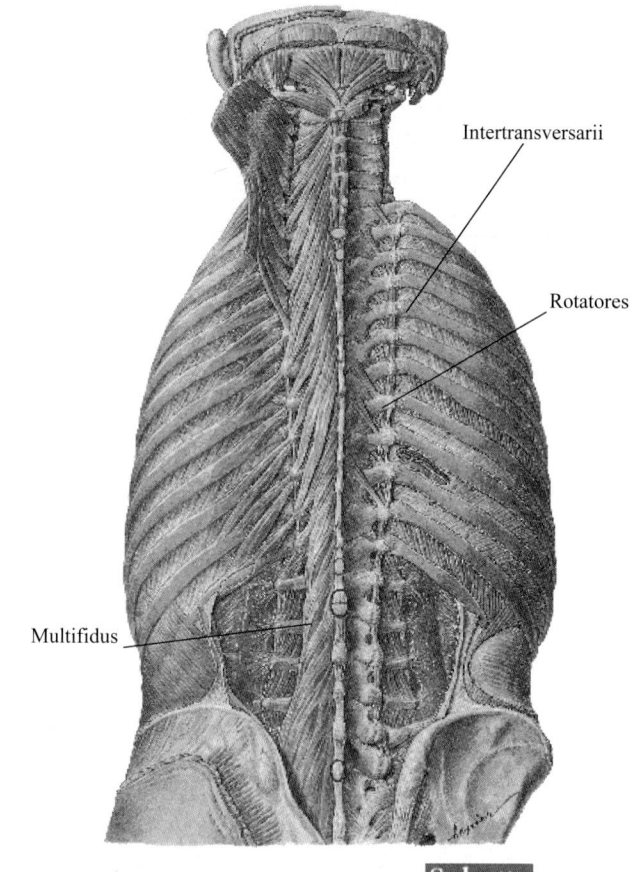

Figure 3-9: Deep muscles of the spine.

such as the abdominals, glutei, hamstrings, and latissimus dorsi.

Posterior Muscles

The posterior muscles affecting the spine are known collectively as the *extensors*. The extensors stretch from the head, shoulder, and trunk down to the sacrum and pelvis. The extensor muscles occupy the broad gutters posterior to the vertebral bodies and transverse processes (TrPr's) on each side of the spine. These can be divided into three groups, from the most medial to lateral (Bogduk Twomey *ibid*).

Superficial Group

ERECTOR SPINAE. The erector spinae is the most superficial group. It arises from the iliac crest and sacrum through a strong aponeuroses (a flat fibrous sheet of connective tissue).

The erector spinae are composed of three columns (Figure 3-8). *Spinalis* and *semispinalis* are the most medial. *Longissimus thoracis* and *capiti* are lateral to spinalis and semispinalis. The *iliocostalis* is the most lateral. The iliocostalis and longissimus arise from the ilial crest and the thoracolumbar fascia, but with the exception of a few medial fibers from the longissimus, they do not attach to the lumbar vertebrae.

The sacral connection of the erector spinae can pull the sacrum forward, inducing nutation in the SI joints and tensing ligaments such as the interosseous and sacrotuberous (Vleeming et al 1995).

THORACOLUMBAR FASCIA. The thoracolumbar fascia envelops the entire erector spinae in the lumbar spine. This strong fascia is connected anteriorly to the transverse processes and is continuous with the abdominal fascia, thereby forming a tube around the spine. When the erector spinae broaden during extension, the thoracolumbar fascia tightens, and with contributions from the latissimus dorsi, multifidus, gluteus maximus, and biceps femoris, the spine is extended (Vleeming et al *ibid*).

Deep Muscle Group.

TRANSVEROSPINALIS. The transverospinalis is the deep muscle group lying deeper than the erector spinae and running along most of the spine. This deep group includes the *rotatores, intertransversarii* and *multifidus* (Figure 3-9). These extensive muscles cross each other in different layers to construct a system of *supporting trusses*. When weak or spasmed on one side of the spine a functional retroscoliosis can result. Various functions have been assigned to intrinsic muscles of the spine, on the assumption that they actually move vertebrae; however, the arrangement and position of the muscle bundles that make up this group seem to make it improbable that they have much to do in this regard (Isaacson 1980).

MULTIFIDI. The multifidi have significant attachments to the spinous process, interspinous ligaments, laminae, and articular capsules of the vertebrae. In the lumbar spine they attach to the medial, intermediate and lateral sacral crests, the sacropelvic surface of the ilium, and the thoracolumbar fascia.

The connection to the sacroiliac joints and ligaments integrates the multifidus into the ligamentous support system of the sacroiliac joints (Willard 1995). Bogduk and Twomey (*ibid*) noted that, out of the dorsal muscles, only the multifidus could contribute significantly to the extension of the lumbar spine. The thoracolumbar fascia and other contributing muscles also aid in extension. Many of the deep dorsal muscles function instead as stabilizers and proprioceptive sensory receptors, that facilitate the coordinated activity of the vertebral complex. Thus (Chaitow *ibid*) the vertebral column and the body must be viewed as a functional unit and not as a collection of parts and organs that function independently of each other. This is a concept which, while obvious, is often neglected in practice.

The Anterior Muscles

The anterior muscles, or flexors, are important for spinal function and stability. The anterior prevertebral musculature lies in close proximity to the vertebrae and is disadvantaged mechanically, especially in the lumbar and thoracic spines. Flexion, therefore, must be assisted by other muscles.

FLEXOR MUSCLES. In the lumbar spine, the *psoas* (which functions more as a trunk flexor) and the *abdominal* muscles function as the major flexors.

In the cervical spine, the *paravertebral* muscles of the neck function as primary flexors. The flexors of the cervical spine are the *longus cervicis, longus capitis* and the *scalenes*. The SCM and other muscles also assist with the flexion of the neck.[25]

In the cervical spine the longus colli and dorsal neck muscles are complementary and the longus colli counteracts the lordosis increment related to the weight of the head and to the contraction of the dorsal neck muscles. The longus coli and posterior cervical muscles form a sleeve that encloses and stabilizes the cervical spine in all positions of the head (Mayoux et al 1994).

STABILITY AND MUSCLE FUNCTION/DYSFUNCTION. Myofascial structures are essential for load transfer, and, according to Vleeming, force closure of the ilia on the sacrum. This contributes to the general stability of the spine and the lumbosacral regions. Forces between the spine and legs are transferred through the thoracolumbar fascia, both ipsilaterally and contralaterally. Electromyographic studies during isokinetic lifting and trunk bending movements demonstrate that the *erector spinae, latissimus dorsi, abdominal* and *gluteus maximus* muscles act in parallel and simultaneously, showing that these constitute a complex system. The muscular functions of the *latissimus dorsi, contralateral gluteus* and *hamstrings* are coupled as well. Together, the above muscles, the *transverse* and *internal oblique abdominal* muscles, as well as *psoas major*, contribute to transferring forces as well as contribute to stability of the SI joints, by "force closure" (Vleeming, Stoechart and Snijers 1994).

Bergmark (1989) and Richardson et al (1999) have categorized muscles as having *local* (central) or *global* (guy wires) functions.

- *Local central* muscles are the intertrasversarii, interspinales, multifidi, transversus abdominis, the posterior portion of the internal oblique, the medial fibers of quadratus lumborum, and the central portion of the erector spinae.
- *Global "guy wire"* muscles are the anterior portion of the internal obliques, external obliques, and rectus abdominis, the lateral fibres of the quadratus lumborum and the more lateral portions of the erector spinae.

Global/guy wire muscles are considered to function like ropes supporting a ship's mast. The local/central muscles are deep lying ones affecting the elements that attach to the spine. Global/guy wire muscles are seen as having the ability to control the spine's resistance to bending. They can influ-

---

25. The psoas and scalenes are often dysfunctionally coupled.

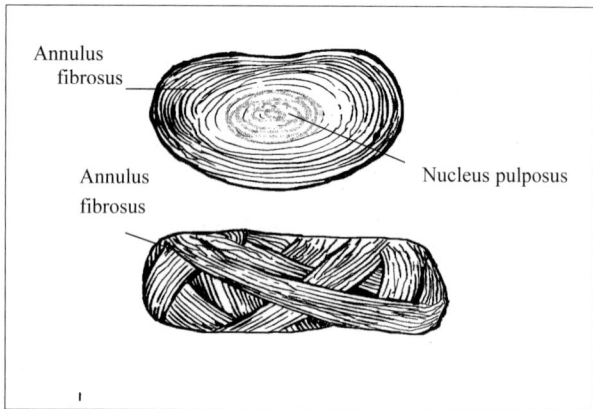

Figure 3-10: Intervertebral disc.

ence spinal balancing and alignment, and can accommodate to the forces imposed on the spine (Chaitow *ibid*).

The Anterior Vertebral Column

The anterior vertebral column is composed of the vertebral bodies and discs. From a reductionist viewpoint, the anterior column is the major resilient, weight-bearing, and shock-absorbing structure of the motion segment (a motion segment is two adjacent vertebrae).

Intervertebral Disc

The intervertebral disc, lying in the center of the anterior spinal column, is one of the larger avascular structures in the body. It is, therefore, liable to develop chronicity once injured, possibly making this pathoanatomically the weakest part of the motion segment (Bonica *ibid*). The disc is radiotranslucent and therefore inadequately evaluated by x-ray. The discs make up about 1/4 of the length of the entire spine and are roughly 1/5 to 1/3 as thick as the neighboring vertebral body. In the lumbar spine the discs encompass about 30% of the length of the column, in comparison to 20-25% in the thoracic and cervical spine. With weight bearing, the discs shrink and dehydrate, and, at night, they usually rehydrate and regain their thickness (Bogduk and Twomey *ibid*).

In the cervical spine, the discs are relatively thicker than in the thoracic spine, broader posteriorly and higher anteriorly. This is perhaps to accommodate the excessive strains on the disc from extensive cervical movements. In the thoracic spine, the discs are relatively thin, probably due to the stability provided by the rib cage. In the lumbar spine, the discs are quite large, as they bear considerable strain, even though rotation and sidebending is restricted by the bony and articular arrangements (Bogduk and Twomey *ibid*). Despite this lumbar architecture and minimal rotational capability the lumbar disc is commonly injured.

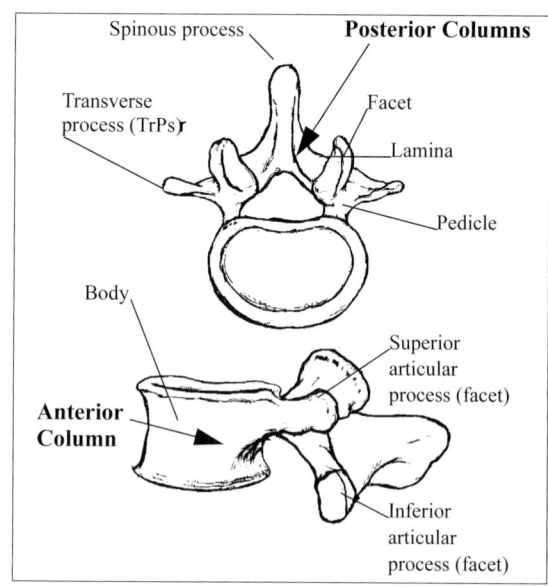

Figure 3-11: Lumbar vertebra.

Nourishment of Discs

In adults, the disc receives virtually all of its nutrition by diffusion through the vertebral end-plates and peripheral vessels. This makes motion of the vertebral column critical for maintaining disc health (Brown *ibid*). Smoking inhibits nutrition to the disc and may explain why patients who smoke often develop chronicity (Holm and Nachemson 1988; Battié et al 1991).

Disc Anatomy

The discs are made of an external capsule of fibrocartilage, the *annulus fibrosus*, and a soft *nucleus pulposus* in the center (Figure 3-10).

Annulus Fibrosus

The annulus fibrosus is made up of twenty concentric collar-like rings (lamellae) of fibers that crisscross each other to increase their strength and accommodate the torsional movements of the spine. The thickness of each lamellae increases from the nucleus outward (Farfan 1973). Its dry collagen mass is 60%-70% (Ombregt et al *ibid*). Because of its fiber arrangement, the annulus has a low tolerance of injury due to shearing, translation, and displacement forces (Kopell and Thompson 1976). (The annulus fibers contribute to torque resistance, and, when deferentially removed, (at appropriate angles), rotation increases by 2° [Krismer, Haid, Rabal 1996]).

Traditionally, the discs were not thought to contain nerves. However, the peripheral posterior aspect of the annulus fibrosus is innervated by nerve fibers from the sinuvertebral nerve. The lateral aspect of the annulus fibrosus is innervated peripherally by the anterior rami and gray rami

The Spine

Table 3-7: Movement Characteristics

MOVEMENT	CHARACTERISTICS
FLEXION	Posterior aspect of the spine becomes increasingly convex. Spaces between vertebrae increase posteriorly. Spaces at the anterior aspect decrease. Superior vertebra glides forward on adjoining inferior. Nucleus pulposus of the disc shifts backward.
EXTENSION	Convexity increases anteriorly. Superior vertebra glides backward in relation to inferior. Nucleus pulposus shifts forward
SIDEBENDING	*Si*debending always occurs with coupled rotation. "Coupling" occurs in same or opposite direction. Nucleus pulposus shifts toward convexity.

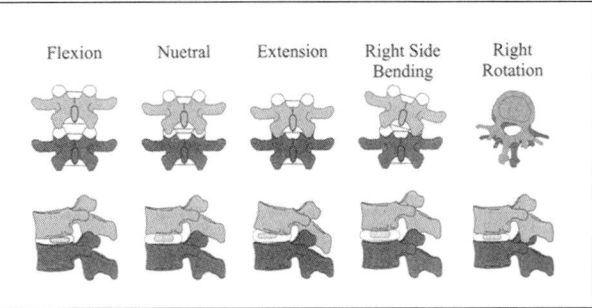

Figure 3-12: Vertebral and disc motions (From Gimmatteo and Gimmatteo Integrative Manual Therapy for Biomechanics Application of Muscle Energy and "Beyond" Technique Vol III, North Atlantic Books 2003. Drawn by T Gimmatteo).

communicantes. Chronic inflammation can cause an increase in the number of these pain fibers (Bogduk, Tynan and Wilson 1981; Bogduk, Windsor and Inglis 1988).

Nucleus Pulposus

The nucleus is approximately 85% water. Its metabolism is anaerobic, with an oxygen concentration of as little as 5%-10% of that at the surface (Holm 1981). The dry mass of collagen is 10%-20% (Ombregt et al *ibid*). The pressure within the nucleus pulposus keeps the annulus fibers taut and prevents the disc space from collapsing, and therefore has the highest proteoglycan content in the body (Brown *ibid*). This allows for rotary, translatory, and rocking movements between adjacent vertebrae. With aging, the disc becomes less elastic and the nucleus dries up, reducing the likelihood of the nucleus to rupture (Cyriax *ibid*).

The Posterior Column

The posterior column of a vertebra is united by a thick pedicle to the vertebral body. The column/arch is created by the connection of the *spinous process*, *laminae*, and *transverse processes* (TrPrs).

The Facet Joint (Zygoapophyseal Joints)

Connecting two adjacent vertebrae are facets (zygoapophyseal joint or articular processes) that arise from the vertebral pedicle. The triangular posterior vertebral column is believed to have minimal weightbearing function. Adams and Hutton noted that about 20% of the entire load of a motion segment is taken up by the facet joints (Brown *ibid*), although the tensegrity model postulates that loads are distributed throughout. By their architectural design, the facets govern motion available in a vertebral segment, and they limit the mechanical range of the discs. In "normal" cadaverous spines, when the lumbar facet joints are removed, rotation increases by 2°(Krismer, Haid and Rabl 1996).[26]

The role of the facet joints in pain has been controversial. For example, osteopathic and chiropractic schools emphasize the facet's essential contribution to vertebral motions. When a dysfunction interferes with their opening or closing, normal motion may be altered, leading to mechanical strains and pain. Cyriax, on the other hand, challenged this because he could not devise a system of examination to distinguish a "syndrome," and, secondly, because he claimed that two parallel surfaces cannot become blocked. Lately Bogduk (*ibid*) has shown the facets to be a common source of pain.

Facet Anatomy and Innervation

The facets are a true synovial joint and have a capsule that is well innervated from the dorsal rami. There is diffuse overlapping innervation to the lumbar facets from three root levels. This may explain part of the controversy, as it leads to poor localization and highly variable pain (Brown *ibid*).

Biomechanics of the Spinal Joints

Movement in the spine is produced by the coordinated action of nerves, muscles, and levers. Elastic energy stored in the fascia and ligaments provides momentum (spring). Prime mover muscles (agonists) initiate and carry out movement, whereas antagonist muscles often control and modify it (Lindh 1980). Spinal movements are always a combination of the actions of several segments, and sidebending is always coupled with rotation and translation. During active gait, the spine responds mostly passively to the primary propellants, the lower extremity, and the pelvic system (the body almost falls forward; Dorman *ibid*).

The spinal column is comprised of a series of vertebrae and joints that are capable of different motions at various levels. These are mainly determined by the facets and their

---

26. When both the facet and the appropriate annular fibers are removed, rotation increases by 7.6°.

angulation. Vertebral movements are described in three basic ways:

- The relationship of a superior vertebra to the corresponding inferior vertebra.
  For example, in flexion, the superior vertebra rotates and glides forward in relation to its inferior vertebra.
- The direction of movement of the anterior aspect of a vertebra.
  For example, in rotation to the right, the anterior aspect rotates right and the posterior aspect (spinous process) moves to the left.
- Rotation around an axis, or translation (gliding) along an axis.
  This kind of description specifies the horizontal (X), vertical (Y), or anteroposterior (Z) axes, around which the vertebral body moves. For example, in flexion, the superior vertebra rotates around a horizontal (X) axis and translates forward in relation to the lower vertebra, along the anteroposterior (Z) axis (Panjabi and White *ibid*; Figure 3-12).

For more information see chapter 9.

The Pelvic Girdle

The pelvis is a three-part bony ring with two sacroiliac (SI) joints posteriorly and the pubic symphysis anteriorly. The role of the sacroiliac joint in musculoskeletal pain has been controversial. The older literature stated that the SI joints are functionally fused and that, therefore, no dysfunction could occur.[27] It is now well-established that the SI joints are true synovial (diarthrodial) joints with an articular capsule, joint space, and cartilage in which movement occurs. A controlled study of low back pain has shown that 30% of patients had pain related to the SI joints. In these patients, tears of the ventral capsule were documented (Schwarzer, Aprill and Bogduk 1995).

The pelvis and sacroiliac joints are key pivots in which there is interaction between the downward gravitational force of the trunk and the upward reaction forces from the ground. The pelvis must withstand great forces in various directions. Pelvic motions are essential for increasing the functional rotation of the spine. The joints are rich in mechanoreceptors, which probably function as proprioceptors amidst these forces.

Several rotational axes in the SI joint (Figure 3-32) and translation or gliding motions have been described in the literature (Kapandji 1974; Colachis et al 1963; Egund 1978; Lavignolle et al 1983; Vleeming et al 1992). In the osteopathic literature, specific motions and dysfunctions of the sacroiliac joints are described as well as techniques to restore normal position and function (Greenman 1989).

---

27. This error was probably due to early anatomical studies that were done on very old subjects with pathological joints.

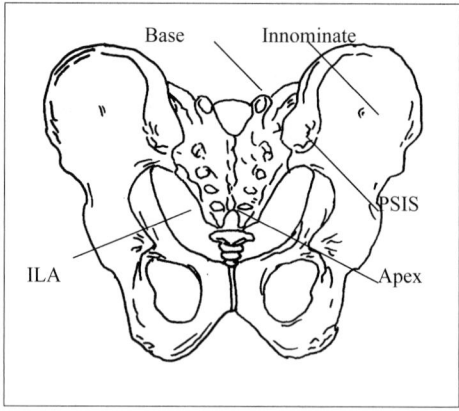

Figure 3-13: Sacrum and innominates.

No primary muscle movers are responsible for SI motions. The two muscles that contribute to sacral movement are the piriformis—the only muscle that crosses the sacrum—and the aponeurosis of the erector spinae, which attach to the posterior surface of the sacrum. Occasionally, a few fibers of the gluteus maximus also cross the joint (Willard *ibid*). The abdominal, latissimus dorsi (through the thoracolumbar fascia), perineum, quadratus lumborum, iliopsoas, gluteus maximus, gluteus medius, pelvic diaphragm and other lower extremity muscles all contribute indirectly to sacroiliac motions via their connections to the pelvis.

Vleeming describes the SI joints as compression joints that rely for stability on forces adducting the ilia onto the sacrum. He calls this *force closure*. The sacrum has also been described by Grant as being suspended in the ilia by the interosseous, posterior SI, and the sacrotuberous and spinous ligaments, and therefore being vulnerable to shear. The stability of the joint is achieved primarily by these ligaments. Vleeming also has evidence that self-bracing against shear is provided by the interaction of the rough surfaces of the joint with ligaments, muscles, and fascial forces on the joint. It has been suggested that in the sitting position, the force closure contributed by the muscles is reduced (Snijders, Vleeming and Stoeckart 1992). This may lead to increased instability in the seated patient and may explain the increased pain often seen after prolonged sitting (a disc is a common cause as well).

Depending on posture, several muscles can either increase the loads on the sacrum or contribute to self-bracing. These are the gluteus maximus, erector spinae, quadratus lumborum, abdominal (oblique and rectus), latissimus dorsi, and psoas muscles. The gluteus maximus and piriformis muscles are thought to increase friction forces and self-bracing. Weakness of the above muscles is thought to cause mechanical pelvic dysfunction (Snijders, Vleeming and Stoeckart *ibid*).

According to Snijders, Vleeming and Stoeckart (1992) the biceps femoris, piriformis, coccygeus and gluteus maximus muscles and the deep layer of the lumbodorsal fascia can influence the ligamental tension that regulates SI joint stability. The lumbodorsal caudad fascial fibers and latissimus dorsi extend to the contralateral side, and function synergistically with the contralateral gluteus maximus muscle. The gluteus maximus can compress the SI joints directly and also indirectly by its firm connections with the sacrotuberous ligament (Vleeming et al 1997).

In forward bending, for example, the transverse and oblique abdominal muscles, and the gluteus maximus muscles in particular, are important in providing stability by increasing force closure of the ilia onto the sacrum. Tightness of the biceps femoris or gluteus maximus will restrict sacral flexion (nutation) whereas weakness will allow increased flexion of the sacrum (Vleeming 1989). This can increase and add to the gravitational forces from the upper body pushing down on the sacral base (the Z-axis or sagital plane) when subject is standing. The erector spinae can pull the sacrum forward, inducing nutation in the SI joint and tensing ligaments such as the interosseous, sacrotuberous, and sacrospinal (Vleeming et al *ibid*).

Tightness or weakness of the piriformis can effect either sacral torsional, or sidebending movements and will influence the tone of the sacrospinous ligament, as they share a common attachment at the anterior sacrum. Both movement and sacrospinous ligament tone are necessary in normal mechanics and stability.

Structural and functional integrity are important physiologically for normal pelvic and spinal function. This integrity is essential for the storage of elastic energy. Dysfunction of this integrity increases oxygen consumption during normal walking. Correcting the dysfunction and the accompanying ligamentous laxity remedies this excess oxygen consumption (Dorman 1995).

Even in people who have "normal" structure and functional integrity, the two SI joints are never symmetrical. However, with joint dysfunction or pathology, one usually can detect loss of motion and functional asymmetry. The pelvis is also important in the osteopathic respiratory and circulatory models because of the relationship of the pelvis to the urogenital diaphragm, and in the osteopathic craniosacral system (Kuchera and Kuchera *ibid*).

The sacrum is most frequently formed by five (though it can be two to six) fused vertebrae and ossified intervertebral discs in a triangular shape. Situated with its base (the wider aspect) superior, its first vertebra has a prominent, oval upper surface with a significant forward slope. Attached to it is a thick disc that unites the sacrum to L5. The inclination of the superior surface of S1, results in L5's tendency to slide inferiorly and anteriorly (Bogduk and Twomey *ibid*), often resulting in spondylolysis.

The sacrum is suspended between the ilia (Figure 3-14), with its base (superior aspect) anterior to its apex (the inferior end), like the platform of a suspension bridge. There-

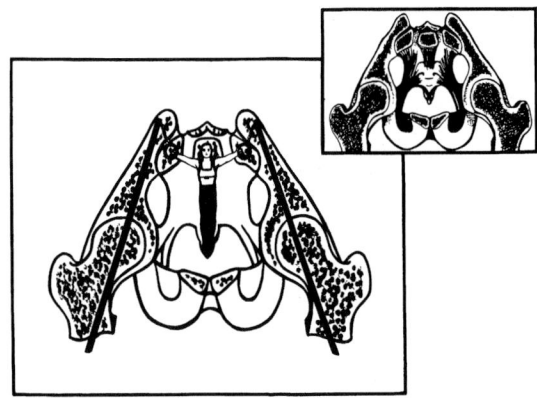

Figure 3-14: Suspended sacrum (courtesy of Dorman and Ravin 1991).

fore, the narrow apex is positioned posteroinferiorly. The apex articulates with the coccyx. The two bony edges inferior and lateral to the apex, just lateral and inferior to the fifth vertebra and sacral cornu, are the sacrum's *inferior lateral angles* (ILA). The ILAs are important landmarks for sacral function and position assessment. Developmentally, the ILAs are the transverse processes of S5 (Mitchell *ibid*). The sacrum is viewed as part of the spinal vertebral (trunk) axis in the osteopathic literature (Figure 3-13).

The Innominates

The innominates (hip bones) are each formed of the fused ilium, ischium, and pubis. In the osteopathic literature they are viewed functionally as part of the lower extremities. The femur is connected to the innominate anteriorly via the hip joint. It is also anterior to the innominate's axis of rotation, believed to be at S2. Therefore, viewed from the side, any rotation at the innominate influences the apparent leg length (Greenman *ibid*).

The Symphysis Pubis

The symphysis pubis is an amphiarthrosis[28] with strong superior and inferior ligaments and a thinner posterior ligament. Movement of the pubis occurs during the normal walking cycle. This movement has been described as the rotation of one pubic bone on the other around a transverse axis. Vertical movement (shear) has been described by some writers as abnormal for the symphysis pubis during walking (Kapandji 1978); however, others consider this motion normal, especially during prolonged standing on one leg. The

---

28. An intermediate joint between diarthrosis and synarthrosis in which the articular bony surfaces are connected by an elastic cartilaginous substance.

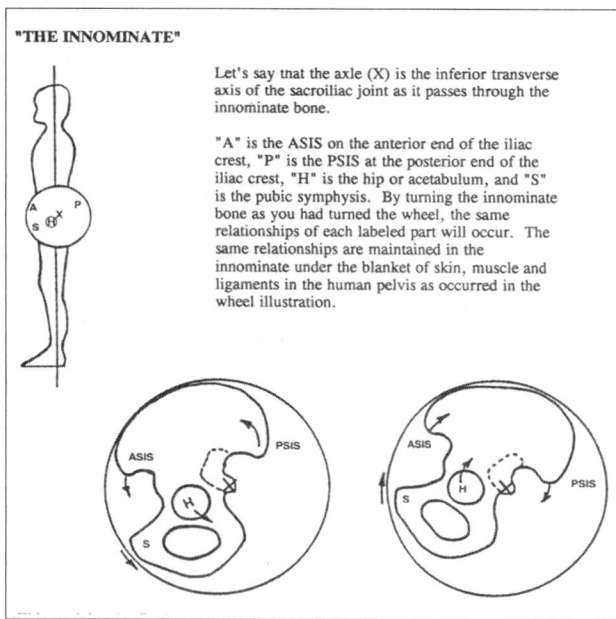

Figure 3-15: Innominate rotations (From Kuchera WA and Kuchera ML, Osteopathic Principles in Practice, KCOM press 1993, with permission).

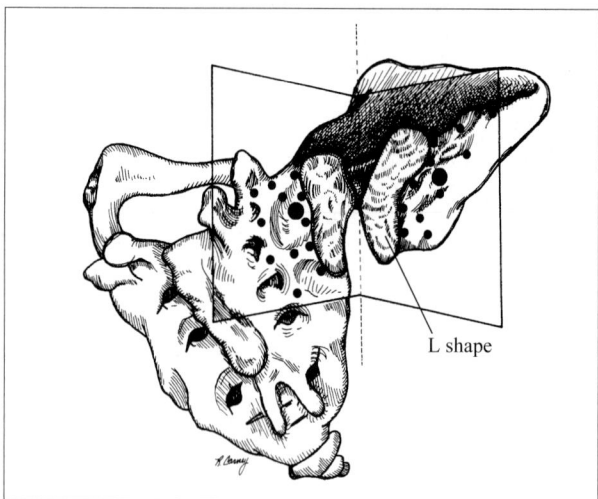

Figure 3-16: L-shaped SI joint surface (courtesy of Dorman and Ravin 1991).

joint realignes when weight is put on the other leg (Dihlmann 1980; Mitchell *ibid*).

Dysfunction and laxity of the symphysis pubis is common during pregnancy under the influence of the hormone relaxin. It has been suggested that use of a sacral belt in the last months of pregnancy prevents such dysfunctions (Vleeming 1994). The abdominal and leg adductor muscles can influence pubic joint function and can maintain dysfunctions that are often due to abnormal nervous input from dysfunction at T11-L2 (Mitchell *ibid*).

The Sacroiliac Joint

The SI joint is derived embryologically from a number of segments. An L-shaped joint (Figure 3-16), its upper and lower limbs have different orientations. The upper is broader posteriorly and the lower broader anteriorly. With its irregular articular surfaces, the joint has a convex/concave relationship between the sacrum and the ilia. It is relatively flat compared to other, more stable joints. This bony configuration is thought to provide some stability as the sacrum wedges in the ilia, and as it leads to an interlocking (wedging in) at S2 (Greenman *ibid*). Because of this structure, the sacrum has been described as the keystone of an arch. However, since its base is anterior to the lumbar spine, and certainly, when one's weight is on one foot as in walking, the SI joints cannot function as a true architectural keystone, which is stable by compression alone. The sacrum is most likely held stable by compression from bones and from the tension of soft tissues. (For this reason, it has been compared to the platform of a suspension bridge.) Additional forces are needed to achieve what a come-along (tie-beam) does. This is accomplished by tension elements and possibly force closure from soft tissues on the ilia and from ligaments that cross the joint. According to Greenman, in about 10-15% of all individuals, the opposing joint surfaces are quite flat, and the function of bony compression is lacking. This leaves the soft tissues completely responsible for joint stability, leaving the joint vulnerable to shear forces.

Ligaments

Body weight is thought to be transmitted from the sacrum to the innominates chiefly by the sacroiliac ligaments, which are thick and strong posteriorly and thinner anteriorly. (Through tensegrity, other tension and compression elements are involved, as well.) The sacrum is suspended from the iliac portion of the innominate by these ligaments (Dorman *ibid*).

ILIOLUMBAR LIGAMENTS. The iliolumbar ligaments are attached to the anterior surface of the ilia and to the transverse processes of the lower lumbar vertebrae. The lower fibers extend anteriorly and join the anterior SI ligaments. Superiorly, they join the transverse processes of L4 and L5. This superior band passes from the transverse processes of L5 to the posterior surface of the medial part of the iliac crest, where the quadratus lumborum also originates in part (Dorman *ibid*). The iliolumbar ligaments were thought to be formed during adolescence from the quadratus lumborum muscle; however, newer information shows the ligament to be present in infants as well (Willard *ibid*). The iliolumbar and the lumbodorsal fascia are important restraining and stabilizing structures in all lumbosacral movements. The iliolumbar ligaments function as guy wires and give lateral stability to the lumbosacral column.

Sprain of the iliolumbar ligament is common, often due to torsional injuries or an unleveled sacral base. It is often the first ligament to cause back pain, as it may be affected by both spinal and innominate sprains (Kuchera and Kuchera *ibid*). The quadratus lumborum is frequently involved as well. Pain from the iliolumbar ligaments is felt in L1-4 sclerotomes (Dorman *ibid*; Figure 3-17).

LUMBOSACRAL LIGAMENTS. The lumbosacral ligaments are a common cause of low back pain in the midline. Pain (posain) from the lumbosacral and interspinous ligaments is provoked by prolonged standing, sitting, or lying. Often the pain spreads symmetrically across the low back and is aggravated by prolonged sitting and flexion to full range. Rotation often is normal. At times extension is painful, as fibers may be squeezed between the spines (Dorman *ibid*; Figure 3-17).

POSTERIOR (DORSAL) SACROILIAC (SI) LIGAMENTS. These ligaments can be divided into three layers (Kapandji *ibid*; Dorman *ibid*):

The *upper layer* and most posterior ligaments span the sacral crest vertically and attach to the ilium. The superficial long ligament fibers are more vertical and blend with the sacrotuberous ligament, which is continuous with the tendon of the long head of the biceps femoris.

The *intermediate layer* overlies most of the posterior aspect of the SI joints and runs from the posterior arches of the sacrum to the medial side of the ilium.

The *deep layer* of interosseous ligaments attaches laterally to the medial aspect of the PSIS and to the anterior foramina of S1 and S2. They are strong and form the principal union between the two bones (Figure 3-17).

The *short fibers* of the posterior SI ligaments are oriented transversely and are intertwined. Therefore, when pulled upon, they tighten (like a rope), approximating the two ilia. They form the major support for the sacrum. These ligaments are an important part of the force closure mechanism of the ilium on the sacrum. When gravitational forces from the trunk push on the sacrum, the dorsal SI ligaments pull the ilia closer to the sacrum.

SACROSPINOUS LIGAMENT. The sacrospinous ligament runs under the sacrotuberous ligament. It attaches medially by its broad base to the sacrotuberous ligament and to the anterior surface of the sacrum. Laterally it attaches to the spine of the ischium (Figure 3-17).

SACROTUBEROUS LIGAMENT. The sacrotuberous ligament is attached superiorly by a wide, flat base to the posterior, superior, and inferior iliac spines. Then the ligament runs inferiorly to the lower sacrum and is attached to the ischial tuberosity. This ligament is connected with the posterior SI ligaments at the PSIS. The lower fibers of the gluteus maximus are attached to the sacrotuberous ligament as well. Below, it is, in part, connected to the tendon of the biceps (hamstring) muscle, which directly affects its tension (Vleeming *ibid*), (Figure 3-17).

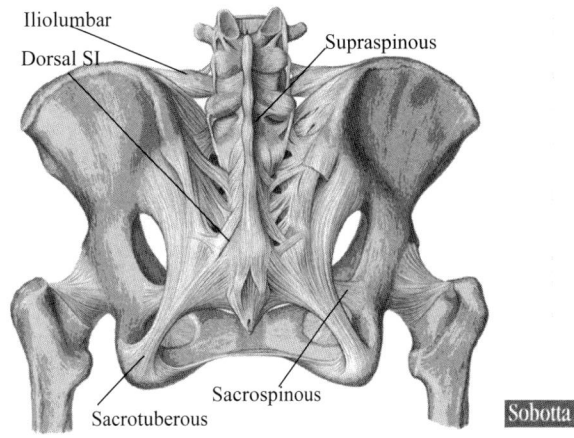

Figure 3-17: Lumbopelvic ligaments.

The sacrotuberous and sacrospinous ligaments function to oppose upward rotation of the sacral apex (bottom of sacrum) under the downward force of the spine on the anteriorly positioned sacral base (top of the sacrum; Figure 3-13).

Motion In The Pelvis

Motions of the pelvic ring have been studied, and there is much disagreement among researchers. Analysis of walking shows that counter-rotations of the two innominates is an important part of normal walking. This movement can occur only if the pubic symphysis can rotate around a transverse axis. The sacrum rotates toward, and sidebends away from, the side on which the innominate rotates posteriorly. This type of movement is called *anterior torsion* (Mitchell 1948; Figure 3-18). Other movements occur as well. Any restriction in these motions renders the walking cycle abnormal. Restrictions can thus affect function and lead to pain in the back and legs. Dorman hypothesizes that during walking, the SI joint must lock and unlock on alternating sides, allowing for maximal efficiency of the pelvic "differential-like mechanism."

When the patient is standing on the right leg, the left innominate is pushed posteriorly by the weight of the trunk, pushing the SI joint caudad (inferiorly) while the supporting

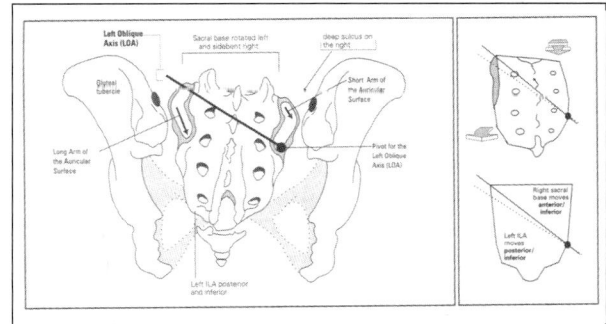

Figure 3-18: A left sacral torsion on a left oblique excess (courtesy of Mitchell *ibid*).

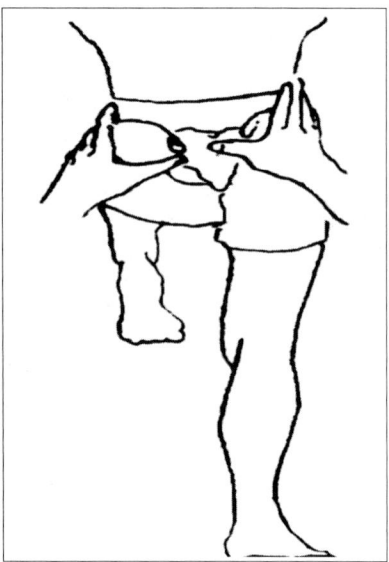

Figure 3-19: Gillet's Stork Test. In assessing SI joint mobility, normally the finger at the PSIS moves downward when the leg is flexed on the same side. Shown here as a negative test on the left side.

Table 3-8: Approximate Loads at L3 in a 70kg Individual

Activity	Approximate Load (kg/cm2)
Lying Supine	30
Sitting	100
Coughing; Jumping	110
Laughing; Bending Forward to 20%	120
Hyperextending Actively while Supine	150
Doing Sit-Ups	180
Lifting a 20kg load with Straight Back	210
Lifting a 20kg load with Back Forward Bent	340

leg pushes the hip superiorly. The hanging leg (left in this example) will pull and rotate the left innominate anteriorly. These motions are used to evaluate the SI joint with the Gillet's-Stork Test, (Figure 3-19), (Brown 1995).

Lumbar Spine

The usual lumbar spine has five vertebrae. The wide part of the vertebral body is situated anteriorly, and the dorsal arch is situated posteriorly. There is a disc between adjacent bodies. The vertebral bodies are thicker anteriorly and wider transversely. Together with the discs, which are also thicker anteriorly, they give the lumbar spine its lordotic curve. L5 is much thicker anteriorly, as is the disc at this level, accounting for the angular lumbosacral junction. In some people, L5 is fused with the sacrum; this is called *sacralization*. The nucleus pulposus in the lumbar spine is located centrally within the disc. This allows for rocker-like movement (Kapandji *ibid*).

The posterior arch, which is united with a thick pedicle to the vertebral body, is composed of a thick and broad spinous process and two transverse processes (TrPs). The arches of L1 through L3 originate from the juncture of the pedicles and laminae, and are horizontal. The TrPs of the lower two vertebrae arise from the pedicles and posterior portion of the body, and are inclined posteriorly (Bogduk *ibid*; Kapandji *ibid*).

The articular facets, in the upper lumbar region, are oriented in a vertical sagittal (vertical and anteroposterior) plane that permits flexion and extension but which resists sidebending when the spine is in a neutral position (the lumbar lordosis is maintained but is not excessive). However, a very small amount of rotation and sidebending is present throughout the lumbar spine and increases when there is slight flexion. Flexion/extension and rotation are greatest at L5-S1. Sidebending is greatest at L3-4 (White and Panjabi 1978). The orientation of the lumbar facets do not permit compression and are not designed for weight bearing (Figure 3-11), (Brown 1995).

The anterior portion of the functional units of the spine (vertebral bodies and the discs) are considered to be weight-bearing, shock-absorbing structures. The discs in the lumbar spine account for about 30% of the column length. Approximate pressure loads at L3 in a 70 kg individual have been measured (Nachemson and Elfstrom 1970) and are summarized in Table 3-8.

The posterior portion (posterior arch) of the functional units are triangular structures composed of two vertebral arches, two transverse processes, a central posterior spinous process, and paired articular facets. The posterior portion is believed to be non-weight-bearing; and the facets within them regulate motion available in the lower spine. Muscles and ligaments which attach to the transverse processes and spinous processes act as tension members and contribute to lumbar mobility and stability. Abnormal disc function, ligamentous weakening, and excessive lordosis may weaken the integrity of the lumbar spine and shift weight bearing to the posterior portions of the vertebral unit, which are not as suitable for carrying this load (Brown *ibid*).

Lumbar Spine Movement: Flexion

Flexion in the lumbar spine consists of the rotation, coupled with translation, of one vertebra on its adjoining inferior vertebra. Usually, it involves simultaneous movement of the

Table 3-9: Muscles of The Thoracic Spine

Function	Muscles
Flexion	Rectus abdominus, external and internal abdominal obliques (bilateral contraction)
Extension	Spinalis thoracis, iliocostalis thoracis (bilateral), semispinalis thoracis (bilateral), longissimus thoracis (bilateral), multifidus (bilateral), rotators (bilateral) and interspinales
Rotation and Sidebending	Iliocostalis (to same side), longissimus thoracis (to same side), internal abdominal oblique (to same side), semispinalis thoracis (to opposite side), multifidus (to opposite side), rotators (to opposite side), external abdominal obliques (to opposite side) and transverses abdominus (to opposite side)

lumbar spine and pelvis in the same plane. Each superior vertebra glides anteriorly, compressing the disc anteriorly. The posterior aspect of the disc is unloaded and therefore widens. During forward bending, the nucleus pulposus moves backward, and the axis of rotation is thought to move with it, and therefore called instantaneous axis of rotation (i.e., the axis of rotation is not fixed; Kapandji 1974).

The effects of flexion on forces exerted by the lumbar back muscles were studied by Macintosh, Bogduk and Pearcy (1993). In flexion, the lever arm length produced by the spine decreases slightly (because the spine is closer to the trunk). This results in up to an 18% decrease in the maximum extensor magnitude exerted across the lumbar spine. Compression loads are not significantly different from those generated in the upright subject. However, there are major changes in shear forces, in particular a reversal from a net anterior to a net posterior shear force at the L5/S1 segment. Flexion causes a substantial elongation of the back muscles, which results in a reduction of their maximum active tension. However, when the increase in passive tension is considered, it appears that the compression forces and tension exerted by the back muscles in full flexion are not significantly different from those produced in the upright posture (Basmajian and Nyberg 1993).

Flexion is limited by the arrangement of tissues: the ligamenta flava, the facet (zygoapophyseal) joint capsules, the interspinous ligaments and, except for the lower vertebrae, the supraspinous ligament. The annulus of the disc also limits forward flexion (Bogduk *ibid*).

During flexion, the erector spinae muscles elongate and help to decelerate forward flexion by eccentric contraction. At the end of flexion, the erector spinae muscles are inactive (based on EMG). Heavy lifting or unguarded movement with the spine flexed may strain structures stressed by flexion, or which help restore the body to the upright posture (the extensor muscles and related tissues). During heavy lifting, the pelvis often rotates first, with the ligaments of the lumbar spine bearing the brunt of the stress. At 45° (based on EMG), the muscles of the back become active (Bogduk 1980). The quadriceps femoris, iliotibial, and gluteal muscles assist in flexion and may be strained.

Cailleit (1981) has designated the movement during flexion the "Lumbo Pelvic Rhythm." Initially the lumbar portion flattens. As flexion continues, a gradual reversal of the lumbar curve occurs, most prominently at the lower portion of the spine. With back pain, guarding often does not allow for normal pelvic rhythm.

Extension

Extension is achieved through a combination of pelvic and extensor muscle shortening, and support through the thoracolumbar fascia and latissimus dorsi (Bogduk 1980). The pelvis rotates backward, and then the spine extends. The body of the superior vertebra rotates and translates posteriorly, compressing the posterior portion of the disc. The nucleus is pushed anteriorly. Extension is limited by the geometry of both tissue and bones of the vertebral arch, and by tension that develops in the soft tissues anteriorly (Kapandji *ibid*).

The sacrospinalis (erector spinae) muscle is ensheathed by the thick lumbar part of the thoracolumbar fascia, which is attached medially to the lumbar vertebrae, and which becomes continuous laterally with the aponeurosis and fascia of the latissimus dorsi and anterior abdominal muscles (Bogduk and Twomey *ibid*). These form a tube around the spine, adding protection and stability when the fascia tightens and expands due to the broadening of the extensor muscles during extension.

Bogduk, Macintosh, and Pearcy (1992) showed that, in the upright position, the thoracic fibers of the lumbar erector spinae contribute 50% of the total extensor movement exerted on L4 and L5. The multifidus contributes some 20%, and the remaining extensor tension is exerted by the lumbar fibers of the erector spinae. At upper lumbar levels, the thoracic fibers of the lumbar erector spinae contribute between 70% and 86% of the total extensor tension.

In upright posture, the lumbar back muscles exert a net posterior shear force on segments L1-L4, but exert an anterior shear force on L5. Collectively, all of the back muscles exert large compression forces on all segments.

Loss of extension has been shown to correlate with low back pain more closely than flexion (Troup 1987).

Sidebending/Rotation

Sidebending to any extent (even though slight) in the lumbar spine is always coupled with translation and rotation. During sidebending the upper vertebra tilts ipsilaterally, compressing the disc on the same side. The nucleus is displaced contralaterally.

When the lordotic curve is intact, sidebending is coupled with rotation to the opposite side (neutral or type I motion). According to Fryette, if the facets are engaged during flexion or extension, sidebending will be coupled with rotation to

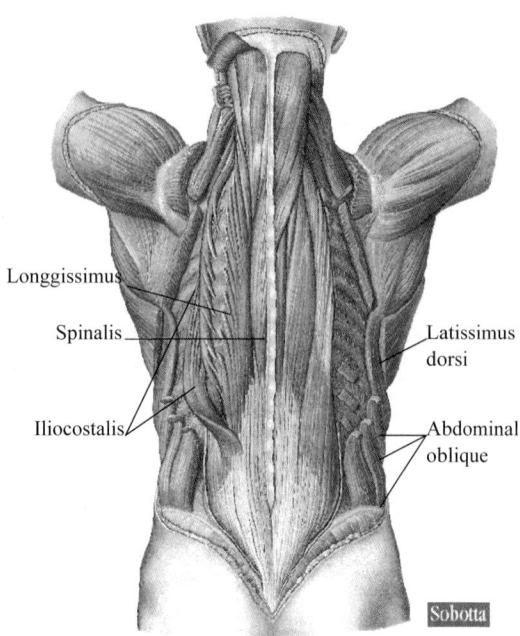

Figure 3-20: Superficial and Intermediate Muscles.

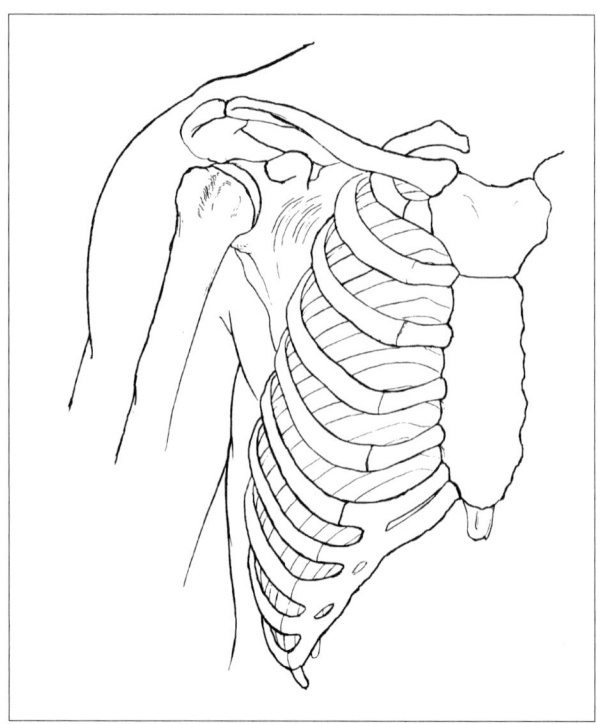

Figure 3-21: Rib cage.

the same side (non-neutral type II motion). With non-neutral (Type II) lumbar mechanics, the spine is less stable, and injury is more likely to occur (Greenman *ibid*). During rotation, the back and abdominal muscles are active on both sides of the spine.

The maximal single fascicle of axial torque generated by the lumbar back muscles was studied by Macintosh et al (1993). Torque was measured in the longissimus thoracis, iliocostalis lumborum and the lumbar multifidus in subjects during standing, in both the upright position and full flexion. The above muscles in upright subjects exerted no more than 2 N/m of axial torque. The collective torque of all muscles acting on a single segment did not exceed 5 N. All torques were considerably reduced in full flexion. From these measurements the lumbar back muscles appear to exert very little torque on the lumbar spine, and contribute only about 5% of the total torque involved in trunk rotation. According to Macintosh, none of the lumbar back muscles should be considered rotators. The abdominal oblique muscles appear to be the principal rotators of the trunk (Macintosh, Pearcy and Bogduk 1993).

The deep, tightness-prone *rotators* and *intertransversarii* muscles function as proprioceptors and probably inhibit and regulate multisegmental and *phasic* muscles. Somatic/vertebral dysfunction often results in loss of this inhibitory functions. It may lead to pain and trigger-point formation in larger muscles, since it appears that the rich proprioceptive innervation of these tiny monoarticular muscles of the spinal joints function to suppress the transmission of pain (Mitchell *ibid*).

Sidebending is limited by the geometry of both bony and soft tissues. The ipsilateral facet closes and the contralateral facet opens, and soft tissues are stretched (Kapandji *ibid*).

Restrictions in sidebending and rotation have been shown to correlate with the degree of low back pain (Mellin 1986).

Thoracic Spine and Rib Cage

The thoracic spine comprises one of the primary curves of the spine. It exhibits a mild kyphosis (posterior convexity). The thoracic spine consists of twelve heart-shaped vertebrae that have vertically oriented facets, with a 60° inclination around the horizontal axis and a 20° inclination around the vertical axis (White and Panjabi, 1978).

The remainder of the bony thorax consists of twenty-four ribs, costocartilages, and the sternum (Figure 3-21). A thoracic vertebra has ten separate articulations, any one of which can become dysfunctional. The spinous processes in the thoracic spine are different from those in other regions in

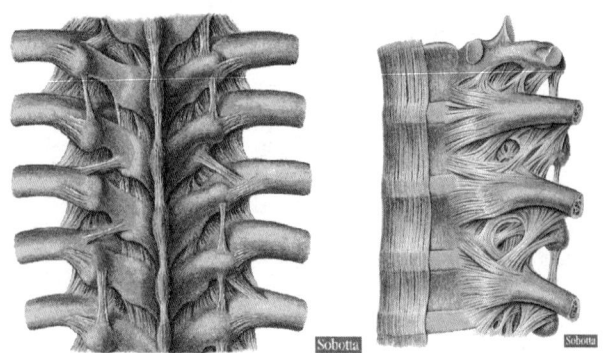

Figure 3-22: Ligaments of thorax

The Spine

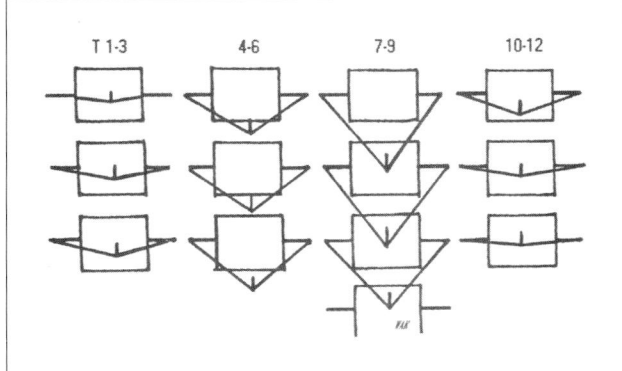

Figure 3-23: Arrangement of the spinous processes in the thoracic spine in relation to the transverse processes (From Kuchera WA and Kuchera ML, Osteopathic Principles in Practice, KCOM press 1993, with permission).

that not all are above their own vertebra. It is important to understand that the thoracic spine and rib cage essentially work as a single unit. Dysfunctions in the thoracic spine affect rib cage function and vice versa.

Thoracic spine and rib cage function can also affect the respiratory and circulatory systems. The diaphragm can be regarded as the "heart" of the venous system (Figure 3-24). Because the thoracic cord supplies sympathetic innervation to the arms, to 50% of the legs, and to the heart, lung, GI tract, kidneys, adrenals, gonads, and mucous membranes of the head and neck, pain from internal organs can refer to the thoracic spine and rib cage, and somatic dysfunction in the thoracic spine and rib cage can affect functions of these organs.

Thoracic Inlet and Outlet

The thoracic inlet is formed by a ring bound by:
- Manubrium;
- First rib;

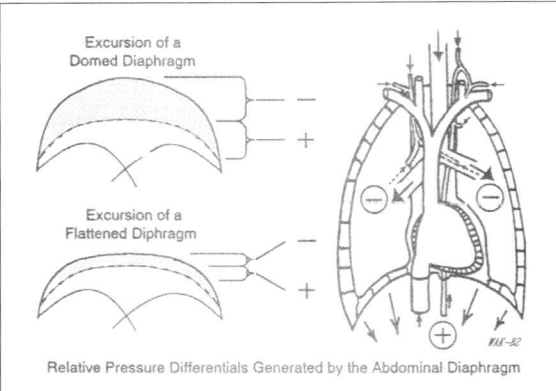

Figure 3-24: The "heart" the of venous system (From Kuchera WA and Kuchera ML, Osteopathic Principles in Practice, KCOM press 1993, with permission).

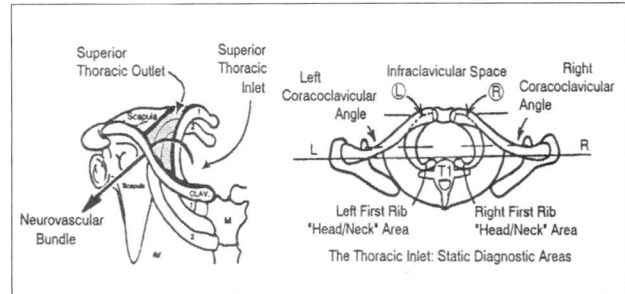

Figure 3-25: Thoracic inlet and outlet (From Kuchera WA and Kuchera ML, Osteopathic Principles in Practice, KCOM press 1993, with permission).

- Cartilages;
- Body of T1.

Structures that pass through are: esophagus, trachea, major blood and lymph vessels.

Motions in Thoracic Spine and Rib Cage

Flexion and extension in the thoracic spine consists of the rotation, coupled with the translation, of one vertebra on its adjoining inferior vertebra. Usually it involves the simultaneous movement of the lumbar spine. In flexion, the superior vertebra glides anteriorly, compressing the disc anteriorly. The posterior aspect of the disc is unloaded and therefore widens. During forward bending, the nucleus pulposus moves backward, and the axis of rotation is thought to move with it. The process in reversed by extension (Kapandji 1974). Sidebending is coupled with rotation and both type-I and type-II motions are seen. Many of the same muscle groups affecting the lumbar spine also affect the thoracic spine.

RIB CAGE MOTIONS. Rib cage movements have been described as: pump handle (ribs 1-6), bucket handle (7-10) and caliper motions (11-12), while all ribs move with a combination of all the above motions (Figure 3-26 and Figure 3-27). The scalene muscles that are attached to the upper ribs (1-2) and pectoralis minor (ribs 3-5) and major (ribs 2-8) are said to contribute to the pump handle motions seen mostly in the upper ribs. The serratus anterior attachments to ribs 2-8 contribute to the bucket handle motions which are the predominate motions in the middle ribs. The influence of the external intercostalis varies (Mitchell *ibid*).

BREATHING. As stated earlier, the diaphragm can be regarded as the "heart" of the venous system. During exercise, the secondary muscles of respiration move three quarters of the total blood volume. *During inhalation*:
- The cranium and whole body rotate externally;
- The quadratus lumborum relaxes;
- The diaphragm tightens and flattens.

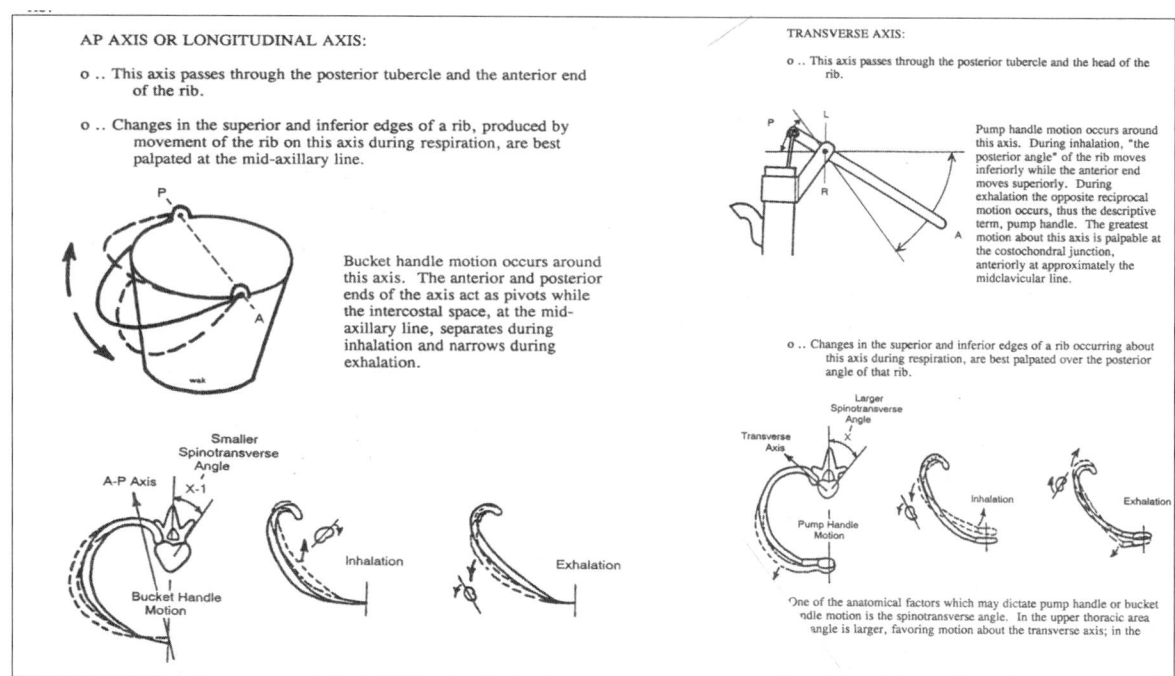

Figure 3-27: Bucket and pump handle rib motions (From Kuchera WA and Kuchera ML, Osteopathic Principles in Practice, KCOM press 1993, with permission).

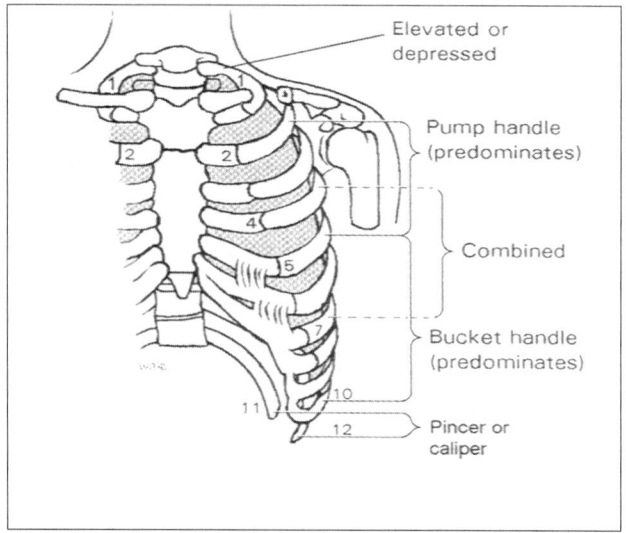

Figure 3-26: Rib motions (From Kuchera WA and Kuchera ML, Osteopathic Principles in Practice, KCOM press 1993, with permission).

During exhalation the process is reversed.

Ligaments

Stability in the thoracic spine is maintained by the costovertebral, costotransverse, and sternal articulations. The costovertebral and transverse articulations are stabilized by the strong ligamentum capitus costae radiatum, costotransverse ligament, and ligament of the tuberculi costae (Figure 3-22).

Muscles

Muscular functions are summarized in Table 1-9 on page 191.

Cervical Spine

The cervical spine can perform a wide range of movements that are necessary for normal function and visual accommodation. It is highly mobile due to the facet arrangement—oblique at angles of 45° (anterosuperior to posteroinferior) at the C2-3 joint, tapering down to 10° at C7-T1. This part of the spine regularly takes part in intricate motions that strain the neck's musculoskeletal structures (Kapandji 1994). The head alone requires complex movements for balance and rotation. One consequence of the cervical spine's flexibility is that the structure can become unstable easily. Degenerative changes and associated pain occur frequently.

The cervical spine has two functional segments: the *typical vertebrae* (C3-C7) and the *atypical vertebrae* (C0-C2), (Figure 3-29).

The Typical Segments (C3-C7)

The typical cervical spine segments are the C3-C7 vertebrae. The inferior facets of C2 have typical orientation as well. Described as a universal joint, a typical vertebra has a body, two laminae, two pedicles, two vertebral arches, and a spinous process. Each of the C3-C6 vertebrae has a foramen

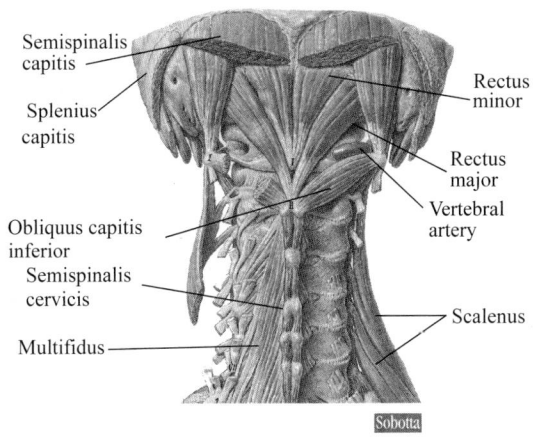

Figure 3-28: Neck muscles.

for the vertebral artery. Each C3-C7 transverse process has an anterior tubercle and a posterior tubercle that serve as attachments for the scalene muscles anteriorly, and for the longus capitis and longissimus cervicis muscles posteriorly. The cervical nerve roots run under the transverse processes through a trough in front of the facets (Bogduk and Twomey *ibid;* Kapandji *ibid*).

On the typical cervical vertebrae, the zygoapophyseal (facet) joints face backward and upward at an angle of about 34° from the horizontal. These joints allow for flexion, extension, translation, and sidebending, with coupled ipsilateral (type II) rotation. The greatest range of motion (ROM), about 17°, is at C5-6 (Kapandji *ibid*) where the most strains and disc herniation occur.

Adjacent vertebrae are linked by a disc, posterior and anterior longitudinal ligaments, facet joints, ligamenta nuchae, ligamenta flava, and the interspinous and intertransverse ligaments (Kapandji *ibid*). From a reductionist viewpoint, the anterior column of the lower cervical vertebrae is believed to function as a shock absorber, and the posterior column of the lower cervical vertebrae is believed to function as a guide for motion.

The Atypical Segments (C0-C1-C2)

The *atypical* segments of the cervical spine are the occipitoatloid joint (occipital bone and atlas) at C0-C1, and the atlantoaxoid joint (atlas and axis) at C1-C2.

The Occipitoatloid Joint (C0-C1)

The head-to-neck junction at C0-C1 is called the *occipitoatlantoid* or *occipitoatloid* joint. Articulation at this junction is of a modified spherical type. Primary movement, which takes place in the transverse axis through a gliding motion of the upper surface of the joint, occurs posteriorly on flexion and anteriorly on extension (Greenman *ibid*).

On the average, motion across the transverse axis (about 24°) is limited by the bony and soft tissues that surround this joint. Sidebending takes place around the sagittal axis (z-axis) and measures about 5°. Occurrence of coupled sidebending and rotation at this joint is minor, but loss of these movements can be significant clinically. The total range of flexion and extension is 15° (Kapandji *ibid*). The principal component of the occipitoatloid joint is the atlas (C1), a solid ring of bone that does not have a body and that articulates with the axis and the odontoid (dens) process. Other components of C1 are two oval-shaped, lateral pillars that run obliquely, anteriorly and medially and that bear the bi-concave articular surfaces (facets). They also bear an arch that, anteriorly, provides a small, cartilaginous, oval-shaped articular facet for the odontoid (Kapandji *ibid*).

The rotator muscles of the head are attached to the transverse processes of the atlas. Since the atlas has no vertebral body, its facet (zygoapophyseal) joints are the only weight-bearing compression members at the joint (Kapandji *ibid;* Bogduk and Twomey 1991).

The Atlantoaxoid Joint (C1-C2)

The nerve roots of the first and second spinal nerves lie superiorly and posteriorly to the articulating lateral masses of C1 and C2. C2 (axis) also called the *odontoid* (dens) vertebra, is a solid ring of bone from which the odontoid process rises vertically and to which the rotator muscles of the head are attached. The facets of the C2, which are located at the anterior aspect, articulate with the atlas. The splenius cervicis muscle attaches at the transverse process of the axis (Bogduk and Twomey *ibid*).

ATLANTOAXOID JOINT MOTION. Motion at the C1-C2 joint is primarily rotation to the right and left. Other motions are slight flexion, extension, translation, and sidebending. Motions occur in four articular vectors:

- Flexion and Extension at this level are about 10°.
- Rotation, the total range of which (about 50°) accounts for about 50% of rotation in the cervical spine.
- Sidebending, 10° on the average, is possible only with coupled rotation. On sidebending, C1 rotates to the contralateral side while C2 rotates to the ipsilateral side of the bending (Kapandji *ibid*).[29]

The Uncovertebral Joints

The uncovertebral joints, found only in the cervical spine, are pseudojoints that do not contain articular cartilage and synovial fluid. They are thought to add lateral stability to the anterior column. The uncovertebral joints are a common cause of neuroforaminal narrowing due to degenerative arthritis (Brown *ibid*).

---

29. Descriptions of the range of motions at this joint vary considerably.

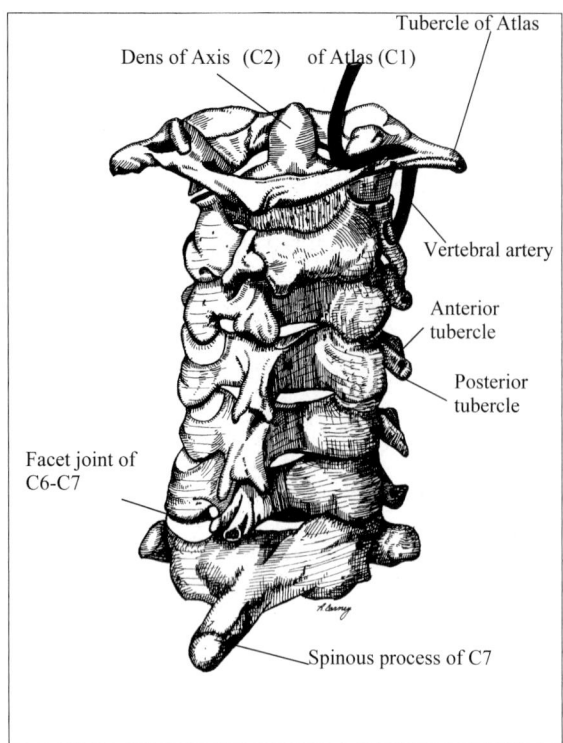

Figure 3-29: Cervical Spine (courtesy of Dorman and Ravin 1991).

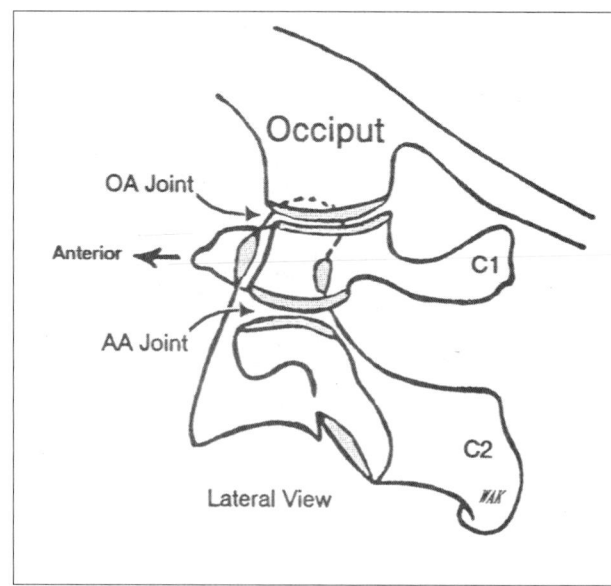

Figure 3-30: Upper cervical joints (From Kuchera WA and Kuchera ML, Osteopathic Principles in Practice, KCOM press 1993, with permission).

Cervical Spine Flexion

Cervical spine flexion takes place in two phases: first at the C0-C1 which accounts for some 50% of movement, and then at the C2-C7 joints which accounts for the other 50%.

Restriction of flexion in the C0-C1 and C1-C2 joints is produced by the nucal ligament, posterior longitudinal ligament, longitudinal fasciculus of the cruciform ligament, tectorial membrane and posterior muscles (Kapandji *ibid*). Flexion of the head and neck depends on the anterior muscles of the neck.

Extension

In the cervical spine, the posterior muscles of the neck perform the extension function. Extension is limited by bony limitation, anterior muscles, alar ligaments, and the anterior longitudinal ligament. Most of flexion-extension at the lower cervical spine takes place at the C3-C6 joints (especially C5-C6) (Kapandji *ibid*).

Sidebending

The sidebending muscles of the head and neck achieve their action mostly by unilateral contraction of cervical muscles.

The total range of movement for the entire cervical spine in sidebending is approximately 45°. From C0 to C3 the ROM measures about 8°. When the neck is in extension, usually no sidebending of significance occurs, due to mechanical restrictions and the alar ligaments. Sidebending is greatest when the neck is in slight flexion. Coupled sidebending and rotation occurs, and is greatest at C2-C3. It decreases at the lower cervical segments (Kapandji *ibid*).

Normal Gait

Basic gait is described as having four phases: stance, double-leg, single-leg, and swing. It is summarized in Table 3-10. Any forward advancement of any organism in its own medium, be it flight, swimming, or walking, is by a process of cyclic movements. This usually involves more than one organ, whereby energy is restored into the system rhythmically through oscillation. Momentum is achieved either through the recoil of elastic tissues or the oscillation of a weight-like pendulum. In walking, humans swing their arms, which act as pendulums. These short pendulums store and release antigravitational energy and contribute to the overall efficiency of the locomotor mechanism, which, in reality, is the whole of the body. The arms swing fore and aft alternately, thereby creating torque through the upper girdle. In brisk walking, the upper girdle rotates alternately with each step opposite the pelvis. This torque represents the storage and release of elastic energy in the fascial layers of the trunk, *particularly the paraspinal ligaments* (Dorman 1998).

In normal gait, one leg moves forward while the weight of the body is supported by the opposite leg (called the swing phase). In that phase the foot goes from plantar flexion to dorsal flexion. The knee is flexed and then extended, the hip moves from extension to flexion, and the pelvis rotates and changes its tilt. This movement of the lower limbs back and forth also serves as pendulums. An easy way to appreciate their role as pendulums is to watch an individual walking on

Normal Gait

Table 3-10: Basic Aspects of Gait

DEFINITION

PHASE		
Stance	Allows for: support weight, advancement of body over supporting limb, 62% of cycle	
	Heel strike	Initial contact: weight-loading period, one foot accepting body weight/absorbing shock
	Flat foot	Load response
	Single leg stance	Mid-stance: midstance of single leg, support entire body, about 40% of cycle
	Heel-off	Terminal stance
	Toe-off	Pre-swing: weight unloading period, about 10% of cycle and both feet in contact with floor
Double-Leg	Parts of both feet in contact with ground. Occurs twice per gait cycle, about 25% of cycle and almost disappears with running	
Single-Leg	Only one foot on the ground. Occurs twice per gait cycle, about 30% of cycle	
Swing	Foot non-weightbearing and moving forward: allows toes to clear floor, leg length adjustments, 38% of cycle	
	Three segments: • acceleration • mid-swing • terminal	In initial phase: foot is lifted off floor, rapid knee flexion and ankle dorsiflexion Legs parallel: the instant when swing leg is adjacent to weight-bearing leg During deceleration: swinging leg decelerates allowing smooth landing of the foot

a treadmill. In this situation the body is stationary against the surrounding room. Its easy to see how each leg rises and falls alternately. The advancement of the trunk of the walking person is not continuous, but oscillates, depending on the phase in the cycle of movement of the legs. As the swing-leg accelerates, the trunk slows relatively. The leg then decelerates, is planted, and the trunk speeds up. The trunk accelerates and decelerates with each leg swing cycle. This phenomenon is repeated when the other leg takes over the pendular-swing function. It is self-evident that the legs have the additional function of stance, and that these functions alternate sides within the cycle (Dorman *ibid*).

During walking, the two innominate (hip) bones rotate alternately forward and backward. During classic cross-patterned gait, the entire pelvis rotates from one side to the other around a vertical axis, with the shoulder girdle rotating in the opposite direction. This rotation occurs around an anterior axis at the symphysis pubis and a posterior axis on the side of the sacroiliac joint. The sacrum appears to move alternately in "wobbling" fashion, with side-bending and rotation coupled to opposite sides. ("In left-on-left and right-on-right oblique axis" is the osteopathic terminology.) These movements follow the induced pelvic rotations. The lumbar spine side-bends and rotates to the opposite sides, probably at L4, in an alternating fashion (Greenman 1997). Walking is an activity of daily living. Assuming only eighty minutes per day of weight-bearing performance, an average adult repeats 2500 stance/swing cycles per limb. That amounts to almost 1,000,000 steps per limb per year (Dananberg 1997). Table 3-11 summarizes the biomechanics of feet.

Kinesiology of the Gait Cycle

Walking combines *phasic actions* of the gluteus maximus, biceps femoris, rectus femoris, gastrocnemius and tibialis anterior muscles, with *tonic stabilizing* functions of the piriformis, gluteus medius, medial hamstrings, vastus medialis and peroneus muscles. The sequential firing of the piriformis and quadratus lumborum muscles in the gait cycle is important in the *Mitchell model* (the "muscle energy" osteopathic model). It can be extrapolated from the general concept that the muscle firing sequence progresses up the leg, through the pelvis, and into the contralateral lower back (Mitchell 1999). The piriformis, being a tonic stabilizer muscle, is prone to tightness and shortening, usually on the right side (Janda *ibid*). Unilateral tightness may inhibit function of the opposite piriformis, rendering the contralateral sacroiliac joint less stable during its stance period.

The human gait can be analyzed in terms of its components: *heel strike, bipedal support, contralateral toe-off, propellant stance, ballistic stance, mid-stride* and *contralateral swing*, and *toe-off*. According to Mitchell, the propellant stance is the first part of the stance period when the gluteus maximus muscle acts to pull the pelvis forward. The gluteus maximus can also affect the sacroiliac joints, both directly and indirectly, by straining the sacrotuberous ligament. This further stabilizes this joint (Vleeming et al *ibid*). Following the propellant stance, the pelvis glides forward by inertia through mid-stride and contralateral swing. The bipedal support is a small fraction of the total cycle. It occurs when both feet are on the ground and ends shortly after the onset of propellant stance. Running essentially eliminates the bipedal support phase. The first step taken from a stationary stance is different in several ways from the steps taken when walking is already in progress.

In describing the walking cycle beginning with right heel strike, Mitchell (1999) states that at *right heel strike* the right innominate is completely posterior, the left innominate is almost completely anterior and the sacrum is straight. The *right piriformis* is then stabilizing (by tonic/eccentric action)

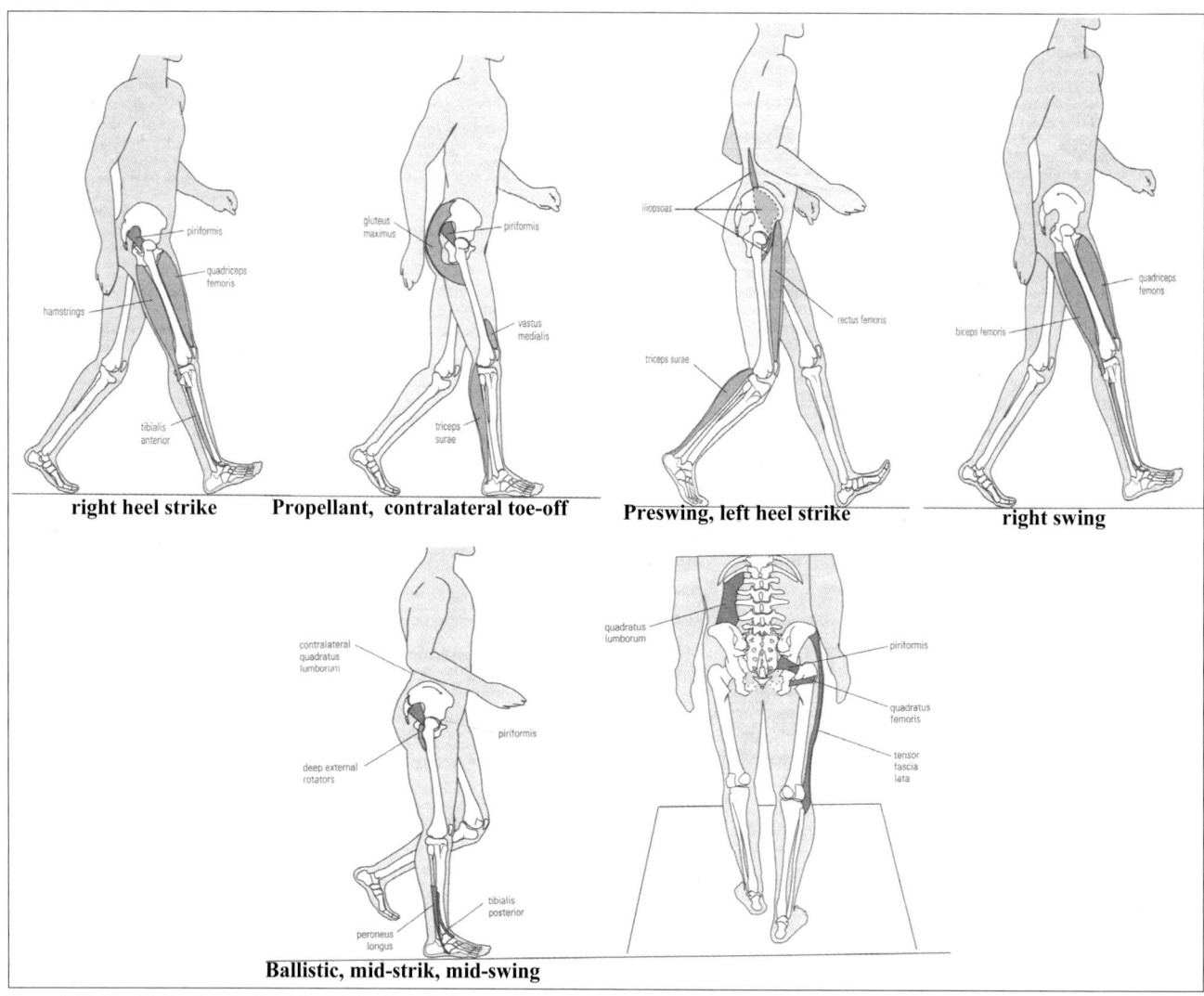

Figure 3-31: In *right heel strike* the right piriformis tonically contracts reflexly to stabilize the sacrum, thereby establishing the left oblique sacral axis. The right tibialis anterior fires eccentrically to prevent toe-slap. During *contralateral toe-off (Prpellant stance)* the right piriformis contraction persists throughout the stance phase. The primary kinesiologic propellant, the right gluteus maximus, fires phasically to pull the pelvis forward and then rests through the ballistic phase. *Contralateral toe-off* assists propulsion through sural muscle action. The hamstring, sural, and vastus muscles continue to stabilize the knee. In *mid-stride (mid-swing)* the stirrup muscles - tibialis posterior and peroneus longus - fire myotatically in response to plantar stretch. The deep rotators turn the femur externally, stabilizing the acetabular joint, and close packing the knee and tarsal joints. The right tensor fascia lata, along with right gluteus medius and left quadratus lumborum prevent Trendelenburg sagging of left hip. In *right swing* the right piriformis remains relaxed (from preswing toe-off, left heel strike) through the ballistic phase. The tonic hamstring and quadriceps stabilize hip and knee (courtesy of Mitchell 1999).

the inferior pole of sacrum, creating a left oblique axis just before *torsioning* commences. At contralateral toe-off, the left innominate reaches maximum anterior rotation. Left swing rotates the left innominate posteriorly. Through the left swing phase, the left *quadratus lumborum* contracts, first concentrically and then eccentrically. This contraction sidebends the spine to the left. It pushes the sacrum into *left torsion on the left oblique axis,* and lifts the right hip so that the foot can clear the ground. During the eccentric contraction of the *quadratus lumborum*, the sacral torsion gradually straightens, becoming perfectly straight at left heel strike. Stated otherwise (Vleeming et al *ibid*), in the right-sided swing phase, the right sacral base inclines forward relative to the iliac bones. Nutation increases, enlarging the ligament tension and sacroiliac joint compression.

A few milliseconds prior to right heel strike, the phasic right *gluteus maximus* begins its contraction, which persists through the propellant stance phase. The contraction reaches maximum a few milliseconds after heel strike and relaxes shortly thereafter. After initiating hip extension and propelling the pelvis and body forward, the gluteus maximus relaxes and allows for ballistic inertia to complete the forward pelvic translation during the stance period.

The *gluteus medius* begins its contraction two or three milliseconds before gluteus maximus and does not reach maximum contraction until mid-stance, after which it begins to relax. The gluteus medius functions tonically to abduct the hip through the mid-stride, holding the opposite side of the pelvis up to prevent the swinging foot (on the opposite side) from dragging on the ground

Normal Gait

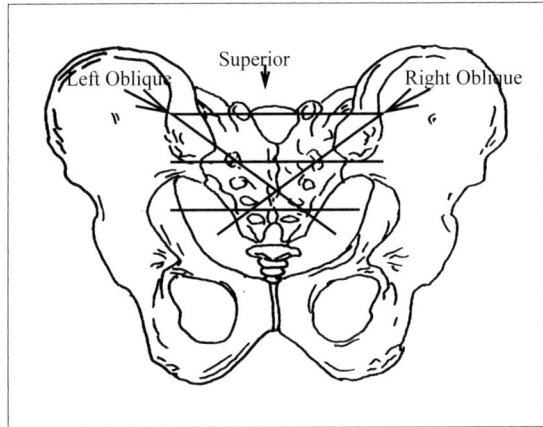

Figure 3-32: Sacral axis: right oblique, left oblique, superior (cranial), middle (sacral) and inferior (innominate) axis.

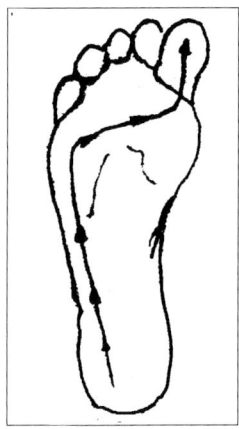

Figure 3-33: Weight transfer across the foot during gait.

Immediately after toe-off, the *rectus femoris* (on the toe-off side), a phasic muscle, contracts forcibly. This throws the femur (on the same side) into flexion as the gait cycle proceeds to the swing phase. As the swing leg gains inertia (in the swing phase) the tonus of the muscle gradually reduces in a controlled, eccentric, isotonic contraction. The inertia of the swinging leg is transmitted to the pelvis through the hamstring, rotating the innominate crest posteriorly on the transverse pubic axis. The *vastus medialis* begins to contract at mid-swing to straighten the knee and persists through heel strike, propellant stance, and mid-stride. This muscle is assisted by the dwindling tonus in the *rectus femoris*. Part of the *quadriceps* muscles, *vastus medialis* (a weakness-prone muscle) acts to stabilize the straightened knee. It fires strongest after heel strike. The *rectus femoris* fires at the beginning of the swing phase.

Starting in terminal swing phase (or just before heel strike), the *biceps femoris* and the *medial hamstrings* (on the same side) sustain their contractions through the first half of the stance period, which includes the phases of heel strike, bipedal support, propellant stance, and mid-stride. The biceps predominate to assist in the lateral rotation of the tibia as the knee extends. Working together, the knee flexors and extensors stabilize the knee. The *hamstrings* limit knee extension, and tension of the *sacrotuberous ligament* increases due to *biceps femoris* activation and sacral nutation.

In anticipation of heel strike, the *tibialis anterior* contracts through mid-stride, when it is joined by the *tibialis posterior* and *peroneus longus* in a myotatic reflex jerk to close-pack the tarsal arch for increased weight support. The foot and ankle are everted by the externally rotating leg. The connection of the *tibialis anterior* and *peroneus longus* at the planter side of the large first metatarsal bone forms a muscle-tendon-fascia sling. Because the *biceps femoris* connects to the head of the fibula and to the *strong fascia* of the *peroneus* muscles at its distal end, when the fibula moves downward during heel-strike,[30] this further loads the already tensed *biceps* muscle and sacrotuberous ligament. The coupled function of the *biceps femoris* and *tibialis anterior* can serve to load the longitudial sling, which could also store energy.

In the single support phase, the release of stored energy and the coupled action of the *gluteus maximus* and contralateral *latissimus dorsi* results in the arms swinging fore and aft, thereby creating torque through the upper girdle. Through the combined actions of the *latissimus dorsi* and the *gluteus maximus*, an oblique dorsal muscle-fascia-tendon sling becomes active. This crosses the spine and probably functions to store elastic energy. The tension of the *gluteus maximus* is partly transferred downward into the *iliotibial tract*. Also, the iliotibial tract can be tensed by expansion of the *vastus lateralis*. During the single support phase, the *vastus* counteracts flexion in the knee. As a result, the *iliotibial tract* is pushed aside laterally and is further stretched. The distal part of the iliotibial tract is part of the outer lateral capsule of the knee. Therefore, during the single support phase of gait, when the knee is fully loaded by body weight, forward shear of the femur in the knee joint can be limited by the tensions which spans through the *thoracolumbar fascia*, *gluteus maximus*, and *iliotibial tract* (Vleeming et al *ibid*; (Mitchell *ibid*).

Although not consistent with the Mitchell model, Lee (1997) states that, during the single-leg stance phase the innominate on that side begins to rotate anteriorly relative to the sacrum. Lee claims this results in a unilateral sacral extension (counternutation).

Oriental Medicine and Gait

While gait as not been elaborated on in the classic OM literature, all movement is understood to take place via the Sinew channels. In its most basic components, gait can be viewed

---

30. As gait proceeds, the ankle needs to dorsiflex, which requires an opening of the ankle mortis to accommodate the talar dome. This expansion is dependent on a translation motion of the fibula, which moves upwards and laterally, reorienting the fibers of the syndesmosis that connect it to the tibia (Dananberg 1987).

Table 3-11: Foot Biomechanics

HEEL CONTACT TO MIDSTANCE	• Heel hits the ground inverted causing the ground to push up on the lateral side.
	• Subtalar joint pronates from ground reactive force.
	• Midtarsal joints unlock (becoming a loose bag of bones) due to pronation. This results in energy accumulation and allows the foot to clear the ground.
	• The leg internally rotates.
	• The lateral side of the foot hits the ground and loads.
	• The first-ray plantarflexes bringing the forefoot to ground and cushioning foot slap.
	• Toes grip the ground.
MIDSTANCE TO TOE OFF	Process reverses:
	• Swing leg moves forward (the opposite side).
	• Support leg rotates externally.
	• Subtalar joint supinates.
	• Midtarsal joint locks due to supination and foot becomes rigid for normal stable weightbearing.
	• Knee straighten.
	• Heel comes off the ground.
	• The first-ray and toe dorsiflex for toe off.

as alternating and contralateral movements into flexion-rotation and extension-rotation of the lower and upper limbs (*Biomedical: when we step forward with our left leg, the right arm also goes forward because the extensor muscles that pull back on the right arm are "turned off." This "turning off" is controlled by and dependent upon getting the correct messages from the nerve endings in the left foot. When we step down on the left foot, the joint receptors there send a message that shuts off the right shoulder [Blaich ibid]*). The trunk both follows and drives the cyclic movement between Yin and Yang Sinew channels. Since the exact muscular composition of each of the Sinew channels is not known, the discussion that follows cannot be absolute. When the left foot is moved forward (in swing phase), a combination of Sinew channel actions must flex and raise the hip, and propel the leg forward. This is probably done mostly by the activity of deep flexors of the hip and trunk Shao-Yin Sinew channel, together with action of the Yang-Ming sinew channels. When the left foot begins to plant on the ground, the leg must become a stable strut firing the Tai-Yang Sinew channel of the weightbearing leg, which locks the knee in extension. Control of the foot as it bears weight from the lateral aspects to toe off (on the medial aspect of the foot) is achieved by the combined action of Yin and Yang Sinew channels. First the lower leg Yang-Ming muscles contract. They remain so until mid-strike when the Foot Tai-Yin, Shao-Yang and Yang-Ming muscles fire to close-pack the foot and support the body weight.

In left swing phase, the right upper limb is thrust forward by a combined Sinew channel activity that flexes the shoulder. The trunk is twisted and the hip is raised and abducted by activity of the Show-Yang, Shao-Yin, and Tai-Yin Sinew channels. Their counterparts in the upper extremity fire synergistically as the arm moves from extension and external rotation into flexion and internal rotation.

Up to now we have looked at various elements and sub-elements constructing the human body from reductionist (Newtonian) and some systemic points of view. Reductionist methods have, and do, dominate the biomechanical and orthopedic literature. Muscles and joints are viewed as levers that can be understood by simple rules of mechanics and engineering. Most students study the attachments of muscles and their "function" in open chain mechanics. However, even a cursory review of actual body movements in space shows these methods to be of limited use and even wrong in some instances. The following section, "A System Science Model for Biomechanical Construction," written by Stephen M. Levin, MD, challenges some of the reductionist models. Dr. Levin points out that all subsystems of the musculoskeletal system are united and are part of a metasystem that is independent and interdependent at the same time. This is true from the smallest cells to large systems within all living things. The body functions has a whole, constructed by tensegrity systems that connects every cell, organ, and system to each other. These tensegrity systems composed of tensional-continuity-supporting compressive elements may function as semiconductor vibratory-information networks and may explain many OM channel perspectives. Although there may be local and specific variations, the underlying principles cannot be violated (*OM: Yin Yang principals*). This systemic view is consistent with many manual therapy concepts and OM.

A Systems Science Model For Biomechanical Construction
by Stephen Levin MD, FACS, FACOS

When given an apparently complex problem, engineers search for the simplest elements of the problem, find a solution, and extrapolate to the whole, more complex design. This usually serves us well, as most constructions in the non-biologic world are Lego Set™ constructions built up block by block to completion of a pre-existing design. This method has been adopted by bio-engineers to explain biologic mechanics. The design used by most bio-engineers to calculate the mechanical forces in vertebrates is the skyscraper (Schultz 1983), with the girders acting as the skeleton and the soft tissue draped like the curtain walls on the building.

The simplest elements of the skyscraper model are the pillar, beam, and lever. But skyscrapers are immobile, unidirectional, gravity-dependent structures that, mechanically, are Newtonian, Hookian, and linear (Gordon 1988) in their behavior, with high energy requirements. If we were constructed like a skyscraper, the forces necessary to stabilize a human would be *bone breaking, muscle ripping,* and energy depleting (Gracovetsky 1988). Much like the creationist's concept of biologic organisms, skyscrapers do not evolve, but must be conceived as a whole. The design is from the top down. They are obligatorily vertically-oriented and rigid, with rigid joints. Otherwise they would collapse.

In the skyscraper / body frame analogy, similes that would seem obvious do not work well. Any brick mason will tell us that stacked building blocks cannot function as a horizontal beam in a building. Neither can stacked vertebral blocks function as a spinal beam in a quadruped or a biped bending over. Nor do blocks, pillars, and beams model the spineless worm, the soaring eagle, the swimming eel, or the writhing snake.

Biologic structures are self-generating and evolutionary (Gordon 1988). They must be independent structurally and functionally at each instant of their development. Nature has no temporary scaffolds to support the emerging organism. The design is from the bottom up, with a functioning lesser structure evolving into a more complex being.

Organic chemistry is structural chemistry. Subcellular structures must exist as *structures* before they are integrated into a cell. A cell must have its own stable construct before it joins with other cells. When removed from the organism, organelles and organs are not amorphous blobs on the dissecting table, but they have individually stable forms of their own. The joints, both intracellular or interstructural, are flexible. The structures must overcome the mechanical paradox of being able to convert from rigid to highly flexible and back again within an instant. It is apparent that, over time, biologic structures evolved that are self-generating, self-replicating, hierarchical, low energy-consuming, stable (even with flexible joints), ominidirectional, and able to function independent of gravity. They are instantly rigid or flexible, depending on their needs. The structural components are, for the most part, nonlinear, non-Hookian, and non-Newtonian (Gordon 1978) in their mechanical behavior, with low energy requirements.

A system scientist seeks a more global, holistic, and deductive solution than do other engineers. All subsystems are part of a metasystem that is independent and interdependent at the same time. Although there may be local and species-specific variations, the underlying principles cannot be violated. A subsystem that is incompatible with the metasystem cannot exist.

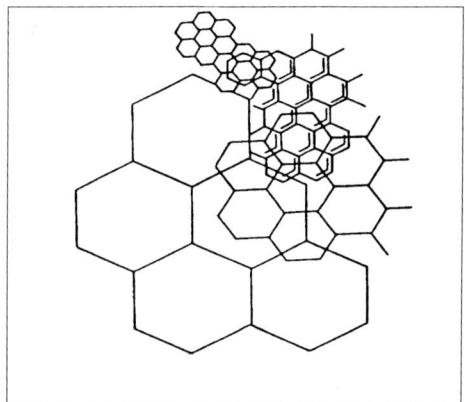

Figure 3-34: A self-generating hierarchy of hexagons.

Biologic structures must build themselves. Any "scaffolding" must be a functioning organelle before it evolves. An "ear" may not start out as an "ear," but it did start out as some functioning organ. Like an evolving beehive (Figure 3-34), each cell packs into place in a self-generating, hierarchical, energy-efficient pattern that is structurally stable at every step. The mechanical laws of beehive construction such as close packing, triangulation, and unidirectional stability are universal and apply to biologic construction as well.

Thompson (1969) proposed a truss model as the support concept in biologic modeling. He suggests that trusses (Figure 3-37) can be analogous models for structural support in vertebrates. For biologic tissue, trusses have clear advantages over skyscraper, post and lintel construction as structural support systems. They have flexible, even frictionless, hinges, with no bending moments about the joint. The support elements are in tension and compression only. Loads applied at any point are distributed about the truss, as tension or compression (Figure 3-36).

In post and beam construction, the load is locally loaded and creates leverage. There are no levers in a truss; the load is distributed *through* the structure. A truss is fully triangulated, is inherently stable, and cannot be deformed without producing large deformations of individual members. Since only trusses are inherently stable with freely moving hinges, it follows that any structure that has freely moving hinges and is structurally stable must be a truss. Vertebrates, meeting these criteria, must therefore be constructed as trusses.

When the tension elements of a truss are wires, ropes, soft tissues, ligaments etc., the truss usually becomes unidirectional. The element that is under tension will be under compression when turned topsy turvy. The tension elements of the body (the soft tissues—fascia, muscles, ligaments, and connective tissue) have largely been ignored as construction members of the body frame, and have been viewed only as the motors.

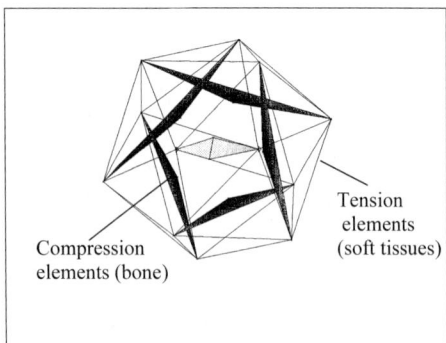

Figure 3-35: Tensegrity icosahedron compression elements suspended within tension elements.

In loading a truss, the elements that are in tension can be replaced by flexible materials such as ropes or wires, or in biologic systems, by ligaments, muscles, and fascia. However, soft tissue can function only as tension elements, and this truss will only function when oriented in one direction. There is a class of trusses, termed "tensegrity" (Fuller 1975) structures that are omnidirectional. The tension elements always function in tension, no matter what the direction of applied force. A wire cycle wheel is a familiar example of a tensegrity structure. The compression elements in tensegrity structures "float" in a tension network, just as the hub of a wire wheel is suspended in a tension network of spokes.

To conceive of the evolution of the metasystem construction of tensegrity trusses that can be linked in a hierarchy, that start at the smallest subcellular component, and that have the potential, like beehives, to build themselves, the structure would have to be one integrated tensegrity truss that evolved from infinitely smaller trusses and that could be, like the beehive cell, both structurally independent and interdependent at the same time. Fuller (*ibid*) and Snelson (1965) described the truss that fits these requirements: the tensegrity icosahedron (Figure 3-35).

The tensegrity icosahedron is a naturally occurring, fully triangulated, three-dimensional truss. It is an omnidirectional, gravity independent, flexible hinged structure. Its mechanical behavior is non-linear, non-Newtonian, and non-Hookian. Fuller and Snelson independently use this truss to build structures. Fuller's familiar geodesic dome is an example, and Snelson (*ibid*) has used it for artistic sculptures that can be seen around the world. Naturally occurring examples

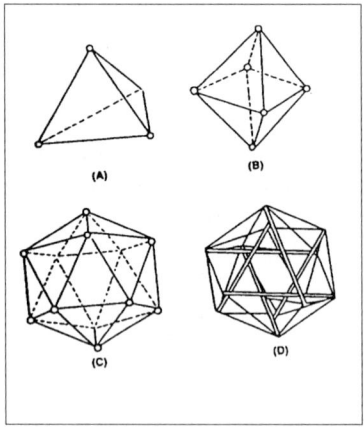

Figure 3-37: Three-dimensional trusses. (A) Tetrahedron; Four faces. (B) Octahedron; eight faces. (C) Icosahedron; Twenty faces. (D)

that have already been recognized are the self-generating fullerenes (carbon$_{60}$ organic molecules) (Kroto 1988), viruses (Wildy and Home 1963), clethrins (de Duve 1984), cells (Wang, Butler and Ingber 1993) radiolaria (Haeckel 1887), pollen grains, and dandelion balls (Levin et al 1986).

Because of the icosahedron's ability to fill space (Brandmuller 1992) and form self-organizing systems with stable carbon molecules (*ibid*), the icosahedron seems to be the space truss most suitable for biologic structures. The tensegrity icosahedron was first conceived by Kenneth Snelson (1965). The outer shell is composed of tension elements separated by compression elements suspended within the tension network. It appears to be the most, if not the only, suitable structure that can model the endoskeleton of cells (*ibid*) or the multicellular organisms that evolve from those cells. Icosahedron trusses are omnidirectional. Once constructed, tension elements are always loaded in tension, and compression elements are always loaded in compression, no

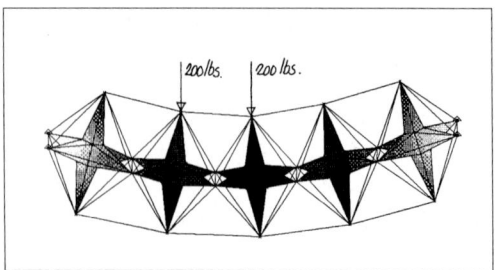

Figure 3-36: Load applied to a three dimensional truss.

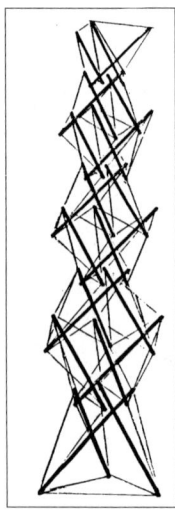

Figure 3-38: A tensegrity column (by Kenneth Snelson, with permission of the artist.)

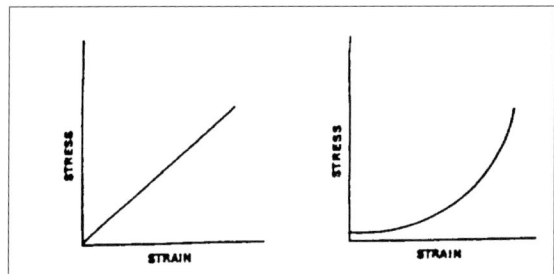

Figure 3-39: Linear and nonlinear stress-strain curves.

matter what the point of application or direction for load. Icosahedra are stable even with frictionless hinges. At the same time they can easily be altered in shape or stiffness merely by shortening or lengthening one or several tension elements. The icosahedron can be linked in an infinite variety of sizes and shapes in a modular or hierarchical pattern. The tension elements, the muscles, ligaments, and fascia, form a continuous interconnecting network. The compression elements, the bones, are suspended within that network. Such a structure would always maintain the characteristics of a single icosahedron so that a shaft, such as a spine, may be built. Being omnidirectional it can function equally well in tension or compression with the internal stresses always distributed in tension or compression with no bending moments and, therefore, lowest energy costs (Figure 3-38).

A unique property of a tension icosahedron as a structure is that it has a J-shaped, non-linear, stress-strain curve when loaded. Therefore, as a structure, the icosahedron seems to be a non-linear dynamic system unto itself (Figure 3-39).

This property is not demonstrated in mechanical systems such as post and lintel construction, or lever construction, or when using cubic or any other polyhedral shapes. J-shaped, non-linear, stress-strain curves seem to be the sine qua non of biologic tissue (Gordon 1988). This property has been demonstrated in bone, muscle, disc, fascia, nerve, composite biologic structures (White and Panjabi 1978), and just about any other biologic tissue studied.

Summary

It seems sensible to use a structure that has analogous mechanical properties to biologic tissue for biologic modeling. Viewed as a model for the spine of man or any vertebrate species, the tension icosahedron space truss, with the bones acting as the compressive elements and the soft tissues as the tension elements, even with multiple joints, will be stable in any position, be it vertical or horizontal, whether the posture is ramrod straight or a sigmoid curve or in any configuration between. Shortening on a soft tissue element has a rippling effect through the structure. Movement is created and a new, instantly stable shape is achieved. This type of structure is highly mobile, omnidirectional, and low energy-consuming. It is a unique structure that, when applied as a biologic model, would yield constructs that conform to the natural laws of least energy, the laws of mechanics, and the apparent peculiarities of biologic tissues. The result is a model which is able depict the fact that *joints of the body are suspended* and may even lift vertebral segments off the ones below (Robbie *ibid*). The icosahedron space truss has been shown to be present in biologic structures at the cellular, subcellular, and multicellular levels. In the spine, each subsystem (the vertebra, the disc, the soft tissues) would be subsystems of the spine metasystem. Each would function as an icosahedron independently and as part of the larger system, as in the beehive analogy. In a non-linear dynamical system, an icosahedron would be a stable "attractor" (Gleick 1988): an underlying form of least energy that the non-linear system seems to be seeking.

The icosahedron-space-truss-spine model is a universal modular hierarchical system that has the widest application with the least energy cost. As the simplest and least energy-consuming system, it becomes the metasystem against which all other systems and subsystems must be judged. If they are not simpler, more adaptable, and less energy-consuming, they should be rejected. Since this system always works with the least energy requirements, there would be no benefit to nature for spines to function sometimes as a post, sometimes as a beam, or sometimes as a truss; or to function differently for different species, conforming to the minimal inventory-maximum diversity concept of Pierce (1978) and evolutionary theory.

The icosahedron-space-truss-model could be extended to incorporate other anatomic and physiologic systems. For example, as a "pump" the icosahedron functions remarkably like cardiac and respiratory models, which have been shown to be non-linear dynamical systems. Therefore, it may be an even more fundamental metasystem for biologic modeling. As suggested by Kroto (1988), the Icosahedron template is "mysterious, ubiquitous, and all powerful."

As this model is universally adaptable to all biologic constructs and mimics function and form, it is proposed here as the metasystem model for biologic constructs, from viruses to vertebrates, including their systems and subsystems.

4

FOUNDATIONS FOR INTEGRATIVE ORTHOPAEDIC AND PHYSICAL MEDICINE ASSESSMENTS

This section presents concepts that are principally from Western Orthopaedic and Osteopathic Medicine. Often integrated within OM/TCM, they can be important for the assessment and treatment of musculoskeletal disorders. Physical examination following TCM principles is limited and often cannot lead to a *tissue specific* diagnosis. Also, since TCM knowledge of anatomy/physiology is limited and the practitioner can only use palpation and symptoms to make a diagnosis, many conditions that are deeper than one's fingers may be unpalpable and therefore inaccessible (such as calcification of tendons, spurs, inflamed bursae, disc disease, etc.). Thus added information from modern diagnostics can aid in treatment; for example, by adding softening, dissolving, and breaking herbs for calcified tendons and bony spurs. Lack of information only limits one's clinical options. Biomedical evaluations are helpful not only in making a "Western" biomedical diagnosis, but also in designing treatments using acupuncture and other TCM methodologies. A biomedical diagnosis is also important for prognosis and safety. The five tools of physical diagnosis (in both TCM and Western biomedicine) are: history, observation, auscultation, palpation, and percussion. (In TCM there is a sixth tool: smelling.)

Before engaging in a full discussion of these diagnostic tools, we must understand how one evaluates the worthiness of any particular tool. This requires a short discussion of the concepts of *reliability, validity, sensitivity, and specificity*.

Reliability

Reliability scores measure how readily two or more people will be able to perform the same test on the same patient and agree if the test is positive or not. This agreement must be greater than that arrived at by chance. The observed agreement is therefore deducted from what could be attributed to chance alone, and only that figure is used to convey agreement beyond chance. Reliability is measured and reported as the *Kappa* score. The range is usually 0-1 (or 0-10). A Zero Kappa score indicates a complete lack of agreement and a score of one (or 10) indicates complete agreement. Good reliability scores should be above 0.6 (or 6).

Table 4-1: Schematic Outcomes of Diagnostic Test

TEST RESULTS	DISEASE PRESENT	DISEASE ABSENT
Positive	True positive	False positive
Negative	False negative	True negative

Validity

Validity is a measurement of the accuracy of a test. Does the test really show what it is said to show? For this, in biomedical research, you need some kind of "objective" criterion or standard, such as an MRI, x-ray, surgical finding, post mortum finding, etc. The test/exam is either positive or negative. And the criterion or standard (sometimes referred to as a "gold standard") is either positive or negative (which is used as a comparison). There are two additional criteria for the validity of a test/exam, *sensitivity* and *specificity*.

SENSITIVITY: Sensitivity is the proportion of cases that the test identifies as positive and which should be positive (i.e., correctly identifying positive tests). This score should be high.

SPECIFICITY. Specificity is the ability to identify the absence of the disease. These parameters are calculated by the use of a simple 2 by 2 table (Table 4-1). If a practitioner, for example, diagnoses every case of acute abdominal pain as appendicitis, he will never miss a patient with appendicitis. On the other hand he will miss all other cases in which abdominal pain is due to other causes. His testing will have high sensitivity but no specificity. You need both for a good clinical test.

LIKELIHOOD RATIO. An additional parameter, the *likelihood ratio*, which uses both sensitivity and specificity, gives an even better indication of the test's performance. The likelihood ratio is calculated as:

$$\text{Likelihood ratio} = \frac{\text{Sensitivity}}{1 - \text{Specificity}}$$

This is needed because the epidemiology for a particular condition can influence the degree of diagnostic confidence. If, for example the epidemiologic likelihood for a lumbar disc herniation is to occur at the L4-L5 levels is over 90%, any test that checks for disc level must have an accuracy higher than 90%. Therefore, the likelihood ratio must be much greater than one. To achieve 80% confidence for a test, one needs to get a likelihood ratio score of at least six.

There are many reports on the validity and reliability of the tests to be described in this text, and some seem to support their use. For example, Page-Echols, Retzlaff and Mitchell at the Michigan State University-College of Osteopathic Medicine have shown good inter-rater reliability in the diagnosis of the respiratory kinematics of the ribs and sacrum (*Journal of the American Osteopathic Association* 1982). Another pilot study reported on the inter-rater reproducibility of diagnosis in a well-defined protocol. Three similarly trained Osteopathic practitioners evaluated the lower cervical and upper thoracic spine (C2-T8) in fifty-four volunteers at Ohio University College of Osteopathic Medicine. The results showed Kappa coefficients of 0.12 and 0.56 (chance agreement of 0.0051) between various tests and examiners (*Journal of Bodywork and Movement Therapies* 2001).[1] Boland and Adams have shown good reliability in the affects of ankle dorsiflexion on range and reliability of straight leg raising (*Australian Journal of Physiotherapy* 2000). However, not all reports are positive. Recently there has been a steady series of published papers which cast doubt on inter-and intra-rater reliability and accuracy in the performance of manual forms of assessment. In the October 2001 issue of the *Journal of Bodywork and Movement Therapies,* an editorial raised questions as to the value, validity, and accuracy of palpation methods in assessing musculoskeletal dysfunction.[2]

The following section is based on a lecture given by Prof. Nikoli Bogduk (University of Newcastle, New South Wales) who claims to have reviewed a large data base of published articles on back examinations. (He does not state the size of his review.) He presented this review in a talk in 1997 to the *American Back Society*. He cynically entitled the talk, "Nothing Works It's All A Ritual." I will base the coming remarks upon that lecture. Though his views do not necessarily negate the use of the examination techniques that will be described in this chapter, it does remind us to always keep an open and curious perspective. According to Bogduk, all medical "truth" comes in the form of two by two tables. The need for *evidence-based medicine*, is said to be due to the necessity to control for opinion, beliefs, epidemiology, and the placebo effect. Statistics rely on mathematics and therefore are thought to be "objective." According to Bogduk, a review of current literature shows physical examination of the spine to be mostly unreliable.

Evidence For Spinal Physical Examination

According to the review of the literature done by Bogduk, the evidence for agreement in examinations of the lumbar spine is as follows:

- Inspection: In general, inspection has fairly good likelihood ratios. Two examiners can agree about a patient's *conspicuous* lordotic curve. Physical therapists are fairly good at agreeing whether a patient has a list or not, though many MDs are said to be poor at it. Looking for asymmetries can result in fairly good agreement.
- Questioning: If we ask the patient whether it hurts to move, there is very good agreement.
- Checking for spasm: The results of checking for spasm or guarding are extremely bad. In one study by Waddell, the results were too poor to publish.
- Palpation: Practitioners finding tenderness in patients *anywhere* can achieve good agreement. But since these are patients with back pain that means very little. If the site of tenderness is specific, the agreement score is from 0.1 to 3.8 (from poor to fair). The best agreement is for tenderness over the iliac crest. Trying to find trigger points in the low back results in Kappa scores from fair to poor. For deep palpation of deep perivertebral muscle, physical therapists can achieve fairly good agreement on segmental tenderness. MDs are said to be very poor at it.
- Motion testing (Maitland testing): Testing for passive accessory intervertebral motions attain Kappa scores no greater than 0.23, and half of the practitioners had negative scores; that is, they disagreed if the patient had any abnormalities at all.
- General mobility of lumbar segments: Physical therapists are fairly good at agreeing about general segmental mobility, but MDs are said to be often inconsistent at it.
- Sacroiliac joint: There may be a high Kappa score (agreement) for some tests (mostly provocation of pain tests).
- Neurological examinations used in lumbar spine: Very poor Kappa and likelihood ratios are found for almost all neurological tests used in lumbar spine assessments. The Kappa scores barely reach one. For some tests, like sensory examination and atrophy, the scores are below one. This means that after you perform these tests "you are more ignorant" than before you started!

Besides the very poor agreement data on many of the above tests, the validity data is often lacking as well. For

---

1. For information on Osteopathic related clinical examinations see chapter 9.
2. It has been pointed out that the results of statistical methods are highly dependent on the way they are setup. Many of the statistical models used in medicine are based on Newtonian and Cartesian principles, ideas that have been shown by modern physics to be of limited use. The questions are often set-up using the reductionist "lens" of biomedicine, and, therefore, they may not be the best way to study complex systems. There are newer models that emphasis multidimensional complex evaluations and that have been used in the psychological and social sciences. These, however, have not been widely accepted in the US. They have been accepted more in Europe (Marcus personal communication) and may be more appropriate in the study of OM.

example, there is no "objective" criterion with which to study trigger points. There is no valid criterion for spasms. There is no physical examination that can provide reliable data on facet joint pain, disc pain, or spasms.

Keeping the above mentioned reservations in mind, one must never the less attempt to make as accurate a diagnosis as possible. Physical examination must be part of the process, especially because imaging is often misleading.

The Diagnostic Process

Before treating musculoskeletal disorders, the practitioner:

1. interviews the patient for a history;
2. examines the patient;
3. assesses symptoms and signs;
4. performs a differential diagnosis, which should be as precise as possible. Vague "diagnoses" such as "rotator cuff syndrome," "periarthritis," "tennis elbow," "back pain" etc., should be avoided. Instead, the practitioner should try, for example, to identify the exact location of a lesion in a case of shoulder tendinitis, such as: the superior aspect of the subscapularis tendon. He/she should ask, is back pain discogenic or not? If it is, is it annular or nuclear? etc. (Cyriax *ibid*).

The accuracy of a diagnosis depends on a composite of the history, the clinical findings, and the practitioner's understanding of referred pain.[3] If a soft tissue lesion is deeply seated, discrepancies can often exist between the location of the pain and the location of the culprit lesion (cause of pain). Often the number of "objective signs" present is not sufficient to suggest a diagnosis, and the practitioner must correlate a set of subjective and objective data. Another problem is that many of the "orthopedic tests" used in the literature and daily practice, have not been proven to be accurate. Many are old and have not been tested against any gold standard. Technical investigations such as imaging are often not helpful and may even be misleading (Cyriax *ibid*). Unusual symptoms and sign patterns are a warning. When they are present, technical evaluations may be needed to rule out a medical origin. The diagnostic process is, for all these reasons, complex, and the "art" of medicine must be applied.

Determining the Origin of Symptoms

To determine the origin of a symptom or set of symptoms, a thorough screening and a full differential diagnosis are paramount. *System/functional*-oriented schools such as Osteo-

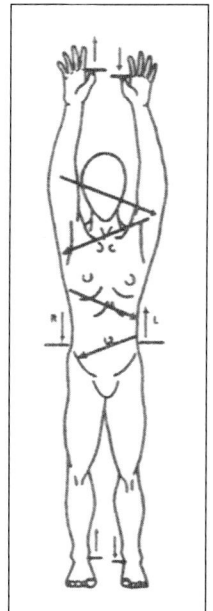

Figure 4-1: Screen for fascial tensions (From Kuchera WA and Kuchera ML, Osteopathic Principles in Practice, KCOM press 1993, with permission).

pathic medicine (and to some extent TCM in musculoskeletal practice) often perform screening/examinations of the entire body. These approaches to examination hold that restrictions of motion are the primary origin of many painful conditions. In TCM the restrictions/obstructions are primarily of Qi, Blood, Fluids, and channel functions.[4] In Osteopathic medicine, the presence of joint and soft tissue restrictions (which are expressed as channels, Qi and Blood in TCM) are more important than the presence of pain and/or the provocation of pain by movement (Greenman 1989). Frequently, Osteopathic and TCM consider the *biomedical lesion* to result from motion and circulation restrictions with localized congestion and malnourishment. Adaptation (physical, postural, or systemic) leads to compensation, which may lead to pathology (the "medical" lesion).

Evaluation Emphasis: Orthopaedic

In *"Orthopaedic Medicine"* (Cyriax style orthopedics), the emphasis in evaluation is on joint and tissue *function and provocation of pain*, not tissue tenderness.

Palpation should be used only after identifying a suspected structure through selective tension methods (when possible) and through functional assessments.[5] Selective tension is a process by which each tissue is isolated and tested

---

3. Pain can be felt along the entire length or in a part of any structure that is innervated by the same spinal nerve (i.e. dermatome, sclerotome or myotome). Analogous to pain along a TCM channel.

4. In TCM, however, the location of pain often correlates to the location of the restriction/obstruction, but Organic and other "holistic" factors play a critical role.

5. Cyriax's Orthopaedic Medicine selective tension method is very helpful for assessing the extremities but is limited for diagnosis of the spine.

separately, when possible. Palpation alone is often misleading as to the location of a *medical lesion*. Many areas in the body are tender in most people, the lesion may lie too deeply, and *referred* pain and tenderness are all too common. When the patient presents with a condition that affects moving parts of the body, some movement or posture *must* be capable of eliciting or aggravating the pain; if not, a medical origin must be suspected. The practitioner's task is to:

- isolate the involved tissue by breaking complex movements into simplified elements;
- test each element separately when possible.

To demonstrate an abnormality, the practitioner must compare all tested structures with similar but unaffected structures, in order to ascertain what is "normal" to that patient. If the location of pain/symptoms is suspected to be the same as the culprit lesion (source of pain), and the tissues are pressure sensitive, the practitioner must demonstrate that this is *the* pain the patient is seeking help for and is not merely secondary to normally sensitive tissues, a *secondary painful condition* (i.e., another pain as opposed to *the* pain), and/or due to *referred tenderness*. To do this the practitioner uses functional test *not pressure for local tenderness*. This process, which is at the heart of selective tension, yields *a nociceptive* (pain generating), lesion-oriented diagnosis.

The practitioner tests movement to assess for pain and limitations. The significance of pain and limitation and the significance of painless movement (with or without limitation) are equal, because they suggest different pathologies or dysfunctions. Since an involved structure cannot always be isolated, the practitioner must consider other information, such as that resulting from an analysis of several motions, followed by a deduction process as to the significance of the findings. Good patient cooperation and clear instructions are important. When a *painful area* does not seem to respond to functional examination (testing for movements and joint motions) the pain is most likely to be referred from a proximal structure, which may be visceral, nervous, somatic, or psychogenic in origin (Cyriax *ibid*).

The Patient History and Presenting Complaint

A comprehensive patient history is imperative for the *medical* diagnosis of musculoskeletal pains. It is the *subjective* part of the progress notes and the patient's experience. In many instances a good history is sufficient for making a medical diagnosis, although (Mitchell 1995) the nature of somatic dysfunction and/or joint dysfunctions will not have been elucidated. The history can help the practitioner not only in diagnosing the "disease," but also in avoiding catastrophic mistakes. In some situations, such as lesions of the knee and spine, a good history can often be relied upon to yield a diagnosis, while if the lesion is in the shoulder, for example, an examination is the only process which will produce a diagnosis (Cyriax *ibid*). It is also important to document the patient's magnitude of pain and functional capacity, as often patients do not acknowledge or recognize improvements (and are poor historians). It is also important to note the duration of flare-ups and how long it takes for them to ease or to settle down, and what activity leads to such flare-ups (e.g., how long can the patient sit, walk, how much can he/she lift, etc.). The amount of analgesic use should be noted. Patients' memory of their pain and functional capacity is often distorted and many tend to focus on their current pain. It is helpful to show them old pain drawings and self-assessment questioners to demonstrate improvement. This type of information can be used to create goals and set benchmarks for progress as well.

The practitioner must learn, and continue developing, a crucial diagnostic skill: listening. The practitioner must also avoid asking leading questions, because, in a subconscious effort to please the practitioner, many patients give the "expected or pleasing" answers. This is true also when evaluating treatment success. Many patients do not want to offend their practitioner and so minimize treatment failures. Patients should be asked precise questions and should be able to describe their symptoms fairly clearly. If not, neurosis or malingering should be suspected. Questions should be neutral or even put in the negative: "Your elbow does not hurt does it?" "Your pain does not spread down your arms, or does it?" Or one can use an open-ended question: instead of asking, "Does your pain spread down your arms?" ask, "Does your pain spread at all?" If the answer is "Yes," ask, "Where to?" In general, the history begins with the patient's chief complaint: the date the symptoms first appeared and their duration. What makes them better? What makes them worse? Any related symptoms? What treatment was given? Who is treating the patient and the results obtained from the treatment should all be recorded. Other information to be recorded is: the family history, previous illnesses, injuries, stressful events, surgeries, accidents, abnormal moods or activities, allergies, and review of systems.

Age/Occupation/Sex/Risk Factors

Having recorded the patient's personal information, the practitioner notes the patient's sex and inquires about age, occupation, handedness, and social history, including past occupations. Age, occupation, and sex can point to risk factors such as:

- ligamentous and postural syndromes, mostly ages twenty to sixty-five;
- disc problems, mostly ages twenty to fifty;
  — sciatica from disc can start during adolescence;
  — primary sciatica more common in males;
  — cervical root pain is extremely unlikely under the age of thirty-five.
- symptoms from spodylolisthesis can start at age fifteen;
- ankylosing spondylitis can start at age fifteen to thirty-five;
  — more common in males.

- A teen with symptoms of knee derangement probably suffers from osteochondritis, but the same symptoms of knee locking and painful twinges in an adult patient suggests a meniscal problem. In elderly patients, the same symptoms suggest a loose body. It is the same with hip trouble: at the age of five it is probably due to Perthes' disease; at fifteen it may be due to slipped epiphysis; at age thirty, ankylosing spondylitis is a possibility; and at age fifty arthrosis is more likely.
- Reiter's syndrome usually starts at ages between twenty and forty and is seen mostly in male patients.
- de Quervain's disease and thoracic outlet syndrome is more common in females.

IN GENERAL PATIENTS OVER FORTY YEARS OF AGE MAY HAVE:[6]

- Traumatic arthritis
- Osteoporosis
- Degenerative diseases
- Loose body in knee (rather than meniscus)
- Osteomalacia
- Cancer
- Paget's disease.

IN GENERAL YOUNG ADULTS MAY HAVE:[7]

- Neurofibromatosis
- Repetitive motion injury
- Strains
- Osteochondritis dissecans.

TRUCK DRIVERS, OTHER PATIENTS EXPOSED TO VIBRATIONS AND NIGHT SHIFT WORK:

- Disc disease[8]
- Deconditioning/postural syndromes.

PATIENTS EXPOSED TO CHEMICALS/TOXINS/DRUGS/MEDICATIONS:

- Neuropathies
- Fibromyalgia.

A patient with an injury to his/her left arm or hand and that is left handed is rated with greater disability than one that is right handed.

---

6. Most of which are related to the TCM Kidneys, Liver, Essence, obstruction, stasis, toxic accumulation, and Pathogenic Factors.
7. Most of which are related to TCM Qi-stagnation, Blood-stasis, and other Pathogenic Factors.
8. Although a recent study showed no difference in disc disease in twin pairs who had different patterns of occupational driving during their life (Battie et al 2002).

Pain/Complaint Inquiry

The practitioner asks about the location of pain/complaint, whether the patient has suffered a trauma or other direct injury, and other questions that help focus on the possible source of the pain/complaint.[9] The following are important aspects of the pain/complaint to ascertain when taking a history:

CHRONOLOGY, PROGRESSION, AND FORCES. The practitioner should inquire about the onset, past behavior, and chronological progression of symptoms. For example, initially the patient feels pain close to the culprit lesion *(OM: Sinew channels)*. During later stages, the pain is likely to be referred *(OM: possibly as pathology enters the Connecting/vessels and Main channels)*, so an account of where the pain started and to where it has progressed is helpful. This, however, does not apply to "pins and needles," which are mostly felt distally in the limb from wherever a nerve is affected.

In general, when pain is diminishing, the condition is improving, although some conditions such as nerve root atrophy and in certain cases of mononeuritis, the pain may disappear long before the condition has resolved. Pain that is becoming worse may indicate a worsening condition. Metastatic pain is usually of short duration with an insidious onset, while other worsening conditions such as a neurofibroma may take a long time to develop (Ombregt et al *ibid*).

Pain shifting form one side of the body to the other can occur due to a shifting lesion in a central structure (i.e. discs), or in changing and multiple lesions. Inflammatory conditions may result in different joints flaring at different times. Pain that is *expanding* and grows but does not leave the original area suggests a serious expanding lesion that should be medically evaluated. Many conditions come and go, and a good history often elucidates the cause. *(OM: Multiple-Bi [Zhong-Bi] is said to shift from side to side but not to change in longitudinal dimensions)*.

In cases of trauma, the practitioner must be familiar with the forces affecting the patient, such as the direction and type of forces. This is especially important in cases where compensation may be claimed. Traumatic events may prevent one from being able to conduct a good examination, and a good history may provide the information needed to suggest a diagnosis.

TIMING OF SYMPTOMS. Joints that have quickly filled with

---

9. Some practitioners use the acronym "OPQRST" for organizing their questions:

    Onset.

    Provoking and palliative factors.

    Quality and character of pain.

    Radiation and referral of pain.

    Site of pain.

    Timing of pain.

fluid or have suddenly swelled-up suggest the presence of bleeding (or infection) and should be aspirated quickly when possible; whereas, in joints that swell-up slowly, the effusion is usually of serous fluid, and usually there is no need to aspirate. Sprained ligaments develop pain progressively over several hours. Fractures, dislocations, and internal derangements are painful at the onset. Muscle and tendon tears usually cause sudden pain during a particular movement. In repetitive micro-trauma such as overuse tendinitis, however, the onset of pain is often insidious. Pain following overuse often suggests tendinous disorders. Night pain, especially of insidious onset, suggests inflammation and *serious* conditions (*OM: Blood-stasis, Heat*). Inflammatory disorders often result in frank stiffness early in the morning, while mechanical conditions (e.g. joint dysfunction) are often characterized by pain and stiffness only at the beginning of movement. Fever developing some time after an injury, or invasive procedure can suggest an infection. A sudden back pain that in a day or two is felt at an extremity or that develops gradually in a few days strongly suggest a *nuclear* disc protrusion, while immediate back pain suggests *annular* pain or disc derangement (Cyriax *ibid*). (*OM: it said that when pain is felt first and then swelling appears, it is due to Qi damaging the Blood. When swelling is noticed first and then the patient feels pain, it is the Blood damaging the Qi. A pain that occurs or increases at a particular time of day may indicate a specific channel's being affected*).

THE RELATIONSHIPS OF POSTURE, ACTIVITY, REST, AND EXERTION. The relationships of posture, activity, rest and exertion can provide important information. A patient that has a musculoskeletal condition *must* have some relationship between the above and their pain. If none are seen, this is a sign of a medical origin rather than a musculoskeletal one. The only other medical conditions that have a strong relation to movement and rest are angina and intermittent claudication (Ombregt et al *ibid*).

Ligament pain is commonly increased by inactivity and relieved by subsequent movement, although heavy work will exacerbate the pain. Rest will characteristically relieve pain due to joint dysfunction (in the absence of discrete pathology), overuse syndromes, and disc disease.

Activity often aggravates pain arising from vertebral (somatic) dysfunctions, typically with certain movements being worse than others. Aggravation of pain by activity is seen also with muscle strain, overuse syndromes, and disc disease. The activity of pathological joints may initially alleviate pain, but, later, it will usually aggravate the pain.

AFFECT OF COUGHING: Pain aggravated by coughing, especially if the pain is felt in the upper limbs, suggests an intraspinal (space occupying) lesion. Increasing back and leg pain when coughing is seen often with disc disease. A cough can increase upper back pain from pleuritis and in the low back and buttock from the sacroiliac joints due to a momentary increase in intra-abdominal pressure which results in a broadening of the sacroiliac joints.

PINS, NEEDLES, BURNING, AND PARESTHESIA. "Pins and needles," "tingling," or other non-painful sensory disturbances suggest nervous system involvement, either primary or secondary but may also suggest metabolic or vascular involvement (trauma, pregnancy, RA, anemia, MS, tumors, etc.).

Vague tingling, pins and needles, and numbness can be caused by a peripheral nerve, a nerve root, a nerve trunk, and the central nervous system. Pins and needles in the feet are an early symptom of pressure on the spinal cord and may be experienced before the plantar response becomes extensor (Babinski sign, see below). Tingling and numbness can also be caused by circulatory disturbances (e.g. Raynaud's disease) and diabetic neuropathy. With circulatory disturbances, the skin of the limb often changes color. The proper differential diagnosis lies in understanding segmental references and performing a good patient history and examination (Cyriax *ibid*).

Peripheral nerve lesions affect the integument supplied by that nerve, for example, meralgia paresthetica which is a lesion of the lateral cutaneous nerve, will affect only the skin directly innervated by it (the front of thigh).

Pain from a ligamentous source is frequently described as "a vague numbness" (nulliness), which, in contrast to neurological tingling, is alleviated by stroking or massaging the area. Stroking often aggravates neurological pain. This (nulliness) is not true numbness, and the patient has no difficulty in differentiating between dull and sharp stimulation, or between stimulation to the affected and unaffected areas (all of which feel the same on sensory testing).

Central nervous system pain (i.e., upper motor neuron) is characterized by *spontaneous* burning or aching pain, hyperalgesia (excessive sensitivity to pain), dysesthesia (pins and needles, numbness, burning) and other abnormal sensations and is usually not related to movement.

TWINGES AND GIVING-WAY. Painful twinges and giving-way often suggests instability, joint block (internal derangement), or tendinitis. Painful twinges (sudden short bouts of severe pain) can occur as a result of mechanical as well as inflammatory conditions. Internal derangement of a joint is suspected when there are symptoms of locking, sudden twinges, and a history of such occurrences. Symptoms of internal derangement are characterized by irregularity: sometimes the joint feels normal and sometimes not. When internal derangement affects a facet or intervertebral disc (IDD), the joint most frequently locks in flexion (Cyriax *ibid*). The typical antalgic posture seen in these patients can also be due to spasm of the psoas and the deep aspect of the quadratus lumborum, FRS spinal dysfunction, and backward torsions of sacroiliac joints (with/out disc disease).

PAINFUL TWINGES OCCUR IN FOUR DISORDERS (Cyriax *ibid*):

1. "Loose body" in the joint space;
2. Discogenic pain;
3. Tendinitis, which frequently follows overuse. Often the patient describes a painful transitory loss of strength which may be due to mechanical stress on the lesion or due to adhesions;
4. Disorders of neurological origin, such as post-herpetic neuralgia, Morton's neuroma, and trigeminal neuralgia;
5. Joint instability. Often a momentary loss of strength accompanies the pain.

ILLNESS, TRAVEL, DIET, SWELLING, PAIN, AND PERSPIRATION.

- A *history of heart* disease can suggest rheumatic disease.
- *Constitutional symptoms* such as weakness, fatigue, loss of weight and perspiring can be due to serious conditions. *Perspiration* may suggest sympathetic nervous system involvement, pain, or a serious condition such as heart disease and lymphomas.[10]
- *Rich diets* may cause gout and obesity, which can result in musculoskeletal complaints.
- *Recent travel* may suggest infection.
- Painful conditions of *ambiguous origin* or of short duration suggest a possible internal medical condition but also common in orthopedic conditions.
- The presence of *swelling* is indicative of an inflammatory process, which can stem from an autoimmune, infectious, neuropathic, or musculoskeletal disorder.
- The presence of a *rhythmic increase of abdominal pain* unrelated to movement, or severe pain felt ventrally should raise suspicion of an internal medical disorder, especially when the abdominal pain is located at the same level as back pain. When concomitant abdominal pain is at a level lower than the back pain, an orthopedic origin is more likely (Mennell 1964). Abdominal pain may be referred from the spine, thorax, pelvic organs, and genitalia. Abdominal pain can be caused by exogenous, endogenous, metabolic, or neurogenic disorders.[11] Patients with abdominal symptoms should be asked: Does taking a deep breath aggravate your symptoms? Does twisting your back aggravate your symptoms? A positive answer to either often indicates a musculoskeletal origin for abdominal symptoms. Patients should also be asked: "Has there been any change in your bowel habits since the onset of your symptoms?" "Does eating foods aggravate your symptoms?" "Has there been any weight change since the onset of symptoms?" "Do you have any urinary burning or discharge?" Positive answers to any of these question should arouse a high degree of suspicion that the symptoms have a visceral origin.

- *Kidney, bladder, prostate, and intestinal diseases* often cause low back pain.
- *Pelvic* and *rectal diseases* often give rise to sacral area pain.
- Disorders of the *gallbladder, liver, heart, lung, pancreas, stomach,* as well as *ectopic pregnancy* often produce back and shoulder pain.
- Disorders of the *esophagus and heart* can refer pain to the neck, jaw, arm, or back.

The use of the acronym CAUTION may be used to remind the practitioner of the symptoms and signs to look for when considering cancer:

Changes in bowel and/or bladder habits.
A sore that does not heal.
Unusual bleeding or discharge.
Thickening or lumps in the breast or elsewhere.
Indigestion or difficulty swallowing.
Obvious changes in a wart, a mole, or skin.
Nagging cough or hoarseness.

MEDICAL CONDITIONS TO KEEP IN MIND. Neurofibromatosis (von Recklinghausen's disease), Schwannoma and other benign and malignant tumors, metabolic destructive lesions, vascular disorders, organic diseases, infections, depression and anxiety disorders, among others, should always be kept in mind (see "Medical Conditions" on page 681.)

In summary, a comprehensive history is imperative in the diagnosis of musculoskeletal conditions and can both aid in the diagnosis/treatment and help avoid catastrophic mistakes.

Physical Examination

An understanding of several examination approaches can be helpful for making an accurate diagnosis. For example, in evaluating soft tissue pain, the selective tension approach is most useful for identifying the pain's *anatomical* source (medical lesion or location of largest nociceptive/pain output). Other examination techniques focus more on function. The evocation and interpretation of physical signs, an art that requires a considerable amount of practice, is best learned by apprenticeship. This section includes several examination methods.

One sequence used for a standard orthopedic examination is:

1. Vital signs
2. Observation

---

10. Excessive perspiration and/or night sweat is often the first symptom in many serious medical conditions, especially lymphomas and tuberculosis, which can result in pain when bones are affected.

11. For more details, see the author's text *Acute Abdominal Syndromes: Their Diagnosis and Treatment According to Combined Chinese-Western Medicine*, Blue Poppy Press, 1991.

3. Palpation

4. Percussion

5. Auscultation

6. Range of Motion/Movement Testing (which is part of the general orthopedic examination)

7. Special Orthopedic Testing (not extensively covered in this text)

8. Neurological Testing

9. Examination of Related Areas

10. Laboratory and Radiological Testing.[12]

In general, clinical orthopedic/neurological examinations follow the following sequence:
Active movements performed by the patient.
Passive movements performed by the practitioner.
Resisted muscle tests.
Sensory assessments.
Deep tendon and other tests for reflexes.

In this text, range of motion/movement testing is included under "orthopedic testing." In Orthopaedic Medicine, palpation is performed last, except for heat and swelling. In this segment on examination, the term:

- *Motion* is used to describe manual medicine concepts of joint play and joint barriers;
- *Movement* is used to describe active movement;
- ROM can refer to either motion or movement, depending on the context.

Vital Signs

The practitioner measures the patient's blood pressure, respiration, pulse, temperature, weight, and the so-called "new" vital sign, *pain*.

After trauma, an unusual drop in blood pressure may signify a micro-hemorrhage which was missed during previous examinations, a CNS dysfunction, or the beginning of post traumatic depression. Asymmetric pressure often results from visceral, osteoarticular, or tissue problems. A rapid, indiscrete pulse accompanied by significant pallor, nausea, and fainting indicates a serious problem requiring a careful medical evaluation, or perhaps referral for emergency care. A difference between the two radial pulses often indicates an osteoarticular problem affecting the balance between the parasympathetic and sympathetic nervous systems. The problem is located usually on the side where the pulse is least noticeable. Another common reason for this type of phenomenon is a decrease in the functional lumen of the subclavian or axillary arteries. This compression can be due to

---

12. It should be pointed out that the following chapter does not follow this list and additional categories are discussed.

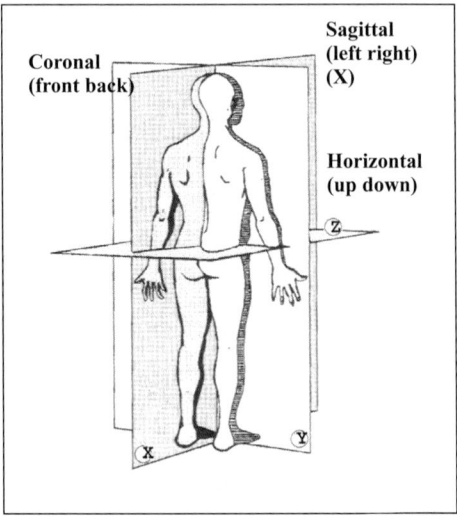

Figure 4-2: Planes of body. Sagittal plane divides the body left and right sides. Coronal plane divides the body anteriorly posteriorly. Horizontal plane divides the body superiorly inferiorly.

an anatomical compression or a change in the sympathetic tone affecting them. Exaggerated abdominal aortic pulse usually signifies intense anxiety, but very rarely may be a sign of a spontaneous or post-traumatic aortic aneurysm. When this is the cause, the pulse is easily felt and sometimes seen throughout the abdomen. One of the first signs of an aortic aneurysm is a *low-grade thoracic* or *lumbar pain* that arises spontaneously without any mechanical cause-and-effect relationship (Barral and Croibier 1999).

Fevers can be caused by infections, trauma, malignancies, infarctions, blood disorders (such as acute hemolitic anemia), and immune disorders (such as drug fevers and collagen diseases). The chief cause of hypothermia is exposure to cold, but some acute illnesses may also produce it. Elderly people are especially susceptible to hypothermia and are less likely to develop fever (Bates 1983).

Observation

The observation process is predominately visual. The interpretive vocabulary is critical to this process. To recognize whether a presentation is normal or abnormal, the practitioner must have a sufficient observational lexicon and knowledge of "normal." Visual observation is used to assess the patient's gait and posture. The practitioner looks for asymmetry, joint or soft tissue swelling and other deformities. Lastly, the patient's reaction to questions and palpation are closely observed.

Observation may allow the practitioner to recognize ruptured tendons, dislocated joints, atrophy, hypertrophy, and neurological problems. For example, when the long head of the biceps brachii ruptures, the practitioner can usually see a lump-like bunching up of the muscle. When there is multiple directional instability at the shoulder, a *sulcus sign*

Physical Examination

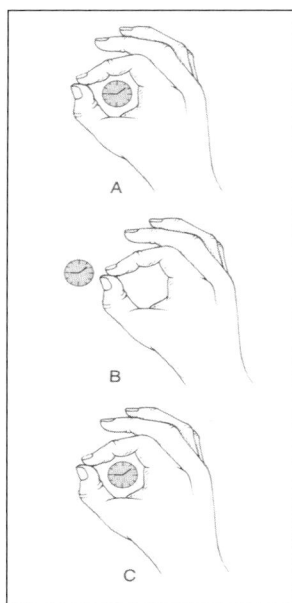

Figure 4-3: Determining eye dominance (From Kuchera WA and Kuchera ML, Osteopathic Principles in Practice s 1994, with permission).

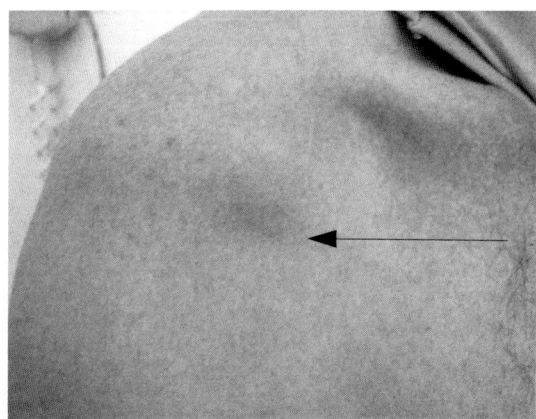

Figure 4-4: Sulcus sign at the shoulder due to multidirectional instability.

can be visualized as a shelf or step deformity below the acromian (Figure 4-4). A separation of the acromioclavicular joint can be easily visualized as a *step deformity*. A sulcus sign or step deformity can also be seen in the knee when the cruciate ligament is torn. The tibia will fall backward showing a shelf between the patella, femur, and tibia. A spondylolysis can also result in a step deformity. Nerve root palsy affecting the long thoracic nerve can result in *winging* of the scapula.

Direct and indirect vision serve as tools for different types of observation. *Peripheral vision* is best for assessing movement. For example, to compare general gait or bilateral movements of the respiratory rib cage, the practitioner gazes at the center of the patient's body and uses peripheral vision to assess symmetry. *Central vision* is effective for evaluating small vertical or horizontal planes. (The practitioner's dominant eye is at a right angle to the plane being observed.)

To determine eye dominance:

1. The practitioner arm is extended, then a circle is made with thumb and index finger and a point across the room such as a clock is positioned within the circle.
2. Now close one eye. If the object is still inside the circle, that is the dominant eye. Sometimes one eye is dominant for near vision and the other is dominant for far vision (Figure 4-3).

Cutaneous and Trophic Changes

Trophic changes pertain to lack of nutrition in the affected area or tissues. Cutaneous trophic changes such as loss of hair, scaly skin, pimples, localized pigmentary changes, puffy skin (as opposed to acute swelling), and dimpling of the skin due to a pull of the fibrils from a chronic increase in subcutaneous interstitial fluids, may occur in a segmental, somatic, and sympathetic distribution *(OM: channel distribution)*. The practitioner can also consider which organ is innervated by the same sympathetic or somatic nerve and may need to treat the affected organs (Kuchera and Kuchera *ibid*).

Myofascial dysfunctions and a variety of symptoms, such as local or referred pain, tingling and burning, can result from scars. Muscle atrophy can be due to neuropathy, to a primary muscle disease, or from disuse.

Posture

An optimal posture may be defined as one in which postural muscles are at their resting tone and no additional energy beyond this basal level needs to be expended for the person to remain upright (Kuchera and Kuchera 1992). The *theoretical* central line of gravity has been described as a plum line which passes from the mastoid process, just in front of the shoulder joint, to a point in front of the knee and on to a point in front of the ankle joint. Deviation from this plum line is often significant when making *mechanical* assessments. Any compensation is then defined as the counter balancing of any defect of posture or function (Figure 4-5). It must be stated, however, that minor postural deviation and minor leg length discrepancies do not seem to have any *predictive* value in neck and low back pain (Andersson 1991; Pope et al 1985; Dieck et al 1985). In a failed back population and other back pain patients, however, Greenman (1992), Friberg (1985) and others *did* find a higher percent of patients with leg length differences.

In *Foundations for Osteopathic Medicine* (Ward 1997), Kuchera and Kuchera describe what they see as an *optimal posture,* highlighting its realistic impossibility.

> Optimal posture is a balanced configuration of the body with respect to gravity. It depends on normal arches of the feet, vertical alignment of the ankles, and horizontal orientation (in the

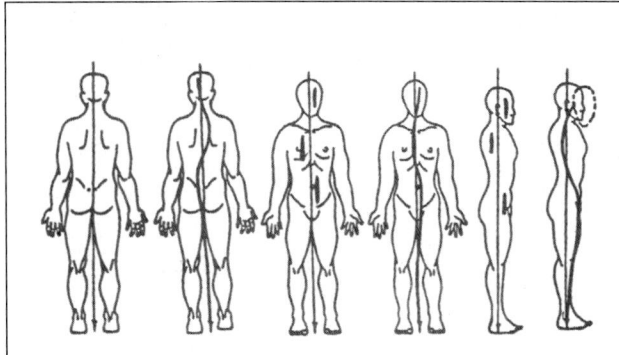

Figure 4-5: Recording a patient's posture (From Kuchera WA and Kuchera ML, Osteopathic Principles in Practice, KCOM press 1993, with permission).

coronal plane) of the sacral base. The presence of an optimal posture suggests that there is a perfect distribution of the body mass around the centre of gravity. The compressive force on the spinal discs is balanced by ligamentous tension; there is minimal energy expenditure from postural muscles. Structural and functional stressors on the body, however, may prevent achievement of optimum posture. In this case homeostatic mechanisms provide for "compensation" in an effort to provide maximum postural function within the existing structure of the individual. Compensation is the counterbalancing of any defect of structure or function.

Compensatory changes of the spine are often named according to their most prominent postural feature. Compensatory curves in the sagittal plane are called *kyphotic* or *lordotic* curves; compensatory curves in the coronal plane are called *scoliotic* curves; and compensations in the frontal plane are called *rotations* or *torsions* (Kuchera and Kuchera *ibid*). Functionally poor posture, which usually results in forward drooping due to gravity, may lead to slack abdominal muscles and diaphragm. These then fail to support the abdominal viscera which become *stagnant*. The disturbances of circulation resulting from a low diaphragm and ptosis may give rise to chronic passive congestion in one or all of the organs of the abdomen and pelvis. All these organs receive fibres from both the vagus and sympathetic systems, either one of which may be disturbed by poor posture and somatic dysfunctions. It is possible that many functional digestive and other organ disturbances may occur, and, if continued long enough, dysfunction may lead to diseases later in life (Chaitow *ibid*).

Posture and TCM

In TCM, posture is mainly controlled by constitutional Essence. Most postural disorders such as scoliosis and excessive lordosis or kyphosis are associated with deficiency of Kidney-Essence. Acquired scoliosis is associated also with Kidney-Essence as well as Spleen-Stomach weakness, Blood-stasis, and retention of Wind-Dampness or Phlegm in

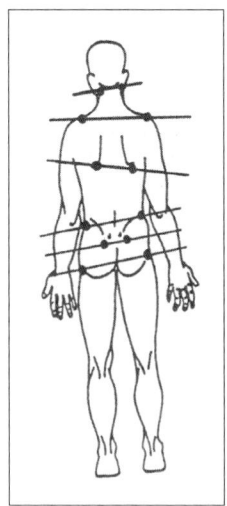

Figure 4-6: Recording a patient's posture (From Kuchera WA and Kuchera ML, Osteopathic Principles in Practice, KCOM press 1993, with permission).

the channels. A list or flattening of lumber lordosis (often due to discogenic disease) are often associated with Kidney and Liver disorders, mostly Liver-Qi-stagnation, Kidney-deficiency (Yin, Yang or Essence), Blood-stasis (often with Liver-congestion), and Cold or Hot pathogens. In patients with severe spasms and a list, Wind may play a role as well.

The *upper back* is influenced mainly by the Governing (Du), Urinary Bladder, and Lung channels. The *lower back* mainly by the Governing (Du), Urinary Bladder, and Kidney channels. The *pelvis* is influenced mainly by the Girdle (Dai) channel that circles the spine and connects to the Kidney Divergent channel, which also ascends alongside the spine, the Kidney Main channel and Organ that control the spine and bone, the Governing (Du) and Kidney, which enter the sacrum, and the Sinew channels of mainly the Kidneys and Spleen. The Sinew channels of the legs as well as the Yin and Yang Motility (Qiao) channels that control balanced muscular control of the lower extremities are important as well. The connecting channels of the Governing (Du) and Kidneys also connect and spread through the spine.

Palpation

Palpation can be very useful in aiding the diagnostic process and is greatly dependent on the style of therapy being used. When diagnosing a patient Orthopaedically, palpation (except for temperature) should follow the functional exam. If performed too early, an incorrect diagnosis is likely (Figure 4-9). The accuracy and value of palpation and manual evaluations are controversial (Morscher and Finger 1977; Panzer 1992; Matyas and Bach 1985; Hardy and Napier 1991) even though they are necessary for the type of therapies advocated in this text. Jull and Bogduk (1988) compared *manual diagnosis* to the criterion standard of local anaesthetic blocks. The authors found the sensitivity and

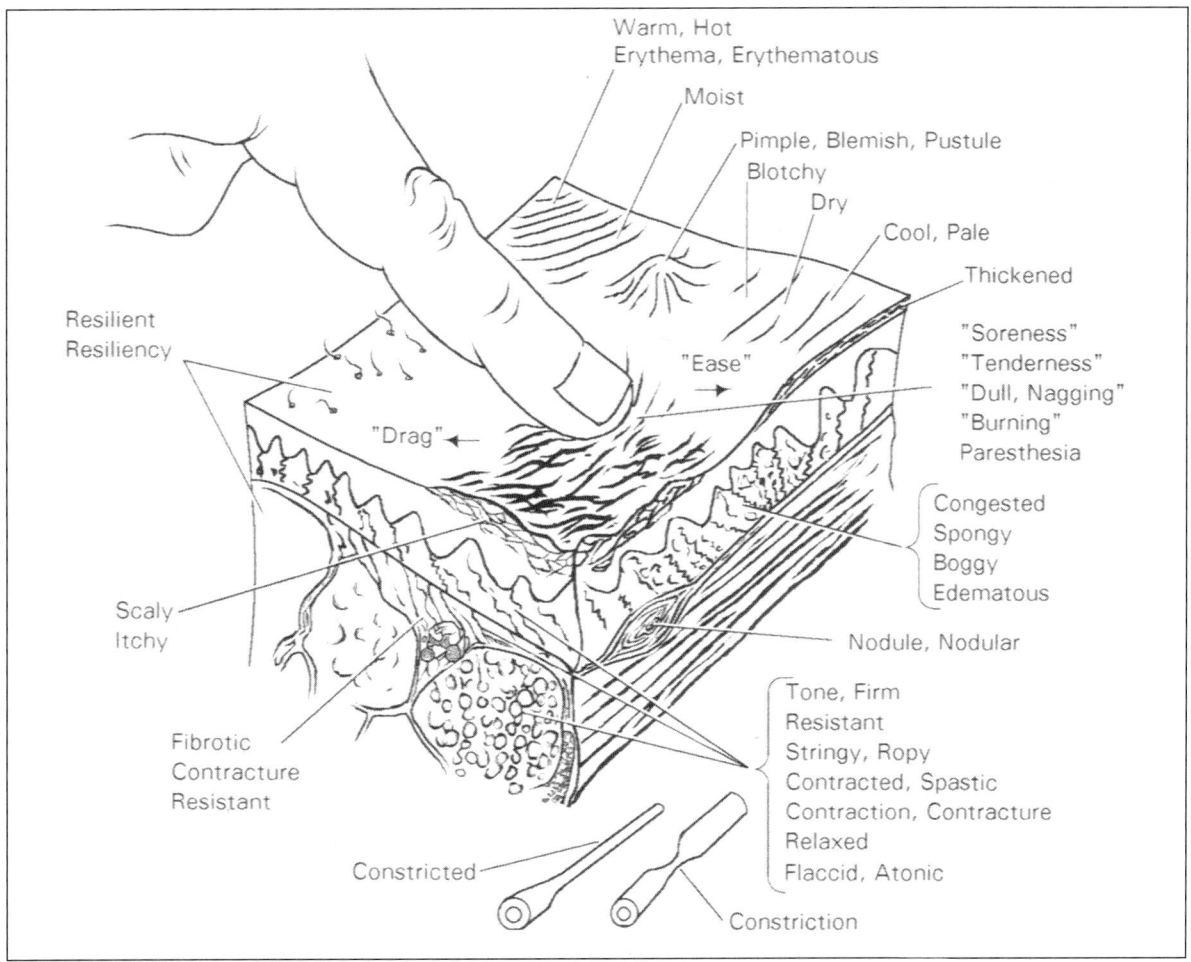

Figure 4-7: Soft tissue palpation (From Kuchera WA and Kuchera ML, Osteopathic Principles in Practice, KCOM press 1993, with permission).

specificity of the manual examination technique to be 100%. The manual therapist correctly identified all patients with proven joint pain, the symptomatic and asymptomatic segments. As this study shows, a skilled therapist is able to localize dysfunction. This suggests that isolating a segment or joint which is dysfunctional is possible by manual therapy techniques. At the same time, as stated in the beginning of this chapter, Bogduk's review of physical assessments of the spine show very poor reliability.

To assess by palpation, the practitioner must have a good three-dimensional perception of anatomy, knowledge of physiology, an ability to read the patient's expressions, and sensitive fingers. When palpating, the practitioner checks mainly for, asymmetry, tissue texture abnormality, temperature, and pain. Palpation requires the practitioner to *feel* with the hand on the patient; *see* the structures under the palpating fingers through a visual mind-image; *think* what is normal or abnormal; and *know* with an inner confidence (which comes with practice) that what one feels is real and accurate (Kuchera and Kuchera *ibid*). Using one's dominant hand is helpful. To find out which is the dominant hand, clasp both hands together; the one in which the thumb is on top is the dominant hand (and is not necessarily one's handedness)

Command of palpatory vocabulary is essential for recognizing normal and abnormal findings, not to mention for notation. The most common mistake when palpating is applying excessive pressure. This leads to guarding, elicits tenderness in normal tissues, and distorts the practitioner's perception. Pressure must remain within normal physiological range for the tissue being assessed. Too much pressure results in a false interpretation. When feeling for inert tissue movement, such as cranial or channel rhythms, it is often helpful to touch the patient's structure with as little pressure as it takes to feel, as though the palpating fingers and patient tissues were one. When palpating deeper tissues, it is helpful to just take-out slack of the more superficial layers and then "listen" to the deeper structure.

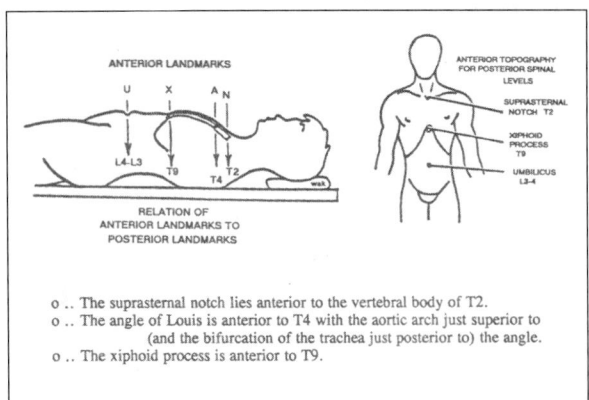

Figure 4-8: Anterior/posterior landmarks (From Kuchera WA and Kuchera ML, Osteopathic Principles in Practice, KCOM press 1993, with permission).

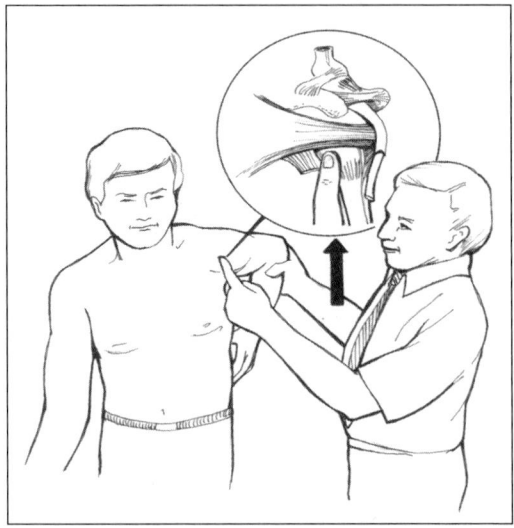

Figure 4-9: Palpation for tenderness is performed only after the functional examination. For example, here the practitioner palpates the anterior shoulder only after resisted internal rotation was found to be painful (courtesy Dorman and Ravin *ibid*).

Palpating for Temperature and Swelling

Before beginning dynamic assessments, the practitioner uses the *dorsum* of the hand (especially middle phalanges) to detect variations in the patient's skin temperature and feels for obvious swelling with the pads of the fingers.

Palpating for Movement

Palpating for joint movements is an important part of functional assessment and for many manual therapies. At times it is difficult to feel bony structures, and palpating for movement between adjacent bones may be easier when touching both bones simultaneously with one finger/hand. When trying to ascertain which of a pair of bones moves first, it is often more sensitive to allow the bone to come toward the palpating fingers rather then to hold the pair of bony structures firmly. Light pressure is almost always preferable.

Progression of Palpation

Palpation should progress layer-by-layer, "taking up the slack" of each layer while proceeding inward with minimal pressure, in this order:

1. Above the skin to sense the body's temperature radiation, or to make a thermal diagnosis. This often should be conducted several centimeters above the skin and is said to reflect the body's vitality, or, in *OM*: some aspects of *Defensive-Qi*.
2. Superficial tissues (skin), for thickness, moisture, ease of displacement (turgor), and tenderness.
3. Subcutaneous fasciae.
4. Intramuscular fasciae.
5. Muscular and tendinous tissues.
6. Joint capsules.
7. (When possible) bones.

The practitioner might sense the patient's breathing, pulsations, cranial rhythm, organ and tissue vibrations/rhythms, bogginess, swelling, masses, resiliency, ropiness, increased tone, resistance, crepitus or the movement of joints.

In Orthopaedic Medicine, the practitioner palpates first for temperature, pulses, and swelling, identifies a possible lesion through selective tension and motion evaluations, and then palpates for tenderness all tissues that have been determined to be the *cause* of pain to further localize the lesion.

Palpation: Findings

A skilled practitioner can obtain a wealth of information from palpation. Tissue texture alteration, a semi-objective finding, is more important than pain and tenderness. The latter is subjective and can easily be misleading.

SKIN AND SUBCUTANEOUS MOBILITY. Skin mobility should be part of any examination. Skin mobility (turgor), which can be evaluated by rolling a skin fold or stretching the skin, is performed along the entire length of the spine *(OM: along the UB and GV channels;* Figure 4-10). Frequently, the skin roll points to dysfunctions that underlie a positive finding. Various authors have shown skin fold tenderness to corollate with musculoskeletal dysfunction and pathology (Baker 1951; Campbell 1983; Hirschberg Lynn and Ramsey 1994). Signs often include changes in thickness of skin and subcutaneous tissues, with accompanying tenderness. Positive findings are common above a joint or dysfunctional motion segments (adjacent vertebrae). Unilateral findings

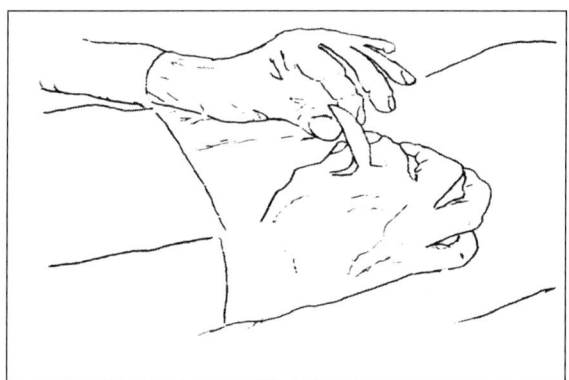

Figure 4-10: Skin roll.

are seen with vertebral (somatic) dysfunction. Bilateral and extensive findings can suggest a serious condition. Ward (1997) states that "tightness suggests tethering, while looseness suggests joint and/or soft tissue laxity, with or without neural inhibition."

The skin roll is both diagnostic and therapeutic. To perform skin rolling, the practitioner grasps a skin fold between the thumbs and index fingers and rolls the skin superiorly: toward the neck, over the center of the spine, and at the sides of the vertebrae. Skin rolling (and cupping as a diagnostic procedure) can also be done over peripheral joints.

SKIN OVERLYING ACTIVE LESIONS. Skin that overlies inflamed structures can be hypomobile and moist, and it may feel warm (OM: Damp-Heat, Wind-Heat, Blood-stasis). If the patient has a chronic disorder, trophic changes such as: reduced skin mobility, increased (or more often decreased) moisture, change in appearance of skin pores, temperature, goose bumps, and hair loss might be present and might be segmental (dermatomal), sympathetic, or somatic nerve in distribution. These changes can point to segmental dysfunctions, a "facilitated segment"[13] or a sympathetic system involvement.[14] A light and quick touch over the skin often reveals increased friction at the level of the lesion. An application of alcohol to the skin can dramatize this finding in acute type dysfunctions and/or injuries. The fingers often glide just as easily over the dry skin in a region of chronic problem as they do over normal skin areas. The skin affected by chronic disorders, however, often feels slightly rough, scaly, or cool.

In the spine, this process can be used to identify joint dysfunctions and the neurologic level (*OM: channels and Organs*) involved.

---

13. A "facilitated segment" causes a vicious cycle of pain, tension/spasm, and increased neural activity due to somatic/vertebral dysfunction or other causes (see chapter 2).
14. Skin alterations in a chronic patient often reflect OM Blood and Lung systems. The distribution of the alteration points to the channel or Organ involved.

ASYMMETRIES: Asymmetries may be seen either during movement or with the patient still. They can point to:

- congenital abnormalities (e.g., short leg);
- compensatory changes (e.g., secondary rotoscoliosis due to sacral subluxation);
- degenerative changes (e.g., facet arthropathy);
- functional disorders (e.g., facet locking and muscle tension).

Although normal body development is never completely symmetrical (even the two sides of the sacrum are never symmetrical), the relationships among symptoms, function, and symmetry become significant clinically and are important for successful manual therapy and some acupuncture techniques.

When the position of a joint is faulty, some ligaments are stretched permanently and some are shortened. Because ligaments are not designed to tolerate continuous stretching and are subject to hysteresis, they can elongate, weaken, and become sensitive. If a joint is hypermobile, the ligaments may be palpably thin and long. In hypomobile joints, the ligaments may feel thick and short.

EXCESSIVE WARMTH/HEAT. Excessive warmth or heat means that an acute condition (acute inflammatory process) is active, or that a chronic condition is in an active phase/flare-up (such as rheumatoid arthritis or subacute lumbago). Heat is palpable in the initial stages of torn tissue, e.g., superficial sprains and strains, hemarthrosis (blood in the joint), and broken bones (as long as they are superficial enough). In the initial stages of torn tissues, rest does not affect the resulting heat. With hemarthrosis the heat remains constant, and movement is extremely limited. If adhesions and/or loose bodies lie in an obstructive position, palpable heat follows exertion and abates quickly with rest (Cyriax ibid). Malignant tumors that are superficial may also produce local warmth.[15]

EXCESSIVE COLD. Cold skin may occur in an area affected by a nerve root palsy *(OM: blockage, Cold, deficiency, or severing of channel and collaterals/network-vessels)*. This is true also in conditions that affect vascular functions, such as complex regional pain type-I and type-II, intermittent claudication, facilitated segment, and other conditions in which increased sympathetic tone accompanies the disorder (such as chronic pain, anxiety). A cold foot that occurs only after exertion suggests an iliac thrombosis. Heat or coldness of tissues or subjective sensing of either are an important aspects of selecting the appropriate TCM treatment methods.[16]

---

15. Thermography may be a sensitive test to pick up some tumors, such as breast cancer, earlier than other tests.
16. In general, skin over thoracic areas is warmer than skin over lumbar areas. The buttocks are often cooler than lumbar areas. This is due to the large number of capillaries in the lung tissues. The buttocks are often covered by significantly larger amounts of adipose tissues.

Table 4-2: Palpation of Contractile Tissues

LOCATION/TYPE OF TISSUE	TECHNIQUE/CONSIDERATION
TENOPERIOSTEAL JUNCTIONS	Carefully. They can be a site of trouble.
MUSCLE BELLY	Perpendicular to the muscle fibers; stroking the fibers gently as if they were the strings of a musical instrument.
WHEN SEEKING DEEP-LYING MUSCLES	Slowly and progressively deeper, keeping overlying muscles relaxed. Begin perpendicular stroking only after reaching desired depth.
TENDER TENDONS	Along the direction of their inserting fibers. Perpendicularly when defining their borders.

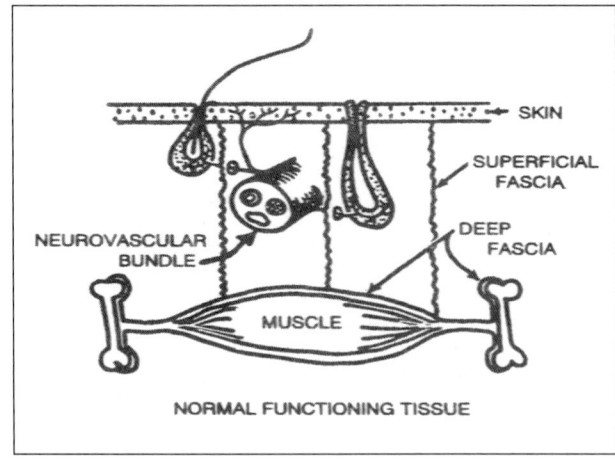

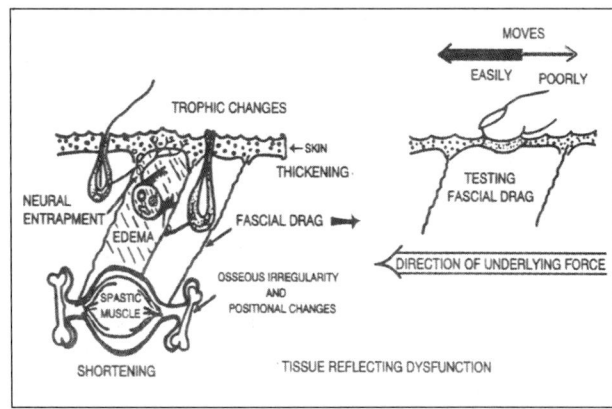

Figure 4-11: Tissue palpation. Normal functioning tissues (top), abnormal tissue (bottom) (From Kuchera WA and Kuchera ML, Osteopathic Principles in Practice, KCOM press 1993, with permission).

RESTRICTIONS OF TISSUES OR MOVEMENTS. The practitioner can detect restrictions of tissues or movements by palpating structures during their arc of motion. By understanding vertebral motions and by following a pair of transverse processes, the practitioner may identify restrictions and design treatments for restoring normal function. See Figure 9-8 on page 464.

SWELLING. Swelling may be palpated as a result of articular/cellular reaction to a lesion and may be local or general. Often fluid fluctuation can be demonstrated in acutely inflamed joints. In a local swelling, the consistency should be ascertained: a soft swelling indicates subcutaneous clear fluid or a thickened bursa, a fluctuating mass may result from a haematoma or from a mucocele, and a hard but still flatulent swelling is typical of a cyst or a ganglion. When the consistency is bony, the cause is usually a callus, a bony subluxation, an osteophytic outcrop, or any other bony deformity which results from destructive processes. A thickened synovial membrane is found in rheumatoid, bacterial or other inflammatory type arthritis. It is not found in mechanical conditions such as traumatic arthritis, post-immobilization arthritis, and arthrosis. To palpate capsular thickening, the practitioner seeks the reflection of the membrane where it overlies a bony prominence (Ombregt et al *ibid*). Trophic edema is often found in chronic conditions with neuropathic involvement.

PALPATION OF CONTRACTILE TISSUES. Following an examination of the superficial integument, the practitioner palpates deeper fascia and muscles, looking for severed tissues, fibrotic changes (found in chronic conditions), taut muscular bands, and trigger points. The practitioner palpates as indicated in Table 4-2.

To determine whether tenderness lies in a superficial or deep structure, the practitioner can palpate the area during contraction and relaxation of the superficial muscle. Pain that is more pronounced when the muscles are tense suggests that the superficial muscle is at fault (*OM: Sinew channel*).

To demonstrate muscle "spasms" and/or triggers, the practitioner finds:

- indurated tissues—tight bands—that lie parallel to the uninvolved fibers;
- thickening of spindle-shaped tissue (contraction knot);
- cross-fiber, stroking-evoked muscle twitch;
- tenderness and referred pain.

Objective tissue changes are more significant than the elicitation of pain. The practitioner must establish the *source* of pain, because referred tenderness is a common phenomenon. It is common to feel palpable looseness over painful areas, particularly in chronic cases. Typically, there is little or no muscle spasm or tightening. The associated muscles are often weak and inhibited. It is necessary to ascertain if such looseness is due to hypermobility from ligamentous laxity or reactive weakness from inhibition from other tighter areas. Inhibition or laxity may leave the affected joints vulnerable to repeated injury and sprain.

PERIPHERAL PULSES AND THE VASCULAR SYSTEM. The practitioner should also palpate peripheral pulses, because arterial pathology is a common cause of pain. The most common areas checked are the femoral pulse at the thigh, the

Table 4-3: Regional Pulses

POINT	ARTERY	INDICATION
ST-5	Facial	Condition of mouth and teeth
ST-9	Carotid	Condition and balance of head and/or channels (compared with radial pulse)
TAIYANG	Zygomaticoorbital and deep temporal	Condition of the forehead
TW-21, 22	Superficial temporal	Condition of eyes, ears, head, neck, urinary system
GB-2	Superficial temporal	Condition of head, neck, ear, eyes, hypochondrial region, Gall Bladder
SI-16	Cervical	Condition of Small Intestine channel, head, urinary system
LU-1 TO LU-4	Axilary	Condition of Lung channel
H-1	Axilary	Condition of Heart and Heart channel, and/or chest
H-7	Ulnar	Condition of Heart and Heart channel
LU-9	Radial	Condition of Lungs and vessels
P-8	Common palmar digital	Condition of chest, Pericardium, and mental
LI-4, 5	Pollicus, radial	Condition of chest and Lungs, the Large Intestine channel
SP-11-12	Femoral	Condition of Spleen/pancreas channel
UB-40	Popliteal	Condition of the head, neck, back, and urinary system
ST-42	Dorsal metatarsal	Condition of head, teeth, gums, epigastric area, Stomach channel and Organ
LIV-3	Dorsal metatarsal	Condition of head, eyes, abdominal area, and Liver Organ and channel
K-3	Posterior tibial	Condition of the Kidneys, Bladder, and reproductive organs, head and neck

dorsalis pedis pulse on the top of the foot (which may be congenitally absent), the popliteal pulse at the back of the knee, and the posterior tibial pulse at the medial malleolus area. The carotid and temporal pulses are checked often as well. Important areas for palpating pulses in TCM assessment are summarized in Table 4-3.

CAPILLARY REFILL TIME: The time it takes the capillary bed to fill after it is occluded by pressure can give some indication of the health of the vascular system. The practitioner blanches the nail bed with a sustained pressure of several seconds, on a toenail or fingernail. The time it takes for normal color to return after releasing the pressure is noted. Normally, it should return in less than two seconds. A slow return may indicate arterial occlusion, hypovolemic shock, or hypothermia.

VASCULAR INSUFFICIENCIES: Vascular insufficiency can result in musculoskeletal like pain. In general, *arterial insufficiency* results in symptoms that come on during exercise and are quickly relieved by rest. Pain in the calf muscles is often due to the superficial femoral artery, in the thigh from common femoral or external iliac artery, and in the buttock from the common iliac artery, or the distal aorta. Pain in the upper extremities is unlikely to be due to peripheral arterial occlusion (cardiac vessel disease can result in arm pain). *Venous insufficiency* comes on during or after several hours of exercise. It is relieved by rest but sometimes only after several hours or even days. The pain tends to be constant.

CREPITUS, SNAPS, POPPING, AND CRACKS. Crepitus (grinding, creaking and rough sounds) always indicates a pathological condition in that they indicate a change in the tissues, but may be clinically irrelevant. These sounds may originate from articular, tendinous, muscular, osseous, or bursal in origin. Crepitus sounds are heard, and often felt, by the palpating hand placed over a moving part during active or passive evaluations. Sometimes crepitus may be heard during resisted movements. A snap sometimes occurs when a tendon catches against a bony prominence and then slips over it. Because snaps are not necessarily painful, if a patient has a pain and a snap, the two may not be related. Popping and clicks can be heard with meniscal lesions and in joints that are hypermobile—especially, the clavicular joints, shoulder, or in a rupture of the medial collateral ligament at the knee. A click can also be heard with joint derangement or with loose body in the joint, as is frequently seen in the jaw, knee, elbow, and spinal joints. A crack may be heard when manipulating or mobilizing a joint and is usually due to an intra-articular air bubble from the synovial fluid as a result of the partial vacuum created by traction (Ombregt et al *ibid*).

ARTICULAR CREPITUS. This crepitus originates from the joint surfaces. Fine crepitus indicates a slight roughening and occurs in mild arthrosis or in longstanding rheumatoid arthritis (RA). RA gives rise to the characteristic "silken" crepitus. A coarse grating is felt in more advanced cases.

TENDINOUS CREPITUS. Crepitus from tendons is seen with tenosynovitis. Fine silky crepitus occurs in acute mechanical cases, while coarse crepitus is felt in chronic rheumatoid or tuberculous tenosynovitis.

MUSCULAR CREPITUS. Muscular crepitus is seen in two situations only. The first is together with tenosynovitis of the two extensors and of the long abductor of the thumb at the distal end. The second is in lesions of the musculotendinous junction of the tibialis anterior muscle.

OSSEOUS CREPITUS. A fracture may crepitate when the limb is moved and is accompanied with much pain.

BURSAL CREPITUS. The subdeltoid bursa often leads to crepitus when inflamed. Creaking on moving the arm is felt sometime after the effusion has subsided.

SCAPULOTHORACIC CREPITUS. The posterior thoracic wall can become roughened and lead to crepitus when moving the arm. It is usually painless and requires no treatment. When associated with pain it can be due to bursitis or osseous projection (Ombregt et al *ibid*)

TCM and Palpation

In TCM palpation is often done over the body surface, chest, abdomen, channels, points, and pulses. Palpation can proceed from the superficial thermic layer (Defensive [Wei] Qi), superficial skin (Fu), deep skin (Ge), subcutaneous (Ji), spaces between the skin and muscles (Cou Li), the fat and muscle (Fen Rou), the muscles and flesh (Rou Ji), and the bone (Gu) using increasingly stronger pressure. In general, one palpates for temperature, tissue texture, and pressure pain. Palpation along the Sinew (or Main) channels for Ashi-tender, Kori-indurated (or rough skin and muscles) and "slack" points or areas are of utmost importance in the treatment of musculoskeletal disorders. Distal points as well as visible cutaneous or vascular changes are said to reflect more the Connecting channels, while proximal points reflect more the condition of the Main channel (or Organ) associated with the tender point. Indurated points (tight bands, fibrous muscle tissues, etc.) often reflect the Sinew channels. The distribution of these palpatory finding is essential in making channel diagnosis and in selecting distal and local acupoints for treatment.

In general, firm and strong muscles are associated with health and strength. Soft muscles and excess fat is associated with Deficiency and Phlegm. Ashi-tender points are said to be associated with a lack of movement of Qi and Blood, induration (and roughness of skin or muscle) with stasis of Qi, Blood or Phlegm. Areas or points which lack tone, are dry or non-resilient are associated with Deficiency. It is common to find all of the above qualities within a single channel or body area. This may reflect interactions between blocked circulation with accumulation and consequent lack of nourishment in other areas within the same channel or vessels.

Palpable radiant-heat, especially if stronger in Yang areas than Yin areas, is considered to be caused by Excess/Full conditions. If radiant-heat is stronger in Yin areas than Yang areas, it may be due to Empty-Heat. If the radiant surface heat is strong as one first touches the skin but abates with extended palpation, the Heat is said to be at the Exterior (skin and muscles); if, however, the radiant-heat increases with prolonged palpation, the Heat pathogen is said to come out of the Interior (Organs, bones, and Yang-Ming). It may be caused by Dampness "raping" Heat (i.e., Damp-Heat with Dampness being predominant). If in acute febrile disease of recent onset the skin is palpably dry, then the condition is said to be due to Excess; while, if the skin is Damp, the condition may be due to Deficiency. Radiant-Heat with dry skin in a chronic condition is often associated with deficient-Blood/Yin or Fluids. Radiant-Heat with wet skin in chronic conditions is often associated with excess-Heat and Damp-Heat.

The most common cause of cold hands and feet is Yang-deficiency. Lung or Heart-Yang-deficiency can cause cold hands only. Kidney-Yang-deficiency will cause coldness of the feet and lumbar region. Spleen-Yang-deficiency tends to cause cold hands, while Stomach-Yang-deficiency may cause both cold hands and feet. When both Kidney and Spleen/pancreas are Yang-deficient, all the limbs tend to be cold. When only the hand and feet (the toes and fingers) are cold, Qi-stagnation may be the cause. Qi and Blood deficiency can also result in cold hands and feet. When only one limb is cold, the cause is often obstruction of Qi and Blood by Phlegm (or Phlegm-Heat). Phlegm (or Phlegm-Heat) may also obstruct Qi and Blood in both limbs and cause cold hands and/or feet. In severe-Heat, the hands and feet may be cold but the forehead and trunk are often warm.

A medium degree of pressure is used along the muscles and channels to ascertain the presence of stagnation and Pathogenic Factors, while deep pressure is often used to palpate the Organs and bones. When heat is felt with strong pressure, it is often due to Yin-deficiency Empty-Heat, especially of the Liver and Kidneys.

A strong dislike of pressure is associated with Excess, while relief of pain with pressure is associated with Deficiency.

Distention, swelling, lumps, and nodules may be caused by Deficiency, Excess, substantial (Blood-stasis, Phlegm) or sometimes by insubstantial (Qi-stagnation, Deficiency) conditions. Well- defined, hard, and fixed masses are often due to Blood-stasis. Well defined masses that are movable or softer are often due to Phlegm accumulation. Poorly defined swellings that are not fixed or that change in location or character are often associated with Qi-stagnation. A subjective sense of swelling but without objective findings is often due to Qi-stagnation or Deficiency of Qi or Blood.

Arthritic conditions that are characterized by articular signs, swelling, and spurs are often due to Pathogenic Factors entering the sinew and bones with Qi/Blood stagnation

Physical Examination

Table 4-4: TCM Palpation

FINDINGS	MECHANISM
ASHI-TENDER POINTS	Lack of movement of Qi and Blood
INDURATION (AND ROUGHNESS OF SKIN OR MUSCLE)	Stasis of Qi, Blood or Phlegm
LACK TONE, ARE DRY OR NON-RESILIENT	Deficiency
RADIANT-HEAT • Stronger in Yang areas than Yin areas • Stronger in Yin areas than Yang areas • Abates with extended palpation • Increases with prolonged palpation • Recent onset skin is dry • Recent onset the skin is Damp • Dry skin in a chronic condition • Wet skin in chronic conditions	• Excess/Full conditions • Empty-Heat • Heat is said to be at the Exterior (skin and muscles) • come out of the Interior (Organs, bones, and Yang-Ming). It may be caused by Dampness "raping" Heat (i.e., Damp-Heat with Dampness being predominant) • due to Excess • due to Deficiency • deficient-Blood/Yin or Fluids • Excess-Heat and Damp-Heat
HEAT FELT WITH STRONG PRESSURE	Yin-deficiency Empty-Heat, especially of the Liver and Kidneys
HEAT OR COLD WITH MEDIUM DEGREE OF PRESSURE	Ascertain the presence of stagnation and Pathogenic Factors in muscles and channels
COLD HANDS AND FEET • Cold hands only • Coldness of the feet and lumbar region • Only the hand and feet (often only toes and fingers) are cold • Only one limb is cold • Hands and feet cold but the forehead and trunk warm.	• Most common Yang-deficiency; also Qi and Blood deficiency; Stomach-Yang-deficiency; Kidney and Spleen/pancreas are Yang-deficiency; or Phlegm (or Phlegm-Heat) obstructing Qi and Blood (may be only one hand or foot, etc.) • Lung or Heart-Yang-deficiency; Spleen-Yang-deficiency • Kidney-Yang-deficiency • May be caused by Qi-stagnation • Obstruction of Qi and Blood by Phlegm (or Phlegm-Heat) • May be severe-Heat
DISTENTION, SWELLING, LUMPS, AND NODULES WELL-DEFINED, HARD, AND FIXED MASSES ARE OFTEN DUE TO BLOOD-STASIS.	• May be caused by Deficiency, Excess, substantial Blood-stasis or Phlegm, or sometimes by insubstantial (Qi-stagnation, Deficiency) conditions
WELL DEFINED MASSES THAT ARE MOVABLE OR SOFTER	• Often due to Phlegm accumulation
POORLY DEFINED SWELLINGS THAT ARE NOT FIXED OR THAT CHANGE IN LOCATION OR CHARACTER	• Often associated with Qi-stagnation
A SUBJECTIVE SENSE OF SWELLING BUT WITHOUT OBJECTIVE FINDINGS	• Often due to Qi-stagnation or Deficiency of Qi or Blood

and Kidney/Liver weakness. Pitting edema is often due to water accumulation and/or Kidney-Yang-deficiency.

Percussion

Percussion of the abdomen and lungs is part of a general physical examination. It can be used to determine the state of solidity and the size of organs. Percussion of bone is part of the orthopedic examination. The practitioner can use a reflex hammer to tap a symptomatic and tender bone. Findings of severe bone pain upon direct percussion is suggestive of fracture and/or cancer. Percussion of the spinous processes may help identify a facilitated segment. The practitioner percusses using a reflex hammer with one hand while monitoring the adjacent muscles for activity. Muscles around a facilitated segment would become active. At times, these same muscles are active even when the spine at other levels are percussed.

Auscultation

The auscultation of bowel and breath sounds is part of a general physical examination. Auscultation for a bruit in the arteries is important in musculoskeletal medicine, because, as stated above, arterial disease can be the cause of muscular-like pain. Arterial blockage can result in a swirling of blood which becomes audible, called a bruit. Normally one cannot hear the blood rush through the arteries using a stethoscope. An audible bruit is most evident over large blood vessels such as: carotid, vertebral, temporal, cardiac vessels (murmurs), aorta, and femoral artery. When heard over the abdomen, a bruit may indicate an aortic dissection, aneurysm, or thrombosis. It may also indicate a dissection or aneurysm of the splenic, renal, or iliac arteries. A bruit over the carotid artery may result from local or transmitted sounds. Transmitted sound include: murmurs resulting from valvular aortic stenosis, ruptured chordae tendineae of the mitral valve, or severe aortic regurgitation. Local sounds may indicate obstructive disease in the cervical arteries (which means absolutely no manipulation should be done to the cervical spine), such as atherosclerotic carotid arteries, fibromascular hyperplasia, arteritis, or small emboli. Mild obstruction produces a short, but not particularly strong, localized bruit; greater obstruction lengthens the duration and heightens the pitch. Complete obstruction eliminates the bruit (Bates *ibid*).

General Orthopedic Testing: Joints

To use the examination this text describes, the practitioner must understand the *joint barrier* and *end-feel* aspects of joint assessment:

Joint Barriers

Joint barriers are physiologic and anatomic barriers that the practitioner can see or sense. Joint barriers are described as:

- Anatomical (Total Range of Movement).
  — This specified the extent of movement possible without injury at a joint, from one anatomical barrier to the other. Movement beyond the anatomical barrier always results in injury.
- Physiologic.
  — This aspect of the barrier describes the extent of active movement (movement performed by the patient) available in the joint.
- Elastic.
  — This is the next-level range of movement, available only by passive assessment (through movement conducted by the practitioner). Thrust manipulations are active within the elastic barrier, in this "potential space."

  (OM: the potential space at the elastic barrier is an area where "Qi force" can be stored. Martial artists learn to

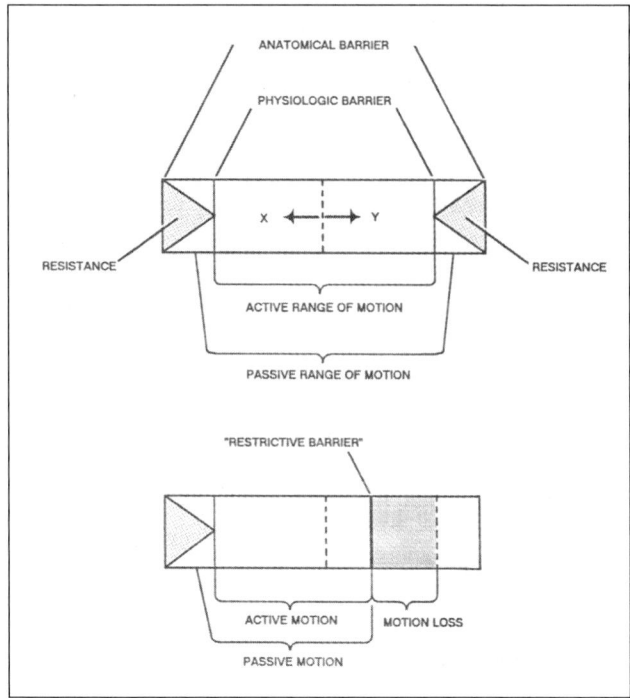

Figure 4-12: Joint barriers (From Kuchera WA and Kuchera ML, Osteopathic Principles in Practice, KCOM press 1993, with permission).

control the opening and closing [pumping] of these spaces to both cultivate and release "energy.")

- Restrictive.
  — This is a pathological barrier that interferes with the normal physiologic barrier. Usually this is found in one or more directions.

Direction of Bind

The more the joint is moved from midline neutral toward the elastic barrier (toward the end-range of a joint), the more tissue resistance (bind) the practitioner can feel. This resistance, called "direction of bind," is due to soft tissue stretching.

Direction of Ease

The farther from the elastic barrier toward the midline neutral (loose-packed position), the easier the movement becomes, and the less resistance is felt. This is called "direction of ease."

Techniques that are designed to correct *pathological barriers* by moving a joint through the restrictive barrier are called *direct techniques*. Techniques that are designed to correct *pathological barriers* by moving a joint way from the restrictive barrier, are called *indirect techniques* (or functional techniques, when movement is incorporated).[17]

Table 4-5: Evaluation Using Selective Tension

Motion Tested	Target
Active Range of Movement and Associated Sensations	Ability / willingness of patient. Degree of muscular strength. Direction of painful movements.
Resisted Movements (Isometric Contractions)	Evaluation of contractile units.
Painful Arc	Seen in pinchable lesions.
Passive Range and Sensations	Evaluation of elastic and anatomical barriers. State of inert (non contractile) tissues.

Midline Neutral

Normal joints and tissues have ranges of movement in which there exists, *approximately* in the midrange of motion, an area of "ease" or balance, where the tissues are least tense. When there is a restriction in normal function, whether of osseous or soft-tissue origin, the now limited range will almost always still have a place, a moment, a point, which is neutral, of maximum comfort, or ease, that is lying somewhere between the new restricted barrier in one direction, and the physiological barrier in the other direction. Finding this balance point, also known as "dynamic neutral," is a key element in functional Osteopathic technique (Chaitow 2002). Midline neutral is *not* necessarily located in the *middle* of the available active or passive range. Midline neutral is somewhere within the total range of movement or motion and can shift with dysfunction or pathology. Midline neutral can be different in different joints. *Joint play* is best appreciated at the midline neutral (loose-packed) position.

Dysfunction

Dysfunction usually includes a mixture of some restricted movements and some full movements. The area of motion loss, as defined by the restrictive barrier, becomes the new physiological barrier. Dysfunction is also defined by loss of normal joint play.

End-Feel

End-Feel is the characteristic sensation the practitioner perceives at the end of the patient's passive ROM. Normal end of range for soft tissues is felt as a progressive build-up of tension, leading to a gradually reached barrier, as all slack is removed. The best technique for establishing the cause of restriction is assessing the end-feel; the results may even suggest a diagnosis. Passive movements are performed by the practitioner and must reach the end of range. A slight overpressure at end-range is performed to assess the end-feel. The end-feel also has therapeutic implications, for example, for deciding whether to manipulate the spine or stretch a joint. Different pathological conditions give rise to different end-feels (Table 4-6).

Rubbery, Leathery

The normal end-feel of the joint capsule when stretched is rubbery or leathery. In this state, the sensation is like stretching a thick rubber band. This end-feel can be found, at times, in non-acute arthritis or arthrosis (in the absence of significant muscle spasm and where the anatomical barrier is not engaged). Arthritis and arthrosis, however, are more frequently associated with a hard end-feel. *(OM: Normal end-feel suggests that the Liver, Blood, Kidneys, and channel and vessel functions, as they pertain to the joint, are essentially healthy).*[18]

Boggy, Spongy, Soggy

Boggy or spongy end-feel occurs in the presence of edema. It also occurs in some early joint effusions in which movement of the joint comes to an abrupt stop but resistance fades slightly with sustained pressure. The soggy end-feel is somewhere between a soft and an empty feeling. It is typical of rheumatoid arthritis in the upper cervical spine. *(OM: This end-feel suggests a diagnosis of Dampness and/or Phlegm).*

Hard

This end-feel occurs when bone-to-bone contact causes the restrictive block or when adhesions cause the restriction. It can also occur when strong muscle spasms restrict movement. A hard end-feel can be normal for some joints, such as elbow extension in which engagement of the olecranon process in the olecranon fossa and strong ligaments suddenly limit the range of motion in that vector. Muscle spasm, in

---

17. The same principle can be used with acupuncture needling technique, where it is called "indirect needling technique" by the author. The needle is inserted at a local or distal point with the palpating hand monitoring at the joint for ease. The needle is gently moved in all possible directions that increase *ease at the joint* (not at the needle site) and surrounding tissues.

18. It may be a mistake to look for "systemic Organ dysfunctions" instead of looking at joints and soft tissues to ascertain Organ functions as they apply to the musculoskeletal system. The Organs, Blood, Qi, etc. may become dysfunctional in their musculoskeletal sphere of influence alone.

Table 4-6: End Feel

Sensation	Indication	Main OM Indication
Boggy, Spongy	Edema. Early joint effusions.	Dampness and/or Phlegm,
Hard	Bone-to-bone contact causing a restrictive block. Adhesions. Strong muscle spasms. Capsular pattern. Can be seen in hypermobile joints.	Spleen/pancreas, Divergent or Extra channels and/or Kidney, Essence and bone disorders, mostly deficiency and excess combined with weak sinews and Organs and excess Pathogenic Factors.
Rubbery or Leathery	Normal examination of joint capsule when stretched. Non-acute arthritis or arthrosis.	Liver, Blood and Kidneys joint functions are healthy.
Springy Rebound	Internal derangement. Loose body.	Phlegm. Damp-Heat. or "Stone" (congealed Phlegm and Blood).
Empty, Soft	Acute or serious diseases. Psychosomatic causes.	Damp-Heat abscess. Latent-Heat and or Toxin. Trauma.

severe active lesions such as inflammatory arthritis or fractures can also give rise to a hard end-feel. (The restriction may be in the capsular pattern. See below.) If fibrotic tissues and/or adhesions are responsible for a reduction in range with a hard, rapidly ensuing end-feel, the tissues will still have a slight elasticity remaining. This end-feel often accompanies limitation of movement from capsular contracture, osteopathic outcrops, myositis ossificans, or a malunited fracture close to the joint. *(OM: A hard end-feel suggests Sinew channel, Kidney, Essence, and bone disorders, and/or Blood-stasis with Deficient disorders, and/or congealed Phlegm and Blood).*

Abrupt Hard Stop

This is a hard end-feel which occurs rather abruptly following a smooth, frictionless movement with some loss of end-feel resiliency (normal rubbery sensation) and is associated concomitantly with increased range of motion. This end-feel is seen often when the joint is hypermobile. In some hypermobile individuals or structures, the end-feel will be "loose" and the range greater than normal. *(OM: Abrupt/hard stop suggests Spleen/pancreas, Liver, Blood, Divergent or Extra channels and/or Kidney, Essence, and bone disorders—mostly Deficiency and Excess combined; weak sinews and Organs and Pathogenic Factors).*

Springy Rebound

A springy end-feel is found in the presence of internal derangement or a loose body in a joint. The sensation is as though something were pulling back at the end of the range of passive motion. Springy end-feel is also encountered when a spinal joint is localized correctly before manipulation; however, in this situation the end-feel is typically less springy than is felt with a loose body. *(OM: Springy rebound suggests Phlegm, Blood-stasis, Damp-Heat, Damp-Cold, or "stone" [congealed Phlegm and Blood]).*

Empty, Soft

An empty, soft end-feel occurs when the patient halts the movement because of severe pain before normal tissue resistance occurs, indicating that the physiologic or elastic barrier has not been reached. An empty, soft end-feel can be an indicator of acute or serious diseases that must be ruled out, such as an extra-articular abscess, acute bursitis, or cancer. Psychosomatic causes should be considered as well. A soft end-feel can also be due to a loose body blocking movement, as may be seen at the elbow when extension is limited by a few degrees with a soft end-feel. It may also be seen with dislocated joints. *(OM: empty/soft end-feel suggests Damp-Heat abscess, Latent/Warm-Heat and/or Toxins and trauma.)*

Selective Tension

Selective tension, the heart of the Cyriax approach to Orthopaedic Medicine, is a process by which the practitioner isolates and tests tissues for pathology. This method is very helpful for identifying lesions in the extremities. Table 4-5 summarizes the four aspects of a selective tension examination.

During the examination both active (patient initiated) and passive (practitioner initiated) motion/movements can be painful. Since the active assessment stresses both contractile and inert (noncontractile) structures, and the passive assessment stresses mostly inert structures, the significance of these examinations does not come to light until after the resisted movement tests are performed.

Active Movement

The end points of active movements are due to the "physiological barrier." Active movements indicate:

- ability and willingness of the patient to perform the movement;
- range of movement possible;

Table 4-7: Passive Evaluations

Symptom/Sign	Indication
Pain at Full Range	Often caused by the stretching or pinching of affected tissues. Also can be caused by the squeezing of tissues such as the bursa between two surfaces (e.g., subdeltoid bursa by the acromion and humerus, the Achilles between the tibia and calcaneus on full passive plantar flexion). The localization of the pain will very often be indicative. Tendinitis. • Usually the patient has full passive range of motion unless: —the inflammation has started spreading to the capsule or —pain restricts movement. Found commonly in joints in which the tendon contributes to formation of the capsule (such as the shoulder) or where stretching of the lesion is painful, as in some muscular and musculotendinous lesions.
Sudden Halt, Short of full range	Most likely caused by a bony block and/or adhesion of soft tissues. Bony end-feel is found in the presence of arthrosis and in joints that have bone spurs.
Full Passive Range Without Ability to Perform the Movements Actively	Suggests loss of muscle function due to either mechanical or neurological causes.
Hypermobility Excessive Range	Can occur: • following injury, especially in joints not under muscular control, such as: acromioclavicular, sternoclavicular, sacroiliac, sacrococcygeal, symphysis pubis (and knee); • if ligaments around a joint are loose due to degeneration; • if joint space is decreased, such as with loss of disc height; • in presence of several connective tissue disorders, such as: — Marfan's syndrome (patient taller than average with arm span greater than height) — Ehlers-Danlos syndrome (skin excessively pliable). Asymptomatic hypermobility can be a normal variant, especially in women, and is then bilateral.
Immobile Joint	May be secondary to severe muscle spasm, septic arthritis, or fibrous or bony ankylosis.

- degree of muscular strength;
- direction of painful movements.
- (OM: Mostly function of Sinews channels, network-vessels, Spleen/pancreas and/or Liver and/or Blood and Kidney condition).

The practitioner uses active movement to observe the ergonomics of function and the presence of functional substitution and compensations. This kind of assessment serves as a screening tool that may indicate the area of dysfunction quickly or indicate an area that should be examined more closely. The practitioner compares the results with the results of the passive motion and resisted movement examinations. When a normal range is found on passive testing and normal muscle strength is apparent when tested against resistance, there should be no reason for any abnormality or restriction of active movement.

Passive Motion and Inert Structures

Evaluation of passive range of motion tests elastic and anatomical barriers (end-feel) and the state of the *inert tissues* of a joint (tissues that are noncontractile and are moved only passively): Capsule and ligaments, bursae, fasciae, bony aspects of a joint, nerves and dura.[19] *(OM: Function of Sinews channels, network-vessels, Extra channels, Divergent channels, Connecting channels/vessels, Spleen/pancreas, Liver, and/or Blood, Essence/ Kidneys and Pathogenic Factors).*

Passive testing can provide useful information about individual joints, and it may indicate the nature and stage of pathology (such as acuteness, inflammatory nature, restriction and/or elasticity). Although passive motions are performed mostly to test inert structures, it is important to remember that they also stretch muscles and therefore can stimulate pain arising from them. When evaluating the passive ROM and end-feel, the sequence in which the pain and limitations occur should be noted. Every joint has a unique end-feel, although most have an elastic soft tissue stretch feel. The end-feels at the elbow for example have the following characteristics:

- Elbow extension is limited by strong ligament tension and engagement of the olecranon process in the olecranon fossa that feels like bone-to-bone contact at full extension. This yields a hard end-feel. Full extension of the knee also feels hard, but less so, since it is limited by the posterior cruciate ligament.

- Elbow (full) flexion is limited by soft tissue approximation (the biceps muscles), which yields a soft muscular end-feel. This *extra-articular* end-feel does not occur in patients with poorly developed muscles: they present an articular end-feel, either hard or elastic (Ombregt et al *ibid*).

---

19. Some new evidence suggests that many of these structures are not completely inert and may be capable of inert motion.

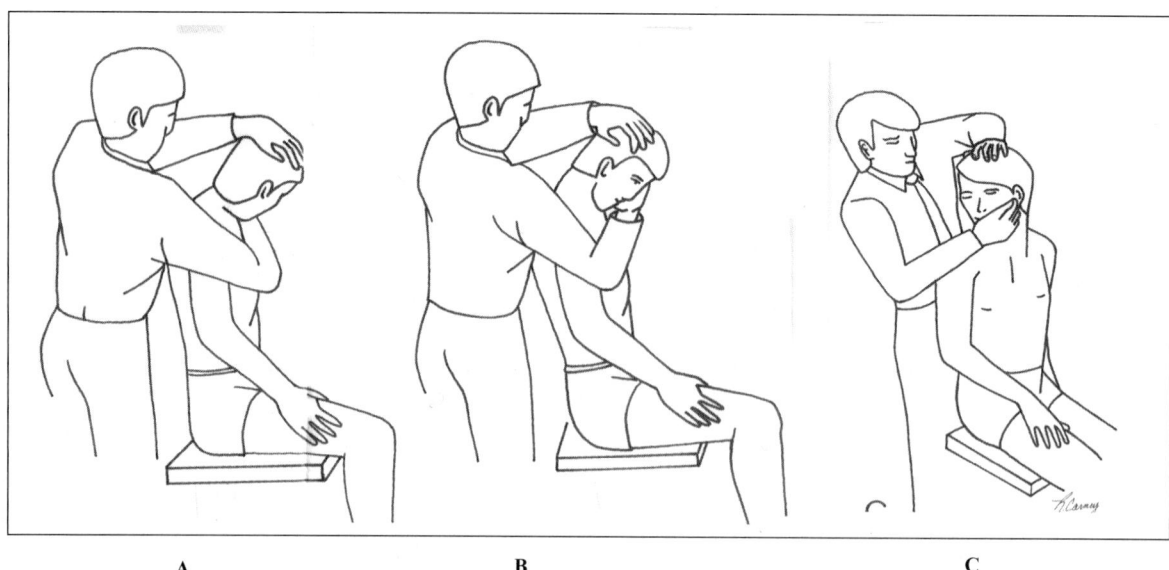

Figure 4-14: A passive flexion-rotation-extension test for cervical spine. The head is moved from a flexed and rotated position into an extended and rotated position. Flexed and rotated position (A) tests the upper cervicals, extended and rotated position (C) tests the lower cervical spine. Pain and/or resistance to movement is assessed and can quickly point to an area of dysfunction, which is then assessed carefully (courtesy of Dorman and Ravin *ibid*).

Assessment of Passive Motions

For passive motion assessment, the patient must be relaxed and allow the practitioner to perform all the movements. This relaxed state eliminates conscious control and muscular effort by the patient and makes it possible for the practitioner to evaluate the end-feel at the joint.

When engaging the physiological barrier the practitioner applies a little quick over pressure, paying special attention to the end-feel and noting abnormalities. For each joint, the practitioner must be familiar with the normal degrees of movement. Comparison with a similar but unaffected joint is useful for identifying variations specific to the patient. At times, to assess a painful arc, the practitioner must complete passive motions even though the patient feels pain and/or resists Figure 4-20.

In nerve root pain it is important to remember that passive movements of adjacent joints can stretch the nerves/dura (analogous to straight-leg raising) and cause pain to come from the spine. Often there is no limitation in range except for pain.

DRAWER TESTS. Drawer tests are passive tests used to assess excessive range of motion due to ligamentous laxity or tear. The joint is held by the practitioner and pulled or pushed to assess range (Figure 4-13).

APPREHENSION SIGN. The apprehension tests are used to assess the patient's reaction to extreme movements. These are often positive when the joint is unstable. The patient resists movement and is apprehensive, feeling the joint is going to sublux, a clunk may be heard (Figure 4-17).

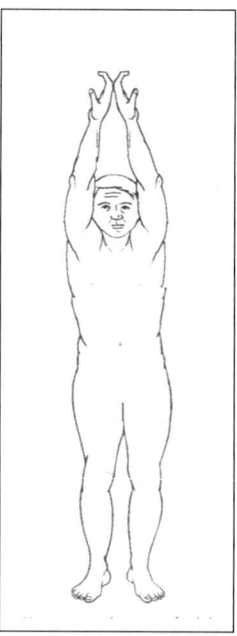

Figure 4-15: Upper extremities active movement screen. This movement requires motions in shoulder girdle, elbow, and wrist joints (From Kuchera WA and Kuchera ML, Osteopathic Principles in Practice, 2ed rev Graden press 1994, with permission).

General Orthopedic Testing: Joints

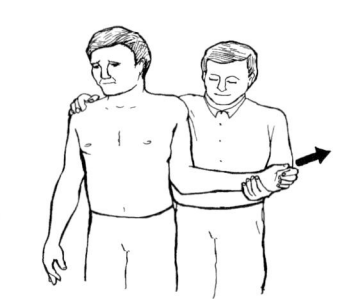

External rotation at the shoulder. A slight over pressure is exerted at end-range and the end-feel assessed.

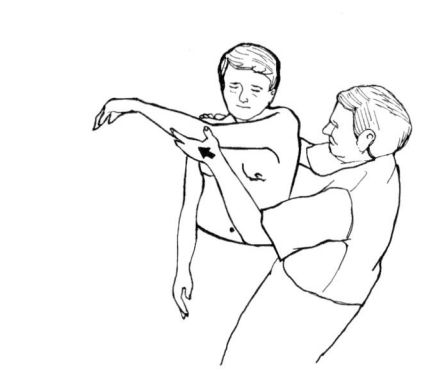

Passive adduction across the front. Slight over pressure is exerted at end-range.

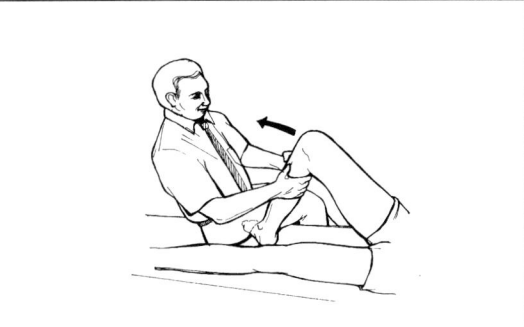

Drawer test for knee stability and cruciate ligaments. Excessive movement indicates ligament laxity or tear.

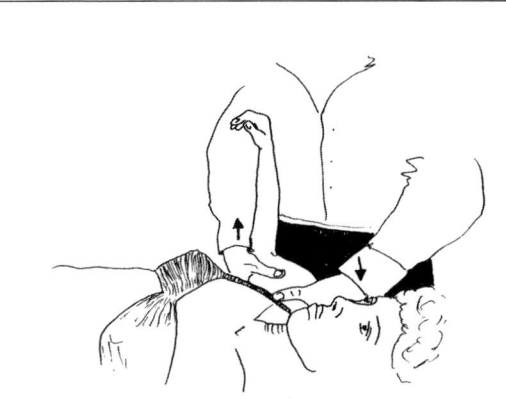

Drawer tests at shoulder. Excessive movement or lag in movement between humoral head and scapula indicates instability.

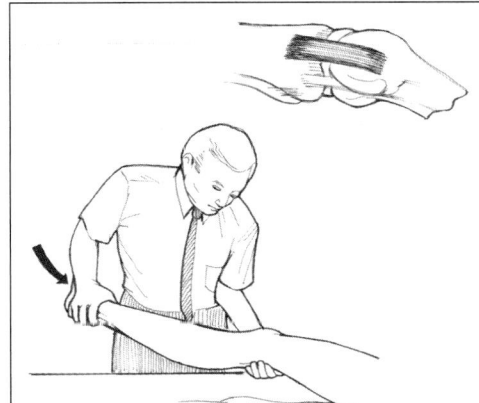

Valgus over pressure at the knee. Pain or excessive movement indicates a lesion in the medial collateral ligament.

Figure 4-13: Examples of passive tests.

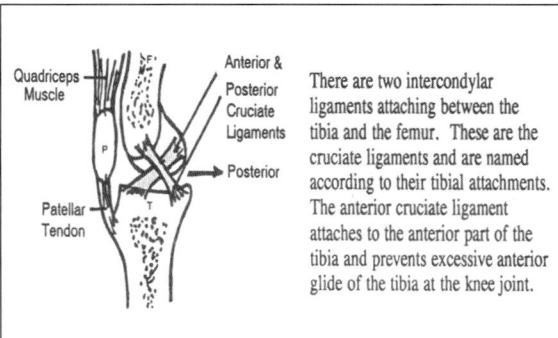

Figure 4-16: ACL and PCL. Drawer tests are often used to test for excessive movement due to tears (From Kuchera WA and Kuchera ML, Osteopathic Principles in Practice, KCOM press 1993, with permission).

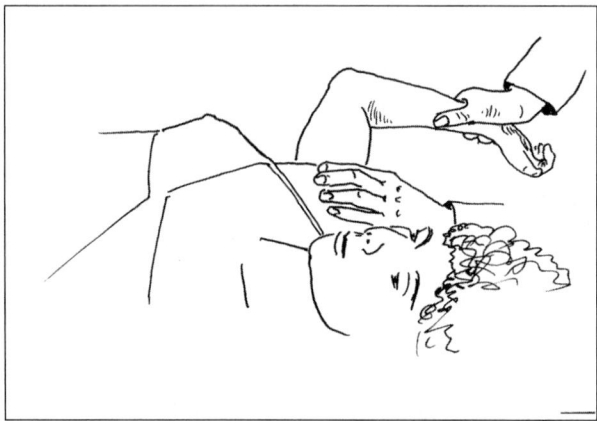

Figure 4-17: Apprehension test for the anterior capsule of the shoulder. The test is positive when the patient apprehensively resists this movement with a sense that the joint is going to "go out." There may be a clunk as well.

Types of Limitations

During passive assessment, limitations of movement and motion can be in the capsular pattern or the noncapsular pattern.

- A *capsular pattern*, which is a specific pattern of limited movements, is found in conditions that affect the entire joint, such as arthritis, arthrosis, or capsular irritation. It is found only in joints under muscular control (i.e., it is not found in the acromioclavicular (AC), sternoclavicular (SC), sacroiliac (SI), sacrococcygeal, lower tibiofibular and symphysis pubis joints) (see page 230).

- A *noncapsular pattern*, which is a restriction of movements not in a capsular pattern (also called a *partial articular pattern*), is found with ligamentous adhesions, internal derangements, vertebral/joint dysfunctions, and extra-articular lesions.

Table 3-7 on page 225 summarizes the indications suggested by some symptoms and signs found in passive testing.

Contractile Unit Testing

Testing of a contractile unit (a muscle and its attachments) requires the isolation of the muscle. Therefore, the practitioner who is assessing muscle strength must have an understanding of muscle function.

The testing of individual muscles is useful for evaluating peripheral nerves, spinal nerves, and contractile unit function and their disorders. Resisted movements (fixed isometric contractions) which help the practitioner assess the contractile unit, may provoke pain and/or demonstrate weakness.

To prevent movement during isometric (resisted muscle) testing, the test is performed with the joint at mid-range and stabilized. This stabilization is achieved by the correct positioning of joint and practitioner during the examination; which allows the practitioner to be stronger than the patient, preventing unwanted movement.

Testing can involve:

- Isometric contraction with resisted muscle testing (resistance against a movement performed by the practitioner);
- Isotonic/active motion performed against resistance, gravity, or modified gravity.

A measure of muscle strength should be charted periodically. Several grading scales are available for documenting muscle strength. A simple grading scale for active movements is:

	GRADE	INDICATES
N	Normal	A complete range of movement against maximal resistance.
G	Good	Complete ROM against moderated resistance.
F	Fair	Complete ROM against gravity.
P	Poor	Complete ROM with gravity eliminated.
T	Trace	Evidence of some muscle contractility but no joint motion.
0	Zero	No palpable contraction.

Table 3-8 on page 230 summarizes findings of contractile unit tests.

Resisted Movement Testing

When testing isometric contraction (resisted movement), (Figure 4-18), the practitioner encourages the patient to pull or push with maximal effort while the practitioner applies enough counterforce to prevent movement. Although the practitioner cannot eliminate movement of the joint completely, this kind of movement should be kept to a minimum. Some inert tissues are stimulated by the resisted movement, and minor shear movements may occur (thereby stimulating noncontractile tissues), but such instances are usually minimal.

General Orthopedic Testing: Joints

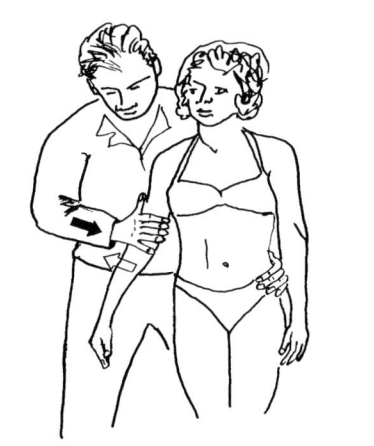

Resisted muscle testing, shoulder abduction. The patient abducts the arm against unyielding resistance by the practitioner.

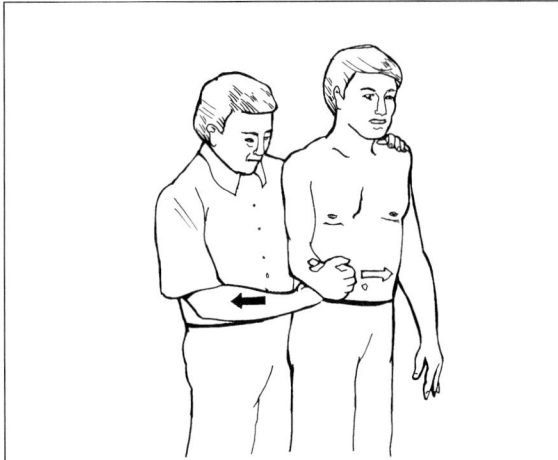

Assessment of resisted internal rotation at the shoulder. The patient internally rotates the arm against unyielding resistance by the practitioner.

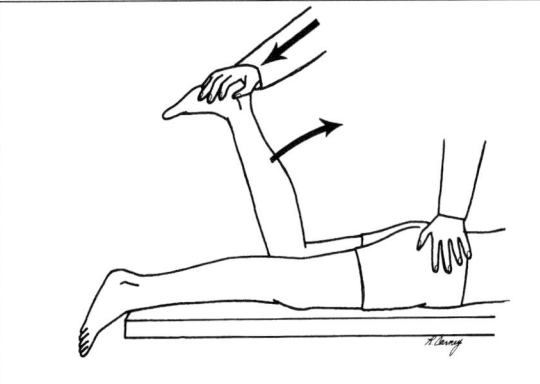

Assessing resisted flexion of the knee for hamstring lesion. The patient flexes the knee as hard as he/she can while the practitioner resists and does not allow any movement.

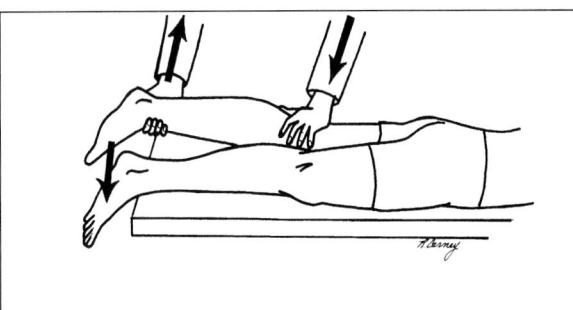

Assessing resisted extension of knee for quadriceps lesions. The patient extends the knee as hard as he/she can while the practitioner resists and does not allow any movement.

Figure 4-18: Examples of resisted testing for contractile structures.

To obtain useful information, the practitioner must isolate the muscle that is to be tested. If several resisted movements are painful, or if incompatible movements hurt, the pain is unlikely to be of contractile (muscle-tendon) structure origin.

In the presence of arthritis and conditions that affect inert structures, resisted movements are generally painless. However, resisted movements can be painful if a lesion lies directly under or near the muscle, and during muscle contraction the muscle broadening stimulates that lesion. Lesions affected most commonly from this kind of secondary stimulation are bursae, abscesses, and inflamed lymphatic glands. Resisted movement may be painful in the presence of fractures, metastases, and psychogenic pain (Cyriax *ibid*).

Sometimes during an examination, even though resisted motions are painless, discomfort occurs when the patient relaxes the tension (lets go). This can occur if the tested muscle/tendon is minimally affected or if a joint is unstable, such as is commonly seen with unstable acromioclavicular (AC), or glenohumeral joints. Thus, when a joint is unstable, pain may be felt when the patient "lets go" and may present with any of several types of muscle contractions. If only one resisted movement is painful (either when letting go or dur-

Table 4-8: Contractile Unit Testing: Findings (Cyriax *ibid*)

A Finding That Is	Suggests
Strong and Painful	Minor contractile lesion. In tendinitis usually there is a full ROM. In muscular lesion there may be limited ROM.
Weak and Painless	Complete rupture of muscle or tendon. More often a nervous condition (palsy), in which case it may be painful.
Weak and Painful	Possible major disorder: sepsis, cancer, fracture. If only one movement is painful and weak and joint moves normally, then possibly there is a contractile unit problem (tendinitis or muscle lesion).
Two Movements Painful	Two contractile structures are affected. One muscle is affected but has combined functions.
Pain on All Resisted Movements	Transmitted stress from muscle contraction, often seen in severe condition. Underlying general sensitivity, a mental state.
Pain following Sustained or Repetitive Contractions	Intermittent claudication (poor blood supply). Tendinitis in a strong patients or minor lesion.
Painless	Arthritis; conditions affecting inert structures.

ing contraction), then the muscle or tendon is likely to be at fault.

When testing resisted movements, the practitioner makes note of abnormal sensations, both when the muscle is contracted and when the muscle is relaxed. The practitioner may need to repeat resisted movement tests several times in order to elicit pain from a minor lesion, especially in stronger patients. To facilitate the eliciting of pain, the practitioner can place the muscle in a position that is mechanically disadvantaged, with the joint and muscle at other than mid-range. This may help demonstrate minor lesions that are not detected using regular examination techniques.

Common Patterns of Passive and Resisted Movements

Passive and resisted examinations are highly effective for determining the source of musculoskeletal pathology, which often presents in common patterns.

Capsular Pattern. The capsular pattern is a specific standard of range of motion restrictions seen when the joint is inflamed. (There is a specific pattern for each joint, e.g., the shoulder.) The capsular pattern is a limitation (to a relative degree) of specific movements in specific directions when a joint has arthritis, arthrosis, or when the capsule is inflamed. Regardless of whether the inflammation is of the synovial membrane, the fibrous capsule, or both, a capsular pattern is seen (Cyriax ibid).

In the presence of a capsular pattern:

- Some movement has some degree of limitation.
- All movements may be limited, but usually to different degrees.
- Arthritis, arthrosis, or capsulitis of each joint has its own pattern of limitation. For example: the capsular pattern in the *shoulder* is some limitation of scapulohumeral abduction (Figure 4-19), with the greatest limitation being in lateral rotation and the least limitation in internal rotation. In the *elbow*, there is usually more limitation in flexion than extension, although equal limitation may be seen. In the *wrist*, equal limitation of flexion and extension is seen. The *fingers* are usually equally limited in flexion and extension, while the *thumb* is limited more in backward movement and extension than in flexion. In the *hip*, internal rotation has the greatest limitation, while less limitation is seen in flexion, abduction, and extension, and external rotation is not limited. In the *knee*, flexion is much more limited than extension. The *ankle* would be slightly more limited in plantiflexion than in dorsiflexion. In the foot, the capsular pattern of the *subtalar* joint is fixation (complete absence of movement) in full valgus. The *midtarsal* joints fixate in full abduction and external rotation. At the *first metatarsophalangeal* joint slight limitation of flexion together with a marked limitation of extension is seen (Table 4-9).

When active and passive movements elicit pain in the same direction, and if the discomfort emerges near or at the limit of range, and if resisted movements are painless, the lesion is likely to be of an inert structure. This pattern occurs with arthritis, capsulitis, bursitis, and instability. The entire joint is affected only if the limitations are in the specific capsular pattern for that joint. Bursitis does not cause a capsular pattern.

In the initial stages of arthritis, a patient might not have the entire capsular pattern. In such a case, the movement

Table 4-9: Capsular Pattern

JOINT	PATTERN
SHOULDER	Some limitation of scapulohumeral abduction, greatest limitation in lateral rotation and least limitation in internal rotation
ELBOW	More limitation in flexion than extension, equal limitation may be seen
WRIST	Equal limitation of flexion and extension
FINGERS	Equal limitation of flexion and extension
THUMB	More limitation of backward movement and extension than in flexion
HIP	Greatest limitation of internal rotation, less limitation of flexion, abduction, and extension. External rotation is not limited
KNEE	Much more limitation of flexion than extension
ANKLE	Slightly more limitation of plantiflexion than in dorsiflexion
SUBTALAR	Fixation (complete absence of movement) in full valgus
MIDTARSAL	Fixation in full abduction and external rotation
FIRST METATARSOPHALANGEAL	Slight limitation of flexion together with marked limitation of extension

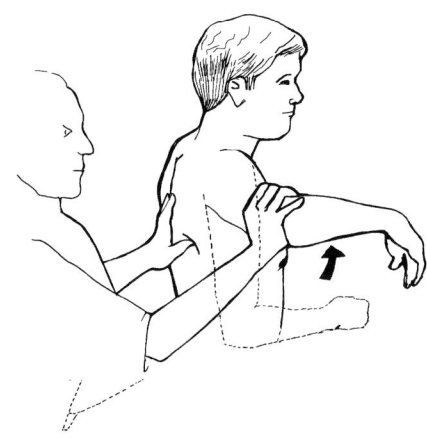

Figure 4-19: Assessing scapulohumeral abduction. The scapula should start moving when the arm is at about 90 degrees obduction.

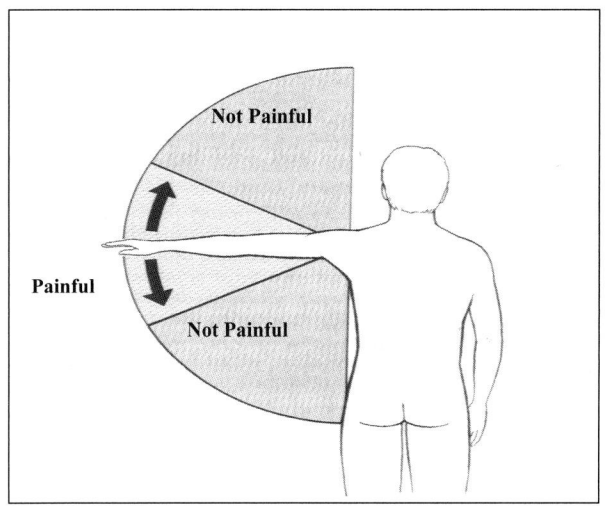

Figure 4-20: Painful arc.

may be limited in only one *predictable* direction, such as lateral rotation in the shoulder and internal rotation in the hip.

In capsulitis of acute onset, muscle spasm is usually responsible for the limited ROM, stimulated by the hypersensitive capsule; whereas, in chronic arthritis, the cause of restriction can be from a tight capsule and ligaments. When secondary adhesions form, the limitation may change and become one of a noncapsular pattern (Cyriax *ibid*).

NONCAPSULAR PATTERN. When a patient presents with limitation of movement that is not in a capsular pattern (i.e., there is only a partial articular pattern), the responsible lesion does not involve the whole joint. These conditions may be due to internal derangement, vertebral and joint dysfunctions, ligamentous adhesions and lesions, or extra-articular lesions. In the presence of ligamentous adhesions and extra-articular lesions, the patient feels pain when the adhesion or lesion is stretched. Therefore, some movements can be painful while others are not (Cyriax ibid)—i.e., joint dysfunction.

INTERNAL DERANGEMENT. Internal derangement is found when a loose fragment blocks some aspect of the joint. The onset of pain is often sudden and may give rise to pain and limitation of movement in the direction that engages the block. Typically one or more movements are limited and painful while at least one movement is free. The restriction may be disproportionate in one direction. This occurs commonly when a partially-torn anterior horn of the meniscus blocks the knee joint, blocking extension markedly but with

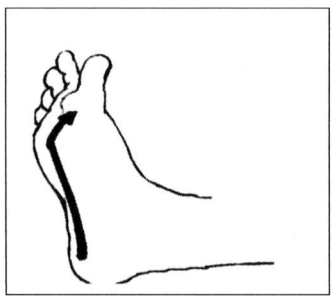

Figure 4-21: Positive Babinski sign. When the bottom of the foot is stroked, the big toe points up.

little flexion restriction. A small displaced fragment that lies in a position that does not greatly hinder the function of the joint, may cause a small proportionate limitation.

The joints that are prone to developing a loose body are: the vertebral facet, knee, jaw, and spinal vertebral discs. Joints that develop a loose body less frequently are the hip, elbow, and tarsal joints (Cyriax *ibid*).

EXTRA-ARTICULAR LESIONS. Extra-articular lesions are suspected when only one direction of movement is grossly limited but all other movements are full and painless. This state can be found in the presence of bursitis, partly torn muscles, or other contractile lesions, and in situations in which a particular movement stimulates a cyst or other lesion (Cyriax ibid).

PAINFUL ARC. "Painful arc" refers to pain that the patient feels during part of the active or passive movement but that abates as the movement continues (Figure 4-20). A painful arc implies the presence of a compressible lesion (Cyriax ibid). For example, when pain is felt upon rasing the arm only during part of the motion this is often caused by part of an inflamed tendon getting pinched between the acromian and the humeral head. When the inflamed portion moves on the pain subsides.

Neurological Testing

Neurological tests are design to assess the condition the peripheral and central nervous systems. In general, clinical neurological testing (in musculoskeletal practice) includes evaluations called:

- Motor
- Sensory
- Reflex.

Motor Tests

Motor tests are basically resisted muscle tests and are performed in a way similar to the orthopedic evaluation, except that weakness (or true spasm) is what is looked for. A weak-

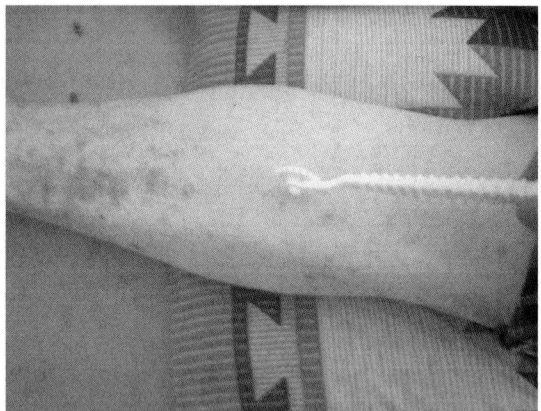

Figure 4-22: Pinwheel assessment.

ness of a muscle or muscle group may result from disruption in the nerve supply from a nerve root, which often affects the myotome with multiple muscles. It may also result from the disruption of nervous supply by a peripheral nerve. In mild nerve root compression, such as in a small disc lesion, muscle weakness may be only demonstrable in the small muscles of the myotome. For example, in mild impingement of L5 root (which supplies the gluteus medius, peronei, and extensor hallucis muscles), clinical motor deficit (muscle weakness) may only show when comparing left and right resisted extension of the big toe (Figure 4-23). Frank spasms are most often due to upper motor lesions.[20]

Sensory Tests

Sensory examinations basically involve stroking the skin to see if there is altered sensation. It is best to test both the symptomatic side and the non-symptomatic side at the same time so that the patient can tell if there is a difference between the two. A pinwheel can be used to ascertain the exact borders of sensory deficits (Figure 4-22). A storke with a cotton ball and a poke with a needle can be used to ascertain if the patient is able to tell the difference. A patient with true numbness would not be able to tell the difference between the dull sensation from being stroked with a cotton ball and the sharp sensation felt by needle pokes.

Understanding peripheral as well as dermatomal distributions is needed to interpret the findings. Dermatomal distributions are determined by the skin areas innervated by a nerve root (Figure 4-25), while peripheral distribution is determined by the peripheral nerves.

---

20. Neurons of the upper motor neuron system contribute to the formation of the pyramidal (corticospinal) and corticobulbar tracts, which may be affected by trauma and by vascular, neoplastic, and other diseases. Lesions often result in hyperactive reflexes.

Neurological Testing

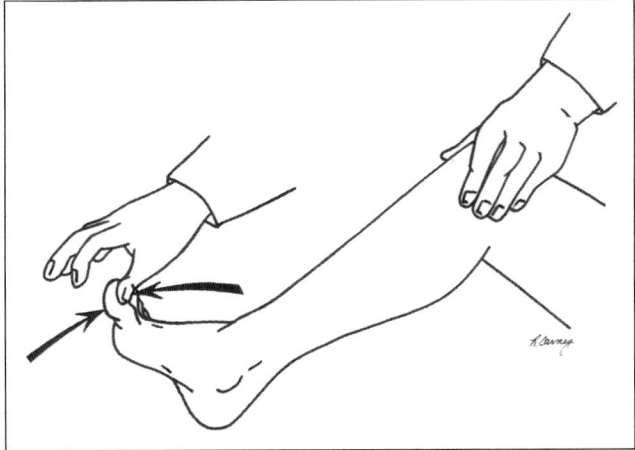 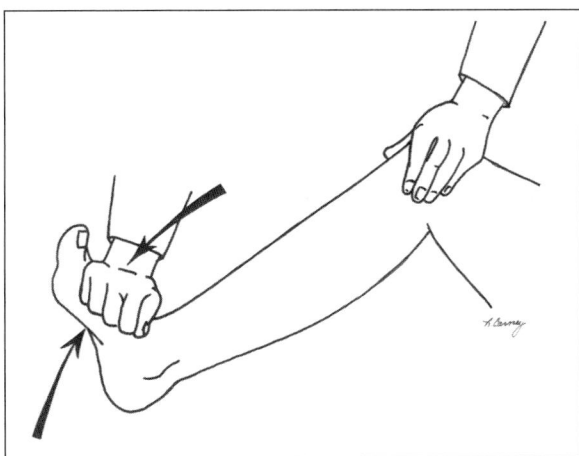

Figure 4-23: Both resisted toe extension and resisted ankle dorsiflexion test the same nerve root. In mild cases one may see weakness when testing toe extension, while ankle dorsiflexion remains strong. This is so because the small muscles which are also down steam may be affected first.

Reflexes

Reflexes are inborn stimulus-response mechanisms that can be classified according to the level of their representation in the central nervous system. The essential neural portion of a reflex includes a sensory neuron and a motor neuron. (Other structures are involved as well.) In its simplest form, the reflex arc contains a primary afferent neuron in a ganglion and a centrally located motor neuron connected by a synaptic junction. Because only one synapse separates the input from the output, this circuit is called a "monosynaptic reflex." In orthopedics, the superficial, deep, and/or pathological reflexes provide an objective indication of the state of the peripheral nerves and of the nerve roots that supply the reflex. The reflexes also provide information on the status of the upper motor neuron system.

A distinction is made as to whether reflexes are normal, weak (absent or diminished), or excessive (exaggerated or clonus). Diminished or absent reflexes can result from any lesion that interrupts the reflex arc or nerve root, or can occur in the presence of peripheral nerve disease and cerebellar disease. Excessive reflexes are seen when lesions of either the cortex or the pyramidal tract (the descending cortical tract or upper motor neuron) result in decreased inhibition of normal reflexes.

The clinically most important reflexes are:
- Superficial (skin and mucous membrane)
- Deep (myotonic)
- Visceral (organic)
- Pathological (abnormal).

Grading of reflexes is usually as follows:
- 0 Absent
- 1 Diminished
- 2 Average (normal)
- 3 Exaggerated
- Clonus (causing repeated jerks).

Warning: Hyperactive reflexes can also be seen in the presence of strychnine poisoning and in some functional disorders. This must be remembered when prescribing Semen Strychnotis (Ma Qian Zi).

Deep Reflexes

The deep reflexes, also called "the deep tendon reflexes" (jerks), are the most commonly assessed in biomedical musculoskeletal medicine.

With practice, the practitioner can elicit reflexes (jerks) from almost any tendon (or muscle). Table 1-10 on page 236 lists the most common tendon reflexes assessed.

Superficial Reflexes

Table 3-11 on page 237 describes the superficial reflexes, subdivided here as mucous membrane reflexes (which are not highly relevant in orthopedics) and skin reflexes (which are considered in orthopedics occasionally).

Visceral Reflexes

The visceral reflexes are considered only occasionally in the musculoskeletal patient (generally after trauma). Table 3-12 on page 237 lists the visceral reflexes.

Pathological Reflexes

Medical science has identified numerous pathological reflexes such as Babinski (Figure 4-21), and Huntington's. A review of all of these reflexes is not within the scope of this text; however, several that are applicable clinically are mentioned in corresponding sections.

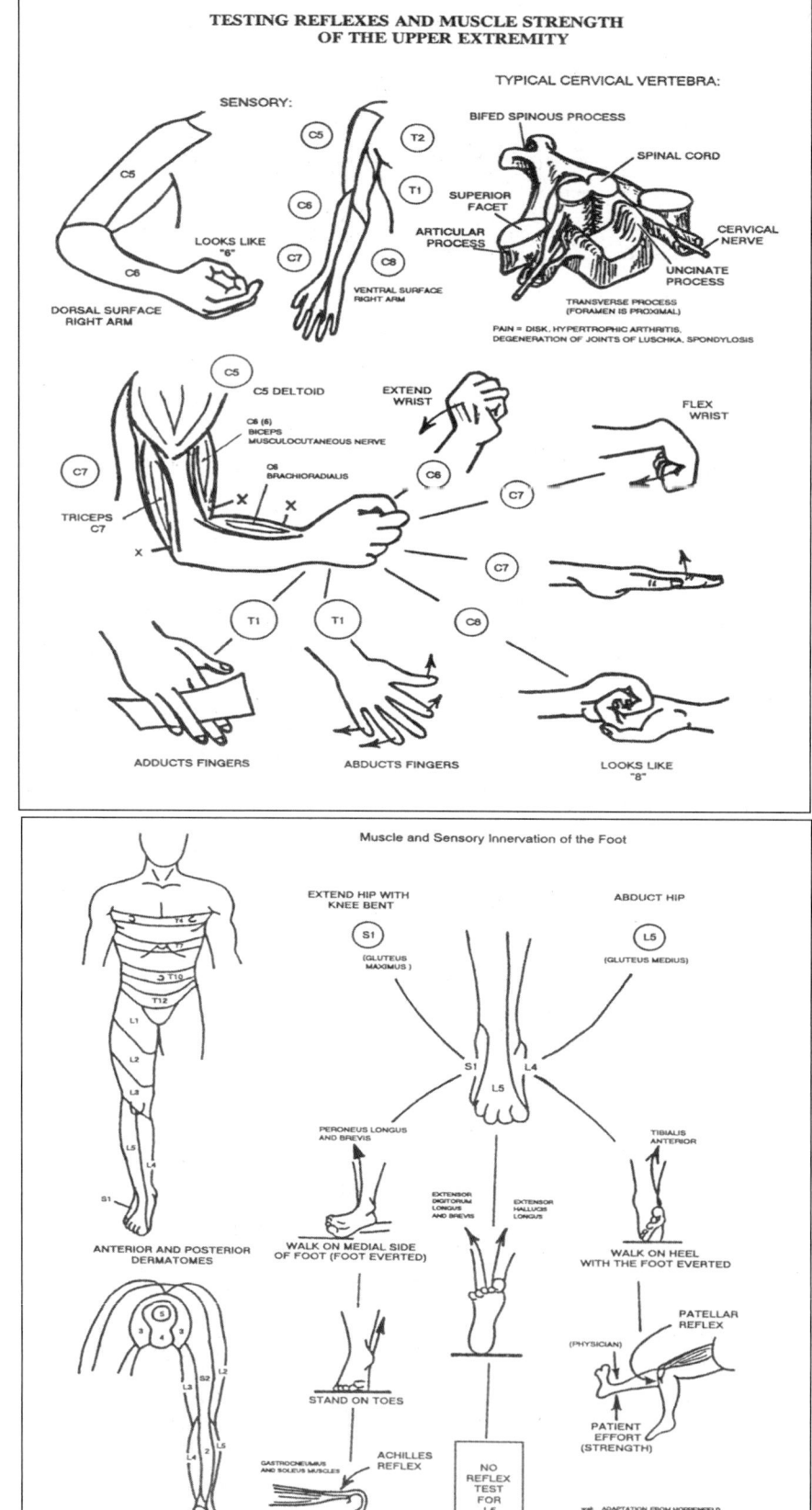

Figure 4-24: Neurological examinations. Upper extremities fand cervical spine top. Lower extremity and lumbar-sacral spine bottom. (From Kuchera WA and Kuchera ML, Osteopathic Principles in Practice, KCOM press 1993, with permission).

Neurological Testing

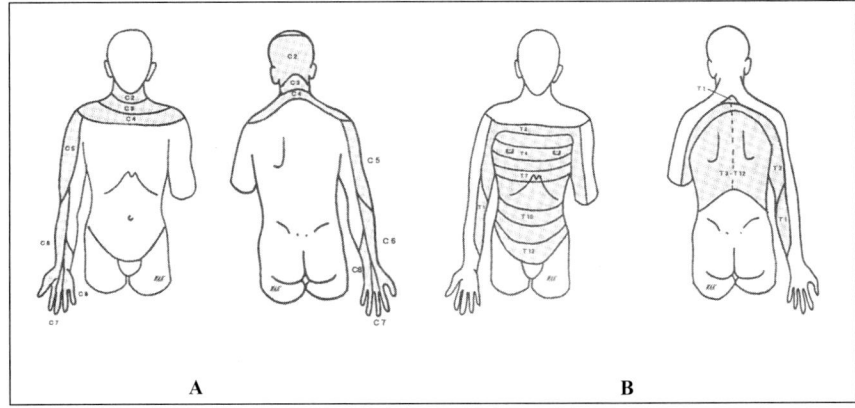
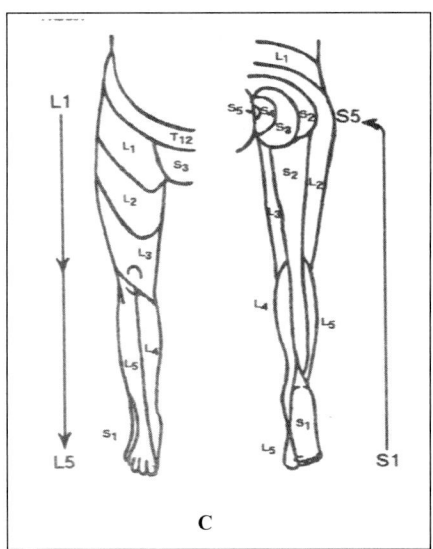

Figure 4-25: Dermatomes: (A) cervical, (B) thoracic, (C) lumbosacral (From Kuchera WA and Kuchera ML, Osteopathic Principles in Practice, KCOM press 1993, with permission).

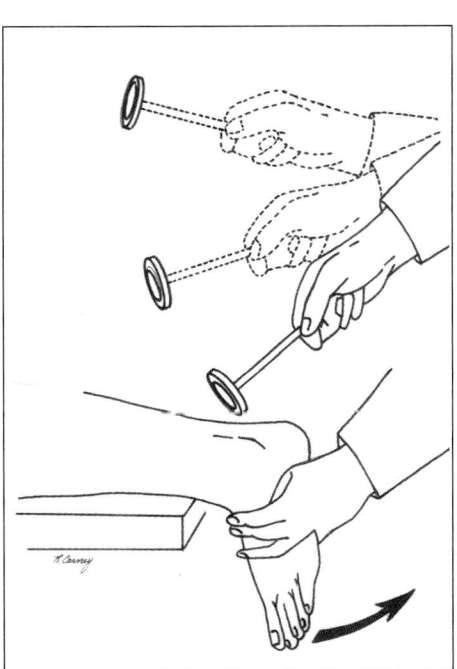

Figure 4-26: Deep tendon reflexes (courtesy of Dorman and Ravin *ibid*).

Neurological Examination of Patients with Neuropathic Pain Syndromes

In addition to performing a standard neurologic examination, several specific bedside sensory and motor tests should be used with patients suspected of having neuropathic pain (Galer and Dworkin 2000).

Sensory Tests

1. Mechanical allodynia: pain caused by mechanical stimuli to the skin *that are normally not painful* are tested as followed:
   A) Static Allodynia;
   — Application of light pressure to one local region results in pain;
   — Slowly applying perpendicular pressure with a blunt-tipped device (pencil eraser, cotton swab) results in pain.
     —Thought to reflect sensitized C-nociceptors.
   B) Dynamic allodynia;
   — Lightly rubbing the skin evokes pain;
   — Can use finger, cotton ball, or hair brush.
     —Thought to reflects A-β (nonnociceptors) afferent fibers.

2. Thermal allodynia: pain caused by thermal stimuli to the skin *that are normally not painful*.

Table 4-10: Deep Tendon Reflexes

REFLEX	DESCRIPTION	NERVE TESTED
MAXILLARY	Jaw reflex. A sudden closing of the jaw upon striking the middle of the chin when the mouth is slightly open.	Cranial V
BICEPS	Flexion of the elbow when the biceps tendon or muscle is tapped.	C5-6
BRACHIORADIALIS	Flexion of the elbow and/or pronation of the forearm when the tendon or musculotendinous junction is tapped.	C5-6
TRICEPS	Extension of the elbow when the triceps tendon or muscle is tapped.	C7-8
PERIOSTEORADIAL	Flexion and supination of the forearm when the styloid process of the radius is tapped.	C6-8
PERIOSTEOULNAR	Extension and ulnar abduction of the wrist when the styloid process of the ulna is tapped.	C6-8
PATELLAR (KNEE JERK)	Extension of the knee when the patellar tendon is tapped.	L3-4 / L 2-4
HAMSTRINGS SEMIMEMBRANOSUS; BICEPS FEMORIS	Flexion of the knee when the hamstrings tendon or muscle is tapped.	L5-S1 / S1-2
TIBIALIS POSTERIOR-PLANTAR	Flexion and inversion of the foot when the tibialis posterior tendon behind the medial malleolus is tapped.	L 4-5
ACHILLES TENDON	Plantar flexion of the foot when the Achilles tendon is tapped.[a]	S1-2

a. A bilateral sluggish (slow to return) Achilles tendon reflex can suggests hypothyroid function.

Neurological Testing

Table 4-11: Superficial Reflexes

REFLEX	LEVEL TESTED	DESCRIPTION
Mucous Membrane Reflexes (Not commonly relevant in orthopedics).		
Corneal	N5.	Conjunctival.
Nasal	N1.	Smell.
Pharyngeal	N9-10.	Gag.
Uvular	N8.	Palatal.
Skin Reflexes (Assessed occasionally in orthopedics)		
Upper and Lower Abdominal	T8-12.	Tensing of muscles beneath the skin area. Stroking causes the umbilicus to move in the direction of the stimulated skin area.
Cremasteric	L1-2.	Elevation of the scrotum and testicle of the same side in response to stroking of the inner aspect of the thigh or the skin over Scapa's triangle.
Anal	L1-2.	Contraction of the sphincter ani in response to stroking of the perianal area, or upon inserting objects such as a gloved finger into the rectum.
Plantar	L4-S2. also upper motor.	Plantar flexion of the toes upon stroking the lateral sole of the foot (known as Babinski sign).

Table 4-12: Additional Neurological Tests

REFLEX	DESCRIPTION	NERVE TESTED
OCULAR REFLEXES		
Light.	Constriction of the pupil when light shines on the retina.	Midbrain Cranial II, III.
Accommodation	Group of three closely-associated reflexes that facilitate production of a sharp image on the corresponding points of the retina. When the eye looks at near-by objects, these reflexes are accompanied by constriction of the pupils.	Central commissural connections that involve the occipital cortex and Cranial II, III.
Ciliospinal	Dilation of the pupils when painful stimulation is applied to any sensory area, usually by pinching the neck.	T1-2, Cervical sympathetic and sensory.
Oculocardiac	Slowing of the heart rate produced by pressure over the eyeballs.	Medulla, Cranial V and X.
OTHER VISCERAL REFLEXES (PARTIAL LIST)		
Carotid Sinus	Slowing of the heart and decrease in blood pressure (by vasodilation) due to pressure over the carotid sinus in the neck.	Medulla, Cranial IX and X.
Bulbocavernosus	Contraction of the bulbocavernosus muscles after: • stroking the dorsum of the glans penis. or • pinching the skin of the penis.	S2-4, pudendal, pelvic autonomic system
Bladder	Also called "urinary reflex," "vesicle reflex," "micturation reflex." Contraction of the walls of the bladder and relaxation of the trigone and urethral sphincter in response to pressure within the bladder.	pelvic autonomic system
Rectal	Impulse to defecate, caused by entrance of fecal matter into the rectum.	pelvic autonomic system

A) Warm allodynia;
— Warm (not hot) stimuli evokes pain;
— Can use warm test tube or tuning fork;
— Quantitative sensory testing (QST) devices can provide accurate thresholds.
—Thought to reflect sensitized C-nociceptors.
B) Cold allodynia;
— Cold stimuli evokes pain;
— Can use cold test tube, tuning fork, or ice;
— Quantitative sensory testing (QST) devices can provide accurate thresholds.
—Thought to reflect central sensitization.

3. Hyperalgesia: an *exaggerated* pain response caused by *normally painful stimuli.*
A) Clinically, can be evoked by two different stimuli;
— Single pinprick;
— Multiple pinpricks.
B) Can manifest itself with two distinct abnormal sensations;
— Summation: the perception of painful stimulus may start as sensory deficit or as a normal sensation, but with persistent stimulation (pinpricks) it heightens to become an exaggerated pain;
— Aftersensation: the sensation that the area of pain spreads ("like a starburst") and lingers for seconds or minutes after stimulus ceases.
—Thought to reflect pathophysiologic alteration in the dorsal horn; i.e., windup.

Motor Tests in Patients with Neuropathy

Although not generally recognized as a characteristic of neuropathic pain syndromes, abnormal motor function can be an important aspect of the patient's overall status that may require therapy. *Neuropathy* often results in: Motor weakness, ataxia (impaired coordinated movement), apraxia (impaired ability to perform purposeful acts), and decreased endurance. *Complex regional pain syndrome* often results in: Motor weakness, decreased endurance, motor neglect that can be tested by comparing how the patient moves the limbs (i.e., movement initiation, frequency, and amplitude) when looking away from the involved limb vs when looking directly at the limb. The patient has motor neglect if the limb is moved significantly better with direct visualization.

Myofascial Tests

Many neuropathic pain patients develop secondary myofascial pain syndrome (tight, spastic, painful muscles, ligaments and tendons) that can become a significant source of pain and disability. Myofascial dysfunction often occur proximal to the area of neuropathic pain. These local tight and spastic soft tissues can result in two distinct pain sites:

1. Locally at the site of myofascial dysfunction.

2. Distally at sites of referred pain. It is common that the complaint of spreading pain is due to secondary myofascial pain and not a spreading of the neuropathic pain syndrome itself. For example, neuropathic pain in the hand can result in myofascial dysfunction in the shoulder girdle muscles and neck, which can then refer back even more pain to the hand, or arm, and head. And, neuropathic pain in the foot can result in myofascial dysfunction in the hip girdle and low back muscles, which can refer pain back to the foot and leg.

Examinations findings include:

• Reduced active range of movement in the involved region.
• Evidence of trigger point; that is, focal tight bands and nodules of muscle that reproduce the patient's focal and referred pain when gently palpated (Galer and Dworkin *ibid*).

Screening Examination

This section describes screening examination geared mainly toward orthopedic and mechanical diagnosis. Screening test geared towards Osteopathic and functional diagnosis are covered on page 470. The musculoskeletal screening has four main objectives:

1. Exclude a remote-area, orthopedic and neurological condition that might be responsible for the presenting symptoms.

2. Establish priorities and help direct one to more specific tests.

3. Find mechanical dysfunctions.

4. Save time.

In general, screening examinations (and general movement tests) are more sensitive for compensatory and adaptive patterns than for detailed joint dysfunction. The practitioner must conduct further specific testing to identify joint (somatic) dysfunctions or other pathologies. When viewed functionally, the body is a dynamic structure that must change and adapt. Therefore, if there is a change in one area of the body, all other parts of the body will have to adapt to this change. However, if some area is not capable of change, an adjacent or mechanically/neurally related area will begin to change. For example, a change in the lower extremity can have far reaching consequences in the neck and cranium (Ursa 1996). Since pain can result from abnormal adaptations and reactions to a primary dysfunction elsewhere, and since the primary dysfunction can be found anywhere, the screening examination helps the practitioner identify and be led to areas that require further investigation. Orthopedic screen tests usually look for gross movement limitations and the provocation of symptoms and pain, starting proximally to the presenting symptoms. They inform us if the pain arises at the painful site or elsewere. Osteopathic screen tests are geared towards dysfunctions and not pain.

Gait Analysis

The first step in the screen tests is a gait analysis (Figure 9-31 on page 198). A patient's gait patterns can be very informative as to pathology in the lower extremities, the spine, and the central and peripheral nervous systems. Table 3-10 on page 197 describes the most basic aspects of the gait examination.

The practitioner must pay particular attention to a few details concerning stance.

NORMAL STANCE AND GAIT DIMENSIONS:
- Distance between feet while standing is 2-4 inches.
- Distance between feet while walking is 2-4 inches.
- Stride length (length of one gait cycle) about 28-32 inches.
- Step (gait) length (equal on both sides) 14-16 inches.
- Vertical pelvic shifts are symmetrical and approximately 2 inches.
- Lateral pelvic shifts are symmetrical and approximately 1 inch to the weight-bearing side.
- In the swing phase, the pelvis rotates 40° forward. The opposite hip joint (which is in stance phase) acts as a fulcrum for this rotation.

Table 4-16 lists gait observations from front and back. Table 4-14 lists gate observations from the side.

ABNORMAL GAIT. Table 4-15 describes a few of the many abnormal gait patterns.

GAIT OBSERVATION. The practitioner begins the musculoskeletal screening by evaluating the patient's gait and other movements. Observation of gait from a distance, from where the pelvic, spinal, and extremity movements can be seen more easily, can be helpful. It is also helpful to ask the patient to walk briskly. Severity of pain can be detected readily by looking at the patient's movement pattern and amount of guarding. A patient who moves slowly and carefully is much more likely to have pain of a severe musculoskeletal origin.

This examination is best performed from front, back, and side, a combination that usually gives succinct clues about the location of the dysfunction. For additional information on clinical interpretations see "Analysis of Findings" on page 476.

Table 4-14 through Table 4-18 summarize general musculoskeletal observations.

Table 4-13: Observation of Gait

LOCATION	OBSERVE FOR
Pelvic Area	Symmetry of laterality, height, and rotation.
Trunk	Swaying. Whether the upper trunk and extremities rotate to the opposite side of the pelvis and of the lower extremities.
Lower Extremities	Bowing, varus, or valgus.
Feet	Base width, during gait and when still. Symmetry of stride, toes out or in, heel and toe strike, toe off.
Ankle	Flexion. (The distal and proximal tibiofibular joints must function well for normal toe-off).
Rearfoot Midfoot Forefoot	Whether the weight transfers from the heel to the lateral side of the foot and back across the metatarsal phalangeal joints to the great toe for push-off. Normal toe-off.
Arms Shoulder Girdle	Swing of the arms and behavior of the shoulder girdle.
Patient's Footwear	Pattern of wear.

Table 4-14: Gait Observation from Side

LOCATION	OBSERVE FOR
Spine	Curves
General	Coordination of movements
Hip Knee Ankle Mid-Foot Fore-Foot	Ability to extend and flex
Gait	Gait length, Duration of gait cycle segments, Limp

Table 4-16: General Observation from Front

Location		Observe for
Pelvis		Underwear is at the same level on both sides of the pelvis (help visually), levelness of pelvis. Muscle tone
Posture (Customary, relaxed)	Plumb Line.	Head straight. Eyes level and pupilary line level. Neck line vertically straight. Nose in line with the sternum and umbilicus. Shoulders, clavicles, and upper limbs level and equal (dominant side might be slightly lower). Arms equidistant from the trunk, and rotated equally. Hip bones (ilia), knees, head of fibula, malleoli and arches of the feet level and equal.
Rib cage		Symmetry.
Facial features		Symmetry.
Knee		Position of patella relative to position of feet. Quadricep size.
Skin		Evidence of segmental trophic changes. Cutaneous lesions and scars.

Table 4-17: General Observation from Back

Location	Observe for
Shoulders Scapula Head	Levelness, rotations, flattening, scapular winging, muscle tone.
Spine	(Spinal curve) kinks, flat areas, scoliosis, step deformity, muscle tone.
Hips (ilia) Buttocks Gluteal Folds	Levelness, muscle tone.
Knees	Swelling, varus or valgus.
Achilles Tendons	Straightness, varus or valgus.
Skin	Evidence of segmental trophic changes. Cutaneous lesions and scars.

Table 4-18: General Observation from Sides

Location	Observe for
Entire Side	Plumb line. Increased/decreased spinal curves. Step spinal deformity. Flat spinal segments. Hunched, flat-back or sway-back postures.
Knees	Hyperextended or flexed (should be straight).
Feet	Flatness. More than 50% of the weight should be on the balls of feet.
Head	Position.
Scapula	Winging.
Skin	Evidence of segmental trophic changes. Cutaneous lesions and scars.

Table 4-15: Some Abnormal Gait Patterns (Hoppenfeld 1976; Mitchell 1995)

PATTERN	DESCRIPTION	COMMENTS

Antalgic	The patient tries to avoid weightbearing or pressure on the affected site.
	
	A patient walking bare-foot on a rocky surface is a good example of an antalgic gait.
		• Generally a self-protective mechanism for pain avoidance.
		  —Results from spinal, hip, knee, ankle, or foot lesion.
		• The patient might list away from the lesion, or position the body in a way that minimizes pain.
		  —However, if a hip is painful, the patient might position the body weight over the painful hip vertically, decreasing the load on the femoral head.
		• The stance phase on the injured limb is shorter. The patient might try to support the affected area with one hand. The opposite arm might be outstretched, acting as a counterbalance.
		• Associated with Painful Obstruction (Bi) and Pathogenic Factors, Cold, Blood-stasis, Heat.

Arthrogenic	The patient's limb swings in a circular, cone-shaped arc (circumduction) around the affected joint or for toe clearance.	• Due to pathology of a single joint; stiffness, laxity, deformity. • Painful or not. • Associated with Painful Obstruction (Bi) syndromes.

Short Leg	Lateral shift toward the short leg and a downward pelvic tilt with a possible limp-like gait.	• Often patient compensates by rotating the innominate posteriorly on the long side and anteriorly on the short leg side (to equalize the leg length);
		  —With a premature heel lift on the short leg side in mid-stance.
		  —Often the short leg is externally rotated.
		  —Long leg pronates.
		• Associated often with Kidney-Essence and Yin and Yang Motility (Qiao) channels.

Gluteus Medius (Trendelenburg)	Often results in an increase of lateral shift.	• Can be seen in the presence of L5 root lesions. • The patient lists laterally to keep the center of gravity over the stance leg. —If the lesion is bilateral, the patient has a wobbling gate ("chorus girl" swing). • Associated often with Wei-atrophy, Kidney-Essence, Gall Bladder, Kidney and Urinary Bladder Sinew channels, and Pathogenic Factors.
Gluteus Maximus	The patient thrusts the thorax posteriorly at heel strike in order to compensate for the weak gluteus maximus.	• Often seen in patients who have a backward tilt (center of gravity moved posteriorly) from S1 lesions. • Associated often with Wei-atrophy, Kidney-Essence, Kidney and Urinary Bladder Sinew channels, Kidney Divergent channel, and Pathogenic Factors.
Steppage; Foot Drop	Foot slapping the ground. Patient lifts knee (flexes leg and hip) higher to compensate and prevent toes catching.	• Weakness of foot dorsiflexor muscles mostly due to radicular disease. • Peripheral neuropathy. • Associated often with sever Kidney and Liver Yin deficiency or Qi and Blood deficiency, internal-Wind, Wei-atrophy.
Psoatic	Lateral rotation, flexion and adduction of hip. Patient exaggerate movement of pelvis and trunk to flex thigh.	• Hip disease. • Associated with Painful Obstruction (Bi), Liver and Kidney deficiency, Essence-deficiency, Pathogenic Factors, Gall Bladder, Urinary Bladder and Liver Sinew channels.
MEDICAL GAITS		

Ataxic	Seen in patients who have bad coordination or poor sensation. The patient may appear to be intoxicated.	• Can be seen in patients who have cerebellar or peripheral/sensory lesions, and in patients who are intoxicated or in multiple sclerosis (MS).
		  —Often in central nervous system lesions, all movements are exaggerated (lurch or stagger).
		  —In sensory or peripheral lesions the gait may be irregular, swaying and jerky (unsteady). The patient may look down to see placement of feet and have broader base.
		• Associated with Phlegm, Blood-stasis obstructing leg vessels, severe deficiency of Kidney and Liver Yin or Essence, obstruction of Clear-Yang.

Table 4-15: Some Abnormal Gait Patterns (Hoppenfeld 1976; Mitchell 1995)

Pattern	Description	Comments
Hemiplegic	Leg is swung outward and ahead in a circle, or will push leg ahead. Upper limb is carried across trunk for balance.	• Patient with hemiplegia due to various causes. • Associated with Phlegm, Dampness, and Wind obstructing the channels, Liver-Wind, Liver, and Kidney Yin-deficiency, Blood-stasis.
Parkinsonian Hypokinetic	Neck, trunk, and knees are flexed (stopped posture). Shuffling or short rapid steps at times. Stiff arms with little movement. May look like falling forward. Difficulty in initiating movement.	• Parkinson's disease or syndrome. • Associated with severe deficiency of Liver and Kidney Yin, Wind, Phlegm, severe deficiency of Qi and Blood, internal-Wind.
Scissors	Spastic gait. Legs are swung forward with great effort. Slow walking.	• Spastic paraplegia. • MS. • Associated with severe deficiency of Liver and Kidney Yin, Wind, Phlegm, severe deficiency of Qi and Blood, internal-Wind, Dryness.

For additional information of functionally oriented tests, screen test, and interpretive information "Osteopathic and Functional Tests" on page 470.

Laboratory and Technical Testing

We live in an age of technology, which promises not only a deeper understanding of the human body, but also a better ability to identify the pathophysiologic sources of symptoms, thereby promoting improved therapy for illness. This promise may be true for some medical conditions, but has yet to be fulfilled in pain medicine. Both patients and their practitioners (as well as the legal system) must realize that no diagnostic test can identify the source of pain with great accuracy or measure the amount of pain felt by an individual. It is always important to remember to *not relay* on test results and when appropriate to validate the patient's symptomes. (Galer and Dworkin *ibid*). In Orthopaedic Medicine, technical examinations are not routinely used but are, instead, ordered only when necessary to refine the clinical diagnosis, to exclude certain lesions, or to clarify differential diagnosis. They are always used if the functional evaluation and/or history reveal warning signs. However, the practitioner should not ascribe too much to these technical tests when positive or negative (especially imaging). For example, it is quite common to see abnormal disc MRI studies in asymptomatic populations. It is also quite common to see partial thickness and full thickness tears of the rotator cuff in asymptomatic populations. Therefor all positive technical examinations must correlate with the clinical presentation. Some musculoskeletal pains can be due to medical conditions that can be detected through laboratory testing. Therefore, laboratory tests can be especially prudent for patients that have chronic or acute pain of unknown origin.

The practitioner orders tests based on clinical presentations. For example, patients suffering from fatigue and generalized muscle pain (fibromyalgia) may be suffering from thyroid deficiency. A sensitive TSH, T3, T4 and thyroid antibody tests should be ordered. In musculoskeletal practice, the following tests *may* be needed:

- Complete Blood Count (CBC) with differential count
- SMAC 24 (a series of several tests)
- Sensitive Thyroid Stimulating Hormone (TSH), T3, T4 and thyroid antibodies
- Urine Strip Analysis
- (Men over 50) Prostate Specific Antigen (PSA)
- (Patients with extensive symptoms) Highly Sensitive C-reactive Protein.

In the presence of joint pain and swelling:
- CBC
- Erythrocyte Sedimentation Rate (ESR)
- Rheumatoid Factor (RF)

- Antinuclear Antibodies (ANA)
- Uric Acid Level
- Urinalysis
- (Possibly) Synovial fluid culture (aspiration of fluid to check for infections or crystalline disease).

The sections, "Blood Tests," "Urine Tests," "Saliva Tests," "Stool Test," "Hair Analysis" and "Some Additional Tests," contain brief descriptions of applicable tests in musculoskeletal medicine.

Blood Tests

Blood tests are often used to exclude medical conditions that either are responsible for or are contributing to pain.

Erythrocyte Sedimentation Rate (ESR)

Erythrocyte Sedimentation Rate (ESR), a nonspecific screening test, is an indicator of inflammatory processes that can be useful for diagnosing patients who have involvement of multiple areas from a systemic disease. For many of these conditions this test can also be used to follow the level of activity.

The ESR increases with aging. Normal values vary with the specific techniques used and the laboratory that performs the test. ESR is a nonspecific marker. A persistent increase can be due to conditions other than those mentioned here.

- The ESR is increased in rheumatic fever, rheumatoid arthritis, and the rheumatoid variants: systemic lupus erythematosus (SLE), polymyalgia rheumatica (PMR), temporal arteritis, and acute infections. Extremely high ESRs (greater than 100) can be found in temporal arteritis, tuberculosis, and cancer.
- The ESR is not increased in degenerative arthritis and in crystalline diseases such as gout, except during severe, acute attacks.

Complete Blood Count (CBC)

Peripheral leukocytosis can be seen with acute infections. However, just as with the ESR, a normal white count (leukocyte) reading does not rule out the presence of infection.

- Decreased white blood count (WBC) can be seen in immune deficiency. An overwhelming infection can cause a decrease in the WBC as well.
- A high WBC usually indicates an infection.
- A finding of a low red blood cell count (RBC), low hemoglobin (Hg), and a low hematocrit is seen with anemias and can also be a clue to the presence of a systemic illness such as lupus erythematosus (SLE), several neuropathies, and internal bleeding.
- A high RBC with high Hg and hematocrit is found in polycythemia.

- The differential of the cell types present (ordered as CBC with differential) can indicate the type of inflammation present (bacterial, viral, or allergic).

Rheumatoid Factor (RF)

Rheumatoid Factor (RF) tests for IgG antibodies in rheumatoid arthritis (RA). RF is negative in a fair number of patients who have rheumatoid arthritis, especially in early or mild stages. Usually the rheumatoid factor is negative in the presence of rheumatoid variants. RF is positive in a significant percentage of patients who have systemic lupus erythematosus (SLE) and in patients who have some other conditions, such as syphilis. It may be positive in asymptomatic populations as well.

Antinuclear Antibodies (ANA)

Antinuclear Antibodies are antibodies to various nuclear constituents (such as DNA and nucleoproteins) found in patients who have autoimmune diseases such as lupus erythematosus (SLE). The test also can be positive in patients who have scleroderma or Sjogeren's syndrome, drug-induced lupus-like syndromes, and in about one-fourth of patients who have RA.

Uric Acid Level

The higher the uric acid level in the blood, the more likely the patient is to have attacks of gouty arthritis. Demonstration of a serum level of uric acid above defined normal limits, however, does not unequivocally prove that joint symptoms are due to gout.[21] Uric acid levels can be increased in cases of renal insufficiency, hypotensive (diuretic) drug therapy, and decreased in acute hepatitis.

Serum Calcium

Serum calcium often increases in the presence of hyperparathyroidism and bone metastasis. Serum calcium can decrease in hypoparathyroidism and hyperthyroidism. Normal levels in children and adolescents are much higher than those in adults.

Phosphorus

Phosphorus increases in the presence of hypoparathyroidism, severe kidney diseases, acromegaly, and patients who have an excess of vitamin D. Phosphorus decreases in the presence of rickets, osteomalacia, malabsorption, and hyperparathyroidism. Normal levels in children and adolescents are much higher than in adults.

Alkaline Phosphatase

Alkaline Phosphatase is a phosphatase that increases with bone growth and disease, biliary and liver disease, and in Paget's Disease. Decreased levels can result in growth retardation in children. Normal levels in children and adolescents are much higher than in adults.

Acid Phosphatase

Acid Phosphatase is a phosphatase that increases in the presence of metastatic prostate cancers. Normal levels in children and adolescents are much higher than in adults.

Serum Glutamic-Oxaloacetic Transaminase (SGOT)

Serum Glutamic-Oxaloacetic Transaminase, an enzyme present in large amounts in muscle and liver tissue, is used primarily as an indicator of acute myocardial infarction and liver disease. SGOT is increased in cases of musculoskeletal disease, especially in the presence of muscular injury and dystrophies, and in heart and liver disease.

Sensitive Thyroid Stimulating Hormone (TSH)

Sensitive Thyroid Stimulating Hormone, a test for thyroid function, reports an increased TSH level in hypothyroidism and a decreased TSH level in hyperthyroidism. Thyroid dysfunction is a common cause of myofascial pain syndromes. More sophisticated tests may be needed to show abnormalities. Blood levels of free T3 (active thyroid) and T4 should also be ordered.[22]

Prostate Specific Antigen (PSA)

Prostate Specific Antigen, which tests for prostate pathology, should be performed on men over fifty years of age, especially those who suffer from back pain. Manual palpation of the entire prostate is not possible and therefore, small early carcinomas might escape manual detection that can be discovered by abnormal levels of serum PSA. Prostate cancer can cause low back pain.

HLA-B27 Antigen

HLA-B27 Antigen is a marker found in 90% of patients who have ankylosing spondylitis, and in about 70% of patients who have Reiter's syndrome, psoriatic spondylitis, or enteropathic arthritis. HLA-B27 antigen can be present in asymptomatic (normal) patients, as well.

---

21. Gout should be diagnosed by the aspiration of synovial fluid that contains uric acid crystals.

22. It is important to understand that functional hypothyroidism can be seen in patients with normal TSH, T3 and T4. T3 is often borderline low. The Achilles tendon reflex is often sluggish. Treatment with whole thyroid tissue (i.e., both T4 and T3) is often helpful.

Sensitive C-Reactive Protein

Sensitive C-reactive protein is a test for inflammation. When high, patients often do not respond to orthopedic treatments. It should be lowered using nutritional and medical methods.

Urine Tests

Urine tests can be helpful for assessing musculoskeletal disorders, especially back pain.

Urine Dip Stick

The Urine Dip Stick Test is important especially for patients who have low back pain.

- In cases of urinary tract infection (UTI), the dip stick can be positive for white cells, nitrites, leukocyte esterase, and possibly protein.
- Kidney stones often present with blood in the urine.
- Diabetes presents with glucose in the urine.

Bence Jones Protein

This is an abnormal urinary or plasma protein that has unusual solubility attributes. Bence Jones Protein is found in patients who have multiple myeloma and osteosarcomas, and sometimes in patients who have reticuloendothelial system diseases (RES).

Osteomark—NTX

The Osteomark—NTX assay measures the urine levels of a compound linked to bone-breakdown (crossed-linked N-telopeptide of type I collagen). Hence, this test can be used to monitor the rate of bone loss and success of therapies used for osteoporosis.

Neurotransmitter and Amino Acid Levels

Testing urine for neurotransmitter levels can be helpful when treating patients suffering from chronic pain and/or secondary psychiatric effects. Anti-depressant and/or nutritional and herbal intervention can then be used based on the test. Proper neurotransmitter levels also help to restore normal function to the pain sensory systems. Urine tests can also be used to measure amino acid levels which may be neurotransmitter and peptide related markers.

Saliva Testing

Saliva testing is especially helpful in the assessment of hormonal levels and adrenal function. Abnormal levels and functions are often associated with chronic pain and poor healing. These tests are mostly used to test sex hormone levels and adrenal functions, but can also be used to assess thyroid function.

Compressive Stool Analysis and Intestinal Permeability Test

The comprehensive stool analysis is used to evaluate the condition of the digestive system and/or the presence of infection. This test evaluates the efficiency of digestion, the presence of normal and abnormal flora or infections and offers important clues about the gut's ability to keep toxic chemicals out of the body. It assesses the ecological balance of the intestinal microflora (i.e., normal and abnormal flora), the adequacy of digestive enzymes and acid production, the capacity of the gut's immune system to defend itself, and screens for parasitic infections.[23] Poorly functioning digestive system has been associated with "leaky gut syndrome"[24] which is said to contribute to a state of "systemic inflammation," and allergies. Many chronic pain and fibromyalgia patients are thought to suffer from a leaky gut which may increase their general sensitivity to painful simuli. Poor digestion is also thought to result in functional nutritional deficiencies which may result in poor healing as well as increase sensitivity.

Intestinal permeability is very simple to measure, is economical, and provides information that is vital in terms of assessing the potential extent to which the body is challenged to cope with toxic and allergy provoking chemicals. To check for a leaky gut the *intestinal permeability test* can be used. This study tests for absorption of a large and small sugar molecules. The larger sugar lactulose is not supposed to pass through the intestinal wall and if present in the urine after the patients drinks it, suggests intestinal permeability. The smaller sugar mannitol should be present in the urine after consumption. If low levels are seen than a malabsorption is suspected.

---

23. The presence of dysbiosis is said to be capable of: deactivation of digestive enzymes, consumption of vitamin B12 and amino acids, saturation of the essential omega 3 and 6 fatty acids, disruption of the intestinal lining, sensitization against translocated bacteria and their fragments, cause irritable bowel syndrome and inflammatory bowel diseases, and the deconjugation of bile acids and estrogens that might potentially induce bowel or breast cancer. Dysbiosis may be caused by: dietary factors, inflammatory conditions, infections, meldigestion, stress, medications (antibiotics, NSAIDs, steroid medications, H2 blockers and other antacids, birth control pills, and chemotherapeutical agents), xenobiotic exposure, immune dysfunction, and by miscellaneous conditions. Dysbiosis has also been associated with rheumatoid arthritis and ankylosing spondylitis.

24. The intestinal lining has the dual role of selectively letting into the body those chemicals which it needs, and keeping out what is toxic. The permeability of this barrier is an especially important factor in maintain the integrity of these critical function. Leaky gut syndrome exists when some factor makes the spaces between the small intestinal epithelial cells wider than normal. This may allow the breach of macromolecules (often large proteins), bacteria and bacterial fragments as well as other toxic substances to go through the gut into the blood stream. Leaky gut syndrome is said to be self-perpetuating by: food allergies, malabsorption and malnutrition, dysbiosis, and unbalanced liver detoxification.

Hair Analysis

Hair analysis can be helpful as a screen test for heavy metal toxicity. Provocative urine test can then be used in patients that show toxicity, to both evaluate kidney function and heavy metal levels in tissues. Normal kidney function is imperative when using oral chelation for heavy metals. Heavy metal toxicity has been associated with chronic pain syndromes, neural dysfunction, and clinical failure of musculoskeletal interventions.

Detoxification Profile

There are urine, blood, and saliva tests said to assess the patients detoxification efficiency. The reserve capacity and balance of the two liver detoxification phases can be revealed by challenging the system with small doses of aspirin, acetaminophen, and caffeine, and measuring how the liver metabolizes them.[25]

Poor detoxification has been associated with non-specific pain syndromes as well as neuropathic pain. It must be remembered that therapies that alter or improve detoxification can alter blood level of medicine and therefore care and close monitoring may be needed in patients using pharmaceutical therapies.[26]

Additional Tests

Neurophysiologic studies provide a way to categorize muscle and nerve damage. They measure the integrity of the nerve muscle relationship and do not, by themselves, offer a specific etiologic diagnosis. Two tests that are very helpful in differentiating the possible causes of muscular weakness, numbness, and paresthesias are electromyography (EMG) and nerve conduction velocity (NCV) (Garrick and Ebb *ibid*). Quantitative sensory testing (QST) are more accurate as they can measure both small and large fiber functions, but are currently used mostly in research settings (Galer and Dworkin *ibid*).

Electromyography (EMG)

Electromyography studies evaluate motor unit potentials by testing the functions of the nerve roots and the way that the nerves affect muscle function. It does this by assessing how well the electrical currents in the nerves and spinal pathways are being transmitted to the muscles. Compression of nerves will slow down electrical conduction along the nerve's pathway. Many abnormal potentials and potential patterns are seen with denervation of the muscle. From the pattern of involvement of several muscles for which innervations are known, the specific location of the pathology can be surmised. Examples include root compression, compression of a specific peripheral nerve at a specific site such as median nerve entrapment (carpel tunnel entrapment*)*, and a polyneuropathy. Intrinsic muscular disease and myasthenia gravis present with very specific electromyographic patterns (Garrick and Ebb *ibid*).

In *Single Fiber Electromyography* (SFEMG), a specially designed needle electrode is used to record and identify action potentials from individual muscle fibers. These recordings are used to calculate the neuromuscular jitter and the muscle fiber density. Increased jitter, blocking, or both, may occur in a variety of conditions, including primary disorders of neuromuscular transmission (Brill *ibid*). To perform an EMG the physician:

1. Inserts thin electrode needles into specific muscles;
2. Observes the elicited motor unit potentials on an oscilloscope screen.

Surface EMG (SEMG) employs a scanner with self-contained electrodes and/or surface electrodes that are applied to the skin, to record the electrical potential of a specific muscle or a group of muscles. SEMG has been used in the evaluation of low back pain based on the direct relationship between muscular pain and elevated myoelectrical behaviors (Brill *ibid*).

Nerve Conduction Velocity (NCV)

A nerve conduction study is used to evaluate the integrity of the peripheral nervous system. These studies measure the conduction velocity, latency, amplitude, and shape of response following electrical stimulation. To measure nerve conduction velocity, the physician:

1. Stimulates a peripheral nerve at a specific site;
2. Measures the time necessary for muscle action potentials to be transmitted distally;

---

25. There are two main liver detoxification pathways called phase I and phase II (oxidation and conjugation). Phase I serves to "biotransform" substances through oxidation, reduction or hydrolysis. It is achieved using the cytochrome P450 mixed-function oxidase enzymes that metabolize many substances as well as medications. This process increases the solubility of molecules and prepares them for Phase II reactions which will further increase their solubility. There is often reactive oxygen produced by Phase I detoxification which can be quite damaging. The use of pharmaceutical medications as well as some herbs can tax the cytochrome P450 systems making them less efficient and result in increased blood levels of the drugs. In Phase II, congugation reactions add a polar hydrophilic molecule to the metabolite or toxin, converting lipophilic substances to water-soluble forms for excretion and elimination. Phase II does not necessarily follow Phase I and may be the primary form of detoxification for some substances. As long as Phase II can quickly metabolize the load of free radicals and carcinogens formed by Phase-I, by their chemical conjugation with glycine, glutathione, glucuronide, or sulfate, there is no problem. These inert conjugated products are simply secreted into the bile, which then pass into the stool, and are excreted from the body.

26. For patients with nonspecific pain syndromes such as fibromyalgia the Whitaker Wellness Center routine is to test: Chem 24, CBC, candida anti-bodies, DHEA-S, testosterone, thyroid panel, ESR, RF, CRP, and comprehensive stool analysis (CDSA). Considered also: lyme titer, cortisol, H pylori, CMV and EBV, mycoplasma, chlamydia pneumoniae, heavy metals, celiac panel, and intestinal permeability.

3. Compares the time with the normal value listed for the age and sex of the patient.

A delay implies peripheral nerve compression somewhere along the nerve. This technique is especially useful for confirming a clinical impression of the location of nerve compression and is used to assess pinched nerves in the neck, back or extremities. It is useful for confirming carpal and tarsal tunnel syndromes, peripheral neuropathy, injury from metabolic diseases such as diabetes mellitus, uremia, or chronic alcohol abuse, or other nerve entrapment syndromes. (Brill *ibid*). Some polyneuropathies slow the conduction velocity, some do not. A comparison with normal nerve values helps differentiate these entities from compression neuropathies (Garrick and Ebb *ibid*).

Both EMG and NCV test are often overutilized in the clinical care of neuropathic pain patients. Although they can accurately measure how a nerve conducts electricity and whether a demyelinating or oxonal injury is present, EMG and NCV test rarely assist in the diagnosis or treatment of neuropathic pain. For example, the diagnosis of peripheral polyneuropathy is most commonly based on history and examination findings; electrophysiologic test may add confirmatory data, but most often are unnecessary. In addition, it is important to recognize that these tests measure only the status of large nerve fibers and cannot assess small-fiber function. Many painful neuropathies affect only the small nerve fibers, so EMG and NCV test will be normal. These tests are painful, unpleasant, and expensive and should be used sparingly and only when they will assist in diagnosis (Galer and Dworkin *ibid*), or change the patient's care.

Quantitative Sensory Testing (QST)

Quantitative sensory testing (QST) can be an important diagnostic test but is currently used more frequently in research on the mechanisms of neuropathic pain. QST measures the functional status of both large and small nerve fibers by obtaining the detection threshold of vibration (large nerves) and cold and warm thermal sensation (small nerves). In addition, measures of pain thresholds and abnormal perceptions elicited by these stimuli, such as aftersensations, can be examined using QST methods. Although more innocuous than EMG and NCV, QST is rarely needed in the diagnosis and treatment of most patients with neuropathic pain (Galer and Dworkin *ibid*).

Somatosensory Evoked Potentials (SSEP)

Somatosensory evoked potentials (SSEP) are ordered to assess the speed of electrical conduction across the spinal cord. If the spinal cord is significantly pinched, the electrical signals will travel slower than the norm. The test is done by stimulating a peripheral sense organ and measuring conduction velocities for central somatosensory pathways located in the posterior columns of the spinal cord, brain stem, and thalamus, and the primary sensory cortex located in the parietal lobes.

SSEP augment the sensory examination and is most useful in assessing the spinal nerve roots, spinal cord, or brain stem for evidence of delayed nerve conduction. SSEPs are altered by conditions that affect the somatosensory pathways, including both focal lesions (e.g., tumors, cervical spondylosis, strokes, and syringomyelia) and diffuse diseases (e.g., vitamin E deficiencies, subacute combined degeneration, hereditary systemic neurological degeneration). SSEP may help document abnormalities in multiple sclerosis (MS) patients with other concurrent demyelinating lesions that may not be clinically evident. SSEP abnormalities are also produced by other diseases affecting myelin (Brill *ibid*).

It must be stated that in many neuropathic pain patients all tests are normal and this should not be used as evidence for lack of illness, or that the symptoms are psychogenic, or that the patient is malingering. It is more likely to reflect our current lack of good diagnostic testing, technology, and understanding of chronic pain syndromes.

Imaging and Radiology[27]

Medical Radiographic Imaging

Medical radiographic imaging remained relatively unchanged from the original way Roentgen did it until the 1960s. The use of x-rays was confined to the x-ray machine emitting radiation and the image being recorded on photographic film. In the 1960s the development of more sensitive ways of detecting radiation became available. The development of nuclear medicine and computerized imaging began. Computerized axial tomography or CAT (CT) scanning combined this new way of detecting radiation that did not use film.

Musculoskeletal imaging can be done usually with plain x-ray imaging. This has considerable advantages. X-rays use low doses of radiation, and the cost to benefit ratio is high. MRI/CT can assist in the diagnosis of some musculoskeletal problems, but they need to be correlated with the routine x-ray to be really useful.

The major emphasis in this text is on clinical methods which are low tech yet useful clinically. The use of radiology and other imaging techniques is ubiquitous and probably has detracted from clinical evaluation overall. The tendency to treat x-rays is a health hazard in the opinion of the author. Judicious use of imaging can, however, support the soft tissue clinician.

---

27. Most of the images are provided by Thomas Ravin MD.

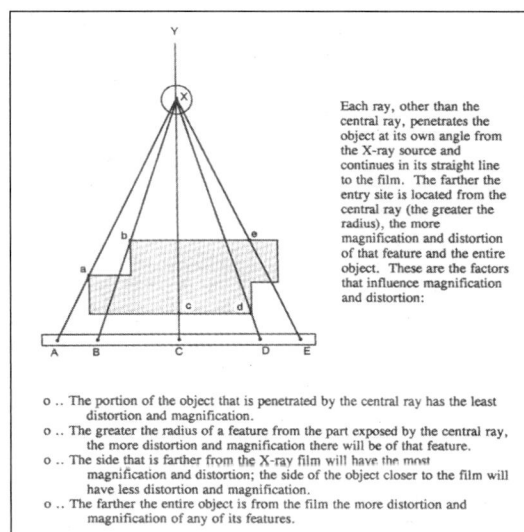

Figure 4-27: X-ray penetration (From Kuchera WA and Kuchera ML, Osteopathic Principles in Practice, KCOM press 1993, with permission).

Safety of Imaging

Medical imaging has continued to raise some safety questions such as: what is this magnetic spectrum doing to the individual and is it fundamentally safe? The radiation doses created by modern X-ray equipment using modern film and film screen technology deliver doses which are very low and may not be much in excess of background levels. Of unknown impact on the body is MRI and ultrasound. Ultrasound can create some tissue warming at the frequency and doses used in the average human, but probably represent no significant threat to the body. The question as to whether an MRI is free of harm is less well known. The effects on the human body of intense magnetic fields and multiple radio frequencies is hard to demonstrate. MRI is probably safe in the doses administered, but possible harm cannot be ignored.

It seems that all of these imaging techniques appear on the surface to be quite safe, and their use in the holistic/complementary practice should not be abandoned because of questions of safety, particularly when health needs are to be addressed. It should not be forgotten, however, that even the lowest radiation doses may create some trauma to genetic material in the ovaries and testes. The impact of high intensity electromagnetic fields and the radiation associated with many of these instruments lead one to approach the imaging modalities with some wariness, constantly keeping the risks versus the benefit ratio in mind. Modern imaging technology has made the risk to benefit ratios favorable, and particularly so in the extremities and axial skeleton in adults.

Basic Principles

An x-ray is ordered and labeled by the direction and relations the x-ray beam has to the patient. For example, a film labeled "anterior-posterior view" (AP), means that the x-ray beam is centered on the anterior portion of the part being filmed and the film is behind the patient. The lateral view has the central beam on the inside or medial aspect of the patient, with the film outside or lateral to the patient. The areas that are closer to the film show greater detail. So, for example, to assess the spine, an anterior-posterior view film is usually ordered (AP view, versus a PA). The films are displayed on the view box as if the practitioner were looking at the patient or the film's right side represented the viewer's left. MRI, CT, and ultrasound images are displayed the same way. If there are axial images (as if slicing a piece of salami), they appear as if the practitioner were looking from the feet to the head.

X-ray films are, in fact, negatives. The film, which is exposed by radiation, causes the silver crystals in the film to change shape and to stay on the film when it is developed. The unexposed portions of the film turn white. This results in denser tissues appearing more white than less dense tissues. (Bones appear whiter than soft tissue, and air appears darkest.) Body substances, in order of descending degree of density (and ascending degree of darkness) are as follows: metal, bone, soft tissue, water, fat, and air.

Basic imaging usually is ordered to exclude medical conditions such as cancers, infections (such as osteomyelitis), and metabolic and inflammatory bone diseases such as osteoporosis and ankylosing spondylitis. They should, therefore, be evaluated by a board-certified radiologist to ensure that no subtle but significant pathology is missed. In acute trauma, films may show fractures and, if the patient is short of breath, the presence of pneumothorax.

With experience, the radiologist can detect not only bony but also many important soft tissue changes, such as joint effusion, tendinous calcification, ectopic bone or muscle, tissue displaced by a tumor, and the presence of air or foreign body.

In general the radiologist inspects for:

1. overall size and shape of bone;
2. local size and shape of bone;
3. thickness of the cortex;
4. trabecular pattern of the bone;
5. general density of the entire bone;
6. local density of bone;
7. margins of local lesions;
8. any break in continuity of the bone;
9. any periosteal change;
10. any soft tissue change;
11. relation among bones;
12. thickness of the cartilage (joint space).

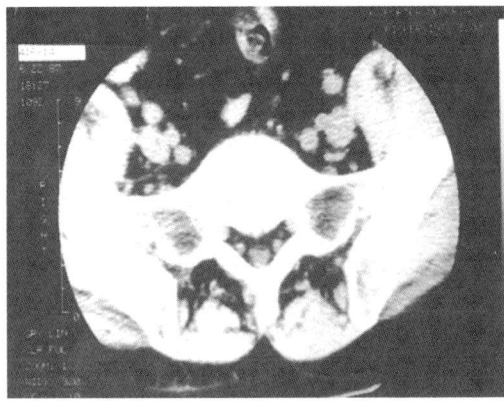

Figure 4-28: CT scan of the pelvis.

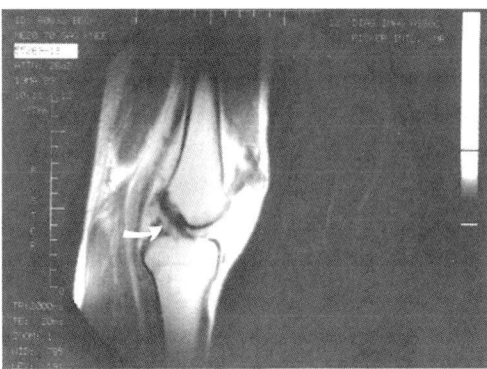

Figure 4-29: MRI image of knee.

Bony Architecture

The opacity of bones on x-ray varies. The apparent density of the bone depends in part on radiographic technique. Although appearances may suggest abnormalities of mineralization, it is known that these appearances often are misleading; hence, it is wise to defer evaluation of mineralization to densitomery, dual photon absorptometry, single photon absorptometry, and CT scanning absorptometry. For osteoporosis to be evident on plain film, approximately 30-35% of the bone must be lost. These observations do not fall within the purview of soft tissue management.

Limitations

Rentgenograms cannot be focused like a light beam. They display a two-dimensional view of three-dimensional structures, and there is superimposition of the several layers.

When joints are visualized, the joint space may be identifiable if the joint is seen head-on and if the space is planar. When seen at an angle, curved joint spaces cannot be assessed reliably; hence, the assessment of degenerative joint disease is based primarily on associated phenomena such as osteophyte formation, the degree of subchondral bone sclerosis, subchondral cyst formation, and soft tissue swelling.

Dynamic Studies

Ideally, imaging should reproduce abnormal physiological movement. Stress views and flexion/extension views are used in an attempt to visualize abnormalities at the end range of movement. Such views should be obtained with the patient just on the threshold of pain aggravation.

Magnetic Resonance Imaging and Computer-Reconstructed Radiographic Tomography

Magnetic Resonance Imaging (MRI) does not use x-rays to create the image (Figure 4-29). It uses radio signals created by nuclear polarity changing directions in strong magnetic fields and is analyzed in many different planes of the body, making it useful in many different areas. Since it does not use x-rays to create the images, it is a safe imaging technique, even near the eyes and gonads.

Radio waves that echo off magnetically charged protons, are the source of MRI images, which, therefore, comprise the best technique for imaging these parts (affecting water molecules present in the soft tissues). When a practitioner wants to look at a bulging disc or the position of a nerve or tendon, MRI is best. The technique can help estimate any increase in water and occasionally also give some indirect information on how acute the process is. Recently, MRI technology has been developed that permits more direct assessment of total cartilage content, integrity, and possibly the state of the matrix itself. MRI permits evaluation of cartilage as a positive image as opposed to radiographic techniques in which articular cartilage is represented as merely the space between the opposing joint margins. By obtaining multiple images across an entire joint, a quantitative determination of the total space occupied by the articular cartilage can be made; additionally, it is possible to define regions of interest and focus on weight-bearing areas if desired. With the identification of specific landmarks, repeated images can be aligned to allow a more precise determination of change. The introduction of more powerful magnets and the use of image-enhancing agents should permit an even more precise definition of change (Schnitzer 2004).

Magnetic Resonance Neurography is a special MRI scan with sensitivity to special biophysical properties of nerves. It is promoted for the diagnostic evaluation of conditions thought to be due to nerve compression or impingement, trauma involving peripheral nerves, and repetitive strain injuries (Brill 2004).

There are also *Magnetic Resonance Angiography* and *Venography* which are used to assess circulatory disorders.

Computer-reconstructed radiogaphic tomography (CT) (Figure 4-28) and MRI provide an enhanced scope of visualization of the interior of the body. The clarity and verisimilitude of the pictures are seductive, but image reconstruction by computer is not analogous to photography. Adjustment in gain and other parameters can both create and ablate appearances; nonetheless, obtaining such images may be helpful in some cases and may be prudent in the current medicolegal jungle. CT is best for imaging bones, because the calcium absorbs x-rays, although the patient's exposure to radiation triples with their use compared to simple x-rays. They also image soft tissues.

Usually CT images are created in transverse sections. The stored information can be displayed as an image of cuts in other planes and even in three dimensions; however, there is loss of detail. In contrast, with some planning, MRI studies can show any plane without loss of detail. This is an important advantage. CT can be used to assess discs, spinal cord and nerve roots, and to rule out tumors. The technique is used often to image lungs and abdominal organs. CT can also be used to pickup small body fractures.

CT with an myelogram consists of injecting a radiographic opaque dye into the sac around the nerve roots and can show how bone is affecting the root and provides excellent information about subtle signs of pressure to the spinal cord or nerve roots. This procedure can result in spinal fluid leak thus causing a spinal headache.[28] This test for the most part has been replaced by MRI. CT is often done in conjunction with a discogram which allows the image to show internal fissures within the disc.

Nuclear Medicine

Nuclear medicine is an imaging technique that takes advantage of the radiation generated by the radioactive decay of the atom's nuclear material. Nuclear medicine is a powerful tool for evaluating physiologic functions as the radiation dosage is small. The radioactive material can be attached to various molecules which go to various tissues in different amounts depending on health and sickness. Bone scanning, a nuclear medicine imaging technique, can be helpful in identifying lesions (cancers, fractures, and metabolic diseases) which do not show under regular x-ray imaging.

Bone Scans

In certain disease conditions the metabolism of bone is accelerated. The rate of incorporation of calcium phosphate taken from the circulating pool is increased. Tagging some of the circulating phosphate with a radioactive marker (technetium-99) leads to the concentration of some of the radioactivity at sites of increased metabolism and blood flow. These sites can be identified by obtaining a body scan of the radioactive emissions. Many conditions of bone show an increased uptake, hence the test is nonspecific but still sensitive.

After injuries, the clinician may want to exclude fractures, and x-rays should be used first. Unfortunately, fractures are not always visible. This applies particularly to hairline fractures of long bones and fractures in vertebrae that have other abnormalities or have had prior partial collapse, as well as the small bones of the wrist and ankle. The process that heals fractures involves an increased metabolism of bone, including the incorporation of pyrophosphate; therefore, even cryptic (hidden) fractures show up with bone scans. Therefore, if an x-ray is negative a bone scan can still be used to exclude a fracture.

In young patients, deposition of calcium and phosphate after a fracture begins promptly. Under the age of sixty-five, acute fractures can be identified within twenty-four hours with 95% accuracy. Delays occur in persons who have slow metabolic rates caused by age and disease; however, within three days virtually all fractures show (Matin 1988; Rupani 1985). If a fracture is not seen but still is suspected, a bone scan can be used.

Like hairline fractures, stress fractures are sometimes invisible on plain x-rays, and bone scanning can clinch a diagnosis. The cortex of certain bones consists of several layers; stress fractures typically involve only some layers. The amount of radioactive uptake, therefore, helps grade stress fractures as well (Matin 1979). Compression fractures of the vertebrae show an increased uptake for up to two years after injury (Daffner *ibid*).

Osteitis pubis, particularly in women, is sometimes visualized on bone scans better than on x-rays. Malignancies and myeloma occasionally can be identified with bone scans.

Medical Ultrasound

Medical ultrasound was developed from a military tool refined in World War II for identifying submarines known as "sonar." Ultrasound Imaging does not use x-rays to create the image. It uses sound waves that are sent into the body. The returning echoes are listened for, just as in sonar. The sound waves are then converted into a visual image. Ultrasound, except for assessment of vascular circulation, is not commonly used in musculoskeletal medicine. This is slowly changing, and a highly trained technician can use ultrasound to visualize most musculoskeletal tissues quite accurately. This can be used in the diagnosis of soft tissue lesions as well as in guiding procedures such as injection into a bursal sac.

Thermography

Thermography is a tool that can be used to measure skin temperature very accurately. It does not involve any radiation or transmission of energy to the patient. It is especially useful in assessing sympathetic nervous activity and blood flow. The four most commonly used devices to measure heat

---

28. A spinal headache, which can also result from other procedures that puncture the spine, is usually treated with bed-rest and caffeine. If the headache does not resolve after a few days blood can be withdrawn from the patient and injected into the epidural space in the back. This usually resolves the pain immediately and is called a blood patch.

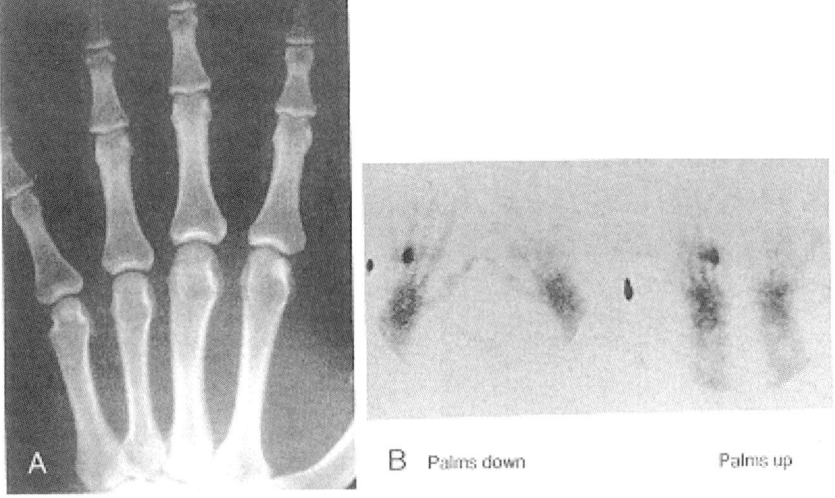

Figure 4-30: Fracture positive on bone scan (B), negative on x-ray (A)

are electrical thermistores, contact thermography, video/TV-thermography, and infrared beam thermography (Figure 4-32). Video-thermography is the most commonly used in clinical practice and can give real-time measurements differentiating between temperatures as little as 0.1 degrees Celsius apart, and can image areas ranging from four square millimeters to the entire body. Infrared hand held devises are essentially the same as used to take body temperature via the ear. They can only measure small areas at a time. So many measurements are needed to be made to get useful information and reconstruct regional views. Contact thermography is not very sensitive or accurate. Thermisters are rarely used clinically.

In general, healthy human bodies exhibit a contralateral temperature symmetry. Some nociceptive and most neuropathic pain pathologies are associated with an alteration of the thermal distribution. Thermography can be used to differentiate between CRPS (RSD) and radicular pain. In CRPS patients the distribution of temperature abnormalities is seen in a multisegmental patterns, while with discogenic or radicular pain a segmental presentation is usually seen. Thermography is also used to document soft tissue injuries. Thermography has been shown to detect pneumothorax rapidly and accurately (Dulabon et al 2004). Thermography has also been shown to be useful in Reynaud's syndrome, phantom limb pain, phantom body pain, stress fractures, and tendinitis (Sherman, Tan and Shanti 2004). Interexaminer and intraexaminer reliability in assessing paraspinal skin temperature patterns is very high (Owens et al 2004). Computerized assisted techniques to assess the image are available as well (Herry and Frize 2004). Thermography is also useful when

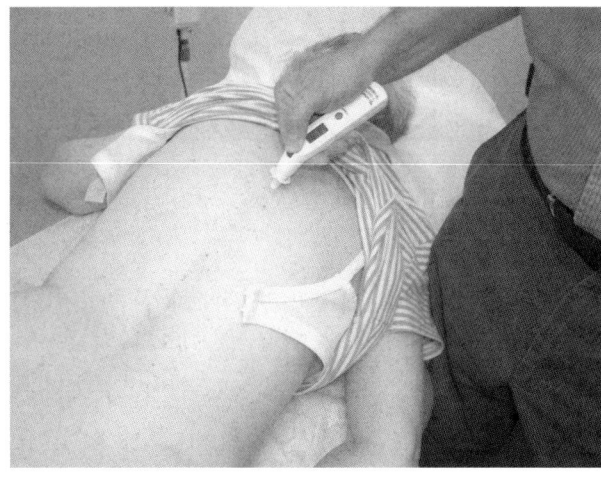

Figure 4-32: Infrared beam thermography.

integrated during laser or photonic therapy to both document change and to guide probe placement (Figure 4-31).

Visceral Imaging

While not commonly associated with musculoskeletal practice, visceral imaging spans the entire spectrum of imaging technology. The use of plain radiographic imaging of the viscera can be discussed briefly, but visceral imaging is the heart and sole of the newer imaging modalities, CT, MRI, ultrasound, and even nuclear medicine.

Plain film imaging of the chest is the standard to which all other modalities are compared. Imaging of the chest for

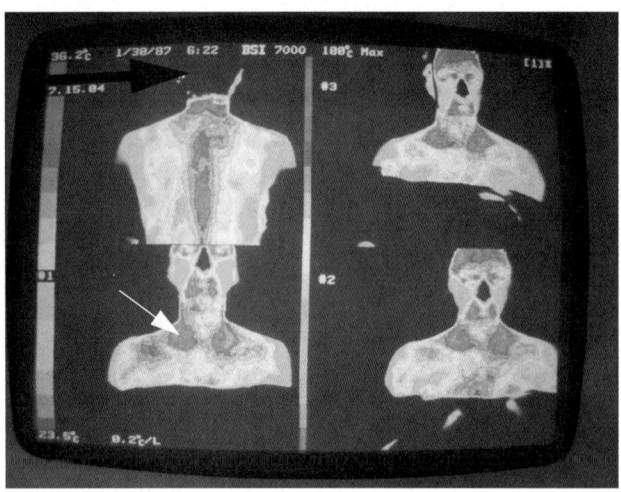

Figure 4-31: Thermography image. Darker colors indicate higher temperatures white arrow).

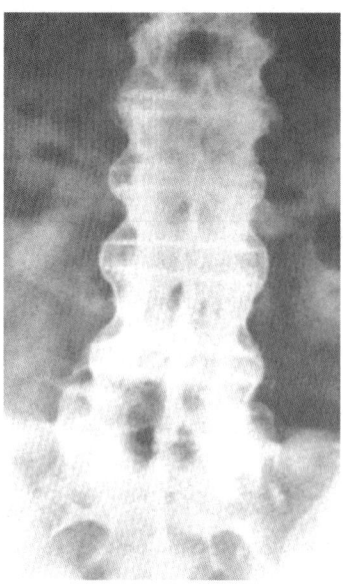

Figure 4-33: Ankylosing spondylitis.

cardiac size and clarity of the lung fields has remained a standard of care for almost the entire 100 years of radiography. The routine chest x-ray is the gold standard for people with coughs, chest pain, and pleurisy.

Plain film imaging of the abdomen is also of value when looking for gas patterns or fluid levels as indicators of obstruction and large abdominal masses. These films are, in many cases, supplemented by other imaging technology, particularly CT scanning, which can better define the organs and nature of masses in the abdomen. These other technologies can be used to exclude visceral pathology when abdominal pain is suspected of being of spinal origin.

ULTRASOUND of the female pelvis is extremely safe and quite informative. The use of this in the evaluation of female pelvic pain and for examinations during pregnancy is now the preferred technique. Pelvic organ disease can refer pain to the low back and sacral areas, and ultrasound may be used when such an origin is suspected.

MAMMOGRAPHY, still being hotly debated, is perhaps the best single way of detecting early breast cancer. As with many costly screening tests, the cost of finding an individual tumor may never be rationalized, but in any individual it may be particularly helpful and valuable, even though statistically mammography may not increase early detection and clinical outcome. As breast cancer spreads to bones, pain is a common complaint.

It should be noted that thermography may be a more accurate technology to pick up early breast cancer and can also reduce the false-negative/positive rates of mammography (Ng and Sudharsan 2004).

Imaging the Spine

X-ray imaging of the spine (and feet) needs to be performed standing or while the subject is bearing weight. If its performed in any other way it is of limited value. This cannot be over emphasized, as, in fact, routine spine imaging is often performed non-weight bearing, and therefore little information about mechanical disorders and joint dysfunction is acquired. Weight bearing studies should therefore be specified when ordering x-ray studies of the spine and foot. Assessment of x-rays for possible causes of, and contributors to musculoskeletal dysfunctions and pain, should be undertaken by the holistic/complementary doctor. This type of analysis usually is not performed by the radiologist, and it is best done with knowledge of the clinical situation. It should therefore follow the assessment by the radiologist, not instead of it. Disc space narrowing and the presence of somatic changes that impact function all need to be assessed on an individual basis. The use of x-ray imaging, particularly in the low back, is frequently misunderstood, but can be a powerful therapeutic tool.

Congenital Abnormalities

Many abnormalities, such as unequal leg length, unlevel sacral base, facet orientations, Ferguson's angle, and kissing spinous processes, can only be shown by taking an x-ray. These abnormalities are clinically significant and may determine appropriate treatment.

Spondylolisthesis, which can be congenital in nature, but of which trauma seems to be the most common cause, can be demonstrated by several views. This lesion of the pars interarticularis can be identified on the AP and lateral x-ray.

Imaging the Spine

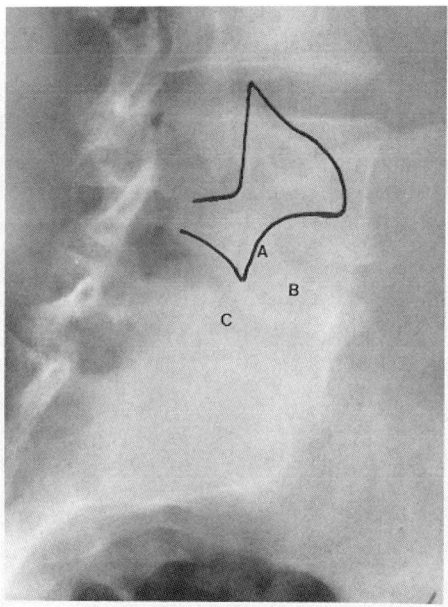

Figure 4-34: Oblique views showing collar of a scotty dog.

These views are require relatively high radiation and should be used sparingly and with forethought. The oblique image demonstrates the lesion and is identified as the "collar of the scotty dog" (Figure 4-34). In degenerative spondylolisthesis the degree of anterior displacement is usually not more than about a fourth of the lower vertebral body width (which is first or second degree spondylolisthesis). For more information see page 647.

Degenerative Disc and Joint Disease

Several degenerative processes in the spine and sacroiliac joints can be demonstrated by x-ray. Spondylosis or degenerative joint disease which can create abnormal joint mechanics is demonstrable by x-ray. The identification of the osteophytes adjacent to vertebral facets is evidence of persistent mechanical problems and is not directly correlated with pain. This condition is, however, correlated with ligamentous laxity.

The sacroiliac joints are frequent sites of degenerative joint disease and instability. The presence of osteophytes, subarticular sclerosis (osteitis condesans), and joint space narrowing are indicative of abnormal joint mechanics. Increased movement in the sacroiliac joint causes an increase in bony architecture of the ilium, called "osteitis condesans ilii." The earliest changes are a fuzziness of the subarticular bone. Eventually the joint space becomes *narrower*.

The radiological assessment of disc space height is sometimes helpful. But the fact that the degree of degenerative disc disease does not correlate with pain makes this assessment of marginal value. The discs, which are made of fibrocartilaginous material, are radio-opaque and do not show an x-ray shadow. A *vacuum* sign can develop—due to collections of nitrogen gas in nuclear and annular fissures—and is seen with an incidence of 2% to 3% in the general population (Figure 4-35).

Assessment of disc disease is best done by MRI, which can display the disc in the sagittal and transverse planes. This allows for assessment of nerve root compromise and internal disc disruption, especially with a T2 image. Disc fissures can be demonstrated as high intensity zones (HIZ) on a T2 image.

Provocative discography is often needed to ascertain if a disc is truly symptomatic, as MRI findings correlate poorly with clinical findings and are often misleading. The underlying premise of discography is that this applied stimulus replicates the clinically noxious stimulus responsible for the patient's symptoms, and that the reproduction of the patients clinical symptoms during the injection confirms the disc as the source of pain. Annular fissures originating in the nucleus and extending to the outer annulus, which is where the majority of the discs' nerve endings reside, can be a cause of pain. During discography, contrast is injected (under radiological imaging) into the nucleus. If there are no fissures, the contrast will be confined to the nucleus (Figure 4-36). Both cadaver and clinical studies have demonstrated that discography is more sensitive than MRI in detecting disc degeneration, particularly when post-discography CT scanning is added (Derby 2004).

Joint Dysfunction

Radiography of the spine can demonstrate persistent mechanical joint dysfunctions. Radiographic evaluation of the spine for somatic joint dysfunctions has remained a challenge since the first osteopaths began evaluating these structures by x-ray. The difficulty has been the correlation of the physical examination of a specific mechanical joint dysfunction with a specific radiographic finding. The problem has been that clinicians trained to assess joint function usually are not as adept at interpreting x-rays, and radiologists are not trained in assessing joint function. The clinician who takes the time to develop skills of reading x-rays for mechanical dysfunctions is rewarded by aiding his diagnosis and demonstrating the effects of treatments. To assess function by x-rays, the films should be taken standing and in flexion, extension, and sidebending.

Ideally, the vertebrae are stacked in perfect geometric formation. Deviations from this ideal should be catalogued and evaluated in the quest for somatic dysfunction. Whether the spinous processes are aligned and whether they divide the spaces between the pedicles symmetrically should be assessed. If there is asymmetry, the relevant spinal level should be noted and the variations between the asymmetries surveyed. The presence of a lateral spinal curve or scoliosis indicates vertebral dysfunction. The nomenclature of the findings and the ascription of clinical significance have pro-

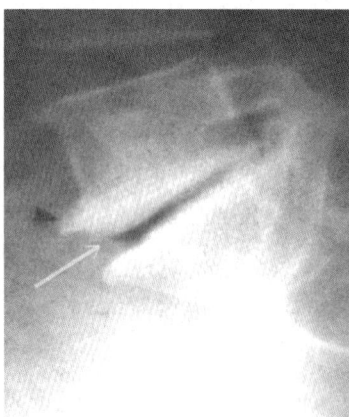

Figure 4-35: Degenerated disc with vacuum phenomenon (white arrow). Note osteophyte formation (black arrow head).

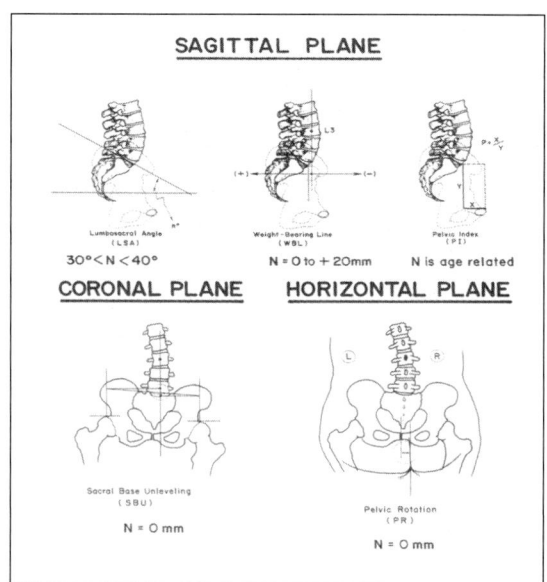

Figure 4-37: Measurements done on pelvic x-rays (From Kuchera WA and Kuchera ML, Osteopathic Principles in Practice, KCOM press 1993, with permission).

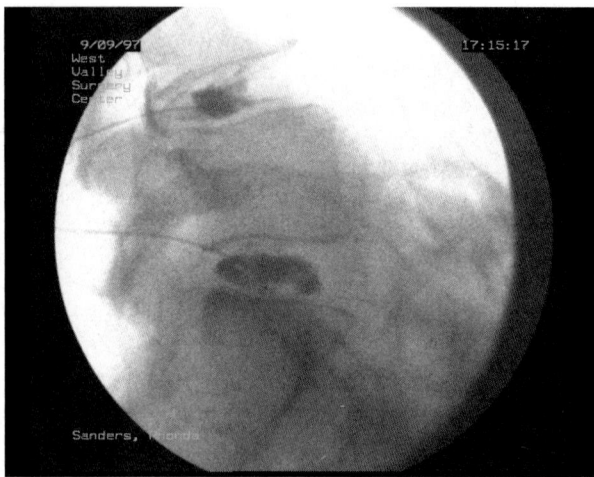

Figure 4-36: Discography of L4-5 discs. Dye is injected into the nucleus of the disc. Pain and leaking are noted. L4-5 is positive and seen as a dark crescent shape of contrasting material at the outer posterior annulus. L5 is normal.

gressed through a number of classifications, mostly in osteopathic circles. The present comments are based on Greenman's classification. The position of each vertebra is described in relation to the one below it. Motion is described as seen from above and in front of the vertebrae. This means that in rotation, the anterior surface of the vertebral body is used for definition rather than the posterior elements, which are available to palpation, and which are used in Chiropractic literature (Greenman *ibid*).

Radiography of Vertebral Rotation

The spine functions as a unit. The short and long "Stays" regulating its interconnected movements consist of the intervertebral ligaments and joint capsules, the fascial sheets at all layers of the paravertebral muscles, and, in fact, the whole sausage of the trunk. Compensatory scoliosis—which seems to be reactive to a distant abnormality—occurs over at least three vertebrae and is often S-shaped and smooth. Vertebral intersegmental movements consist of side bending and rotation in opposite direction (Veldhuizen 1987). This is *type one scoliosis* (neutral dysfunction). An unlevel sacrum (sacral base) is one common cause (Nash 1969). The sacrum may be unlevel because of a geometric factor (i.e., leg-length discrepancy or asymlocation). The somatic dysfunction of the sacrum itself also can be classified.

The extent of scoliosis is commensurate with the amount of unleveling. The spinous processes rotate to the inside of the curve and the anterior surfaces face the outside of the curve. On lateral films, the spinous processes fan out normally in flexion; the scoliosis is not seen. This type of scoliosis is usually secondary and does not cause back pain (Figure 4-38).

The rotation and sidebending of one vertebra on its fellow below *to the same side* is defined as a *type two somatic dysfunction (*nonneutral dysfunction). The findings are those of a *short-curve scoliosis* or a vertebral curve involving only two (or at most three) vertebrae. It is thought that type two somatic dysfunction is often caused by local factors, or at least local stiffness. The radiographic description of a type two lesion requires standing films, which should include erect anteroposterior and lateral films, taken in flexion and extension as well.

An alteration in the AP curve (fanning of the spinous processes) is seen in flexion, extension, or both. The stuck joint prevents the adjacent vertebrae from moving into flexion or extension. (In the lumbar spine, flexion lesions are more common.)

Because the vertebrae concerned retain a fixed position in side bending, they develop a two-segment, *short-curve scoliosis* (Hayes 1989), as seen on the AP x-ray view.

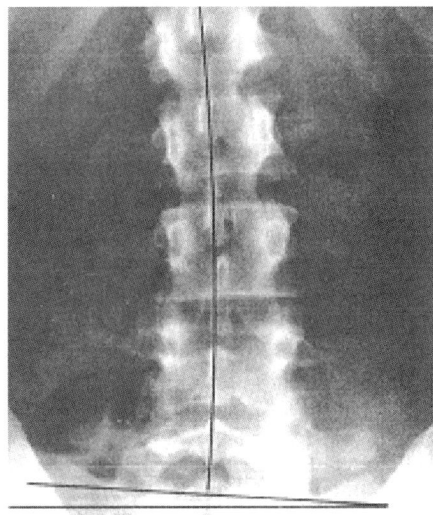

Figure 4-38: Scoliosis from sacral base unleveling.

The clinical description of type two somatic dysfunction is based on altered vertebral motion, as judged by palpation; the radiological description is based on still films, hence views at the extreme range of movement are needed (Figure 4-39).

In the radiographical analysis of type two somatic dysfunction the following should be noted:

- the way in which the concerned vertebrae are side bent and rotated;
- the response to flexion and extension.

The radiographic evaluation thus requires analysis of the spine, vertebra by vertebra.

The position of the spinous process between the pedicles on the AP film defines rotation (Cobb 1958). The *bony appearance of the pedicles* can give clues about rotation as well.

The short-curve scoliosis is created because the lumbar vertebrae in the dysfunctional segment cannot rotate without side bending; therefore, the two transverse processes will *appear* to approximate each other on the concave side (Greenman *ibid*).

Objects are magnified in radiography the farther they are from the film. This can be used as a clue to vertebral rotation. If one transverse process *appears* larger, it is probably *farther* from the film (Figure 4-39).

In summary, in type two somatic dysfunction the radiographic findings might include:

1. a spinous process rotated out of the mid-vertebral position;
2. pedicles that appear to have different sizes or shapes;
3. transverse processes on the inside of the curve spread farther apart and seeming larger;
4. transverse processes on the outside of the curve spread farther apart and seeming larger;
5. a possible *flat spot* on the flexion/extension films (Figure 4-40).

Changes on Magnetic Resonance Imaging and Computed Tomography

Type two somatic dysfunction might be suspected from the appearance of asymmetry in MRI and CT images. Since the upper vertebral body of the "short-curve scoliosis" is side-bent and rotated in the transverse plane, the changes will be reflected in the images. The rotation will appear to be a spinous process of the upper vertebra *not* in line with the rest of the spinous processes. The transverse processes will be inclined relative to the bottom of the film. The side bending will appear to be one transverse process, seeming to be more "imaged" than the other, or not equally sliced. Disc bulging may be seen posteriorly on the inside of the curve of the side bending. Zygoapophyseal joint asymmetry may be present in marked cases, and in chronic cases, osteoarthritis changes develop (Figure 4-41).

It is not possible to see changes with flexion and extension on MRI or CT because the gantry always is horizontal. The clinician will have noted if the patient has difficulty lying flat, but when the patient is made to lie as flat as possible for the study, a number of incidental observations may give graphic clues to the presence of type two somatic dysfunction. This dysfunction, as previously mentioned, causes side bending and rotation at one level, and, because the patient may not be able to lie straight, the spine will not image symmetrically, the pelvic ring will be affected with asymlocation, and the coronal views might slice the sacrum tangentially. It should be remembered that the spine functions as a whole, including the pelvis. Through tensegrity the artificial straightening of the dysfunctional segment distorts the alignment of remote parts—in this case, the pelvis—which, although not weight-bearing, might be more easily repositioned in space.

It is a tautology that somatic dysfunction in the pelvic ring concerns the position of the three bones. It also concerns the position of the three bones within the trunk. This is why computer-assisted reconstitutions of the anatomical relationships in the supine torso can be a source of abundant information, which has so far remained untapped. For instance, the presence of an ilial upslip or downslip is reflected on the transverse images, one side appearing to be sliced lower than the other (Figure 4-42)..

It so happens that type two somatic dysfunction is common at L4-L5 but is hard to evaluate on plain films. With MRI and CT images there are, however, many findings. (It is unlikely that these studies would be requisitioned for confirmation of somatic dysfunction in Osteopathy or Orthopaedic

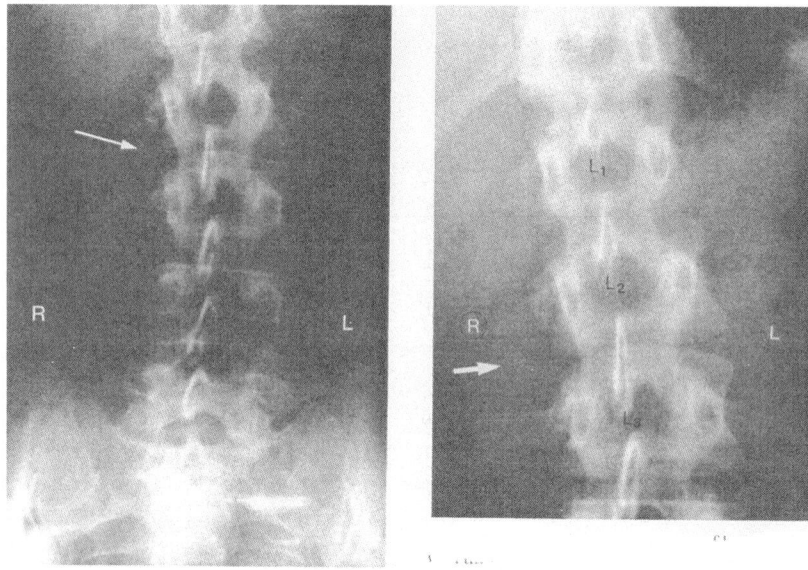

Figure 4-39: **A**; Type two dysfunction. The L2 vertebra is rotated right, side-bent right or "RSR." If the vertebra is stuck in flexion, the lesion is "flexed, rotated right, and side-bent right" Note right transverse processes are closer together and smaller. **B**; Anterior-posterior view of lumbar spine with the closed arrow pointing to the short curve scoliosis at L2-3.

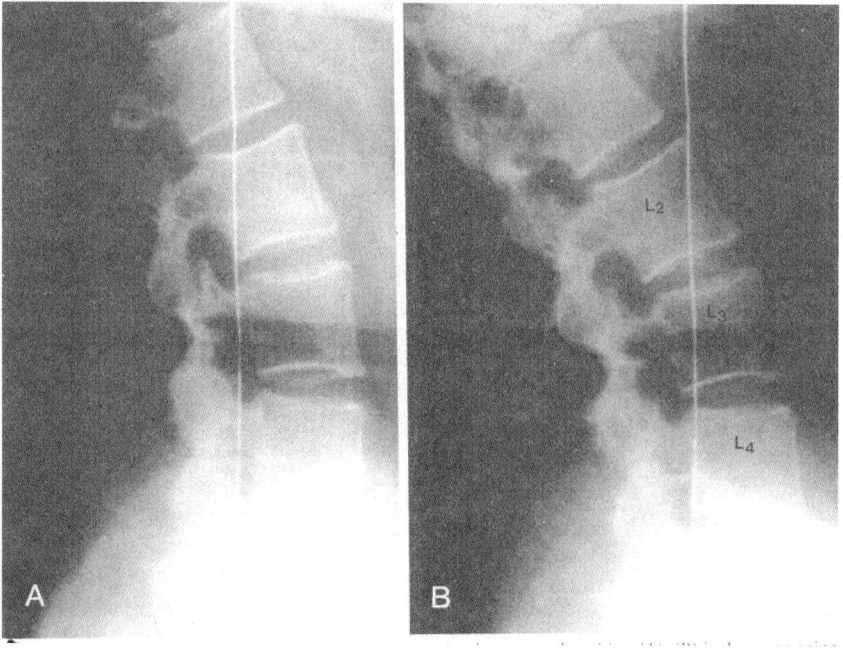

Figure 4-40: Lateral standing view of lumbar spine in a neutral position (A). (B) is the same spine in extension. Note that most of the movement is from L3 and above. L4 vertebra moves only slightly and is therefore "fixed" in flexion.

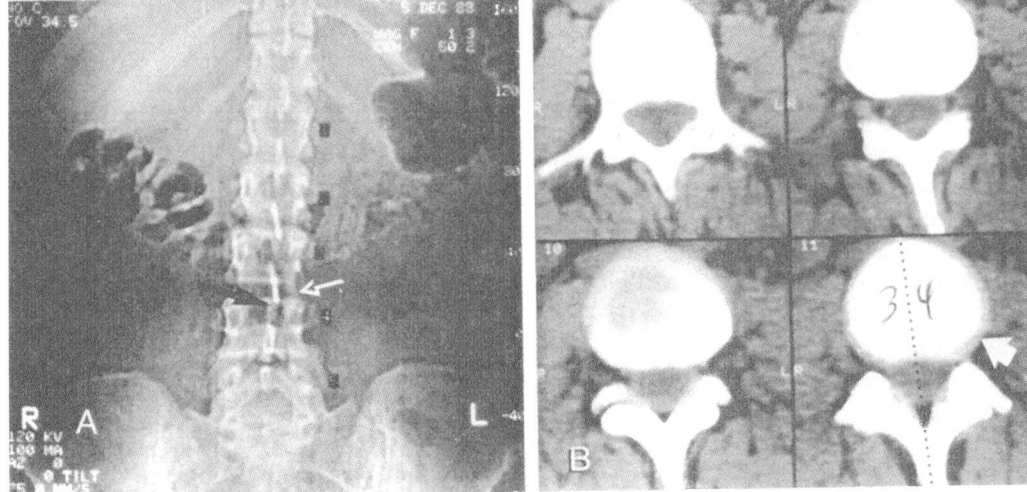

Figure 4-41: (A) is an anterior-posterior computer reconstructed image showing a type II somatic dysfunction at L3-4. The L3 vertebra is side-bent left and rotated right. The black arrow points to a spinous process that is out of line, and the white arrow points to the disc space, which is compressed on the left side. In (B) note the disc bulging (white arrow). The vertebral bodies appear rotated, and this is not an artifact but an essential observation. The dotted line is drawn on the long axis of the L3 vertebra and demonstrates the right rotation in axial plane.

medicine, but the images may be available through serendipity from the search for a disc pathology.)

Wrist Imaging

Lateral imaging of the wrist for the presence of ligamentous injuries is probably the most useful and powerful tool in diagnosing somatic joint dysfunctions and ligamentous laxity in all radiography. Other films of the wrist, including the radial and ulnar deviation views, also contain significant information regarding the presence of joint dysfunctions. This information should not be overlooked in any individual with upper extremity pain. Often a wrist dysfunction impacts both the elbow and the shoulder. Resolving pain complaints in these areas can become particularly difficult unless wrist joint dysfunctions are treated.

The lateral wrist film can demonstrate the presence of significant ligamentous injuries just by calculating the radio-scaphoid and the radio-lunate angles. The radio-scaphoid angle is a reflection of the integrity of the scapa-lunate ligament. Laxity of this ligament usually follows a fall with an outstretched hand and a dorsi-flexed wrist. Injury to this ligament can have a significant impact on the dynamics of how the entire wrist works. The radio-lunate angle defines the relationship of the lunate to the radius and provides information regarding the status of the bony architecture of the entire wrist.

The posterior to anterior (PA) wrist films also contain important information on the presence of somatic joint dysfunctions, and, again, attention should be paid to the position of the scaphoid and the lunate (Figure 4-43). The scaphoid should appear to become bigger between radial and ulnar deviation. Lack of changes in its size is a significant finding and suggests the presence of joint dysfunctions of the wrist and possible ligamentous injury.

Ankle Imaging

Ankle imaging is as important as wrist imaging. Sprained ankles, any inversion injury, and almost any ankle injury is capable of creating a tremendous number of somatic dysfunctions and ligamentous injuries. Injuries to the ligament holding the tibia and fibula together (the syndesmosis) are frequent, particularly in sprained ankles. This slight widening of the ankle mortise creates a moderate amount of ankle instability that can sometimes be treated by conservative measures.

Also, since sprained ankles are so common and frequently create joint dysfunctions, assessment of the foot is particularly important. Assessment of foot imaging can best be performed by looking at the lateral film for the cyma line. The cyma line is the combination of the curved linear line and the mid tarsal joint line. If this line is present and intact, there are no major foot faults or joint dysfunctions. If however, this line is broken, then either manipulative care, orthotics, injection, acupuncture therapy, or, at times, surgery is indicated (Figure 4-44).

The lateral film is also capable of generating considerable information about other joint dysfunctions, including the talus and cuboid. During gate, the talus rotates medially and inferiorly to accommodate the tibia. This particular motion of the talus is controlled by powerful ligamentous

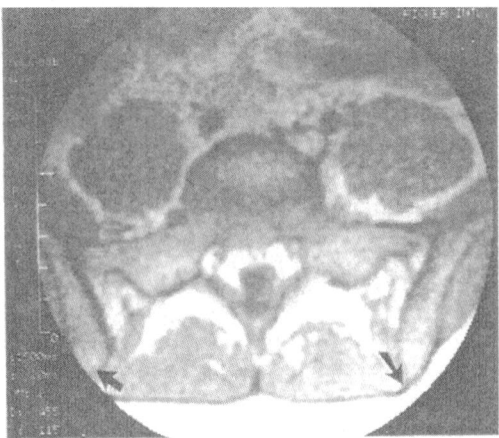

Figure 4-42: MRI scan with ilia cut unequally indicating sacral somatic dysfunction (even though the picture is centered on the disc). Note that the ilii (arrows) are unequal in size and are at different heights from the table top.

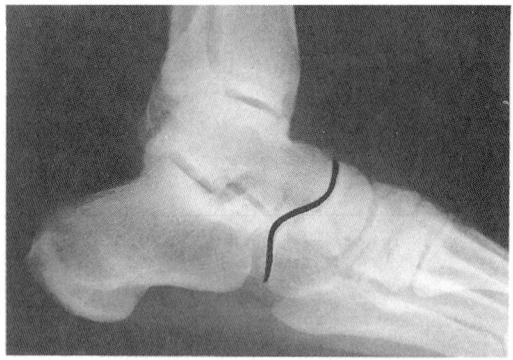

Figure 4-44: Lateral view of foot with cyma line drawn on it.

these two findings are present, the bone is in good position and offers the foot considerable stability.[29]

Knee Imaging

The knee is frequently imaged by plain films, but generally only for identifying major dysfunctions and the presence of degenerative osteoarthritis (Figure 4-46). However, an MRI of the knee has proven to be worthwhile (Figure 4-47).

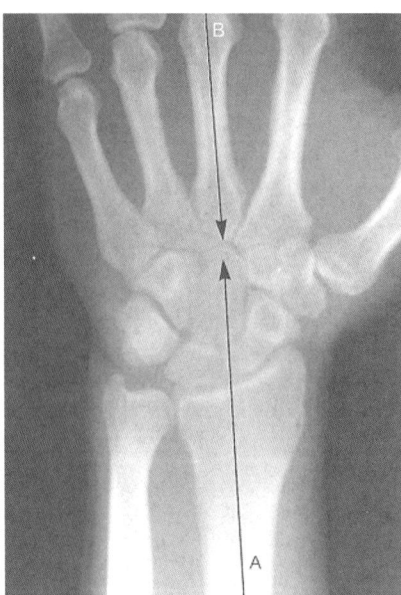

Figure 4-43: Wrist with normal alignment.

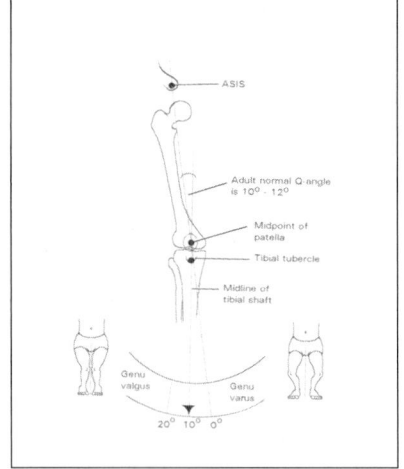

Figure 4-45: Q angle (courtesy of WA Kuchera).

structures. Injuries to these structures due to sprained ankles frequently allow this bone to go into internal rotation and slight extension very early in stance phase, and create a very unstable foot. On the normal film, this bone should be horizontal. If tipped into a more vertical position, this is an indication of ligamentous laxity and talar instability, which could also be interpreted as foot instability.

The cuboid is also quite important in identifying the presence of joint dysfunctions. When in an incorrect position, the cuboid can create a myriad of abnormalities. The correct position demonstrates a clear peroneus longus line, and the calcaneal-cuboid joint lines should align. When

---

29. The cuboid which is the "keystone" of the lateral arch is frequently displaced in sprained ankles and other ankle and foot injuries. Think for a moment of all of the dysfunctions which are created by this single bone dysfunction. The peroneus longus is now being stretched. This causes it to fire early and longer than normal, causing "shin splints." A process of the cuboid lies above the long plantar nerve, so when the bone rotates internally, this process begins to stretch the nerve. This creates pain, which is referred to the distal foot and can sometimes be mistaken for a Morton's neuroma. These foot dysfunctions (also common after motor vehicle injury) and pain create a limp, which can cause pain in the neck, back, and shoulder.

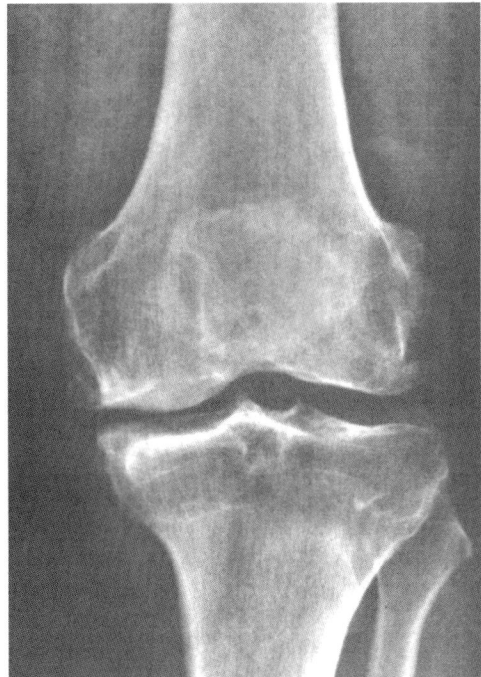

Figure 4-46: Degenerative joint disease of the knee.

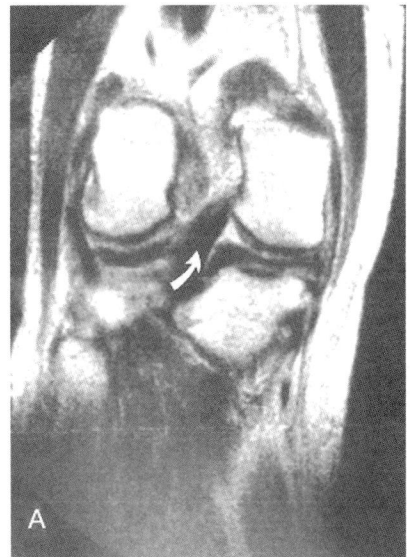

Figure 4-47: MRI image of normal knee.

Assessment of the meniscus, anterior cruciate ligament, posterior cruciate ligament, the cartilaginous and bony structures adjacent to them can all be made using the MRI. Numerous "blind" areas on an MRI of the knee occur, but the only other option is arthroscopic evaluation, which is much more invasive. An MRI of the knee appears to be the least expensive and perhaps the best overall way to evaluate the knee

Anterior knee pain, which is a frequent musculoskeletal complaint, can and often does leave radiographic "tracks" that can be found on an x-ray. The Q angle of the femur and the tibia is an important measurement and is easy to evaluate on an x-ray. The sunrise view of the patella is also helpful in the evaluation of anterior knee pain. Anterior knee pain can be due to many causes that leave little or no radiographic changes, so the use of radiography should be used only after a careful physical evaluation has been performed.

Shoulder and Elbow Imaging

The shoulder and elbow are frequently talked about as areas to be imaged by plain radiography. However, the physical examination in these areas is so superb, and the imaging modalities so relatively imprecise, that x-rays usually are not needed (Figure 4-48). Acromioclavicular subluxation is shown in Figure 4-49.

In summary, radiographic imaging can aid the clinician in determine the cause of musculoskeletal pain. Radio-

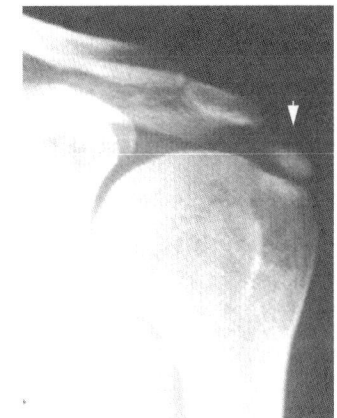

Figure 4-48: Calcification of supraspinous tendon.

graphic imaging is also vitally important in excluding other possible medical causes.

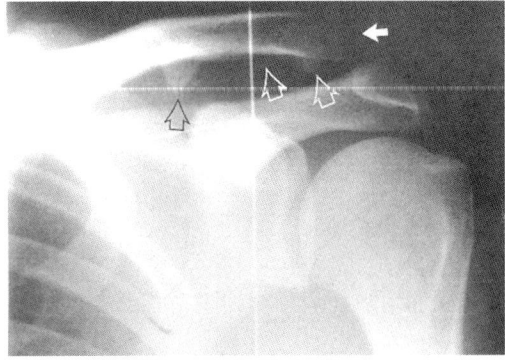

Figure 4-49: AP view of shoulder girdle with subluxed acromioclavicular joint.

5

TREATMENT PRINCIPLES FOR INTEGRATIVE MUSCULOSKELETAL MEDICINE: ACUPUNCTURE AND DRY NEEDLING

Oriental Medicine (OM) has many techniques that can be useful when addressing both systemic and musculoskeletal disorders and that are helpful in the overall management of musculoskeletal disorders. Artifacts have dated acupuncture back to about 1,000 BC, and acupuncture/Chinese medicine was well described as a medical system by about 200 BC in *The Yellow Emperor's Classic of Internal Medicine* which devoted many pages to the treatment of pain. James Cyriax (the developer of Orthopaedic Medicine) used to say that all pain arises from a source, so all treatments must reach that source and be appropriate for *the* lesion. However, many musculoskeletal disorders have combined etiologies and often are not the result of a single identifiable lesion; an integration of ideas is therefore helpful. While Orthopaedic Medicine and most modern biomedical approaches emphasize treatment of a disease (or a lesion), less attention is paid to why this "failure" has occurred in the first place. Other medical paradigms (many of which have been called "energetic" or "holistic" medicines) tend to study *systems* (such as Myers myofascial channels, channels in OM, or Osteopathic integrative models). Their integration can greatly supplement "lesion/disease" oriented approaches. Modern biomechanical or biomedical ideas can be integrated with OM to increase our understanding of the cause of pain. By integrating Orthopaedic Medicine and TCM and/or OM methods, specificity of treatment and successful outcomes can be increased.

Proper application of OM methods requires a full OM medical evaluation. *Spiritual Axis* states, "The superior physician understands the spirit. His understanding of man includes both Blood and Qi, whether there is Excess or Deficiency, whether he could tonify or disperse." Several OM and acupuncture methods, however, can be performed independently or with a minimal knowledge of Chinese medical theory; and many so-called medical acupuncturists have pointed out that it is possible to get "very good results" from what TCM/OM trained practitioners would consider "very bad acupuncture" (Hopwood 1997). In 1997 an NIH Consensus Statement said that:

> Acupuncture as a therapeutic intervention is widely practiced in the United States. While there have been many studies of its potential usefulness, many of these studies provide equivocal results because of design, sample size, and other factors. The issue is further complicated by inherent difficulties in the use of appropriate controls, such as placebos and sham acupuncture groups. However, promising results have emerged; for example, efficacy of acupuncture in adult postoperative and chemotherapy nausea and vomiting and postoperative dental pain. There are other situations such as addiction, stroke rehabilitation, headache, menstrual cramps, tennis elbow, fibromyalgia, myofascial pain, osteoarthritis, low back pain, carpal tunnel syndrome, and asthma, in which acupuncture may be useful as an adjunct treatment, an acceptable alternative or be included in a comprehensive management program. Further research is likely to uncover additional areas where acupuncture interventions will be useful.

Patient characteristics for outpatient treatments with acupuncture in Beijing, China are: The most common condition is Bell's palsy, which represented 20.6% and 25.3% of total cases at the two clinics, respectively. The second most common condition was cerebrovascular accident (CVA) rehabilitation. These treatments represented 11.9% and 12.0% of treatments at the two clinics, respectively. Other trends at the clinics included the following: (1) neurologic complaints predominated; (2) doctors see a large number of patients per day; (3) the majority of patients overall were female; while (4) the majority of patients treated for CVAs rehabilitation were male (Napadow and Kaptchuk 2004).

Musculoskeletal disorders are among the more common conditions for which patients seek relief. It is the stated supposition of this text that integrated medicine benefits patients beyond any single intervention. Many studies seem to support this position. A few examples follow below.

A multidisciplinary approach to chronic back pain has been shown to be beneficial (Elkayam et al 1996). In the treatment of fibromyalgia (FM), Offenbacher and Stucki (2000) concluded that, based on anecdotal evidence and small observational studies, physiotherapy may reduce overloading of the muscle system, improve postural fatigue and positioning, and condition weak muscles. Modalities (ultrasound, diathermy, etc.) and whole body cryotherapy may reduce localized as well as generalized pain in the short term. Trigger point injection may reduce pain originating from concomitant trigger points in selected FM patients. Massage may reduce muscle tension and may be prescribed as an adjunct with other therapeutic interventions. Acupuncture may reduce pain and increase pain threshold. Biofeedback may positively influence subjective and objective disease measures, and TENS may reduce localized musculoskeletal pain. Accordingly, a multidisciplinary approach combining these therapies in a well-balanced program may be the most promising strategy and is currently recommended in the treatment of FM syndrome. Acupuncture and other "alternative" modalities were shown to be helpful in musculoskeletal patients in both hospital-based and outpatient settings. Even inpatients with severe pain such as postsurgical pain can benefit from integrated approaches. Acupuncture can be used for post-surgical pain and other functional complications such as reducing reflex retention of urine, impairment of the drainage function of the bronchi, intestinal paresis, bronchial asthma, vomiting, nausea, pain or itching in the stoma, chills, and hyperthermia. Electrical stimulation and biofeedback may be helpful as well (Tsibuliak, Alisov and Shatrova 1995). Preoperative intradermal acupuncture can reduce postoperative pain, nausea, and vomiting, analgesic requirement, and sympathoadrenal responses (Kotani, Hashimoto, Sato, Sessler, Yoshioka, Kitayama, Yasuda, Matsuki 2001). In patients with cancers of the head and neck, xerostomia is a frequent and potentially debilitating toxicity of radiotherapy. Acupuncture provides palliation for such patients (Johnstone, Peng, May, Inouye, Niemtzow 2001). Acupressure is an effective technique for pain treatment of minor trauma patients and can improve the quality of care in emergency transport (Kober et al 2002). Another important use of acupuncture is aiding in withdrawal symptoms from opiates (commonly needed in chronic pain patients), including rapid opiate detoxification (Otto 2003; Montazeri, Farahnakian and Saghaei 2002). Acupuncture effects in heroin dependence is through the same pathway as the opiate agonist (Procedol) on opiate receptors (Timofeev 1999). Acupuncture effects have been compared to the physiological effects of physical exercise (Andersson 1997) and may be of benefit for sedentary patients suffering from chronic pain. A recent study published in *Spine* compared acupuncture, manipulation, and medications in managing chronic (thirteen weeks duration) spinal pain (Giles and Muller 2003). The highest proportion of early (asymptomatic status) recovery was found for manipulation (27.3%), followed by acupuncture (9.4%) and medication (5%). Manipulation achieved the best overall results on the Oswestry scale (p-158). Acupuncture on the other hand showed the best VAS (p-156) scores for neck pain. Karjalainen et al (2003) found moderate support for evidence of positive effectiveness of multidisciplinary rehabilitation for subacute low back pain and that a workplace visit increases the effectiveness.

The treatment principles of musculoskeletal disorders in TCM are the same as those of other diseases: they are based on pattern diagnosis. The selection of treatment methods should be individualized considering the severity of the disease, the age of the patient as well as how long the patient has been ill, and the general health status of the patient.

There are often great differences between patients, the lengths of their illnesses, their states of health, and, therefore, there are corresponding differences between the natural courses of their conditions and their treatment prognoses. In clinical practice, it is often necessary to adopt multi-layered treatment methodologies. Treatment of Qi and Blood patterns are *usually* the first priority when treating musculoskeletal disorders. Considering both the skeletal and soft tissue systems, the Root and Branch, and both Interior and Exterior are important in all cases. In chronic cases, the length of the disease is particularly significant as it may effect the patient's general health (Zheng), their Organs, and therefore their ability to heal. It may be necessary to improve their Righteous-Qi so that healing can occur. There are many methods that can be used to address musculoskeletal injuries including: manipulation, mobilization, acupuncture, exercise, herbs, and surgery.

The main TCM treatment principles are as followed:

1. Qi and Blood patterns are usually given priority over the appearance of other patterns in the treatment of musculoskeletal disorders as these address pain. Regardless of clinical manifestations, regardless of whether there is visible damage to the Exterior, and regardless even of whether there is infection, the main etiology of symptoms associated with pain is disharmony of Qi and Blood. All pain that is due to soft-tissue injury is from Qi and Blood stagnation. The *Classic of Internal Medicine* (Su Wen) says, "Sickness caused by damage to Qi is invisible, but sickness caused by damage to Form (i.e., damage to bodily tissues or substantial evil such as Blood-stasis or Phlegm) is visible." Therefore, damage to Qi and Blood may manifest variously. While there may be damage to Qi only or to Blood only, in clinical practice both Qi and Blood are usually affected simultaneously, though the severity may manifest more in the Blood or in the Qi.

   In acute sprain/strains and/or contusions, both the Qi and Blood are injured, and one often finds diffuse pain, swelling, and/or hematomas. This means that Form and Qi are damaged, and, therefore, that the main treatment principle is to circulate the Blood to clear stasis, together with regulating Qi to reduce pain. This is the first priority when treating sprains and strains. The characteristic of Qi damage is distention-pain without swelling. Because Qi tends to move, pain from Qi-damage is difficult to localize and often affects large areas. When Qi-damage predominates, the treatment principle would be to regulate the Qi to stop pain, assisted by promoting Blood-circulation to eliminate and/or prevent Blood-stasis. Guiding formulas such as Bupleurum Powder to Spread the Liver (Chi Hu Shu Gan San) and Revive Health by Invigorating the Blood Decoction (Fu Yuan Huo Xue Tang) can be used.

   In contrast to Qi-stagnation, the characteristic of Blood-stasis is to gather and form masses/swellings, and to manifest as sharp and stabbing pain. The pain is easily localized, and the patient can point to the specific site of pain. The main treatment principle would be to promote Blood-circulation, assisted by regulating-Qi to stop pain. Formulas such as Four-Substance Decoction with Safflower and Peach Pit (Tao Hong Si Wu Tang) can be used as a guide.

It must be pointed out that one must also consider factors such as: Heat, Cold, Deficiency and Excess, and that frequent adjustments of treatment methods and formulas (both herbal and acupuncture) are usually needed. There is a TCM saying that applies to musculoskeletal disorders: "Distinguish between Yin and Yang, soft and hard, in the treatment of trauma. Treatment should target Yin for disorders of Yang and Yang for disorders of Yin." Treatment therefore must be based on the cause and origin of the disease and whether Qi or Blood damage dominates. For those with Blood-Excess patterns (Stasis), attacking methods should be used; and for Deficient patients, the tonification of Qi is emphasized.

2. The skeletal and soft tissue systems should be given equal weight because the two are closely related and always affect each other. For example, if a patient dislocates a joint, the bones move out of proper alignment, resulting in the derangement of the soft tissues connected to the affected bones; therefore, impairment of the Sinews (soft tissues) must be considered and treated in conditions such as fractures and bony dislocations. At the same time, primary injury to soft tissues can easily affect joint functions and therefore bony alignment. Here again, treatment of both structures is needed. Only by attending to both, can full function be restored. It is therefore important to learn manual therapies that can treat bony and soft tissue misalignments, as well as acupuncture and the use of herbs to treat underlying patterns and assist in regulating Qi and Blood.

3. The concept of the "Root and Branch" pertains to many ideas in TCM. It is used to explain the relationship between "conflicts" in the cause and manifestations of disease. In regard to the Righteous and the Evil, Righteous is the Root. In regard to the cause of a disease and its symptoms, the cause is the Root while symptoms are the Branch. In terms of location, the inner Organs are the Root and the Exterior is the Branch. In relation to chronicity, chronic disorders are the Root and new ones are the Branch, etc. The basic approach of TCM is the diagnosis and medical management of presenting symptoms and signs (pattern diagnosis). Healing can be achieved only if one is able to identify and treat the cause of the disease as well presenting symptoms. The onset and development of many medical conditions may manifest with a variety of symptoms and signs. These often represent the superficial pathology and may not reflect the Root cause of the disease. Hence, in clinical practice one must closely analyze superficial or Exterior symptoms, as well as history, in order to understand the Root and Branch. Clinically, treatment that addresses superficial symptoms, i.e., pain, takes precedent, as this is the patient's major concern. Treatment of the Root (e.g., Organs, fundamental joint functions) is often performed later in the development of the condition. Nevertheless, the Root must be addressed for the condition to heal.[1]

The patient may present in the clinic with an acute, chronic, or mixed disease, i.e., with both Root and Branch presentations. This may make it difficulty to determine treatment priorities. If the patient presents with the severity of Branch and Root equal, treatment is given equally to both. If symptoms are severe (e.g., pain), the Branch is usually treated first. The Root is addressed when the urgency is reduced. For example, when a patient presents with pain caused by spinal joint derangement, massage and acupuncture may be applied to the muscles to relieve spasm and thus treat the pain, the Branch; and manipulation may be used to treat joint derangement, the Root. This is known as treating the Branch and Root simultaneously. If, however, the pain and spasms are severe, it may be unwise to manipulate the patient's spine until the severity of symptoms is reduced.

The significance of considering both the Interior and the Exterior is that of paying attention to localized tissues as well as the whole body, as opposed to considering somatic (Exterior) or Organ (Interior) systems in isolation. Because musculoskeletal disorders often present with many symptoms and signs, the etiology may be complicated. The condition may be characterized as minor or severe, acute or chronic. The etiology and prognosis may vary depending on the location of trauma, which tissues are affected, and the patient's general condition (Righteous-Qi). Damage to somatic structures will result in the disharmony of Qi and Blood in the Exterior, and, later, in the Interior via the channels and Organs, which will be affected by the tissues they control. This results in loss of communication between Yin (or Ying/Essence) and Wei (Interior and Exterior), and disharmony between the Solid and Hollow Organs (Zhang and Fu). For example, in terms of soft tissue injury, Sinew damage can tax the Liver Organ/channel systems, since these control the health of the sinews. The channels and vessels are the conduits of Qi and Blood, which are always affected; therefore, even localized trauma may result in a whole-body effect, disrupting both the Exterior and the Interior. At the same time, any primary dysfunction within the channels, vessels, or Organs can also result in damage to the sinews. Attention to the whole body is therefore the hallmark of TCM treatment of musculoskeletal disorders.

---

1. While not a part of classical TCM thinking, healing often occurs regardless of treatment and therefore the natural course of different musculoskeletal disorders should be understood.

Depending on the nature of the condition, OM/TCM and integrative treatment of musculoskeletal disorders may include:
- Acupuncture and injection therapies
- Electromagnetic therapies
- Manual therapy—manipulation/massage
- Oral and topical herbal or pharmaceutical medications
- Moxibustion
- Cupping
- Bleeding, scraping, and related techniques
- Stabilization and other exercises
- Nutritional therapy
- Orthotics.

Thus, acupuncture and other "alternative and complementary" therapies should play a role in the management of many medical conditions. This chapter reviews mainly acupuncture treatment techniques used in this text, including both OM/TCM and Western methods. Chapters 6-9 cover the other topics.

Acupuncture and Dry Needling

For the purposes of this book:

> **Acupuncture** is the practice of using acupuncture needling techniques according to Oriental Medicine theories that have evolved throughout its development including developments during the modern period.
>
> **Dry needling** is the insertion of an acupuncture needle according to neuroanatomical concepts.[2]

While dry needling and acupuncture techniques often overlap, or are the same, the rational behind them is quite different. In general, acupuncture and other dry needling therapies have been shown to affect the immune systems, the inflammatory systems, the nervous systems (including autonomic, somatic, central, somatovisceral, and viscerosomatic pathways), the circulatory system, and the endocrine system. Acupuncture can be thought of as a method by which peripheral nervous and mechanical stimulation regulate endogenous mechanisms. The effects of acupuncture, including neurochemical, neurophysiological, anti-inflammatory, and circulatory have been documented in: *The Neurochemical Basis of Pain Relief by Acupuncture* (Han 1987; 2000); *The Vital Meridian: A Modern Exploration of Acupuncture* (Bensoussan 1991); *Medical Acupuncture: a Western Scientific Approach* (Filshie and White 1998); *Acupuncture & Related Techniques in Physical Therapy* (Hopwood, Lovesey and Mokone 1997), and *Clinical Acupuncture Scientific Basis* (2001), among others. Kendall (2002) reviews both Chinese and Western literature and includes some interesting *speculations*. A recently completed document produced by the Council of Acupuncture and Oriental Medicine Associations and the Foundation for Acupuncture Research titled: *Acupuncture and Electroacupuncture: Evidence-Based Treatment Guidelines* (2004) contains the most recent and up to date review on the Western literature.

In the West, acupuncture is often criticized as having "psychological" effects related more to "placebo" and the patient's "psychology" than the treatment itself. Many studies on acupuncture however have shown effectiveness greater than placebo. For example, acupuncture decreases somatosensory evoked potential amplitudes to noxious stimuli in *anesthetized* volunteers in a double blind setting (Meissner 2003). One study (Creamer et al 1999) evaluated the relationship between demographic and psychosocial variables and response to acupuncture as defined by reduction in pain and disability, at the end of an eight-week course of treatment of patients with knee osteoarthritis. Patients with symptomatic knee osteoarthritis who had previously participated in a controlled trial using acupuncture were recalled for an interview approximately one year later. Depression, anxiety, helplessness, self-efficacy, and fatigue were measured by standard instruments. Knee examination and assessment of pain threshold were measured by dolorimetry. The study results showed response at eight weeks was significantly related to duration of symptoms. A statistically nonsignificant trend was found for older and more educated subjects indicating better response for these populations. Anxiety and fatigue were found to be slightly inversely related to response (also statistically nonsignificant). Subjects with localized medial pain had significantly better response in terms of pain and disability than did subjects with generalized knee pain. The authors concluded that other than a weak relationship with anxiety (at eight weeks only), *no evidence* of a link between *psychosocial* variables and response to acupuncture was found.

At the same time, acupuncture, like all types of somatic sensory or other medical interventions has placebo effects, and acupuncture may be particularly effective at activating the positive effects of "placebo." (While many studies show some difference between so-called "sham" acupuncture and real acupuncture, the effects of sham is often higher than when compared to other placebos.) Placebo (mind-body-therapist-patient) effects must be acknowledged as being both potent and physiologically real. Many of the author's acupuncture teachers stated that the practitioner's "intention/Yi," (which is the cumulative effect of one's study, skill, concentration, will and physical condition), can be as important as point selection or physical technique. The skill of the practitioner therefore has effects that cannot be accounted for by the intervention used or by simply calling them a pla-

---

2. Although many "dry needling" techniques in this text are based on "neuroanatomical" concepts, they are supported by TCM theory and needle techniques (see quote from *Simple Questions* on p-605). Interestingly when using neuroanatomical principles to guide needling techniques and placement, often the areas (points) chosen are the same as if one would be using TCM theories.

cebo.[3] The effects of the "ritual" of performing acupuncture procedures did not escape classic TCM literature. The classic *Book Of Difficulties* states: "The practitioner, after harnessing his spirit, must look up to the patient's eyes and harness the patient's spirit. In this way the Qi can move easily."[4]

THE PLACEBO EFFECT. The placebo effect is the response of a patient to a so called *inert* therapeutic intervention. Studies on chronic pain (postoperative pain, diabetic neuropathy, chronic headache, etc.) have shown around a 35% response to placebo interventions (Beecher 1955), while in acutely induced experimental pain the response to placebo is usually around 5%. A study of cimetidine (Tagament) for the treatment of duodenal ulcers has shown the placebo response to be as high as 63%, as compared to a 76% response to the drug (Binder 1978). Recent research shows that the patient's expectations of outcome and beliefs influence the treatment. A recent review article published in the *Journal of American Board Family Practice* (2003) has shown that "mind body" therapies can have significant positive effects in many medical diseases including musculoskeletal disorders. It is clear from such studies that the mind plays a critical role in healing, and, therefore, patient participation is important and should be incorporated into all treatment approaches to maximize such effects. Speaking of the physician patient relationship, Hippocrates stated: "Some patients, though conscious that their condition is perilous, recover their health simply through their contentment with the goodness of the physician."

Acupuncture is probably most effective when used in conjunction with its related traditional systems. However, an understanding of Qi/functional flow, channel harmony and balance, and constitutional and Organ functions requires considerable training and experience. In this section both traditional and modern explanations of acupuncture (needle use) are included. This is done not only for the sake of understanding the mechanisms of acupuncture but also to provide practitioners with the tools to develop *new* understanding and treatment techniques.

---

3. Interestingly Nordenström has observed that the potential difference between the subcutaneous tissues of the patient and the practitioner's fingers from capacitive (stored) flow of current, can eventually equalize the charge. The charge may flow in either direction depending on the relative strength of the practitioner's and the patient's fields. The intention as well as the practitioner's physical state may therefore influence outcome. Other studies have shown that intention or belief of researchers can alter outcome of studies done on animals.

4. The famous acupuncturist Guo Yu explains how intention is hampered by anxiety. "Now when it comes to treating nobles, they look down on me from the heights of their distinguished places, and I am filled with anxiety that I might not please them... Though the acupuncture needles demand precise measure, with them I am often in error. I am burdened with a heart full of trepidation, compounded by a will reduced in strength. Thus intention is not fully there. Consider what influence this has on treating the disorder. This is the reason I cannot bring about a cure" (Scheid and Bensky).

Purposes of Dry Needling

Dry needling is used to strengthen tendons and ligaments, stimulate Golgi receptors and muscle spindles, deactivate trigger points, treat overactive motor points (Table 7-4 on page 611), provide blood and growth factors to hemodynamically disturbed tissues (commonly seen in myofascial pain syndromes), reset motor points and neural control (possibly including replacement of oversensitive tissues with less sensitive tissues), and stimulate other reflex mechanisms.

Strengthen Tendons and Ligaments

Needling may strengthen soft tissues such as tendons and ligaments by inducing a local inflammatory reaction. Fenestration of areas of tendinosis and ligament insufficiency by needling may promote beneficial bleeding into new channels created through degenerated mucoid tissues. This mechanical disruption may transform a failed intrinsic healing to a therapeutic extrinsic one (Figueroa 2002). Electron microscopy shows evidence of tissue injury on the surface of an acupuncture needle: collagen and elastic fibers, fibroblasts, mast cells, and adipocytes can be seen (Kimura et al 1992).

- The mechanical trauma that results from needling may injure cells, including mast cells, blood cells and vessels.
- The current of injury is activated.
- Blood products (such as platelet growth factors and transforming growth factor beta) spill and activate healing.
- Amines and other mediators of inflammation are set free or are newly-formed locally, generating an acute inflammatory reaction (flare).
- Plasma seeps into the tissues, possibly allowing blood to reach poorly-vascularized areas such as ligaments and tendons. After a delay of a few hours, the plasma begins to attract polymorphs. In the absence of significant bacterial infection, this leukocytic infiltration is mild and fades quickly.
- Macrophages migrate into the area of inflammation and work to remove red blood cells, fibrin, dead polymorphs, and other cellular material. At the same time, with granulocytes, the macrophages work to activate fibroblasts.
- Local fibroblasts begin to hypertrophy and to generate collagen and elastic fibers. If foreign matter such as an injection of pumas solution is left in place, or acupuncture suture burial—a TCM surgical technique, it causes a foreign matter response. This response, which includes an invasion of giant cells and a strong fibrous reaction, adds strength to the tissues.

Caution: The healing process can be delayed and may be weakened if the blood supply is poor, if the patient is poorly nourished (particularly in the presence of ascorbic acid and zinc deficiency), and if the patient is treated simultaneously with anti-inflammatory medications. Smoking can also affect healing.

The Stimulation of Golgi Organs and Muscle Spindles

Many acupuncture points are based on nerve arrangement. According to Gunn, two types are found in muscles, principally in motor points and Golgi tendon organs (Gunn 1977). The rotation of a needle in hypertonic muscle tissues can tug on muscle fibers, not unlike the way thread rolls on a spool. This action seems to stimulate stretch-sensitive Golgi receptors and muscle spindles, which may account for the resulting muscle relaxation. The secondary muscle spindles (group II proprioceptors, in the nuclear bag region), which provide static load information, have been implicated with the propagated needle sensation of acupuncture.

The Deactivation of Trigger and Overactive Motor Points

Since many "acupuncture points," muscle trigger points, and motor end-plate zones are identical in location (Gunn 1976, 1979, Bonica *ibid*) needle insertion can result in muscular movements and insertional activity which can be recorded on electromyography (EMG). Insertional activity occurs from the depolarization of innervated single or grouped muscle fiber discharges which are micro-twitches. This may be the basis of pain relief from EMG and intramuscular stimulation methods (Chu 2002). Locally induced micro-twitches from electrical stimulation or insertional activity are capable of producing micro-stretch effects on the adjacent shortened muscle fibers undergoing varying stages of denervation. This reduces the mechanical traction effect produced by these shortened muscle fibers on pain sensitive structures including intramuscular nerves and blood vessels. This concept of stretching shortened muscle fibers to produce pain relief is justified since even more significant musculoskeletal pain relief can be obtained through inducing larger force twitches (Yi 2002; Gunn *ibid*).

Muscle needling may provide blood products and wash away sensitizing substances. It can break fibrotic tissue that has entrapped nerve endings, and it possibly may be able to replace hyperactive nociceptors with nonpainful tissues. Travell has reported that active myofascial trigger points can be treated with dry needling since it often leads to characteristic muscle twitches and stretch effects on the adjacent shortened muscle fibers. The resulting muscle relaxation may reduce mechanical stresses on tissues such as intramuscular nerves, blood vessels, and tendons, thereby allowing more effective healing (Gunn *ibid*, Chu *ibid*).

Muscle motor points are points that are packed densely with sensory end-organs, allowing muscle to be easily excited and become most susceptible to tenderness. In his writings on the relationship of motor points to acupuncture points and their sensitivity to pain, Gunn (*ibid*) states and gives evidence to the affect that needling motor points is affective in treating muscular pain and tension. The proposed mechanism is similar to that of needling techniques in other muscle tissues. Gunn postulates that growth factors released by injured cells and platelets also result in the healing of mildly-demyelinated nerves.

Jessen et al (1989) remarks that even in trigger point injection the most important factor may not be the injected substance; rather, it may be the mechanical effects of needling on the abnormal tissue and the interruption of the trigger point's mechanism. Travell and Simons (1983) state:

> The needle may mechanically disrupt abnormally functioning contractile elements, or nerve endings which are sensor and motor components of the feedback loop believed responsible for sustaining the trigger point activity. Cessation of the neuromuscular dysfunction relieves the tautness of the palpable band of muscle fibers and the hyperirritability of the sensory nerve that is responsible for both the referred phenomena and local tenderness.

Providing Blood and Growth Factors

Chronic muscle tension and spasm can cause reduced oxygen and other nutrient supply. This, in turn, can possibly result in a small area of abnormal function and ectopic muscle facilitation. Bleeding, which can be an effect of needling, can break microscars in these areas and can provide blood and growth factors to facilitate healing. Platelet-derived-growth factor can attract cells and facilitate DNA synthesis as well as stimulate collagen and protein formation. Growth factors may heal localized tissues as well as sensitized nerves. This process may lead to the healing of somatic as well as visceral tissues (Gunn *ibid*).

Altering Neural Control and Reflex Mechanisms

Needling may alter neural control by neurotransmitter and endorphin stimulation. Needling can activate reflexes that stimulate inhibitory fibers by a fusimotor mechanism and may result in transmission saturation or depletion in joint and other receptors. Travell and Simons (*ibid*) also state that the local release of intracelluar potassium due to damage to muscle fibers by the needles can cause a depolarization block of nerve fibers in the area where extracellular potassium reached sufficient concentration.

Needling cutaneous and other tissues can stimulate various spinal reflexes and serotinergic descending inhibitory systems (see chapter 2). Pain fibers (somatic nociceptors) travel to the dorsal root ganglia and are distributed to specific segmental levels in the spinal cord. They also communicate with the afferent sympathetic neurons of the viscera and blood vessels that travel to the same cord segment (Wall *ibid*). This may potentially account for various segmental as well as sympathetic effects seen with needling techniques. Periosteal needling techniques (Lawrence 1987) are believed to regulate sympathetic fibers in and around the periosteum, increasing blood circulation in the area.

Altering Tensegrity

The acupuncture channels have been referred and compared to the fascial plains in the body (Matsumoto and Birch

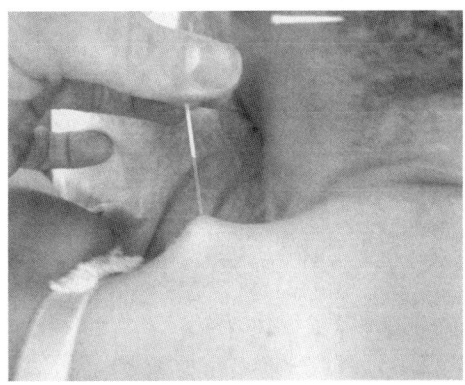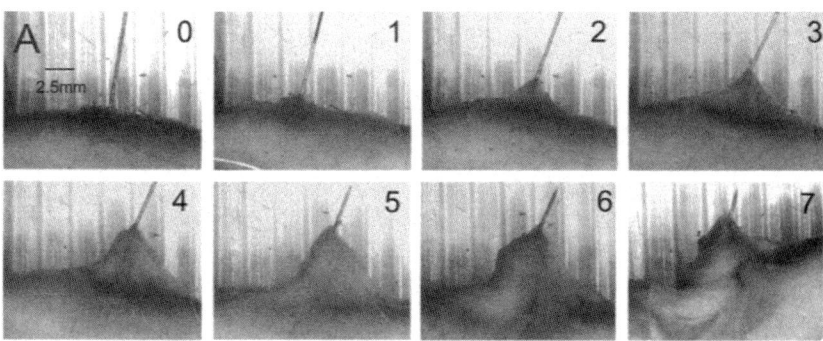

Figure 5-1: Needle grasp by directional twisting and pulling. Right side shows the formation of a connective tissue "whorl" with needle rotation (with permission Langevin and Yandow 2002).

1988). New research has shown a relationship between acupuncture points, channels, and connective tissue (Langevin et al 2001, 2002). Langevin et al propose that acupuncture points may correspond to sites of convergence in the network of connective tissue permeating the entire body. As discussed in chapter 3, the soft tissues of the body form a system of trusses that stabilize, communicate, and integrate the body as a whole. Levin (1997) has described the need for *twelve* degrees of freedom and/or stabilizing restraints, corresponding to the tetrahedron keeping it both movable and rigidly fixed. This principle can be demonstrated in a wire-spoked bicycle wheel which needs a minimum of twelve tension-spokes to rigidly fix the hub in space. The twelve Main and Sinew channels and their relationship to fascia and other soft tissues may therefore represent such a system. Needling strategic points related to fascial planes may influence stability and function and may also explain the propagated effects of acupuncture. Langevin at al have shown that needle twisting and grasp (of soft tissues) can result in a whorl of tissue around the needle (Figure 5-1). Acupoint stimulation therefore may result in altered tension at connective tissue trusses. Also, the placement of a needle in strategic areas may result in a "short-circuit" between nerves and ground substances in tissues and fascia and between the outer and inner epidermal layers, both of which have been shown to possess resting potentials. Needling acupuncture points which are said to be located within neurovascular bundles and that are high in water and chemical contents (and therefore electrically conductive) may result in a kind of short-circuit between the points (conductive systems) and fascia, which is electrically resistant. The epidermal layer has been shown to act as a kind of battery with the outside layer being negatively charged and the inside being positively charged. Acupuncture may thus lead to a change of tension within the systems of biological trusses, via both electrical and mechanical effects. As stated earlier, Dorman (*ibid*) has demonstrated that treatment to the ligamentous fascial organ has multiple effects which result in restoration of tensegritous efficiency.

Acupuncture Mechanisms

It is not the purpose of this section to authoritatively review all the known literature regarding the basic science of acupunture. As stated previously, many excellent texts are available presenting such information. Only the more common information relevant to this text is discussed.

Most modern (Western) studies of acupuncture mechanisms and most clinical outcome studies follow Newtonian principles of cause and effect. It should be remembered, however, that strictly linear, reductionist Newtonian principles are of limited scope when complex systems such as the human body are analyzed. For example, within Quantum mechanics[5] as well as Chaos theory, phenomena are said to *consist of three layers*. The first layer consists of those aspects of our everyday world that may be accurately described by Newtonian physics *(OM: possibly described in part as pertaining to the Earth)*. The third level consists of all objects and phenomena that are best described by chaos theory *(OM: possibly described in part as pertaining to Heaven)*. The second layer, located between the two, is best described as *relative uncertainty*, or "determined chaos," within which all the phenomena of the universe exists *(OM: possibly described in part as pertaining to Man)*. It is in this second, most curious dimension where the observer, simply by the action of observation, influences what is observed.[6] The limitation of Newtonian theory to account for the infinite, peculiar and random possibilities of the second layer establishes the difficulty of

---

5. The Quantum theory was first advanced by Planck at the end of the 19th century, and was further refined by Bohr. Bohr advanced the idea that electrons can instantaneously jump to different orbits through absorbing and dispersing energy, which "connect" all parts of the universe and communicate all parts with all other parts (Royal 1990). Quantum mechanics is used mostly to explain atomic behavior which has been found to be quite unpredictable (nonsmooth, jittery). It cannot however explain gravity. The new "string" (unifying) theory attempts to combine gravity with quantum mechanics. String theory proposes that everything in the universe is made of a tiny unit of energy called strings. It also proposes that the universe has more than one dimension (at least 5). It is these dimensions that are thought to keep the forces of the universe in "tune."

studying the human body, and TCM/OM mechanisms in particular. Research, therefore, needs to be interpreted in context. Very few, if any, multi-centered and large-scale studies on acupuncture exist which even attempt to minimize such effects. At the same time, studies on acupuncture should incorporate appropriate methodologies that allow acupuncture to be used based on TCM/OM principles. Appropriate statistical analysis must be used. For example, a recent study by Vickers (2004) has shown that when reanalyzing 4 trials using analysis of covariance outcomes, showed that prior negative studies have not accurately analyzed the data and in some studies the results were actually positive when the study reported negative outcomes. Often the problem lies in not adjusting for baseline pain scores.

In TCM/OM on the other hand, it is exactly in that second layer, in the therapist-patient relationship, where the invaluably positive part of the medical intervention occurs. In the TCM/OM paradigm, one does not wish to separate the relationship from the procedure effects; rather, these are maximized. Also, it is important to remember that most studies on acupuncture done in the West, control and restrict the therapeutic freedom needed to perform acupuncture as prescribed by TCM/OM methodologies. Because biomedical research follows Newtonian reductionist study designs, the freedom needed to change treatment methods, point selection, and the need to follow what is always seen as a continually evolving and changing diagnosis/condition in TCM, are not allowed. This handicaps acupuncture at the onset and if such study designs are viewed from OM/TCM perspectives, they can be seen as comparing two poor treatment protocols, i.e., sham needling with a poorly fixed acupuncture protocol, which can be seen as just another "semi-placebo." TCM/OM is best evaluated looking at clinical outcomes which can be compared to another excepted therapy. The clinical outcome evaluators can be blinded to which treatments patients have been receiving, fulfilling in part the need for blinding.

Acupuncture points have been described as 2-8mm cylindrical shaped perforations within superficial fascia (e.g., Lu-8 is 2mm and UB-52 8mm), in which a neurovascular bundle runs (Heine 1988, 1997).[7] Kellner (1966) has shown the existence of two types of acupoints, receptor and effector, in *histological* studies. In a review article Sims (1997) suggests that there may be a functional and/or anatomical relationship between acupuncture points, channels (meridians), and the nervous system. Therefore, acupuncture effects are closely related to the nervous system and are achieved by complex mechanisms which integrate peripheral, ascending, descending, and higher centers in the nervous system. Neural blockade by anesthetics and various surgical techniques which interrupt the nervous system completely negate most effects of acupuncture (Han *ibid*), although Lui (1998) has shown that not all of acupuncture effects are blocked by anesthetic neural blockade.

Acupuncture points are said to possess lower skin impedance than surrounding skin (Kho and Arnold 1997), and may be singular points in the surface of bioelectric field epithelia that usually maintains a 30-100 mV deferential. This voltage is said to be the potential difference across cell layers, not membrane potential. Acupoints are also said to be points with high density of *gap junctions* that are hexogonal protein complexes that form channels between adjacent cells. Gap junctions facilitate intercellular communication and increase electric conductivity (Shang *ibid*). Acupuncture points are also said to "store" electric charges to a higher degree than surrounding tissues. (This is called "capacitance," at 0.002-0.5 mF [microfarads, units of capacitance], i.e, the ability to store and slowly release electrical charges; Dumtirescu 1977; 1989, or 01-1mF according to Ionescu-Tiroviste and Pruna 1990). Acupuncture points are also intimately related to the distribution of nerve trunks, motor endplates, and blood vessels (Dung 1984; Gunn *ibid;* Chan 1984*)*. Dung listed ten structure which are said to be found in the vicinity of acupuncture points:

1. Large peripheral nerves. The larger the nerve, the more effective the point.
2. Nerves emerging from a deep to a more superficial location.
3. Cutaneous emerging from deep fascia.
4. Nerves emerging from bone foramina.
5. Motor points of neuromuscular attachments.
6. Blood vessels in the vicinity of neuromuscular attachments.
7. Nerves composed of fibers of varying sizes. This is more likely on muscular nerves than on cutaneous nerves.
8. Bifurcation points of peripheral nerves.
9. Ligaments (muscle tendons, joint capsules, fascial sheets, collateral ligaments), as these are rich in nerve endings.
10. Suture lines on the skull.

Ionescu-Tirgoviste and Pruna (1990) have suggested that the:

Qualities of Superficial Acupoints are:

---

6. Some studies in physics have shown that depending on the observer's expectations, atoms for example behave differently, i.e., the observer changes atomic behavior. Another example is when researchers are told that a group of mice are genetically dumb and then compared to so-called normal mice in learning studies. The "dumb" group performs worse is learning tasks even though the two groups are identical. Therefore the concepts of "objectivity," "linearity" and "cause-and-effect" that dominate modern biomedical thinking may not be the best way to study complex treatment *systems* such as acupuncture and manual therapies. At the same time, this is not to say that medical outcomes cannot be evaluated as they should. The magnitude of such 'observer" effects is usually quite small and therefore clinical efficacy using evidence based research must still be done.

7. Acupuncture points may be translated from Chinese as "transport holes." Traditionally they are said to be a place on the surface where Qi and Blood of the channels and collaterals pass or gather. They are found in depressions called Xue, Xue Wei, or Xue Dao.

- High electric potentials (up to 300mV)
- High electric capacitance values (0.002-0.5 mF)
- Low electrical resistance
- Increased skin respiration
- High local temperature
- Spontaneous visible light emission from Jing (well) and Yuan (Source) points
- Sound signals at the acupuncture points (2-15Hz, with amplitude of 0.1mV, sharp or sine wave);

Qualities of Deep Skin Acupoints are:
- Low deep perception threshold to an electrical stimuli
- Tissue capacitance (storage of charge)
- Electro-resonance with other acupoints
- High conductivity of isotopic tracers.

Acupuncture appears to activate endogenous substances which inhibit nociceptive (pain) transmission. One theory is that the acupuncture analgesia occurs as a generalized "stress response," or as a result of an individual's "suggestibility." However, the choice of stimulation modality may influence the clinical outcome. Different forms of stimulation such as electroacupuncture and transcutaneous electrical nerve stimulation (TENS) can activate different pathways to produce analgesia. Sims (*ibid*) review suggests that neural and humoral mechanisms by themselves do not fully explain acupuncture analgesia.

For *analgesia*, point specificity in acupuncture (especially in chronic pain) seems to be less crucial than when acupuncture is used as a therapeutic intervention for other types of disorders such as vomiting. A recent study has shown that both manipulation (versus no needle manipulation at acupuncture points) and site of needling (acupuncture points versus sham sites) contribute significantly to the elevation of pain pressure threshold (PPT) following acupuncture. However, the difference between non-acupuncture point sites and acupuncture points was minimal. The difference between using needle manipulation and not using needle manipulation was more significant. Therefore, distribution of effects on PPT did not support either neural segmental or TCM channel theories. Psychological and physiological nonspecific effects appeared to play a minimal role in changes to PPT (Zaslawski, Cobbin, Lidums and Petocz 2003).

While some studies have shown little difference between "sham" and "true" points, other studies in both humans and animals have shown superior effects for "true" acupuncture. For acute laboratory-induced pain in human subjects, needling true points produces marked analgesia while needling sham points produces very weak effects. This is interesting because the placebo effect is usually much lower in acute laboratory-induced pain. With the latter population, placebo pills usually work on only 3% of subjects, as compared with 30-35% in chronic pain.

When acupuncture is used to treat depression, (and many other medical disorders (Allen et al 1998, among others) showed that patients receiving specific acupuncture treatments improved significantly more than those receiving a placebo-like nonspecific acupuncture treatments. Results from that (and other) studies suggest that acupuncture can provide significant symptom relief in depression at rates comparable to those of psychotherapy and pharmacotherapy.

Some animal studies support differing functions of specific acupuncture points. For example, in eight hound dogs implanted with one pair of bipolar serosal electrodes 2cm proximal to the pylorus, gastric myoelectrical activity was recorded for three complete cycles of the migrating myoelectrical complex (MMC) in two sessions, one with electroacupuncture at points ST-36 and P-6 and the other at sham points. There was a significant difference in the frequency and power of the gastric slow wave during different phases of the MMC. In comparison with the sham points, electroacupuncture at the acupoints increased the number of spike bursts (Qian et al 1999).

Acupuncture directed at the management of pain, *done correctly*, can increase the oxygenation of cardiac muscles, reduce gastric acidity, and control inflammatory responses (Sims *ibid*). Acupuncture points have also been shown to have region-specific effects in the brain (Chen et al 1986). Inspite of these findings, Pomeranz (*ibid*) states: "The acupoint maps are essential for localizing the sites where the best De-Qi can be achieved (i.e., location of type II and III muscle afferents). In that sense, the points are specific. However, the further claim of traditional Chinese medicine that the points are also target specific may not be true."

A measurement of the force needed to pullout needles at real acupoints vs points 2cm away showed an 18% differential between the two (Langevin et al 2001). Langevin and Yandow (2002) also hypothesized that the network of acupuncture points and channels can be viewed as a representation of the *network formed by interstitial connective tissue*. This hypothesis was supported by ultrasound images showing connective tissue cleavage planes at acupuncture points in normal human subjects. To test this hypothesis, they mapped acupuncture points in serial gross anatomical sections through the human arm. They found an 80% correspondence between the sites of acupuncture points and the location of *intermuscular* or *intramuscular connective tissue planes* in postmortem tissue sections (Figure 5-2). Langevin and Yandow propose that the anatomical relationship of acupuncture points and channels to connective tissue planes is relevant to acupuncture's mechanism of action and suggests a potentially important integrative role for interstitial connective tissue. They also point out that studies suggesting neurovascular bundles, neuromuscular attachments, and various types of sensory nerves that have been described at acupuncture points have not included proper statistical analyses comparing acupuncture points with appropriate "nonacupuncture" control points and that the studies on skin conductance may have been flowed as several factors are known to

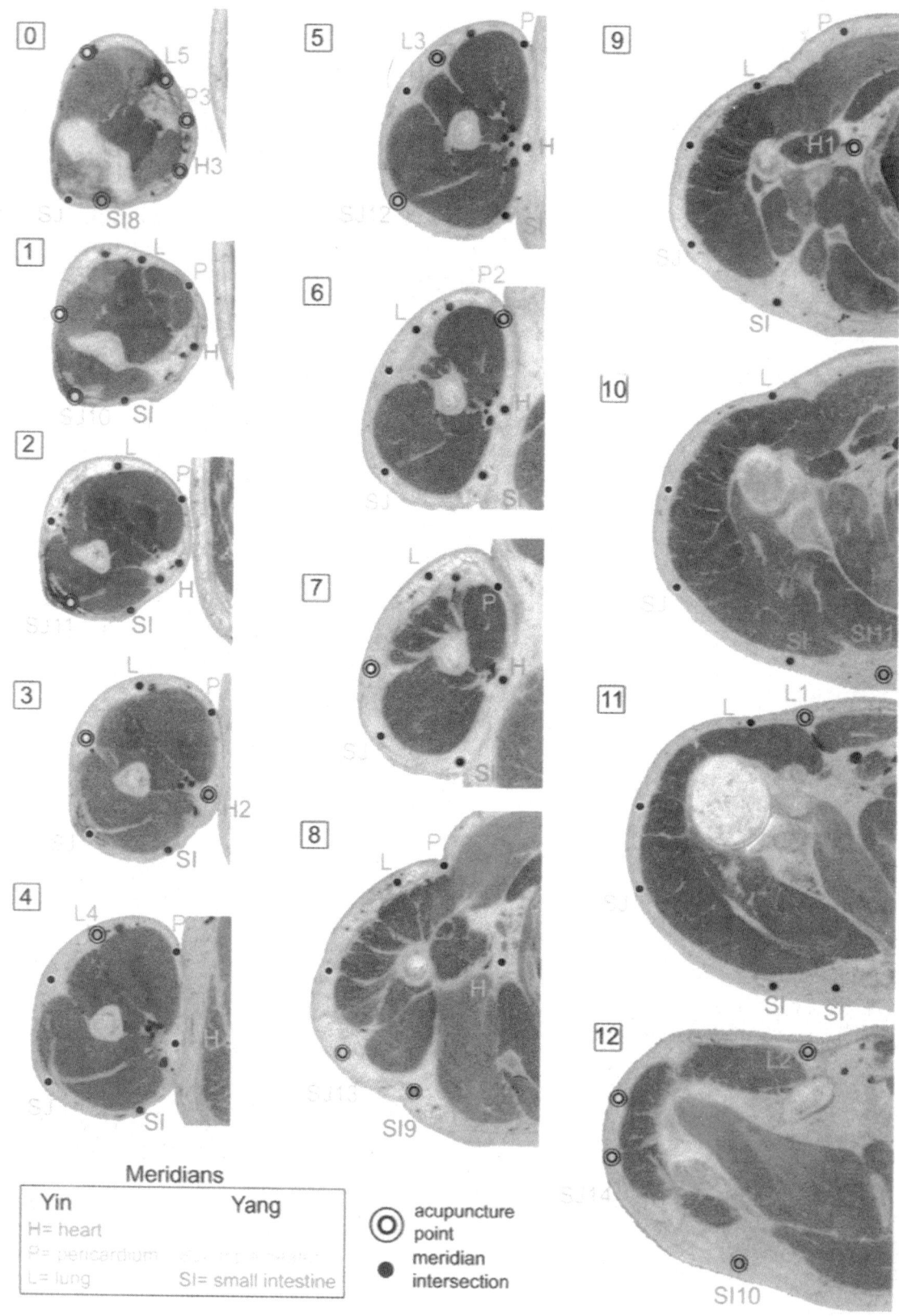

Figure 5-2: Location of acupuncture points and channels in serial gross anatomical sections through a human arm (with permission Langevin and Yandow 2002).

affect skin conductance, and, to date, no study has both controlled for these factors and included sufficient numbers of observations to confirm these findings.

The mechanisms of acupuncture's effects have been summarized as neurochemical and neurophysiologic.

Neurochemical Mechanisms

By and large, acupuncture analgesia has been described as the stimulation of small diameter and medium nerves (A-δ and A-β), in the periphery that then send impulses to the spinal cord. Then, three neural centers (spinal cord, midbrain, and pituitary) are thought to be activated and to release neurochemical substances which are responsible for the analgesic effect (Pomeranz 2001). The fact that acupuncture analgesia can be transferred from a treated animal to a non-treated animal (Han 1992) by cross-circulation and CSF infusion to ventricles supports the hypothesis of a systemic neuropharmacologic effect.

Opioid Systems

Early reports on the analgesic mechanism of acupuncture involved opioid systems.[8] In 1975, the year endorphins were discovered, David Mayer documented that acupuncture affects the opioid system in his demonstration that, in humans, naloxone can block acupuncture analgesia.[9] Naloxone has also been shown to block the analgesic effect of acupuncture on dental pain. The affects are influenced by dexamethasone levels which in turn also affect endorphins (Mayer, Price and Rafii 1977). They implicated the periaqueductal (PAG) and periventricular gray areas in the midbrain. The newly discovered opioid peptide, orphanin, seems to have antagonistic effects on electroacupuncture analgesia (Han 1998). The analgesic effects of acupuncture can be enhanced by D-phenylalanine and D-leucine, which enhance met-enkephalin degradation (Ehrenpreis 1985; Han 1991), or by bacitracin[10] (Zhang, Tang and Han 1981).[11] In a review, Pomeranz et al (1977) concluded that acupuncture analgesia implicate pituitary endorphins. They postulate that this is so, because placebo acupuncture is not as effective, the analgesic effect of acupuncture can be eliminated by ablation of the pituitary gland, and because naloxone is effective in blocking the analgesic effects of acupuncture. Substance P has been implicated with both neural effects and in the stimulation of neurokinin 1 (NK1) receptors and other kinins (Luger, Bhardwaj, Grabbe and Schwarz 1996) and therefore may be implicated with the local inflammatory and immune effects of acupuncture. The peptide cholecystokinin-8 (CCK-8), angiotensin II, and nociceptin have been shown to play a role in acupuncture analgesia acting like the opiate antagonist naloxone (anti-opiates) to block endorphin-mediated analgesia (Han 2000). Perhaps the ratio of CCK to endorphins is the important variable in producing analgesia (Pomeranz *ibid*). The release of anti-opiates and 5-HT may be associated with "acupuncture resistance" (Han *ibid*).

Non-Opioid Systems

Non-opioid systems are affected by acupuncture (also see chapter 2).

- Serotonin (5-HT), norepinephrine, GABA, calcium and magnesium ions, secondary central cyclic nucleotides (Han 1987), and acetylcholine have been implicated in acupuncture analgesia (Guan, Yu, Wng and Liu 1986). Serotonin and norepinephrine can be stimulated by periaqueductal gray (PAG) activation of raphe nucleus located in the caudal end of the medulla oblogata, causing it to send impulses down the dorsolateral tract to release monoamines (serotonin and norepinephrine) into spinal cord cells. Norepinephrine (probably with synergistic effects from serotonin) binds to alpha receptors in the cord to block pain (Pomeranz *ibid*). Electroacupuncture can increase the content of 5-HT in the brain and spinal cord by 15-26% and the 5-HIAA in the brain by 35%. It is postulated that the acupuncture release of 5-HT and subsequent analgesic effect may be achieved by the activation of receptor of $5-HT_{1a}$ and $5-HT_{1c/2}$ (Han *ibid*).

- Dopamine is implicated in inhibition of acupuncture analgesia (Patterson 1986). However, an injection of a dopamine antagonist, haloperidol, antagonizes acupuncture analgesia, while a microinjection of dopamine into the posterior hypothalamic arcuate nucleus induces dose-dependent analgesia. It is possible that dopamine serves as the neurotransmitter interface between acupuncture afferent and efferent pathways (Takeshige 2001).

- Anti-inflammatory/stress system effects have been elicited by stimulation of 17-hydroxycorticosterone, ACTH, and cortisol secretion (Ying 1976; Omura 1976; O'Connor 1981).

  Inflammatory/adrenal/stress mediators can affect pain perception as beta-endorphin levels can be affected by ACTH. This is because ACTH can antagonize the enzyme cleavage from a large, precursor, pro-opiomelancortin (Smock and Fields 1980), which may be one explanation of why needle insertion can stimulate endorphins. ACTH travels to the adrenal cortex, where cortisol is secreted into the blood, which may explain the anti-inflammatory effects of acupuncture. Sin has summarized the anti-inflammatory effects of acupuncture (Sin 1984)

- Acupuncture effects on cholinergic mechanisms may regulate sympathetic tone and pressor effects (Sun, Yu and Yao 1983).

---

8. These reports may have contributed to, and at least supported, the discovery of the endorphin systems (Han 1986).

9. Naloxone is a chemical that can block opioid receptors.

10. Bacitracin is a peptidase inhibitor (a D-amino acid), the injection of which results in increased neuropeptides.

11. Met-enkephalin degradation results in a net gain in opioid-like chemicals.

- Enhanced nitric oxide (NO) concentrations and expression of nitric oxide syntheses (nNOS) in acupuncture points/meridians was demonstrated in adult rats. Enhanced NO in the acupoints/meridians may be generated from multiple resources including neuronal NOergic system, and NO might be associated with acupoint/meridian functions including low electric resistance (Ma 2003). NO seems to be a messenger molecule with a wide range of biological effects within the CNS, peripheral nervous system, vascular system, and endocrine system. It may signal cell aptosis (programed cell death), and account for tonic relaxation of blood vessels and non-adrenergeic and non-cholinergic relaxation of the gastrointestinal tract. Acupuncture seems to modulate NO activity in the hippocampus, brainstem (nucleus gracilis), basal ganglia striatum, and the cerebral cortex (Koslow et al *ibid*; Kim et al *ibid*; West et al 2000; Ma *ibid*).[12]

Neurophysiologic and Other Mechanisms

Neurophysiologic mechanisms involve sensory nerves stimulated at the acupuncture point. The afferent (sensory) systems seem to be important in acupuncture analgesia, and needle sensation (De-Qi) is required for successful treatment of pain (Han *ibid*).[13] Preacupuncture local anesthesia of subcutaneous and muscle tissue abolishes the needling sensation and often abolishes acupuncture's analgesic effects (Chiang et al 1973). This suggests that receptors within the muscle are responsible for the De-Qi sensation, probably due to A-β and A-δ fibers (Pomeranz and Paley 1979; Wang, Yao, Xian and Hou 1985). According to Wang et al (1985), the receptive fields of the acupuncture point relay sensation as follows: group II neurons convey the sensation of numbness, group III distension and heaviness, and group IV soreness.

Low threshold, large diameter mechanoreceptors situated in the skin, muscles, tendons, and joints are activated by innocuous stimuli that may activate the "gate control" mechanism. Acupuncture stimulates A-β and A-δ (small and medium) fibers which enter the spinal cord and arrive at the medial and lateral portions of the dorsal horn. A-β fibers terminate in the nucleus propius and in more ventral regions of the dorsal grey matter. A-δ fibers terminate in the marginal zones of the dorsal grey matter, the ventral portion of lamina II, throughout lamina III, and inhibit dorsal horn cells at laminae I and V (Yaksh and Hammond 1982; Dorman and Gage 1982), all of which are associated with the spinal mechanisms of the "Gate" theory of pain. According to Han (*ibid*), however, the slow onset of acupuncture analgesia precludes the gate theory as being a significant mechanism in electroacupuncture.

Analgesic effects that result from stimulation of small, myelinated fibers are transmitted both segmentally and bilaterally (Chiang et al 1973, 1975). C-fibers (unmyelinated) do not seem to contribute significantly, and application of capsicum which selectively blocks C-fibers does not affect acupuncture analgesia (Yu, Bao, Zhou and Han 1978). When diluted procaine solution is injected into animals (blocking C-fibers) it is still possible to achieve analgesic effects by electroacupuncture. If however a compleat nerve block is achieved an analgesic effect is not obtained (Stacey 1969, Besson et al 1987).

The needling sensation (De-Qi) is important in blood circulatory effects. Sandberg et al (2003) investigated the effects of needle stimulation (acupuncture) on skin and muscle blood flow. Three modes of needle stimulation were performed on the anterior aspect of the tibia: superficial insertion (SF), insertion into the anterior tibial muscle (Mu), and insertion into the muscle including manipulation of the needle in order to elicit a distinct sensation of distension, heaviness, or numbness (De-Qi). Compared to the control, muscle blood flow increased following both Mu and De-Qi for twenty minutes, with the latter being more pronounced for the initial five minutes. Skin blood flow increased for five minutes following De-Qi. However, no increase was found following SF. The results indicate that the intensity of the needling is important, the De-Qi stimulation resulting in the most pronounced increase in both skin and muscle blood flow.

The Brain

Many areas in the brain have been associated with acupuncture including: nucleus raphe magnus, cerebral cortex, cerebellum, head of N Caudatum, Accumbens, N Lateral Habenular and periaqueductal gray matter (Han 2000). Acupuncture seems to stimulate specific regions in the brain many of which are known to influence pain. The thalamus is thought to be the most important area responsible for the processing of pain impulses and/or integration of pain sensation. The centromedian nucleus of the thalamus, the raphe magnus nucleus, and the arcuate nucleus seem to be the main areas related to acupuncture analgesia (Zang 1980; Hamba and Toda 1988; Yin, Duanmu, Guo, and Yu 1984). Peripheral stimulation of an acupuncture point was observed to stimulate thalamic neurons with a similar pattern in a cat (Linzer and Van Atta 1975). Lesions made in the thalamus result in differing effects to low and high-intensity electroacupuncture (Wang 1990, Dong et al 1984)

Removal of the cerebral cortex of different animals have differing effects on electroacupuncture analgesia with some animals being affected and other not (Wang 1990) Lo and Cui (2003) studied literalized motor cortex effects using transcranial magnetic stimulation and acupuncture. Right-sided reduction in motor cortex excitability and a tendency

---

12. NO has important effects in regulating vascular tone, and supplemetation with the amino acid L-arginine may influence circulation. L-arginine may be helpful in the treatment of neuropathies and cold extremities.

13. Many Japanese systems, however, use sensationless (to the patient) techniques.

to the opposite effect on the left side was seen with acupuncture. Sham needle insertions did not result in significant changes of motor cortex excitability. These findings provide neurophysiological evidence of cortical excitability modulation.

Treatment of LI-4 at 2Hz, a point used often for analgesic effects, and a near-by non-classical/non-analgesic point, respectively, in normal subjects and assessed by positron emission tomography (PET) showed that regions activated by acupuncture stimulation at LI-4 included the hypothalamus with an extension to midbrain, the insula, the anterior cingulate cortex, and the cerebellum. Only the stimulation at LI-4 activated the *hypothalamus* under similar psychophysical ratings of acupuncture sensation (De-Qi) as elicited by the stimulation at the two points, respectively. The data suggests that the hypothalamus might characterize the central expression of acupuncture stimulation at the classical analgesic point and serve as one key element in mediating analgesic efficacy of acupuncture stimulation (Hsieh et al 2001).

The effect of acupuncture on thirteen normal subjects studied with PET scans in 3-D mode showed that true acupuncture activates the left anterior cingulus, the insulae bilaterally,[14] the cerebellum bilaterally, the left superior frontal gyrus, and the right medial and inferior frontal gyri. Most of the activated areas are shared with areas activated in acute and chronic pain states as described in the literature. Thus acupuncture appears to function by activating areas also involved in pain. This indicates that acupuncture could relieve pain by unbalancing the equilibrium of distributed pain-related central networks (Biella, Sotgiu, Pellegata, Paulesu, Castiglioni, and Fazio 2001).

Functional magnetic resonance imaging (fMRI) techniques allow for visualization of minute changes in vascularized areas in the brain. It can be used to study regional anatomy and function in vivo (real time live patient). Cho et al (1998, 1999) have shown that needling extremity points known to have specific effects in OM can result in increased activity in related brain regions. For example, GB-37 a point used often for eye diseases has been shown to activate the visual cortex and GB-43, a point used for ear-related diseases activates the auditory cortex. A recent study by Litscher et al (2004) has also shown this to be true when using a laser to stimulate the acupuncture points (showing effects with both fMRI and functional transcranial Doppler sonography).

Descending and Ascending Tracts

Innocuous stimulation of peripheral nerves may excite descending inhibitory serotinergic tracts that, in turn, can inhibit nociceptors (Bowsher 1991). The descending dorsolateral funiculus of the spinal cord seems to be involved in acupuncture analgesia. Lesions made at T1-T3 levels resulted in complete abolition of acupuncture analgesia (Shen, Tsai and Lan 1975). Lacerating the contralateral anterolateral columns eradicated the analgesic effect from stimulation of St-36, whereas laceration of the dorsal column at the level of T-12-L1 or superficial lateral cordectomy did not affect acupuncture analgesia (Chiang et al 1975). Cephalically, impulses produced by acupuncture analgesia are believed to be transmitted through the extralemniscal system, then to the thalamus and the sensory cortex.[15]

"Supraspinal descending inhibition of pain" is the pattern of neuronal activity in the diencephalon,[16] brainstem, and spinal cord during antinociceptive stimulation in midbrain, periaqueductal gray (PAG) or medullary nucleus raphe magnus. The descending systems may not only depress the mean discharge rates of nociceptive spinal dorsal horn neurons, but also may modify the harmonic oscillations and nonlinear dynamics (dimensionality) of discharges. Propriospinal, heterosegmental inhibition may occur by antinociceptive heterosegmental interneurons which may be activated by noxious stimulation or by supraspinal descending pathways (Sandkuhler 1996). Periosteal acupuncture (and any short painful needle techniques) have been postulated to induce the diffuse noxious inhibitory controls (DNIC) systems. DNIC is thought to occur when any noxious stimuli is applied to any part of the body distant from the excitatory receptive field (LeBars, Dickenson and Besson 1979).

Convergence of Visceral and Somatic Innervation

Experimental data that demonstrates the existence of the convergence of visceral and somatic innervation in laminae V-VII may support the rationale for the use of many manual and acupuncture therapies in somato-visceral and visceral-somatic pain (Figure 5-3). The electrical stimulation of the skin (at acupuncture points) has been shown to influence nerves within gray matter (Selzer and Spencer 1969) and so may influence visceral function. Moreover, visceral pain has superficial receptive fields (irritation zones that can be mistaken for musculoskeletal pain) that can be activated by noxious and innocuous stimulation, and by muscle activity beneath the skin (Forman and Ohata 1980; Cervero 1982). Stimulation of acupuncture points at superficial receptive fields may provoke a reflex mechanism that may explain the empirical data about the effectiveness of acupuncture. In both human and animal studies, local anaesthesia by subcutaneous injection at referral zones has been shown to effect organ functions and abolish pain arising from visceral origins (Simons, Travell and Simons *ibid*). Reflex mechanisms may also explain why the use of distal acupuncture points affects visceral pain.

---

14. The central lobe of cerebral hemisphere.

15. The lemniscus is a bundle of sensory fibers in the medulla and pons.

16. Second portion of the brain, or that lying between the telencephalone and mesencephalone.

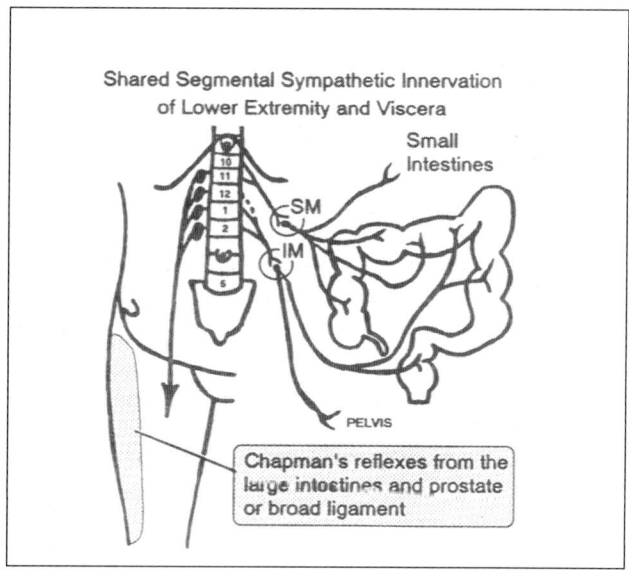

Figure 5-3: Visceral somatic interactions and Chapman's reflexes (From Kuchera WA and Kuchera ML, Osteopathic Principles in Practice, KCOM press 1993, with permission).

The Autonomic Nervous System

The circulatory effects and the decrease of hypersympathetic activity in pain patients is probably one of acupuncture's most important clinical effects. Acupuncture points on the Urinary Bladder, upper Stomach, Large Intestine, and deep abdominal channels are in close proximity to the sympathetic ganglia, stimulation of which may affect the autonomic nervous system. Although the details are still unknown, experimental and clinical evidence suggest that acupuncture can reset the sympathetic system via mechanisms at hypothalamic and brainstem levels. These effects may be due to hypothalamic beta-endorphinergic system inhibitory effects on the vasomotor center (VMC). This effect elicits a decrease in sympathetic tone with vasodilatation and decreased drive on the heart following the initial excitation of the VMC, during exercise or nerve stimulation (Anderson *ibid*). In a study of hemorrhagic hypotension in rats, Sun, Yu, and Yao (1983) have shown that the pressor effects in hypotensive animals was not antagonized by naloxone but was significantly diminished by intravenous injection of scopolamine, suggesting that the effect is mediated by cholinergic mechanism. Many animal experiments and clinical trials suggest that the acupuncture point P-6 is effective in the control of some vegetative functions. Experiments performed on twenty-nine healthy volunteers for basal values of cardiac frequency, systolic and diastolic blood pressure, and sympathetic electrical response was done by Abad-Alegria, Pomaron, Aznar, Munoz, and Adelantado (2001). Readings were taken before and after acupuncture at P-6, non-acupuncture point puncture, supine lying for fifteen minutes, acupuncture at P-3, and bipolar electrical stimulus of the median nerve at the P-6 level in the wrist. The study showed that acupuncture at P-6 *strongly* inhibits sympathetic tone, with reduction of cardiac frequency, systolic blood pressure and an important reduction of the amplitude of the sympathetic electrical response; the latency of the electrical response was also prolonged. Some *weak* effects on blood pressure and cardiac frequency were observed also with nonspecific points and median nerve stimulation. The authors hypothesize from previous anatomical data and this study, that the level of such actions is suprametameric, with strong implication of the diencephalon and cerebral cortex.

Another recent study by Wang, Kuo, and Yang (2002) has shown that acupuncture applied 2mm deep into Sishencong (M-HN-1) points resulted in an increased HF% (high-frequency power 0.15-0.40 Hz) but a decreased LF% (low-frequency power 0.04-0.15 Hz) of precordial ECG signals compared with the before-acupuncture stage. Such effects did not occur when manual acupuncture was applied to the control points. Vagal withdrawal and/or sympathetic overactivity is always accompanied by various kinds of stress and is dangerous to the body. The authors proposed that mild acupuncture on the Sishencong (M-HN-1) points may effectively enhance vagal activities but suppress sympathetic regulations of the heart in humans.

Using thermography, acupuncture's effect of increasing skin temperature locally, contralaterally, and in other regions has been documented (Lee and Ernst 1987, 1983; Ernst and Lee 1985). Ernst and colleagues have demonstrated long-lasting warming effects as well. In some instances the temperature distribution was in a craniocaudal gradient, which they speculated was mediated by the reticular formation via the activation of diffuse noxious inhibitory controls on the convergent cells of the dorsal horn. Liao and Liao (1985) have demonstrated that stimulation of acupoint St-36 affected the leg of a stroke patient, producing a small temperature increase in the normal leg and a marked increase in both hands. Kaada (1982) reported increased skin temperature and decreased pain in patients with Raynaud's disease as a result of transcutaneous electrical stimulation of the hands. Appiah, Hiller, Caspary, Alexander, and Creutzig (1997) reported similar effects with acupuncture.

Most authors agree that acupuncture points possess lower skin impedance (resistence), which is said to relate to the autonomic nervous system (Kho and Arnold 1997); however, the methodologies of most of the studies are questionable. Electrical skin resistance can be demonstrated and measured using simple devices. Increased pseudomotor activity (increased perspiration from sympathetic activity) lowers skin impedance, which has been documented over injured areas, and in segmental distributions, including from visceral disease (Korr et al 1962). Little evidence, however, exists for special affects at acupuncture points. Some acupuncture diagnostic devices (Voll and Vaga for example) use this information in the selection of channels and points to be treated. They even claim to be able to diagnose allergies and most diseases, and to be able to find appropriate homeopathic remedies. However, the reliability of these instruments is questionable for various technical reasons, and because the act of measuring (which involves passing an electrical charge through the skin) actually changes the impedance.[17] According to Pomeranz (*ibid*), only his study accurately measured skin resistance. In this study, Ag/AgCL electrodes were used to avoid polarization from DC currents, microampere current was used to avoid electrical damage to the skin, a spring-loaded probe was used to control pressure, and a very small amount of saline was supplied through a bridge through a Millipore filter to overcome skin moisture variation. Preliminary results to date using this methodology suggest that acupuncture points do, *sometimes*, have lower impedance than surrounding skin.

A study by Li and Chen (1996) suggests that a reflex shortloop outside the central nervous system may be formed directly by a primary afferent neuron and a sympathetic post-ganglionic neuron for the purpose of regulating the activity of the autonomic nervous system. It also suggests that the sympathetic nerve may have a feedback regulation function to the primary afferent and that this may offer partial morphological evidence for the expoundity of acupuncture mechanism.

Different modes of manual acupuncture stimulation differentially modulate cerebral blood flow velocity, arterial blood pressure, and heart rate in human subjects (Backer, Hammes, Deppe, Conrad, Tolle, and Dobos 2002).

In summary, a significant improvement of peripheral circulation can be achieved by electrical and acupuncture stimulation (and electroacupuncture) of nerves innervating an ischemic area. This effect is probably due to local mechanisms with the release of vasodilating substances and the possible inhibition of related sympathetic systems. These effects are useful in the treatment of pain, healing of nerves, and recovery from surgical and other injuries, including diabetic ulcers. Acupuncture effects may also help in the treatment of facilitated segments.

Immune Effects

Sabolovic and Michon have found stimulation of T and B lymphocytes by acupuncture (Sabolovic and Michon 1978). By influencing met-enkephalins, acupuncture can increase T lymphocyte rosette formation from human T lymphocytes (Wybran et al 1979). Acupuncture has been shown to increase beta-globulins, gamma-globulins, lysozymes, agglutinins,[18] opsonins[19] and complement (Dragomirescu et al 1961). Acupuncture influences beta-endorphins and met-enkephalins, both of which may enhance natural killer cell activity (Matthews et al 1984). Electroacupuncture has also been reported to modulate natural killer cell activities (Hahm et al 2002). Acupuncture may exert its actions both on pain and immune processes by the coupling of the immune and pain systems which occurs via common signaling molecules—opioid peptides. It is possible that opioid activation leads to both the processing of opioid peptides from their precursor, proenkephalin, and the simultaneous release of antibacterial peptides contained within the precursor (proenkephalin). Thus, central nervous system pain circuits may be coupled to immune enhancement (Gollub, Hui and Stefano 1999). Acupuncture therapy may normalize both increased light chain K value of IgM and lowered trace element Zn content in patients with Bechet's disease with statistically significant differences, suggesting that acupuncture therapy can elevate humoral immunologic function and improve the metabolism of the trace element in these patients (Yu, Bai, Zhang and Wu 2001). Acupuncture and moxibustion may be as effective as antibiotics in the treatment of gastrointestinal infections (Rogers and Bossy 1981). Acupuncture has been reported to stimulate circulating interferon in humans (Chin, Lin and Wang 1988). Finally, acupuncture like all invasive procedures, injures cells and may initiate inflammatory and immune processes.

Electrical and other Effects

Several electrical and electromagnetic theories have been proposed in relation to acupuncture. Robert Becker associated cellular polarity and DC currents with the growth, healing, and regeneration of tissues, including articular cartilage (Becker and Marino 1982; Becker 1972). Burr (1972) suggested that all events in the body generate electro-dynamic fields. Bioelectrical homeostasis and its relation to acupuncture was reviewed by Zukauskas et al (1988) and Zhu Zong-Xiang (1981).

Bioelectrical fields have been shown to interact with morphogens and guide growth control. The morphogenetic singularity theory suggests that organizing centers have high density of *gap junctions* and *high electrical conductance*. The formation and maintenance of all the physiological systems are directly dependent on the activity of the growth control system, the evolutionary origin of which may have preceded all other physiological systems. The regulation of most physiological processes is through growth control mechanisms such as hypertrophy, hyperplasia, atrophy, and apoptosis. Acupuncture points, which may also have high electrical conductance and high density of gap junctions, originate from organizing centers. This theory can explain the distribution and non-specific activation of organizing centers and many research results in acupuncture (Shang 2001). Bioelectrical signal systems may control extrinsic and

---

17. The instrument applies electrical charge across the skin in order to measure skin resistance. This can change the properties and resistance of the skin, although the Voll instrument ignores the initial peak resistance reading concentrating on the capacitive "fall back" of the reading to a steady-state (usually higher) value. Inconsistent pressure can change the results, and it is quite difficult to have a consistent pressure during each and every measurement. Some newer instruments may be more reliable.

18. An antibody which causes agglutination or clumping of specific antigens (bacteria or cells).

19. A substance which acts upon microorganisms and other cells, facilitating phagocytosis.

intrinsic tissue repair. Monaka described the "X-signal" system representing a "primitive" regulatory system that is different from the classical nervous and hormonal systems (Monaka, Itaya and Birch 1995). This system is said to consist of immeasurably small charges in and around the body that ultimately regulate all life processes, which are said to be measurable only via changes in the pressure sensitivity of acupoints, pulse diagnosis, or kinesiology (so-called O-ring test), none of which have been satisfactorily tested and proven valid.[20] In Monaka's view, the channels form a multi-level network where acupuncture points function as transducers that use pathways within the body's enveloping, electrically active fascia to communicate information through-out the organism. Ho and Knight (1998) have described the water system of the body in relation to acupuncture. Wave and fractal theories may relate to electrical fields as well.

Anti-Stress Effects

Acupuncture is often used and advocated as a preventative medical intervention. It is a common observation that patients undergoing acupuncture become significantly relaxed and many fall asleep during therapy. Akimoto et al (2003) studied responses of immunologic and endocrine markers during athletic competition and the effects of acupuncture on the athletes. The measured parameters included salivary secretory immunoglobulin A (SIgA) level, cortisol level in saliva, subjective rating of physical well-being, and profile of mood states (POMS). The results of the study support the effectiveness of acupuncture for physical and mental well-being. They demonstrated that exercise-induced decrease of salivary SIgA and increase of salivary cortisol can be inhibited by acupuncture. Acupuncture improved subjective rating of muscle tension and fatigue. The POMS score was also modulated by acupuncture.

Acupuncture Therapeutic Systems and Techniques

The channels—the pathways that carry Qi, Blood, and body Fluids throughout the body—provide for the free flow and balance of Yin and Yang and serve as a conduit for communications between all parts of the body. The *Classic of Internal Medicine* states that there are 365 acupuncture points on the Main channels that correspond with the number of days in the year and describes in detail about 160 of them. Over time, the number of points has grown and now stands at several thousand. In practice, however, individual clinicians probably use an average of a hundred points or so.

In this section, the term *channel therapy* is used to describe a variety of ways of treating the body via the channel systems. The Major points described below can be used to activate the channels and are often sufficient to attain a clinical response. The following are a few of the more common systems used clinically.

Channel Treatment Design

Varying methods can be used to choose channels or points. In general, the French systems use theoretical methods while many Japanese therapists rely almost exclusively on palpatory findings. In TCM, so-called Organ (Zhang Fu) diagnosis is often emphasized. It is common in TCM to recommend local, adjacent, distal and proximal (Back-Shu and Alarm-Mu, Transport, etc.) points when treating musculoskeletal disorders. As can be seen from the discussion on acupuncture mechanism, this approach recruits multi-level analgesia by segmental, extrasegmental, descending, autonomic, and somatovisceral reflexes.

Treatment must always follow the individual condition of each patient. The classic literature clearly states that not all patients are candidates for acupuncture or moxibustion therapy. For example, the *Classic of Internal Medicine* states: "[One] should not needle a patient with a muddled (Hun) pulse." *Spiritual Axis* states: "When both Man's Prognosis (carotid artery) and pulse-opening (radial artery) are more than threefold in size...and moxibustion is applied, unusual change [occurs] and another disease [may appear]." In general, acupuncture may not be appropriate in patients that are very weak, when the pulses are "counterflowing" or counter to the patients disease, or when the patient's Righteous-Qi is exceedingly depleted.

The major differential diagnosis questions which always must be considered are whether the disorder is Full or Empty and whether the patient's constitution/condition is weak or strong. *Spiritual Axis* states:

> An insufficiency of Form and Qi with a surplus of diseased Qi indicates that the evil is overwhelming (the anti-Pathogenic Factors) and, subsequently, warrants prompt drainage. A surplus of Form and Qi with an insufficiency of diseased Qi calls for prompt supplementation. An insufficiency of Form and Qi with an insufficiency of diseased Qi demonstrates that Yin and Yang are both insufficient, and, consequently, excludes acupuncture treatment.

Thus, the practitioner must determine the appropriate techniques. In general, information on the patient's health-state/appropriate function (Righteous-Qi) takes precedence over the specifics of the disorder (branch symptom/signs).[21]

---

20. Devises such as SQUID (Sub-quantum interference device) that can measure such low level activity without altering the signal itself have been used by some researchers and may provide more acceptable evidence.

21. This is not a strict rule and opinions differ widely. The more acute or severe the disorder, the more attention is paid to the Branch-disease (manifesting symptoms). However, it is a mistake to think that the Root is always Deficiency and the Branch always Excess. When using acupuncture, treating channel Excesses is commonly done to treat Interior-deficiency, reaching Yin from Yang and vice versa.

Once this has been determined, the channels can be treated from the more superficial Sinew channels and cutaneous regions to the deep Main, Divergent and Extra channels according to the location of the disease and condition of the patient. Many treatment types and approaches can be used. The following are some of the more common approaches regarding, in particular, the sequence of the treatment:

- A simple therapeutic program can be achieved by selecting the main activating points for the particular channel, at the energetic/functional/depth being affected. For example, early after injury or, if the condition results from external Pathogenic Factors, the Sinew channels can be used first. As or if the symptoms progress, or if there is bleeding and/or edema, treatment directed to the Connecting channels/network-vessels can be added. This is also said to prevent further progression of Pathogenic Factors and to eliminate Blood-stasis and edema. If symptoms begin to expand and involve larger areas, the Main channels are integrated into the treatment plan. In late and chronic stages when significant tissue pathology is present, or if the patient is weak and has Organic involvement, the Divergent and Extra channels can be emphasized. Even in acute disorders, it is not uncommon to support the Organ which controls the affected tissue, for instance by adding Kidney tonics (herbs and points) to prescriptions used to treat bone fractures, even when the patient does not show clear Kidney-deficiency symptoms and signs.

- Some practitioners divide all treatments into two main depths: the "superficial" levels are treated at the symptomatic areas usually using the Sinew channels and cutaneous regions (Ashi and Kori points); then "root" treatments are added. These can be directed at the Organ systems or the constitutional patterns of the Extra and Divergent channels.

- Alternatively, root treatments can be applied first. When using mainly palpatory systems (as is preferred by the author) the patient's weakest Organ pulse (or other Organic palpatory findings) may be addressed first by using the tonification point (or four needle technique) for the related Organ. (This is referred to as "deep root treatment.") Then the area of the patient's pain (not necessarily the channels) can be palpated and active points treated. (This is referred to as "superficial" or "branch treatment.") Active points are then sought along the effected channels and treated. Related channels/zones (Yin Yang, same name i.e., Yang-Ming [Stomach and Large Intestine], etc.), can then be palpated and active points needled. A Divergent or Extra channel or zone treatment can be applied to finalize and integrate the treatment. (This is a deep root treatment.)

- Tight abdominal areas can be treated first by directly treating active abdominal muscles, triggers, and points. This can indirectly treat the affected Organs and channel systems associated with abdominal reflexes. The abdominal assessment can be used also to ascertain which Organs or channel systems are involved, i.e., making a diagnosis, and distal points can then be used to treat the patterns found. Symptomatic treatments follow.

- The Back-Shu (or Jia Ji) and Alarm (Mu) points for all affected Organs (ascertained by history, pulse, abdomen, etc.), or that are sensitive to pressure palpation can be treated first to address the root and support the patient for symptomatic treatments.[22] Then the symptomatic area is palpated and active points are treated.

- A simple protocol commonly used by the author is to first treat distal points. Tong-style points or any imaging/reflection systems are used to assess and treat points in relation to the symptomatic area: contralateral points; upper to treat lower; front to treat back, etc. (see p-350). This protocol can be easily combined with concurrent manual therapies or patient exercises. A four needle technique or other root treatment is added at the end of treatment to address the root.

In general, it has been demonstrated that the best *pain relief* is achieved by acupuncture (electroacupuncture) or TENS stimulation in the region of pain (Andersson *ibid*, Han *ibid*).

Orthopedic Integration, Neuroanatomical Acupuncture

Acupuncture (dry needling and transcutaneous electro-stimulation) treatments can also be based on modern orthopedic evaluations, which enable the treatment to be more lesion- or tissue/nerve-specific. Biomedical functional and structural assessments are then used to determine which channel (segment) or local tissue/points are to be treated.

Channel (distal) and local-needle therapy is most effective when based on *palpatory* and *exam findings*. Tissue texture and pressure pain are highly significant in determining which TCM/OM channels or points are affected and which needle techniques are to be used.[23] Therefore, when using Orthopaedic Medicine diagnostic information,[24] needling input becomes tissue/lesion-specific, and depends on provocation and functional testing, and is much less dependent on local or distal palpation for tenderness (in the area of symptoms or referred areas). When using neurological maps of dermatomes, myotomes, sclerotomes, or viscerotomes, palpation for tissue texture, pressure pain, and trophic edema are highly significant in determining which level(s) is affected. The following are some examples of integrative acupuncture techniques:

---

22. Osteopathic motion and other palpatory assessments can be used at the spine as well.

23. This contrasts with Orthopaedic Medicine, in which tenderness is much less important (see referred pain and tenderness, chapter 2).

24. This can yield a lesion-specific finding, i.e., a small lesion which is responsible for a wide range of symptoms and signs.

Table 5-1: Sympathetic Innervation of Organs, Shu, and Mu Points (Teitelbaum 2000)

Organ	Sympathetic Innervation	Shu Point Vertebral Level	Mu Point Dermatome Location
LUNG	C3-4; T2-9	UB-13; T3	Lu-1; C4
HEART	C3-4; T2-9	UB-15; T5	CV-14; T7
LIVER	T5-10	UB-18; T9	Liv-14; T6
GALL BLADER	T5-10	UB-19; T10	GB-24; T7
SPLEEN	T5-11	UB-21; T12	Liv-13; T10
STOMACH	T5-11	UB-21; T12	CV-12; T8
KIDNEY	T10 L2	UB-23; L2	GB25; T11
LARGE INTESTINE	T6-L5; S2-4	UB-24; L4	St-25; T10
SMALL INTESTINE	T5-12	UB-27; S1[a]	CV-4; T12
URINARY BLADER	T11-L2; S2-4	UB-28; S2	CV-2; L1
PERICARDIUM	C3-4; T1-8	UB-14; T4	CV17; T4
TRIPLE WARMER (ADRENAL)	T8-L2	UB-22; L1	CV-5; T11

a. There is no sympathetic output to the small intestine from this vertebra.

1. Points can be used based on innervation (segmental) levels. Dermatomal, myotomal, and sclerotomal levels are assessed and treated (i.e., neurological channels). Trigger and motor-point charts and neuroanatomical maps may be used to evaluate symptoms and to choose segmental levels, and/or TCM channels and points for treatment. Stimulation can include points that affect the peripheral nerve, the spinal nerve, sympathetic ganglia, descending tracts, etc.
  A. For example, points at the L3 segment (UB-22, 23, Jia Ji, and lateral-to-anterior thigh) can be stimulated for a patient with hip or knee pain to induce segmental effects. Deep insertion of points at the T10-12 vertebrae directed at the ganglia may have sympathetic effects, possibly regulating blood flow to the hip and knee. This also affects the "thermatomes;" referred pain related to circulatory sympathetic effects. (Due to the risk of pneumothorax, extra care should be taken or shallow needling used.) If a tibial fibular dysfunction (restriction) is found, (this commonly effect hip function and pain), GB-34 (or local triggers) can be used for the anterior fibula, and UB-38 (or local triggers) can be used for the posterior fibula (Figure 5-4).
  B. Another example is back and hip pain due to *iliopsoas syndrome*. UB-22 and UB-23 can be used, as they are located over areas related to the nerve roots that innervate the psoas and hip. Local points such as Sp-12 through 15 can stimulate the femoral nerve which is the peripheral nerve innervating the iliacus. Other distal points at these levels of innervation can be used, for example: St-32, 33, Team of Four Horses [88.18, 17, 19] or, more often, Three Nine Miles [88.25, 26, 27] all of which are within the L3 dermatome.[25] Liv-10 through 12, which are over the L2 myotome, and periosteal needling of the femur, which is the L3 sclerotome, can be used as well.
  C. While local segmental stimulation usually gives a more intensive analgesia than distal nonsegmental needling, because it can stimulate mechanisms within the spinal cord, midbrain and pituitary (Pomeranz *ibid*), and therefore often used as the primary method. Segmental stimulation combined with extrasegmental stimulation (locations) may increase the duration of pain relief (six months to two years) among patients that have initially responded to acupuncture (Lunderberg, Laurell, and Thomas 1988; Thomas and Lundeberg 1994; Thomas et al 1995). In back and hip pain, for example, extra-segmental points such as Spirit Bone (Ling Gu 22.05) and Great White (Da Bai 22.04) may be added to local segmental points.
  D. It is also possible to needle a single segment. This is often done on distal points. For example, it is common to use

---

25. These are Tong-style points see p-350.

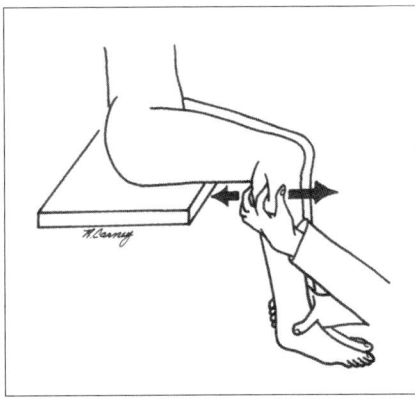

Figure 5-4: Assessment of Tib Fib function.

SI-3 for neck and arm pain of a C8 distribution. It is also possible to needle a nonsegmental point such as Lu-7 (C7 segment), GB-39, or UB-64 in the treatment of similar neck pain. Using a single needle and segment may be helpful in acute pain and resulting stiffness or muscle spasms. The stimulation is usually *strong* and of short duration, and, therefore, is thought to act via the noxious inhibitory controls (DNIC). Distal needles have more general than segmental pain-inhibitory effects (Le Bars 1983). They can also extend the effects of treatment (Andersson 1993).

2. A knowledge of muscle innervation can be helpful. For example, points between Sp-6 and Sp-8 are located over or within the tibialis posterior muscle. The stimulation of these points results in afferent activity in T12, L1, 2 and S1, 2, 3, and 4 (mostly L5, S1) spinal segments. To treat the *diaphragm*, which is often important to regulate fluid and venous blood flow, points at C3-5 can be used.

3. When Organic/organic disorders are influencing musculoskeletal structures (visceral-somatic effects), segmental points can be used as seen in Table 7-1. When treating Back-Shu points to treat Organic/organic disorders, it makes sense to evaluate all the involved levels in the range of sympathetic innervation to the organ. When treating an organ that has not been described in TCM, it makes sense to evaluate the appropriate levels of innervation (see p-136).

   It is often important to treat the involved sympathetic segments and ganglia in musculoskeletal disorders. This not only addresses possible facilitated segments (i.e., the vicious cycle of pain and spasm) but may also increases related blood supply. To achieve sympathetic effects, superficial needle insertion can be tried first, but deep stimulation at the vicinity of the ganglia may be needed. It is this author's experience that very low intensity electric stimulation works best (i.e., results in warming effects at the affected areas, probably by reducing sympathetic tone). The sympathetic chain runs ventrally on the left and right sides of the vertebral column, from the level of the first cervical vertebra to the coccyx. For pain anywhere in the *craniocervical* areas, points around T1-T2, both ventral and dorsal, can be used to affect the related sympathetic nerves and ganglia. For pain in the *upper extremities,* points at T4-9 (UB and Jia Ji points) can be assessed and treated. For pain in the *lower extremities,* points in the regions of T10 through S2 can be used to reach the sympathetic ganglia, with points at T10-L2 being in charge of sympathetic innervation to the lower limbs (T10-12 upper half, and T12-L2 lower half).

A. For example, when treating patients with symptoms in upper quadrant areas that also show evidence of hyperactive sympathetics, such as cold limb, edema, etc., it is often helpful to treat the cervicothoracic ganglion. In the cervical area there are only two or three ganglia which in most patients combine at the lower ganglia to form the stellate ganglion (Figure 5-6).[26] The stellate ganglion (Bosch *ibid*), is 30-100mm long and about 0.3-1mm wide. This ganglion lies on the head of the first rib, about 10mm laterally from the T1 joint, and 25-30mm from the median line of the body. This ganglion is one of the largest neural control centres apart from the CNS. It has afferent and efferent branches leading to the sympathetic thyroid and parathyroid plexuses, the phrenic, recurrent, and vagus nerves; it has vascular branches to the vertebral, subclavian, and interior mammary arteries, and, on the accelerant nerve to the cardiac plexus. It also provides the autonomic innervation of the whole upper quadrant of the body. The stellate ganglion can be stimulated using anterior or posterior approaches. Points such as St-9 through 11 and UB-11 are situated in areas particularly suitable to stimulate this ganglion. St-9 and UB-11 are often recommended for the treatment of pain in general, and in the upper quadrant in particular. St-9 or 11 should be stimulated unilaterally in order to avoid excessive effects on blood pressure (the patients should be lying down).

B. When treating the lower extremities, it is often recommended to treat the femoral artery at the groin. Because the sympathetics run down the leg with the femoral artery, treatment of the artery may influence blood circulation which is particularly important in conditions such as diabetic neuropathy.

4. When treating an affected vertebra (or referral pattern), it may be a good habit to assess and treat all three vertebral levels, since a nerve root innervates the muscles and tissues above and below its place of emergence (Bogduk and Twomey 1987). The secondary (related) segments are assessed and treated if necessary.

---

26. While Jenkner (1980) reported that TENS-like electro stimulation can affect the stellate ganglia, Larsen et al (1995) were not able to reproduce his findings and did not find sympathetic effects using their protocol.

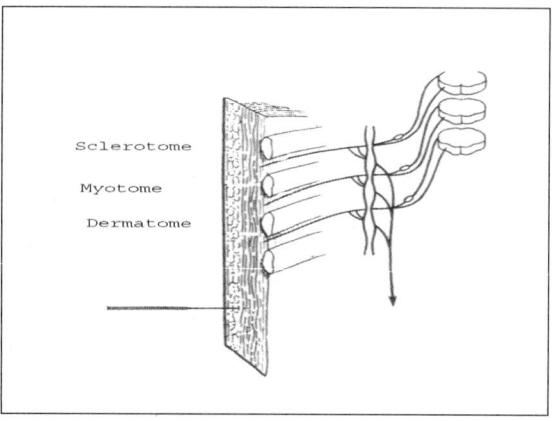 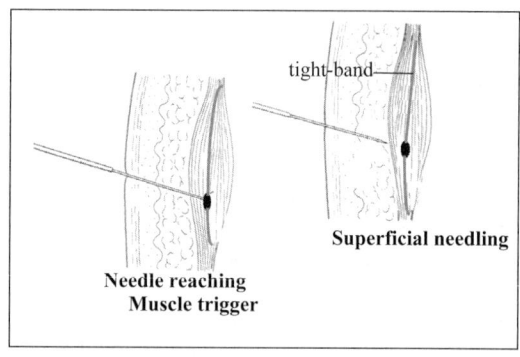

Figure 5-5: Depending on the depth of needle insertion, different segmental levels may be stimulated. Superficial stimulation will mostly influence the dermatome and A-beta (II) and A-delta (IIIa) fibers, muscle stimulation of the myotome and type III and IV nerve fibers, and deeper stimulation to bone and ligaments of the sclerotome as well as sympathetic fibers and type IV fibers (after Bekkering and Bussel 1998). Remember that many tissues receive their innervation from the same segmental level, i.e., the dermatome, myotome, and sclerotome of the same nerve root. However, conscious perceptions of sensation from these tissues do not overlap and may be separated by considerable distance. This means that when assessing the patient's symptoms based on pain distribution and characteristics one needs to understand that the dermatomal, myotomal, and sclerotomal distributions are different. Pain in a L3 dermatomal distribution that arises from ligaments may actually indicate lesion at higher levels than L3.

5. Needle depth and placement can be based on the neurological and somatic levels to be treated. For example, in a patient with *nuclear* disc pain (which usually follows a clear dermatomal distribution), it is often best to first treat the locally involved spinal level (UB and Jia Ji points) with a thin 36-38 gauge needle inserted *only* 2-4 mm on the *non-painful side* (i.e., skin or dermatomal level) and the distal points in the pelvis and legs (or shoulder and arms) *on the painful side* (again, inserted to the depth of 2-4 mm, dermatomal level). This can activate the appropriate "gate control" systems and is less likely to increase the patient's symptoms (by causing a flare) and more likely to affect the *dermatomal* distribution of pain. If one needs to needle the related myotome or sclerotome (i.e., deeper tissues), points on higher vertebral levels may be chosen and needles inserted more deeply (Figure 5-5).[27] *Superficial* needling, which mostly stimulates A-β (II) and A-δ (IIIa) fibers and inhibit sympathetic fibers, is often more appropriate when sympathetic fibers are facilitated in conditions such as post-surgical pain and complex regional pain syndrome (CRPS or RSD).[28]

6. *Selective tension assessments* can be used to choose points and channels. Pain on resisted internal rotation of the shoulder is a common clinical finding in tendinitis of the subscapularis. Pressure tenderness (and patient's symptoms) may be demonstrated anywhere in the C5 dermatome and would not be helpful in determining where the lesion lies. Knowing that the subscapularis is the culprit can lead one to assess more appropriate TCM (and neurological) channels and vertebral level points at C4-5 and T4-5. Local needles at the lesser tuberosity of the shoulder may be emphasized regardless of where the patient feels his/her pain. Local laser or other stimulation can be used directly over the lesion with proper interpretation of selective tension tests showing if the lesion is at the superior, middle, or inferior part of the tendon. The antagonist muscles and shoulder girdle stabilizers may be treated as well.

When resisted abduction of the shoulder is painful, the supraspinatus tendon is often the culprit. To treat this muscle/tendon, a needle can be threaded from LI-16 under the acromian towards LI-15, or greater tuberosity of the humerous (the insertion site for the supraspinatus). This can be done regardless of which areas are pressure-sensitive and regardless of the location of the patient's pain (which, again, can be anywhere in a C5 sensory distribution because the shoulder sensory innervation is from C5). Proper interpretation of selective tension tests can reveal if the lesion is at the tenoperiosteal junction, the tendon body, or the musculotendinous junction, and, therefore, local laser or other stimulation can be very specific.

---

27. It is this author's experience as well as his observation of practitioners in US and China that severe nuclear disc pain (especially with clear dural-radicular interaction) often does not respond to TCM interventions satisfactorily. An integrated approach should be used and may include: acupuncture, injections, intra-discal procedures, manual therapies, traction, herbs, pharmaceutical medications, and, if needed, surgical interventions.

28. It is often better to use only distal points (i.e., away from disc or painful nerves) when treating severe discogenic or neuropathic pain.

Acupuncture Therapeutic Systems and Techniques

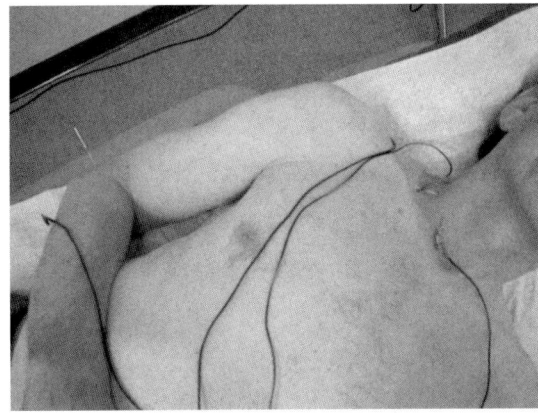

Figure 5-7: Monopolar microamp electroacupuncture used to treat weakness of finger extensors following brachial neuritis. The positive electrode is used to stimulate the stellate ganglion and negative electrode at the finger extensors.

7. Muscle strength (resisted) and tension (passive) testing can be used to identify weak and tight muscles (and related Sinew channels). Related neurological areas,

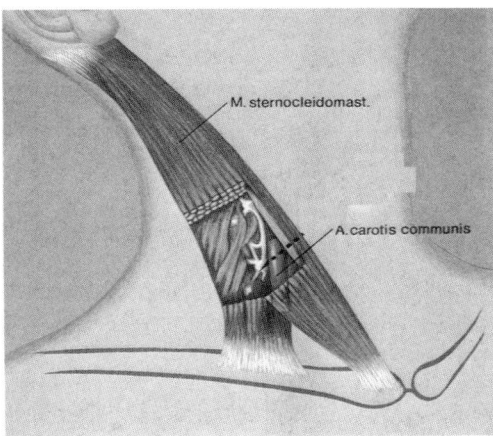

Figure 5-6: Stellate ganglion (After Dosch 1985).

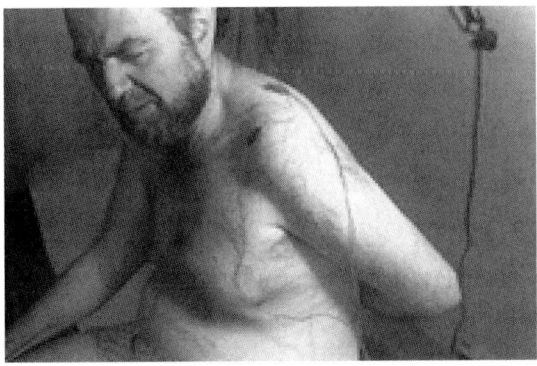

Figure 5-8: Proper position for needling supraspinous tendon at the tendinous attachment and tendinomuscular junction.

reflex points as described by Goodheart (often on muscle attachments or AK sedation points see p-512), motor points, trigger points, and Chapman's reflex points (see p-498) may then be used to restore balanced muscle activity. Treatment is then applied based on biomedical anatomy instead of Sinew channel distribution.

A. For example, when *passive* shoulder abduction is painful and limited one assesses and treats adductor muscles such as: teres major and minor, pectoralis and latissimus dorsi, or often also the anterior capsule of the joint (and subscapularis muscle, an internal rotator muscle). To facilitate relaxation, points at C5 and C6 can be genitally needled or moxaed before local points on the tight muscle are needled. The motor points, active triggers, and points over the musculotendinous junction are emphasized. They can be needled or heated with moxa. Abnormal fibrous tissues are carefully sought, needled and heated. H-7 may be used to sedate the subscapularis, TW-10 the teres minor or infraspinatus, St-45 the pectoralis muscles, or Liv-2 the pectoralis major (Goodheart's muscle sedation points, p-512).

B. *Weak* muscles are often stimulated gently at active attachment points, gently along muscle (parallel to) fibers next to motor points, active triggers, and at Goodheart or Chapman's reflex points. The stimulation is mild using thin needles.

8. In the spine, when a segment is fixed/stuck extended on one side and does not flex (i.e., on that side the facet will not open), it will usually also be rotated to the same side when the spine is flexed. In other words, the anterior part of the vertebral body will rotate to the same side, and the *spinous process* will appear to be rotated toward the other side only when the spine is flexed (and will look even when the spine is extended) (Figure 5-9, A). This dysfunction and rotation may be maintained by a shorting of the deep rotator muscles, preventing the facet from opening. Needling these deep muscles, which run from the *spinous process* of the rotated segment toward the *transverse process* of the vertebra below (or above), can often effectively release such dysfunctions. Anatomical position is used to optimize needle insertion as apposed to "acupuncture" point location. The patient can be positioned on the treatment table to maximize normalization of function as seen in Figure 5-11.

If the restriction is of extension (i.e., the facet on one side does not close), the deep intertansvesai muscles can be needled (Figure 5-9, B). These muscles run from the tip of one transverse process to the next. Thus needle placement is usually slightly more lateral and inferior to that used to flexion restriction. Also in a flexed segment (restriction of extension) the muscle on the apposite side of the openly stuck facet is needled (Figure 5-12). In general, flexed segments (extension restriction) are more difficult to treat using needling alone.

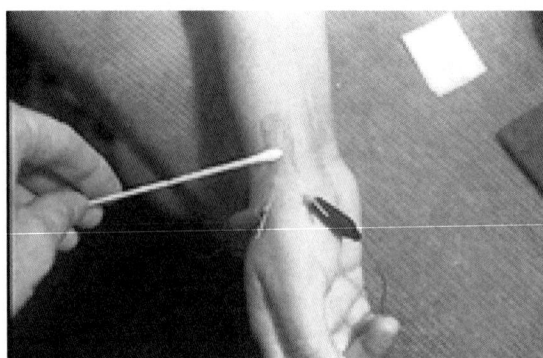

Figure 5-10: Topical herbal application with local monopolar electroacupuncture for the treatment De Quevain tenosynovitis.

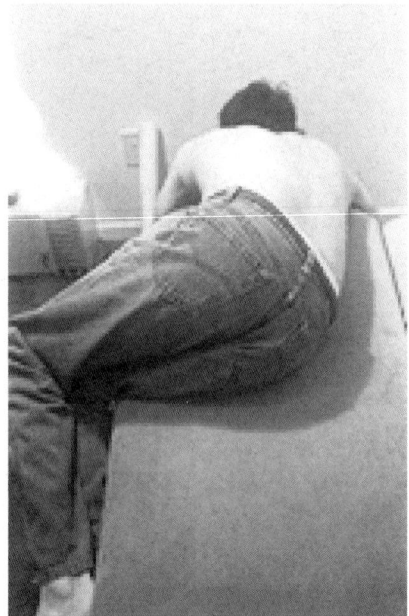

Figure 5-11: Patient treated in the Sims position for vertebral fixation in extension. In this case the left side is fixed and resists flexion.

9. In pelvic torsion, when pain and/or sacral asymmetry increases with lumbar extension (Figure 5-9, C; such as in left on right torsion see p-463), the piriformis (GB-30) and lumbar sidebenders (UB-23 and 52) are needled on the same side, with the spine placed in some extension. If the patient has an anterior sacral torsion such as left on left, the piriformis and lumbar sidebenders are needled on opposite sides and the patient is placed in the Sims position (Figure 5-11).

10. When ligamentous laxity is demonstrated, strong periosteal/ligamentous stimulation may be appropriate even though the patient may be weak, which would otherwise (in TCM) suggest that strong techniques may be contraindicated.

According to Kendall (*ibid*), strong stimulation with short retention time (two to four minutes) is used to enhance the inflammatory phase of the needling response and to reduce (sedate) an acute condition (although no reference or rational is given). Short retention with strong stimulation is also used to treat visceral function (Yang) deficiency, as found in conditions such as hypothyroidism. Long insertion times (fifteen to twenty-five minutes) enhance the controlling phase of the tissue

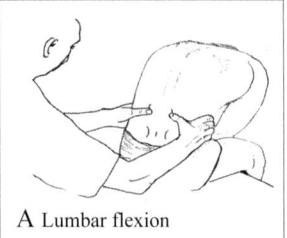

A Lumbar flexion

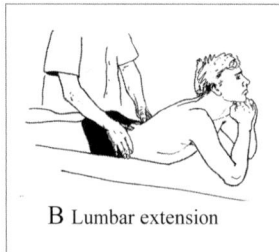

B Lumbar extension

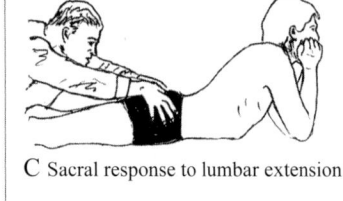

C Sacral response to lumbar extension

Figure 5-9: Evaluation of spinal and sacral functions

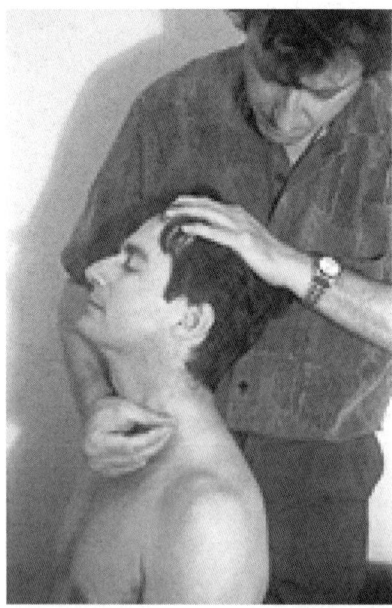

Figure 5-12: Needling position for treatment of extension restriction. The segment is positioned at the stretch barrier and the muscle (or cutaneous area or motor point) is needled gently. After each needle stimulation, the neck is moved to its newly gained restricted barrier.

reaction and produce anti-inflammatory responses to treat false Heat due to visceral substance (Yin) deficiency and to promote tissue repair and reduce pain.

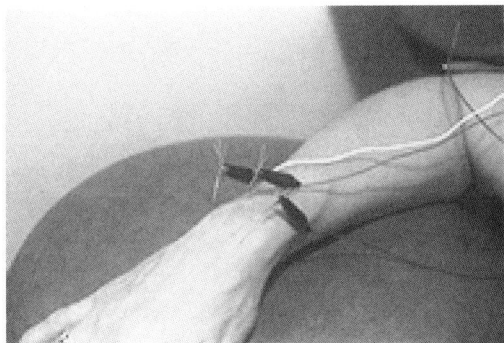

Figure 5-13: Periosteal acupuncture to stabilize the dorsal wrist ligaments. All needles are touching bone and monopolar electrostimulation is added.

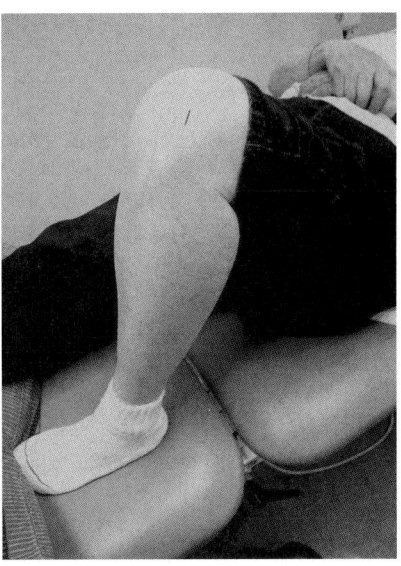

Figure 5-14: Knee flexed to allow the needle to reach the ACL attachment.

11. Integration of TCM/OM theories can be used to address biomedical lesions. For example, when a spinal joint somatic dysfunction reoccurs, frequently the TCM Organ/channel that is associated with the level of dysfunction can be assessed and treated. If dysfunction reoccurs at L4-5, the Large Intestine channel can be assessed and treated if appropriate,[29] especially for flexion restriction and if the patient also suffers from Large Intestine related symptoms. Dietary advice may prove very helpful. For extension restrictions, the coupled Lung, or Ren/Yin Qiao channels may be assessed and treated when appropriate.[30] One can also integrate knowledge of modern segmental innervation to organs with TCM Organ diagnosis and assess and treat these levels using TCM Organ diagnosis (Table 7-1).

In summary, understanding the pathology from TCM/OM and biomedical perspectives gives the practitioner more choices when using acupuncture and has proven to be effective in the author's clinic.

Positioning of Patient

Patient positioning is very important when treating musculoskeletal disorders with acupuncture. In general, when needles are retained for long periods, the patient should be positioned comfortably so that the injured area has a minimal nociceptive output. (The muscles in the treated area should be at maximum relaxation and comfort.) Proper positioning allows the practitioner to reach the needed area (Figure 5-14), facilitates joint movement in the desired direction, and helps avoid aggravating the symptoms. When treating myofascial triggers or joint dysfunctions, positioning the muscle or joint at the *tension barrier* and sequentially needling and stretching the muscle or joint is helpful. This results in an increased painless range of motion. Shallow needling often works best, but not always.

When treating discogenic pain, one needs to differentiate between *nuclear* and *annular* pain. Patients with annular pain often do better if positioned in slight extension as long as needles are retained, while patients with nuclear pain need to be positioned so that no further stimulation of the nerves occurs. Patients with nuclear pain often need to be positioned in slight flexion and sidebent away from pain. Many patients with discogenic pain do better when treated standing, or seated *with in-and-out* needle retention (and often do best when using only distal points; i.e., no vertebral points).

TCM literature for the most part discusses patient positioning as it relates to acupuncture points, for example, *The Systematic Classic of Acupuncture & Moxibustion* states.

> Upper Gate (TW-3) should be needled with the patient's mouth open rather than shut, while Lower Gate (St-35) should be needled with [the patient's knee] bent rather than extended, while Inner Gate (P-6) should be needled with [the patient's elbow] extended rather than bent.

Qi Circulation

Circulation of Qi throughout the channel system is essential for health. The loss of it leads to disease and pain. Without proper circulation, the channels can become empty of Qi and Blood, or they can develop areas of stagnation and stasis. Because of the Yin and Yang laws of nature, a Deficiency state is usually accompanied by an accommodating Excess. The opposite is true in the presence of Excess. Both should be addressed.

---

29. The back Shu (Transport) point of the Large Intestine is at L4. Such a patient is more likely to respond to Ling Gu, Da Bai (LI-4 1/2, LI-3 1/2).

30. The author has treated somatic dysfunction using these principles successfully.

CHANNEL OBSTRUCTION. In TCM, most pain results from obstruction in the channels. As the old saying goes: "Tong ze bu tong; Bu tong ze tong." (If there is free flow, there is no pain; If there is no free flow, there is pain.) Therefore, mobilization of Qi and Blood (or the affected structure) is the treatment most likely to unblock the channels and treat pain.

Some of the channel-subchannel therapies in this section can be performed without extensive OM/TCM diagnostic evaluation or extensive knowledge of specific acupuncture point functions. However, although these methods are highly effective for musculoskeletal applications by themselves, without OM/TCM diagnostic and treatment techniques, they are less effective for addressing *root* causes and may result in only temporary improvement, unless they treat the "lesion" or biomechanical dysfunction directly, in which case long term reduction in symptoms is still very likely.

It is the author's practice to attempt to treat both root causes (not to be confused with Deficiency) and branch/symptomatic presentation when possible. TCM/OM root treatments can be applied by balancing the patient's pulses and abdominal presentations, and, by and large, are achieved by treating distal channel points. Symptomatic (branch) treatments may be applied using channel therapies (distal points) or "local" points. Again, however, if local needle placement is based on specific lesion-tissue diagnosis, even local treatments may become root treatments since they address the *specific* cause of pain.[31] Local treatments are especially important in chronic cases and often are more likely to achieve a lasting effect. Orthopaedic Medicine principles and not pressure tenderness should then guide the practitioner.

CHANNEL ACTIVATION/DOWNWARD DRAINING. Channel activation is probably the most common acupuncture therapy used for musculoskeletal disorders. The technique can be used by itself or in conjunction with other methods. The practitioner

1. needles tender and abnormal points in and around the painful area.;
2. usually needles one or two points further downstream (usually on the extremity) on the affected channels, most often, the Accumulating, Connecting, and/or Spring/Ying points;
3. needles empirical or regional points such as LI-4 for head, SI-3 for neck, etc. These are often combined with Command points to activate the appropriate channel, the Well point to activate the Sinew channels, Reflex points (ear, wrist/ankle, cranial etc.) to activate analgesia of affected area.

Or the practitioner

---

31. Not a classical idea.

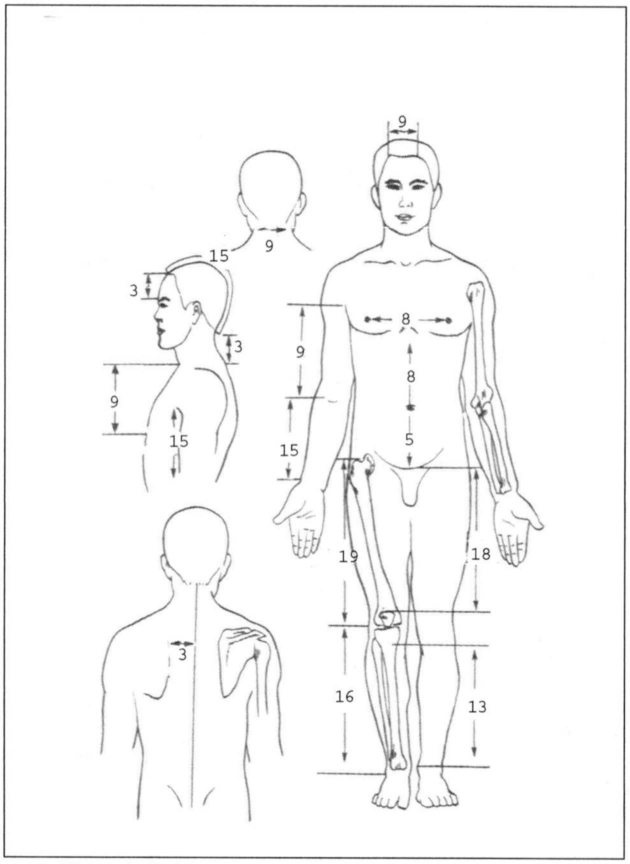

Figure 5-15: Cun measurements.

1. uses a contralateral point or opposite point imaging (front/back, up/down left/right, etc.);
2. uses the Spring/Ying point on the affected channel and a paired Stream/Shu point on the contralateral-diagonal channel (e.g., P-2 on the affected channel with a contralateral Liv-3);
3. uses the Spring/Ying or Steam/Shu on the affected side and a contralateral Yin/Yang point (e.g., P-8 on the affected side with GB-41 on the contralateral side).

Locating Channels and Points

Locating points is an acquired art. As with all physical medicine arts, it demands palpatory vocabulary and finger sensitivity. The *Spiritual Axis* states:

> Ask above and below the point, because each person's channels are not the same...If you want to get the point or examine them, you will have to rub them. Inside [the point] there will be some reaction or pain.

In some Japanese traditions points may be considered "Live" only when active, and only then are responsive to treatment. According to Sodo Okabe (Hayden 2001), there are five types of changes associated with acupuncture points:

1. Induration—a small nodule is felt at the point, which may produce a dull pain when pressed.
2. Tenderness—a hard area which produces a strong pain when pressed.
3. Hyperesthesia—pain felt on the surface of the skin when stroked or lightly pinched.
4. Depression—a small area into which the finger falls, often at source or tonification points.
5. Congestion—a superficial, slightly bloated, pillow-like stagnation often found on the abdomen.

Indurations tend to come in three types: Soft/spongy, medium, and hard. In the Toyohari association (p-339), the names given to these are *Kyoro* (moving), *Gomu* (rubber) and *Karebone* (bone-like). The softer indurations are less chronic and easier to treat. If a person has significant amounts of hardened tissue, their prognosis is accordingly much worse. Depressions and sticky congestions are usually felt when looking for tonification points on Yin channels. Points on Yang channels usually have more tenderness or indurations.

The pulse can be monitored for changes when palpating around acupuncture points, especially for tonification points. If the pulse improves while lightly touching the point, then the point should be good for tonification.

It is the author's practice to look for, categorize, and treat muscular induration and tightness as Sinew channel points, and "holes" and depressions as other channel points.[32] Thus Main (Extra, Divergent) channel acupuncture points are often located on the body surface in depressions between muscles, tendons, and other soft tissues. Frequently these points have a different tissue sensibility. The depression may have a firm or soft texture; the area may feel damp or relatively dry. At times, heat or some type of vibration can be sensed just over the point. Pathological (congested) points (which are often non-channel points i.e., Kori [hard], Ashi [sensitive], trigger points [both sensitive and hard] on Sinew channels) may feel indurated and hard.

Since bodily dysfunctions are often unilateral, it makes sense that tissue sensibility is different on the left and right channels. It is this author's practice to lightly touch/palpate major activating points (such as command points) bilaterally and compare their tissue resiliency. Often, one side is tighter and feels fuller than the other and may be treated with sedating techniques. The other side can be moxaed. Other palpatory sensations can be felt as well. For example, when palpating or holding the feet (or any part of the body) one can feel rhythmic external and internal rotation movements that correspond to the primary respiratory system (cranial-sacral rhythms). Other *endogenous* motions can be felt as well and may correspond to an array of conditions/functions and tissues. For *channel palpation*, one can hold two points on the same channel with two fingers of one hand and the same two points on the other side with the other hand. A rhythmic movement can be felt. Sometimes both sides move in unison, while at other times one side feels as though movement is in a proximal direction while the other side moves distally. One side may feel as if it were moving with a higher frequency than the other. These subtle channel/point palpation techniques can be used to assess both function and treatment. The multitude of sensations are yet to be classified. A sense as though the body pulls toward an area is often felt in the presence of somatic or organ dysfunction (local dysfunction).

Sliding a Finger Lightly Over a Surface

Spiritual Axis states: "First, attentively observe and differentiate Fullness and Emptiness of the channel by pressing with the fingers, using sliding techniques, and also rubbing and flicking the points."

One way for the practitioner to locate a Main channel acupuncture point is, therefore, to slide a finger over the surface around the anatomical region where a point is said to be located (about 5cm on either side), until one feels a depression. Little force should be used when making contact with the patient's skin, because the depression may present either as a physical trough or as a sudden loss of tissue elasticity. Note if the finger stops anywhere along the channel. Is there a depression? a sticky feeling? a puffy feeling? a nodule? fibrous tissues? tight-band? etc. The patient's face is observed for wincing, or to see if their breathing changes. Active acupuncture points are frequently tender.

Subcutaneous Points

To assess the condition of acupuncture points at the subcutaneous level, the practitioner presses the skin, taking up the slack between the skin and subcutaneous tissues, and moves the skin over the subcutaneous tissue. This may reveal indurated pathological areas, fibrous tissues, and acupoints.

Point Location and Reactivity

Textbooks describe the location of acupuncture points as "fixed," in positions measured in body inches (*cun*) from body landmarks that often are skin creases and/or bony, tendinous, and muscular sites.[33] Figure 5-15 illustrates regional cun measurements. These point locations should only serve as guides. Points move constantly, and personal variations occur. According to Dr. Shima, text-book locations of chan-

---

32. The word "acupoint" in Chinese means a hole or depression. This differentiation between indurated and hole points is not classical as far as I know.

33. A body inch (cun) is defined as the width of the patient's thumb, or as the distance between the ends of the patient's interphalangeal creases on the radial surface of the middle finger. The distance between the outer edge of the index finger and the outer edge of the little finger is said to be three cun.

nel points pertain to healthy people only. In Deficient conditions points are said to move proximately, and, in Excess conditions, points are said to move distally.

By and large, however, doctors at modern Chinese hospitals treat points at their "text-book" locations, whereas Japanese acupuncturists emphasize palpation to identify locations specific to the patient.[34]

Principles for Selecting Techniques and Points

Creating a treatment plan is an intellectual and a tactile process. *Spiritual Axis* says:

> The principles of using these fine needles are easy to say but difficult to master. Ordinary skill of acupuncture maintains the physical body; high skills maintain the spirit, use the spirit to reveal the spirit and the guest [evil] at the door...The unskilled physician grasps only form when using acupuncture. The superior physician understands the spirit...To know the Qi and how and when to treat it, one must know its comings and goings, its flow and couterflow, as well as its fullness and emptiness. The importance of cycles must be understood in the timing of obtaining Qi. The doors are closed to the unskilled physician.

The practitioner's attitude, therefore, must be confident and enlist all available tools during therapy. He/she should be calm and focus his/her attention on the needle as well as the patient. Verbal communication and assurance to the patient can alleviate anxiety and harness the patients "healing powers," confidence, and conviction that acupuncture therapy is appropriate, all of which will increase effectiveness. Eye contact may be useful.[35] It is said that one must quickly grasp the Qi with the needle or the Qi will "retreat." The practitioner, therefore, must be attentive to feedback from the patient and the needle. Sensing the Qi is said to be mysterious, subtle, and without form.

In general, the practitioner selects points and techniques that correspond to the patient's general condition as well as the local disorder. *Spiritual Axis* says: "A mild disease requires shallow (needling), while a serious one, deep [needling]. A mild disease requires fewer [points], while a serious one, more [points]." Sensitive points and channels should be emphasized over theoretical functional points.[36] The following (mostly traditional TCM/OM) guidelines should be followed with flexibility.

- The practitioner may needle the appropriate level and reach the lesion or related tissue;

---

34. This is a generalization, as many Chinese doctors palpate as well.

35. As stated earlier, all medical interventions have placebo effects and harnessing and maximizing them is by no means negative.

36. This statement reflects the author's opinion. TCM style acupuncture, which has been criticized as "herbalized" acupuncture because functions for points were borrowed from Chinese herbal medicine. Organ diagnosis is often emphasized rather than palpatory based point selection.

— needle superficially for superficial syndromes (in muscle and skin), when there is swelling, active inflammation, spasms, and when the patient reacts strongly to light pressure, or if the pulse is floating. If there is swelling, shaking the needle is said to be appropriate.

For superficial muscle Obstruction syndrome use an oblique insertion from the edge of the affected muscles toward the center, or use five needles with one in the center of the affected muscle and four placed obliquely toward the center needle.

A shallow insertion is said to remove Pathogenic Factors from the Exterior and to promote blood flow. It is also thought (Kendall *ibid*) to preferentially influence viscerosomatic responses.[37]

— The practitioner may needle deeply if a lesion is deep (e.g., in ligament or bone) and there is no *active* inflammation or spasm, if the patient likes deep pressure, if the pain is only reached by deep pressure, or if the pulse is submerged. For bone or joint Obstruction syndrome, use lifting and thrusting techniques or rapid insertion and withdrawal. For deep muscle Obstruction syndromes, use three needles inserted deeply. Deep insertion is thought to reach the bone (and marrow) and Ying (Nutrient) levels. Needling to the "middle" depth is said to remove Yin Pathogenic Factors (Dampness, Blood-stasis, etc.); however, it is common to use various depths for similar reasons.[38]

— The practitioner may needle tissues corresponding to or associated with Organs (not necessarily the injured site). To treat muscles, Spleen, and Stomach, needle the muscles. To treat the tendons and Liver, needle a tendon. To treat a ligament and Liver, needle a ligament. To treat the skin and Lungs, needle the skin. To treat the vessels and Heart, needle a vessel (or near a vessel). To treat bone and Kidneys, needle the bone.

---

37. However, no support is provided.

38. In discussing needle depth and retention, the *Spiritual Axis* also states: "Those in the prime of their life and of strong build have abundant Blood and Qi with solid and strong skin. Therefore, when they are affected by an evil, they should be needled by means of deep insertion and retention of the needle. This holds true for fat persons [as well]. Those with broad shoulders, axillae and napes, thin flesh, thick skin, dark complexions, and drooping lips have black, turbid Blood and choppy Qi and move slowly. They are not enterprising and generous in nature. In needling such a person, the needle should be inserted deeply and retained to the maximum degree possible...Those thin individuals having thin skin with little color, lean flesh, thin lips, and soft voice have thin Blood and slippery Qi. Consequently, their Qi is liable to desertion and their Blood is subject to damage. In needling them, the needle should be inserted shallowly and extracted rapidly...[For] average people...they are possessed of strong muscles, mobile joints, and sturdy bones. If these people behave in a serious manner, their Qi is choppy and their Blood is turbid. In needling them, the needle should be inserted deeply and retained to the maximum degree possible. However, if they behave in a rash manner, then their Qi is slippery and their Blood thin, and the needle should be inserted shallowly and extracted rapidly."

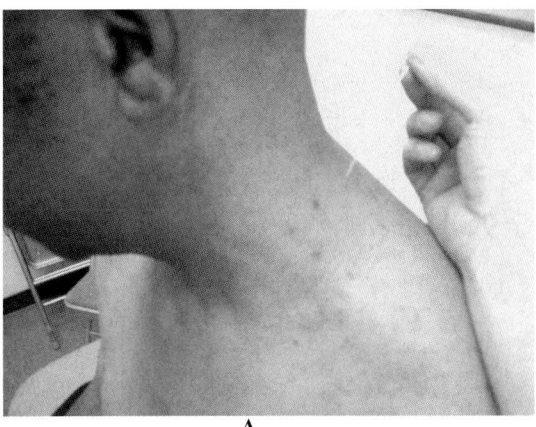 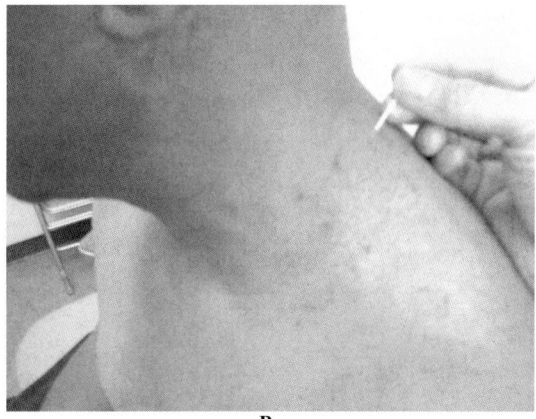

Figure 5-16: Needling over the scalene muscle cross fiberally using a three inch needle. A) shows beginning needle position and B) shows inserted needle. Care must be taken not to puncture the lungs.

- The practitioner may needle superficially and use bleeding techniques for Heat, Blood-stasis, or acute injuries when strong muscle spasms (or pain) are present.
  — If the pulse is quick the practitioner may remove the needle after obtaining Qi, or retain until redness around the needle fades.
  — For Blood-stasis and Excess conditions, the practitioner may bleed deeper vessels as well.[39]
- The practitioner may needle deeply and use moxibustion for Cold and Deficient conditions.[40] Insert needle slowly with pressure (i.e., hot-needle technique), withdraw quickly.[41]

---

39. As with most suggestions on needle technique, there is often contradictory information even within the same text. *Spiritual Axis* states, "Needle all fevers like one using the hand to touch boiling water. Needle Cold wasted diseases like a man who has no desire to move." At the same time, *Spiritual Axis* also states, "In needling [a patient with an] urgent [pulse movement in the vessels] (usually meaning Heat), the needles [should go] deep inside and be retained for a long time; needling the moderate [pulse should be] superficial and with quick removal of the needle;...in needling the big [pulse] Qi [should] slightly be drained and no Blood [should] spill out; in needling the slippery [pulse], remove [the needles] quickly and needle superficially; in needling the rough [pulse] the needle [should] reach the middle [level] of the vessel and, according to rebellion and smoothness [needles should be] retained for a long time, first press the finger while following and when the needles are removed, the hole (acupoint) should be closed by pressing, to not let Blood spill out;...When the pulse is excessive, needle deeply;...when the pulse is deficient, needle superficially."

40. In *The Systematic Classic of Acupuncture & Moxibustion*, however, moxibustion and harsh herbal formulas are forbidden in patients that are both Yin and Yang deficient (Shou-Xiong and Chace *ibid*).

41. There is, however, an interpretation of the classic statement: "If the Qi of the five viscera is expiring in the Exterior and the practitioner replenishes the Interior this results in what is called counterflow inversion...sure to result in death...," interpreted to mean Yang-deficiency in which deep insertion and long retention is use, tonifying Yin, may result in overwhelming Yang even more (Shou-Xiong and Chace *ibid*).

- The practitioner may use pressure to direct the propagated needling sensation (PS) to the affected area. Studies have shown that pressure can block PS (Wu et al 1993), and, therefore, can be used to direct sensation proximally from the pressure point. Warming-up the area (channel) prior to needling can help as well.
- When the channels are depressed and sinking, or knotted firm, and solid, use fire-needle or moxibustion.
- The practitioner may needle contralaterally in the spaces (valleys) between the muscles for pain of unfixed location and or pain that moves around (Wind), or "chase" Ashi/tender points from superior inferiorly.
- The practitioner may needle and tonify between divisions of the muscles/flesh (often where nerve trunks are located) to treat flaccid, weak, and sluggish muscles from Stomach weakness. Follow by tonification at St-36.
- The practitioner may needle across (transversely) muscle fibers for Sinew channel tightness (Figure 5-16) and along muscle fibers for Sinew channel weakness.
  — "Through and Through" acupuncture (i.e., connecting more than one point or channel with one needle) can be used to treat tightness and inhibited movement.
  — Needling along muscle fibers can be used to treat weak and sluggish (slow to react) muscles.
- The practitioner may bleed the collaterals/network vessels (superficial and deep blood vessels, Connecting points) and then needle St-36 for a chronic Painful Obstruction Disorder (Bi) that has been refractory to other treatments.
- The practitioner may needle above swellings caused by Wind and then use a sharp needle locally (shaking it), after which one should press the swollen area to "push out" pathogenic-Qi.
- Treating a single channel for acute disorders may be sufficient. One should treat several channels in chronic disorders.

- The practitioner may treat local reactive points for chronic or mild, subacute pain.
- The practitioner may needle below to treat above and vice versa, especially for chronic and/or acute and subacute disorders (or when using manual therapies or mobilization). The diaphragm is considered the separation of upper and lower.
- The practitioner may needle the right to treat the left and vice versa, especially for acute and subacute disorders (or when using manual therapies or mobilization).[42]
  — For inflamed tendons needle the opposite-side tendon, selecting points on each side of the tendon with strong stimulation.
  — Other examples of cross needling are: sedate the affected channel using Well (Jing/Ting), Spring (Ying), or accumulation (Xi) points, and tonify the *contralateral* channel extremity point with moxa or gold needles; or choose opposite analogous points: lower/upper, Yin/Yang, etc.
- The practitioner may needle front to treat back and vice versa, especially for acute and subacute pain (or when using manual therapies or mobilization).[43]
- The practitioner may needle diagonally on analogous areas (e.g., left foot and right hand), especially for acute and subacute pain, (or when using manual therapies or mobilization (see Table 5-5 on page 348). "Cross needling" is said to treat the Connecting channels and network-vessels.
  — The above techniques that treat areas away from the pain are quite common and may be tried one after the other until the pain improves.
  — The practitioner may strongly stimulate the point (with as almost as, or more intensity than the patient's pain), while asking the patient to move the affected area. This may activate the so-called *diffuse noxious inhibitory control system* and result in a non-specific analgesia.
- The practitioner may needle proximal points first and distal second for chronic disorders. Needle distal points first and proximal second in acute disorders.
- The practitioner may use mid-day mid-night rules (see p-306).
- The practitioner may choose points that have a wide therapeutic range and activate multiple systems, such as:
  — P-6, the command point for the Yin Wei channel regulates the Pericardium channel, opens the chest, calms the spirit, and regulates the autonomic nervous system;
  — Sp-6, which connects the three leg Yin channels;
  — TB-8, which connects the three arm Yang channels;

  — Extra channels command points and Sp-21 for widespread pain.
- The practitioner may use Divergent channels if pathological tissue *changes* are present, or if there is deep and lurking pathogens.
- The practitioner may combine Back-Shu with Alarm-Mu or appropriate influential points for the tissues and Organs.[44]
  — Combine Liver and Gall Bladder for sinews; Spleen and Stomach for muscles; etc.
  — Use traditional points such as GB-34 to treat the sinews, Lu-5 and LI-10 to "moisten sinews," (usually Lu-5 on opposite side for lower body and same side for upper body); St-36, Sp-3, 4, 6, and 10 for muscles; UB-11, 23, K-3, and 7 for bones, etc.
  — The practitioner may use traditional points for the conditions or regions such as: GB-31 for Wind; St-40 for Phlegm; UB-17 for Blood; TW-4 for ankle; or LI-5 and St-41 for wrist/ankle; GB-39 and SI-3 for neck; and St-38 for the shoulder, etc.
- The practitioner may choose extremity points for their dynamic and activating properties.
  — The more distal the point the farther its effect up the channel.[45]
  — Use Transporting points such as Shu-stream for musculoskeletal pains, swelling, heaviness, and for the joints. Spring-Ying points can be used to increase the Qi-dynamic and then used on upper/lower and opposite lower/upper extremity on the same "energetic" level (e.g., GB and TW).
- The practitioner may use points unilaterally to vitalize Qi and Blood, thereby alleviating pain and facilitating movement. This works best on Yang Ming channels as they have more Qi and more Blood (e.g., Ling Gu and Da Bai, see Tong-style acupuncture).
- The practitioner may use points bilaterally to tonify and strengthen. The "great needling" method is said to treat the Main channels.

---

42. This technique has been shown to increase the firing rates of neurons lying in the bulbar structure in the reticular formation (Bing et al 1991).

43. *Spiritual Axis* also states, "When inspection shows the front is painful, that must be treated first."

44. The Alarm (Mu) points are anatomically located in dermatomes that are consistent with segmental sympathetic output for their organs. There are no exceptions to this among all the Alarm (Mu) points. The word "Shu" can be translated as "transport," and the word "Mu" as "to collect." Since the vertebral nerves can be described as transporting neurologic information from the spine to the organ, the concept of Shu-Transporting points may be similar to the biomedical understanding of efferent stimulation, since the Mu points are located in dermatomes that "collect" neurologic input and transfer that input to the spine for processing. The Mu points may describe some of the concepts called the afferent system in biomedicine (Teitelbaum 2000). Thus a Mu-Shu treatment may have effects primarily through direct efferent and afferent input.

45. Bing et al (*ibid*) showed (in rats) that a higher release of opiates in the cervical region than lumbar region can be produced by stimulation of a lower extremity point St-36, thus having a nonsegmental effect.

- The practitioner may tonify the Deficient channel on one side and disperse the Full channel on the other side, or the paired channel.
- The practitioner may use four needle technique with tonifying point on one side and dispersing on the other side, or use same points and technique bilaterally.

• The practitioner may disperse indurated, hard, and sensitive points.

• The practitioner may tonify or apply moxa on soft unresilient and depressed points.

• For severe pain, one can use two (double) needles 2-3mm apart for local stimulation.

• The practitioner may use microsystems such as auricular, wrist/ankle, etc., for acute trauma/injuries or to enhance general analgesic effects. They can be used to regulate functions as well.

• The practitioner may treat points generally from Yang to Yin, i.e., from back to front, from top to bottom. The needles can be withdrawn in the same way. However, in Deficiency, one should needle from bottom up and front to back.
- Treat Alarm-Mu points first followed by back-Shu points. In many acute disorders, however, distal points may be chosen first.

Acute (Yang) Disorders

For acute (or Yang) disorders such as in patients who have constant pain, inflammation (tenderness, swelling and warmth) and guarding, or in patients who have local pain and otherwise are strong and healthy, the practitioner uses acupuncture, electroacupuncture, or ion cords as described in Table 7-2. If points on Yang channels are strongly sedated, it is a good idea to tonify a point on the paired Yin channels, in order to protect the patient's vitality, especially in old and weak patients.

Chronic (Yin) Disorders

For chronic (or Yin) disorders in patients who have intermittent pain, no obvious inflammation, pain mostly during some movement but not during others (as seen with joints dysfunction), pain worse after activity and better with rest, and/or mild local tenderness that pressure seems to relieve, the practitioner uses acupuncture or electroacupuncture as indicated in Table 7-3.

Balancing of Yin and Yang

In general, the goal of acupuncture is to harmonize (balance) the Yin and Yang. The balancing of Yin and Yang has several aspects, such as balancing top and bottom, left and right, anterior and posterior, Qi and Blood, etc.

BALANCING TOP AND BOTTOM. *Spiritual Axis* states, "If the disease is located in the upper body, treat the lower body. If disease is located in the lower body, treat the upper body." Points, therefore, can be chosen away from pain or may be treated in a balanced fashion. For example, when treating tennis elbow, the practitioner can balance LI-11 and TW-10 (local excess points) with contralateral needles at St-36, GB-33, 34, or points on leg Yin channels such as Sp-9, or Kidney gate (77.18). This combination (on similar "energetic" levels, both being on Yang Ming/Shao Yang, or related Yin/Yang) can both strengthen the treatment and balance the top/bottom Qi imbalance (especially in chronic cases). In treating upper/lower imbalance the Girdle (Dai) channel is particularly helpful.

NOTE: Some systems do not combine top and bottom points and consider it detrimental at times. The thought is that by using top and bottom point, the Qi collides disturbing the Qi dynamic.

When using many points which are either on the upper or lower parts of the body, the practitioner may want to balance these with a point on the opposite level (often to prevent dizziness). Balancing top and bottom is not usually necessary in acute conditions when mobilization of Qi/Blood is more important. Mobilization of Qi/Blood can be accomplished by choosing a point contralateral on opposite limb, on the same channel level, or a Yang point for a Yin area of symptoms—thus vitalizing Qi and Blood through the affected area (for more detail see p-350).

Another aspect of top/bottom balancing is the affects of channel obstruction on its own channel balance, as well as other channels up and downstream. When the channel is obstructed, Qi and Blood tend to accumulate upstream (from the lesion) leading to Fullness, and Emptiness develops downstream from the obstruction which reduces overall circulation. This imbalance has to be addressed within the channel. Since the direction of Qi flow within each channel system is not clear (due to different theories), palpation and symptoms should be used to determine which areas, within a channel, are Full and which are Empty.

BALANCING LEFT AND RIGHT. Left and right imbalances are common, as both stagnation and deficiency can manifest on the same side of the channel and result in a Yin Yang reaction. Disorders that affect the left side are considered Yang; disorders that affect the right side are considered Yin. Therefore, it is common to choose points on the left side for men (men are more Yang) and on the right side for women (women are more Yin). Some Tong-style acupuncturists needle men primarily on the left and women primarily on the right (or begin needling on these sides respectively). *The Systemic Classic of Acupuncture & Moxibustion* states that the balancing of left and right, especially the removal of Blood-stasis, is the most important aspect of treatment in chronic diseases. It also states that males should be needled shallower than females in order to restrain True-Qi and prevent evil-Qi from penetrating.

Table 5-2: Acute (Yang) Disorders

Acupuncture	1. Use many local needles at the site of pain. Use stronger stimulation or positive[a] pole electrostimulation.
	2. Apply a sedating needling technique.
	3. Treat tightness in muscles with cross-fiber through and through (entire muscle width) needle stimulation, but not if muscle is acutely painful and/or spasmed. If acutely painful and spasmed, needle superficially over active triggers. Insert the needle is a 60 degrees oblique angle to the muscle fibers.
	4. Leave the needles in place until local erythema diminishes.
	5. Use bleeding techniques.
	6. Use silver needles.
	7. Cup and stretch fascia after removing the needles.
Electroacupuncture	Indicated frequently. Use strong stimulation, usually at the connecting point, to activate the channel and drain the area. • Apply the anode (+) pole locally and the cathode (−) pole distally. or • Use the cathode (−) pole locally to push Qi through. • The frequency can be set to 100-5000 Hz (to induce nerve blockade), alternating with a low 2-4 Hz (for prolonged effects).
Ion Cords	Can use ion cords to direct Qi through the channel. Use the open side of the diode locally.

a. This author often prefers the negative pole if close to bone or affected tissues to reduce swelling.

Table 5-3: Yin Disorders

	1. Use few local needles at the site of pain.
	2. Apply a tonifying needling technique (mild stimulation, moxa or negative[a] pole electrostimulation).
	3. Needle along muscle fibers.
	4. Leave needles in place for no more then 10-30 minutes.
	5. Use moxa to warm and push the Qi and Blood through the channel, especially after needles are removed.
	6. Use gold needles.
Electroacupuncture	• Uses mild stimulation: the cathode (−) pole locally, the anode (+) distally on the channel on painful side or on opposite side; or cathode (−) at source or tonification point to add local energy and anode (+) at connecting point to activate the painful area; or • Uses mild stimulation: the cathode (−) pole distally (or at beginning of channel), the anode (+) proximally (or downstream) to activate the channel. • Frequency can be set to 2 Hz, if needed, alternating with 75-100 Hz but very low intensity.
Ion Cords	Can use ion cords to direct Qi through the channel. Uses the closed side of the diode locally.

a. This author often prefers the positive pole, especially on local tissues that need to be proliferated.

In treatment of left/right imbalances, the Extra and Divergent channels are particularly useful, especially the Yang Motility (Qiao), Yin Motility (Qiao), Conception (CV) and Governing (GV) channels. When treating men, the practitioner can choose an extra channel command point on the left and its coupled point on the right. When treating women, the practitioner can choose an extra channel command point on the right and its coupled point on the left and vice versa for men.

Needling sensitive and indurated points on one side and applying moxa on less sensitive and lax-tissue points on the other side can be useful. Using a Yang channel on one side with its Yin pair on the other side is common, as Excess in one often results in Deficiency of the other. The French ear point Master Oscillation is useful as well.

BALANCING ANTERIOR AND POSTERIOR. To balance the dorsal and ventral aspects of the body, the Urinary Bladder and Governing (Du) channel can be treated first, followed by ventral/anterior channels. Treating back Transport (Shu) and Alarm (Mu) points and connecting them with an ion-cord or electrical stimulator is a good way to balance the anterior and posterior somatic aspects.

Treating the Connecting channels, which connect the Exterior aspects of the channels with the Interior aspects, also balances the ventral and dorsal aspects.

The Girdle (Dai) channel encircles the trunk and balances the ventral/dorsal, and top/bottom somatic aspects.

BALANCING QI AND BLOOD. To balance Qi and Blood, the practitioner can combine points on channels that have more

Table 5-4: Channel Qi/Blood Balance (Simple Questions)[a]

CHANNELS	BALANCE OF QI AND BLOOD
Tai Yin LU and Sp	More Qi and Less Blood
Yang Ming LI and St[b]	More Qi and More Blood
Shao Yin H and K	More Qi and Less Blood
Tai Yang UB and SI	Less Qi and More Blood
Jue Yin Liv and P	More Blood and Less Qi
Shao Yang GB and TW	More Qi and Less Blood

a. In *Spiritual Axis,* Tai Yin has more Blood, less Qi; Shao Yin has more Blood and less Qi; and Jue Yin more Qi, less Blood.
b. St-36 is probably the most used point in acupuncture as it is the Sea and lower He point of Stomach channels which contains more Qi and more Blood. Being the sea and He point make it useful for Organic disorders. Being on the Stomach channel makes this point important in digestion and therefore nourishment.

Qi, with points on channels that have more Blood. Points on channels with more Blood may be bled when Excessive, or moxa may be used to build the Blood when Deficient. Adding a point on the Yang Ming channel makes it possible to balance both Qi and Blood, as Yang Ming channels have more Qi and more Blood. Treating Source points on a primary affected channel and its coupled Yin-Yang Connecting (Luo) point can regulate both Qi and Blood as the Source points regulate Qi (of the channel and Organ) and Connecting (Luo) points regulate the Blood. Table 7-4 lists the channel's balance of Qi and Blood.

Pain All Over

Vague and defuse pain (other than that accompanying infections) is commonly due to Blood-deficiency, together with Penetrating (Chong) channel disorder. Dampness/Phlegm and Wind as well as Qi-stagnation can also be a cause. Blood-deficiency can result in the "drying" of Sinews and the formation of endogenous-Wind. Symptoms are chronic and associated with paleness, dizziness, and thready or choppy pulse. Treatment is aimed at tonifying the Qi and Blood and subduing, or tracking Wind. Points such as:

- St-36, 37, Sp-6, 10, 4, 21, LI-11, Lu-7, UB-11, 17, 20, GB-34, and 20 can be used.
- For Dampness, St-40, Sp-9, 21, 6, CV-9, 12, GB-34 and P-6 can be used.
- For Wind, GB-20, 31, 34, UB-62, 11, 16, LI-4 and TB-5 can be used.
- SP-21, which is the master of all the Connecting channels, is used often for any of the above conditions. St-18 is used in the same way.
- Sp-4 and P-6 are used to activate the Penetrating (Chong) channel, i.e. Blood. Lu-7 and K-6 can be used as well.
- Liv-3 and LI-4 (Four Gates) and Ear Shenmen can be used to calm the patient and treat pain.

Frequency and Number of Treatments

The ideal frequency of acupuncture treatments for musculoskeletal and other conditions has not yet been established. The half-life of acupuncture *anaesthesia* (from high frequency stimulation) is fifteen to seventeen minutes in humans and five to thirteen minutes in rabbits (Han 1986; Han, Zhou and Xuan 1983; McLennan, Gilfillan and Heap 1977). Other studies show the analgesic effect of acupuncture to last around 30-40 minutes with a slow onset (30 min) and a slow offset, suggesting a chemical dynamic. In other animal studies, some *analgesic* effects (usually from low frequency stimulation) can last upto about 48 hours. An additional treatment after forty-eight hours has a cumulative effect. In humans acupuncture to LI-4 produces significant increase of the pain threshold with a peak at 20-40 minutes after needle insertion. A stronger effect is achieved if LI-4 is combed with St-36.

Too frequent low-frequency (Hz) electroacupuncture treatments may result in tolerance/resistance and may even interfere with opioid medications. There is evidence that electroacupuncture induces tolerance. Han et al reported that repeated electroacupuncture at 30-minute intervals produced a gradually blunted analgesic effect. Alternating the site as well as frequency and type of electro-stimulation can postpone the onset of tolerance (Lin et al 1993, Han *ibid*). Other effects such as circulatory often last for shorter durations, although long-term effects have been demonstrated as well (Han *ibid*). It therefore makes sense to treat the patient every other day for the first few treatments. *Spiritual Axis* states:

> For disease of nine days, three acupuncture treatments. For disease of a month, ten treatments. More or less, far or near, treat in accord with the dimensions of the disease...When the body is first diseased but it has not penetrated to the viscera, the needle [treatments] should be as half. If the viscera is first diseased and then the body responds, needle double...A chronic disease is when the evil Qi as penetrated deeply. To

needle this disease, insert deeply and retain for a long time. Every other day repeat the needling. One must first harmonize the body's left and right to remove disease from the Blood and Channels.

In China, patients are frequently treated daily for long periods, and perhaps this is the reason for the high success rates reported in the Chinese literature. It is possible that frequent treatments reinforce physiologic memory, as frequent sensory experiences can result in a strengthening of synaptic connections and the sensitization phenomenon.[46] When treating patients every day or every other day, it is better to alternate points, as overusing a point is said to deplete its Qi and Blood. (In animal studies, daily treatment does not offer any advantage over treatment every other day, Han *ibid.*) Early in the treatment phase, the patient should be seen on a frequent basis (twice or three times per week). As symptoms improve, the frequency can be reduced. If this is not done, cumulative positive effects from acupuncture may be negated and only short-term benefits seen. Later, the frequency can be reduced first to once per week, then once per two weeks, once a month, etc. When strong myofascial, ligamentous, and capsular dry needling techniques are used, a frequency of once per week to every other week (or even once per month) often result in satisfactory effects.

Generally, patients show some improvement within four visits; however, some do not until ten or so visits. Patients who do not show significant improvement by that time would probably not benefit from any further treatment. Some nonresponders (in pain treatments) can be converted to responders by treatment with the amino acid DL-phenylalanine, which potentiates endorphins (Pomeranz *ibid*).[47]

NOTE: The above guidelines do not apply when techniques that rely on the regeneration of soft tissues (after strong periosteal acupuncture for ligaments and tendons) are used. In these cases it may take up to several months before the results can be assessed, as many patients report improvement two to three months later (and often increased symptoms initially), even in difficult cases with chronic mild instabilities. The treatment course is usually ten to fifteen visits and occasionally more.

A study which recorded somatosensory-evoked potentials (N19) in patients with chronic pain undergoing electroacupuncture showed that the absolute peak latency of N19 was significantly delayed ($p < 0.05$) in chronic pain patients when compared to the control group. This increase in latency of N19 persisted after the first electroacupuncture treatment ($p < 0.05$) but tended to revert to normal after the fifth treatment ($p > 0.05$) and *reverted completely to control values* after the tenth treatment ($p > 0.05$).[48] Visual analogue scores also decreased significantly ($p < 0.05$) after the fifth and tenth sessions. These observations suggest that there is an interaction of the neural mechanisms of electroacupuncture with the thalamic generator of somatosensory-evoked potentials, i.e., N19 (Kumar, Tandon, Bhattacharya, Gupta, and Dhar 1995). This study may support the idea of having ten sessions as one treatment course.

Adverse Effects and Complications from TCM

The practice of TCM is generally safe and very few serious complications have been reported. It must be mentioned, however, that one study showed that medical practitioners (MDs [the largest group], nurses, physiotherapist, naturopaths, and chiropractors) may have a higher rate of complications than primary TCM trained practitioners. The difference may reflect disparity in relevant education, different reporting behaviors (Bensoussan et al 2000) or possibly less fear of using more invasive techniques. Complications from acupuncture are quite rare, although they have been known since the time of the *Classic of Internal Medicine*:

> Whenever one needles the chest and the abdomen one must not puncture the five solid Organs. If one punctures the Heart, this leads to death within a circulation [period]. If one punctures the Spleen, this leads to death within five days. If one punctures the Kidneys, this leads to death within seven days. If one punctures the Lungs, this leads to death within five days.[49]

The most common side effects are *needle pain, drowsiness,* and *fatigue* immediately following a treatment. These effects can be minimized by reducing the number of points and the duration of the treatment. Patients should be warned, and, if need be, should be advised to take some time before driving or operating dangerous equipment. In rare cases, some patients experience an energizing effect that can result in a euphoric and almost manic state. These patients report

---

46. Long-term potentiation (LTP) is characterized by enhanced transmission at synapses that follow high-frequency stimulation. Frequent treatments may also stimulate "windup/winddown" for treatment of sensitization phenomenon when a therapeutic stimulus is repeated at a frequent rate (see chapter 2).

47. D-phenylalanine may work even better.

48. p values are used to describe statistical significance and to ascertain if observed clinical effects are actually produced by the independent variable (therapy) or whether the differences are more likely to have been the result of random or chance fluctuations (or placebo). By tradition, and some logic, the usual standard value that must be reached for a difference between the experimental and control groups to be considered significant must be $p=0.05$. This is the so-called "p value" and is a measure that takes into account the variability of the data and the number of subjects in the study, among other things. The p value is essentially an estimate of the probability that the study will show a difference as great as, or greater than, observed difference purely by chance. Thus a p value equal to 0.05 means that only one in twenty or five in one hundred subjects would have a difference as great or greater than that observed by chance alone, if the experimental variable actually had no effect. Thus, p values greater than 0.05 are considered probably due to chance fluctuations in measurement or to weak effects of the experimental variable (therapy). It is a mistake, however, to assume that if the data show a p value "approaching" 0.05 ($p=0.056$, for example), that the data are "almost" significant (Patterson 2003).

49. This section also points out that the Organs were also seen as physical entities and not just as "officials" and channels as interpreted by some.

difficulty sleeping after treatments. In these patients needling St-36, P-8, and moxa on K-1 at the end of the treatment session can prevent such complications.

Vasovagal Reactions

Vasovagal reactions (lightheadedness, fainting, and nausea) are frequently encountered with new patients, especially when treating the upper body (GB-21, and arias around the thoracic inlet). It is more common in slender, young, dehydrated patients, or patients that are suffering from a cold or flu. It is rare in the elderly. They should therefore be treated lying down. Strong pressure on the lower abdomen is helpful and extract powder of Ginger, Ginseng, and Bamboo made into tea quickly resolves any residual feelings of nausea and lightheadedness.

Bleeding and Bruising

Bleeding and bruising can result from deep and strong techniques (and may be induced on purpose). These are almost never severe or bothersome. A history of a bleeding disorder or use of anti-clotting medications may be a relative contraindication. Ginseng and Pseudoginseng (Tian Qi) can be prescribed for such patients, to minimize the risk of bleeding, with only minimal effect on thrombin time or blood viscosity.

Serious Complications

More serious complications, such as *pneumothorax*, *punctured viscera* (spinal cord injuries, nerve damage, burns from moxa), and *infections* (endocarditis, septicemia, hepatitis B, osteomylitis, myositis, peritonitis, and human immunodeficiency virus) can occur. There have also been allergic reaction to certain needles. However, with proper technique, these risks are minute. A Medline computer search at Copenhagen University's library of medicine, after deleting reports with inadequate or questionable descriptions and duplicate articles, showed forty-one published reports of adverse effects attributed to acupuncture for the years 1980 through 1995. These were pneumothorax (most frequent), bacterial endocarditis, hepatitis, cardiac tamponade, and injury due to broken needle tips (Rosted 1996).

One estimate indicates that pneumothorax might occur once in 120 years of full-time practice. An Australian survey estimated that sixty-seven out of 100,000 may have experienced an adverse effect from acupuncture. In another survey, two cases of pneumothorax were observed in 140,000 treatments, and two cases involved a broken needle that had to be removed surgically. A second survey of 28,000 treatments in a Taipei clinic noted only fainting in fifty-five cases. In another survey of 65,000 treatments of acupuncture in a Japanese college, the serious adverse events were twenty-seven cases of failure to remove needles, and one deep moxa burn. Another survey in Singapore reported no serious adverse events in 12,000 treatments. Taking these surveys together, the risk of serious adverse events occurring in association with acupuncture is approximately 0.14 per 10,000, which is minimal.

Contraindications for acupuncture include patients with bleeding disorders, patients during the first trimester of pregnancy except for treatment of nausea (possibly), and electrical stimulation in patients with a cardiac pacemaker. Patients should not drive or operate machinery after acupuncture, especially following their first treatment. Acupuncturists need to be concerned about hepatitis B and should be tested for hepatitis B surface antigen (White and Ernst 2002).

Considering the sheer volume of acupuncture treatments performed per year, acupuncture can be considered extremely safe.

Adverse Events Reported on TCM Herbs

While some serious events have been reported after the use of TCM herbs, these by and large have not occurred when the herbs have been prescribed by professionally trained TCM practitioners. Bensoussan et al (2000) reported about one adverse event every eight or nine months of full time practice or one adverse event for every 633 (0.16%) cases treated with TCM (both herbs and acupuncture). A prospective study of hospital admissions during an eight-month period in Hong Kong showed that 0.2% of hospital admissions were related to Chinese herbs while 4.4% were related to pharmaceutical medications (Chan et al 1992). There have been direct toxic reactions, interactions with other medicines, allergic reactions, hepatic damage, kidney failure, idiosyncratic reactions, and death reported (Chan 1994; Maheux et al 1989; Kane et al 1995; Bateman et al 1998; Cheng 1995; Perharic et al 1995; Vanherweghem et al 1993; Depierreux et al 1994; Vanhaelen et al 1994; Cosyns 1994; among others).

Ideal Conditions for Treatment

In general, patients should not be too exhausted, hungry, dehydrated, or depleted when receiving acupuncture. *Spiritual Axis* recommends sweet and neutral herbs before treating depleted patients. It also recommends to treat the patient in a quiet inner room so that the patient can receive Spirit and Essence. *Spiritual Axis* also states,

> Fresh from sexual intercourse, do not needle; fresh from needling do not have intercourse. Already drunk, do not needle; already needled, do not drink. Fresh from labor, do not needle, already needled, do not labor. Already full of food, do not needle, already needled, do not eat in excess. Already starving, do not needle, already needled, do not fast. Already thirsty, do not needled, already needled do not make thirst. For great surprise or great anger, one must center the patient's Qi, then needle. If the patient rides a carriage to come, have him lie down and rest for a time equal to eating a meal, then needle. If the patient comes by walking, have him sit and rest for a time equal to walking ten li (five kilometers), then needle.

Needling Techniques

Inserting and manipulating needles is a skill that demands practice. The insertion and manipulation can be performed in many ways, using techniques that vary according to tradition and personal preference. Though acupuncture is often thought of as the stimulation of *specific points* at or near the skin, the classic literature often refers to the needling of deep anatomical tissues and channels (see quote from *Simple Questions* p-605). *Spiritual Axis* states, "If the hands can bend and not stretch, the disease is located in the sinews. If they can stretch but not bend, disease is located in the bones. When at the bones, treat the bones. When at the sinews, treat the sinews." The early Han dynasty text, *Prescriptions for Fifty-two Diseases* mentions only channels, not points. The modern saying, "hitting the point is not important as long as you are on the channel" was repeated to this author frequently in China.[50] As Hsu points out in *On the Origin and Further Course of Medicine,* there are many different indications, techniques, and shapes of needles. He writes:[51]

> According to the *Simple Questions,* the methods of needling may undergo nine variations and may be divided into twelve sections. The *nine variations* include the needling of transport [points alone]; needling from a distance; needling channels; needling network [vessels]; needling [the space] between [the skin and flesh]; needling to induce drainage of large [amounts of pus or blood]; needling [of the skin as cautiously as with a hair]; square needling [contralateral]; and cauterization needling [heated needles]. The twelve sections include *paired needling* [two sides on front and back into painful site]; *retaliation needling* [multiple] insertions at pain sites [for migratory pain which moves; using needles at the painful site and then palpating for a new painful site and moving the needle there and so forth]; *broad needling* [used next to cramped or painful sinew to widen space and to relax the sinews; using a perpendicular insertion and repeatedly lifting and thrusting forward and backward]; *combination needling* [needle to the left and right of a center needle used for treating localized, small accumulations of deep cold/hot]; *scattered needling* [four needles around a center needle all needled shallowly for chills and fever]; *direct needling* [needling under skin without injuring flash, drawing up the skin and needling obliquely for treatment of shallow lying cold-Qi]; *transport needling* [fast and deep perpendicular insertion and withdrawal for treatment of Excess and Heat]; *short needling* [deep insertion close to bone, and gentle shaking of the needle as it is inserted. The needle is then repeatedly lifted and thrust to rub against the bone, to treat bone-Bi]; *surface needling* [slanted/oblique superficial insertion, to treat sinews that are tense and cold]; *yin needling* [needling foot Shao Yin channel on posterior malleolus, both on left and right sides of the body to treat Cold Inversion due to Cold in Center]; *sideways needling* [needling to the side of a already inserted needle at the affected area, to treat long-standing fixed/Damp-Bi]; and *supportive needling* [shallow insertion to drain blood using multiple insertion and withdrawals to treat swelling and pain]....In ancient times the needles were shaped in nine [different ways including] the chisel needle, the round needle, the arrow-head needle, the lance-point needle, the sword needle, the round-sharp needle, the hair needle, the long needle, and the large needle.

Spiritual Axis states: The chisel needle has a big head with a sharp tip. It may be used to disperse the Yang Qi. The round needle has the shape of an egg. It is used for rubbing and massage, to divide and to separate so as not to injure the muscles and flesh. It divides and disperses the Qi. The spoon needle has a point which is as sharp as a grain of millet. It controls the channels by touch, not by penetration, so as to bring about the Qi. The lance needle has three cutting edges and may be used to affect chronic illnesses. The sword needle tip is like a sword. It may be used to press out large pustules. The round and sharp needle is as large as a tuft of hair. It is both round and sharp. The center of its body is a bit larger. Its use is to seize the abrupt, cruel Qi. The hair-fine needle has a tip like a mosquito or a gadfly's beak. It can be inserted slowly and quietly and detained for a long time to nourish true Qi. It may be used also to reach the sickness of painful Bi syndrome. The long needle has a lancet-like edge and a thin body so that it may be used to reach distant paralysis and deep Bi syndrome. The big needle is tipped like a stick and its point is slightly round. It may be used to disperse water by moving gates. These are the nine needles.

When disease is located on the skin without a definitive location, treat by using the engraver's needle for this disease, except at the white regions of the skin. When disease is located at the divisions between the flesh, treat using the round needle. When the disease is of the main channels, chronic illness, or Bi syndrome, use the lance needle. When the disease is in the channels and the Qi is sparse, tonify at that point. Treat using the spoon needle at the well, spring, stream, and river shu points. When the disease makes large pus-filled ulcers, treat by using the sword needle. When the disease is Wind-Damp with abrupt and cruel Qi coming forth, treat by using the round needle. In the case of persistent Wind-Damp and pain, treat using the hair-fine needle. When the disease is located in the center of the body, treat by using the long needle. When the disease is edema, which causes blockages at the gates and joints, treat using the big needle. When the disease is located in the five viscera and is solidly established, use the lance needle. Disperse the well, stream, dividing, and shu points, and treat in accord with the four seasons.

The Systematic Classic of Acupuncture & Moxibustion states: The choice of these standardized needles is totally important in needling treatment. Each of the nine types of needles has its own use. Whether they be long or short, large or small, they each have their specific applications. If used inappropriately,

---

50. This certainly complicates the idea of "sham" acupuncture used in many Western studies on acupuncture.

51. Some additions by the author from *Systemic Classic of Acupuncture.*

the illness cannot be removed. If the illness is shallow and one needles deeply, this will only injure the healthy flesh and cause yong in the skin. On the other hand, if illness is deep but one employs a shallow needle insertion, the disease Qi will not be drained. On the contrary, this will result in grand purulence. If a disease is mild and a large needle is used, this will drain the Qi too rapidly, ultimately causing further harm. If the disease is a major one and a small needle is used, the (evil) Qi will not be drained off and this too will result in failure. The most appropriate manner of needling is to apply major drainage in the case of a major (illness) and to avoid drastic (therapies) in the case of minor illnesses...

Even a beginner can achieve a painless needle insertion by using a guide (a hollow tube, usually supplied with the needles); the practitioner quickly taps the needle into the subcutaneous layer. After the needle is inserted, the practitioner can manipulate the needle until the De Qi is sensed.

Obtaining De Qi

Obtaining De Qi is necessary for Chinese-style acupuncture treatment to succeed. The patient senses the arrival of Qi as a dull ache, tingling, heaviness, warmth, chill, distention, electric-like movement, or other "strange" sensations. Japanese acupuncture systems often use sensationless (to the patient) techniques, especially when tonifying or strengthening.

Generally, the practitioner decides whether the desired stimulation is to be supplementing or dispersing. This determines the depth, direction, and technique of needling. This decision however, is dependent in part on information the practitioner receives from the needle. Stimulation is then continued until the practitioner feels the De Qi sensation as tissue resistance to needle manipulation (necessary with Japanese techniques as well), and until the patient indicates feeling the arrival of Qi. Normally, unless electricity or stronger stimulation is needed, once De Qi arrives, no further needle stimulation is needed. The classic literature greatly emphasizes the practitioner's attention, concentration, intention (Yi) and sensitivity when treating patients with acupuncture.[52] In writing on the power of Intension and Touch, Upledger (1997) states:[53]

> I saw that some of us could do acupuncture with great success and others didn't get the same degree of success, even on the same patients. At first I thought it was suggestion, so we tried to control any positive or negative comments about expectation...The strong correlation seemed to be in the unspoken attitude of the therapist. Those of us who had seen acupuncture work and believed in it got much better results than those who did not necessarily believe or disbelieve that it would work...I also think that the energy you supply the patient through your well-intentioned touch (which shows up as voltage increase in the patient) helps activate that patient's self-correcting mechanisms.

A technique commonly used by the author is to palpate the *affected area* (joint, muscle, etc.) with a sensing hand while gently exploring different needle techniques (on local or distal points) in various directions, rotations, and pressures to achieve a sense of tissue compliance and increased sense of ease with the non-needling hand. This often results in De Qi type sensations (but not always) that the patients can feel as well.

Tonification and Sedation

Many techniques are available for achieving tonification and sedation. Throughout history the methods described have contradicted each other (O'Connor and Bensky 1981). Some studies show that needle technique can be important in determining outcome. For example, a study conducted at the Institute Zhongda Hospital affiliated to Dongnan University Nanjing (2003) showed that acupuncture with attention to tonification and sedation techniques has significant effects in the treatment of hypertension, measured by a Doppler ultrasonic blood-flow monitor, as well as other clinical therapeutic effects. In the classic texts, consideration is given to the day of the month, the patient's date of birth, and to respiratory cycles, among other factors that may not be practical or credible in modern practice. For example, in the classic *Spiritual Axis,* sedation/dispersion is said to be contraindicated at the time of the new moon, and tonification/supplementation contraindicated when the moon is full. It also states, "Therefore, it is said one must know the astrological avoidances to speak about the theory of acupuncture."

Recently, a Japanese physician, Professor Nishijo Tanaka (1996), suggested that superficial needling during exhalation, in a sitting subject, results in long-lasting parasympathetic activation evident in longlasting reduced heart rate. (Exhalation is a parasympathetic-dominated phase of respiration; the heart rate slows down.) This technique can be

---

52. The practitioner intention (Yi) should not be underestimated. Experiments show that the observer's *expectation* can influence an experiment's outcome. The human body generates electrical fields that have been described by touch therapists (Qi Gong practitioners, for instance) that may influence the patient. For example, when a group of researchers were given two groups of rats, one that was said to be composed of "smart" rats and the other retarded, and asked to study their learning, the so-called smart group learned much quicker even though both groups were actually identical (Frost *ibid*). In another study Grinber-Zylerbaum and Ramos (1989) reported on "nontouching, silent communication" between two or more individuals. Electroencephalgrapy (EEG) was used to study silent communication patterns. Partners who reported feelings of being blended with one another altered their EEG pattern to the point of being virtually identical. This may explain why some patients do better with one practitioner as opposed to another when both use the same treatment. At the same time, the fact that some large studies comparing MD-administered acupuncture (which has been criticized since many MDs have minimal training in acupuncture) and sham acupuncture show little difference between the two (both achieve fairly high positive outcomes that cannot be simply explained by "placebo") does bring into question the magnitude-effect of intention, assuming that acupuncture-trained MDs believed in acupuncture and had full intention and expectation that "real" acupuncture would perform better than sham.

53. John E. Upledger DO is a well known Osteopathic physician and the developer of CranioSacral Therapy™.

thought of as *tonification*.[54] The sympathetic system is said to be activated by needling more deeply with the patient lying down, and during both inhalation and exhalation (i.e., under continuous stimulation). Low-frequency, 1 Hz electro-stimulation can be added. The points used are said to be irrelevant.[55] Imai and Kitakoji (2003) investigated the difference in transient heart rate reduction associated with brief acupuncture in twenty healthy subjects at rest in a supine and in a sitting position. Acupuncture needling using the sparrow-pecking method, in which the needle is moved vertically lifting and thrusting, was performed for one minute at LI-10. The procedure was carried out with the subjects in a supine position and in a sitting position. The results showed that the average heart rate reduction associated with stimulation in supine subjects was 3.6 +/- 0.19 (mean +/- standard error (SE)) beats per minute (bpm), while that for sitting subjects was about 7.0 +/- 1.07 (mean +/- SE) bpm, indicating that stimulation reduces heart rate to a greater degree in subjects who are sitting ($p<0.05$, Mann-Whitney test). These results would be consistent with a mechanism involving reduced sympathetic drive to the heart, as sympathetic nerve activity has more influence on the heart rate in the sitting than in the supine position

TONIFICATION/SUPPLEMENTATION. The most accepted guidelines for tonification are:[56]

1. Use a thin needle.

2. Prepare the point by massaging in the direction of the channel.

3. Insert the needle:
   along the direction of channel flow;
   as slowly and as painlessly as possible;
   during exhalation;
   superficially first, then slowly more deeply only after obtaining Qi.[57]

4. Leave the needle in position up to fifteen minutes. Longer retention is possible, but the patient may become fatigued.

5. Withdraw the needles quickly (from the inferior to superior points), during inhalation.

6. Immediately apply pressure to the point to prevent Qi from escaping.

---

54. Or sedation when correlated to *Spiritual Axis* relations concerning breath and reduction in heart rate. Reduction of heart rate is usually considered a Yin effect.

55. The author finds this technique helpful, at times, in the treatment of painful disorders (especially in RSD), using normal point selection. It is also helpful when surrounding inflamed tissues or active scars.

56. Some consider all acupuncture techniques to have sedating effects and moxibustion to have tonifying effects.

57. Japanese practitioners often emphasize painless/sensationless and shallow techniques with little stimulation.

7. Use gold needles.

Electrical stimulation with the cathode (-) pole at the point can be used. (Place the anode (+) upstream on the channel.)

SEDATION/DISPERSION. The most accepted guidelines for sedation are:

1. Use a thicker needle.

2. Insert the needle:
   in the direction against the channel flow;
   quickly and deeply;
   during inhalation.

3. After obtaining De Qi, pull the needle out somewhat slowly with a circular movement to pull out Qi.

4. Leave the needle in position from ten to forty-five minutes. (Stimulate stronger and longer than for tonification.)

5. Withdraw the needle slowly (from superior to inferior points) during exhalation.

6. Do not apply pressure to the point (allow Qi to escape).

7. Use silver needles.

Electrical stimulation with the anode (+) pole at the point can be used. The cathode (-) can be placed up the channel.

According to Ionescue-Tirgoviste (1987), classical needle techniques can influence action potentials between distal and proximal points. Needle techniques as well as the patient's condition influence measurements taken by electroacupuncturgram (EAG). He studied clockwise and counterclockwise twirling, back-and-forth twirling, and lifting and thrusting techniques. He found that the distal points had negative potential in comparison with the abdominal needles in all cases, but the degree of potentials varied between -25 and -250mV according to the needling techniques and the health of the patient. Counterclockwise twirling/lifting/thrusting increased electro-potential the most. Healthy patients recovered their basal readings soon after discontinuing stimulation, while unhealthy patients recovered more slowly or not at all. Different metals are also said to have differing ability to stimulate action potentials in acupoints, and having the needle handle made of or wrapped by various metals (copper, gold or brass) has been said to polarize the needle, making the tip positive.

Point Injection (Fluid Acupuncture)

Point injection is a common and important modern TCM technique used for both its systemic and local effects. Both modern pharmaceuticals and traditional herbs are injected.[58]

---

58. In China point injection is used commonly for treatment of musculoskeletal and other disorders.

Table 5-5: Main Channels: Tonification and Sedation Points

Channel	Tonification Point		Sedation Point	
Lung	Lu-9	Earth	Lu-5	Water
Large Intestine	LI-11	Earth	LI-2	Water
Stomach	St-41	Fire	St-45	Metal
Spleen	Sp-2	Fire	Sp-5	Metal
Heart	H-9	Wood	H-7	Wood
Small Intestine	SI-3	Wood	SI-8	Earth
Bladder	UB-67	Metal	UB-65	Wood
Kidney	K-7	Metal	K-1	Wood
Pericardium	P-9	Wood	P-7	Earth
Triple Warmer	TW-3	Wood	TW-10	Earth
Gall Bladder	GB-43	Water	GB-38	Fire
Liver	LIV-8	Water	LIV-2	Fire

These techniques can greatly enhance clinical outcomes. The practitioner:

1. selects a point in the vicinity of the lesion;
2. injects directly into the lesion;
3. injects Shu points to strengthen.
   For injection, commonly used medicines are:[59]
   Radix Angelicae Sinensis (Dang Quai)
   Flos Carthami (Hong Hua)
   Radix Ligustici Wallichii (Chuan Xiang)
   Human Placenta (Zi He Che)
   Dextrose or Alum (Ming Fan)[60]
   Procaine
   Steroids/Licorice
   Autologous Blood.

Biomedical injection therapy can be used to reduce inflammation in arthritis, bursitis, ligamentous and nerve problems, and lesions of contractile structures. It may also be used to treat instability.

Prolotherapy/Regenerative Injection Therapy

Prolotherapy, also known as sclerotherapy and regenerative injection therapy, is a biomedical technique that uses injections for the purpose of tightening and strengthening loose or weak ligaments, tendons, or joint capsules through the multiplication and activation of fibroblasts. It is used to treat chronic pain due to connective tissue diathesis. The most common proliferant used is a 15% dextrose solution. When injected into ligaments or other connective tissues it results in an osmotic gradient and cell dehydration.[61] This activates inflammation and a fibroblastic healing response. Before and after biopsy and strength studies show increased ligament size and strength (not scar tissue) in both animals and humans (Figure 5-17, Dorman *ibid*). Although according to the *Department of Health and Human Services* there is not enough evidence to support the use of prolotherapy, *The Florida Academy of Pain Medicine* has recently published a review of studies from 1937 through 2000. They reviewed reported case studies, retrospective, prospective, and animal experiment studies. The calculated number of patients reported in those studies exceeded 530,000. Improvement in terms of return to work and previous functional/occupational activities was reported in 48% to 82% of patients. The resolution of pain symptomatology was evaluated differently in various studies and ranged from zero to 100%. Complications included twenty-eight pneumothoracies, two requiring chest tubes, twenty-four allergic reactions, one grand mal seizure, and one aseptic meningitis (Linetsky et al 2001). A newly high quality article published in *Spine* (Yelland et al 2004) has also shown long-term benefit for ligamentous injections; however, no difference was found between injection of dextrose (the proliferant) and saline. Significant reduction in pain and disability was shown in both groups. In this study the addition of flexion extension exercise was not shown to improve outcome. Other studies using stronger proliferent solutions such as P25G (Phenol 2.5%, Glucose

---

59. For more information on herbs used for fluid acupuncture injection therapy, see chapter 7.
60. A 5-8% Alum solution is used to inject hemorrhoids as well to necrotize them.
61. Dextrose (in various strengths) injected into ligaments and acupoints is used in modern TCM for similar conditions.

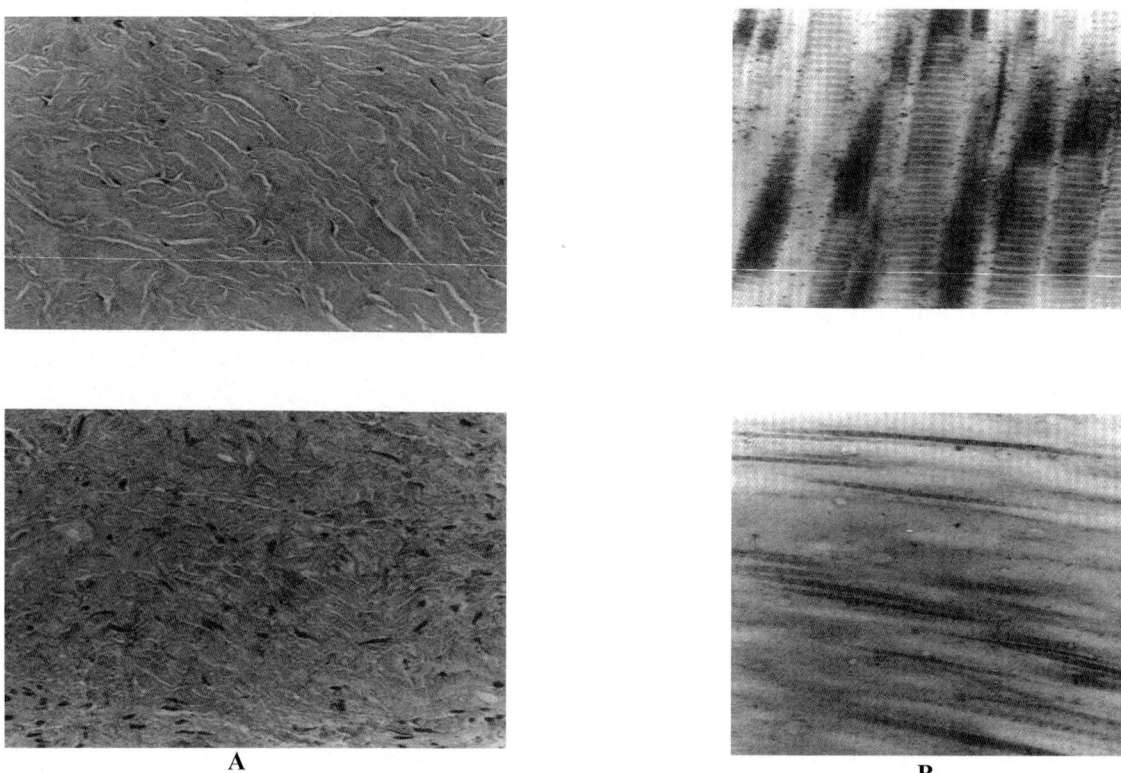

Figure 5-17: Top of figure (A) shows light microscopy H and E stain before prolotherapy x 250. Bottom shows after prolotherapy. Top of figure (B) shows EM micrograph of collagen fibers before prolotherapy, bottom shows it after prolotherapy. Note increase in number and size of collagen fibers (courtesy Dorman *ibid*).

25%, Glycerine 25%, Pyrogen-free water to 100%) have shown greater effects than saline (Dorman *ibid*).

The author finds it necessary to refer patients to prolotherapy often if symptoms of instability are recurrent, and if periosteal acupuncture and other stabilization therapies have failed. Prolotherapy is especially helpful for low back pain due to SI ligaments and/or facet joints, and neck/shoulder pains from degenerative or traumatic causes. It is also helpful in wrist pain due to repetitive use injuries, and for many other symptoms which can result from ligamentous laxity. It can also be used to treat tendinosis. Prolotherapy can be especially important when restoration of proper tensegrity of the musculoskeletal structure is needed and has been shown to have systemic effects beyond reduction of pain and improved musculoskeletal function, such as more efficient oxygen utilization and need during exercise. Dr. Dorman has also documented measurable structural changes in both knee and pelvic symmetry and stability (Dorman *ibid*).

Skin Preparation

While the use of alcohol to "disinfect" the skin is generally advocated, studies have shown that it cannot *sterilize* the skin (Dan 1967). Experience also shows that acupuncture does not result in infections in the absence of alcohol disinfection. Many diabetics routinely self-inject without the use of alcohol swabbing, with no adverse effects even in this vulnerable population (Korista and Felig 1992). To achieve skin sterilization a surgical scrub left in place for two minutes is needed. This may be considered when treating immunologically vulnerable patients, when using large bore needles in periosteal acupuncture, and for medicolegal reasons.

General Precaution with Acupuncture Treatment

Acupuncture has a very good record for safety as long as certain precautions are followed. As with all other invasive techniques the practitioner must have a good working knowledge of the relevant anatomy. Before inserting a needle, the skin overlying the area must be examined for signs of infection. If there is any such signs the needle should not be inserted. Needling the extremities caries much less risk of injury than areas on the trunk. Some points are located in potentially dangerous areas and increased caution is needed when inserting needles at these regions.

All the points around the base of the neck are in close proximity to the apex of the lung and therefore the danger of a pneumothorax must be kept in mind. Lifting and holding the appropriate tissues with one hand while inserting the needles can decrease such dangers. This is also true for points over the chest. While Hua Tuo Jia Ji (paravertebral) points are generally safer than UB points, because they lie over the vertebral bodies, care still needs to paid as the needle can slip between spaces and reach the lung. Some patients have a congenital opening in their sternum and therefore the thoracic cavity can be penetrated in these patients, and damage to the heart has been reported. An oblique needle insertion may reduce such risks. When inserting needles in the abdominal areas it is possible to puncture the underlying organs. Clinical experience, however, shows that this is rarely a problem even though probably done quite often (and often purposely as, for example, penetrating the urinary bladder to achieve a propagated sensation to the groin). A potential extra risk would occur if one were to puncture the liver or spleen. To avoid this, the abdomen should be examined for abnormally enlarged viscera.

Occasionally an acupuncture needle may break in situ. If this occurs, the point of entry should be clearly marked and immediate surgical help sought. If local irritation is caused by acupuncture, a metal allergy should be considered.

Electroacupuncture should be avoided in a patient with a pacemaker or other implanted electromagnetic devices.

Main Channels

Treatments that use the Twelve Main channels vary depending on style and tradition and on the patient's condition. Points on the Main channels can be used in Five Transporting (Phases) treatments and in other channel therapies as well.

The practitioner can select points on the Main channels based on the points':

- Traditional functions (e.g., strengthen the Spleen, eliminate Dampness, move the bowels)
- Connecting points (Table 7-8)
- Source, Entry, Exit and timing (Table 7-9 on page 305)
- Accumulation points (Table 7-11 on page 307).
- Influential points (Table 7-12 on page 308)
- Alarm and Back-Shu points (Table 7-14 on page 314)
- Placement within the channel energetic/Qi flow (e.g., Well (Jing), Spring (Ying), Stream (Shu), River (Jing), Sea (He) points), (Table 7-13 on page 310)
- Main activating points (Well [Jing] points for Sinew channels, commend points of Extra channels, etc.)
- Five Phases theory and Four Needle techniques (Table 7-16 on page 315)
- Empirical points (p-314).

Connecting Channels/Network Vessels

The Connecting channels/network-vessels are important in disorders of circulation. (The Connecting channels/vessels are part of the vascular system.) Swelling (Dampness, Phlegm or Blood-stasis), masses, spider veins, and changes in skin colorations are all signs of Connecting channel/network vessel disorders. Often an area near dysfunctional articulations shows congested and dark blood vessels. The vessels and the Connecting (Luo) points can be bled.

External Pathogens

The Connecting channels can be affected also by invasion of Exterior Pathogenic Factors (Wind), giving rise to pain. Symptoms will manifest in the Connecting channels before entering the Main channels. For such conditions the practitioner needles the Connecting (Luo) point on the affected side. When Pathogenic Factors enter the Connecting channels, pain may begin to radiate/expand.

Theoretically, incorrect treatment of the Connecting channel can result in further movement of Pathogenic Factors into the Main channel. In practice, however, this *probably* does not occur.

In general the Connecting channels are treated with shallow acupuncture, cupping, bleeding, seven star needles, moxibustion, and herbs.

Painful Obstruction/Bi Syndromes

Correct treatment to the Connecting channels (vessels) is said to prevent further movement of Pathogenic Factors and therefore prevent the development of Painful Obstruction (Bi syndrome).[62] The Connecting channels are therefore important in preventing the development of chronicity and should be used early in the course of acute or subacute disorders.

Treatment of Lesions Outside the Channels

The Connecting (Luo) points can be used to treat disorders that fall between the defined somatic arrangement of Yin and Yang Main channels as blood vessels cover the entire body.

The Spleen Great Connecting (Luo) Channel/Collateral

This channel separates at Sp-21 (Figure 5-18), six cun below the axillary fossa spreading to the chest and hypochondriac regions. It is said to be useful in treating "whole" body pain, polyarthritis, whole body weakness and muscular atrophy. For whole body pain such as seen in fibromyalgia, polyarthritis, multiple sclerosis etc., Sp-21 is often combined with GV-14, UB-11, 65, SI-3 and Liv-8. For whole body weakness and muscular atrophy Sp-21 is combined with St-36, CV-4, 6, UB-17, 43 and UB-23.

It is interesting to note that Sp-21 lies near the latissimus dorsi muscle which has a direct connection from the upper extremity across to the opposite lower extremity.

---

62. Ling Shu (*Spiritual Axis*).

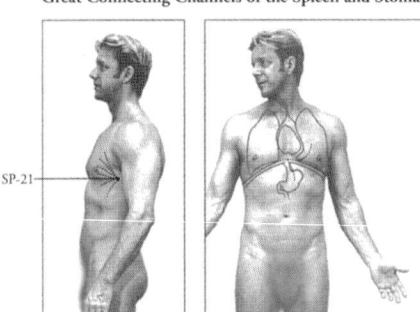

Figure 5-18: Sp-21.

Divergent Channels

The Divergent channels can be reached and activated through their Access points, both on the channel and on the paired Yin-Yang point. Treatment usually includes needling the Return point and a Directing/Focusing (local) point to channel the Qi/Blood to the injured area (Helms *ibid;* Shima *ibid*). Table 7-6 lists the Access and Return points. According to Shima and Chase, to treat the Divergent channel one must treat the Return point (Master/upper head or neck point) with one or more Transport (back Shu) points, and Source (Yuan) or connecting (Luo) points on the extremities. The Occidental Institute of Chinese Studies suggests that to treat these channels one must first:

1. Needle the local area and Ashi points on the symptomatic side;
2. Needle the Well/Jing point on the *nonsymptomatic* side;
3. Needle channel supplementation points on symptomatic side;
4. Needle Stream/Shu point on symptomatic side;
5. Needle Sea/He point on symptomatic side;
6. Needle GV-20.

Shima and Chase list many other Japanese style treatment variations including Shima's own use of Akabane testing. They also list possible herbal formulations to be used for the Divergent Confluences.

Pathological Tissues

Since the Divergent channels connect directly to the Organs (and Original and Nutritive-Qi), they are used to treat visceral and Yin (substance) disorders. Therefore, the Divergent channels are used to treat pathological (beyond dysfunction or energetic) conditions, or to reinforce the channel and Organ functions.

Prevention of Chronicity

The connection of the Divergent channels with the Main and Sinews channels (Internal/External) are said to be capable of preventing the materialization of Exterior/Qi (energetic functional) disorders, i.e. becoming Yin/structural. Therefore, the Divergent channels may be used to prevent chronicity and in disorders of Shao Yang, between Internal and External. (The Connecting channels may be more appropriate if exogenous factors are involved.)

Other Uses

The Divergent channels can be treated when Internal/External coupled (Organ/Channel) disorders are present and in left/right imbalances. When symptoms keep moving from one side to the other, the Divergent channel is often used together with Yang Ming (Stomach and Large Intestine) channels. They are also particularly important when treating deep-lying (lurking) pathogens. Because the Divergent channels connect the Interior to the Exterior they can be used to guide pathogens to the Exterior.

The Sinew Channels

The Sinew channels are best employed within the first seventy-two hours after an injury, but they can become the principal treatment up to two weeks after injury occurrence. Sinew channels are used as an adjunct to other channel therapies at later stages as well. They are activated by a point one fen proximal to Well points, (or the Well points themselves), the most distal of the Main channel points. Most often, treatment is employed unilaterally on the painful side. When the Sinew channels are used to address more chronic dysfunctions of locomotion, gait, and/or pain, they are combined with the Main, Extra, and Divergent channels.

Pain associated with:

- movement away from the body is treated using the Tai-Yang (UB/SI) channels;
- movement towards the body is treated using Yai-Yin (Lu-Sp) channels;
- rotation of the arm, shoulder, hip or trunk when these are kept straight is treated using Shao-Yang (GB/TW) channels;
- rotation movements with arm or leg bent is treated using Shao-Yin (H/K) channels,
- paralysis, weakness or atrophy is treated using Jue-Yin Liv/P) channels.

In general, the Sinew channels and Twelve Cutaneous Regions are treated with shallow needling (or deep when needed), scraping (Gua Sha), cupping, moxibustion, or fire-needle, bleeding, seven star needles, interdermal needles, and herbal medicines.

Table 5-6: Divergent Channels (Helms *ibid*, Shima *ibid*)

CHANNEL	ACCESS POINTS			RETURN POINT
Lung Large Intestine	Lu-1 or Lu-5(+)	and	LI-15 or LI-11(+)	LI-18 or St-12 (-)
Spleen Stomach	Sp-12 or Sp-9 (-)	and	St-30 or St-36 (-)	UB-1 or St-1 (+)
Heart Small Intestine	H-1 or H-3 (+)	and	SI-10 or SI-8 (+)	UB-1 or St-1(-)
Kidney Urinary Bladder	K-10 (-)	and	UB-40 (-)	UB-10, UB-11 or UB-1 (+)
Pericardium Triple Warmer	P-1 or P-3 (+)	and	TW-16 or TW-10 (+)	GV-20 (-)
Liver Gallbladder	Liv-12 or Liv-8 (-)	and	GB-30 or GB-34 (-)	GB-1(+)

THE SINEWS CHANNELS CAN BE USED BY:

- Tapping one fen proximal to Well (or Well) point and the first four painful (or Ashi) points, main joints along the Sinew channel, or Main channel points quickly with a burning incense stick or fire-needle. This can be used as part of an Akabane test and/or treatment.[63] In *Spiritual Axis* the Sinew channels are mainly treated with fire-needle techniques, techniques which may be helpful in the treatment of fibrous tissues (scars);[64]

- Needling one fen proximal to Well points. Electrical stimulation can be used; however, it is often painful.

- Bleeding one fen proximal to Well (or Well) points.

- Needling the termination points on the head or trunk:
  CV-2 or 3 for the **Yin-Leg** Sinew channel as the three Yin of the leg all connect to the genitalia;
  SI-18 for the **Yang-Leg** Sinew channel as the three Yang of the leg connect at the face (zigoma);
  GB-22 for the **Yin-Arm** Sinew channel as the three Yin of the arm connect at the diaphragm;
  GB-13 for the **Yang-Arm** Sinew channel as the three Yang of the arm connect at the corner of the head (temprofrontal area);

- Bleeding the related Connecting/Luo point.

- Tonifying/moxa the opposite Source/Yuan point, and areas on the channel that feel depressed, cold, and/or non-resilient;

- Needling the Jing/River points on the channel (where the channel is said to "bind");

- Treating the Liver Sinew channel (Liv-1), which is said to connect with all of the other sinew channels *(Spiritual Axis)*;

- Treating local points at the painful areas, especially indurated (Kori) and trigger points (see chapter 10).
  — *Spiritual Axis* says, "The fourth [method] is called adjacent valleys acupuncture. Adjacent valleys acupuncture is to needle left then right from the same hole [acupoint], like a chicken's foot. Needle the division between the flesh. This treats Painful Obstruction of the muscles."

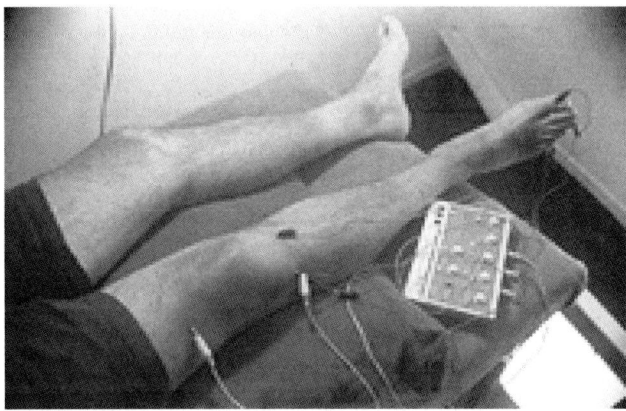

Figure 5-19: Sinew channels activated for the treatment of acute knee strain.

---

63. Akabane test is used to evaluate the balance of the channels by stroking the Well/Jing/Ting points with an incense stick and seeing how many strokes it takes before the patient reports that the heat is excessive. In general, 5-10 strokes is considered normal, above 10 stokes Deficient, and below 5 is considered Excess. This test can be used in diagnosis of the Main, Sinew, or Divergent channels. Channels that take longer (above 10) may be treated by repeating this stimulation at the Well points. Other points such as back-Shu points on the Deficient side, or Divergent activating points can be moxaed. It should be pointed out that this test can not be done in such a way that results in consistent heat at the tip of the incense stick. Having a small difference in the amount of ash, or slight differences in pressure results in greatly varying temperatures. Modern equipment that can deliver a more consistent heat is available.

64. Most acupuncture needles are made from stainless steal and are very poor conductors of heat. If one is to hold the needle *shaft* while heating the needle *handle* till red hot, very little of the heat transfers to the shaft. The effects of heating needle handles therefore may not be via an actual significant rise in tissue temperature. Fire needle is done by actually heating the needle shaft and then quickly inserting and withdrawing it. If the effect sought is to soften soft tissues, it is helpful to use diathermy, which does penetrate deeply and raises tissue temperature. Diathermy cannot be performed with the needles or any other metal in situ.

- (Using reflex points as described by George Goodheart in Applied Kinesiology (see p-509), at attachment points of weak muscle chains (Sinew channel), at acupuncture points, and at Chapman's reflex points are often helpful as well, (see p-498)).

A technique often used by the author is to first evaluate the affected area by passive motions, noting all abnormal or painful movement, and assessing range (and muscle tension). Resisted testing is used to determine which Sinew channels (functional muscle groups) are weak or painful when made to work (contract). The patient is then positioned comfortably so that painful movements (or appropriate muscles) can be *gently engaged*. Palpation using massage strokes cross-fiberally is then used to identify all tight bands, which are then explored for tenderness (using as much pressure as is necessary, which can be quite significant). Painful areas are significant only if abnormal fibrous tissue is sensed.[65] Many areas and muscles in the body are pressure-sensitive and will feel painful when strongly pressed or squeezed. When a painful point is found but the tissue feels normal and pliable, this may be considered normal and ignored. Once all abnormally fibrous muscles and areas are identified, the Sinew channel(s) is activated by quickly stimulating the Well point and the head or trunk termination point. Then each active site is explored slowly with the muscle(s) at its stretch barrier (just at the tension or discomfort stretch barrier) by slowly inserting a needle (Figure 5-20). The patient is instructed to report any discomfort and to relax into the procedure. It is often helpful to ask the patient to concentrate all his/her attention at the tip of the needle and to breath slowly. The stimulation continues at the edge of pain. The patient should understand that *pain occurs only at abnormal tissue* (which can be demonstrated to him/her by inserting a needle into healthy muscle tissue), and that stimulation to such tissues is therapeutic *and not injurious* even though uncomfortable. Fear decreases the pain threshold, prevents progression of the therapy, and is probably detrimental to good outcome. When dense fibrous tissues are engaged, the needle can be warmed using a moxa stick or any other heat source (fire needle). The procedure is repeated for all movements that have been shown to result in pain or abnormal function. Areas that result in muscle twitches are stimulated several times. All tight bends are followed to their bony attachment and the periosteum is stimulated. It is advisable to preheat the area before treatment commences. A TDP (or other) heat lamp can be used, but diathermy (shortwave stimulation) works best.[66] Usually treatment once a week to once every two weeks for three to ten times is all that is necessary to achieve maximum benefit.

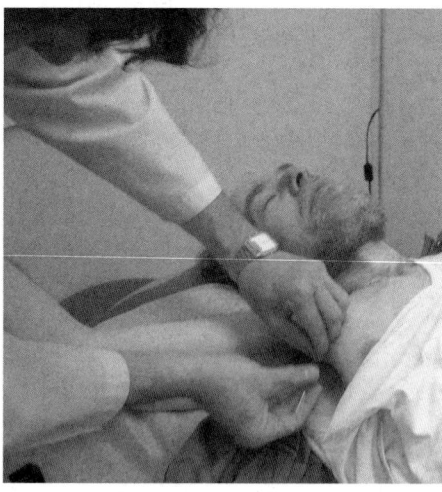

Figure 5-20: Shoulder adductor muscle needled at stretch barrier.

This treatment technique results in soreness, and the patient is told that the "healing" discomfort may last a day or two, and that it shows that his/her healing mechanisms are active. Heat and massage can be used to minimize such soreness. The patient is instructed in appropriate stretching and strength exercises. Usually activity is kept at a minimum for twenty-four hours following the treatment. To minimize pain and possibly abnormal scaring, the following formula can be taken:

> Radix Pseudoginseng (Sheng San Qi) 12g
> Pollen Typhae (Pu Huang) 6g
> Radix Puerariae (Ge Gen) 25g
> Radix Astragali (Huang Qi) 9g[67]

It must be understood that this kind of technique is not appropriate in all cases, especially when treating an *actively* inflamed joint or neuropathic pain. With active arthritis (especially if severe) it is not the muscular tissues that result in pain, muscle tension, and reduced range of motion. Muscles are functioning to protect the joint. Positioning the joint at stretch often only aggravates the pain and does not result in any real improvement. Other techniques which address the capsule should be used first.

Fullness

Acute disorders often result in Sinew channel Fullness. Local triggers (Ashi-sensitive or Kori-altered texture points) are carefully located and needled superficially. The related Main channel is tonified by use of moxa at the tonifying

---

65. Muscle testing as described in Orthopaedic Medicine or in Applied Kinesiology can also be used to determine what areas of the contractile units are at fault.

66. Some diathermy instruments can interfere with electrical and phone circuits and are therefore problematic in the office.

67. Typhae and Pseudoginseng have a mild anti-inflammatory activity, and, therefore, if the goal of treatment is to induce an inflammatory response (which is needed often in patients with instability), this formula *may* theoretically be detrimental. While modern NSAIDs clearly interfere with clinical outcome in prolotherapy and some dry needling techniques, the author has not been able to confirm detrimental effects for these herbs. The fact that they do seem to decrease soreness following such treatments, does, however, suggest possible reduction in inflammation, which therefore may decrease some healing effects.

Table 5-7: Extra Channels (Vessels)

VESSEL	MASTER POINT	COUPLED POINT	ACTIVATING POINT	ACCUMULATING POINT
Governing	SI-3	UB-62	GV-1	—
Conception	Lu-7	Ki-61	Ki-1	—
Penetrating (Chong)	Sp-4	PC-6	Ki-3/St-30	—
Girdle (Dai)	GB-41	TW-5	GB-26	—
Yang Motility (Qiao)	UB-62	SI-3	UB-62	UB-59
Yin Motility (Qiao)	Ki-6	Lu-7	Ki-6 (Ki-8)	Ki-8
Yin Linking (Wei)	PC-6	Sp-4	Ki-9	Ki-9
Yang Linking (Wei)	TW-5	GB-41	UB-63	GB-35

point. If after treatment the patient's symptoms have moved but are not resolved, the process is repeated. If the pain follows a wide distribution, the Connecting (Luo) point is used.

Emptiness

Chronic disorders often result in Sinew channel Emptiness (Defensive-Qi depleted). The pain is dull and poorly localized. Treatment emphasis is on moxa of local sensitive (Ashi) points, especially if they lack tone. Needling of local points is superficial and mild, or deep if indicated. The related Main channel may be sedated. If the pain follows a wide distribution the Connecting (Luo) point is used.

Extra Channels

The Extra channels are used with various treatment methods, usually for persistent chronic disorders (Table 7-7 on page 303). Selection can be based on channel indications, by diagnosis of an abnormality using palpatory techniques, involvement of several channels (widespread pain/symptoms), abdominal pattern, pulse, and trajectory of the channel.

Musculoskeletal Use

The decision to use Extra channels in musculoskeletal medicine can be based on a combination of the indications, topical organization, and abdominal signs. For example, the Yang Linking (Wei) channel, which combines aspects of the UB, GB, St, TW, SI and GV channels, is indicated for cervical pain with headache that radiates from the base of the head (GB-20) to the forehead or behind the ipsilateral eye. This channel is effective also for musculoskeletal disorders that affect the sides of the body (unilaterally) or that radiate to the side of the body, such as sacroiliac joint disorders radiating to the hip. The Yang and Yin Linking (Wei) channels together with the Girdle (Dai) channel can also be used for structural instability with symptoms in UB, GB, St, TW, SI, and GV areas. The Yang and Yin (Motility) Qiao channels are often used to treat muscle "spasms" and tension/hypertonisity. If muscles are hypertonic on the Yang sinew channel(s) the Master (Meeting) point of Yang-Qiao (UB-62) is sedated and the Master point of the Yin-Qiao (K-6) is tonified. Conversely, if muscle hypertonicity is found in a Yin sinew channel or channels, then K-6 is sedated and UB-62 tonified. The Extra channels should be used in all chronic disorders—especially in Deficient patients (for more detail see p-69).

Channel Activation

The Extra channels are activated by the superior and inferior Master (Meeting) points and a Coupled point (of the paired Extra channel).[68] Four of the Master (Meeting) points are also Connecting (Luo) points of a Main channel. Each of the Extra channels has an Activation point and a Departure point. Four Extra channels have lower Accumulating (Xi) points (Table 7-7). Often related Back Shu points are integrated as well.

Herbal Therapy

Although by and large the Eight Extra channels are treated with acupuncture, herbal medicine can be used as well (Table 7-3.) Governing (Du) channel herbs that warm Yang can be used in patients with Governing channel related symptoms when associated with Yang-deficiency. Herbs used for Conception (Ren) channel are mainly those that nourish Liver, Kidney, and Blood and may be used for patients with Conception channel symptoms and appropriate signs. Herbs used for the Girdle (Dai) channel are often astringent, strengthen the Kidneys and Blood, and can be added for the patient's Girdle-channel-related symptoms and appropriate signs. Herbs used for Yang (Wei) Linking channel harmonize the Nutritive and Defensive levels and can be added for patient's Yang-Linking-related symptoms and appropriate signs. Herbs that enter the Yin (Wei) Linking channel can be used to guide other herbs to the channel. Herbs used for Yang (Qiao) Motility channel often clear Wind and Dampness or tonify Liver and Kidneys and can be

---

68. Each Extra channel is coupled with another channel in a Yang-Yang and Yin-Yin relationship.

added to treat patients with Yang Motility related symptoms and appropriate signs. Herbs used for Yin (Qiao) Motility often treat Phlegm, calm Spirit, move Qi, clear Empty-Heat, and can be used to treat patients with Yin-Motility-related symptoms with the appropriate signs. Herbs used for Penetrating (Chong) channel often treat rebellious-Qi, nourish and move Blood/Qi, warm Kidneys, clear Phlegm, and can be used for patients with Penetrating-channel-related symptoms and appropriate signs.

Point Gateways and General Treatment Methods

This section addresses some of the major point gateways used in OM/TCM to treat patients through the channel systems.

Source (Transport) Points

Source (Transport) points are said to contain and release the Phasic (Elemental) quality of the Organ/Channel systems. They are the place in which the Original-Qi resides within the channel. These points are used often, either when tapping into the Organ/channel's "energetic" quality, or when directing the Qi of one channel—with the Connecting (Luo) point—to its Yin-Yang pair.

The Source points on the Yin channels have a direct effect on their own Organ—especially tonifying. The Source points on the Yang channels, however, affect their channel more so than the Organs and are able to dispel Pathogenic Factors.

The classic, *Spiritual Axis*, tells us that when the five solid (Zang) Organs are diseased, one can find an abnormal reaction at the twelve Source points.

> When the five yin organs are sick, they respond and come out to the twelve source [points]. The twelve sources each have places where they come out. [If one] clearly understands the sources and observes their responses, one is able to know the extent of the damage to the five yin organs...

Thus, the Source points are used as diagnostic indicators as well—and utilized by many modern diagnostic skin resistance instruments. The Source points are the main points to treat the *joint*s.

Connecting (Luo) Points/Vessels

The Connecting channels (vessels) leave the Main channels, in part, at the Connecting (Luo) points (Table 7-8). Clinically they are used mainly when there is coupled Interior-Exterior (channel-Organ) disorders, and to treat the Connecting/network-vessels. Disorder of the Connecting-vessels is seen frequently when there is musculoskeletal pain with no Organic symptoms or signs. A third important and common use is to re-route Qi and Blood from one channel to its pair.

Table 5-8: Connecting/Luo Points

CHANNEL	CONNECTING/LUO POINTS
Lung	LU-7
Pericardium (Master Heart)	P-6
Heart	H-5
Spleen	Sp-4
Liver	LIV-5
Kidney	K-4
Conception/Ren	CV-15
Large Intestine	LI-6
Triple Warmer/Heater	TW-5
Small Intestine	SI-7
Stomach	St-40
Gall Bladder	GB-37
Urinary Bladder	UB-58
Governing	Gv-1
Great Spleen Connection	Sp-21

All of the above can be accomplished by needling the Source point on the primary affected channel and its coupled Yin-Yang Connecting (Luo) point.[69] This then regulates both Qi and Blood as the Source points regulate Qi (of the channel and Organ) and Connecting (Luo) points the Blood. The source point is used on the channel which was affected first and the Connecting (Luo) on the channel affected later. This technique may be used for *somatic pain originating from the Organ systems* (viscerosomatic reflex and pain).

The practitioner can also reverse the Source and Connecting (Luo) points. For example, Excess or Stagnation of Qi or Blood in a channel (painful location or swelling along the channel) can be treated by needling a point upstream and a point downstream of the lesion, and at the same time needling the Connecting (Luo) point and the Source point on the paired Yin-Yang channel. In chronic disorders, local points can be tonified (by needle technique or addition of moxa) and the Connecting (Luo) point (most often on a Yang channel) sedated. The paired Source point is tonified.

Entry and Exit Points and Channel Flow

The idea of *continuous* Qi circulation throughout the Main channel system originated in the *Spiritual Axis* were it says, "The main channels are mutually connected like a circle without end."[70] The Entry Point is where the channel Qi enters, the Exit point is where it exits. Entry and Exit point combinations may be used when other treatments have failed and when the physical findings are of excessive/inflated

---

69. Also known as the guest host technique.
70. This has been interpreted by Kendall (*ibid*) to mean vascular circulation.

Table 5-9: Source, Entry, Exit points

Main Channels[a]	Source Points	Entry Points	Exit Points	Circadian Time	Tonification Points[b]	Sedation Points[c]
Lung hand Tai Yin	Lu-9	Lu-1	Lu-7	03 am - 05 am	Liv-8	Lu-5
Large Intestine hand Yang Ming	LI-4	LI-4	LI-20	05 am - 07 am	Lu-9	LI-2
Stomach leg Yang Ming	St-42	St-1	St-42	07 am - 09 am	St-11	St-45
Spleen foot Tai Yin	Sp-3	Sp-1	Sp-21	09 am - 11 am	St-41	Sp-5
Heart hand Shao Yin	H-7	H-1	H-9	11 am - 01 pm	Sp-2	H-7
Small Intestine- hand Tai Yang	SI-4	SI-1	SI-19	01 pm - 03 pm	H-9	SI-8
Urinary Bladder- leg Tai Yang	UB 64	UB-1	UB-67	03 pm - 05 pm	SI-3	UB-65
Kidney leg-Shao Yin	K-3	K-1	K-22	05 pm - 07 pm	UB-67	K-1
Pericardium arm Jue Yin	P-7	PC-1	P-8	07 pm - 09 pm	K-7	P-7
Triple Warmer arm Shao Yang	TW-4	TW-1	TW-23	09 pm - 11 pm	P-9	TW-10
Gall Bladder leg Shao Yang	GB-40	GB-1	GB41	11 pm - 01 am	TW-3	GB-38
Liver leg Jue Yin	LIV-3	LIV-1	LIV-14	01 am - 03 am	GB-43	Liv-2

a. The leg and arm channels are related: arm Tai Yin is related to leg Tai Yin etc. Dysfunction is often related to one of these three systems or circuits.
b. These are special tonification points to be used at the channel's circadian time.
c. These are special sedation points to be used at the channel's circadian time.

pulse or when there are other symptoms/signs of Excess in a principal Main channel combined with a weak pulse or other symptoms/signs of Deficiency in the next channel on the circadian flow. In a constitutionally weak person the pulse may be flat instead of inflated. The blockage is often caused by trauma, especially when scars are formed. Table 7-9 lists circadian (diurnal) flow of Qi and Source, Entry, and Exit points for the Main channels. The table also shows the three systems of related channels. Four arm channels with four leg channels are often used as connected systems/circuits when choosing points. A study on the timing of acupuncture treatments has shown that acupuncture and moxibustion at SP-6 can significantly elevate T-lymphocyte transformation rate and the rosette formation rate of erythrocyte C3b receptors compared with the control without treatment. The elevation was greatest in the rabbits treated at 9:00A.M.-11:00A.M., the next at 3:00 P.M., and the least at 9:00 P.M.-11:00 P.M. This provides experimental bases for investigating mechanisms related to the timing of needling.

In general "channel circulation" is said to *begin in the chest* from the Lung channel going outwards to the upper extremities and back to the face/chest via the next channel (Large Intestine) and outwards to the lower extremity (via Stomach), and then up to the face/chest again, repeating this cycle from channel to channel until the Qi returns from the Liver channel to the Lungs.[71]

A blockage in the Urinary Bladder channel, for example, (that is said to travel from the face downwards to the little toe via the posterior/exterior aspect of the body), may then result in obstruction of Qi and accumulation/stagnation in the Urinary Bladder channel, with decreased (or blocked) circulation to the next channel, the Kidney channel, which goes from the foot back upwards to the next channel. Thus symptoms of Excess such as pain, tightness, and muscle spasm may be palpated at the Urinary Bladder channel (Yang muscles), while weakness is demonstrated in deeper/

---

71. Defensive-Qi is said to begin flowing in the Exterior when the eyes are open.

anterior in (Kidney, possibly) channel muscles. In discussing Organ Bi (Painful Obstruction) the *Classic of Internal Medicine* describes regional effects of blocked Qi and Blood:

> If in case of a black [complexion] the pulse arrives firm and big above, accumulated Qi exist in the lower abdomen and in the Yin Region. This is called Kidney block (Bi).

Treatment for such conditions can be undertaken using the entry and exit points. For the above example, UB-1 and K-22 or UB-67 and K-1 may be used depending on symptoms and signs. It is also possible to use the Source and Connecting points for these channels.

Treatment Timing, Stems, Branches, and Numeric Systems

Channel "energy" circulation, especially Ancestral-Original Qi circulation, is said to take twenty-four hours to complete one full cycle. There is a period of two hours at each channel in which the channel's Qi reaches its zenith. Symptoms that occur regularly at particular times are often considered to be consequences of this circadian (diurnal) system. Symptoms of Excess may appear during peak hours (zenith of circulation); symptoms of Deficiency may appear during peak-out (nadir of circulation) time of Qi flow (twelve hours after the peak hour, the so-called "*mid-day mid-night*" rule). According to Barral and Mercier (1993) when an organ/Organ reaches its zenith in the TCM circadian clock, it's *palpable* "vitality and amplitude" of mobility (not "rhythm") increases, thus providing support to the TCM circadian clock.[72]

When other types of treatment have failed, sometimes treatment during special times may prove effective. The time most opportune strengthening Qi is just after a channel peaks. The most opportune time for dispersing Qi is during or prior to the peak period.

The Qi circulation that follows this sequence travels from one Main channel to the next through the Entry and Exit points.[73] The prescribed source, entry, exit, tonification and sedation points can be used at the appropriate time, or channels can be treated with the following relations:

- Lung<—>Liver
- Large Intestine<—>Stomach
- Spleen<—>Heart
- Small Intestine<—>Urinary Bladder
- Kidney<—>Pericardium
- Triple Warmer<—>Gall Bladder.

The mid-day mid-night rule can be used to treat pain in a channel regardless of the time of the day. *Tender* channel points are chosen with the following relations:

- Lung<—>Urinary Bladder
- Large Intestines<—>Kidneys
- Stomach<—>Pericardium
- Spleen<—>Triple Warmer.
- Heart<—>Gall Bladder.

Numeric systems ("magic Square/Cube" Table 7-10, arrangement of *I Ching* trigrams, etc.) or heavenly stems and terrestrial branches are systems that also involve the timing of worldly phenomena, including channel and point functions. They may be used to design treatment combinations and point selection. Organs (and body regions) are assigned numbers, and combinations that result in the number 5 (or 15 with cube) are used. For example, pain along the Urinary Bladder channel can be treated using Heart channel points. If the pain is in the neck, H-4 is treated, while, if it is in the low back and leg, H-7 can be used, or LI points such as Great White (22.04) [LI-3 1/2] and Spirit Bone (22.05) [LI-4 1/2] can be used (see Tong/Lee acupuncture below for more information on using the Magic Square).

Many of the stems and branches systems were based on the movement of the stars, the timing of so called "open" points, and the patient's birth date.[74] The terrestrial branches which correspond to months of the year are:

1. Gall Bladder (Zi)
2. Liver (Chou)
3. Small Intestine (Yin/Lung)
4. Heart (Mao/Large Intestine)
5. Stomach (Chen)
6. Spleen (Szu)
7. Large Intestine (Wu/Kidney)
8. Lungs (Wei/Small Intestine)
9. Urinary Bladder (Shen)
10. Kidneys (You)
11. Pericardium (Hu)
12. Triple Warmer (Hai).

Ten-Stems combinations (with the number 5) are used as follows:

- Gall Bladder<—>Spleen
- Small Intestine<—>Lung

---

72. Barral is a French osteopathic practitioner skilled in visceral manipulation techniques.

73. In contrast to other theories, such as the Five Transporting Points theory, in which Qi in all of the channels flows proximately. Dan Bensky DO, in discussing meridian palpation, also states that channel Qi flows proximally. The theory of Five Transporting Points may however pertain to Original (Yuan) Qi as compared to Channel (Jing) Qi.

74. The author does not have any experience with the use of "Open Point" timing or the use of the *I Ching (Book of Changes)* and birth date systems and cannot confirm their benefit. There are several systems used to calculate which point is open at any moment in the day. Like many theories in TCM, they do not agree with each other.

Table 5-10: Magic Square/Cube

4	9	2
3	5	7
8	1	6

- Stomach<—>Kidney
- Large Intestine<—>Liver
- Urinary Bladder<—>Heart.

Accumulating/Cleft/Xi Points

The Accumulating (Cleft/Xi) points (Table 7-11) are areas in the channels where channel Qi and Blood, which flow relatively superficially along the channels from the Well points, are said to concentrate and accumulate. These points are usually located in the middle half of the leg or forearm. The Qi is said to slide deeper into the channel at the Accumulating (Cleft/Xi) points. There are sixteen Accumulating points, one on each of the twelve Main channels and one each on the Yin Motility, Yang Motility, Yin Linking and Yang Linking channels. On palpation, these points are felt easily as clefts or depressions in the muscle. The Accumulating points are often tender if a disease is acute; they are almost always tender when circulation in the channel is obstructed. These points can be used for both diagnosis and treatment and are very important in the treatment of pain. If channel stagnation is severe they may become indurated, very sensitive, and pressure-induced pain may radiate. These are usually signs of Excess. If these points are only mildly pressure-sensitive, the condition is often one of Deficiency.

Although the Accumulating points are used commonly in acute disorders including pain, and have been referred to as emergency points, they can be used in chronic disorders (and in weak patients) when there is painful channel obstruction. They are often used in chronic and stubborn diseases involving the channels and Organs, particularly if there is also pain. The approach of using Accumulating points in Deficient patients is similar to the attacking methods used in herbal medicine. The theory is that by the elimination of Pathogenic Factors, the patient's condition is strengthened. These points can be used for the symptomatic treatment of pain in the *channels, vessels, or Organs*. They are often used for musculoskeletal pain

As Accumulating points do not have a *phasic* property, they can be used to treat the channel without having any secondary Five-Phase related effects. The points on the Yin channels can treat Blood disorders. The Accumulating (Cleft/Xi) points most commonly utilized by this author for musculoskeletal disorders, are Lu-6 for mid-back pain, SI-6 for upper back periscapular pain, St-34 for knee pain, and UB-63 for sudden pain of unknown cause.

Table 5-11: Accumulating Points

CHANNEL	ACCUMULATING (CLEFT, XI)	COMMON USES
LUNG	Lu-6	Mid/upper back pain and pain along the Lung channel. Blood-stasis/bleeding (Lungs), hemorrhoids.
PERICARDIUM	P-4	Blood-stasis, chest pain.
HEART	H-6	Blood-stasis, Heart pain—chest arm pain, headache.
LARGE INTESTINE	LI-7	Painful obstruction along LI channel, heat and swelling of the face.
TRIPLE WARMER	TW-7	Not commonly used.
SMALL INTESTINE	SI-6	Painful obstruction along channel, shoulder, scapular and neck pains. Low back spasm.
STOMACH	St-34	Knee and chest pain.
GALLBLADDER	GB-36	Painful obstruction and/or atrophy along channel.
URINARY BLADDER	UB-63	Sudden intense painful. Obstruction and mental disorder.
SPLEEN	Sp-8	Blood-stasis (abdominal).
LIVER	LIV-6	Blood-stasis (abdominal).
KIDNEY	K-5	Blood-stasis and deficiency (abdominal).

Influential/Meeting/Gathering Points

The Influential (Meeting/Gathering) points (Table 7-12) are empirical points that have been found particularly effective for the treatment of the tissue/Qi they influence from either Deficiency or Excess. They are used to access the broad sphere of each system they influence (e.g., GB-39 for marrow, brain, nervous system, spinal cord, blood, sinews and bone). These are sites where the Organs and channels and their Qi, Blood, Essence, bones, and Marrow collect and meet. Therefore, they can be used to influence all the above body milieu, especially when treating chronic disorders with related Deficiencies. For example, when treating arthrosis and bony osteophytes (congealed Phlegm and Blood-stasis), UB-11 (GV-14) may be used to influence the bones; GB-39, the influential point of the marrow, can be used to stimulate bone strength and eliminate Wind-Dampness; UB-17 is used to vitalize and strengthen Blood needed to heal related soft tissues; Liv-13 is used to strengthen the related Yin Organs, which are often depleted in cases of arthrosis; and GB-34 is used to effect the involved soft tissues and eliminate Pathogenic Factors.

Back Shu (Transport) Points

Back Shu (Transport) points (Table 7-14; Figure 5-21), are

Table 5-12: Influential/Meeting Points

INFLUENCE	POINT	USE
YIN ORGANS	LIV-13	Tonify Spleen and all Yin Organs.
YANG ORGANS	CV-12	Treat Stomach and Yang Organs.
QI	CV-17	Regulate Chest (Zong) Qi. All Qi disorders. Lungs, Heart, and respiration.
BLOOD	UB-17	Most important Blood point for stasis, Heat, or Deficiency.
SINEWS	GB-34	General treatment of sinews—stiffness, tightness, and pain. Painful obstruction, GB channel symptoms.
BLOOD VESSELS	Lu-9	Blood vessel disorders and pain. Blood-stasis pain. Chest (Zong) Qi weakness (weak pulses).
BONES	UB-11 (or possibly GV-14)	Bony painful obstruction (deep chronic), various bone diseases, spinal pain.
MARROW/BRAIN/ SPINAL CORD	GB-39	Strengthening the sinews and bones—weakness, paralysis, spasticity. Brain and nervous system disorders. Chronic cases.

located on the Urinary Bladder channel, from the third thoracic vertebra to the second sacral vertebra, through which the Qi of the Organs is said to circulate. Many are named after their corresponding Organ and lie at the level of the Organ. Other back Shu (Transport) points correspond to the Governing channel (UB-16), Diaphragm/Blood (UB-17), Qi (UB-24), Source/Origin Gate (UB-26), Midspine (UB-29) (although used more for lower spine), White Ring/pelvic ring (UB-30), and Vital region/deficiency (UB-43). Organ disorders can cause tenderness, swelling, indurations, or any abnormal manifestation, reflexively, at the back Shu points. Therefore, these points are often used to diagnose and treat Organic diseases. It is said that when pressing the correct point, with resulting reduction of symptomatic pain, the point is accurately located.

The back-Shu points are situated in depressions in the erector spinae muscles, about midway between the medial edge of the scapula and the midline (1-1/2 cun from midline). Although several texts have stated that the back Shu points are used for Yin diseases (Organ), a review of their indications clearly shows that they can be used for both Yin and Yang disorders. In musculoskeletal medicine, the back-Shu points are used in segmental and facet joint disorders and to affect the somatic-visceral systems. Needles are best left in back-Shu points for no more than ten to fifteen minutes to avoid fatiguing the patient, although, if much redness is created around the needle, it may be necessary to leave the needle in until the redness disappears. (This is often seen in patients with Heat, facilitated sympathetic system, histamine excess.) The back-Shu points with their associated channels are often used to treat vertebral dysfunctions.

The back Shu points may relate to the spinal and autonomic innervation of somatic and visceral structures. Some interesting work on this subject was accomplished by Kenyon et al (1992). Table 7-8 on page 152 lists the embryological segments; Table 7-6 on page 136 lists sympathetic segments.

Hua Tuo Jia Ji Points

Hua Tuo Jia Ji (paravertebral) points are located in the first paravertebral trough, about 0.5-1 cun lateral to the Governing channel and level with the lower border of the spinous processes. These points overlie the intrinsic spinal muscles and facet joints and therefore are very useful in the treatment of vertebral joint dysfunctions and fixations. They can be used for both diagnosis and treatment and often their use is based on the same principles as back Shu points. In a normal segment one can needle the intrinsic muscles with a 32-38 gauge needle without much reaction by the patient or sensation of tightness at the needle tip. At restricted segments these muscles are tense, and reactions to the needle are frequently elicited. These points often have stronger effects than the Back Shu (Transport) points, and, in general, are safer to needle deeply.

Alarm/Collecting (Mu) Points

The Alarm (Mu) points (Table 7-14; Figure 5-21), are situated ventrally in the chest and abdomen and are said to connect directly to the Organs and to reflect Organic health. The word "Mu" means to *collect* and these points are said to collect Organic-Qi and prenatal-Essence. Only three of the Alarm (Mu) points are located on there own channel; Lu-1 (Lung), Liv-14 (Liver), and GB-24 (Gall Bladder). As with the back-Shu points, the Alarm (Mu) points are said to become tender in reaction to Organic disease and may develop abnormal tissue texture such as lumps, depressions, and indurations. The Alarm (Mu) points are located in the appropriate somatic/neurologic areas particular to the sympathetic innervation of the organ they represent. The Daoist conception of these points is that they collect Essence (Jing) at the moment of birth and therefore reflect constitutional conditions.

The Alarm (Mu) points are used often for the treatment of Heat or Yang disorders; however, a review of their indications shows that they can be used for Yin disorders as well. Various authors have described varying uses for these points; for example, Mann used them for Yin disease with cold, depression, weakness, and says that they are usually tonified but can be sedated. Maciocia states that they are mostly used for acute disease but can be used for chronic diseases as well and then tonified. In combination with Sea (He) points, the Alarm (Mu) points can be used to treat acute

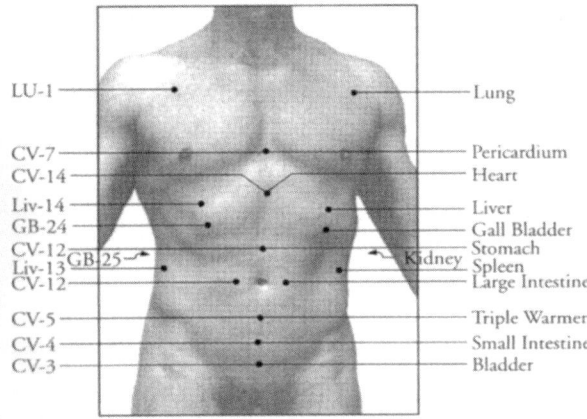
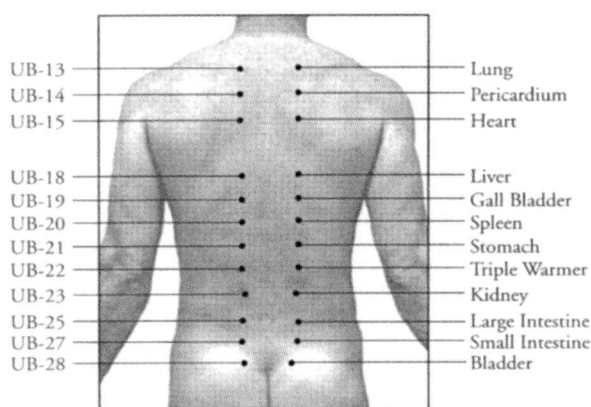

Figure 5-21: Alarm (Mu) and Back Shu points.

Excesses. It is often helpful to moxa these points if the patient reports that pressure on them feels good.

The Alarm (Mu) points can be combined with Influential (Meeting) or other points such as:

- Liv-13 (Yin Organs) and GB-34 (Sinews) for sinews and joints.
- CV-12 (Hollow Organs) and Lu-9 (Vessels) for the Vessels and circulation.
- CV-17 (Qi) and Lu-9 (Vessels) to support and regulate Qi and Blood of the entire body.
- CV-17 (Qi) and St-9, GV-15, 14 for sea of Qi-excess (chest fullness, red face, difficult breathing).
- CV-17 (Qi) and UB-17 (Blood) for Blood and Qi disorders.
- CV-5 (Triple Warmer) and UB-11 for Kidney and bone weakness.
- GB-25 (Kidney) and GB-39 (marrow) for brain, Kidney and bone disorders.

BACK SHU AND ALARM/COLLECTING POINTS COMBINED. The Back Shu and Alarm points are often combined in the treatment of Organic disorders and when balancing the dorsal and ventral channels. Their combination may represent treatment via efferent and afferent neural systems. The Back Shu and Alarm points can be used to treat Defensive and Nutritive-Qi (Wei and Ying) disharmony as well.[75] Treating the back Shu and Alarm points for five minutes at the beginning of treatment can be helpful for weak and fatigued patients (especially with Kidney-related ailments).[76] Connecting an electrical stimulator with the (-) pole at the Alarm (Mu) point and (+) pole at the back Shu point may facilitate the treatment (Figure 5-22). The appropriate Source point and moxa is often added. The following are commonly combined:

- CV-17 and UB-11, 23 for disorders of bones.
- CV-17 and UB-13, 14, 15, 17 for weak Chest (Zong) Qi, poor circulation and diaphragmatic function.
- Liv-14 and UB-18 for Sinews.
- Liv-13 and UB-20, 18 for Muscles.
- Lu-1, CV-17, and UB-23 for Excess above Deficiency below.
- CV-12 and UB-20, 21 for Phlegm/Damp disorders.
- CV-14 and UB-15 for Heart and spirit.

Five Phases Points

Within each channel system resides a five-phasic and quality representation of Qi that is said to be concentrated and/or influenced at the associated phasic point (also called "transport," "elements," or "command" points). These points are used to manipulate the channel's "phasic" qualities and are said to be particularly potent in general.

The Five Phases points are located on the extremities of the Main channels (Figure 5-23). They are used to treat specific "energetic/phasic" disease processes and to manipulate the phasic qualities of the Main channels and Organs. These points, which depict the growth of Qi from small and shallow to large and deep,[77] can be compared to the flow of a river from its origins to its merging with the sea. The Qualities of Qi evolve as the Qi travels down the channel:

---

75. Commonly seen in musculoskeletal disorders with symptoms of changing pain, Heat (inflammation), and Cold (or alternating) and symptoms of hyper-sympathetic tone—excessive perspiration. Use with a variation of Cinnamon Combination (Gui Zhi Tang+-), Jade Windscreen Powder (Yu Ping Feng San+-) or Minor Bupleurum (Xiao Chi Hu Tang+-).

76. The Divergent channel can be used in the same way, with Monaka's Kidney return being especially useful.

Table 5-13: Five Phasic Points: Influence

Point	Phasic Quality	Channels	Location	Governs/Affects
Well/ Jing/Ting	Wood---> Metal---->	Yin Yang	Finger/Toe Tips	• Visceral disease. • Uppermost channel symptoms. • Fullness below heart. • Release of Fullness and Heat. • Restoration of consciousness. • Emotional disorders. • Activation of Sinew channels —at the body surface; —in musculoskeletal disorders; —acute disorders. —in diseases of the sinews and bones due to Solid (Zhang) Organs.
Spring/ Ying	Fire ----> Water--->	Yin Yang	Hands/ Foot	• Heat and Fullness (fever). • Change in complexion (not just face). • Disorders of the surface and channels. • Disorders of the Yang channels. • Diseases of Solid Organs (with Shu/Spring). • Pain. —Qi blood stagnation; accelerates and pushes Qi through channel.[a] —Diseases of the sinews and bones due to Hollow (Fu) Organs. • Chaotic Qi.
Stream/ Shu	Earth----> (source-point) Wood---->	Yin Yang	Wrist/Ankle	• The main point for joints. • Prolonged disease (Qi begins to internalize). • Diseases that come and go (intermittent). • Bodily heaviness, Joint pain (Painful Obstruction). • Activation of defensive and original Qi (regulates Internal/External, Deficiency/ Excess).
River/ Jing	Metal ----> Fire ----->	Yin Yang	Arm/Leg	• Diseases of sinews and bones. —Structural and channel disorders, especially on extremity (helps nourish joints and sinews), paralysis or spasms, "binds" to sinew channel. • Dampness of muscles, joints, bone (Painful Obstruction). • Diseases affecting the voice. • Dyspnea, asthma, cough. • Chills and fever (malaria).
Sea/He	Water----> Earth ----->	Yin Yang	Elbow/Knee	• Painful obstruction, spasm or paralysis. • Bleeding. • Organ disease, especially stomach. • Regulates flow between Channels and Organs (Divergent channels). • Irregular appetite. • Rebellious-Qi (reflux) and diarrhea. • Deep-seated disorders. • To induce generalized balance.

a. Can be used instead of Well/Jing points.

---

77. As stated before, the theory of proximal flow of channel Qi predates the 24-hour Qi flow theory according to which Qi flows from one channel to the next and in which flow alternates from proximal to distal. This is another example of how TCM has no difficulties with conflicting ideas.

- *Well/Jing/Ting* points have the *greatest* Yin-Yang *polarity* and the least amount of energy/Qi. They are located at the nail area where each channel's Qi emerges.
- *Spring/Ying* points are where Qi begins to trickle and accumulate. It takes shape with the image of a gushing

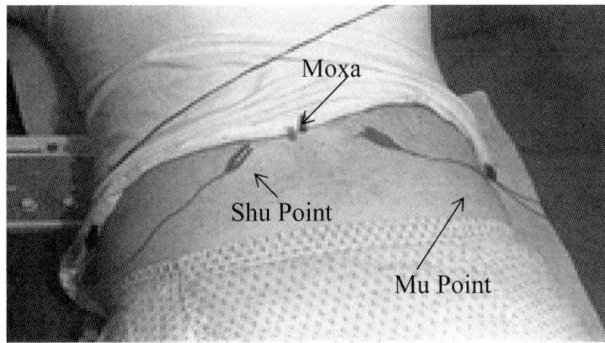

Figure 5-22: Patient's Kidneys strengthened by electroacupuncture with (-) pole on the Alarm points and (+) pole on the back Shu points. GV-4 is needled and Moxaed.

babbling brook. Here, Qi *gains* a great deal of *momentum* and begins to surge; however, since the channel is still constricted in size, the Qi's transporting power is limited.[78]

- *Stream/Shu* points are where flow grows and becomes large enough to *carry* and *transport*.
- *River/Jing* points are where Qi and channel size and momentum are great enough to *traverse* great *distances*.
- *Sea/He* points are where the channel's Qi *unites* with the Qi of the associated *Organ* and enters *deeply*.

In this system, the Qi flows from the Well points on the fingers and toes (first points) to the Sea points on the elbows and knees (last points) in a proximal direction.

Each of the Five Phases (command) points has in its region on the channel a characteristic quantity of Qi and a phasic/elemental quality. These points can be used to manipulate the channel's phasic quality and quantity. For example, in patients with abdominal pain due to Liver Spleen disharmony, the Wood point on the Spleen channel can be sedated while the Earth point on the Wood channel can be tonified. In order to activate a phasic quality within the patient, the phasic point in the channel that is currently most active (in circadian circulation) can be stimulated. For example, to activate a Wood phasic quality in a patient seen between nine and eleven a.m., Sp-1, the Wood point of the Spleen channel, can be stimulated.

Each Main channel has a principal tonification point and a principal sedation point that can be used to supplement or drain Qi from the channel. This is summarized in Table 7-5 on page 297. Table 7-13 describes the main indication for the Five Phases points. Table 7-13 and Table 7-15 on page 315 list the Five Phases points for the Yang and Yin channels.

---

78. Is also said, however, that the farther down (distal) the point is located, the farther its effect up the channel. Jing and Ying points are often used to treat the head, while He points have greater effect on the trunk/Organs and large joints.

Other Important Uses

The Five Phases (command) points are used quite often when treating musculoskeletal pain. In general, the Well/Jing points are used for *acute injuries, Heat,* and *stasis*; the Spring/Ying points are especially important for disorders of the *body Exterior*, the *muscles,* and *skin*; the Stream/Shu points are the main points for *joints* and are also used for *chronic disorders* and for diseases that *come and go*; the River/Jing points are used for the *bones and sinews;* and the Sea/He points are used in *Painful Obstruction* (Bi) syndromes and the associated *Organs*. The Well/Jing and Spring/Ying points can also be used for diseases of the sinew and bones that are due to the Solid (Zhang) Organs. The Stream/Shu points can also be used for diseases of the sinews and bones that are due to the Hollow (Fu) Organs.

Examples of other uses are: two Stream/Shu points on opposite sides can be chosen, one on the arm and the other on the opposite leg. Usually, the first point is needled on the affected side followed by the other on the opposite lower/upper extremity. One can also use the Spring/Ying point on the affected side, while using the Stream/Shu point on the contralateral lower/upper extremity. The Well/Jing points are of particular interest as they activate the Sinew channels; the point on the affected channel is needled or bled while the Well/Jing point on the other side of the same channel is tonified.

Supplementing or Draining Energy: The Four Needle Technique

The Five Phases points are used also to supplement or drain Qi through the Four Needle technique. This method uses the channel's sedating and tonification points, and, on related channels, it uses points that either supplement or deplete the intended channel. For each Organ/Channel system, regardless of whether the intention is to tonify or to sedate, two points are tonified and two are sedated. Table 7-16 and Table 5-17 on page 315 list the points used in the Four Needle sedation and tonification techniques.

The Five Phases points can be used also to warm or cool the channels. Table 7-18 on page 316 and Table 7-19 on page 316 describe techniques to warm and cool the channels.

Group Connecting Points

The Group Connecting points are four points on the extremities where several channels intersect.

- P-5 connects all the arm Yin channels and therefore can be used in disorders of the Lungs, Heart, Pericardium and chest. P-6 is often substituted. P-5 is an important point for the treatment of Phlegm and to calm the spirit.
- TW-8 connects all the arm Yang channels. TW-8 is one of the "forbidden" points for needling, and, therefore, many practitioners use TW-5 instead. It can be used in disorders of the Small Intestine, Large Intestine, and Triple

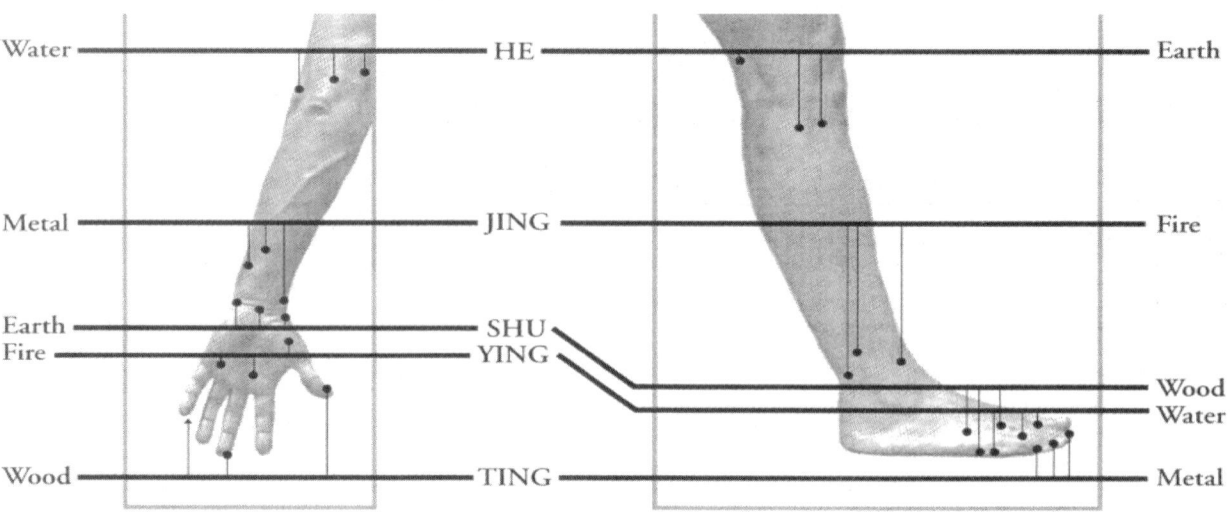

Figure 5-23: Five Phases (Transport) points.

Warmer, and in painful disorders of the arm, neck, and shoulder. It can also be used for lumbar sprain.

- Sp-6 connects all the leg Yin channels and therefore can be used in disorders of the Liver, Spleen, and Kidney. This point is often used in weak and Deficient patients. It can resolve Dampness, invigorate the Blood, and activate the channels to alleviate pain.

- GB-39 connects all the leg Yang channels and therefore can be used in disorders of the Gall Bladder, Urinary Bladder, and Stomach. It is often used in disorders of the lower extremity and *neck*. It can benefit the sinews and bones, clear Wind-Damp, and activate the channels to alleviate pain.

Lower Sea (He) Points

The lower Sea (He) points connect the three Yang channels of the upper limbs with the three Yang channels of the lower limbs. They are usually used to treat the Organ that is related to them (mostly in Excess disorders). They are:

- Stomach—St-36
- Large Intestine—St-37
- Small Intestine—St-39
- Gall Bladder—GB-34
- Urinary Bladder—UB-40
- Triple Warmer—UB-39.

General Reunion Points

The general reunion points are areas of reunion of several principal channels that are said to be important in balancing Yin and Yang:

- LI-4 reunion of Yang
- GV-13 reunion of Yang channels of the foot
- GV-19 reunion of Yang channels of the hand
- GV-14 reunion of all Yang channels
- UB-17 reunion of Yin and Blood.

The Barrier (Guan) Points

The barrier points are a group of points that are located mostly around major joints. These are areas where the circulation of Qi is commonly said to be obstructed. They all contain the word "Guan" in their name and are used to treat painful disorders of the extremities and trunk. They are: St-31, 22, 7, CV-4, GV-3, TW-1, 5, P-6, GB-3, 33, 37, UB-46, 26, K-18, 5, Liv-8, and Liv-7.

Another group of Barrier points has been assembled by French acupuncturists that relate to four aspects of "energy" manifestation: state, space, mutation, and time (Helms 1995; Figure 5-24). These points are used within the Eight Principles diagnosis system:

- Wrist: SI-6, LI-9, P-4, and Lu-6
- Elbow: H-6, TW-7 and 13
- Shoulder: LI-15, SI-11, P-2 and Lu-2
- Hip: UB-29, St-31, Sp-12 and Liv-11
- Knee: GB-33, 36 and K-5
- Ankle: St-37, UB-63, Sp-8, and Liv-6

Regional Command Points

Some points are said to have strong activity for general regions of the body, for example (Figure 5-25):

- St-36 for abdominal and ventral body regions
- Lu-7 for head and neck (posterior and/or anterior) regions

Point Gateways and General Treatment Methods

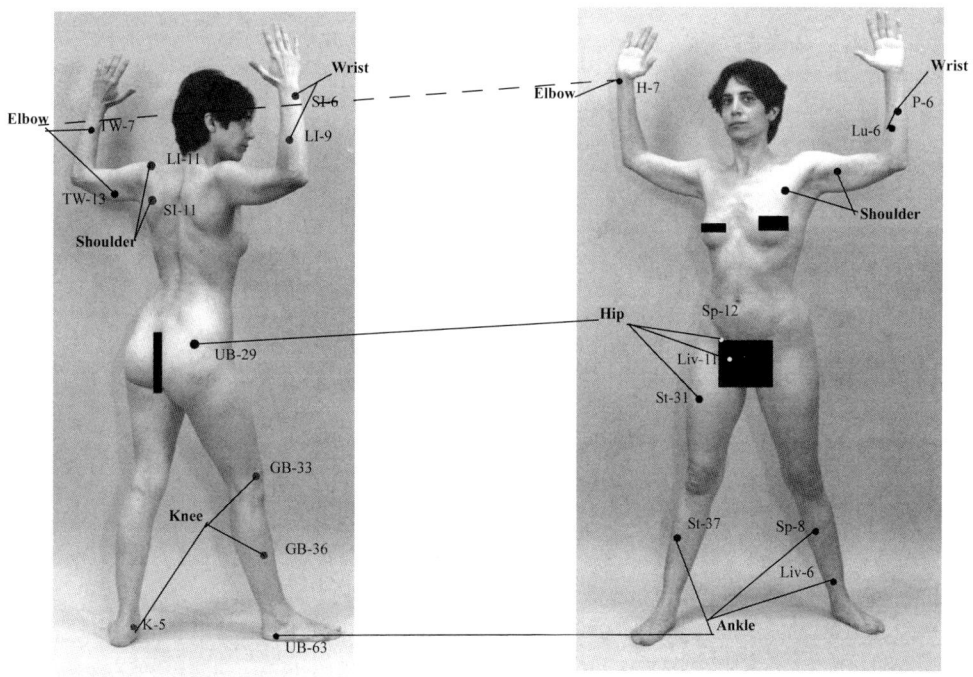

Figure 5-24: French Barrier Points (after Helms 1995).

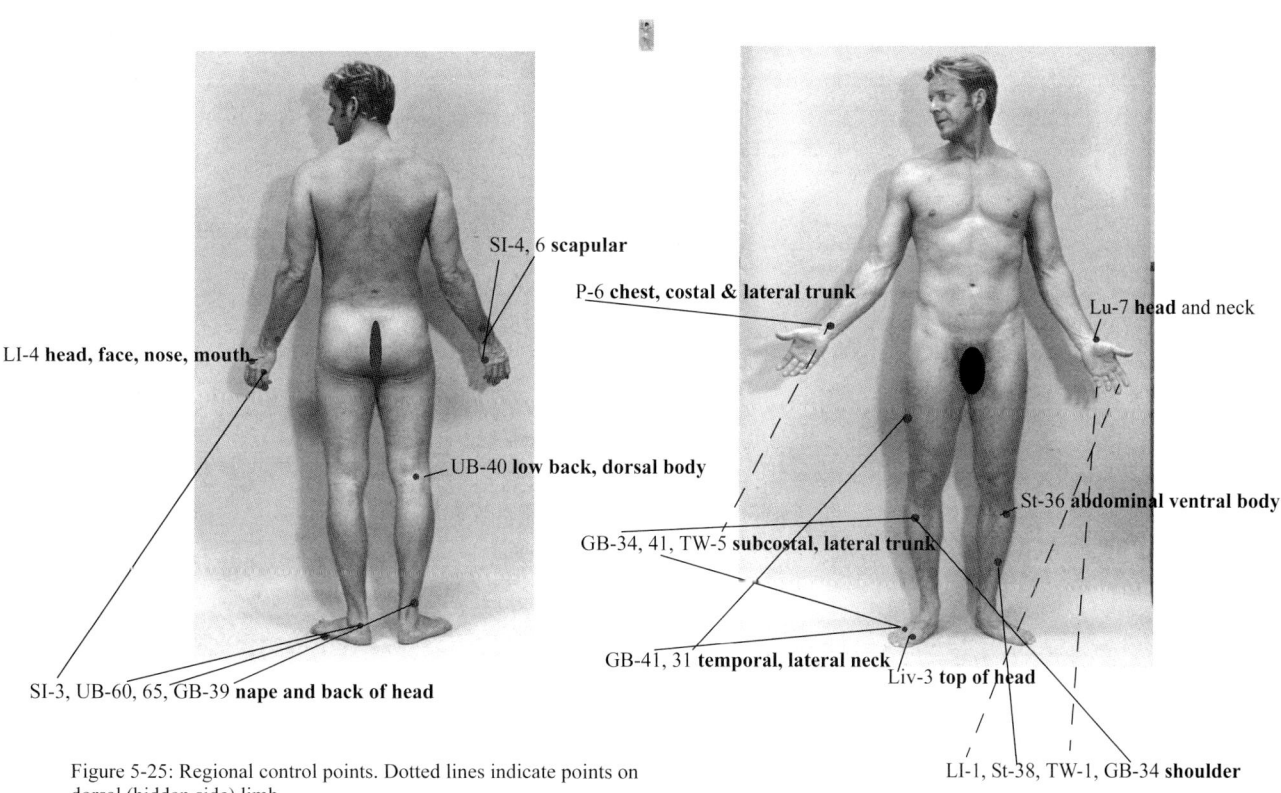

Figure 5-25: Regional control points. Dotted lines indicate points on dorsal (hidden side) limb.

- Liv-3 for top of the head region
- UB-40 for low back and dorsal bodily regions
- LI-4 for face, head, nose, and mouth regions
- P-6 for chest and lateral costal/trunk regions
- GB-34, 41, TW-5 subcostal and lateral costal/trunk regions
- SI-4, 6 for scapular region
- SI-3, UB-60, 65, GB-39 for nape and back of head region
- GB-41, 31 for temporal and lateral neck region
- LI-1, St-38, TW-1, GB-34 for shoulder region.

These points are usually used in combination with other points and are said to direct the treatment toward the specific area.

Rescue Points

Rescue points are used to treat the collapse of Yang and symptoms such as loss of consciousness and coldness. H-8 is used often by the author for the treatment of vasovagal reactions. It can also be used for treating other complications during an acupuncture treatment. The rescue points are: LI-4, St-36, Sp-6, K-1, K-3, H-8, GB-30, GV-15, and CV-12.

Commonly Used and Auxiliary Points

There are many acupuncture points and point combinations that can be used in the treatment of musculoskeletal disorders, which are said to have specific effects. *It must be emphasized, however, that better clinical outcomes often depend on palpatory rather than theoretical selection of points*; therefore, the practitioner should palpate each proposed point for reaction before using it in treatment.[79] Table 7-20 on page 316 summarizes the points and combinations most commonly utilized by the author. Management of musculoskeletal disorders often requires attending to other systems and to mental states. Table 7-21 summarizes points for mental conditions. Table 7-22 on page 323 summarizes points used for the endocrine system. Table 5-23 on page 324 summarizes points to regulate the nervous system. Table 5-28 on page 327 through Table 5-35 on page 332 present additional commonly used points in musculoskeletal medicine. In general, acupuncture points and herbs can be chosen based on the location and type of symptoms. Table 7-4 on page 402 summarize points and herbs commonly used in musculoskeletal disorders. Table 7-6 on page 404 summarizes the most frequently used herbal formulas and their indications. Table 7-7 summarizes combinations of herbs commonly used in musculoskeletal disorders. Table 7-8 on page 417 summarizes the pharmacological actions of commonly used herbs. Chapter 7 covers in more detail many of the important herbs used to treat musculoskeletal disorders.

---

[79]. This is not universally accepted and many acupuncturists and systems of acupuncture use minimal palpation and choose points more from theoretical frameworks.

Table 5-14: Back Shu and Alarm (Mu) Points

Organ	Back Shu (Transport) Points	Alarm (Mu) Points	Manaka Alarm (Mu) Points[a]
Lung	UB-13	Lu-1	Lu-1 to Lu-2
Pericardium	UB-14	CV-17	P-1
Heart	UB-15	CV-14	CV-17 (Pericardium), K-23, Sides CV-14
Liver	UB-18	LIV-14	LIV-14 to GB-26
Gall Bladder	UB-19	GB-24	GB-24 to -29
Spleen	UB-20	LIV-13	GB-26 to -21
Stomach	UB-21	CV-12	CV-12 to St-21
Triple Warmer	UB-22	CV5	St-25 Upper Warmer CV-17 Middle Warmer CV-12 Lower Warmer CV-5
Kidney	UB-23	GB-25	K-16, occasionally GB-25
Large Intestine	UB-25	St-25	St-27 or slightly lateral to St-27
Small Intestine	UB-27	CV-4	St-26 or slightly medial to St-26
Urinary Bladder	UB-28	CV-3	K-11

a. The late Dr. Manaka was a contemporary Japanese physician.

Table 5-15: Five Phases Points Yang Channels.

CHANNEL	WELL (JING) METAL	SPRING (YING) WATER	STREAM (SHU) WOOD	RIVER (JING) FIRE	SEA (HE) EARTH
LARGE INTESTINE	LI-1	LI-2	LI-3	LI-5	LI-11
TRIPLE WARMER	TW-1	TW-2	TW-3	TW-6	TW-10
SMALL INTESTINE	SI-1	SI-2	SI-3	SI-5	SI-8
STOMACH	St-45	St-44	St-43	St-41	St-36
GALLBLADDER	GB-44	GB-43	GB-41	GB-38	GB-34
BLADDER	UB-67	UB-66	UB-65	UB-60	UB-40 (54)

Table 5-16: Four Needle Technique Sedation

CHANNEL	SEDATING TECHNIQUE		TONIFYING TECHNIQUE	
Lung	Lu-5	K-10	Lu-10	H-8
Large Intestine	LI-2	UB-66	LI-5	SI-5
Stomach	St-45	LI-1	St-43	GB-41
Spleen	Sp-5	Lu-8	Sp-1	LIV-1
Heart	H-7	Sp-3	H-3	K-10
Small Intestine	SI-8	St-36	SI-2	UB-66
Bladder	UB-65	GB-41	UB-54	St-36
Kidney	K-1	LIV-1	K-3	Sp-3
Pericardium	PC-7	Sp-3	PC-3	K-10
Triple Warmer	TW-10	St-36	TW-2	UB-66
Gallbladder	GB-38	SI-5	GB-44	LI-1
Liver	LIV-2	H-8	LIV-4	Lu-8

Table 5-17: Four Needle Technique Tonification

CHANNEL	TONIFYING TECHNIQUE		SEDATING TECHNIQUE	
Lung	Lu-9	Sp-3	Lu-10	H-8
Large Intestine	LI-11	St-36	LI-5	SI-5
Stomach	St-41	SI-5	St-43	GB-41
Spleen	Sp-2	H-8	Sp-1	LIV-1
Heart	H-9	LIV-1	H-3	K-10
Small Intestine	SI-3	GB-41	SI-2	UB-66
Bladder	UB-67	LI-1	UB-54	St-36
Kidney	K-7	Lu-8	K-3	Sp-3
Pericardium	PC-9	LIV-1	PC-3	K-10
Triple Warmer	TW-3	GB-41	TW-2	UB-66
Gallbladder	GB-43	UB-66	GB-44	LI-1
Liver	LIV-8	K-10	LIV-4	Lu-8

Table 5-18: Four Needle Technique to Treat Cold Symptoms

Channel	Tonifying Technique		Sedating Technique	
Lung	Lu-10	H-8	Lu-5	K-10
Large Intestine	LI-5	SI-5	LI-2	UB-66
Stomach	St-41	SI-5	St-44	UB-66
Spleen	Sp-2	H-8	Sp-9	K-10
Heart	H-8	K-2	H-3	K-10
Small Intestine	SI-5	UB-60	SI-2	UB-66
Bladder	UB-60	SI-5	UB-66	SI-2
Kidney	K-2	H-8	P-3	H-3
Pericardium	P-8	H-8	P-3	H-3
Triple Warmer	TW-6	UB-60	TW-2	UB-66
Gallbladder	GB-38	SI-5	GB-43	UB-66
Liver	Liv-2	H-8	Liv-8	K-8

Table 5-19: Four Needle Technique to Treat Hot Symptoms

Channel	Tonifying Technique		Sedating Technique	
Lung	Lu-5	K-10	Lu-9	Sp-3
Large Intestine	LI-2	UB-66	LI-11	St-36
Stomach	St-44	UB-66	St-36	UB-54
Spleen	Sp-9	K-10	H-7	K-3
Heart	H-3	K-10	H-7	K-3
Small Intestine	SI-2	UB-66	SI-8	St-36
Bladder	UB-66	SI-2	UB-54	St-36
Kidney	K-10	H-3	K-3	Sp-3
Pericardium	P-3	H-3	P-7	Sp-3
Triple Warmer	TW-2	UB-66	TW-10	UB-54
Gallbladder	GB-43	UB-66	GB-34	UB-54
Liver	Liv-8	K-10	Liv-3	Sp-3

Table 5-20: Commonly Used Points in Musculoskeletal Disorders

Points	Uses
SI-3	Strengthens the spine and relaxes muscles. Neck pain needle on same side (combine with H-4 for middle trapezius [Shao Yang] or UB-64, 65 for upper trapezius [Tai Yang]. Upper back and neck pain (occipital area) with UB-60. For temple region with TW-5 and GB-43. For periscapular pain with SI-6 or Double Child 22.01 and Double Immortal 22.02. For ERS spinal somatic dysfunctions with UB-62 and local points.
UB-11	Tightness of the upper spine. Weakness in one or all bones and joints in body. General weakness with UB-40, 23, K-10. Trapezius, levator scapula, and rhomboid disorders.
UB-18	Tightness and tension of the mid-back. General tightness due to stress and/or Blood-deficiency. For contracted sinews with GV-8.

Table 5-20: Commonly Used Points in Musculoskeletal Disorders (Continued)

POINTS	USES
UB-20	Pain and weakness of the thoracolumbar area. Weakness of the extremities with or w/out digestive system weakness.
UB-23	Weak or stressed patient with/out Kidney weakness symptoms. Adrenal weakness with UB-52, GB-25, and TW Divergent channel treatment.
UB-55 through UB-58	General area for pain anywhere in UB sinew channels; look for skin discoloration; treat as trigger points. Find Kori-Ashi-triggers; treat mostly on pain side for low back pain. Calf pain, or Achilles pain; treat on same or opposite side (with Lu-2 or Ashi in area for Achilles, needle same side). Upper back pain with UB-57 treat opposite side (can bleed). Leg and foot sprain/strain with UB-57, K-2.
UB-62	Relaxes the muscle channels over the entire body with symptoms of spinal stiffness, painful obstruction syndromes, and/or stiffness anywhere. Myofascial pain radiating to head (parietal) and eyes. Exterior Wind.
GV-26	Mid/central-spine pain and weakness; acute sprain/strain of lumbar spine.
GV-16	Insensitivity of the feet. If also hot in soles of feet and difficulty walking (pain) with Sp-6.
St-36	Strengthens weak patients, tonifies Qi and Blood. Strengthens all skeletal muscles. General soreness and weakness with LI-11, GB-38. To treat leg problems, needle 0.5-1 cun deep; Heart trouble, 2-3 cun deep; Stomach trouble, 1.5 cun deep (Miriam Lee). To treat neck, needle 0.5 cun deep; abdomen, 1 cun deep; to reach CV-12, needle 1.5 cun deep; throat, 2 cun deep; to bring blood of the vertex down, needle 3 cun deep (Wang Le-ting).
CV-6	Weak patient, especially with a "slipped" disc (use with CV-4). Tonifies Qi and Kidneys. (If CV-4 pressure sensitive, also good for knee pain).
P-6	Hyperactive sympathetic nervous system with Sishencong (M-HN-1). Chest, upper thoracic, lateral trunk tightness, and/or pain. Medial knee pains (needle opposite side with Liv-3 on the pain side, or LI-11, 10 opposite side, and/or Sp-4 on painful side). Nervousness and nausea. Phlegm and rib/chest sprains and other Phlegm trouble with St-40. Intercostal muscle strain TW-6. Neck and shoulder muscle tension and headaches TW-4.
GB-38	Aches and pains throughout the body. Muscular spasm in general. Pain and stiffness of the neck. Pain and soreness in the calf and lateral aspect of the lower extremities.
Lu-6	Muscle spasms. Thoracic or upper lumbar pain (needle opposite side).
CV-9	Tension in the spine and abdomen from disc disorders in T12-L2.
Liv-5	Back stiffness with loss of flexion. Coldness. Aching and pain in the lower leg and feet and difficulty flexing the knee.
GV-4	Exhausted weak patient, especially with symptoms of unstable Yang or Yin-Fire (use moxa).
H-8	Any complication due to an acupuncture treatment, such as, pain, dizziness, nausea, etc. Mid-back pain
Sp-21	Whole body pain with GV-14, UB-11, 65, SI-3, Liv-8. Whole body weakness with St-36, CV-4, 6, UB-17, 23.
GB-34 (or Beside Three Miles)	Fatigued muscles, weakness, and/or pain/tightness of tendons, ligaments or bones. Pain in the lateral costals/trunk or head.
LI-10 connected to LI-14	Scapular dysfunction and stiffness.
LI-11 connected to H-3	Elbow dysfunction and stiffness.
LI-4 connected to P-8	Metacarpophalangeal dysfunction and stiffness.
GB-30 connected to GB-31	Hip dysfunction and stiffness (needle superficially).
GB-34 connected to Sp-9	Knee dysfunction and stiffness.

Table 5-20: Commonly Used Points in Musculoskeletal Disorders (Continued)

POINTS	USES
GB-39 connected to Sp-6	Ankle dysfunction and stiffness.
GB-40 connected to UB-62	Ankle dysfunction and stiffness. Spastic inverted foot dysfunction.
Sp-5 connected to K-6	Spastic everted foot dysfunction.
St-41 connected to Liv-4	Foot drop. Ankle region paralysis.
St-35 connected to Liv-7	Muscular paralysis of knee region.
LI-15 connected to H-1	Inability to raise shoulder (frozen shoulder).
SI-9 connected to SI-10 and then 11	Difficulty in external rotation of shoulder (reaching behind to back pocket).
K-3 connected to UB-60	Heel pain (needle opposite side).
SI-11, 13, GB-21, then tap with seven star needle and cup to draw blood at SI-13	Chronic shoulder, periscapular pain from shoulder joint or neck. Levetor scapulae insertional bursitis.
K-6 and Lu-7	Poor abdominal muscle tone. FRS spinal somatic dysfunctions (with local point on anterior channel). Medial side muscle spasms, loosening of lateral muscles. Foot inversion with UB-62, K-8, Liv-3, 8, GB-34, Sp-6.
P-6 and Sp-4	Medial side problems. Medial knee pain with Liv-3. Whole body fatigued Sp-4 (red) IP cord.[a] Problems with the diaphragm.
UB-62 and SI-3	Regulates muscular activity along the posterior and lateral aspect of the spine, especially in patients with flaccidity of the muscles of the medial aspect of the lower extremity and spasm of the lateral aspect. Strengthen the spine. Drop-foot. Pain in the inner canthus, neck front and back, ears and shoulders. Functional hallux limitus with piriformis irritation (GB-40—>UB-62), GB-30. Lateral muscle spasms, loosening of medial muscles, eversion of foot with K-6, UB-59, Liv-3, GB-34, St-36. General joint pains and Exterior symptoms with UB-59, 40, GB-29, 34, SI-10, LI-15, 10, GV-3, 9.
TW-5 and GB-41	Lateral trunk pain, lateral knee pain. Also pain at outer canthus, behind the ears, shoulder and neck (frontal). TW-5 (alone) Rib pain, Rib/lateral-trunk pain needle on same side or opposite side with GB-34, 35 or [Beside Three Miles 77.22 and 77.23]). General excess-Yin TW-5 and LI-4 (can also use P-6, Sp-4, K-6, Lu-7 sedating all points). GB-41 (alone) Spinal weakness, weakness and paralysis of extremities, ligamentous laxity with GB-26, 27, 28, 34, St-36, 32, LI-11. TW-5 (red), GB-41 (black) IP cords for whiplash; with GB-26, 34, Liv-3, Sp-3 for spasms, numbness, pain of extremities. Pain of joints and bones; hip, hypochondriac region and neck both points with GB-35, 21, 14, 39, TW-15, UB-11, 65, Liv-3. Low back pain with coldness both points with GV-4, UB-23, K-3.
UB-11, St-36, 37, 39, 30, GB-26, 34, LI-15, 11, 4, Liv-3	Atrophy (Wei syndrome), muscle weakness and wilting especially of lower extremities.
Sp-4, Lu-7, UB-11, St-37 and 39	Fibromyalgia. For distortion of body image, sensation of swelling w/out swelling, sensation of shrinking w/out shrinking etc. Difficulty describing symptoms.
Lu-5 and LI-10	General stiffness, "dryness" of sinews. Facilitate movement of joints. Lu-5 (local vessel) can be bled for frozen shoulder on painful side. Lu-5 also good for knee pain on opposite side.
St-36, CV-4, GB-39	Moxa to strengthen body, sinews and bones.
GB-20, UB-17, Liv-3, Sp-3, LI-4, GV-16, and 14	Wandering Painful Obstruction (Bi). Changing arthritis.
UB-20, 23 and 18	Whole body Painful Obstruction (Bi).

Table 5-20: Commonly Used Points in Musculoskeletal Disorders (Continued)

POINTS	USES
Liv-3 and 2	Spasms, cramps, and pains, especially in a neurotic patient. Used together to strengthen the Heart. Headaches, dizziness, groin/testis pain, lumbar pain with radiation to abdomen (T-11 to L-2 lesions). TMJ syndrome. L5 lesions with lower extremity pain and coldness. Trunk and lateral costal pain due Blood-stasis with Liv-14, 13, TW-6, GB-34, Sp-6.
Liv-10, 11	Muscle fatigue, paralysis especially lower extremities.
LI-15, LI-11 and LI-4.	Pain, numbness and weakness along LI sinew channel. Lateral knee pain LI-11 with TW-10, LI-11 with St-43 for Painful Obstruction Bi syndromes. Lateral hip pain LI-15 with TW-14. Face area symptoms LI-4 (or 4 1/2 Spirit Bone [22.05]) for any pain, but mostly opposite lower back buttock and leg pains (combine with LI-3 1/2 [Great White 22.04]). Upper limb weakness LI-10. Both hands and wrists aching pain and weakness with SI-4.
LI-16 connected to LI-15 (under acromian)	Supraspinatus tendon problems.
GV-8, 3, 24, Liv-3, LI-4, GB-34, H-5	Neuropathies, neuromuscular diseases, nervous tension.
LI-11, 14, GV-17, LI-15, TB-14 and SI-9	Inability to raise shoulder (frozen shoulder).
GB-21, TW-6, SI-11 and 12	Shoulder scapular pain.
TW-5, 4 and LI-4	Five finger pain.
SI-2, TW-2 and 3	Elbow, arm, and wrist pain.
LI-11, Lu-5 and SI-4	Finger and wrist weakness.
LI-2, SI-2 and P-7	Finger cramping.
LI-11 connected to H-3, Shou Jian (M-MU-46), LI-10 and TW-10	Elbow joint pain.
LI-11, GB-34 and St-35 (needle first) Liv-7, Xi Yan (M-LED-16a), GB-33 and St-36 (needle second)	Advanced Knee arthrosis/arthritis. "Crane Knee Wind."
GB-30, 31 and St-33	Foot and Knee aching and pain, difficulty standing and walking.
Sp-5, St-40 and GB-41 "Three Ankle Points"	Leg and Foot problems.
GV-4, UB-23, K-3 and CV-4	Supports the weak patient (Kidney-deficiency). Adrenal weakness. Disc disease.
Liv-3 and LI-4 "Four Gates"	General bodily tension, especially in women. Insomnia. Regulate Qi Mechanism (flow), circulate Qi in a "figure 8" throughout, balancing updown/left right. Trunk and lateral costal pain with Liv-14, 13, TW-6 and GB-34.
GV-14 and CV-4	Warm Yang. General Coldness (best to moxa).
St-36, Sp-6, LI-11, 4 and Lu-7 Or "Old Ten Needles" CV-13, 12, 10, 6, St-25, 36 and P-6 Dr. Lee version of old ten needles St-36, 25, Sp-6, P-6, CV-12 and 9	General weakness. Recurrent chronic diseases. Deficiency below Excess above. Especially if with respiratory or immune system symptoms.
LI-4, 11, P-6, St-36, GB-34, CV-12, Liv-3, 13, Sp-6 and CV-4 "10 Completely and Greatly Tonify Formula"	General weakness. Recurrent chronic diseases. Deficiency of Qi, Blood, Yang, Spleen and Kidney.

Table 5-20: Commonly Used Points in Musculoskeletal Disorders (Continued)

Points	Uses
LI-4, 11, P-6, Sp-6, St-36 and GB-34 "Hand and Foot 12 Needle Formula"	Regulate functions and open channels. General arthritis or chronic diseases. Paralysis or atrophy. For upper limb or lower limb joint pain, first treat the healthy side, then painful side (use both upper and lower points). Knee pain with St-35 and 34. Ankle pain with St-41. Shoulder pain with LI-15. Wrist pain with TW-4. Inflammatory arthritis with Ba Feng (M-LE-8) or Ba Xie (M-UE-22).
UB-13, 15, 18, 20, 23 and 17 "Five Viscera Transports Plus Ge Shu"	Chronic disease, weak patient. When other treatments fail. Strengthen sinews and bones.
GV-20, 16, 14, 9, 8, 6, 5, 4, 3 and 1 "Governing Vessel Thirteen Needles"	Paralysis. Atrophy.
St-36, 44, LI-11, 4, 17, UB-40, 57, 60, Liv-3, GB-30, 34, H-5 Ma Dan Yang's "Twelve Points of Heavenly Star," most important points	Regulate functions and open channels. General arthritis, acute or chronic diseases. All diseases.
GB-39 and TW-8 (on right side) Sp-6 and P-5 (on left side)	Yang-excess on left side of body. For excess on right side of body, switch sides.
P-5 and Sp-6 (on left) TW-8 and GB-39 (right side)	Yin-excess on the right side. For excess-Yin on the left side, switch sides.
Sp-4, K-6 (first) then TW-8	Excess-Yang in the lower part of body.
P-6, Lu-7 (first) then GB-39	Excess-Yang in upper part of body.
GB-41, UB-62 then P-5	Excess-Yin in lower body.
TW-5, SI-3 then Sp-6	Excess-Yin in upper body.
CV-6, ST-36, Sp-10, SP-4, UB-20, CV-12	Tonifying both Qi and Blood. Bleeding with Qi-deficiency, taxation, prolonged disease, insomnia, painful obstruction of the chest, atrophy disorder, dizziness, blurred vision, general lassitude, shortness of breath, reluctance to speak, palpitations.
CV-4, Lu-9, GV-20, Sp-4, 1, 8, ST-34	Tonifying Qi to Hold Blood. Taxation leading to the impairment of Spleen with hemorrhage, petechiae, uterine bleeding, nosebleed, bleeding gums, vomiting of blood, coughing of blood, blood in the urine and stool, shortness of breath, general lassitude.
ST-36, CV-12, UB-20, 21, CV-6, Sp-10, UB-17, LI-4, Liv-3 Apply tonifying method on ST-36 and CV-6, even method on the other points	Tonifying Qi and Invigorating Blood. Deficiency of Qi fails to move Blood, prolonged disease, taxation, stroke, painful obstruction, fixed stabbing pain, numbness of the limbs or hemiplegia, deviation of the mouth and eye
CV-4, GV-4, UB-23, Shixuan (M-UE-1), SP-6, GB-34, 39, LI-10, TW-5, SP-10, UB-17, LI-4, Liv-3. Apply tonifying method on CV-4, GV-4, UB-23, Sp-6, and sedation method on the other points	Warming Channels and Dispersing Cold. Obstruction of both Qi and Blood, exogenous pathogenic Cold in Blood level, Painful Obstruction, Raynaud's disease, Shen disorder, fixed stabbing pain, cold limbs, cold pain in the genital region which radiates to the inner thigh, numbness or discharge of blood and pus.
GV-26, 20, K-1, CV-8	Tonifying Qi to Rescue Collapse. Collapse of both Qi and Blood due to heavy bleeding.
CV-6, Sp-10, UB-17, LI-4,11, SP-6, Liv-3, Ashi points Apply sedation or even method on all points	Moving Qi and Invigorating Blood. Emotional stress resulting in stagnation of Liver Qi and subsequent blood stasis, traumatic injury giving rise to stagnation of Qi and blood. Qi stagnation and blood stasis can set up a vicious circle, both eventually causing stagnation of both Qi and blood. This pattern is often seen in headaches, painful obstruction of the chest, stomach ache, flank pain, painful obstruction, dysmenorrhoea, fixed and stabbing pain.

Table 5-20: Commonly Used Points in Musculoskeletal Disorders (Continued)

Points	Uses
GV-14, LI-11, 4, St-44, Liv-2, Shixuan (M-UE-1) Apply sedation method on all points	Clearing Heat, Detoxifying Fire Poison, and Cooling Blood. Toxic heat at both Qi and Blood levels, warm-febrile diseases, purulent sores, carbuncles, high fever, restlessness, convulsion of the limbs.
GV-20, Liv-2, GB-43, 20, 5, Taiyang (M-HN-9), UB-58 Apply sedation method on all points	Subduing Rebellious Yang, and Regulating and Pacifying both Qi and Blood. Anger, invasion of Pathogenic Factors, stroke, epilepsy, trigeminal neuralgia, distending headache, red complexion, high fever, propensity to anger, forgetfulness, coma, delirium, deviation of the mouth and eye.
GV-13, UB-10/GB-20, TW-15, LI-15, SI-9 and UB-39	General "Control Loop" for cervical syndrome.
LI-14, 11, 10. 4, SI-8, 9 and TW-5	General "Control Loop" for arm.
Sp-6, Liv-8, 12, St-36, GB-37 and UB-58	General "Control Loop" for blood supply in the lower extremity.
TW-22, 17 and GB-17	General "Control Loop" for blood supply in the head.
Sp-5, 6, 9, Liv-8, TW-4 and 5	General "Control Loop" for connective tissue.
GB-34, St-36, LI-10, 11, K-8, P-6 and UB-23	General "Control Loop" for musculature.
LI-14, 15, SI-9, 2 and local sensitive points	General "Control Loop" for shoulder.
GV-4, UB-31, GB-30, 26,/27/28, UB-23 and 50	General "Control Loop" for lumbago.
TW-5, UB-23, 47 and Liv-8	General "Control Loop" for inflammation.
LI-4 1/2 (Spirit Bone 22.05) and LI-3 (1/2) (Great White 22.04)	Good for any pain, especially with Lung weakness or lower body. Ischial bursitis, back pain, sciatica, buttock pain, anterior hip pain (inguinal), upper limb pain (esp elbow). Needle opposite side for lower body and same side for upper body.
DT-1 and 2 (SI-9 area)	L5 sciatica (GB channel). Bleed and cup.
Heart Door 33.12	Inner knee pain, groin pain.
Shoulder Center Middle (44.06)	Knee pain, patellar pain, shoulder pain.
Three nine miles (a combination of three points) (88.25-26-27)	Upper and/or lower back pain with leg pain or nulliness (numb-like with inactivity). Tightness of the iliotibial tract with weakness of abdominal muscles. Pain at ilial areas, add tender points between LI-11 and LI-10 right against the radius bone. Unilateral headache or back pain (for unilateral pain, needle contralaterally). Vertebral hypertrophy (any level).
Correct tendons (a combination of two points) (77.01-02) and Upright scholar (77.03)	Central or bilateral upper back and/or neck pain. Disc pathology (chronic). Plantar fasciitis (tight heel cord). All disorders of the tendons.
Fire Complete (88.16)	Vertebral dysfunctions and pathology with upper back, foot, and heel pain.
Heaven Emperor Quasi (77.18)	Shoulder pain especially with Kidney-deficiency. Pain on shoulder abduction Hand numbness with K-7.
Passing through Upper Back (88.11)	Shoulder pain and general swelling.
Hand Five Gold (33.08) Hand Thousand Gold (33.09)	Sciatica with UB channel distribution (S1). Lower body neuropathy.
State Water (1010.25)	Low back pain (midline).
Five Tigers (11.27)	Ankle pain. Polyarthritis.
Water Passing Through (1010.19) Water Gold (1010.20)	Joint and/or back pains with Kidney-Essence weakness. Pain aggravated by coughing.

Table 5-20: Commonly Used Points in Musculoskeletal Disorders (Continued)

Points	Uses
Flower Bone Three (55.04) Flower Bone Four (55.05)	Sacral or SI joint pain. Thoracic paravertebral pain. Sciatica and leg or foot numbness.
Two yellow 88.12, 88.14 and UB-40 (bleed)	Spondylitis (vertebral hypertrophy, especially Liver and T12 through L4 related).
Three yellow 88.12, 88.13, 88.14	Weakness of Heart, Liver, Spleen, and Kidney. Arthritis and fatigue (especially if points are very tender).[b]

a. Ion pump clip.
b. For additional Tong-style points see below.

Table 5-21: Commonly Used Points: Mental Conditions

Indications	Point Group/Major Points
Madness, psychosis, mania, "possession", epilepsy	Ghost points: GV-26, Lu-11, Sp-1, P-7, P-8, UB-62, GV-16, St-6, CV-24, GV-23, CV-1 LI-11, Hai quan (below tongue) (bleed).
Any mental disease	GV-26, 24, 23, 16, St-6, 40, UB-15, CV-15, LI-11, 4, P-8, 5, H-7.
Psychoemotional disorders, disorders of sense organs, disharmony between Qi of Body and Head with Qi or Blood rushing upwards Excess above, Deficiency below: Anger, irritability, insomnia, agitation. Sharp headaches relieved by cold compress. Cold feet, nightly muscle cramp. Weakness in legs, hemorrhoids Deficiency above, Excess below: Mental confusion, difficulty concentrating, loss of memory, sequelae to CVA, hot feet, strong physique	Windows of the Sky:[a] LI-18, St-9, Lu-3, TW-16, UB-10. Minor Points: SI-17, SI-16, CV-22, P-1, GV-16, TW-17.
Anxiety or Irritability Anxiety and/or depression with weakness	GV-19, 20 and CV-15, Wood Anger (11.17).[b] GV-15 (black) and P-6 (red) ion cords. Yin Teng (M-HN-3), GV-20 and CV-4.
Insomnia	LI-4 and Liv-3. For difficult falling asleep, add Liv-1; much dreaming add St-44, 36; early awakening add K-2, 3; elderly patient add Two Emperors (77.18 and 77.21); restless sleep add St-45, Sp-1; Heart and Kidney not harmonized add K-2, H-3.
Insomnia, thought disorder, agitation, anger, labile, depression, any mental stress	H-7, Yin Teng, LI-4 and Liv-3. Yin Teng (M-HN-3) and GV-20 with electrical stimulation. P-6 (black) and Sp-4 (red) ion cords. Ear: Shen Men, Tranquilizer/Valium, Internal secretion, Master Cerebral, Stress Control/Adrenal.
General "control loop" for depressive state	H-3, CV-6, UB-39.
General "control loop" for exhaustion, mental and physical	CV-6, Liv-13, 3; CV-4, UB-39, GB-37.
General "control loop" for sleep	UB-62, K-6.

a. Windows of the Sky points are found as a group only in modern Western texts, although there are references to them in the *Spiritual Axis*. They are located in the neck area and most have the character for heaven (tian) in their name.
b. A set of two Tong-style points located on the left hand only. On the palmer side of the index finger 4 fen from the median line of the proximal phalanx and 3 fen up and down from the midpoint. Used for any Liver-Fire associated symptoms.

Table 5-22: Points: Endocrine Dysfunctions

Adrenals	Pancreas	Parathyroid	Pituitary	Ovaries	Testes	Thymus
K-7	Sp-3	UB-11	CV-15	K-13	K-11	Sp-2
UB-47	K-3	UB-58	CV-16	UB-67	CV-3	St-11 (EAV)
CV-10	UB-20	GB-30	CV-19	K-7	CV-4	
Sp-6	TW-3	St-36	K-13	GB-37	CV-5	
GV-6	Liv-2	GV-2	Sp-6	Sp-6	UB-47	
CV-6	CV-3	Liv-3	K-11	K-2	St-30	
CV-16	LI-13 (EAV)	GV-15	UB-47	GV-4	GV-3	
P-7		UB-3	GB-37	Liv-3	GV-4	
UB-22 (EAV)		P-7	GB-5	St-31 (EAV) Sp-11 (EAV) LI-11 (EAV)	UB-60	
		St-9 (EAV)	UB-60		St-31 (EAV)	
		St-10 (EAV) thyroid	CV-10			
			SI-15 (EAV) anterior GB-20a (EAV) medial GB-12 (EAV) posterior		Sp-11 (EAV)	

Table 5-23: Points: Nervous Regulation (Wong 1999; Leonhardt 1980)

Neural Structure	Points
Frontal Lobe	GV-21-24, UB-3-7, GB-4-18, St-8
Parietal Lobe	GV-18, 19, UB-8
Temporal Lobe	GB-6-10
Occipital Lobe	GV-17, UB-9, GB-11, GB19
Rhinencephalon	UB-2, Yu Yao, TW-23, Yin Teng
Cerebellum	GV-16, GB-20, GB-12, (GV-19 EAV)
Thalamus	GB-14, Thalamus point, (GB-4 EAV)
Hypothalamus	Yin Teng (M-HN-3), GV-20, (TW-20.3 EAV)
Medulla Oblongata	GV-26, GV-16, (UB-10 EAV)
Sympathetic/Parasympathetic Central Control	GV-20, Sishengcong
Sympathetic Mid-Brain Control Parasympathetic Medulla Oblongata	GV-26, GV-16
Sympathetic Cervical Ganglia	SI-17, St-10, St-11, (GB-20 EAV sympathetic nerve)
Sympathetic Outflow in Spinal Cord	GV-14, HJ at C8/T1 GV-4, UB-23, HJ at L2/L3 GV-1
Parasympathetic Cranial Control	3ed CN: UB-1, St-1 7th CN: TW-17 9th CN: CV-22, 23 10th CN: St-10, CV-22, CV-24, Shenmen (auricular)
Parasympathetic Sacral Control	S1-S4, UB-31-34
Autonomic System Crisis Brain Attack	GV-26 and GV-16
Increase Oxygen Uptake In Brain	St-9, GB-20, UB-2, CV-22, GV-20 and Sishengcong
Cerebral Edema Reduce Brain Inflammation	Yin Teng (M-HN-3), LI-4 and St-36
Vagus Nerve	Shenmen (ear), CV-22, St-10 and 9
Spinal Accessory	GB-20, 21 and LI-18
Stellate Ganglion	St-11
Diencephalon	GB-7 EAV
Autonomic Nervous Control of Head	Sympathetic UB-2, GB-20 Parasympathetic: UB1, St-1, TW-17, CV-24 Control from neck: SI-17, St-9
Autonomic Control in Neck	Sympathetic: GB-20, GV-14, SI-17, St-10, 11 Parasympathetic: CV-22, St-9
Major Sympathetic Control for Lower Extremity Major Parasympathetic Control for Lower Extremity	Liv-3, St-36 Sp-6, UB-40
Major Sympathetic Control for Upper Extremity Major Parasympathetic Control for Upper Extremity	LI-4, 11 P-6, H-7
Major Sympathetic Control of Back Major Parasympathetic control of Back	UB-23, GV-4 UB-32, UB-60

Table 5-24: Points: Treating Cervical Extension and/or Flexion

Symptom	Points
Resistance to cervical extension and/or flexion	UB-11.
Resistance to cervical extension and/or flexion also good for neck pain and headache	UB-64 and UB-65.
Increased symptoms and signs with extension and/or flexion movement	UB-64 and UB-11.
Relieves pain and stiffness in the head and back of the neck, especially painful extension	UB-64, 11 and CV-24.

Table 5-25: Points: Treating Cervical Movement Restrictions and Rotation

Symptom	Points
Resistance or pain with cervical rotation	GB-21. TW-5 (red) and GB-41 (black) IP cord[a] LI sensitive channel points (especially LI-3 1/2 and LI-4 1/2)
Torticollis Restricted Sidebending/rotation	GB-20 (towards the opposite GB-20), GV-16, GV-14 and P-6.
Sudden neck muscle spasm with limitation of neck rotation	UB-10.
Acute shoulder pain with resistance to cervical rotation	St-38.
Sudden neck muscle spasm with limitation of neck rotation	UB-37,10, SI-3 and GB-21.

a. Ion pomp clips.

Table 5-26: Points: Treating General Cervical Stiffness

Symptom	Points
Stiff neck	TW-16 and SI-3.
Stiff neck	SI-3 and UB-65 (both bilateral).
Stiff neck	CV-24, GV-16, and SI-3.
Stiff neck	Laozhen (on affected side) and Ashi (tender) points (especially between SI-16, 17), SI 3, and GB-3.
Stiff neck	CV-24, SI-3, GV-16.
Stiff neck	UB-64, 37, 11, 10, GB-21, TW-16, and SI-3. LI sensitive channel points (especially LI-3 1/2 and LI-4 1/2).
Stiff neck with superficial syndrome	UB-65, 10.

Table 5-27: Points: Treating Neck, Shoulder, and Head Pain

Symptom	Points
Neck, shoulder, and/or head pain and stiffness	GB-20—>GB-20. and/or UB-10—>UB-10.
Severe neck and shoulder pain especially in levator scapula reference pattern	UB-62, SI-3.
Shoulder pain with difficulty raising arm	GB-26.
Severe neck and shoulder pain	SI-6, UB-10.
Neck and shoulder pain	TW-14.
Neck pain that radiates into the back and shoulder	TW-10 (medial-inferiorly).
Levator scapula muscle reference pattern; neck and periscapular	SI-1 (moxa) and SI-3 1/2 (rotate for 2 minutes), or Double Son with Double Fairy.
Immobile, severely painful neck	SI-1, 2, 3, 5, UB-2, 60, GB-12 and H-3.
Radicular Pain Cervical Spondylosis	SI-17 (inferior-medially), SI-9, 10, 11 (superiorly), LI-15 (inferiorly), 13, 10, 4 and TW-14 (inferiorly).
Pain due to supraspinous and interspinous ligaments	GV-26 and SI-3—> LI-4.
Pain of lateral part of vertebra, radiating periscapularly	SI-3 and 6.
Neck pain radiating to the upper border of scapula	TW-5 (proximally) and GB-39 (proximally).
Pain and spasm of SCM muscle	LI-4, Lu-7 (proximally), K-6, Ashi in-out and cup 3-15 minutes.
Midline pain, occipital pain, disc pain	Correct Tendons (deep to bone.)

Table 5-28: Points: Treating Headache

Symptom	Points
Frontal	GV-23; LI-4, 7; ST-36 (1/2), 44 and Yinteng (M-HN-3) —> UB-2, Sp-4 and 9. GV-24, Yinteng (M-HN-3), GB-14 and UB-2. GV-23 (black), LI-4 or Lu-7 (red) IP cords.[a]
Corners of Forehead	St-8, GB-5 and Lu-7.
Parietal	GV-21, 20, UB-64 and 65. Tai Yang (black), TW-5 or GB-41 (red) IP cords.
Left-sided	TB-23—>GB-8, GB-20—>GV-16, Sp-6, GB-34 and Liv-3.
Posterior parietal	Liv-3 and SP-6.
Occipital	Taiyang (EX-HN-5), St-7, 8, TW-5, GB-38, UB-10 and 64, 65. GV-15 (black), SI-3 or UB-60 (red) IP cord).
Temporal	TW-1 through 5, GB-1, 14, 38, 41, LU-7 and St-43. Beside Three Miles. Taiyang (EX-HN-5), GB-7 and LI-4. Tai Yang (black), TW-5 or GB-41 (red) IP cord.
Vertex or Deficient	K-1 and UB-65. Liv-2 and 3. GV-20, 24, Taiyang (EX-HN-9), GB-20 and LI-4. GV-20 (black), LI-4 or Liv-3 (red) IP cord.
Occipital radiating to Forehead or Eye	GB-41, 35, 20, TW-5 and UB-63.
Head and Eye	UB-1, 2, GV-24 and St-8.
Behind the Eye	Four Flowers (Stomach channel lower leg sensitive points needled on same side of pain to a depth of 2 cun.
Migraine	Taiyang (EX-HN-5), GB-8, GV-20 (backwards) and GB-20. TW-6; GB-37, 20 and 4. Taiyang (EX-HN-5) St-8, TW-5, GB-7, 38, 41 and H-8. UB-64 and 65. GV-24, Taiyang (EX-HN-5) and UB-2 (vomiting and vertigo). Beside Three Miles (temporal). Four Flowers Middle (if with eye pressure). GB-14, 15, Taiyang (EX-HN-5) and TW-17 (towards mandible).
Felt as a band around the head	UB-62, 63
With TMJ syndromes	Taiyang (EX-HN-5), St-7 and LI-4. Or with Liv-2 and 3. Points on bottom of heel.
Head and Teeth	CV-24, GV-16, LI-2, St-36 and K-3.
General Tension	Taiyang (EX-HN-5), GB-20 (to opposite GB-20), GB-8 (backwards) and P-6. Liv-2, 3, LI-4.
Comes and goes	CV-12 moxa 50 cones.

a. Ion cords.

Table 5-29: Important Points and Point Combinations for the Thoracic/Shoulder Areas

Points	Uses
Pain and weakness in the arm and shoulder regions Pain in the chest and lateral costal regions Pain and/or neuralgia and numbness in the scapular and the posteromedial aspect (SI channel) of the arm and elbow Levator scapula, infraspinatus, supraspinatus and upper posterior trapezius lesions	SI-11 and SI-6 (proximally).
Upper back and shoulder pain especially due to muscle channel dysfunctions Spasm of the upper anterior trapezius, scalenus anterior, and the deltoid muscles	LI-15 (direct needle toward lesion).
Anterior chest pain Rib dysfunctions	St-44.
Anterior chest and rib pain and dysfunctions Costochondritis Fourth through twelfth rib pain Pain in the ventral aspect of the arm and forearm	P-6.
For intercostal neuralgia	with GB-34 and Ashi.
Anterior chest and rib pain Dysfunctions of the upper two ribs and clavicle Lesions in the scalenus muscles	Lu-8-9-10 (may connect with one needle).
Upper chest, rib, and neck pain with inability to raise the arm	Lu-5 (on painful side, bleed) and LI-10 (opposite side).
Anterior chest and rib pain Dysfunctions of the second third and fourth ribs Lateral costal pain	H-8 and 7.
Lateral trunk pain Thoracic joint dysfunctions	TW-5 (proximally), Ashi, Jie Ji and UB-40.
Mid back pain	Lu-6, TW-3.
Upper back, neck, shoulder, and arm pain Trapezius lesions	GB-21 (toward tight band).
Acute upper back and neck pain and tightness	GB-39 (proximally).
Lower and/or upper back pain Rib dysfunctions, costal pain, and flank pain in a weak patient	Team of four horses (88.17-18-19) (for unilateral pain needle contralaterally).
Local pain, numbness, and weakness in upper thoracic and shoulder regions	SI-14 (inferiorly) and GB-21 (toward tight band).
Musculoskeletal pain in the upper and lateral back, chest and upper limbs	St-36, St-32, Sp-10, GB-30, 31 and 34.
Upper back pain with degenerative disc and joint disease in fatigued patient Spinal deformity	Two+ yellow (a combination of three points) (88.12, 88.14) and Passing Heaven (88.03).
Upper chest, neck, and arm pain from scalene muscle lesions	Lu-7 —>Lu-8 and subcutaneous needling along superior border of the clavicle Or in the direction of skin drag restriction.
Bursitis at shoulder	Ashi under AC joint, LI-15 (downwards), LI-11—>H-3 (subcutaneous) and SI-10.
Supraspinatus tendinitis	LI-16—>LI15 (under acromian).

Table 5-29: Important Points and Point Combinations for the Thoracic/Shoulder Areas (Continued)

Points	Uses
Supraspinatus Tendinitis	LI-11, SI-15 (medially), GB-21 (inferiorly) and Ashi.
Infraspinatus Tendinitis	With SI-10 and SI-8 (proximally).
Subscaularis Tendinitis	With Lu-5 (proximally) and Lanwei (EX-LE-7).
Shoulder Capsulitis (Frozen)	LI-15, SI-10, St-38—>UB-57, Lanwei (EX-LE-7), Taijian (N-UE-11), Jubi (N-UE-10) and Shoulder-ear. Kidney Gate (Sp-8 1/2).

Table 5-30: Points: Low Back Sprain and Strain

Symptom	Points
General acute sprain/strain	LI-3, LI-4 1/2 (Ling Gu and Da Bai), with UB-65 for UB type or unilateral pain, or GB-42 for GB pain. GV-26, K-2 and bleed UB-40. Next, stimulate local ashi (trigger) points quickly without needle retention. State Waters (1010.25), GV-20 and UB-7 ask patient to mobilize the back. SI-3 (opposite pain), Du-26, Hand lumbar and leg pain (Yaotongdian N-UE-19) #1 and #2 (on painful side). Cup area with patient seated. Move cups with muscle stretched. Lu-5, UB-40, GV-26, UB-60, UB-65, TW-6 and GB-34.
Pain More Central, Supra/Interspinous Ligament Sprain	SI-3—>LI-4 and UB-40. UB-65. Sp-9 superficially upward, or bleed and cup.
With Acute Costal/Subcostal Pain	Lu-5, LI-11—>10, LI-4, Sp-6, Sp-9, Liv-2, and St-36 (deep).
Acutely Stiff Back and Spine	UB-11, UB-41 and CV-9. GV-11, GV-6, GV-2, and GV-1. UB-17, CV-9, GV-4, UB-20, UB-27 and UB-28. UB-47 and GB-25.
Upper Low Back/Thoracic	H-8, TW-3. Hand lumbar and leg pain (Yaotongdian N-UE-19) #1 and #2.
Sudden Pain aggravated by deep breath/cough	Water Gold and Water Passing Through (1010.19-20).
Spasm of Quadratus Lumborum (seen often with Kidney deficiency)	Double Child Immortal (internal Hoku, LI-4) on the contralateral side. Or moxa Lu-10.
Acute/chronic pain with inability to stand for long	GB-25, Liv-2.

Table 5-31: Points: Other Spinal Conditions

Symptom	Points
Vertebral Hypertrophy	Bleed UB-40. Bright Yellow (88.12), Three 9 Miles (88.25-27) and SI- 3½.
Coccydynia	GV-20 and Hua Tuo points at C5-7, UB-67. If needed, add UB-34, 35 and GB-30. Lu-8 (if St-27 is tender).
Sacroiliac Dysfunction and Pain	State waters (1010.25) plus a needle ½-inch laterally to the contralateral side of the painful joint. Flower Bone Three and Four bilaterally; mobilize the joint at the same time. If needed, palpate and treat Hua Tuo point at T-10 through L1. UB-32 and 34 contralaterally. Liv-8, local Ashi or tight areas, K-6, UB-62. Hua Tuo and UB points from L2 to L5.
Pubic Dysfunction and Pain	Active Hua Tuo Jia Ji points from T12 through L2 and CV-6. Sp-9 and trigger points in adductor and abdominal muscles. Hormonal dysfunction add Liv-8 and 3 Emperors (77.18-21).
Central stenosis, cold, numbness of limbs	St-12 (first), GV-1, UB-31, 32, 33, 34.

Table 5-32: Points: Based on Location of Back Pain

Symptom	Points
Anywhere from Thoracolumbar Junction to Lumbosacral Junction	UB-40, 60 and UB -18 through 25. Hua Tuo point at these levels. Sensitive areas on calf (UB-58 areas). UB-point on left —> UB-point on right.
More Central	Moxa UB-67. SI-3, GV-16 (or State Waters), LI-4 1/2 and 3-1/2 and 3-Emperors (77.18-21). Bleed Flower External (77.14) local Hua Tuo and GV points. Bleed UB-40 and needle UB-60.
More Lateral	GB-41 and TW-5. Beside Three Miles (77.22-23). GB-19, 29, 30, and 31.
Sacral area	Liv-8, local Ashi or tight areas, K-6, UB-62. Jia Ji and UB points from L2 to L5. Correct Tendons (77.01), UB-57, 60, LI-4, 2 (follow by cupping). Flower Bone 3 and 4 (55.04, 05).
At Lumbosacral Junction	State Waters (1010.25) plus points ½-1cm lateral to them on the contralateral side of the pain. Local points through and through from one side of UB channel—>other side, UB-24—>UB-24, UB-25—>UB-25 and UB-32—>UB-32. UB-25 through 34, GV-3 and 4. UB-57, 60, LI-4, 2 (patient raises and lowers leg 300 times).
More Lateral, at Lumbosacral Area	GB-19,18, 31 and Nine Miles (88.25-27). GB-41 and TW-5.
At Iliac Crest	GB-31, Ashi at LI-11-10 areas close to bone.
With Shoulder and Upper Back Pain	UB-58.
Mixed GB and UB channels	UB-59 and GB-30. Flower Bone 3 and 4 (55.04, 05).
Both Lower and Upper Back	UB-60, 40 and GB-30. GV-4, UB-23, 18, 19 and 28. UB-25, 26 and 40 for inability to look-up and down.

Table 5-32: Points: Based on Location of Back Pain (Continued)

FIXED LOCATION LONG-TERM	Bleed UB-40, 17 and followed by local cupping.
CHRONIC LOW BACK AND LEGS (ARTHRITIC)	GV-2 (moxa), GV-4 and UB-23. UB-31-34, 40 and 60.
LOW BACK PAIN RADIATING TO LOWER ABDOMEN, INABILITY TO FLEX/EXTEND,	Points at sacral base, UB-34, treat right for left pain.
THORACOLUMBAR, TIGHTNESS, LOWER ABDOMEN TOUGHNESS (L2-3)	UB-47, TW-3.

Table 5-33: Points: Based on Low Back Movement

SYMPTOM	POINTS
RESTRICTED EXTENSION PAIN **OR** **PAIN AGGRAVATED BY EXTENSION**	UB-41,53, GV-2, 3 and 26, Liv13 and 14 and CV-2 through 6. UB-29, 28, 34.
PAIN AT MIDLINE AGGRAVATED BY FLEXION AND/OR EXTENSION	GV-26 and SI-3, Bleed UB-40. K-2, UB-47 and Liv 3 also can be used for extension and/or flexion restrictions. UB-29, 28, 34. Sp-9.
RESTRICTED FLEXION **OR** **PAIN AGGRAVATED BY FLEXION**	GV-26, UB- 23 and 52. Bleed UB-40. Point at sacral base (UB-25—>UB-25). Moving cups on the patient's back muscle with patient seated and forward bent.
RESTRICTED ROTATION **OR** **PAIN AGGRAVATED BY ROTATION**	UB-62 and SI-3 especially with Ion cords. GB-41 and TW-5.
GENERALLY RESTRICTED LUMBAR MOVEMENT	Moxa UB-67 and 60. Bleed Liv-13 and UB-40.
EXTENSION RESTRICTIONS ESPECIALLY WITH FLACCIDITY OF MUSCLES OF LATERAL ASPECT OF LOWER EXTREMITY AND SPASM OF MEDIAL ASPECT	K-6 and Lu-7.
FLEXION RESTRICTIONS AND PAIN ALONG POSTERIOR AND LATERAL ASPECT OF SPINE, ESPECIALLY IF MEDIAL ASPECT OF LOWER EXTREMITY MUSCLES ARE FLACCID, AND LATERAL ASPECT IS SPASMED	UB-62 and SI-3.
DIFFICULTY IN TURNING ONTO THE SIDE **UB AND GB CHANNEL PAIN**	LI-11, GB-30 and UB-40. Severe pain inability to turn over Liv-13.

Table 5-34: Points: Acute and Chronic Disc or Back and Leg Pains

Symptom	Points
Disc Pain General	Ashi points at midline and 1/4 to 1.5 cun lateral to midline on opposite side of pain. GB-30 and UB-40 on painful side. Ashi points at midline and 1/4 to 3 cun lateral to midline (deep in-out puncture, intertransversei and rotator muscles, only in chronic mild cases), GB-30, UB-54, 37, 40 and 57 on painful side. GB-38.
L2 and L3 Disc Lesions	Passing through Kidney and Upper Back (88.09-11) and H-8.
L4 and L5 Disc Lesions	GB-31, GB-38, Liv-3 and 2. LI-4 1/2 and TW-3 1/2. GB-34, St-36, 38 and Liv-3. SI-9 bleed and cup.
S1 and S2 Disc Lesion	Five Thousand Gold (33.08-09) opposite side of pain, with UB-40, GB-31, GB-38, H-4 (painful side) and GV-26.
Foot Drop	GB-34, St-36, 38, Liv-3 and UB-62.
Acute Flashes/twinges of Pain in Lumbar Spine due to any level disc lesion	GV-26 and UB-40 (bleed).
Pain Radiating to Buttocks	Flower Bone Three and Four (55.04-05).
Chronic Disc Lesions	Correct Tendons (77.01-02). CV-4 and 6. GB-30 strong stimulation. Hua tuo jia ji in painful areas, on the painful or none-painful side. Hua tuo points needled with patient sitting, standing or prone, without needle retention.
Limb Numbness	LI-11 and GB-30.
Low Back and Thigh symptoms	Sp-10, GB-31, 30 and 34.
Sciatica	Five Thousand Gold (33.08-09). Four Flower Below (77.11) and Four Flower (77.10). Bowel Intestine (77.12) (with additions of disc points as needed). Stimulate ipsilaterally to painful side GB-30, GB-31 and St-36 then, stimulate contralaterally painful side UB-27 and UB-25 or affected level. Follow with moxibustion at St-36, K-3, UB-23, 59 and 32, and GB-31 and 32. Pain down Shao-Yang channel (GB) TW-23. First St-38—>UB57 (10 minutes), then UB-30, 34 and GB-39. Left-sided pain use Bowel Intestine (77. 12). Right-sided pain use Four Flower Quasi (77.10).
Sciatica: other common prescriptions	Pain that radiates down lateral aspect of leg GB-30, GB-34, GB-39, St-36 and St-4. Pain that radiates down posterior aspect of leg UB-40, UB-56 and UB-57. For back pain with sciatica UB-23, UB-30, UB-50, GB-30, UB-51, UB-54 and GB-34. UB-31, UB-32, UB-49, UB-57, GB-39, UB-60, GB-41.

Table 5-35: Dr. Yoshio Monaka's Ion Cord Treatment for Low Back

Symptom	Points
Lower Back Pain	UB-47 (black clip) and UB-57 (red clip).
Lumbar Pain	UB-23 or UB-47 (black clip) and SI-3 or UB-62 (red clip).
Lumbar and Thigh Pain	GB-30 or UB-51 (black clip) and GB-35 or GB-34 (red clip).
Lateral Low Back Pain	UB-23 (black clip) and GB-29 or GB-34 (red clip).
Numbness	Tender points on affected limb, with black clip connected to Yin points and red clip on Yang points.

6

ADDITIONAL ACUPUNCTURE SYSTEMS AND RELATED TECHNIQUES

Several systems of acupuncture are helpful in the management of musculoskeletal disorders. This section describes some of the more commonly used systems.

Abdominal Assessment

The model of abdominal assessment and treatment that was developed mostly in Japan follows the basic principles found in the classic *Book of Difficulties*, the oldest book in which abdominal topography is mentioned (Matsumoto and Birch 1988). As seen in *Book of Difficulties* Chinese medicine considers the abdomen to be a location imprinted with the function and dysfunction of many Organ system, i.e., it is a somatotopic area that reflects the patient's health. The treatment of abdominal points may have effects on the fascial system as it relates to the Organs as well as Somatic structures. (*Biomed: Travell and Simons (ibid) have stated that treatment to abdominal trigger points (TP) in muscles, skin, and fascia can relieve symptoms that are often associated with visceral problems such as diarrhea, gas, belching, urinary problems, etc. They state that viscerosomatic responses (TPs) are quite common with diseases such as peptic ulcer, intestinal parasites, dysentery, ulcerative colitis, diverticulosis, diverticulitis, choleithiasis, kidney stones, stress, trauma, and infections. These are said to frequently activate myofascial trigger points. At times these medical disorders are said not to "heal" until the trigger points are inactivated. Therefore, the abdomen can be evaluated as a myofascial organ and treated regardless of OM interpretations.*)

The areas of the abdomen correspond to different channels and Organs. The practitioner uses several maps to interpret the findings of the examination. The fact that each map is slightly different invites criticism; however, the practitioner can use the physical findings (without a "diagnosis") and treat the abdomen *directly* to affect both local (abdominal wall) tissues, and the Organ/organs systems. Therefore, the differences in the maps are not critical, and abdominal palpation and direct treatment is useful even for those that are not familiar with the more detailed traditions. In many Japanese systems, distal channel points are used to address the abdominal findings.

It is common to find tender and active spots (triggers) at the abdominal wall. Frequently these spots are found on the rectus abdominis, oblique muscles and their aponeuroses, and on the linea alba or its tendinous intersection with the rectus muscle. When assessing by palpation, the direction of the varying abdominal muscles must be kept in mind. Treatment of the abdomen frequently results in deep relaxation of the patient and may influence fascial planes. (*Biomed/Osteopathy: Collateral ganglion inhibition (by carefully applying midline abdominal pressure until a fascial release is palpable) can be applied over the abdominal collateral sympathetic ganglion that is related to the dysfunctional organ with hypersympathetic activity. These ganglia are located between the xiphoid process and the umbilicus and lie just anterior to the aorta. Ventral abdominal (or visceral) manipulation applied to relieve congestion around the nerves, plexi, and receptors in the affected abdominal tissues or organs is also useful to reduce visceral afferent input to the spinal cord and to treat sympathetic hyperactivity [Kuchera and Kuchera ibid]).*

Abdominal treatments can be used at the end of musculoskeletal treatment, when this relaxing-effect facilitates the integration of the newly established post-treatment sensory patterning, or at the beginning of treatment to prepare and relax the patient. Meridian balancing through evaluation of the pulse (page 341) or Extra Channel treatment can be incorporated at the same time, and all may be considered a "root" treatment in OM.

Status of Patient's Constitution

In OM, treatment techniques used in musculoskeletal disorders depend often on the patient's constitution/condition as well as the local pathology. Diagnosis by abdominal palpation is particularly useful when determining the patient's constitution or general condition. The practitioner feels for temperature variations, tightness, or looseness of the skin, tension of the muscles, pain or tensing on light pressure, fluid movements during palpation, sensation of movement and draft across an abdominal region, any lumps, swellings, induration, or depressions, and lack of normal flexibility.

While knowledge of the patient's constitutional type cannot substitute for the actual diagnosis of the presenting disharmony or pattern diagnosis, understanding the patient's basic constitution can apprise us of his/her tendencies to certain disharmonies or dysfunctions, and therefore can help in forecasting and possibly preventing the development of such problems. It can also put the pattern diagnosis in perspective,

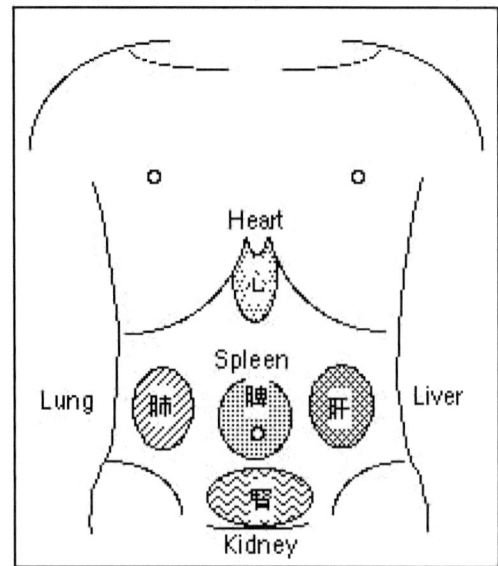

Figure 6-1: Abdominal topography according to *Book of Difficulties* (courtesy of Robert Hayden).

gauging severity and urgency (i.e., whether the pattern or the constitution should be treated first). It can also aid in understanding the patient's "root" condition and can guide underlying treatments.

A healthy abdomen should be relaxed and flaccid above the navel, while the area below the navel should be fuller, tighter, and more resilient. The rectus abdominus muscles should not be rigid. If the abdomen is full and rounded with a wide costal arch, the patient is considered to be strong (Yang constitution). Presence of these normal signs suggests a strong patient who can be treated more aggressively. The classic, *Spiritual Axis,* states that patients with thick and strong muscles (not just abdominal) can be treated with stronger needling and moxa techniques and can tolerate larger and stronger herbal interventions.[1]

If the abdomen (especially below the navel) is weak and flaccid, without resilience, and has a narrow costal arch, the patient is considered weak, especially in Kidney-Qi (basic vital energy). This type of patient must be treated less aggressively, and the poor constitution must be addressed. If this does not occur, the treatment outcome may be poor. Both acupuncture and herbal medicines should be prescribed. Some acupuncturists assess the umbilical area for so-called "birth trauma," which is then considered the patient's root pattern.

Yang-deficient (Abundant Yin) Constitution

Patients who are constitutionally Yang-deficient tend to be flabby (fat, and/or with poor muscle tone); the abdominal muscles are poorly developed, and the lower abdomen and flanks are cold. They may have loose muscle with thick or thin skin and always prefer heat and warm clothing. They are often of a *Tai-Yin (Spleen/pancreas)* body type, being overweight especially in their lower body (endomorphic), and their muscles are flaccid and weak. These patients fatigue easily, are often listless and low in spirits and slow to move. They may have a shallow, pale, shiny, bluish or dark complexion, and their tongue tends to be pale or bluish and swollen (with teeth marks). Their pulses are soft, yielding (not tense), weak, and deep. They often lack "moons" under their finger nails.[2]

Patients that are Yang-deficient tend to develop excess-Yin pathogens such as: Cold, Dampness, Phlegm, and Blood-stasis. They can also develop Yang disorders such as Qi-stagnation and Transformative-Heat.

Yang-strong Constitution

A patient who has reddish complexion and is strong, with firm and compact flesh (muscles), who is generally well-developed, especially in the upper body (holding head high while standing), who prefers cold, is intolerant of heat, prefers light clothing, is lively and talkative, and has strong pulses, is said to be of *Yang-strong* constitution and tends towards Excess (including Phlegm) and Heat syndromes. This type of patient is often said to be of a *Tai-Yang (or Shao-Yang) body type.*[3]

Patients with a Yang-strong constitution tend to develop Yang pathologies such as Heat, Fire, or deficiency-Yin with Empty-Fire.

---

1. Some TCM ideas on constitution such as that having short earlobes indicates weak Kidneys and a short life span are questionable and should be scientifically evaluated. At the same time it should be noted that ear morphology is one of the most sensitive indicators of malformations in other organs.

   Spiritual Axis states: "Yellow Emperor said: There are persons who can endure pain and others who cannot endure pain, yet it is not due to being courageous or timid. The brave soldier who cannot endure pain will act without fear in a difficult and dangerous situation, but will stop and cannot endure pain. The timid soldier who can endure pain, will act with fear when faced with difficult and dangerous situations but can endure pain...Shao Yu said: A person who can endure pain or cannot endure pain will have either a thick of thin skin, muscles and flesh which are firm or weak. Their pain tolerance cannot be determined by their bravery and timidity...People with firm muscles, strong bones, sinews are light and skin is thick can endure the pain of the stone needles as well as the heat of cauterization...Additionally if his complexion is black and he has excellent bones, he can endure the fire of cauterization...Firm flesh but thin skin does not endure the pain of stone probes nor the heat of the fire of cauterization...If Stomach is thick, the complexion is black, the bones are large, and the body fat, he will not be injured by the poisons of medicine. Therefore, he who is thin or with a thin Stomach will be injured by the poisons of medicines."

2. The eggs of a black chicken (or black chicken patent pills) are said to be capable of building up the moons and strengthening the patient's constitution.

Abdominal Assessment

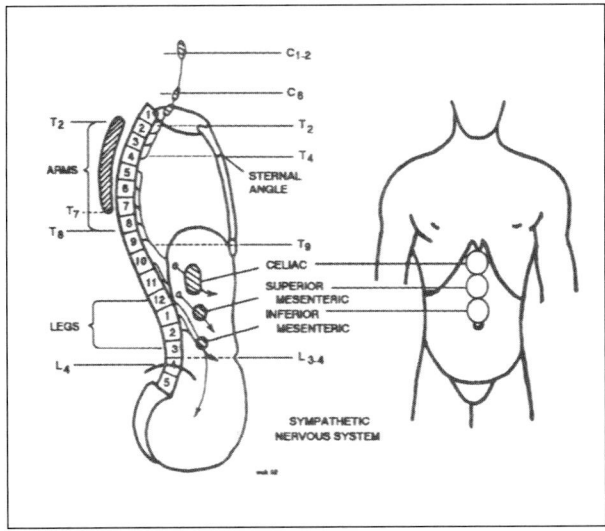

Figure 6-2: Abdominal ganglia (From Kuchera WA and Kuchera ML, Osteopathic Principles in Practice, KCOM press 1993, with permission).

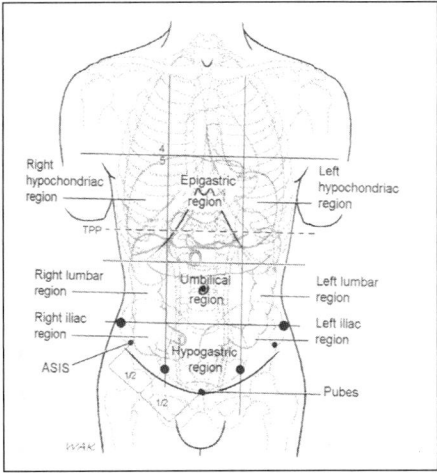

Figure 6-3: Abdominal regions and related organ (From Kuchera WA and Kuchera ML, Osteopathic Principles in Practice, KCOM press 1993, with permission).

Yin-deficient Constitution

Patients who are constitutionally Yin-deficient tend to be thin; the abdominal wall is thin, is often tight and weak, and may feel warm, especially at the upper abdomen. Their abdominal extensor muscles are floating and ticklish when pressed. Their bodies tend to be thin (ectomorphic) and are often nervous but with a weak disposition. They have an excited look and a restless expression on their face and in their eyes. They may move nervously and quickly. Their complexion may be flushed (especially cheeks and lips), grayish or yellowish, and their tongue thin and red. The shape of their head is said to be "long" with a long neck and narrow shoulders. They tend to stand bent forward. Their pulses tend to be tense, wiry, or floating and quick.

They tend to feel warmer. This can affect the quality of their sleep. They often develop Liver-congestion Qi-stagnation symptoms. They also tend to develop patterns related to Yin and Essence deficiency with hyperactive-Yang, Dryness and Empty-Heat.

Lung Disorders

The condition of the Lungs for Lung/metal disorders is palpated mainly in the upper thoracic areas around Lu-1, 2. If the skin is dry and the flesh is soft, or if the upper ribs can be easily seen or felt, the Lungs are constitutionally weak. Tenderness or indurations can be palpated at GB-20, GB-21, UB-13, UB-43, GV-12, Lu-1, and Lu-5. The right periumbilical and rectus muscles are said to relate to the Lungs. The Lung pulse may be felt to move more medially than the classical location and show qualities associated with weakness (as described by Dr. Shen).

Metal-type patients are said to have a pale white complexion, a square-shaped face with a relatively small head. Their shoulders and upper back are relatively small and they have a flat abdomen. They have small feet and hands. Their voice is strong and they move quickly (both physically and mentally). They are trustworthy, tend to be quiet and calm, and are good leaders.

Metal-type patients tend to feel good in autumn and winter, but may become sick in spring and winter by invasion of Pathogenic Factors.

The *Chapman's* upper lung anterior (diagnostic) *reflex points* are located between the third and fourth ribs near the sternum. The lower lung anterior points are located between the fourth and fifth ribs near the sternum.[4] Posterior (treatment) points are between the third and fourth transverse process (TrPr,) midway between the spinous process and the

---

3. *Spiritual Axis* states: "Those with tough muscular masses and replenished skin are [classified as] oily. Those with muscular masses which are not tough and skin that is slack are [classified as] greasy. And those in whom the skin and flesh cannot be separated are [classified as] fleshy...As for the greasy [type], those with tender flesh and coarse skin texture have a Cold body, while those with fine skin texture have a Hot body. As for the oily [type], those with tough flesh and fine skin and texture have a Hot [body], while those with coarse skin texture have a low [body temperature/Cold body]...The greasy [type] have an abundance of Qi. Those who are abundant in Qi are Hot, and those who are Hot can endure the cold. The fleshy [type] have abundance of Blood. Those who are abundant in Blood have a full form, and those who have full form possess well-balanced [Qi]. The oily [type] have Blood that is thin and Qi that is meager and slippery. Therefore, they cannot grow bulky. The above distinguishes those types from "the general populace"...The majority of people possess no superfluous skin, flesh, or fat, nor do they have any superfluity of Blood and Qi. Accordingly, their forms are neither small nor large, with their various parts in good proportion to their trunk. [That is why] they are called the general populace."

4. For information on Chapmen's reflexes see page 498.

tips of the TrPr of the third and fourth vertebrae. The lower lung points are at the level of the fourth and fifth vertebrae.

Heart Disorders

Heart/fire disorders often result in palpatory findings in the epigastric region. The areas between CV-15 and CV-14 are assessed carefully. If there is a strong pulsation or if the area is hard, the Heart may be deficient. Tenderness or indurations may develop at CV-15, CV-14, UB-15, P-6, H-3, and H-6 in both Excessive and Deficient disorders.[5]

Patients that are of the Fire-type are said to have a red complexion, have *pointed* features and small head, and have well developed muscles. Their hands and feet are said to be relatively small. They also tend to be active, energetic, but are short-tempered. They tend to "shake" as they walk. While they tend to have good judgment, they are not trustworthy (*Spiritual Axis*). The tongue tip and Heart pulse shows qualities associated with Heart problems.

They tend to feel healthy in spring and summer, and are likely to feel sick in the autumn and winter from the invasion of Pathogenic Factors. They often develop emotional problems and may suffer from sudden death.

The *Chapman's anterior myocarditis* reflex points are located in between the second and third ribs close to sternum. The posterior treatment points are found at the same level.

Liver Disorders

Liver/wood disorders can result in a darkening of the skin along the lower border of the costal arches and in abdominal palpatory findings on the right side. (Early writings, however, state the opposite, with Liver changes palpable on the left). *Difficult Issues states*: "Palpation on the left side below the ribs conveys the condition of Liver/wood."[6] The areas on the sides of the abdomen anterior to GB-26 are assessed carefully. Lack of muscle tone in the flanks or in the subcostal areas, especially at the right Liv-13 area (and diaphragm) reflect a Liver-deficiency and may predispose the patient to a "stroke." Tenderness or induration can be palpated at GV-20, GV-22, UB-18, CV-4, Sp-6, and Liv-8. The tongue edges and Liver pulse show signs of Liver weakness.

A Wood-type person is said to be tall, thin, and have a "sinewy" body. He/She may have a small head and a long-shaped face, broad shoulders, and a straight back.

Even though they look strong, their physical strength is often poor, and they tend to develop diseases caused by Pathogenic Factors in the autumn and winter. They may feel best in the spring and summer.

The *Chapman's anterior* reflex points for *congestion* of *liver* and *gallbladder* are located in the intercostal space from the mid-mammillary line up to the sternum on the right side between the sixth and seventh ribs. They may be palpable under the ribs on the right side. Soreness in the gallbladder area is common. The posterior treatment points are found at the same levels.

Spleen/pancreas Disorders

Spleen/pancreas/earth disorders may result in a somewhat yellow skin along the lower border of the costal arches, and in abdominal palpatory findings on the left side. (The classic of *Difficult Issues*, however, states the opposite, with changes of Spleen/Lung palpable on the right.) The area between CV-12 and CV-9 is assessed carefully. The Spleen/pancreas is deficient when this area feels "mushy," when it feels bloated as if full of fluid, or if the patient is extremely ticklish. Tenderness, pulsation, or indurations may be palpated at the periumbilical area, CV-12, CV-13 (14), Liv-13, UB-20, and Sp-8.[7]

Earth-type people tend to have a yellowish complexion, a round-shaped face with a relatively big head and wide jaws. Their shoulders and back are well-developed with strong musculature throughout the body. They may have a large abdomen. Their gait is firm and they lift their feet high while walking. They tend to be calm and generous. The tongue body and center and Spleen pulse show signs of Spleen/Stomach problems.

The *Chapman's anterior* reflex points are located in the intercostal space between the seventh and eighth ribs on the left side near the junction of the cartilages. Posterior points are on the same level.

Kidney Disorders

Kidney/water disorders often result in the hypogastric area, around CV-6, being cold and depressed with a tight band of tension that can be palpated deeply. Excessive pulsation[8] at this area results from Kidney-deficiency. Tenderness or induration can be often palpated at CV-7, CV-9, SI-19, UB-23, UB-52, and K-3 and 7. The tongue root and Kidney pulses show signs of weakness.

Water-Type patients are said to have a relatively dark complexion with wrinkles, a relatively big head, a round face and broad cheeks. Their abdomen is large but the shoulders

---

5. The Heart is considered the most Yang of the Yin Organs and therefore tends to develop disorders related to Excess (and sometimes is not included in the basic Deficiency patterns). However, some say the Heart should never be sedated; instead, the Pericardium is treated (Miriam Lee personal communication). This view is supported by *Spiritual Axis* chapter 71.

6. Some have interpreted this to mean the physician's side.

7. The umbilical region is also said to reflect the Kidney channel (because of the prenatal association), and the Penetrating (Chong) and Conception (Ren) channels. The region should feel elastic but not hard. Fullness or distension may indicate stagnation of Qi and Blood in the Penetrating (Chong) channel. If painful, this may indicate Blood-stasis. If very soft and lacking resiliency, this may indicate deficiency of the Kidneys or in the Conception (Ren) and Penetrating (Chong) channels.

8. One must keep in mind the possibility of aneurysms whenever a strong pulsation is felt in abdomen.

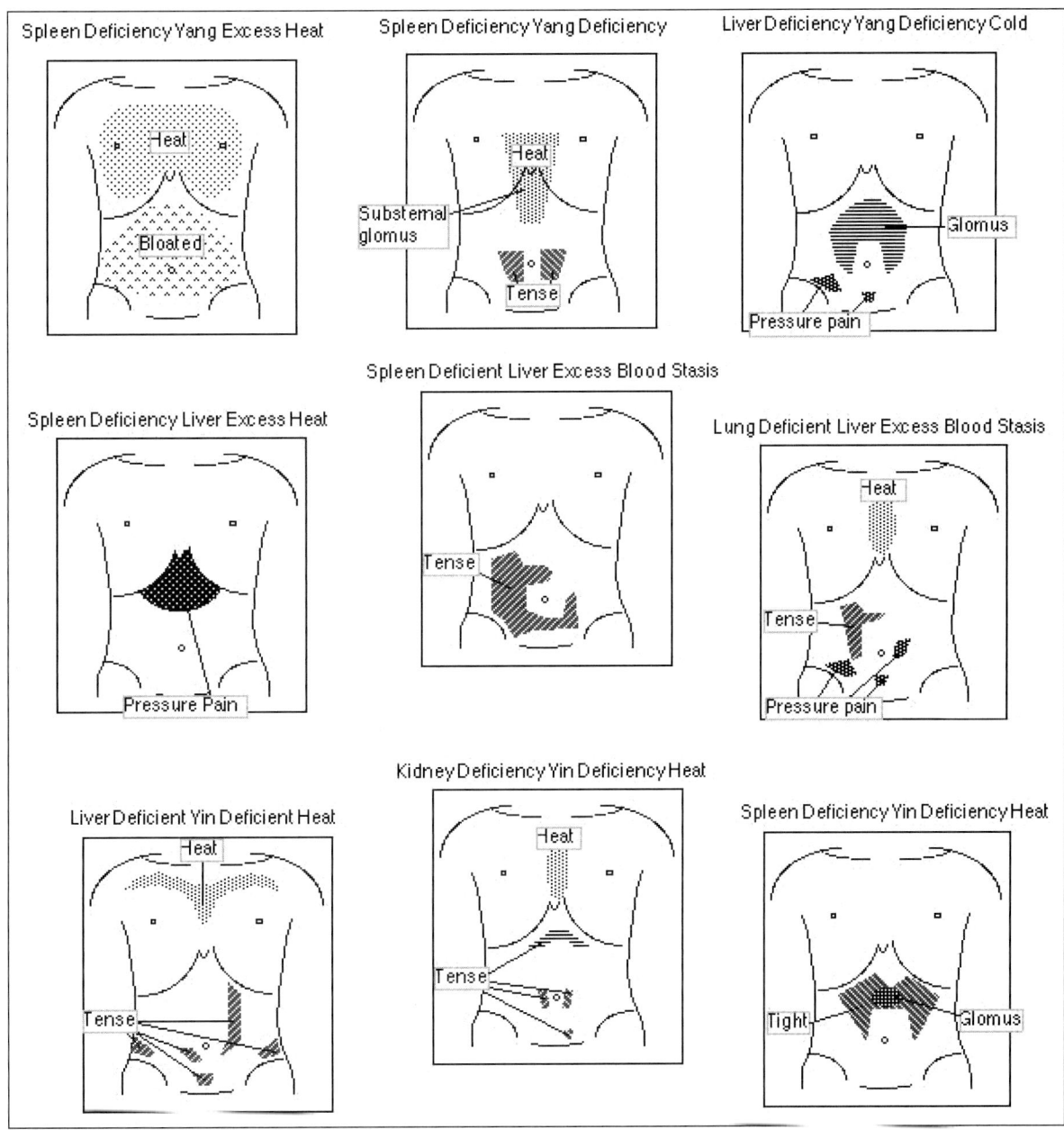

Figure 6-4: Examples of Japanese abdominal patterns (courtesy of Robert Hayden).

are narrow and small and their spine is long. They tend to be restless and keep their body in motion. They tend to "quiver" while walking. They are said to be loyal, good negotiators, and sensitive. *Golden Mirror of Medicine,* however, states that they do not respect anybody, and, while they pretend to be humble, they tend to deceive and mislead.

They tend to feel best in autumn and winter and suffer from Pathogenic Factors in the spring or summer.

The *Chapman's anterior* reflex points are located about an inch above, and lateral to the umbilicus. The points for the *adrenals* are one to one and half inches above the kidney points. The posterior (treatment) points are found between the twelfth thoracic and first lumber vertebrae. The adrenal points are between the eleventh and twelfth vertebrae.

Blood-stasis

Blood stagnation and stasis often result in palpable reactions in the lower left abdominal quadrant. The area may show discoloration, small spiderweb veins, or greenish-blue skin colors. The diaphragm is often sensitive. Liv-4, UB-18, 17

LI-11, and Sp-10 may be sensitive. The tongue and pulse may or not show signs of Blood-stasis.

Excess Dampness/Phlegm

Dampness may result in palpable changes and audible sounds, especially over and in the stomach and intestines. The abdominal wall and other tissues may feel soft and "soggy." St-40, CV-12, and Sp-9 may be sensitive. The tongue body is swollen and coat often thick. The pulse is soft, slippery, or, less frequently, just wiry.

Yin Linking (Wei) and Penetrating (Chong) Extra Channels

The findings of Liver disorders are also true for disorders of the Yin Linking and Penetrating Extra channels. Tenderness may be elicited at Liv-14, GB-24, Sp-21, and P-1.

Yin Motility (Qiao) and Conception (Ren) Extra Channels

In disorders of the Yin Motility and Conception extra channels, the abdomen is thin often, and poor muscle tone may form a trough in the midline. Tightness may be found in the lumbar region. Tenderness may be elicited at K-11 through 16, St-30, and LU-1 and 2.

Yang Linking (Wei) and Girdle (Dai) Extra Channels

In disorders of the Yang Linking and Girdle Extra channels, the ASIS area often has palpatory tenderness, especially on the left (with innominate posterior rotation). Palpatory tenderness can be found also along the Girdle channel, from the navel to the lateral edge of the abdomen.

Yang Motility (Qiao) and Governing (GV) Extra Channels

In disorders of the Yang Motility and Governing channels, palpatory tenderness may exist along the ASIS, K-11 and St-26. Tenderness may be found also at the PSIS, the posterior axilla region (SI 9-10) and the cervical vertebrae.

Examination

In the Japanese system, the abdominal examination is performed with the patient supine and the legs straight. (Because only tension is assessed, no deep muscle relaxation is needed.) The practitioner:

1. prepares the patient by wiping the abdomen dry with a tissue;

2. evaluates the area just above the abdomen, looking for radiating heat;

3. assesses the entire abdomen (using a very light touch) for areas that have abnormally high levels of cold, moisture, hardness or softness, indurations, depressions, excessive sensitivity to pain, and ticklishness or itching;

4. (Addition by the author] observes the direction of tissue preferences to drag (direction in which it is easier to pull skin);

5. pushes the abdomen with medium firmness (just enough to take out the slack between the skin and the subcutaneous tissue) and moves the skin/fat over the subcutaneous tissue, feeling for tissue texture abnormalities such as softness or hardness, small lumps, or depressions.[9]

Normal abdominal skin should be smooth and even in consistency. The abdominal wall should be soft and resilient. The skin should be neither excessively dry nor moist, and neither hot nor cold. Palpation should not elicit point tenderness or indurations, and strong pulses should not be present.

Treatment

Following assessment, abdominal areas that show pathologic findings can be treated directly and without a "diagnostic interpretation." The practitioner:

1. locates abnormal areas;

2. assesses the tissue drag preference within the abnormal areas;

3. inserts a needle shallowly in the direction of tissue resistance;

4. leaves the needle in for ten minutes;

5. in areas where a definite sense of depression is felt, moxa application is appropriate.

The information learned from abdominal palpation can be used also as further diagnostic data. The author often uses abdominal reflexes in Extra channel treatments.

SESSHOKU-SHIN TECHNIQUES. Another, less specific treatment uses Sesshoku-Shin techniques. Sesshoku-Shin is a non-insertion technique where needles are used just to stimulate the skin without penetration. The practitioner:

1. holds a regular needle (or special dull-tipped needle) between the thumb and first finger, so that the tip is exposed only slightly and the skin is stretched lightly by the other hand;

2. stimulates the abdomen by tapping the skin lightly with the needle, crisscrossing the area until a faint redness appears on the skin. This may elicit a reflex action in the desired channels.

Many Japanese acupuncturists use specific distal points to treat specific findings in the abdomen. For example, Kiiko Matsumoto treats low back pain as follows (Magidoff 1999):

---

9. This technique (step 5) can be used anywhere on the channel systems or on the musculoskeletal system to find stagnated acupuncture-Kori, or pressure sensitive-Ashi points.

- For palpatory tenderness and ropiness at the ASIS region (said to reflect sacral twists): GB-26 (local point) and K-7 (distal point).
- For tenderness over the inguinal ligament (said to reflect sacral tilt): St-13, GB-26 and Inner Yin (5 fingers above K-10).
- For tenderness over the inguinal groove or inner thigh (also said to reflect sacral tilt): Liv-4.

Abdominal Confirmation and Herbs

In general, when using Kampo (Japanese style herbalogy), patients with subcostal findings may be treated with Radix Bupleuri (Chai Hu) containing formulas as in Figure 6-5; with epigastric findings they may be treated with Rhizoma Pinelliae containing formulas; with periumbilical findings with Poriae Cocos (Fu Ling) or Rhizoma Atractylodes (Bai Zhu) containing formulas; and hypogastric findings with Radix Rehmanniae (Di Huang) or Semen Persicae (Tao Ren) containing formulas.[10]

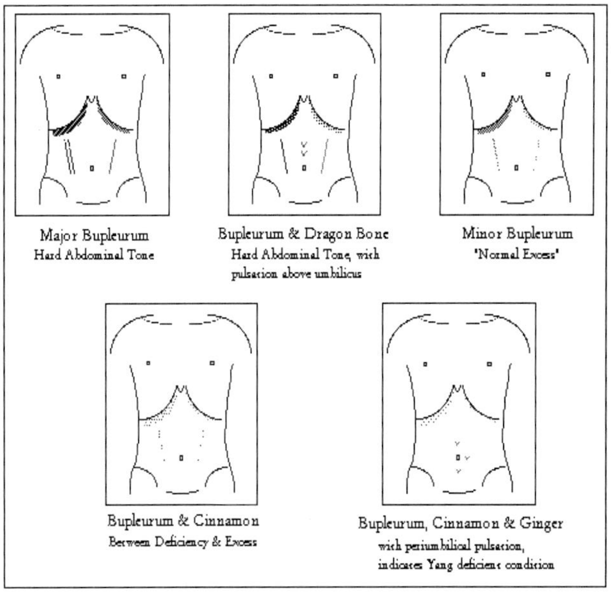

Figure 6-5: Examples of abdominal patterns for bupleri formulas (courtesy of Robert Hayden).

Meridian Therapy (Keiraku Chiryo)

Meridian Therapy is a relatively new style of acupuncture which was developed in the mid-1930s. Meridian Therapy is based primarily on the early classics such as the *Classic of Internal Medicine, piritual Axis,* and *Classic of Difficult Issues.* The primary paradigm used to diagnose and treat is that of the Five Phases. While all of the tools of four examinations are used, it is primarily the pulse that determines the pattern. The basic pattern of imbalance is always defined in terms of a deficiency of a Yin Organ or meridian (channels). According to Shudo and Brown, the meridians (channels) are considered more Yang and tend towards excess (Jitsu), while the Organ systems are Yin and tend towards deficiency (Kyo), especially with aging (Shudo and Brown 1990). The basic Yin Organs or meridians (channels) have a tendency to become deficient and are associated with four basic patterns (Sho):

- Lung Sho: Lung and Spleen Deficient
- Spleen Sho: Spleen and Heart (Pericardium) Deficient
- Liver Sho: Liver and Kidney Deficient
- Kidney Sho: Kidney and Lung Deficient

There is no Heart Sho because the Heart itself will rarely be deficient (it is the most Fire of the Organs, i.e., most Yang), and when diseased would be too serous.

As with most Japanese acupuncture systems, palpation is emphasized not only to determine the pattern (pulse and abdominal palpation), but also in point location. Points are not only considered to move and have locations that vary between individuals, but the practitioner also must palpate to find the "live points." Acupuncture points are considered more than just anatomical landmarks: they are manifestations of a functional problem in the body. As such, they are normally dormant, becoming active only when a pathological condition begins to form, and as stated earlier according to Shima text book location pertain to healthy people. In Deficient conditions according to Shima points move proximately, and, in Excess conditions, points are said to move distally. Robert Hayden (2001) also states that live points not only move, and often some distance away from their anatomical location (frequently seen with connecting [Luo] points), but the same live point on different sides of the body, for example SP-4, may be in very different locations. By the time the patient returns for their next visit, the particular live point will likely have moved or may even have disappeared. Palpation is also used to reassess the quality and appropriateness of the treatment. Live points are discovered by palpating for tissue reactions such as: increase or decrease in skin tension or turgor, changes in skin moisture, temperature, smoothness, thickening or thinning and a sensation of draft arising from the point; changes in subcutaneous tissues such as indurations, puffiness, lumps, adherent tissues; and changes in deeper tissues such as tight bands, induration, tightness or lack of tone, increased or decrease in temperature, etc. In general, treatment to the "root" using the Five-Phases is emphasized.

---

10. This is an over-simplification of the Japanese systems of herbalogy but is still helpful as a guide.

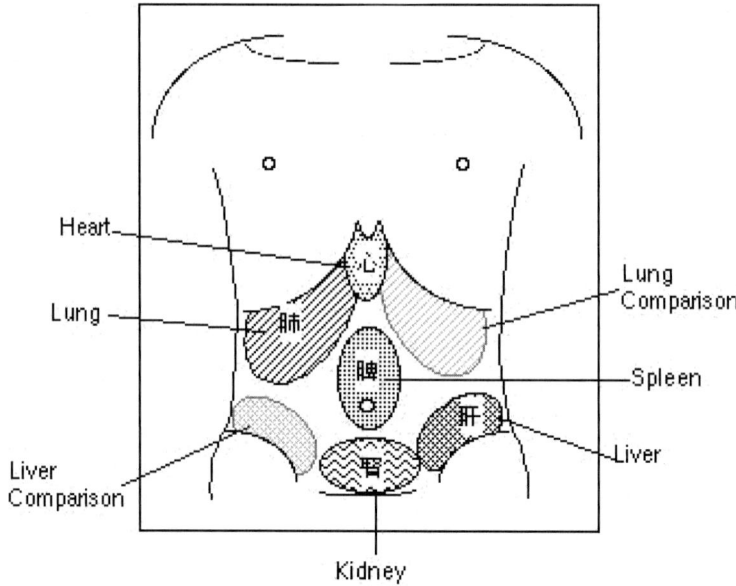

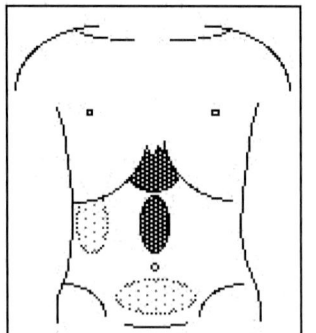 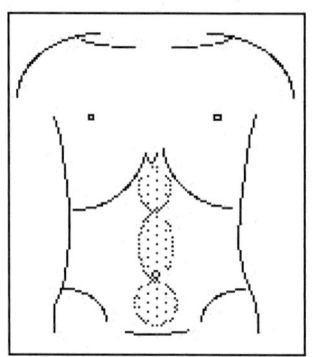 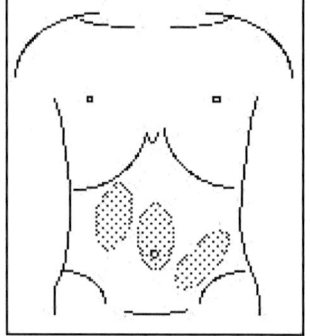

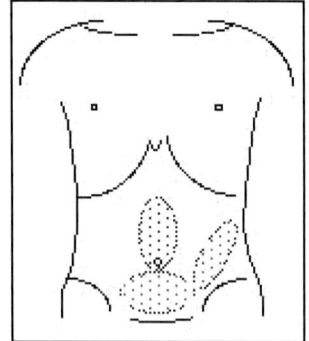 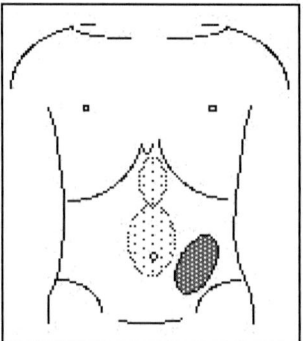

Figure 6-6: Additional examples of Japanese abdominal patterns (courtesy of Robert Hayden).

Meridian Therapy (Keiraku Chiryo)

Table 6-1: Pulses: Organ Associations

Wrist	Position	Depth	Organs
Left	Distal	Superficial	Small Intestine
		Deep	Heart
	Middle	Superficial	Gallbladder
		Deep	Liver
	Proximal	Superficial	Bladder
		Deep	Kidney
Right	Distal	Superficial	Large Intestines
		Deep	Lung
	Middle	Superficial	Stomach
		Deep	Spleen
	Proximal	Superficial	Triple Warmer
		Deep	Pericardium

According to Hayden, Meridian Therapy is not monolithic. There are many different streams of thought coming from a common pool of *Nan Jing*-based theory (*Classic of Difficult Issues* theory). Major variations on this theme have been developed by, among others, Kodo Fukushima's Toyo Hari association and Masakazu Ikeda's Kampo Inyokai. The Toyo Hari association was originally conceived as a study group for blind acupuncturists. As a result, their primary emphasis is on very subtle palpatory skills. Their needling tends to be very light, with non-inserted, or contact needling (sesshokushin) being a characteristic feature. Another strong characteristic of Toyo Hari is that the pulse is used as a system of feedback for virtually all phases of the treatment and is the standard by which a successful treatment is judged. Masakazu Ikeda is a practitioner of Kampo as well as Meridian Therapy.[11] As a result, he has extended the theoretical parameters of Meridian Therapy by the addition of elements from Shang Han Lun theory (an herbal tradition). In addition to these, there are numerous other associations and hundreds of practitioners of Meridian Therapy. Some do straight four-pattern, root-branch types of treatment, while others may combine elements of other systems, such as Extraordinary Vessels (Kikei Hachi Myaku). The theoretical construct on which Meridian Therapy is founded has proven to be quite flexible to adaptation, in addition to its clinical utility. Meridian Therapists account only for about 10-20% of acupuncturists in Japan. The majority of acupuncturist use "scientific" based modern techniques.

Pulse balancing is very helpful in making patients feel generally healthier and stronger. Frequently, however, ortho-

---

11. In Japan, only medical doctors and pharmacists may prescribe herbal medicine.

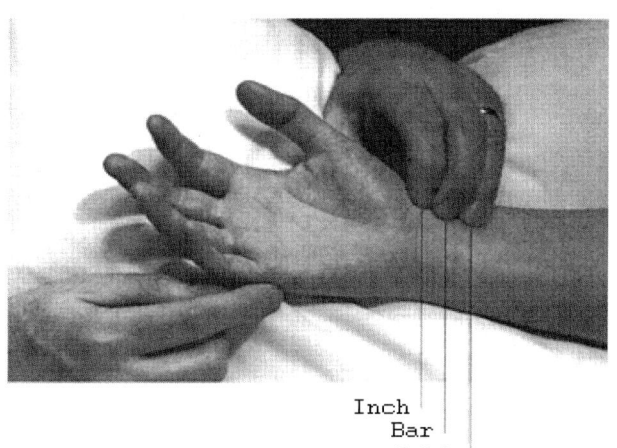

Inch
Bar
Cubit

pedic complaints (and signs) remain and a more specific intervention is needed. The author often uses pulse balancing with four needle techniques, although looking also at other pulse qualities from the those described in Meridian Therapy. Pulse balancing is considered a "root" treatment.

Pulse Diagnosis

Pulse diagnosis, the heart of the OM assessment method, is a complex and highly subjective system of diagnosis. The practitioner assesses six positions of the radial artery pulse (near the wrist) for a minimum of twenty-eight characteristics at three depths. In-depth discussion of these techniques is not within the scope of this book.

A simpler version of pulse diagnosis, used with the Japanese Meridian balancing system, is more easily learned and is a good way to evaluate the patient's meridian/channel balance and so-called "energetic" health. The practitioner evaluates the six positions of the pulse for relative Deficiency or Excess, which reflects the balance of the meridians (channels) and Organs.

Wrist Unit Measurement

The area over the radial artery just above the wrist is divided into three positions: distal (called *inch*), middle (*bar*), and proximal (*cubit*). The locations of these three positions are based on the unit measurement by which acupuncture measures distances and locations of points. The entire anterior aspect of the forearm between the cubital and carpal creases is considered to be twelve units (*cun*), and the quality of the skin along the forearm is said to reflect the same qualities within the pulses.

- The proximal pulse is two units above the crease of the wrist.
- The middle position is located usually next to the radial eminence and is slightly proximal to the highest point of the radial eminence.
- The distal position is located halfway between the middle position and the crease of the wrist.

Finger Placement

The practitioner's finger placement and the patient's wrist position are extremely important for a correct reading. Any inconsistency between the two results in false interpretations. The practitioner's fingers should be arranged in a straight line on top of the patient's wrist positions, with the fingertips resting against the tendon of the flexor carpi radialis.

THREE PALPATION POSITIONS. The practitioner palpates the pulses on both wrists simultaneously. The beginner may find it easier to assess one position at a time, i.e., proximal, middle, and then distal, palpating each position at three depths: superficial, middle, and deep.

- At middle depth the pulse is felt most strongly with medium pressure.
- At superficial depth the pulse is barely palpable with very light pressure.
- At deep depth the pulse just about disappears due to application of strong pressure.

The major qualities of the pulses can be assessed best at the middle depth of pulses, where the "Stomach-Qi" is evaluated. If the Stomach-Qi pulse is very Deficient (especially in the middle right position or Spleen pulse), the patient is said to be seriously ill.

If the skin at the forearm is:

- reddish, warm, slippery, and soft, it may indicate a Heat disorder;
- pale, cold, and tight, it may indicate Cold disorder;
- tense and bouncy, it may indicate Liver/wood disorder;
- dry and rough, it may indicate Lung/metal or Blood disorder;
- soft, "mushy," and damp, it may indicate Spleen/earth disorder;
- cold, slightly moist, and hard, it may indicate Kidney/water disorder.

Strength and Size of Pulse

The meridian balancing system emphasizes the relative strength and size of the pulse for diagnosis. Treatment is then applied to the "weakest Yin" (deep pulse) meridian/Organ system. The relative strength of the pulse at a similar position (distal, middle, and proximal) and the pulses on the control cycle (see Five Phases chapter 1) are assessed and should be equal in strength and size. A pulse that is weak at both the Yin and Yang depth (superficial and deep) is considered balanced, even though weak. For the orthopedic patient, treating the most Excessive Yang (superficial) pulse is some times helpful.

Treatment

The points used for treatment vary. Generally, the Source point on the most deficient meridian may be used first. After needle insertion, the practitioner rechecks the pulse to see whether a positive change has occurred. Only mild and superficial stimulation (between 1-3mm) is advocated. The needle may or may not be retained. If the response is inadequate, either mild stimulation to the tonification point or the Four Needle techniques (Table 5-16 on page 315 and Table 5-17 on page 315) can be used.[12] Excessive pulses should be treated by first draining the accumulation points, and then (if necessary) by applying the Four Needle technique. For the most part, needle insertion is very shallow, especially when the tonifying and stimulation is very mild.

Five Phase treatments are root (initial) treatments intending to treat the patient's central imbalance (Yin Yang House 2003). The Five Phase treatment follows a five-step protocol, and adjunctive techniques may be used within these steps and/or afterwards to address the patient's symptomatology directly:

1. Diagnose and treat the patient's primary Yin imbalance (Sho). The side for initial needling should generally be chosen based on a preponderance of symptoms on one side. One treats the "healthier" side, or, lacking information about that, one bases one's choice on gender:

---

12. Four needle techniques are not necessarily part of Meridian Therapy but are often used by the author.

the left side for men and the right side for women. Use #1 needles retaining, for ten minutes. Points used are:

- Spleen Sho - Sp-3/2 & P-7
- Lung Sho - Lu-9 & Sp-3
- Kidney Sho - K-7 & Lu-5 or Lu-8
- Liver Sho - Liv-8 & K-10.

2. Balance the controlling cycle for the primary Sho selected above. This is diagnosed by using the pulse. In those cases where there is no clear secondary imbalance, you needle the points listed above on the opposite side (treat bilaterally). Use #1 needle for tonification and #2 for dispersion, on the opposite side from Sho, retaining for the remainder of the ten minutes

- Spleen Sho: Earth controls Water—Kidney Deficiency (no K excess) use K-3. If Wood controls Earth—Liver Excess or Deficiency use Liv-3.
- Lung Sho: Metal controls Wood—Liver Excess or Deficiency use Liv-3. If Fire controls Metal, there is no Heart treatments.
- Kidney Sho: Water controls Fire, there is no Heart treatments. If Earth controls Water, Spleen Excess or Deficiency use Sp-3.
- Liver Sho: Wood controls Earth—Spleen Excess or Deficiency use Sp-3. If Metal controls Wood, Lung Excess or Deficiency use Lu-9.

3. Balance the Yang meridians based on the pulse. First treat the most deficient Yang pulse (tonification) and then treat the most excess Yang pulse (dispersion). It is possible to have either no Yang pulse imbalances or only one clear Deficient pulse or Excess pulse. Use #1 for tonification and #2 for dispersion, on the side of the chosen meridian (channel), retaining for one or two minutes for tonification and twenty to thirty seconds for dispersion.

On the right side:
- Large Intestine—Tonify LI-11 or Disperse LI-6.
- Stomach—Tonify St-36 or Disperse St-40.
- Triple Warmer—Tonify TW-4 or Disperse TW-5.

On the left side:
- Small Intestine—Tonify or Disperse SI-7.
- Gall Bladder—Tonify or Disperse GB-37.
- Urinary Bladder—Tonify or Disperse UB-58.

4. Treat the related back Shu points. Choose the Shu points related to the primary Five Phase pattern you selected, adding, if appropriate, the Shu points for the controlling cycle as well. For example, if you treated P-7 and Sp-3 for Spleen Sho and had a Kidney-deficiency secondary, you could treat UB-14 or UB-15 (P or H), UB-20 (Sp), and possibly UB-23 (K). Use #1, #2, or #3 needles, retaining for two to ten minutes.

5. Treat the branch, i.e., symptomatic treatment. This is generally based on the presenting complaint(s) and is aimed at alleviating symptoms. Again, point selection is mainly based on palpatory findings along the affected meridian or body area. Empirical points are used as well. For the symptomatic phase of treatment, the needles used may be thicker and insertion may be deeper. However, usually the needling technique is still very mild in comparison to many of the Chinese systems. Only occasionally-evoked needle sensation (De Qi or Hibi-Ki) is sought. Symptomatic treatments can include moxibustion (Okyuu), blood-letting (Shiraku), cupping, and retention of intradermal needles (Hinaishin or Empishin). Some use Extra channels and Sinew channels.

In summary. the approach of Meridian Therapy can be helpful in that it treats the "root" and is very gentle. To treat the root the practitioner:

- tonifies the deficient Yin meridian (channel) and its mother;
- treats the controlling cycle;
- treats the symptoms (branch) and pathogenic Qi (Jacki, evil-Qi/Ki), usually by using the Yang meridians (channels).

Symptoms are treated using a variety of methods such as: Extra channels, Sinew channels, intradermal needles, cupping, etc. This approach requires highly developed palpation skills. Table 6-1 lists the Organs associated with the wrist pulses.

Auricular Therapy

Auricular therapy is very useful clinically and does not require knowledge of OM/TCM. Auricular therapy is helpful as an adjunctive therapy in musculoskeletal disorders. It is

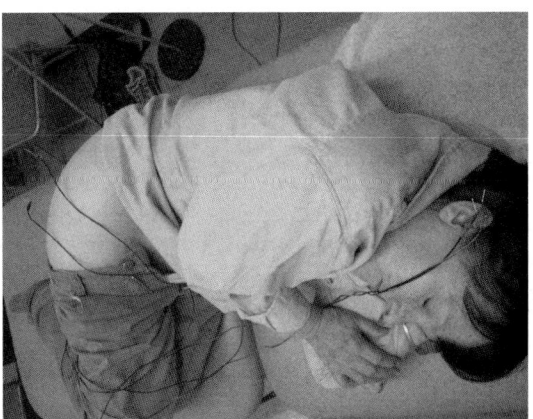

Figure 6-7: Patient treated with combined ear-body acupuncture. The positive pole of a monopolar microstimulator is connected to the ear and the negative pole to hip area motor points.

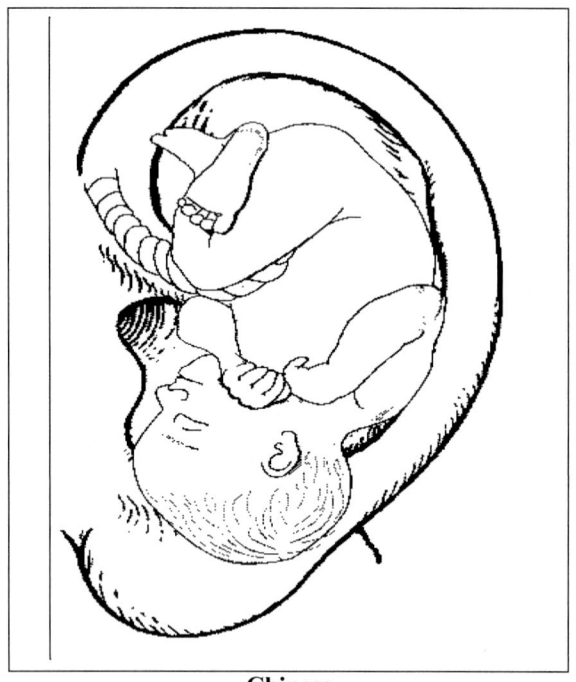
Chinese

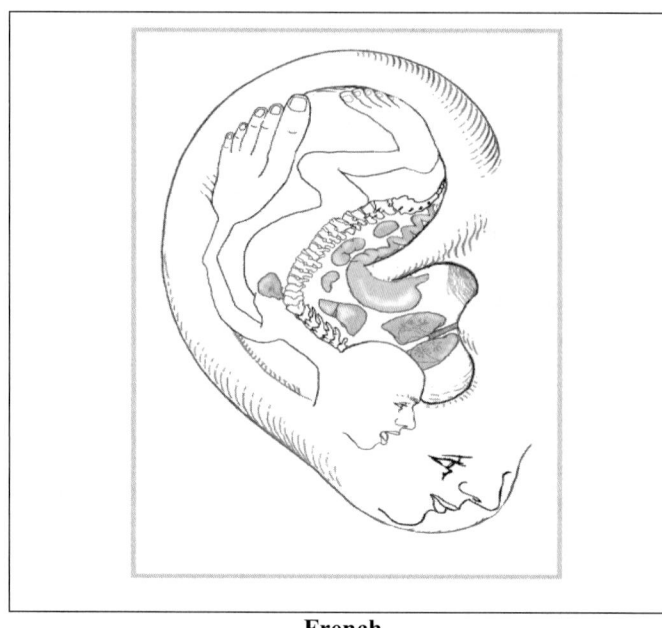
French

Figure 6-8: Ear topographical maps.

the experience of this author, however, that clinical results obtained by auricular therapy are often palliative only, and, therefore, should be used together with other treatment methods. As with abdominal diagnosis, auricular therapy draws on the concept that a singled out part of the body such as the ear can have a somatotopic (fractal) system representation that can show dysfunctions of the entire body bioholographically.[13] The ear has origins that are mesodermal (innervated by cranial V), endodermal (cranial X) and ectodermal (C1, C2, C3) that may represent a somatotopic mechanism of embryonic tissues. Embryological work by Bourdiol (1982) has shown that innervations to the ear come from nerves V_3, VII, IX, X, and from branches of the superficial cervical plexus. These nerves travel from the ear to the cranial nerve inputs and to the reticular formation of the brainstem, and, therefore, connect the ear to cerebrospinal innervation and spinothalamic fibers in the reticular formation[14] which may be responsible for the diagnostic painful response seen in the ear (Helms *ibid*). Auricular morphology is one of the most sensitive indicators of malformations in other organs. Auricular malformation has been observed in Turner's syndrome, Potter's syndrome, Treacher-Collins syndrome, Patau's syndrome, Edwards' syndrome, Noonan's syndrome, Goldenhar's syndrome, Beckwith's syndrome, Digeorge syndrome, cri du chat syndrome, fragile x syndrome, and in maternal diabetes and atherosclerosis (Shang *ibid*).

Origins of Auricular Therapy

Auricular therapy was developed, not through TCM, but by Dr. Paul Nogier, a French physician. In their own development of this type of therapy, the Chinese considered both Dr. Nogier's observations and quotations from *Classic of Internal Medicine* that states that all the Yang channels pass through the ear and the Yin channels meet in the ear. Working in the mode of Dr. Nogier's research, the Chinese developed another topographical map that varies a little from the French map, but is very similar (Figure 6-8).

Historic Uses of the Ear for Treatment

Practitioners in other cultures, such as French folk healers, Persians, Egyptians, and Greeks (Hippocrates) have used the ear to treat various diseases. A blind study at the UCLA pain clinic demonstrated a 92% concurrence in musculoskeletal injury diagnosis between medical and auricular diagnoses (Oleson et al 1980). Differentiable electrical characteristics in different auricular points were shown in cases of cancer and immune disease as well (Bing et al 2001). A recent study

---

13. Miniaturized areas represent reflexively the whole body, much as a fragment of a hologram shows the entire hologram.
14. The reticular formation is a modulating intersection that activates and inhibits cranial, spinal, somatic, visceral, and autonomic impulses (see chapter 2).

Table 6-2: Auricular Master Points

Name of Point	Use
Point Zero/Solar Plexus	Used often at beginning of treatment: • to bring ear and entire body into homeostatic balance; • to activate other ear points.
Shen Men/Spirit Gate	Used commonly: • to treat anxiety and other psychiatric disorders; • to treat pain; • to regulate the nervous system. Almost always active and tender. Can be used as a standard for impedance measurements. Useful for antistress (adaptogenic) treatment.
Endocrine/Internal Secretions	Used often for weak, depleted patients. Important for regulating hormonal system.
Sympathetic	Used: • to regulate autonomic nervous system, blood circulation to limbs, and temperature, and for pain control; • commonly for musculoskeletal disorders.
Thalamus/Pain Control	Used to inhibit spinothalamic (pain) transmission.
Master Cerebral/Psychosomatic	Used for chronic pain and psychosomatic disorders. Anxiety.
Master Sensorial/Eye	Used to treat distorted perceptions, both somatic and psychological.
Master Oscillation/Cerebral Hemispheres	Used to treat problems of cerebral literality (often found with dyslexia). If untreated, literality problems can reduce auricular therapy effectiveness.
Tranquilizer/Valium/Hypertension	Used: • to relieve muscle tension, general tension; • to sedate; • to lower blood pressure; • anxiety.
Stress Control/Adrenal	Used to control stress by regulating the adrenal system.

showed that Nogier's pulse diagnostic technique (VAS) can demonstrate the accurate location of active ear points. By touching an acupuncture needle on an active auricular acupuncture point, the radial artery wall over the styloid process changes in tone more prominently than when inactive points on the auricle are touched. This was demonstrated by objective digitalized measurements (Ikezono and Ackerman 2003).

Examination

A careful inspection of the ear should precede any therapeutic procedure. Frequently, signs such as an edematous, inflamed area, pronounced superficial capillaries, flaking, dryness, and discoloration are seen in reflex-auricular areas that reflect bodily pathology or dysfunction. Active areas are usually tender and have a lower skin impedance. It is important to think of zones rather then "points" when evaluating the ear.

For auricular diagnosis, an electric skin resistance measuring device (point locator) is ideal. The practitioner:

1. cleans the ear with alcohol and wipes the ear dry. (This is not done by many practitioners and may or may not be significant);
2. uses a point locator probe to scan all areas, making sure the pressure used is uniform throughout;
3. treats positive areas as well as functional points.

Chronic, unresolved lesions frequently leave skin changes at their reflex auricular areas. These are tender and often are edematous with superficial capillary clustering. Therefore, they have low skin resistance. Healed lesions often show an area in the ear that has increased electrical conductivity but is not tender.

Treatment

Since the ear is made mostly of cartilage and its blood supply is poor, it is imperative to use appropriate, clean techniques when needling ear points. There have been case reports of infections and cartilage calcification following acupuncture treatments.

Tools

The surface of the ear is very sensitive so a good needle technique is required to minimize pain. The ideal needle (½-inch, 36/38 gauge or Korean hand acupuncture needle) can be

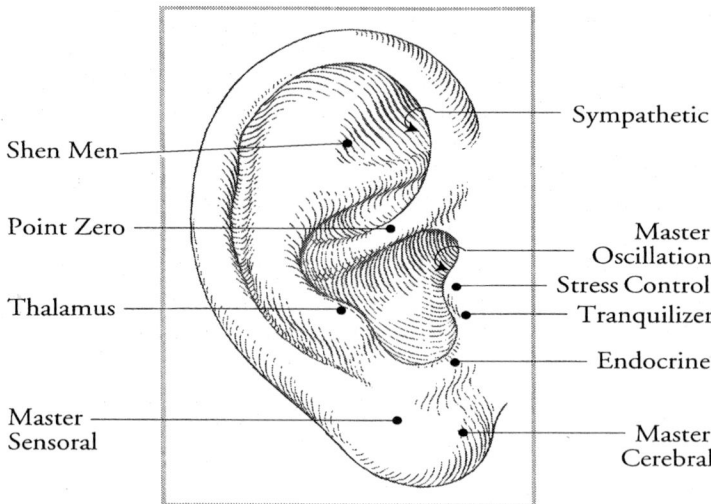

Figure 6-9: Master points

inserted quickly with a twist of the fingers, allowing for minimal discomfort and maximum control. A guide tube may be used. However, controlling the exact site of insertion is more difficult. Also available are semi-permanent needles, magnets, metal balls, and seeds that can be left in place for as long as one or two weeks.

Points

Generally, points are selected on the ipsilateral ear over the reflex area that corresponds to the injured tissue (Figure 6-8). For the treatment to be effective, the point must be active. When treating pain, stimulation to the points at the back of the ear directly behind the active point in the front is helpful. In the French system there are several phases in which representation of bodily areas change at different times. Scanning these may be helpful when the primary points are insufficient.[15]

Frequently several important points called *Master points* are used at the same time. Master points are used on the patient's dominant side (right ear in right-handed patient). Many Chinese practitioners often needle men on the left and women on the right. Table 6-2 lists some uses for each Master point.

Auricular therapy is frequently combined with other channel therapies. Electrical stimulation can be connected between the affected area and the reflex area in the ear (Figure 6-7). Areas in the ear that have clusters of blood vessels can be bled.

Metacarpal Bone Systems

This is also a modern system developed in China. It uses the first metacarpal bone as an holographic image of the body. The first metacarpal bone is divided from its head to the base into twelve sections. The distal end (LI-3) is said to represent the head. The proximal end (Ling Gu) is said to represent the lower body. The practitioner palpates for sensitivity at the related area and needles right against the bone. Points can be chosen on the painful side or on the opposite side. The fifth metacarpal (SI channel) bone can be used in the same way.

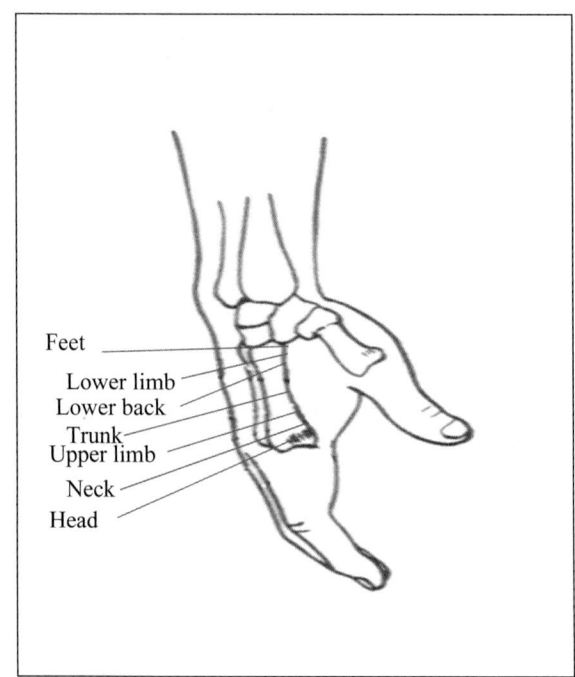

Figure 6-10: Metacarpal system.

---

15. Many such holographic (micro) systems have been described. There are systems using the nose, chin, eye, scalp, hand, and feet.

Wrist and Ankle Acupuncture

Wrist and Ankle Acupuncture (Zhang 1991) is a modern technique developed by a Chinese physician, Dr. Zhang Xinshu. Dr. Zhang's method incorporates longitudinal symptom patterns that are similar, but not identical to, the twelve TCM cutaneous regions. The cutaneous regions are superficial areas on the skin (TCM dermatomes) which are under the influence of the Main channels (Figure 6-12 on page 349). The six wrist points (Table 6-4) and six ankle points (Table 6-3) are located in the centers of their respective regions, a few points on the Yin side of the joint, a few on the Yang side, and a few at the intersecting areas (Figure 6-11).

Wrist Points

The wrist points, labeled *Upper 1* through *Upper 6*, are in a circular shape located about two finger-breadths proximal to the wrist crease.

Ankle Points

The points at the ankle, called *Lower 1* through *Lower 6*, are located in an approximate circle, three finger-breadths proximal to the highest spot on the malleoli.

Selecting Points

Selection of points is based on the location of symptoms and signs (Table 6-3 through Table 6-5). When pain is unilateral, the practitioner needles the point on the affected side (although points can also be chosen on the basis of contralateral and left-right relations). When pain is at midline or if it is on the side but the location of the discomfort is difficult to ascertain, the practitioner needles the points bilaterally.

Wrist points are used for pain in the upper body; ankle points are used for pain in the lower parts. In motor impairment of the limbs (such as paralysis and tremor), Upper 5 is used for the upper limbs and Lower 4 is used for the lower limbs.

Needling Techniques in Wrist and Ankle Acupuncture

During wrist and ankle acupuncture, the needle penetrates only subcutaneously.[16] The practitioner:

1. pulls the skin tight at the site of insertion;
2. introduces a 4 cm, 32-gauge needle at a 30-degree angle, toward the painful site (usually proximally);
3. inserts the needle until sensing the first loss of resistance;
4. verifies that the depth of the needle is correct.

---

16. Subcutaneous needling is used when treating superficial fascial layer restrictions as well.

Table 6-3: Ankle Points

Point	Location	Use
Lower 1	Close to medial anterior border of tendocalcaneus muscle.	Shao Yin distribution. Infrequent.
2	On medial aspect of the leg at edge of tibia.	Tai Yin distribution. Sometimes. For SI, lumbosacral ligamentous, and L3 disc lesions.
3	1cm medial to anterior crest of tibia.	Jue Yin distribution. Seldom.
4	Midway between anterior crest of tibia and anterior border of fibula.	Yang Ming distribution. Frequent.
5	On posterior border of fibula, in groove between border of fibula and tendon of peroneus longus muscle.	Shao Yang distribution. Frequent.
6	Close to lateral border of tendocalcaneus.	Tai Yang distribution. Frequent.

Table 6-4: Wrist Points

Point	Location	Use
Upper 1	Between ulna and tendon of flexor carpi ulnaris muscle. Found by sliding thumb along border of ulna until point is found in a depression between border of ulna and radial side of tendon.	Shao Yin distribution. Very frequent.
2	On ventral side of arm between tendons of palmaris longus and flexor carpi radialis muscles. Treatment may be blocked by a blood vessel. Needle insertion can be aimed proximally to avoid the vessel.	Jue Yin distribution. Infrequent, for thoracic and rib dysfunctions, and for muscular headaches.
3	On the ventral side of the arm on the border of the radius, between the radius and the radial artery.	Tai Yin distribution. Seldom used.
4	At the lateral surface of the radius.	Yang Ming distribution. Sometimes, for cervical lesions.
5	In center of dorsal side of forearm, midway between ulna and radius.	Shao yang distribution. Very frequent.
6	On dorsal side of forearm, 1cm medial to edge of ulna.	TaiYang distribution. Frequent.

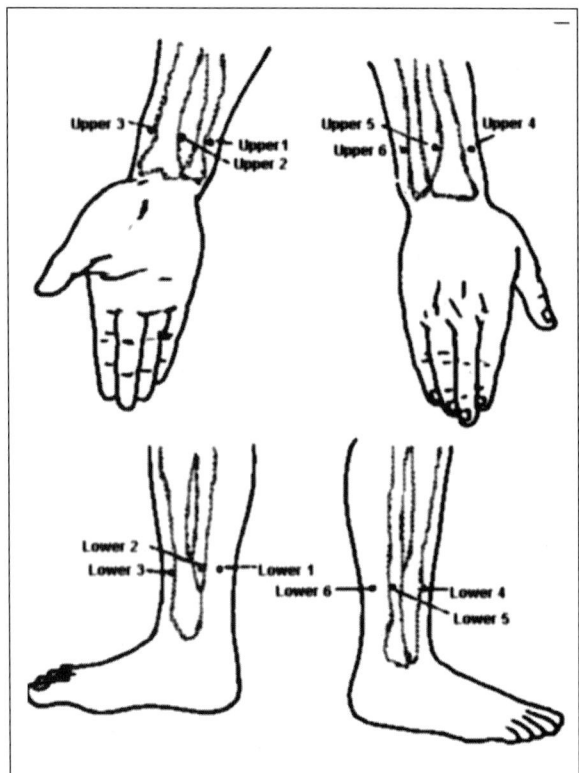

Figure 6-11: Wrist and ankle points.

Table 6-5: Wrist and Ankle Points: Areas and Types of Pain

Area/Type of Pain	Point to be Needled
Unilateral	Affected side
Midline	Bilateral
Location difficult to distinguish	Bilateral
Upper body	Wrist
Lower body	Ankle
Upper limbs: motor Impairment (paralysis, tremor, etc.)	Upper 5
Lower limbs: motor Impairment (paralysis, tremor, etc.)	Upper 4

If the practitioner were to let go of the needle, it should drop and lie flat on the skin surface. If the needle were not to lie flat, the needle would be either too deep or too shallow;

5. advances the needle subcutaneously, about 3.5 cm. This should be painless;

6. (if the patient feels pain) adjusts the needle;

7. (generally) asks the patient to mobilize the affected area;

8. leaves the needles in about one-half hour. (In a few cases the needle can remain for as long as twenty-four hours.)

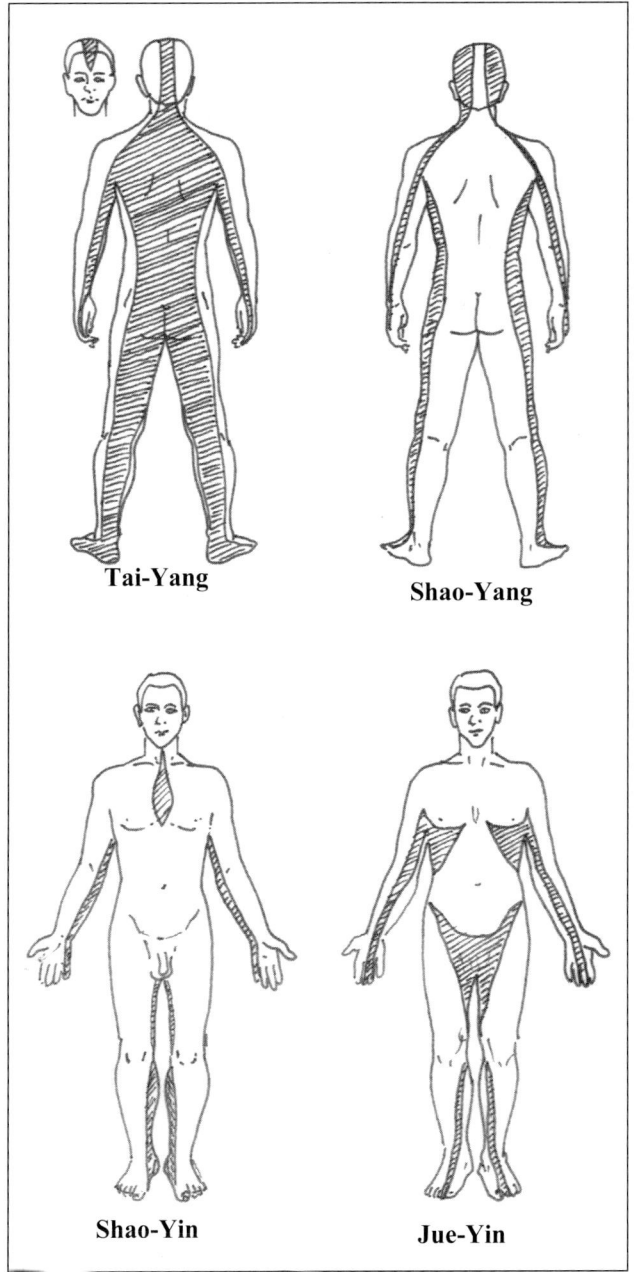
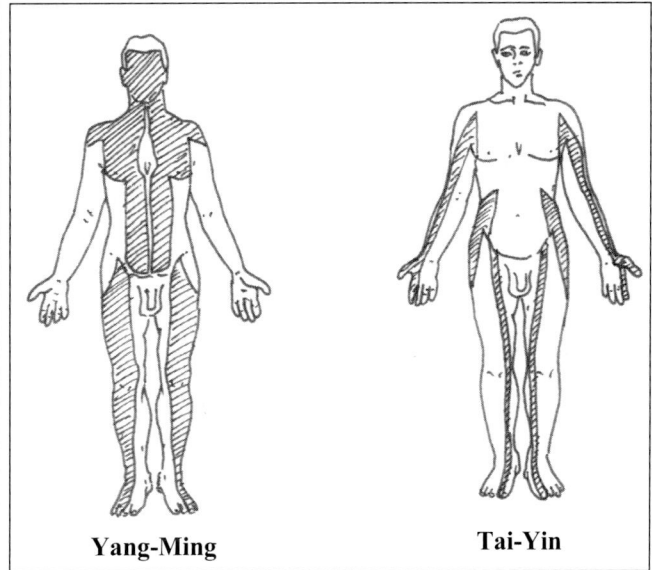

Figure 6-12: OM dermatomes.

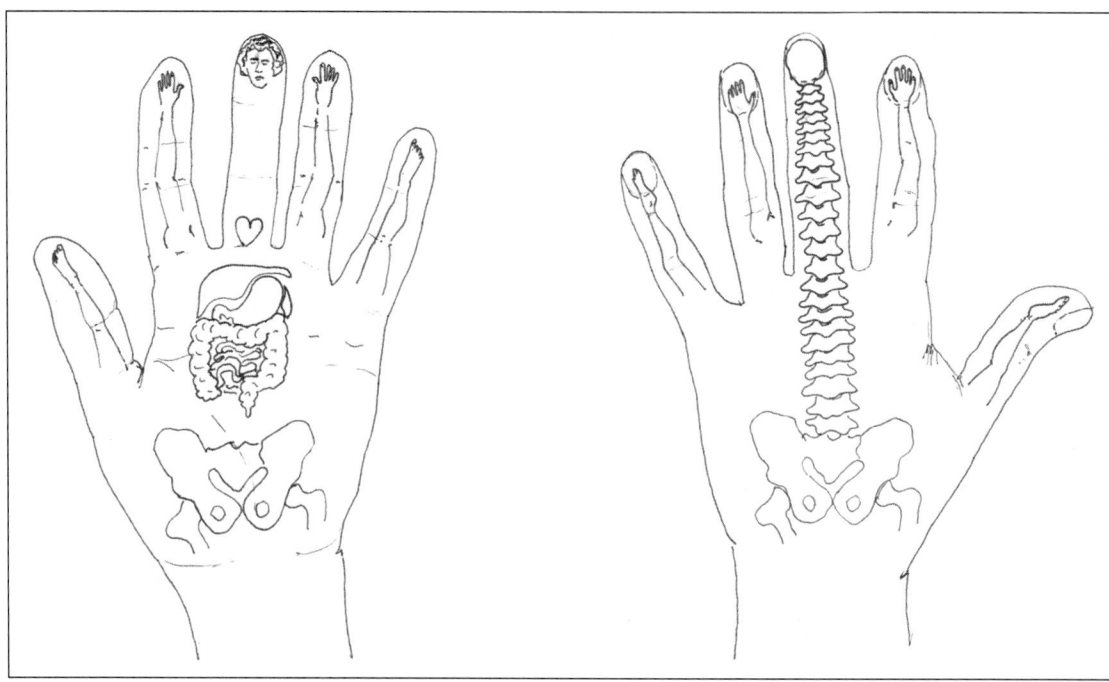

Figure 6-13: Korean hand acupuncture map.

Korean Hand Acupuncture

Korean hand acupuncture is another modern technique that uses the hands as a holographic image of the body. The somatic map can be used by finding a tender spot at the area that corresponds to the patients symptomatic area. Treatment may be achieved using needles, magnets, laser, or electrical stimulation (Figure 6-13).

Tong/Lee-style Acupuncture

Tong-style acupuncture is a style that in part has been passed down within the Tong family (said to be about 300 years old). It is an effective ancillary the technique for management of musculoskeletal disorders.[17] Tong-style is a system that *in part* involves older theories relying on early numerological correspondence systems and the needling techniques described in *Spiritual Axis* that treat points in regions away from the symptomatic areas. It is also said to be related to the Spleen and Stomach school of Li-Dong. The Tong system mainly uses bodily *reflections* (analogous areas) that relate each body area to another area, mainly on the extremities (These are imaging or somatoreflex systems, e.g., the hand and points of the hand reflect and can be used to treat the head, or the foot, etc.) There are eight (or nine) main imaging systems within Tong-style, the most commonly used being the "same name" upper and lower channels systems (i.e., using Yang-Ming points of the lower limb to treat pain in a upper limb Yang-Ming area).

Few of the principal points used in this acupuncture style are on the Main channels and are often said to be between major muscle groups in the intermuscular "valleys." Nonregular channel points, i.e., Tong points, are the main points used. Tong points are located within somatoreflex areas that correspond to specific Organ systems. These regions are unique to the Tong-style system but considered less frequently when treating musculoskeletal disorders than when treating internal medical disorders. At the same time, SI-3 and SI-4, for example, are said to be the reaction area of the Kidneys and are used to treat Kidney-deficiency with symptoms such as back pain, sciatica, and tinnitus and therefore the somatoreflex areas may be significant when treating musculoskeletal disorders as well.

Activating a Wave Through the Channel System

The strengths of Tong/Lee-style acupuncture are its simplicity, its use of a minimal number of points on unaffected areas, and its selection of points mainly on a regional and channel basis (i.e., one just needs to match areas of pain or Organic symptoms with their possible reflection in other

---

17. The author studied Tong-style acupuncture with renowned acupuncture physicians Dr. Miriam Lee and Dr. Yang Wei-Chieh. The information that follows is part of Dr. Lee's (and Dr. Yang Wei-Chieh's) teachings and does not strictly follow the Tong-style. Dr. Lee integrated several methods and was influenced by Wang Le-ting as well as other acupuncture physicians. Late in her career Dr. Lee, used other bleeding techniques that she learned in mainland China.

Table 6-6: Local Contralateral, Same-Name, Point Connections[a]

JOINT/ AREA OF PAIN AND VICE VERSA	LOCAL AREA AND POINT	CONTRALATERAL AREA AND POINT	CONTRALATERAL JOINT/AREA OF PAIN AND VICE VERSA
Shoulder	LI-15 (Yang-Ming)	St-31 (Yang-Ming)	Hip
	SI-10 (Tai-Yang)	UB-36 (Tai-Yang)	
	TW-14 (Shao-Yang)	GB-30 (Shao-Yang)	
	LU-2 (Tai-Yin)	SP-12 (Tai-Yin)	
	H-1 (Shao-Yin)	K-11 (Shao-Yin)	
	P-2 (Jue-Yin)	LIV-11 (Jue-Yin)	
Elbow	LI-11	ST-36	Knee
	SI-8	UB-40	
	TW-10	GB-34	
	LU-5	SP-9	
	H-3	K-10	
	P-3	LIV-8	
Wrist	LI-5	ST-41	Ankle
	SI-5	UB-60	
	TW-4	GB-40	
	LU-9	SP-5	
	H-6	K-5	
	P-7	LIV-4	

a. It is also possible to change a Yin point for a Yang point and vice versa. One may also try a contralateral distal/proximal joint. For example, if the patient has pain around a wrist Lung point, the practitioner can palpate and seek a sensitive point on the contralateral hip on Yin, or related Yang channel. LI-15 was commonly used by Dr. Lee to treat foot pain (so that the proximal/distal areas are switched, foot relating to shoulder and vice versa). The system for choosing remote points, as one can see, is very flexible and is best used based on palpatory findings of sensitive and reactive points (although Dr. Lee rarely palpated for sensitivity). Pain relief should be quick, and, if not achieved, another point should be tried. (See use of the Nine Stars of the Magic Square).

areas of the body and empirically treat points until a desired effect is achieved). Because it is an acupuncture system, an "herbal" type (Zhong Fu/Organ) TCM diagnosis is not needed. Most Tong-style treatments result in little or no aggravation of symptoms and allow the patient to move the affected joint or area during treatment. Points are also chosen based on master Tong's clinical experience as suggested by his (or family style) point indications. These however can usually be explained by their location within one of the bodily imaging systems, or by commonly understood relationships between Yin and Yang. Dr. Lee (who as stated above was the author's Tong-style teacher) also used acupuncture "formulas" such as St-36, Sp-6, Li-4, 11, and Lu-7, nicknamed by her students "Great Lady Great Tonifying Formula, or Ten Great Tonifying Formula" to treat mainly Qi-deficiency. She also used other formulas, such as "Old Ten Needles" (St-36, Sp-6, P-6, CV-9, 12, LI-25) for the treatment of respiratory symptoms secondary to Kidney weakness and/or other inflammatory/immune reactions in a weak patient. These were not based on Tong-style methods. Dr. Lee also used bleeding, cupping, and scraping techniques (see below).

The mobilization of an affected painful joint during an acupuncture treatment, as is attempted in Tong-style, often results in an increased pain-free range of motion. However, *functional* signs and orthopedic or osteopathic test results do not *always* change even when the patient feels less pain. The longevity of such change, when it occurs, is difficult to predict. The effects of the needles are said to last about two or three days, with bleeding techniques having a longer effect. Tong-style acupuncturists therefore like to see patients two or three times per week, with gradually less frequent visits as

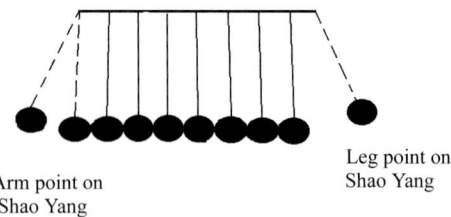

Figure 6-14: Energy activation. Note that one can use a related Yin point as well.

the patient improves. Occasionally, improvements last for a long time. The author has seen occasional cases in which long-standing pain resolved by a single treatment using distal points. This, however, is an exception. In its discussion of "perverse" diseases, the *Spiritual Axis* states:

> Those headaches which occur from blows or falls which cause the sick Blood to remain inside cannot be treated by acupuncture. With injury of the flesh, where the pain does not cease, one can treat by local needling, but not by using distal points. Headaches which are not affected by acupuncture come from the illness of great Bi syndrome. If they are treated daily, one can effect a minor change, but not an end of the problem.

The Tong system and the usage of remote points is particularly helpful while practicing manual therapy at the same time. The combination of manual therapy and acupuncture has several advantages:

- The patient's pain is reduced and so is muscle guarding.
  — This allows for better and more accurate evaluation of joint end-feels.
- There is an increased ability to bring joints closer to their dysfunctional end-range during therapy, with less pain or guarding.
- The combination is clinically synergistic.
- The combination may address different aspects of the patient's symptoms or the root causes of his or her symptoms.

When the practitioner is using remote points, a wave is said to be activated through the channel system (Figure 6-14). The practitioner selects from one to four points on the Qi circulation channel system, often as far from the lesion as possible, as can be seen in Table 6-6, or as is indicated by any of the reflection (imaging) systems. This results in unblocking the channels and the concentration of Qi at the area of the pain. A second rationale for choosing a contralateral point is that pain (stagnation of Qi and Blood) on one side on the channel results in a Yin/Yang reaction with Emptiness and weakness on the opposite side or at analogous

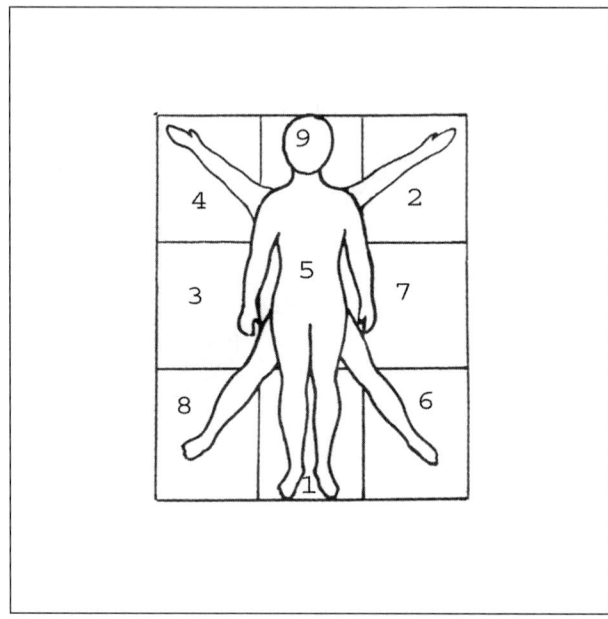

Figure 6-15: Nine Stars of the Magic Square.

areas. While Dr. Lee often strongly stimulated opposite points when treating pain, master Tong is said to have just inserted the needles and not to have stimulated them.

Dr. Lee uses contralateral (or other nonlocal) points extensively, asking, why punish the painful area? The practitioner finds the source of pain and needles at the same level of "energy" on the channel system as far away from the lesion as possible. For example, if the pain is located on the lateral ankle area (on the Gall Bladder channel or in the Shao Yang region), the practitioner needles at the contralateral wrist Triple Warmer channel or Shao Yang region (i.e., using same-name channels on opposite sides). This system of choosing points is applied as follows:

- Lung<—>Spleen
- Large Intestine<—>Stomach
- Heart<—>Kidney
- Small Intestine<—>Urinary Bladder
- Pericardium<—>Liver
- Triple Warmer<—>Gall Bladder

For the preceding example (lateral ankle pain) one can also choose a Yin-related point on the Pericardium channel, i.e., the paired arm Jue-Yin channel to Triple Warmer for pain within a Shao-Yang distribution of the foot.[18] This system of choosing points is applied as follows:

- Lung<—>Stomach
- Spleen<—>Large Intestine
- Heart<—>Urinary Bladder

---

18. Jue Yin is paired with Shao Yang—Liv/GB and P/TW.

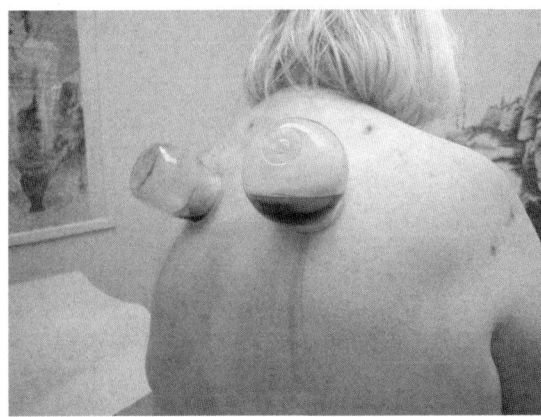

Figure 6-16: UB-43 is cupped and bled for the treatment of knee arthrosis.

- Kidney<—>Small Intestine
- Pericardium<—>Gall Bladder
- Liver<—>Triple Warmer.

Another system involves pairing left-right Yin/Yang relationships with the Internal/External relationships. A Yang point on the left side is used to treat the paired channel Yin area at the same height, e.g., K-10 to treat UB-40. This system is applied as follows:

- Lung<—>Large Intestine
- Stomach<—>Spleen
- Heart<—>Small Intestine
- Urinary Bladder<—>Kidney
- Pericardium<—>Triple Warmer
- Liver<—>Gall Bladder

Another common association used by master Tong is Tai-Yin to treat Tai-Yang (and vice versa), Shao-Yin to treat Shao-Yang (and vice versa), and Jue-Yin to treat Yang-Ming (and vice versa):

- Spleen<—>Urinary Bladder
- Lung<—>Small Intestine
- Kidney<—>Gall Bladder
- Heart<—>Triple Warmer
- Liver<—>Stomach
- Pericardium<—>Large Intestine

Most of the Tong-style reflection (imaging) systems can be summarized form the *"Nine Stars of the Magic Square"* as follows (Figure 6-15):

BOTTOM TO TOP (#1—>#9): For example, use St-44 to treat head; Correct tendons to treat neck and back of head; Flower Bone one (55.02) to treat the eyes; UB-62, 63 to treat headaches felt as a band around the head; and Liv-3, 2 to treat the jaw.

TOP TO BOTTOM (#9—>#1): For example, use State Waters (1010.06) to treat low back pain; and GV-20 to treat the ball of the foot.

OPPOSITE SIDE, BOTTOM TO TOP (#6—>#4). For example, Beside Three Miles (77.22, 23) to treat opposite shoulder/arm; GB-31 to treat opposite elbow.

OPPOSITE SIDE, TOP TO BOTTOM (#4—>#6): For example, LI-3 (1/2) and 4.5 (Ling Gu, Da Bai (22.04, 05)) to treat opposite back and leg pain; P-6 to treat opposite knee; Hand Five Thousand Gold (33.08, 09) to treat opposite UB channel leg pain; Heart Gate (33.12) to treat opposite groin pain; TW-4 to treat the opposite ankle; LI-11 to treat opposite side knee pain; LI-15 to treat opposite side hip and buttock pain; and TW-2 to treat opposite thigh pain.

SIDE TO SIDE (#4—>#2; #3—>#7; #8—>#6): For example, LI-15 (or shoulder triangle three points 1-2 cun below LI-15 in a triangle) for opposite shoulder pain; LI-11 for opposite LI-11; St-36, GB-34; and Sp-9 for opposite knee pain.

ALL DIRECTIONS TOWARDS CENTER (#3—>#5; #9—>#5; #6—>#5; #1—>#5): For example, Four Flowers Middle (77.09) to treat the chest, Lungs and Heart; SI-18, St-4 to treat Urinary Bladder burning pain; Water Gold Water Through (1010.19, 20) to treat the chest and low back; St-43 to treat opposite abdomen; Flower Bone Three and Four (55.04, 05) to treat the sacrum.

UPPER EXTREMITY RELATED TO HEAD AND TRUNK (#3/7/4/2—>#9; #3/7/4/2—>#5): For example, P-6 for chest disease (forearm to treat chest); LI-11 for navel area (arm/forearm for trunk abdomen); LI-4 head area (hand to head disease).

LOWER EXTREMITY related to HEAD AND TRUNK (#8/6/1—>#9; #1/3/8/6—>#5): For example, St-36 to treat naval area (leg to abdomen) and St-44 to treat head and throat area (foot to head).

Any of these imaging relationships can be flipped around. For example, the bottom to top imaging can be used as "the foot being related to the head." St-44 is then used to treat head symptoms. The limb can be flipped. Areas of the hip will then relate to the head. GB-30 and 31 can then, for example, be used to treat symptoms in the head. When treating knee pain Lu-5, LI-11 etc., can be used, as the elbow can be related to the knee. If the image is flipped and the wrist joint is related to the knee, the common use of P-6 to treat the knee can be explained (Figure 6-17). These systems are therefore very flexible and can help guide the practitioner to various areas in the body and to access the channel system in various combinations.

In general, points with any of the above channel relationships on analogous areas or systems are palpated for tenderness (although Dr. Lee rarely palpated for tenderness when choosing an imaging system or points). The practitio-

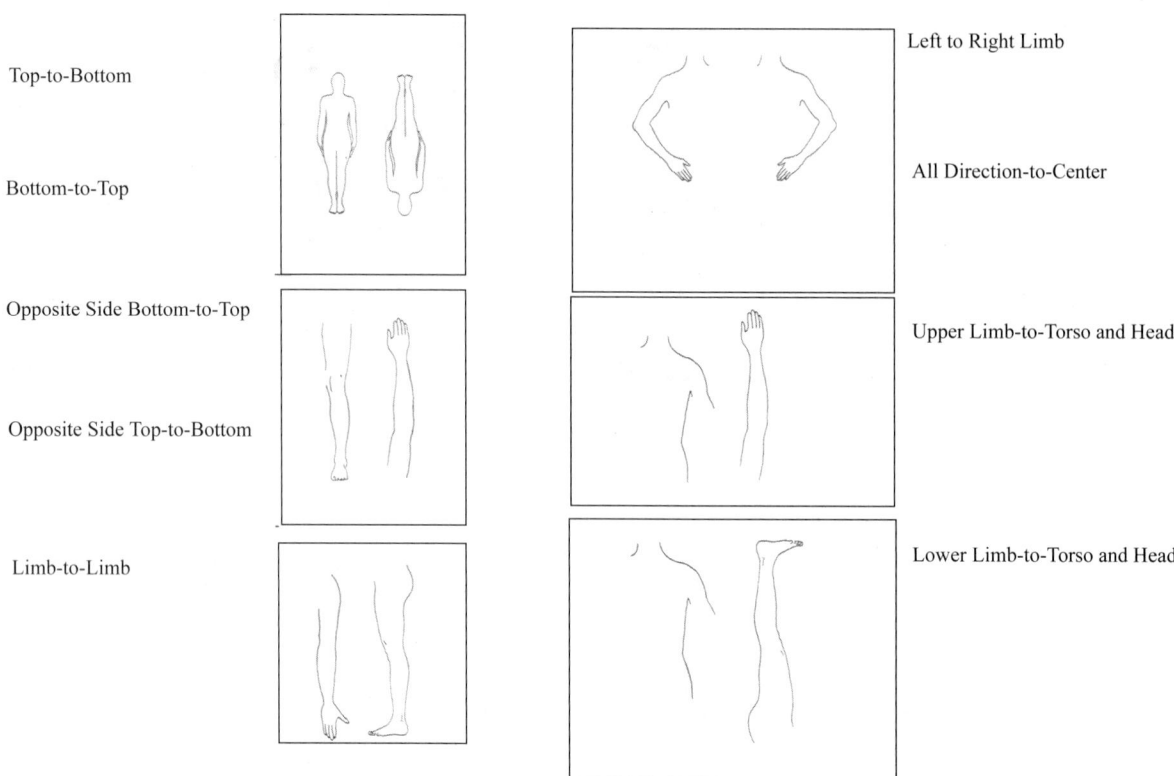

Figure 6-17: Microsystems related to the Nine Stars and Magic Square (courtesy of S Johnson).

ner uses points which yield the most tenderness, or treats empirically to see which gives the best clinical result. For example, for leg pain (or sciatica) opposite side LI-4.5 (Ling Gu 22.04), LI-3.5 (Da Bai, 22.05), and UB-65 can be used. A change in the pain is to be expected *within a minute* or so. If no improvement is seen, another analogous (imaging) area is palpated and needled, such as Hand Five Thousand Gold (33.08, 09) for example. Points can be chosen from any of the systems such as left to treat right, up to treat down, anterior to treat posterior, posterior to treat anterior, Yin to treat Yang, Yang to treat Yang, Yin to treat Yin, mid-day to treat mid-night, magic cube combinations, stems branches combinations, Extra channel command points, Source points, Connecting points, Accumulating points, etc. Any of the regular rationales for choosing points can be incorporated at the same time, such as, points Jing/Ting Well points to treat the Sinew channels, Heat and inflammation.[19]

Tong Points

In the Tong method, the names of the Main channel points differ from (and have different functions than) the standard Main channel points. Points are located on body areas that have special functions and relate to Organs in a unique Tong-style methodology. An understanding of the channel system (and early numeric systems) helps in determining the location to be needled but is not mandatory. Most of the body Tong points are found in the *valleys* between muscle groups, and, therefore, are in close relationships to major nerve trunks and fascial compartments. Tong "channel lines" functions should therefore be understood and accurately located. Points on these lines often share common names and functions.

Commonly Used Tong-Points

Table 6-7 summarizes Tong-style points. Point names and numbers are taken from *Master Tong's Acupuncture* (Blue Poppy Press) and are the most commonly used by Dr. Lee for the treatment of pain. These points are presented in order of use in the treatment of pain, not by body region.[20] These points were originally organized into a book by Dr. Yang Wei-Chieh, one of Master Tong's main students. In general, when treating pain, the points are almost always used on the opposite side of the pain. Occasionally, they are used bilaterally or on the painful side. When treating Organ dysfunction, it is common to treat bilaterally. When treating points on the Stomach channel, it is common to treat points on the same side of symptoms or bilaterally. Needle retention is usually for a minimum of thirty minutes, the approximate time it

Tong/Lee-style Acupuncture

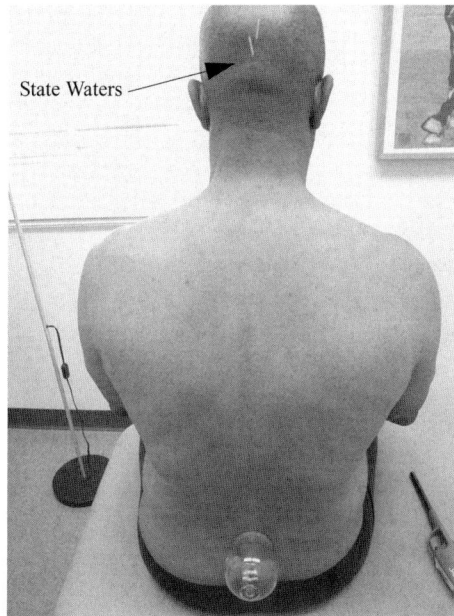

State Waters and local cup used first

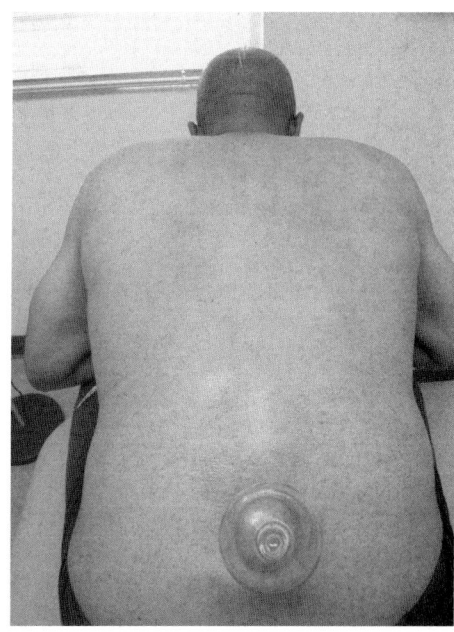

Patient flexes his spine and a moving cup technique is used all over his right and left spinal muscles

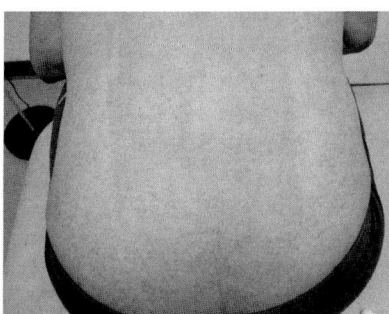

Patient skin following moving cups

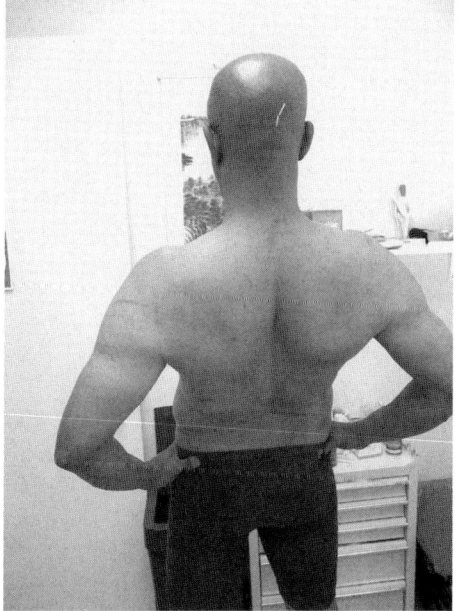

The patient then performs extension exercises while State Waters is retained

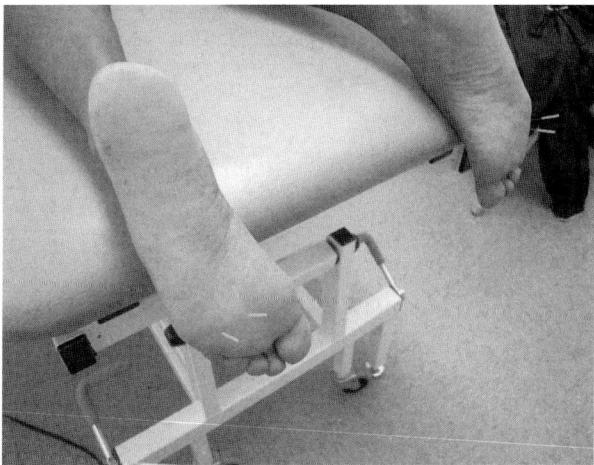

Flower Bone Three and Four is used to address residual sacral area pain

Figure 6-18: Typical treatment of low back pain. This patient came in with acute low back, buttock and thigh pain. His osteopathic diagnosis was FRS(lf) T-12 and posterior sacral torsion. He did not have positive dural signs. He presented with a forward and left sidebent postural list. It was painful for him to stand and therefore he was treated sitting. State Waters and local moving cup was performed. Following this his back pain improved but he still had buttock and thigh pain. He was then instructed to perform extension exercises if these did not aggravate his leg pain. Following the exercises his pain centralized to sacral area (leg and buttock pain improved) and therefore Flower Bone Three and Four was used. At the end of treatment he was pain free.

takes for one cycle of Qi circulation throughout the channel systems. In general, Dr. Lee used longer retention when few points (or Tong-points) were used (forty-five minutes to one hour or more and thirty minutes when using larger groups or normal channel points such as the formulas mentioned above). When Dr. Lee used electroacupuncture (which was not very often) stimulation lasted for twenty minutes.

Bleeding, Cupping, and Moxa Techniques

In addition to needling, Tong-style frequently includes the "bleeding" of blood vessels and Tong's acupoints. Whereas Tong-style needling is often performed distally, Tong-style bleeding is often performed locally. Points on the back (and on UB channel) are bled often as well. Bleeding is said to have effects of a longer duration than needling.

Dr. Lee used bleeding and cupping to vitalize Blood and to clear Heat and other pathogenic influences. Clearing Heat and pathogenic influences by bleeding is often performed for Deficient patients, especially using UB-43. Even though considered a sedating technique, bleeding can be used in Deficient patients because, by eliminating pathogenic influences, the patient is strengthened by a method similar to the attacking method used in herbal medicine.[21] Dr. Lee often bled and cupped UB-13, 17, and 18 to "increase blood circulation" and to treat extremity pains due to poor circulation, e.g., diabetic neuropathy. UB-43 was often bled for knee pain. The retention of cups when used for bleeding is usually around five minutes. For other uses its between five and ten minutes (sometimes longer). She also utilized scarping (Gua Sha) techniques, using Wan Hua oil extensively. Dr. Lee used moxa cans (pots) to treat coldness, deficiency, and to build Blood. These were used to either warm the tissues or to "smock" psoriatic lesions.

When Is Tong-style Best Used?

It is the author's experience that Tong/Lee-style acupuncture, as well as other distal point systems, are best used when local tissue texture abnormalities are not *clearly* demonstrable (e.g., there are no clear tight-bands with triggers to account for symptoms). There is often palpable tenderness, muscle shortening, and possibly limited and painful movement. It is also helpful when joint pathology is involved. When clear, myofascial tight-bands are palpable, it is the author's preference to treat these directly, and then, if needed, to use distal/Tong points (especially in chronic cases). As stated earlier, the use of distal points is very helpful when integrated with other manual therapies. This system is very helpful in acute cases when the patient is in great pain. Tong-style bleeding and cupping techniques can greatly augment the patient's total care, and their use is encouraged.

It is the author's experience that Tong/Lee-Style acupuncture is the most predictable, in terms of analgesic effects, of any of the "traditional" acupuncture systems he uses.[22] While as stated above, this system is often not sufficient to resolve the patient's mechanical dysfunctions and therefore symptoms, this system can be used to reduce the patient's pain almost immediately and can improve total function. Therefore, it is best to integrate joint and tissue specific diagnosis/examinations, which must be reassessed after the Tong-style treatment to ascertain if further manual therapy is needed. It is not uncommon to have the patient report great improvement in pain (and therefore also show increased range of motion) after Tong-style treatments, but for orthopedic and joint play tests (especially provocation tests) to still show little improvement. In such cases it is advisable to integrate other therapies; doing so will greatly improve long-term outcome. Another observation by the author is that Tong-style treatments work better when a thicker gauge (30-32) needles are used. 18 gauge hypodermic needles can be used for bleeding with less pain than would be elicited by lancets or traditional bleeding needles. In general, when bleeding, it is more important to look for congested blood vessels than "point location."

---

19. Considering all the possible rationales available for choosing areas and points for treatment can make one wander if it really matters where one needles (as one can treat any area in the body from all other areas!). As seen in chapter 2 and chapter 3, much of the nervous system is integrated in multiple relationships beyond simple segmental innervations. It's possible that each of the reflection (imaging) systems results in the peripheral stimulation of these diverse neurological connections. Studies have also shown that the activation of reflexes brought on by massage (and presumably acupuncture) and exercise of *contralateral* or adjacent muscles can stimulate the plastic state of the muscle (the ability of tissues to manifest structural change).

---

22. The author prefers to use "neuroanatomical" acupuncture when treating local tissues (i.e., dry needling).

Table 6-7: Important Tong-Style Points Used In Musculoskeletal Disorders

Point	Location	Usage	Illustration
State Water (1010.25)[A]	On the sagittal midline on the back of the head, the first point is located at the external occipital protuberance. The second point is located 0.8 cun above the first.	Used for lower back pain, especially midline pain. Also for weakness or numbness of the lower limbs. Needle downward 1-3 fen in depth. Dr. Lee needled about 0.5-1.2 cun in depth. The lower point is needled first. One may need to pull the skin to needle the upper point. The patient must exercise and stretch while needles are in. Follow with local cupping.	
Beside Three Miles (77.22) **Beside Below Three Miles (77.23)**	0.5-1 cun lateral to St-36 slightly anterior to the GB line. It is found in the intermuscular septum between the peroneus longus and anterior tibialis right over the superficial peroneal nerve. 2 cun below 77.22.	The two points are known as Beside Three Miles and are used mainly for one-sided complaints or conditions for which GB-34 can be used, or for any GB channel pain (mostly upper body). One sided headache, trigeminal nerve or acute shoulder pain (with Liv-3), wrist, elbow and/or shoulder pain or strain. Needle 0.5-1 cun in depth until De Qi goes down leg; if needle sensation stops at ankle, then massage the ankle.[b] For Deficiency, tonify; for Excess, sedate. (Use needle feel to ascertain if Deficient or Excess). Needle opposite side. If bilateral symptoms, work bilaterally.	
Spirit Bone (22.05) **Great White (22.04)**	At the joint of the 1st and 2nd metacarpals of dorsal palm. LI-4 1/2 or at base of 2nd metacarpal. In the shallow area between the 1st and 2nd metacarpals LI-3 1/2 or LI-3.	Usually used together (Ling Gu, Da Bai). Good combination for any pain. Said to move both Qi and Blood in the entire body. Used especially for Lung weakness or for lower body pains. Used for ischial bursitis, back pain, sciatica (with Lung weakness), buttock pain, anterior hip pain (inguinal), upper limb pain (esp. elbow). Needle opposite side for lower body and same side for upper body (although Dr. Lee always needled opposite side of pain). The needles should be right against the bone. Spirit Bone (Ling Gu) is always needled first. Needle 1-2 cuns.	
Correct Straight Tendon (77.01) **Upright Straight Tendon (77.02)**	3.5 cun superior from the base of heel 2 cun above 77.01.	The two points are known as correct tendons and are mainly used for head and neck midline symptoms Said to treat all the tendons of the body.[c] Correct Straight Tendon (77.01) can be used with quick insertion and withdrawal for low back strain and for plantar fasciitis. Combine with UB-40 for acute back pain. Said to correct alignment of spine. Also helpful for cranial and mental symptoms due to whiplash injury. Needle through tendon until touching bone. Leave needles for at least one hour when treating the neck and head regions. Always treat bilaterally.	

Table 6-7: Important Tong-Style Points Used In Musculoskeletal Disorders

Point	Location	Usage	Illustration
Water (Passing) Through (1010.19) Water Gold (1010.20)	0.4 cun inferior to corner of the mouth. 0.5 cun medial and slightly inferior to 1010.19.	Used together for back pain aggravated by coughing with Kidney weakness.[d] Joint pains due to Kidney or Essence weakness. Low back sprain. Crystal joint diseases (e.g. gout). Rheumatic diseases with Kidney weakness. Needle the darkened area about 1-5 fen or upto 1 cun in depth. Needle all four points.	
Three Gold (DT 07)	Same as UB-42, 43, 44.	Used to treat knee joint pain from degenerative arthritis. These points are only used for actual joint pain not surrounding soft tissues. Look for most painful point(s) to treat, or can treat all three as well. Can treat on painful side or bilateral. Use bleeding and cupping and take out several CCs of blood.	
Heaven Emperor Quasi (77.18) [A.K.A Kidney Gate] Earth Emperor (77.19) Human (Men) Emperor (77.21)	4 cun below the knee joint, about 1.5 cun below Sp-9 at the medial epicondyle of the tibia. 7 cun above the medial malleolus on the Spleen line. Posterior to Sp-6 on the Kidney line.	77.18 can be used for upper extremity pain, stiffness and weakness, especially of the shoulder, coccygeal pain, upper back pain, low back pain, headache, elbow pain and inability to raise the arms upward. The three points are known as Three Emperors and are used mainly to treat Kidney weakness and back pain.[e] Needle 1-1.5 cun in depth. For upper extremity pain needle opposite side. For all other indications needle bilaterally.	
Three Nine Miles (88.25-88.27).	The first point is located in the midpoint of the midline on the lateral aspect of the thigh (GB-31). The second is 1.5 cun horizontally anterior to the first. The third is 1.5 horizontally posterior to the first.	These points are used for musculoskeletal pains especially when the patient suffers from fear. Lumbago, leg pain, neck pain, hand numbness. Also for pain which moves around and is difficult to describe. Mostly for problems of lateral body. GB-31 is said to be especially helpful for bone spurs. Needle 0.8-1.5 cun. Needle opposite side of pain. May be used bilaterally. Look for sensitive points.	

Table 6-7: Important Tong-Style Points Used In Musculoskeletal Disorders

POINT	LOCATION	USAGE	ILLUSTRATION
FLOWER BONE FOUR (55.05) **FLOWER BONE THREE (55.04)**	1.5 cun posterior to the web between the fourth and fifth toes on the plantar surface of the foot. 2 cun posterior from the web between the third and fourth toes on the plantar surface of the foot.	Used together for thoracic paravertebral pain, sciatica, and for leg and foot numbness. Can treat leg pain ("sciatica") of any channel distribution including L3, L4, L5, and S1. The patient should exercise the legs while the needles are in. Mostly useful for SI joint or sacral bone pain. The practitioner can mobilize the joint while the needles are in. Needle 0.5-1 cun in depth. Needle bilaterally.	
HEART (GATE) DOOR (33.12)	1.5 cun distal to H-3.	Used for medial knee or groin pain. Also for sciatica, tail bone or sacral pain and inflammatory arthritis. Dr. Lee considers inflammatory knee pain to be caused by Heart, while non-inflammatory knee pain to be caused by the Kidneys. Needle 4-7 fen. Needle opposite side of pain.	
HAND FIVE GOLD (33.08) **HAND THOUSAND GOLD (33.09)**	6.5 cun above the pisiform and to the lateral side of the ulna. 8 cun above the pisiform and to the lateral side of the ulna. Both located 0.5 cun ulnerly from the TW channel (or on the TW channel).	The two points are known as Hand Five Thousand Gold. Used for sciatica with UB channel distribution (S1) which is said to be due to drinking cold drinks, i.e. not due to spine (but can be used for musculoskeletal origin as well). Also helpful in the treatments of neuropathies of the lower extremities. Needle only 3-5 fen in depth (not deeper). Needle opposite side of pain.	
SHOULDER CENTER MIDDLE (44.06)	Located in the center of the deltoid muscle, with the patient supine, 3 (or 2.5) cun below the aromion process.	Used for patellar (knee) pain. Also used on the opposite shoulder to treat shoulder pain. Needle 0.5-1 cun in depth.[f] Needle opposite side of pain.	

Table 6-7: Important Tong-Style Points Used In Musculoskeletal Disorders

POINT	LOCATION	USAGE	ILLUSTRATION
Four Flowers Quasi (77.10) **Four Flowers Middle (77.09)**	10 cun below the inferior lateral edge of the lower border of the patella, 0.5 cun above St-38. 7.5 below the inferior lateral edge of the lower border of the patella and 2.5 cun above Four Flowers Quasi (77.10). All the Four Flower points are on a line just lateral to the first muscle group from the tibia, in the groove between the extensor digitorum longus and the tibialis muscle. At about the medial one-third of the distance between the tibial crest and the head of the fibula. These points are just over the deep peroneal nerve.^g Four Flower Middle was always combined with Four Flower Upper (St-36) by Dr. Lee.	Used for migraine headaches when pain is felt behind the eyes, and only if pressure on the eye feels uncomfortable to the patient. Or when the eye balls feel very tight. Used also for bone deformity. Needle deep to a depth of 1.5-3 cun. Bleed congested vessels. Treat on the painful side.	
Foot Thousand Gold (77.24) **Foot Five Gold (77.25)**	5 fen posterior and 2 cun distal to Beside Lower Three Miles (77.23), more on the GB line. 2 cun distal to 77.24 (about 1 cun posterior and distal to St-40).	Used for painful shoulder with limited external rotation. Needle 0.5-1 cun. Needle opposite side of pain.	
Four Flowers Below (77.11) **Bowel Intestine (77.12)**	5 cun below 77.09. 1.5 cun above 77.11.	Used together for proliferated-Bi syndromes (generalized joint swelling). Needle 2-3 cun in depth. Needle on painful side or bilaterally.	
Passing (Through) Kidneys (88.09)	At the superior medial angle of the patella.	Used for cold and painful lower extremities, in men. Elderly patients with one cold foot. Needle 3-5 fen. Needle on left side (men) or opposite side of pain.	

Table 6-7: Important Tong-Style Points Used In Musculoskeletal Disorders

POINT	LOCATION	USAGE	ILLUSTRATION
PASSING (THROUGH UPPER) BACK (88.11)	4 cun above the medial edge of the patella.	Used for shoulder pain and general swelling. Needle 0.5-1 cun in depth. Needle opposite side of pain.	
PASSING (THROUGH) GATE	1 cun above 88.11.	May be used for inflammatory joint disease with Phlegm (swelling). Needle 0.5-1 cun in depth. Needle opposite side of pain. Can combine both points	
RELEASE (RESOLVE, UNTIE) (88.28)	1 cun above and 3 fen lateral to the outer edge of the patella.	Used to treat post acupuncture or injection pain. Also for any traumatic pain in the first 48 hours. Needle 3-5 fen in depth. Usually short retention but can be as long as 45 minutes. Needle same side of pain or bilaterally.	
BRIGHT YELLOW (88.12)	At the midpoint of the midline of the medial aspect of the thigh. Between the groin and patella. On the Liver channel. In the medial valley on the line just between the vastus medialis/quadriceps femoris and rectus femoris muscles.	Used for low/mid back tension from Liver disorders. Bone enlargement. Use with a point 3 cun above and 3 cun below if with a Liver/liver disorder (called Three Yellows). Arthritis in Deficient patient with fatigue from Spleen, Kidney, Liver, and Heart. Needle 1.5-2.5 cun. Needle bilaterally.	
DOUBLE CHILD (22.1)	In the palmer side of the hand 1 cun proximal from the skin fold between the first and second metacarpals in the thenar eminence.	These two points are mainly used for periscapular pain and for knee pain. Also used for quadratus lumborum pain with Kidney-deficiency. Needle 3-5 fen deep only. Needle opposite side of pain.	
DOUBLE IMMORTAL (22.02)	On the line intersecting the midlines of the first finger and thumb just proximal to Double Child (22.01). These points are found at the edge of (or just within) the thenar eminence which is visualized at the scapula.		
FIVE TIGERS (11.27)	On the radial division between the palmer and dorsal surface of the phalange bone of the thumb. The five points are situated in equal distances on the shaft. Measure 2, 4, 6, 8 fen, and 1 cun from metacarpal-phalangeal joint.	Used for ankle sprains and polyarthritis. Head pain, foot pain, hand pain. Also useful for neuropathies and for toe or forefoot pain. #1 used for Sp-1 area pain. #3 big toe or any toe area. #4 foot ankle pain. #2 supports other points. Dr. Lee often used #4 or all 5 points together. Needle 3-5 fen in depth. Needle opposite side of pain.	

Table 6-7: Important Tong-Style Points Used In Musculoskeletal Disorders

Point	Location	Usage	Illustration
Water Cure (44.17) **Upper Curve (44.16)**	2.5 cun below the posterior aspect of the acromion on the shoulder between the deltoid and triceps. Look for a tender spot. About 1.5 cun inferiorly laterally from Water Cure (44.17).	Used together for any Kidney related pain in the upper or lower extremity and for low back pain or Kidney disease. Strengthens the body. Wrist pain. Needle 3-5 fen in depth. Needle opposite side of pain.	
(Team of) Four Horse Middle (88.17) **Four Horse Upper (88.18)** **Four Horse Lower (88.19)**	6 cun above the top of the patella and 2 cun toward the lateral thigh (between St and GB channels or on St channel). 2 cun above 88.17. 2 cun below 88.17.	Rib pain, sciatica, and lumbago due to Lung weakness, psoriatic arthritis. Needle all three points 0.8-2.5 cun. Needle opposite side of pain. Needle bilaterally for psoriatic arthritis.	
Catching Ball (77.04) **Upright Scholar (77.03)**	Same as UB-57. 2 cun above 77.02 (upright straight tendon) or between UB-57 and 77.02.	Used to treat spasms of the lower leg, low back, soreness, and upper back pain. Needle 1-2 cun in depth. Needle opposite side of pain or bilaterally. May needle any area between these two points using quick insertion and withdrawal. Can be bled if visible vessels are seen. Can be bled instead of UB-40 for low back pain.	
Upper White (22.03)	5 fen proximal from the dorsal metacarpal-phalangeal joint and 3 fen to the radial side of the middle finger.	Sciatica. Needle 3-5 fen. Needle mostly on right side, especially for women. Or needle opposite side of pain.	

Table 6-7: Important Tong-Style Points Used In Musculoskeletal Disorders

Point	Location	Usage	Illustration
Middle White (22.06)	Same as TW-3.	Sciatica due to Kidney weakness. Needle 3-5 fen in depth. Needle opposite side of pain.	
Wrist Normal Flow (Wrist Prosperous One) (22.08) Wrist Normal Flow Two (Wrist Prosperous One Two) (22.09)	Same as SI-3 or 5 fen proximal to SI-3. Lateral side of 5th metacarpal bone 1.5 cun distal to the wrist joint.	Used to treat Kidney-deficiency with: headache, sciatica, exhaustion, enlargement of the bones of the four limbs, waist pain, and/or upper back pain.[h] 22.9 has same indications as 22.08. Needle 2-4 fen in depth only on one side. Needle opposite side of pain, especially for lower body symptoms. May use both points together.	
Heart Knee (11.09)	Symmetrically 4 fen from median line of dorsal of side of middle phalanx of middle finger.	Inflammatory knee pain due to Heart fatigue or over-work. Shoulder pain due to over-work. Needle 0.5 fen. Needle opposite side of pain.	
Fire Scatter (66.12)	Horizontally 1 cun proximally to Sp-4.	Headache (frontal) and sensation of brain soreness, low back pain from Kidney weakness, upper back pain. Needle 5-8 fen in depth. Needle opposite side of pain or bilaterally. Combine with Sp-3 and Sp-4 for brain soreness (brain tumors, etc.)	
Great (Distance) Space (11.01) Small (Distance) Space (11.02) Middle (Distance) Space (11.05)	On the palmer side of the index finger, 3 fen to the radial side from the median line in the center of the proximal phalanx of the index finger. 2 fen distal to Great Space. In the midline of the middle of the proximal phalanx of index.	Used to treat inflammatory knee pain. Pain in corner of the eye (Wind or GB imbalance).[i] Same indications as Great space. Swelling of knee due to Heart and Spleen imbalance. Same indications. Needle all three points only on one side to a depth of 1 fen. Needle on opposite side of pain.	

Table 6-7: Important Tong-Style Points Used In Musculoskeletal Disorders

Point	Location	Usage	Illustration
Wood Fire (11.10)	On the junction center between distal and middle phalanx of the dorsal middle finger.	Paralysis of arms. Hemiplegia. Needle 0.5 fen. Needle opposite side of pain or weakness.	
Lung Heart (11.11)	On the dorsal aspect of the middle finger. The first is 3 fen proximal to the midpoint of the distal phalangeal joint. A second point is located 3 fen distal to the midpoint of the proximal phalangeal joint.	Used for upper back and neck aching and pain, spinal pain and lower leg pain, especially due to varicose veins.[j] Needle 0.5 fen slanting radially. Needle opposite side of pain.	
Two Corner Bright (11.12)	On the dorsal aspect of the middle finger. The first is 3 fen proximal to the midpoint of the proximal joint. The second is 1 cun distal to the midpoint of the metacarpal-phalangeal joint.	Used for low back pain, Kidney pain, flank pain, nose bone pain and supraorbital pain. Especially for sprained low back with difficulty standing straight, moving and breathing. For last indication use with Water Passing Through (1010.19) and Water Gold (1010.20). Needle 0.5 fen slanted insertion. Needle opposite side of pain.	
Fire Knee (11.16)	Same as SI-1. Two fen lateral to nail bed of small finger.	Used for inflammatory knee pain as well as other inflammatory diseases. Needle 0.5 fen. Needle opposite side of pain.	
Recover Source (11.22)	On the palmer aspect of the proximal phalanx of the ring finger. On a line 2 fen to the ulnar side of from midline. The first point is 2.5 fen, the second is 5 fen, and the third is 7.5 fen from the metacarpal-phalangeal joint on that line.	These points are used for arthrosis. Hypertrophic osteoarthritis. Needle 0.5 fen. Needle opposite side of pain.	

Table 6-7: Important Tong-Style Points Used In Musculoskeletal Disorders

Point	Location	Usage	Illustration
Fire Mound (33.05)	On the TW channel 5 cun above the wrist.	Used for chest pain and muscular cramping. Sensation of chest enlargement.	
Fire Mountain (33.06)	On the TW channel 6.5 cun above the wrist.	Needle 0.5-1 cun in depth. Forearm spasm use opposite side while for chest pain use same side of pain.	
Fire Bowel Sea (33.07)	8.5 cun above the middle wrist joint on dorsal forearm.	Sciatica, back pain due to weak Kidney. Fatigue due to Heart weakness. Needle 0.5-1 cun in depth.	

Table 6-7: Important Tong-Style Points Used In Musculoskeletal Disorders

Point	Location	Usage	Illustration
Back Vertebral (44.02) **Head Wisdom (44.03)**	On the TW channel 2.5 cun above the elbow. 2 cun above Back Vertebral (44.02).	Used together to treat upper back vertebral "prolapse and slippage," upper back distension and pain, low back pain and kidney organ inflammation. Used for upper or lower back pain due to vertebral and discogenic disorders. Can treat the whole spine. Needle the more reactive side only (i.e., left or right). Needle 3-5 fen in depth and leave in a long time (1-2 hours or more).	
Man Ancestor (44.08) **Heaven Ancestor (44.10)**	3 cun above the elbow joint between the long and short head of biceps muscle. 9 cun above the elbow joint between the long and short heads of biceps muscle.	Foot pain, arm pain, limb edema (elbow capsulitis) Needle 0.8-1.2 cun in depth. Needle opposite side. Lower leg pain, polio. Needle 1-1.5 cun in depth. Needle opposite side. May be used together.	
Seven Tigers (77.26)	On a line 1.5 cun posterior to the tip of the lateral malleolus. The first is located 2 cun above the tip of the malleolus and the other two are 2 and 4 cun superiorly.	Used to treat shoulder bone pain, clavicular pain, AC joint pain, breast-bone pain with swelling and distension, and costal pleural inflammation. Said to be the only point for clavicular bone pain. Needle 0.5-0.8 cun. Usually only four used at one time (i.e., 2 on each side). Or needle opposite side.	

a. State Waters is the most common point used by Dr. Lee for low back pain; she often followed needling with local cupping. Other points she used are: Flower Bone 3 & 4 for sacral bone or mixed GB-UB leg pain (bilateral); SI-3 with UB-65 (SI-3 opposite side, UB-65 opposite or same side), for one sided pain; Ling Gu (LI-4.5) and Da Bai (LI-3.5) (always on opposite side) also for one sided pain, especially in the buttock area; bleeding of UB-40 on the same side as the pain or bilaterally (in chronic or acute cases); and Water Through with Water Gold for low back pain aggravated by coughing, in the first 48 hours after a sprain, and/or in a patient with Lung and Kidney weakness.
b. While it is often thought of as De Qi, since these points are right over the peroneal nerve, the needle sensation more likely has to do with the stimulation of this nerve. It must also be stated that, at least theoretically, whenever a nerve is stimulated directly, the danger of developing a neuroma at some point in the future is increased (possibly).
c. In Tong-style acupuncture, it is often said that if one needles a tissue, it affects the Organ(s) associated with that tissue. Therefore, treating the correct tendons can affect the Liver as well as the tendons.
d. Pain aggravated by coughing is often due to dural tension. In the experience of the author, these points will not have significant effect when the patient shows true dural signs.
e. Dr. Lee mostly used the upper and lower points (called two Empires) for Kidney Yin-deficiency (especially in men). The use of all three points is said to be more appropriate when the patient suffers from edema or Kidney Yang-deficiency. The author likes to use all three in all cases.
f. Dr. Lee/Yang often used TW-5 for posterior shoulder pain; Beside Three Miles for pain at GB-21 area; Foot Thousand Gold (77.24) and Foot Five Gold (77.25) for painful and limited internal rotation of the shoulder; Kidney Gate (77.18) for painful and limited shoulder abduction; Shoulder Triple on opposite side for whole shoulder pain. Shoulder Triple is located in a triangle about 1 cun inferior and to the right and left of 44.06. These treatments are often followed by local cupping. Dr. Yang recommends bleeding Lu-5 on the painful side for "frozen" shoulder, acute shoulder sprain, or for pain radiating from the neck to the shoulder. For neck and shoulder pain in GB channel areas, Dr. Lee often scraped (Gua Sha) the area using Wan Hua oil.

g. Four Flower Middle is often combined with Four Flower Upper (St-36). Both are needled deeply at least 2.5 cun. Also, because the Four Flower points are on the Stomach channels which have more Qi and more Blood, whenever one sees congested superficial vessels on this line, they should be bled. Because these are on the Stomach channel, these points are often needled on the symptomatic side.
h. Dr. Yang suggests using these points for neck pain in Tai-Yang areas just lateral to the vertebrae or going down between the scapula with SI-6. For pain in the mid-neck (GV channel) he suggests using GV-26, especially if the pain is associated with motor problems. For Shao-Yang pain lateral to Tai-Yang areas, he suggests using TW-5 with GB-39. For Yang-Ming pain such as SCM pain, he suggests using LI-4 with Lu-7. If still painful after treatment, Ashi points are treated with quick insertion and withdrawal. This is followed by cupping for three minutes. For combined Tai-Yang and Shao-Yang pain he suggests connecting TW-5 to SI-6.
i. Dr. Lee divides knee pain into "Kidney knee pain and Heart knee pain." Kidney knee pain is usually non-inflammatory, while Heart knee pain is inflammatory. In general, Dr. Lee uses P-6 (especially if LI-4 is pressure-sensitive) on opposite side and bleeds UB-43 on the same side of the painful knee joint, in most cases. For medial knee pain (such as medial collateral ligament pain), Dr. Lee suggests to palpate the abdomen in the aria just below the naval. If tender, Three Plum Blossom (i.e., CV-4 and St-27 bilaterally, or just above CV-4 and 1.6 cun lateral to CV-6) is needled, then Sp-9, 10 and Liv-8 on the opposite side of the painful knee is needled. The painful area is then scraped or cupped.
j. Dr. Lee considered varicose veins to be mainly caused by Lung dysfunction. She liked to needle these points with UB-17, Liv-2 and 3, and bleed the veins.

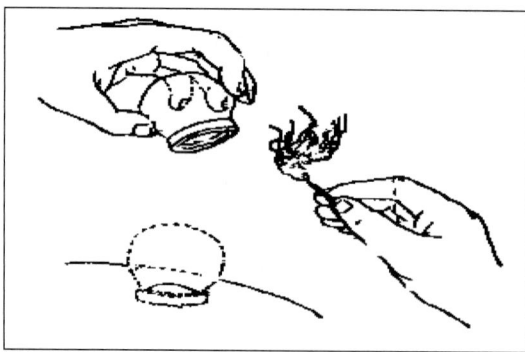

Figure 6-19: Cupping

Other OM and Related Western Therapies

Several techniques are used regularly in OM therapy. Among the more common are ion cords, cupping, scraping, and moxibustion.

Ion Cords

An ion cord is a simple device made of electrical wire with a diode in the middle (patented by Yoshio Manaka). It is used to "direct" the channel flow in one direction and influence "cellular polarity." Ion-pumping cords are said to work on the principle of equalization of charge imbalance in the channels. Some Japanese practitioners use ion cords frequently in treatment of Extra channels, burns, and other conditions. When using ion cords with Extra channel treatments, it is said to "balance and direct" the deepest "energy" layers. There is, however, very little convincing evidence that these cords actually do what they are said to. Supporting evidence often uses unacceptable evaluation techniques such as O-ring tests (i.e., muscle testing) and pressure sensitivity on abdominal or other acupoints. Clinically, however, ion cords do seem to be useful in "root" as well as symptomatic (branch) treatments.

Cupping

Used for centuries in both the East and the West, cupping is a method of increasing superficial circulation by causing local congestion (hematoma) and fascial tissue stretch. In early Chinese medicine, cupping was known as the "horn method" or "fire cup." An early text by Ger Hong (281-361 AD) describes the application of cupping to draw-out Blood as "damp cupping technique." In general, cupping is used to treat Painful Obstruction from Wind-Dampness, Coldness, and Stasis and to treat generalized tightness. Cupping (when a flame is used to create the vacuum), can lead to warming of the affected area and therefore may have thermal effects.

Cups are also capable of creating a blister and are then said to "draw-out" pathogenic-Dampness and to remove deep blockages. Cupping can be helpful in treating both acute and chronic disorders, especially if skin rolling is found to be painful or the skin is found to be tight (see page 217). In chronic disorders, cupping is often combined with bleeding and seven-star-needle techniques to draw-out Blood/blood. Moving cups are often used when treating large areas with thick muscles, such as the chest, back, etc. Moving cups are also useful when treating recurrent *flexed sacrum* due to sacrospinalis muscle tension (see "Joint Dysfunctions and Manual Medicine Models" on page 461). To treat local numbness, "flesh" cupping is used—removing the cup as soon as the cup draws onto the skin until a mild erythema (redness) of the skin is noted. Another method of using cupping is to pre-boil the cup with herbs or to add medicinal liquid into the cup.

The mechanism by which cupping works is not fully understood, but its effects can be generally divided into local and generalized. Locally, the warming effects may increase blood circulation, metabolic rate, and nutrition. The congestion causes an alteration in osmotic pressure, increasing lymphatic circulation. This may help in reducing inflammation in muscular tissues. The generalized effects may be due to the increase in capillary permeability, which produces a local bruise that induces self-hemotolysis. This provides a mild degree of stimulation to the capillary system which may also stimulate sensory nerves.

To apply cups, a flame (Figure 6-19), a cupping instrument, or even by using a breast pump, the practitioner can:

1. Create a partial vacuum in a jar.

2. Apply the semi-evacuated cup to the patient's skin.
   The suction draws up the underlying tissue, thereby stretching the fascia, increasing circulation by forming blood-stasis (which results in the body's trying to maintain its own homeostatic balance thus removing such stasis), and possibly drawing out interstitial fluid. The drawing out of interstitial fluid, which may result in blisters, is thought to increase circulation and to be otherwise therapeutic, especially in patients who have Painful Obstruction (Bi) syndrome from Wind-Damp. If Blood is "impure/bad," the skin tends to become darkened easily (with signs of stasis/bruising). The darker the color, the greater the degree of stasis and impurity there is said to be. Repeated cupping, then, often results in improved signs, and bruising will no longer be seen.

3. To create further stretching, the practitioner can leave the cups in place for from five to twenty minutes. (If they are left longer than ten minutes, there is a greater chance of rasing a blister.)
   And/or he/she can move them up and down, i.e.: pull the cups upward and perpendicular to the affected area; or he/she can swiftly remove the cup and reapply repeatedly; and/or pull the cups in a direction parallel to the affected

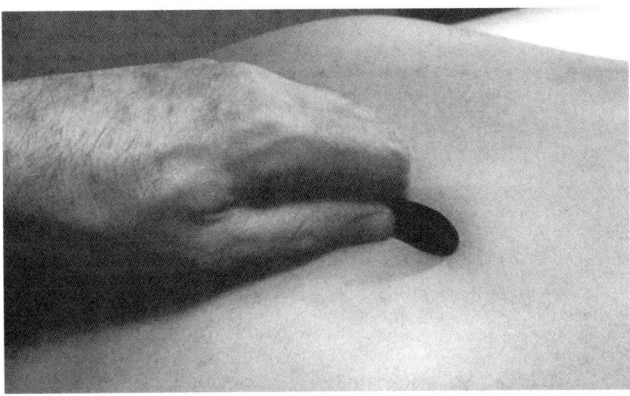

Figure 6-20: Scraping.

area; and/or slide the cups up and down the patient's skin (without breaking the vacuum).

4. For medicinal cupping, bamboo cups are boiled for fifteen minutes within a decoction that usually contains herbs that warm and circulate Blood. Then the cups are removed and their orifices are wrapped with a cool towel. With cups still warm, the practitioner places them over the selected areas. Care is taken to prevent scalding.

Sliding the cups while the vacuum is maintained can be quite painful for the patient. The practitioner can use this technique after having performed regular cupping and pulling cups to minimize pain. Because of the strong mechanical stretching a moving cup produces, it is helpful to preheat the area. Heat helps transform connective tissues from a gel-state (hardened) to a sol-state (more fluid) and encourages tissue softening and lengthening. Heat also increases the local metabolic rate so that nourishment is increased and waste is removed. This may prevent damage to the tissues and minimize soreness.

There are several methods that incorporate bleeding and cupping. The first involves tapping the skin with a seven-star needle and then applying the cups. Another method is to use a lancet (or three edged needle) and then to apply the cup. The last method is to use a lancet on raised papules that are found on the skin following moving cup procedures. This method can be used for various types of internal injury to soft tissues, both in acute or chronic sprains and strains. It is also used for inflammatory conditions of soft tissues or joints (e.g., RA, neruogenic dermatitis, erythema nodosum, etc.). This technique can also be used for psychosomatic and inorganic disorders.

PRECAUTIONS AND CONTRA-INDICATIONS DURING APPLICATION OF CUPPING

- Patient should remain still to prevent the cups from falling off.
- Cups should be applied on smooth and even surfaces. Excessive body hair may be shaved.
- The patient should be protected from cold drafts.
- Care should be taken to avoid scalding the patient by dripping burning alcohol and when using medicinal-cupping.
- During removal, in order to avoid unnecessary pain, one hand is used to tilt the cup and the other to press on the skin next to the cup to break the vacuum. When suction breaks, the cup is removed.
- If an area is to be cupped repeatedly, time should be allowed for the skin to heal.
- Cupping should not be used on patients with severe cardiopathy, haemophilia, generalized edema, generalized dermatopathy, or localized injured skin (ulcers, fissure, etc.), expecting mothers after the first trimester, children under six years of age and elderly patients over seventy years of age (small gentle cups may still be used), and on patients with a high fever or cramps or convulsions.

Cupping can also be used as a diagnostic aid. If a slight bleeding occurs over the cupping area, it may indicate some pathological changes in the capillaries. Cupping can induce the skin rash of measles to appear sooner than otherwise. At times, when edema is difficult to detect, cupping can easily produce blistering. Cupping can also be used for testing several diseases that cause alteration in the permeability of blood capillaries. For example, in endocarditis cupping can induce an increase in the permeability of the capillaries in the treated area. When a few drops of blood are collected for examination, they will show an increase in monocyte count two or three or even as much as five times greater than samples collected from areas that did not under go cupping (Wolldmon's test).

Scraping

Scraping (Gua Sha) is a useful TCM technique for reducing pain and loosening tight muscles. The practitioner applies a medicated oil (or any oil) to the skin and scrapes the area with a porcelain spoon or other instrument until skin erythema (redness) or hematoma (bruise) is created (Figure 6-20). Intense prolonged redness which occurs due to the "red response" indicates an area of poor vasodilation or that the patient is a histamine producer. This procedure, which has both diagnostic and therapeutic value, should be repeated until the skin no longer responds with quick bruising and prolonged erythema (usually two to six sessions). Scraping is used often at the cervical spine and shoulders. Scraping may cause raised papules that may be bled and which are then thought to allow "sand-toxin" from excess-Heat to escape. This may be done after cupping as well. Again, preheating the area is helpful.

Moxibustion and Heat Therapy

A common treatment for chronic musculoskeletal pain, moxibustion tonifies, warms, and vitalizes Qi and Blood. Moxi-

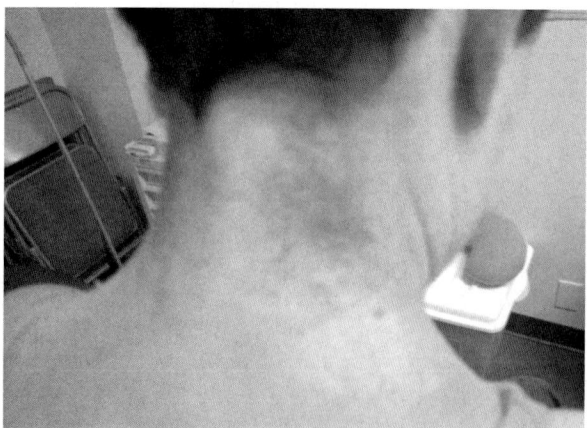

Figure 6-21: Patient's skin after neck scraping.

bustion has warming and supporting effects on Yang; it can be used to move and free the flow of the channels and collaterals, expel pathogenic-Cold, dispel Dampness, and disperse swelling and nodulation. The practitioner ignites a preparation of Artemisia Vulgaris (Ai Ye) and may place it directly over the acupoint, on top of a needle, hold it above the point/area, or use it to warm a needle (Figure 6-22). Moxibustion is usually performed starting on Yang areas and points followed by Yin areas or points (i.e., starting in upper parts and working downwards) to prevent fainting, dizziness, and thirst. Moxa is used most often in chronic disorders and on weak (Yang-deficient) patients or on patients with acute attacks of Cold with strong surface and muscle tension. Moxa is available in various forms: moxa rolls that can be used over the skin to heat large areas, small moxa balls that can be put on an acupuncture needle and are said to result in deep penetrating heat, small threads that can be used directly on the skin, adhesive sticks used directly on the skin, and in several smokeless forms. There are several types of moxa boxes that can be used to heat larger areas. Direct moxa (applied directly to the skin) can result in burns and is therefore rarely used in modern practice. Moxa and heat therapy should not be used on patients with reduced skin sensitivity, as they may not be aware when burned.

Mechanisms of Heat and Moxa

As connective tissues (and blood) are thermoelectric and heat can change them from a gel (solid) to sol (liquid) state, moxibustion and heat therapy may have bioelectrical and mechanical effects. Heat can increase metabolic rate, cell activity, and local blood flow, all of which can encourage healing. The lowered blood viscosity allows for better microcirculation and pain relief. The change of connective tissue to a sol state allows for easier tissue stretching and results in pain relief. Increased metabolic rate results in improved tissue repair and removal of metabolic by-products and therefore faster relief of pain. There are also neural effects such as stimulation of proprioceptors which then decrease muscle spasm and pain. Heat can also encourage the propagated sensation associated with acupuncture. Heat may also stimulate the hypothalamus, a brain region that can effect pain perception.

According to Mussat, currents generated by heating needles can be as high as 20mV (higher than that achieved by using different metals). It must be realized, however, that heating the needle shaft of a modern stainless steel needle probably results in little (if any) increase in the temperature of the needle shaft and therefore of the tissues. This is easily demonstrated when one holds the needle shaft while heating the handle. Even when the handle is red hot, very little temperature change is sensed at the shaft, because the thin-gauge, stainless steel needle is a very poor conductor of heat. Claims that warming needles softens scar tissues are therefore questionable. For more information on thermotherapy see page 541.

Clinical Use in Musculoskeletal Disorders

A whole-body moxa treatment that is said to strengthen the constitution, increase circulation, and help Original and Nutritive-Qi can be performed at:

- St-36
- Sp-6 and 10
- CV-12, 8, 6, 4
- GV-14 and 12
- UB-17, 18, 20, 23, 32 and 52.

These points can be either treated simultaneously in one session or alternately in several sessions.

Following moxibustion it is recommended that the patient not drink tea for fear it will negate the heating effects and not eat for fear the channel Qi will stagnate. The patient should rest quietly for one or two hours. When using moxibustion, it is also recommend that the patient should not eat too much rice, spicy foods, or drink too much alcohol for fear of causing Phlegm.

The following points are said to be contraindicated for moxa treatment:

- Head and Neck: GV-15, 16, 25, UB-1, 2, 10, 6, GB-15, St-8, 9, TW-16, 23
- Chest and Abdomen: Lu-3, Sp-16, 20, GB-22, St-17, CV-15
- Back: UB-15, 30, GV-16, 3
- Upper Limbs: SI-9, TW-4, Lu-11, 10, 8, P-9
- Lower Limbs: Sp-1, 7, 9, St- 31, 32, 33, 35, 38, UB-36, 51, 40, 62, GB-42.

In modern times, heat lamps, hot packs, diathermy, and ultrasound or other heat-generating equipment are often used to substitute for moxibustion. Medicated (herbal) heat packs and steaming an area with an herbal decoction are often used

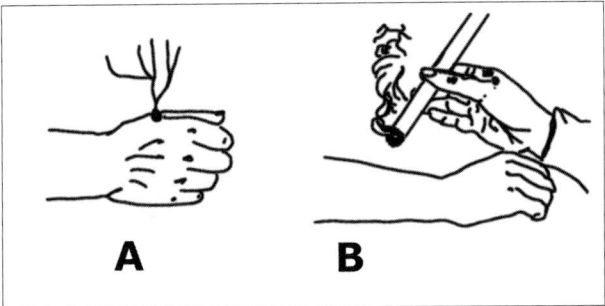

Figure 6-22: (A) Direct moxa, (B) Indirect moxa.

to treat pain as well. Modern steaming instruments are available. Most modern instruments can be easily controlled to give a uniform source of heat.

Warm acupuncture refers to warming the needle after insertion into the body (holding a moxa stick against the needle handle, or placing it on the handle), or prior to insertion (Fire-Needle). Fire-needle is used to treat the Sinew channels and muscle spasm. After applying heat, the body will respond by trying to maintain its own homeostatic thermal balance. In musculoskeletal practice, Moxa is especially helpful when applied over musculotendinous junctions or at points that lie over musculotendinous junctions (e.g., LI-16, 10, 6, TW-5, 10, 14, SI-9, 10, etc.).

Cold Therapy

While the rationale for cold packs to treat inflammation can be easily demonstrated as existing within TCM principles, cold therapy was not used in ancient times. In modern times, ice packs are sometimes recommended in the early stages of sprains and contusions. By and large, however, cold therapy is discouraged by most TCM/OM practitioners, as it is believed that cold can lead to injury, even though studies clearly show benefit when used in the early stage of spain/strain (see page 539). Many TCM/OM practitioners hold the view that cold results in "freezing" connective tissues which leads to "scar" tissues. Cold is also believed to be capable of causing joint pain and leading to the development of arthritis (Bi syndromes). This view, however, is dogmatic, even though the fact that connective tissue can become hardened (go into the gel state) by the application of cold does support the possibility of increased temporary tightness. Cold therapy has been shown to reduce the recovery time of ankle sprains. Cold therapy has been shown to result in a rebound increase of circulation but with rebound lymphatic congestion as well, which may be detrimental.

Blood-Letting Therapy

Bleeding techniques are one of the oldest known therapies in Chinese medicine, and, according to many physicians (Hsu and Miriam Lee, for example), are very important and

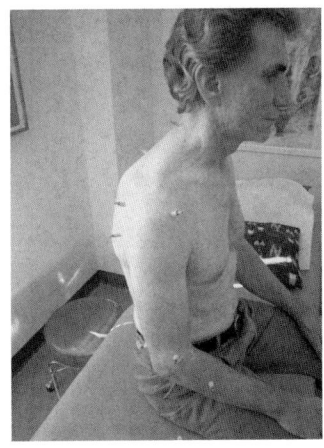

Figure 6-23: Adhesive moxa cones used to treat muscle weakness following brachial neuritis.

should not be ignored. Blood-letting is used mainly to drain Heat or quicken the Blood and Qi and to relieve local congestion. An entire chapter of the classic, *Spiritual Axis,* is devoted to the connecting channels, the network-vessels, and blood-letting therapy. Several needles such as triangular lance and sword-like flat needles are described. It is said that "When the Blood and Qi are both abundant and the Yin-Qi is plentiful, the Blood will be slippery so that needling will cause it to eject." On the other hand, "When much bleeding takes place with needling, but the color does not change and there are palpitations and depression, it is because needling the connecting channel causes the channel to become empty." Blood-letting therapy was mainly recommend to drain fevers, treat Heat, draw "old" Blood, treat fear, convulsions, madness, and to "exhaust" chronic diseases. *Spiritual Axis* also recommends bleeding for the treatment of Heat disease where the whole body feels heavy, the center of the Intestines is hot, when there are spasms around the navel and chest, and the ribs are full. It states: "Whenever in examining the Blood network-vessels they show red, black, and bluish green color, this is Cold and Heat Qi...when needling Cold and Heat always [choose] many Blood network-vessels and absolutely treat every other day. When bleeding is exhausted, the treatment stops, depletion and repletion is then harmonized." Another indication for bleeding therapy is Excess in the Organs: "For excess of the Liver, bleed the Jue-Yin and Shao-Yang channels; for excess of the Spleen, bleed points of the Tai-Yin, Yang-Ming and Shao-Yin; for excess of the Lung, bleed the Shao-Yin channel; for excess of the Kidney, bleed the Shao-Yin and Tai-Yin channels; for excess of the Heart bleed points under the tongue (Jin Jin and Yu Ye) and at H-6." The *Classic of Internal Medicine* states: "When the minute vessels (Sun) are visible upon examination and show abundance and firmness and are bleeding, select all of them [for treatment]." The *Systematic Classic of Acupuncture* also includes much information on bleeding techniques, and bleeding was recommended to drain Heat, treat pain, sore throat, and to dissipate and "drain" chronic diseases. Bleeding of UB-40 is recommended for lower back pain: "The unraveled vessel cause\

s people to suffer from splitting lower back pain with irascibility....Needle the unraveled vessel at UB-40, pricking the binding connecting vessel there which is like a millet grain. Upon being pricked, the vessel will eject black Blood and, once the Blood turns red, the treatment may be stopped."[23] As with all types of treatment, bleeding is not appropriate for all patients. For example, *Spiritual Axis* states: "[In conditions where there is] a mad and urgent pulse, which stands out and bulges, and the vessels in the four extremities are swollen and jumpy, if the pulse is full, prick and let blood out, if the pulse is not full, use moxibustion on the Tai-Yang [channel] at the nape of the neck, on the Girdle/Belt vessel (Dai), three cun from the hip, and all the Transport (Shu) points on the extremities." The *Classic of Internal Medicine* also warns against inappropriate bleeding and the possible harm that can be caused by bleeding the vessels (especially visible vessels such as the popliteal or cubital).

Although most texts mention weakness as contraindications for blood-letting as stated earlier, Dr. Miriam Lee often used bleeding on weak and old patients saying that by eliminating "bad" Blood and Pathogenic Factors the patient is strengthened. She often bled UB-43 for this purpose (mainly in degenerative knee disease). This therapy should *not* be used on patients who have already suffered from hemorrhage (including post-partum) and for those who are extremely weak. Tapping the skin with a seven-star needle (until light bleeding occurs) followed by cupping is often used to increase Blood-circulation and to treat taxation pain, such as chronic epicondylitis, bursitis etc.

Subhuti Dharmananda states:

Peripheral blood-letting today is mainly carried out at the fingers and toes. At the tips of the toes, for example, are the qiduan points, located 0.1cun behind the nails.These are said to be useful for emergency treatment for stroke or for numbness of the toes, also for redness, swelling, and pain of the instep of the foot. Near the toe webbing, there is another set of points, the bafeng (eight wind) points, four on each foot. These can be needled either by standard procedure with shallow oblique insertion, or they can be pricked to cause bleeding. The points are indicated for swelling of the legs, toe pain, snake bite to the foot or lower leg, and swelling and pain of the dorsum of the foot. Similarly, at the tips of the fingers are the shixuan points, located 0.1 cun behind the nails. Pricking these

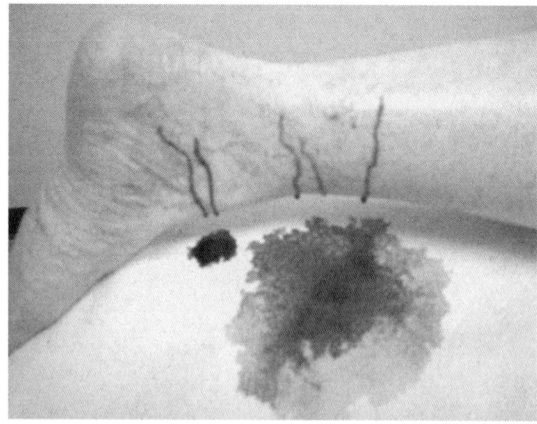

Figure 6-24: Bleeding congested vessels around the ankle.

points to let out blood is said to be useful for coma, epilepsy, high fever, and sore throat. A little further down, at the finger creases (the lower of the two creases along the finger joints), are the sifeng points (four wind points; the thumb, which has only the one crease, is not included). Pricking these to let out plasma fluid that is yellowish white, is said to treat malnutrition and indigestion in children and whooping cough.[24] Finally, points between each pair of fingers, at the top of the webbing joining the fingers, are the baxie points. These can be acupunctured with shallow insertion of 0.5-0.8 cun depth or pricked to cause bleeding, used to treat snakebite of the hand. The terminal jing points, known by some as "ting" points, are also pricked to let out blood. These "well" points, of which there are 12, are mainly located at the tips of the fingers and toes (the exception is KI-1)

It is this author's practice to use blood-letting in acute sprains/strains where there is swelling and throbbing pain. One looks for "congested" dark blood vessels rather than picking predetermined points or channels. Well/Jing/Ting points are bled as well. Blood is squeezed-out until there is a change in color.[25] In chronic conditions, visibly congested

---

23. This technique was used extensively by Dr. Miriam Lee for this and other conditions. Vessels at UB-40, Lu-5, and Tai Yang were bled deeply using a triangle needle until the flow would stop on its own and the blood color would change.

24. Dr. Lee often bled these point in children saying it helps accelerate their growth, especially when small for their age.

25. Dr. Lee used to say that "bad blood" which was described as thick and black was too acidic. As Dr. Dharmananda points out, there is little convincing modern research to support the concept of "bad" blood or the proposed mechanism for bleeding techniques. Nevertheless, when local congestion is evident, bleeding is even used in modern hospitals, usually using leeches. Leech therapy has been shown to be helpful in osteoarthritis of the knee, although this may not only be due to the bleeding effect (Michanlsen et al 2002). Bleeding is used in disorders with excess red-blood cells, as well.
   In this author's experience bleeding congested blood vessels around acutely injured joints (not the bruise itself) often results in immediate reduction of throbbing pains. Some practitioners bleed the bruised area directly; however, this author has had a few patients in which such a technique may (possibly) have resulted in prolonged recovery and hardened local tissues. Many chronic pain patients also respond to bleeding techniques when there is *evidence* of vascular congestion.

and dark small veins can be bled to "improve" circulation and get rid of Blood-stasis. This is often helpful in patients with arthritic and discogenic pain. It is also helpful in older patients with problems of stenosis and neuropathy. In the lateral cases, bleeding is not used over local hyperalgesic tissues.

A related technique is to draw the patient's blood and then inject it into acupuncture points or pathogenic tissues. For example, for lateral epicondylitis (tennis elbow of the tendinosis type), blood is drawn and then injected at LI-11, 10 and at the tendinous insertions. The elbow is then wrapped using a medicated plaster. This may be repeated two or three times.

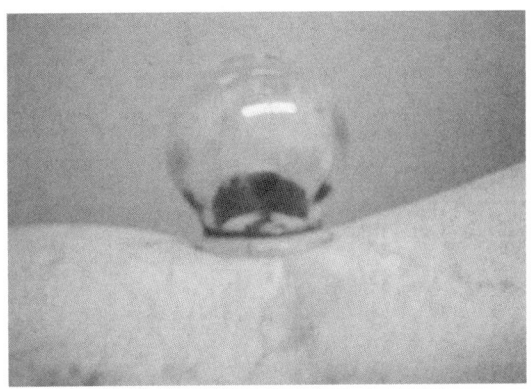

Figure 6-25: Patient's low back is cupped and bled for treatment of annular disc pain.

7

FOUNDATIONS FOR INTEGRATIVE HERBAL MEDICINE

Using herbs in the treatment of most chronic musculoskeletal disorders can be helpful but is usually not sufficient on its own. Herbs are helpful when used topically as well as teas, powders, and pills.

Chinese Herbal Therapy

Herbal medicine has been the core of TCM therapy through most of its history. It was the mythical emperor Sheng Nung, around 2800 BC., who is credited with the discovery and first systematic recording of the healing powers of plants, although the classic text carrying his name did not appear until about 100 BC. Since the time of the classic, *Damage by Cold,* in the third century BC, practitioners have been accustomed to using formulas or combinations of herbs that were categorized in specific groups and assigned to specific diseases/patterns/syndromes. These prescriptions often address the patient's general condition and disease (so called root and branch). In TCM, formulas are designed using four major categories of herbs.

These are:

- Chief or King herb, which is the main herb that is directed against the principal pattern diagnosis or disease.
- Minister or Deputy herbs, which aid the chief in addressing the principal pattern, as well as serve as the main element directed against a concurrent pattern or disease.
- Assistant herbs, which reinforce the effect of the chief and/or minister, balance the effects of the chief and/or minister by having an opposite effect, and moderate or eliminate the toxicity of the chief or minister herbs.
- Guide or Envoy herbs, which direct the formula to the appropriate channel or region and harmonize and integrate the actions of the other herbs.

Although not all formulas contain all these elements, it is this balanced approach to formulation which accounts for the low toxicity and side-effects seen with Chinese herbal therapy. In modern times, practitioners often use a variety of information including historical and modern biomedical research when designing herbal formulations. The proper practice of Chinese herbal medicine *requires* a thorough understanding of TCM/OM theory. Just as in acupuncture, herbal medicine is used with many and differing systems and paradigms within Chinese Medicine. The systems of correspondences and "transliterations" are used in herbal medicine, as well. For example, peels of fruits and barks are said to have effects on the bodies "peel" or Exterior; the twigs of trees enter the channels, the vines and the spongy parts of fruit (that have a network-like look) enter the network-vessels; and seeds with the capability of growth, can move downward and often enter the Kidneys. Other relations can be seen, for instance, herbs or substances that are heavy tend to descend; herbs that are light tend to ascend; pungent and hot qualities are active, making the herb that has them capable of movement, activating Qi and out-thrusting or moving to the Exterior. Cold qualities would make an herb more likely to slow down activity and move inwards. Sourness would make an herb astringent and thus render it capable of helping to reduce swelling.

Treatment of Blood Circulation

The following is a general discussion of the treatment of Blood-stasis as it pertains to sprains and strains, as well as to other musculoskeletal Painful Obstruction disorders. The 18th century practitioner Wang Qing Ren emphasized the treatment of Blood-stasis in chronic diseases and pain, a pathology which often must be resolved when treating Painful Obstruction, especially in trauma and chronic disorders.[1] It is said, "when treatment fails, look at Blood-stasis." Blood flow may be slowed or blocked by any of the Pathogenic Factors as well as Organic and Qi-dysfunctions. In early stages or in mild cases, the Blood moves slower than it should. Later, if there is no improvement, the Blood stagnates and begins to accumulate. In more severe cases, or when no effective treatment has been given, the Blood congeals and may form substantial swelling (mass: Ji, Ju, Jie, etc.), and/or tumor. It is not uncommon at this stage to see Blood and Phlegm masses, especially in late-stage degenerative conditions with bony spurs. Thus, in clinical practice, there are generally three main *levels* or *degrees* of eliminating Blood-stasis. If a method that is too strong is chosen, not only may this cause hemorrhaging (theoretically), but also it

---

1. Wan Men-Ying, also a 18th century physician, emphasized the treatment of Phlegm in late chronic Painful Obstruction.

is said to waste or injure the Blood, Yin, Fluids, and Qi. In general, Blood-stasis herbs are used in four ways:[2]

1. The first level is activating the Blood, regulating-Qi, promoting circulation, and transforming stasis. This method uses medicinals such as Rhizoma Ligustici Wallichii (Chuan Xiong), Rhizoma Corydalis (Yan Hu Suo), Radix Salviae Miltiorrhizae (Dan Shen), Flos Carthami Tinctorii (Hong Hua), Rhizoma Polygoni Cuspidati (Hu Zhang), and Rhizoma Curcumae Longae (Jiang Huang) to promote Blood circulation and to sweep away stasis. It can be used in the *postural/dysfunction phase*[3] of the degenerative cascade with stasis, and Painful Obstruction in the channels. This method can be used in patients where pain increases when tissues are stressed for some time, such as prolonged slouched sitting (where not disc related), or when tissues have been stretched excessively for prolonged periods. This type of pain is due to the poor circulation and nourishment of sinews and to excessive demand from overuse. The condition is not chronic and often relatively easy to treat. Some of these herbs move the Blood by activating the Qi within the Blood (Yan Hu Suo, Chuan Xiong, Yu Jin).[4] Many of these herbs are slightly warm and pungent, which helps move the Blood. However, some are slightly cold, such as Tuber Curcumae (Yu Jin) and Salviae Miltiorrhizae (Dan Shen). This is the least "attacking" of the three TCM methods for treating Blood-stasis.

Rhizoma Ligustici Wallichii (Chuan Xiong) is a very important herb for treating pain. It enters the Liver, Gall Bladder, and Pericardium channels and can move upward, downward, inward, or outward. It is often used in patients with headaches, neuralgias, traumas, and/or arthritis. It can be used for crampy (cold) pain in any part of the body. It can be prescribed for Excess, Deficiency, Cold, or Hot conditions. Because it is pungent and warm it can injure Yin and Qi, and thus should be used with care, especially if a large dosage is used. The extract of this herb can be used for injection to treat musculoskeletal disorders and intravenously for heart disease.

Rhizoma Corydalis (Yan Hu Suo) is very important for treating pain. It enters the Liver and Spleen channels as well as the Qi and Blood levels. This herb can be used for all types of pain; when fried with vinegar its analgesic effects increase. It also has anti-inflammatory effects. The extract of the herb can be used as an injectable analgesic.[5]

Radix Salviae Miltiorrhizae (Dan Shen) enters the Heart and Liver channels, but primarily acts on the Heart. Because it is bitter and cold, this herb can clear-Heat, cool the Blood, and calm the mind. This herb can also promote circulation, remove congealed-Blood, and reduce pain. Although more often used in Heart disease, this herb can be used for musculoskeletal pain, as well. Studies have suggested that it can aid deposit calcium at a bone fracture zone. Clinically, it is often used to treat arthritis or traumatic injuries, especially with swelling and pain due to Heat-type stasis. It can also be added to any formula that deals with Blood-stasis. Extracts of this herb can be used as injectable for myofascial disorders.

Tuber Curcumae (Yu Jin) enters the Heart, Lung, and Liver channels. This herb is cool and pungent and is mostly used to treat Liver and Heart related disorders with pain due to Qi-stagnation and Blood-stasis. It can also treat bleeding from Blood-Heat, and then it is sometimes used in traumatic bleeding. It is sometimes used to treat headaches.

Flos Carthami Tinctorii (Hong Hua) enters the Heart and Liver channels. It can invigorate the Blood and promote circulation. When used in large dosage (10-15g) this herb can break up congealed-Blood and reduce pain. When used in small amounts (1-3g) it can help generate Blood and therefore it can be added to Blood-tonic formulas. It is used very often to treat trauma, reduce

---

2. Mao Xiao (2003) describes four methods of using acrid (spicy) medicinals: 1) Acrid and moistening method is used to diffuse, disperse, to open, and to reach the subcutaneous layers (Cou Li), move the Fluids and free the flow of Qi and Blood. It is used widely to treat hypochondrial pain, stomach pain, stagnation patterns, blood loss, yellowing, etc. Herbs such as: Xuan Fu Hua, Xin Jiang, Qing Cong, Hong Hua, Xi Cao Gen with Dang Gui, Lao Ren, Bai Zi Ren, Yu Jin, Yan Hu Suo, and Cuan Lian Zi and others can be used. 2) Acrid and Warm method is used to disperse Cold. Used often to treat Cold-Damp congealing and stagnation, internal prevalence of Yin-Cold causing network-vessel obstruction; like Accumulations (Ji) and Gatherings (Ju), Stomach pain and other patterns. Medicinals such as: Rou Gui, Fu Zhi, Gui Zhi, Xie Bai, Gan Jiang, Xiao Hui Xiang, etc. with the addition of Pu Huang, Wu Ling Zhi, Tao Ren, and others can be used. 3) Acrid and fragrant method is used to move and penetrate. This method is often used in Heart pain, abdominal and umbilical pain, Stomach pain, hypochondrial pain, Conglomerations (Jie) and Gatherings (Ju) masses and other patterns, especially in chronic diseases. Medicinals such as: Jiang Zhen Xiang, Mu Xiang, Xiang Ru, Bi Ba, Xiao Wu Xiang, Xie Bai, Cang Bai are often combined with Ru Xiang, Mo Yao, Dan Shen, Jiang Huang, Tao Ren, Chuan Shan Jia, and others can be used. 4) Acrid and salty method is used as a harsh and attacking method to treat headaches, stubborn obstructions, pathological conglomerations, accumulations and gatherings, and other chronic diseases that are difficult to treat. Medicinals such as: Qiang Lang, Feng Fang, Meng Chong, Di Long, Quan Xie, Zhenchong, Chuan Shan Jia, Qi Cao, Jiang Can, Shui Zhi, Wu Gong and others can be used.

   The *Classic of Difficult Issues* states that Accumulations are caused by Yin influences and affect the Yin Organs. They may pertain to fixed masses. Gatherings are caused by Yang influences and affect the Yang Organs. They may pertain to movable masses.

3. For more information see "Three Phases of Degeneration," page 556.

4. Some of this discussion is not classically described. These herbs can be used to treat posain. When lying down (or when immobility) causes joint pains, it is considered to be due to the Qi within the Blood not moving.

5. Much of the Corydalis (Yan Hu Sou) available on the market contains alpha toxin in excess of the allowed amount in Europe (but expectable in US). Alpha toxin is liver toxic and can cause cancer.

   To treat pain, Corydalis (Yan Hu Sou), Frankincense (Ru Xiang), Myrrh (Mo Yao), Ligustici (Chuan Xiong), Carthami Tinctorii (Hong Hua), Trogopteri (Wu Ling Zhi) and Notoginseng (San Qi) are the most important Blood-moving herbs.

swelling, stasis, and pain. It can be used for joint as well as soft tissue pains. Because of its strong moving effects and its pungent and warming effects, this herb can increase bleeding if used early post-traumatically, and, therefore, should be combined with other herbs. Extracts of this herb can be used as injectable for the treatment of myofascial disorders or intravenously to thin the blood.

Rhizoma Curcumae Longae (Jiang Huang) enters the Spleen and Liver channels and can vitalize the Blood and promote circulation. It can also "break-up" Blood-stasis. This herb can also clear Wind from the channels and collaterals/network-vessels, thus relieving pain. It is especially important for shoulder or upper limb pain. It has anti-inflammatory effects (COX-2 inhibition).

Rhizoma Polygoni Cuspidati (Hu Zhang) enters the Liver, Gall Bladder, and Lung channels. This herb is used to activate the Blood circulation to stop pain. It can be used to treat traumatic injuries. This herb has anti-inflammatory effects.

2. The second level is to dispel stasis and activate the Blood. These herbs often dissolve and dissipate congealed Blood and open the channels and network-vessels. In this case, the stasis is first dispelled. This results in the activation of Blood circulation, often by opening vessels, thinning blood and increasing microcirculation. Consequently, the Blood can penetrate and dispel stasis and nourish tissues. These herbs are mostly slightly pungent and warm, but some are slightly cold. Radix Millettiae Reticulatae (Ji Xue Teng), Radix Rubrus Paeoniae Lactiflorae (Chi Shao), Fasciculus Vascularis Luffae (Si Gua Lao), Gummi Olibanum (Ru Xiang), Myrrhae (Mo Yao), Fructus Liquidambaris (Lu Lu Tong), Sanguis Draconis (Xue Jie), Lignum Sappan (Su Mu), and Squama Mantitis Pentadactylae (Chuan Shan Jia) are representative herbs for this purpose. They are used often in the *instability* and *stabilization* phases to increase circulation to ligaments and tendons. Pain in the instability stage is often worse when the patient does not move for a period of time (cocktail party syndrome) in the morning, and is better with some movement (i.e., posain). The patient often complains of his/her back being "out" and needs frequent manipulations (adjustments). The condition is chronic and more difficult to treat. For these purposes these herbs are often used with tonifying and tissue-strengthening herbs.[6]

Radix Millettiae Reticulatae (Ji Xue Teng) enters the Liver and Kidney channels, and especially the network-vessels/collaterals. This herb can invigorate the Blood and promote circulation. It can also tonify the Blood and therefore is often used in chronic conditions such as chronic arthritis, neuropathic pain, numbness, stiffness and cramping pain in the limbs. It can open the collateral/network-vessels and reduce pain due to Blood-stasis or Blood-deficiency. It is often used in elderly patients when a large dosage can be used.

Radix Rubrus Paeoniae Lactiflorae (Chi Shao) enters the Heart and Liver channels. Because it is slightly cold and bitter, it can clear excess-Heat from the Blood. This herb also has a mild Blood-tonifying function (although some texts say it has no Blood tonifying effects). It is especially useful in treating Blood-Heat, because it is able to invigorate the Blood and thus less likely to result in stasis by its cold nature. This herb is used often to treat inflammation, swelling, and pain from traumatic or other origins.

Fasciculus Vascularis Luffae (Si Gua Lao) enters the Liver, Stomach, and Lung channels. Because this herb can expel Wind, invigorate the Blood, and clear Damp-Heat, it is useful when treating painful or sore muscles and sinews. It can also be used in acute injuries, especially chest or lumbar, and in other joint disorders. Because it is neutral, it can be used in most cases.

Gummi Olibanum (Ru Xiang) enters the Heart and Liver and can promote both Qi and Blood circulation. Its aromatic nature allows the herb to penetrate and regulate Qi. It "relaxes" the sinews (more so than Mo Yao) and thus is often used for stiff, swollen, and painful joints or soft tissues. This herb is also used often for traumatic sprains, strains, and fractures, because it is analgesic and can disperse swelling and aid in healing.

Myrrhae (Mo Yao) enters the Liver or all twelve of the twelve channels and network-vessels. Like Gummi Olibanum (Ru Xiang) it is used to treat stiff, swollen, and painful joints and soft tissues. This herb is also used for traumatic sprains, strains, and fractures. It can break up congealed Blood and therefore can treat hard masses such as bony outgrowths (spurs).

Fructus Liquidambaris (Lu Lu Tong) enters mainly the Liver and Stomach channels. It is also said to be able to open all the channels and network-vessels. It promotes the movement of both Qi and Blood. Because it can also eliminate Wind-Dampness, it is used for Painful Obstruction (Bi) syndromes. The herb can be added to many formulas that treat pain, especially of the lower back and extremities. This herb has anti-inflammatory effects.

Sanguis Draconis (Xue Jie) enters the Heart and Liver channels. It can dispel Blood-stasis and alleviate pain. This substance is often used to treat sprains, strains, contusions, and fractures. It is used topically to stop bleeding due to external injury. Because it is neutral it can be used in most cases.

Lignum Sappan (Su Mu) enters the Heart, Liver, and Spleen channels. This herb invigorates the Blood, reduces swelling, and alleviates pain. It is used for pain due to sprains, strains, contusions, and fractures. It can also be used for arthritic pain.

Squama Mantitis Pentadactylae (Chuan Shan Jia) enters the Liver and Stomach channels but can reach (and penetrate) the entire body (Organs, channels, collaterals/

---

6. Not classically described.

network-vessels). This substance (animal) is mild and can be used in most patients. It can disperse Blood-stasis, reduce swelling and expel Wind-Dampness in the channels. It is mainly used to treat swelling, stiffness, numbness, and tingling or spasms of the limbs. It is often added to formulas that treat chronic arthritic pains. Because this substance is said to drain pus and treat swellings, it is used also in the treatment of nodules with or without pus. This substance has anti-inflammatory effects. Manitis is an endangered species.

3. The third level is braking stasis and dispersing mass. This is the strongest method of eliminating Blood-stasis. Often combined with Phlegm herbs, these herbs are used for cases of *substantial* stagnant-Blood, such as seen in the *stabilization phase* of the degenerative cascade. In this case, usually, there are palpable masses/nodes or spurs on x-rays. The pain may be independent of movement. It is more related to the location of the hypertrophy and whether there is an impingement of the nerves or whether local congestion is severe.[7] Since it is said that "it takes Qi to move the Qi, and takes Blood to move the Blood," care must be applied when using this method as it can damage Yin, Blood and Qi. If needed Qi, and Blood tonics are added. Semen Pruni Persicae (Tao Ren), Hirudo seu Whitmania (Shui Zhi), Eupolyphaga seu Opisthoplatia (Tu Bie Chong; also called Di Bie Chong), Rhizoma Curcumae (E Zhu) and Rhizoma Sparganii Stoloniferi (San Leng)[8] are commonly used herbs that brake stasis and disperse masses.

Semen Pruni Persicae (Tao Ren) enters the Heart, Large Intestine, Liver, and Lung channels. This herb is important when treating Blood-stasis and accumulations (mass). It can be used for many kinds of pain due to traumatic causes or due to chronic Blood accumulation. Because it is neutral, it can be used in most cases.

Hirudo seu Whitmania (Shui Zhi) enters the Liver and Bladder channels. Because it is a blood socking animal (leech), it is said to penetrate masses to break up and drive out Blood-stasis. This substance is sometimes used in acute traumas.[9] Because it is slightly toxic, it should be used with care.

---

7. Not classically described.

8. Although the last two are not commonly recommended in musculoskeletal medicine, the Guangzhou municipal hospital #2 general use Tie Da (trauma) formula contains: Radix Glycyrrhizae (Gan Cao) 6g, Radix Rubrus Paeoniae (Chi Shao) 10g, Rhizoma Curcumae (E Zhu) 10g, Rhizoma Sparganii (San Leng) 10g, Radix Dipsaci (Xu Duan) 10g, Fructus Psoralea (Bu Gu Zhi) 10g, Tuber Curcumae (Yu Jin) 10g, Radix Angelica (Dang Gui) 10g.

9. Worms, insects, and reptiles are often used for disorders that have entered the collaterals/network-vessels (Blood circulation system). They can also "tract" Wind, i.e., treat Wind of external and internal origin that combine with each other. Live leech therapy placed over painful joints has been shown to be helpful in arthritic joint diseases. Refludan, a newly FDA approved anticoagulant, is structurally based on hiudin, one of the active ingredients in leeches.

Oposthoplatia (Tu Bie Chong) enters the Liver, Heart, and Spleen channels. Because it is an insect (a wingless cockroach), it is said to penetrate masses to break up and drive out Blood-stasis. This substance can also aid in the healing of sinews and bones ("connects sinews and fuses bones"), and is often used for trauma and acute lumbar sprain.

Rhizoma Curcumae (E Zhu) enters the Liver and Spleen channels. It can remove congealed Blood and treat masses. This herb also strongly moves Qi. It is sometimes used to treat old injuries with accumulations or bony spurs. Because this herb can injure the Qi and Blood, it should be used with care.

Rhizoma Sparganii Stoloniferi (San Leng) enters the Spleen and Liver. It is used in the same way as Rhizoma Curcumae (E Zhu) except that it is less potent in activating Qi.

4. A fourth method in which Blood moving herbs are used is known as "dispelling stasis and generating the new." This method is used in cases where Blood-stasis is hindering the generation of fresh Blood. It is also used during recuperation from injuries where a residue of Blood-stasis is said to impede the generation or growth of healthy new tissues or Blood. These herbs often have vitalizing and tonifying effects on Blood. In the treatment of musculoskeletal disorders, this method is often used when Blood "de-stagnating" medicinals are added to other formulas during the recuperative period in weak patients to enhance the clinical effect and in chronic diseases. They are often used in the treatment of fractures as well. These herbs can be used in the *postural, instability,* or *stabilization phases* of the degenerative cascade. Radix Angelica Sinensis (Dang Gui), Radix Rubrus Paeoniae Lactiflorae (Chi Shao), Radix Millettiae Reticulatae (Ji Xue Teng), Radix Achyranthis Bidentatae (Niu Xi), Herba Artemisiae Anomalae (Liu Ji Nu), Pyritum (Zi Ran Tong) and Herba Lycopi Lucidi (Ze Lan) are particularly important, as they can both vitalize and tonify Blood.

Radix Angelica Sinensis (Dang Gui) enters the Heart, Liver, and Spleen. This herb can tonify Blood, invigorate the Blood, reduce swelling, alleviate pain and "generate flesh." It is often used for both chronic and acute disorders.

Radix Achyranthis Bidentatae (Niu Xi) enters the Liver and Kidney channels. It has a weak Blood-moving effect but can tonify the Liver and Kidney, and therefore strengthen the sinews and bones. Because this herb can direct Blood and Heat downwards, it can be used to treat headaches and dizziness with or without epistaxis. This herb is used often to treat chronic disorders, especially with low back ache, weakness of waist and knees, and difficulty walking.

Radix Cythulae Officinalis (Chuan Niu Xi) also enters the same channels but is stronger at moving Blood. It is often used for headaches and dizziness as it can "pull" Blood downwards. This herb can be used also to treat musculoskeletal pains due to traumatic injuries. Like Radix Achyranthis Bidentatae (Niu Xi), this herb can tonify the Liver and Kidney and strengthen the sinews and bones (although less so). It is therefore used to treat chronic weakness and pain of the low back and knees.

Herba Artemisiae Anomalae (Liu Ji Nu) enters the Heart and Spleen channels. It can dispel Blood-stasis and unblock the channels. This herb is sometimes used in trauma, mostly to dispel swelling.

Pyritum (Zi Ran Tong) enters the Liver and Kidney channels. This mineral (copper) can dispel Blood-stasis and unblock the channels. It can also "renew" the sinews and therefore is used for traumatic injuries and instabilities. Clinically, it is mostly used for traumatic injuries with swelling, pain, inflammation, and bruising. It is also commonly used to treat bone fractures.

Herba Lycopi Lucidi (Ze Lan) enters the Liver and Spleen channels. This herb is mild and can both supplement and move Blood and therefore can be used in most patients. It treats Blood-stasis, Blood-deficiency, edema, and joint swelling that occur due to Liver-congestion, Qi-stagnation causing Spleen-deficiency. It can be used for acute injuries as well. Clinically, this herb is often used to treat back or other joint pains from traumatic injuries. It can also be used for chronic arthritic pains with swelling. The extracts of this herb can be used intravenously to treat disseminated intravascular coagulation (DIC).

BLEEDING. Bleeding in musculoskeletal disorders is generally associated with trauma. Trauma and stasis of Blood can result in transformative-Heat. It is therefore common to add some cooling herbs when treating acute traumatic injuries. Many of these herbs are used for their other properties as well. To treat Bleeding there are five major methods:

- Clear Heat from the Blood division/depth (cool Blood).
- Eliminate stasis to stop bleeding.
- Tonify Qi/Spleen to hold the Blood in the vessels.
- Astringent method to stop "leaking" Blood.
- Hemostatics methods that may be warm, cold, or neutral.

Carbonizing (charring) an herb strengthens its hemostatic function. Care must be taken when using hemostatics, as they may cause Blood-stasis and usually treat only the symptoms.

- To cool the Blood, herbs such as Cortex Mountain Radicis (Mu Dan Pi), Radix Rehmanniae raw (Sang Di Huang), Cortex Lycii Radicis (Di Gu Pi), and Radix Paeoniae Rubra (Chi Shao) are often used. Dan Pi and Chi Shao can be used without fear of further stagnating Blood due to being too cold, as they also move the Blood.
  — *Cortex Mountan Radicis* (Mu Dan Pi) enters the Heart, Liver, and Kidney channels. This herb can invigorate the Blood and clear Heat from the Blood. It can be used to treat swelling and acute injuries, and it can be used for both Empty-Heat and Full-Heat. It can also be used to balance Yang-tonics, preventing side-effects. Large doses are especially helpful in inflammatory arthritis such as psoriatic arthritis.
  — *Radix Rehmanniae raw* (Sheng Di Huang) enters the Heart, Liver, and Kidney channels. This herb is cold and moist in nature. It can be used in both Empty-Heat and Full-Heat disorders. As it enters the Blood, it can also clear Heat from the Blood-division and can stop bleeding. This herb is used frequently for inflammatory disorders and to calm the patient's spirit when he/she suffers from irritability and thirst. It can be used to treat acute or chronic disease with Full-Heat or Yin-deficiency-Fire (Empty-Fire). It can also be used to balance Yang-tonics, preventing side-effects especially in patients with Yin and Yang deficiency and a tendency to develop Empty-Heat. For this purpose, a large dosage can be used with warm Yang herbs (as much as ten times the amount of Yang tonic herbs).[10] Raw Rehmanniae (Sheng Di Huang) also has a mild Yin-nourishing effect and is less cloy (causing digestive side-effects) than the prepared variety (Shu Di Huang), which is used to tonify the Yin, Blood, Liver, and Kidneys.[11]
  — *Cortex Lycii Radicis* (Di Gu Pi) enters the Lung, Liver and Kidney channels. It has a strong function of reducing Empty-Heat and can be used to treat bleeding and inflammation. This herb can be used also to treat arthritis and to balance the hot properties of Yang-tonics, preventing side-effects.

- To vitalize the Blood and stop bleeding, herbs such as: Radix Pseudoginseng (San Qi), Rhizoma Rhei (Da Huang), Pollen Typhae (Pu Huang), Lignum Sappan (Su Mu), Faeces Trogopterorum (Wu Ling Zhi) and Herba Lycopodii Serrati (Jin Bu Huan) are commonly used.
  —*Radix Pseudoginseng* (San Qi) enters the Liver and Stomach channels. This herb is quite effective at stopping bleeding (when used as a raw powder), yet can unblock the channels and network-vessels, and

---

10. It is not uncommon to use Kidney-Yang tonics to treat chronic low back pain. Many patients, however, are both Yin and Yang deficient, and Kidney-Yang herbs can easily arouse Empty-Heat or Ministerial-Fire. Large doses of Sheng Di can be used in these patients. Yang-Heartening Decoction (Yang He Tang), although using Shu Di Huang (the prepared variety) is often used in such patients. It contains: Rehmanniae (Shu Di Huang) 30g, Colla Cervi (Lu Jiao Jiao) 9g, Cinnamomi (Rou Gui) 3g, Zingiberis (Pao Jiang) 1.5g, Sinapis (Bai Jie Zi) 6g, Ephedrae (Ma Huang) 1.5g, Glycyrrhizae 3g. This formula is often used to treat bony spurs, degenerative joint disease with swelling and weak wasted muscles as often seen in the knee.

11. In patients with weak digestion, Rhizoma Polygonati (Huang Jing) can be substituted for Shu Di Huang. It can tonify Qi, moisten the Lung and Heart, nourish Essence and Marrow, and support the sinews and bones. Another alternative is to add Sha Ren and Ban Xia, or Ma Huang and Shi Chang Pu (or any one of them) to the decoction to counteract the cloy properties of Shu Di. Fu Zi is also useful.

purge congealed-Blood. It is therefore often used to treat traumatic bleeding and swelling. It is also used to treat chronic arthritis with swelling and is one of the most important herbs for pain. This herb can be used topically to stop bleeding.
— *Rhizoma Rhei* (Da Huang) enters the Heart, Large, Intestine, and Liver channels. This herb can both drain Heat and invigorate the Blood. It is a very important herb to treat Blood-stasis, both chronic and acute. It can be used for traumatic bleeding and stasis. It can also expel Hot-Phlegm through the Intestines. It is also used to prevent accumulation of Heat from tonic herbs. It is commonly used topically as well.
— *Pollen Typhae* (Pu Huang) enters the Pericardium and Liver channels. This herb is mild and can be used for most patients. It has weak anti-inflammatory effects and therefore can be used for arthritis. It is often used to treat traumatic swelling.
— *Lignum Sappan* (Su Mu) enters Heart, Liver, and Spleen channels. This herb stops bleeding, invigorates the Blood, reduces swelling, and alleviates pain. It is often used in acute injuries. It is also used in some chronic disorders, mostly for its Blood vitalizing function.
— *Faeces Trogopterorum* (Wu Ling Zhi) enters the Liver (and Spleen) channel. This is a mild substance that disperses Blood-stasis and alleviates pain. It can also transform stasis to stop bleeding. It is often used in chronic pain patients, both in muscular and articular disorders. It is mainly useful in treating swelling and myofascial pains.
— *Herba Lycopodii Serrati* (Jin Bu Huan) enters the Lung, Liver, and Large Intestine channels. This herb can disperse Blood-stasis, invigorate Blood circulation, and stop bleeding. It is used to treat sinew and bone pains.[12]

- To tonify Qi/Spleen arrest bleeding, herbs such as Radix Ginseng (Ren Shen) and Radix Astragali (Huang Qi) are mainly used in weak patients and chronic conditions.
— *Radix Ginseng* (Ren Shen) enters the Lung and Spleen channels. This herb strongly tonifies Original-Qi and is used in weak patients, especially after hemorrhaging. It is often used in chronic cases. It is also helpful in patients when pain becomes worse after (not during) activity.
— *Radix Astragali* (Huang Qi) enters the Lung and Spleen channels. This herb is often used for patients with Qi-deficiency (pain getting worse after activity). It can lift Spleen-Qi and help arrest bleeding. This function is also important in patients with muscular weakness, as this herb is said to be capable of increasing the strength of the muscles. It can also treat numbness and pain due to insufficient nourishment and circulation of Qi and Blood.

- Astringent herbs to stop bleeding such as: Os Sepiae (Hai Piao Xiao), Stamen Nelumbinis Nucifera (Lian Xu), Semen Euryales Ferocia (Qian Shi), Galla Rhois Chinensis (Wu Bei Zi) and Pericarpium Papaveris Somniferi (Ying Su Ke) are *less commonly* used, except topically.
- Warm hemostatics such as Folium Artemisiae Argyi (Ai Ye) and Lignum Dalergiae Odiforae (Jiang Xiang) are *not commonly* used. Ai Ye is sometimes used topically for Cold-type pains.
- Cold hemostatics such as Cacumen Biotae (Ce Bai Ye) and Rumiae Radix (Qian Cao Gen) are sometimes used.
- Neutral hemostatics such as Ophicalcitum (Hua Rui Shi) and Herba Agrimoniae (Xian He Cao) are *not commonly* used.

Clinical approaches and *formulas* for the treatment Blood-stasis and its complication in patients with musculoskeletal disorders are:

1. Transforming Blood-stasis, opening and regulating channels and collaterals/network-vessels, is used for acute or chronic musculoskeletal pains, joint dysfunction and/or pathology, stiffness, and pain worsening at night or by inactivity. Representative formulas are: Seven-Thousandths of a Pearl Powder (Qi Li San), Trauma Pill (Die Da Wan), and Fantastically Effective Pill to Invigorate the Collaterals (Hou Luo Xiao Ling Dan).

2. Transforming Phlegm, dispelling Wind and invigorating the Blood is used for patients with symptoms of weakness, paralysis, arthritis, fibromyalgia (with fatigue and heavy-pain), swelling, psychiatric symptoms (anxiety and fear) and edema. Representative formulas are: Augmented Ten-Ingredient Decoction to Warm the Gallbladder (Jia Wei Shi Wei Wen Dang Tang); Augmented Pinellia Atractylodis Macrocephalae and Gastrodia Decoction (Jia Wei Ban Xia Bai Zhu Tian Ma Tang); Minor Invigorate the Collaterals Special Pill (Xiao Huo Luo Dan); and Major Invigorate the Collaterals Special Pill (Da Huo Luo Dan).

3. Regulating Qi and transforming stasis is used for disorders with distension/bloating-pain, non-substantial swelling, tension and/or pain mostly in the chest, trunk or subcostal and diaphragm areas, or for mental and emotional/psychiatric symptoms (moodiness, cynicism, paranoia, etc.), functional nervous system disorders, as well as sprain and strains. Representative formulas are: Drive Out Blood-stasis in the Mansion of Blood Decoction (Xue Fu Zhu Yu Tang);[13] Drive Out Blood-stasis Below Diaphragm Decoction (Ge Xia Zhu Yu Tang); and Revive Health by Invigorating the Blood Decoction (Fu Yuan Huo Xue Tang).

---

12. A patent product with the same name, which is a pharmaceutical alkaloid of the herb, has been associated with the development of hepatitis and loss of consciousness when overdosed.

4. Warming Yang and vitalizing Blood is used for patients with Interior Cold and Blood-stasis with symptoms of cold extremities, sensitivity to cold, severe pain aggravated by cold, stiffness especially in the morning (on waking) or due to inactivity, and Painful Obstruction of all four limbs. Representative formulas are: Tangkuei Decoction for Frigid Extremities (Dang Gui Si Ni San); Frigid Extremities Decoction (Si Ni Tang); and Yang-Heartening Decoction (Yang He Tang).

5. Clearing Heat transforming stasis is used in disorders of burning pain, neuropathic pain, acute injuries, inflammation, bleeding, and autoimmune diseases, especially during acute flare-ups. Representative formulas are: Rhinoceros Horn and Rehmannia Decoction (Xi Jiao Di Huang Tang) and Augmented Four-Substance Decoction with Safflower and Peach Pit (Jia Wei Tao Hong Si Wu Tang).

6. Dissipating nodules and transforming stasis is used in patients with nodules and masses (Ju, Jia, Ji etc.) such as enlarged lymph nodes, muscular and other sinew nodules (fibromyositis, arthritic spurs), joint mouse (free body) and vertebral hypertrophy. Representative formulas are: Augmented Reduce Scrofula Pill (Xiao Luo Wan Jia Wei); Against Bony Hyperplasia Tablet (Kang Gu Zeng Sheng Pian); Ginseng and Carapax Amydae Pill (Ren Shen Bie Jia Qian Wan); and Rhubarb and Eupolyphaga Pill (Da Huang Zhe Chong Wan).

7. Stopping bleeding transforming Blood-stasis is used on patients with acute sprains/strains, contusions, and bleeding with purplish or black/brown colored blood (hematomas). Representative formulas are: Ten Partially-Charred Substances Powder (Shi Hui San); Sudden Smile Powder (Shi Xiao San); and Yunan White Medicine (Yunan Bai Yao).

8. Tonifying Qi and Blood transforming Blood-stasis is used in patients with chronic diseases that have not healed despite treatment. Pain aggravated after activity or in afternoon, fatigue, shortness of breath, paleness, prolonged bleeding, sequelae of stroke, weakness due to radicular or peripheral nerve disease, and other muscular atrophy disorders can be treated in this way as well. Representative formulas are: Tonify the Yang to Restore Five [Tenths] Decoction (Bu Yang Wu Tang); Relax the Channels and Invigorate the Blood Decoction (Shu Jing Huo Xue Tang); and Astragalus and Cinnamon Twig Five Substance Decoction (Huang Qi Gui Zhi Wu Wu Tang).

9. Nourishing Yin/Blood, clearing Heat, and vitalizing and transforming Blood-stasis is used in patients with chronic disorders that have damaged Yin-Fluids. This is frequently seen in patients with concomitant internal diseases such as diabetes, phlebitis, deep venous thrombosis (DVT), chronic inflammatory diseases, and autoimmune diseases. This pattern is seen also as a *sequelae to acute neuritis* with weakness and muscular atrophy as in suprascapular neuritis or Parsonage-Turner syndrome for example. Symptoms may present with burning pain (more in the acute inflammatory stage), insomnia, night sweats, tacycardia, warmth of palms, soles of feet, and chest, and night pain.[14] The affected area and face are often dark, blackish, dry, and lusterless, or dry and hot. There is often muscle weakness (or paralysis) and atrophy. Representative formulas are: Argument Great Tonify Yin Pill (Da Bu Yin Wan Jia Jie); Linking Decoction (Yi Guan Jian); Hidden Tiger Pill (Hu Qian Wan); and Four-Valiant Decoction for Well Being (Si Miao Yang An Tang).

10. Purging, cracking and dispersing stasis is used in patients with hard accumulations and swelling of joints, masses, stenosis, spurs, severe inflammatory arthritis and septic arthritis. Representative formulas are: Rhubarb and Eupolyphaga Pill (Da Huang Zhe Chong Wan) and Drain Static Blood Decoction (Xie Yu Xue Tang).

These formulas are often modified using herbs for Qi-stagnation, spicy releasing, Wind dispelling, warming and Dampness resolving.

Commonly-Used Herbs In Painful Obstruction Syndromes

In general, therapies that can unblock flow and thus treat pain incorporate one or more of the following herbal categories:

1. Blood moving (discussed above)
2. Qi regulating
3. Spicy Exterior releasing
4. Wind extinguishing
5. Warming
6. Damp resolving.
   This category includes herbs that clear Heat and dry Dampness; spicy Exterior releasing herbs; purgatives; herbs that are Dampness draining, Wind-Damp dispelling, aromaticaly transforming Dampness, Phlegm

---

13. Xue Fu Zhu Yu Tang can be thought of as the main formula to treat Blood-stasis. While it is said to treat the stasis above the diaphragm, it can be easily modified to treat Blood-stasis anywhere in the body. Four-Substance Decoction with Safflower and Peach Pit (Tao Hong Si Wu Tang) is another formula that can easily be modified to treat stasis in most patients.

14. Night pain (that wakes the patient) always suggests a serious disorder that needs to be considered. It should be considered a red flag. Traditionally (TCM) it is associated with Blood-stasis or Yin-deficiency. This can be due to any turbidity or any pathogenic condition that affects Blood circulation. Thus the root may be Hot, Cold, Deficient, or Excessive.

transforming, as well as Qi moving. Strengthening Yang is often added to address Spleen weakness, promote Yang-movement, and to address underlying Kidney and Liver deficiency.

7. A deficiency of Qi, Blood, and Organs may also lead to pain, i.e., malnourishment-Deficiency type pain and is often seen with chronic syndromes. Herbs that tonify, nourish, and moisten are often used to treat root causes.

A. Qi is often stagnant in a patient that suffers from pain and from life stresses. Commonly used Qi-moving herbs in musculoskeletal pain are: Radix Linderae Strychnifoliae (Wu Yao), Lignum Aquilariae (Chen Xiang), and Flos Rosae Rugosae (Mei Gui Hua), as well as Radix Curcumae (Yu Jin) and Rhizoma Corydalis (Yan Hu Suo) which moves the Qi within the Blood.[15] According to (Chen and Chen 2003) the Taiwanese herb, Folium Cardia Dichotoma (Po Bu Zi Ye), in combination with Caulis Vanieriae (Mo Gu Xiao) and Herba Solidaginis (Liu Zhi Huang) is especially effective in treating *bone spurs*.[16]

For retrograde flow of Qi with nausea, vomiting, hiccups, belching, and sometimes just for *swelling*: Haematitum (Dai Zhe Shi), Pericarpium Citri Reticulatae (Qing Pi), Fructus Immaturus Citri Aurantii (Zhi Shi) and Calyx Diospyri Kaki (Shi Di) can be used. These herbs do not have any primary uses in musculoskeletal disorders.

Radix Linderae Strychnifoliae (Wu Yao) enters the Bladder, Kidney, Lung, and Spleen (Gall Bladder and Triple Warmer) channels. It is a warm herb and may be used to treat lateral trunk and lower Warmer pain. It is helpful for pain referred to the groin or abdomen from ligamentous or myofascial triggers.

Lignum Aquilariae (Chen Xiang) enters the Kidney, Spleen, and Stomach channels. This herb is warm and is sometimes used for patients with back pain who also suffer from asthma or shortness of breath.[17]

Flos Rosae Rugosae (Mei Gui Hua) enters the Liver, Spleen (Gall Bladder and Triple Warmer) channels and is not commonly used to treat musculoskeletal disorders. Because this herb is warm and promotes movement of Qi and Blood and relieves pain, it is sometimes added to formulas that treat Blood-stasis secondary to trauma and when treating females with concomitant menstrual disorders.

---

15. Information on some of the herbs is found in other sections below.

16. The combination of these three herbs is said to be useful as an anti-inflammatory for most musculoskeletal conditions including neuropathies. For bone spurs Dr. Chen recommends Flex (Spur)™: Sebastan (Po Bu Zi Ye), Solidago (Liu Zhi Huang) Hyptis (Mo Gu Xiao), Vanieria (Huang Jin Gui), Mastic (Ru Xiang), Myrrh (Mo Yao), Euonymus (Da Ding Huang), Lonicera (Jin Yin Hua), Citrus (Chen Pi), Angelica (Bai Zhi), Licorice (Gan Cao), Fritillaria (Zhe Bei Mu), Ledebouriellae (Fang Feng), Gleditsia (Zao Jiao Ci).

17. The aromatic quality of this herb is said to be especially helpful for patients with "cotton" pulses (Shen-Hammer style).

B. Pungent Exterior releasing herbs are used mainly for Exterior syndromes, to move Qi and Blood, resolve exterior Pathogenic Factors, lead Pathogenic Factors or other herbs to the surface, assist in resolving Dampness, and to treat the muscles and skin. Commonly used Spicy/Pungent *warm* Exterior releasing herbs for musculoskeletal pain are: Ramulus Cinnamomi Cassiae (Gui Zhi), Radix Ledeboriella [Siler] (Fang Feng), Rhizoma et Radix Notopterygii (Qiang Huo), Rhizoma Ligustici (Gao Ben), Radix Angelicae Dahuricae (Bai Zhi) and Herba cum Radix Asari (Xi Xin). Pungent *cool* Exterior releasing herbs for musculoskeletal pain are: Fructus Viticis (Man Jing Zi), Radix Puerariae (Ge Gen), Fructus Arctii (Niu Bang Zi) and Radix Bupleuri (Chai Hu).

The spicy/pungent character of these herbs also moves Qi outward and therefore is often used to warm the channels and muscles, assist in moving Qi and Blood, and for analgesic effects.

Ramulus Cinnamomi Cassiae (Gui Zhi) enters the Heart, Lung and Urinary Bladder channels. This is an important herb and is often used to treat pain. It can enter the Blood, warming and promoting circulation as well as "traveling" in the superficial layers of the body to warm the muscles and open the channels and collaterals/network-vessels. It is used to treat Wind-Cold, either Exterior or Interior. Because its pungent warming and vasodilating effects, this herb is used to treat many conditions with cold extremities such as Raynaud's disease. It is often added to colder formulas, especially if there is Blood-stasis, to increase circulation and to balance cold-natured herbs. This herb has analgesic effects and the extract can be used in acupoint injection therapies for myofascial pain.

Radix Ledeboriella [*Siler or Saposhnikovia*] (Fang Feng) enters the Urinary Bladder, Liver, and Spleen channels. It is a mild herb and is only mildly warm so that it can treat Exterior pathogenic Wind without damaging Righteous-Qi. It can be used for both Wind-Cold and Wind-Heat presentations. Because this herb enters the Spleen, it is used often to expel Cold and Dampness from the flesh/muscles and subcutaneous regions. Because it enters the Liver channel, it can be used to dispel internal-Liver-Wind with symptoms of muscle spasms, cramps, tetanus, trembling of hands and feet, and for seizures. This herb is also used frequently in treating arthritis and Wind-Type (moving) pain.

Rhizoma et Radix Notopterygii (Qiang Huo) enters the Bladder and Kidney channels. Because this herb is warm, pungent, and bitter, it is used for pain due to both Wind-Cold and Wind-Dampness. It is often used as a guiding herb that leads Qi to the Tai-Yang (Bladder) and Governing channels. Therefore, this herb is used frequently for pain in the back of the neck and head (occipital) and for pain in the *upper* extremities. The pain is characterized by a feeling of heaviness, sleepiness, or lack of desire to move. This herb is used often in arthritic conditions characterized by pain and cramping of the affected area. It has analgesic effects.

Rhizoma Ligustici (Gao Ben) enters the Urinary Bladder and Governing channels. This herb is warm and is used frequently to treat headaches due to Wind-Cold, especially vertex headaches due to Wind-Cold or other causes. It is often used for migraine headaches as well.

Radix Angelicae Dahuricae (Bai Zhi) enters the Lung, Stomach, and Spleen channels. This herb is used mostly for painful disorders in the upper-frontal body areas (Stomach/Yang-Ming channels), especially forehead pain. Because this herb is said to penetrate turbidity (expel pus), and transform Phlegm, it is used in disorders such as ganglion cysts, especially when found on the thumb tendons (because of the connection of Yang-Ming LI and Lu), and/or other Yang-Ming areas. Because it enters the Stomach channel, it is used often for TMJ pain. This herb has anti-inflammatory and analgesic effects.

Herba cum Radix Asari (Xi Xin) enters the Lung and Kidney channel. This herb is very pungent and hot and is very important in the treatment of pain. Because it enters the Kidney channel, this herb is said to penetrate deeply and is useful for bone and sinew/soft tissue pain. It is used often for arthritic pains. Its penetrating qualities are said to "search-out" Wind, Cold, and Dampness. Therefore, this herb is used in chronic and Deficient (especially Kidney) disorders, for acute Painful Obstruction syndromes, and to treat headaches. Even though this herb is pungent and hot, small amounts are often added to cold formulas when pain is due to Damp-Heat. It has anti-inflammatory effects. This herb should be used with care, because it can damage Yin, and because, in patients with kidney (biomedical) disease, it can be nephrotoxic. (Dosage should not exceed 3g in decoction.)[18]

Fructus Viticis (Man Jing Zi) enters the Bladder, Liver, and Stomach channels. This herb is pungent, cool, and bitter and therefore can be used for Wind-Damp-Heat disorders. Although mostly used for pain in the head and eye, it can be also used for Damp-Heat type pain in the extremities, especially for Damp-Heat in the muscles. It can also be used to treat joint pains with cramping of the muscles. It is most useful for treating temporal headaches.

Radix Puerariae (Ge Gen) enters the Spleen and Stomach channels and is said to have an affinity for the neck (shoulder). This herb is light and gentle and can be used in most patients. It is often used when Pathogenic Factors (Wind-Heat or Wind-Cold), have entered the subcutaneous and muscle layers (said to enter the muscles). Because this herb can also raise Spleen-Qi and Clear-Yang as well as nourish Fluids, it can be used for muscular weakness and wasting and for "dryness" in the flesh. Because it enters the Stomach channel, it is often used to treat TMJ pain. It is most frequently used for pain in the back of the neck and shoulder. It has been shown to prevent bone loss in ovariectomized mice.[19]

Fructus Arctii (Niu Bang Zi) enters the Lung and Stomach channels. This herb has a mild anti-inflammatory function, and, according to some traditions, when used in large doses, it can tonify Kidney-Essence. It can be used in the treatment of disc disease.

Radix Bupleuri (Chai Hu) enters the Gall Bladder, Liver, Pericardium, and Triple Warmer channels. This herb is pungent and slightly cool. Its main function is often related to Liver, Gall Bladder, and Qi disorders (although it can enter the Blood as well). It can be used in patients with pain in Gall Bladder channel distribution (chest, subcostal, and trunk), and in patients that are stressed, irritable, and depressed with other symptoms and signs of Liver-congestion. It can also "harmonize" the Exterior and Interior and treat Shao-Yang disorders with conflicting and confusing pain syndromes, especially in stressed patients with lingering Exterior conditions. Because this herb has a strong "opening" effect on the Liver (which treats Liver-congestion/depression), it is used with care, as it may "over" stimulate the patient and damage Qi and Yin. For patients with weakness and muscle wasting, a small dose is often used to raise Spleen-Qi and Clear-Yang. This herb has analgesic and anti-inflammatory effects.

C. Wind can be due to Exterior or Interior causes. Interior-Wind can arise from deficiency of Yin/Blood or from Excess-stagnation transformation-Heat. In general, Painful Obstruction (Bi) syndromes are said to be caused by exogenous Pathogenic Factors; however, endogenous factors also result in painful musculoskeletal syndromes. Commonly used Wind-extinguishing herbs for musculoskeletal pain are: Rhizoma Gastrodiae Elatae (Tian Ma), and insects like Lumbricus (Di Long), Buthus Martensi (Quan Xie), Scolopendra (Wu Gong), and Bombys Batryticatus (Jiang Can). They are often used in patients with muscle spasms, cramps, headaches, and deep-seated obstructions because of their so-called *penetrating* qualities. Nidus Vespae (Lu Feng Fang) is also used for its Wind-expelling properties. (This herb is in the external application category.) Insects and animal substances are often needed in intractable and chronic disorders to penetrate, dredge, and open the Connecting/network-vessels and expel pathogens.[20]

Rhizoma Gastrodiae Elatae (Tian Ma) enters the Liver channel. This herb is one of the most important in treating

---

18. Signs of intoxications include: headache, pressure in head, anxiety, restlessness, vertigo, sweating, pupular dilation, hypertension, increased respiratory rate, elevated temperature, and tachycardia, all of which may be seen one to two hours after ingestion. Early treatment is done with emetic methods, followed by ingestion of milk, egg whites, or activated charcoal.

19. Ge Gen contains a high amount of isoflavonoids such as daidzein and genistein, which are known to prevent bone loss induced by estrogen deficiency.

Wind. It is mild and can be used in most patients. It is useful for both internal and external Wind. It is used most often for symptoms of spasms and tremors. Because it has a neutral and moistening nature (the only Wind herb that moistens), this herb can be used in both Excess or Deficient-Yin/Blood Wind disorders with symptoms of muscle twitching, cramping, spasm, tonic-clonic convulsions, stiffness, numbness, tingling or headache. It is commonly used to treat headaches including migraines, and arthritic problems characterized by pain, numbness, and decreased agility. The extracts of the herb can be used for intramuscular injection in the treatment of various neuritic pains.

Lumbricus (Di Long) enters the Urinary Bladder, Liver, Lung, and Spleen channels. Because this is an earthworm, it is said to be able to "dig-in" and "penetrate" the tiny network-vessels/collaterals and to break up obstructions. This substance is cold so that it is also useful for internal-Liver-Wind with symptoms such as convulsions, seizures, mania, and fever. It is used often for Painful Obstruction with symptoms of stiffness, weakness, numbness, and pain in the limbs (mostly lower limbs). It can free the channels and move Blood so that it is often used for chronic arthritic disorders characterized by Heat with redness, warmth, and swollen joints, and/or pains increasing with exposure to heat. It can also be used to treat arthritic disorders characterized by coldness, numbness, stiffness, and pain that increases by exposure to cold. This substance can be used to treat bone fractures with swelling and pain.

Buthus Martensi (Quan Xie) enters the Liver channel. This substance (scorpion) is usually used for acute or chronic spasms, tremors, or convulsions from Liver-Wind and Heat. It is useful for chronic and stubborn headaches, especially frontal, temporal, and migraines. It can also be used to open the network-vessels/collaterals and treat arthritic disorders with severe pain, numbness, decreased mobility, or paralysis. It is said to inhibit joint destruction and stiffness. Because it is toxic, it is not used for long periods.[21]

Scolopendra (Wu Gong) enters the Liver channel. This substance (centipede) is similar in function to Buthus Martensi (Quan Xie) and is used similarly. It is more suitable for Cold conditions than Buthus Martensi (Quan Xie), and, therefore, it is more commonly used for pain of the sinews and muscles with numbness and stiffness. It is used for joint pains characterized by pain that moves from one joint to another. It is also used for chronic and stubborn headaches. Because it is slightly toxic it is not used for long periods.

Bombys Batryticatus (Jiang Can) enters the Liver and Lung channels. This substance (silk worm) is similar in function to Lumbricus (Di Long) but has a stronger effect on Dampness/Phlegm. It can be used for fascial (and facial) pain, spasm, numbness and paralysis in the extremities. It is used most commonly for head and face pain, and for Wind-Damp arthritis/arthrosis.

Nidus Vespae (Lu Feng Fang) enters the Lung and Stomach channels and is toxic. It can be used to relieve toxicity, expel Wind, dry Dampness and treat pain. It is mostly used for intractable Painful Obstruction Syndromes, often with Heat-Toxin symptoms. Because it is toxic it is not used for long periods.

D. To warm the channels, joints and sinews: Radix Lateralis Aconiti (Fu Zi), Radix Aconiti Carmichaeli (Chuan Wu), Radix Aconiti Kusnezoffii (Cao Wu), Cortex Cinnamomi Cassiae (Rou Gui) and Rhizoma Zingiberis (Gan Jiang) are used in patients with severe pain and cold contraction of tissues (stiffness).

Radix Aconiti Lateralis (Fu Zi) enters the Heart, Spleen, and Kidney channels, and, because of its strength, it is also said to enter all twelve channels, collaterals, and tissues. This herb is very pungent and hot and is therefore used for Cold, Damp, and Yang-deficient disorders. It can dissipate Phlegm and other accumulation. It is used for Painful Obstruction (Bi) syndromes when Cold is predominate with symptoms of severe pain, stiffness, cramping of the muscles and sinews, all of which are aggravated by cold weather. It is also helpful in treating atrophy with spasms and contractures, inability to walk, and cyanotic or dark complexion of the limbs or face. Because it is pungent, hot, and toxic, it can harm Yin and Fluids. Care must be paid when using this herb. If dry mouth, thirst, or tongue numbness develops, the dosage is decreased or the treatment is discontinued, or other herbs are added to counteract these side-effects. In small doses, this herb can be used for prolonged periods. To treat severe pain or stiffness, doses of up to 60g may be needed and may be the key for successful treatment. There is no equivalent substitution for this herb in the pharmacopoeia. At high doses, this herb is also helpful when withdrawing steroid therapy. It has anti-inflammatory effects and can be used also in patients showing signs of Heat when other herbs are added. When used in high doses this herb *must* be cooked for at least three hours to reduce toxicity.[22] Ingestion of honey is said to reduce the toxicity of this herb[23].

---

20. It should be noted that other herbs can be used to treat Interior-Wind as well. For example, to treat Interior-Wind with predominately muscle spasms and/or paralysis, Notopterygium and Ledebouriella Decoction (Qiang Huo Fang Feng Tang) may be used: the two herbs with Radix Ligustici (Chuan Xiong), Radix Glycyrrhizae (Gan Cao), Radix et Rhizoma Ligustici (Gao Ben), Radix Angelicae (Dang Gui), Herba Asari (Xi Xin), Radix Sanguisorbae (Di Yu) and Radix Paeoniae (Bai Shao).

21. Overdose can result in dizziness, fever, perspiration, photophobia, tearing, runny nose, excess salivation, nausea, vomiting, stiff tongue, hypothermia, convulsions, dyspnea, bleeding, heart rhythm disorder, hypertension or hypotension, seizures, unconsciousness, cyanosis, pulmonary edema, and respiratory depression. Overdose can be treated by purging using Natrii Sulfas (Ming Fen) or with herbs that clear Heat and Toxins and purge the bowls.

Radix Aconiti Carmichaeli (Chuan Wu) and *Radix Aconiti Kusnezoffii* (Cao Wu) enters the Heart, Liver, and Spleen channels. They are similar to Aconiti (Fu Zi) but considered to be more toxic. They have stronger effects for expelling Wind and opening the channels and collaterals/network-vessels. Therefore, these herbs are used in treatment of Painful Obstruction (Bi) syndromes with symptoms of severe pain, generalized pain, numbness, stiffness, cramping, and spasms. They can be used for both acute and chronic pain but for short periods only. Besides their use in treating pain, both herbs can be used to reduce swelling and treat abscesses (Yin-abscesses).

Cinnamomi Cassiae (Rou Gui) enters mostly the Kidney channel, but also the Heart, Liver and Spleen channels. This herb is hot and pungent and is used mostly for patients with low back pain, weakness of waist and knees, and difficulty walking due to Kidney-deficiency. It is used also to treat floating-Yang that is due to Mingman-deficiency (Cold and/or false Heat). It can be used to treat edema from Kidney-deficiency and help in "generation" of flesh.

Rhizoma Zingiberis (Gan Jiang) enters the Heart, Lung, Spleen, and Stomach channels. This herb is used to warm the Interior and channels, dissolve Phlegm, and stop bleeding. It has anti-inflammatory effects (via COX-2) and can be used to treat joint pains, especially of the low back and lower extremities. The extract of this herb (and Sheng Jiang) can be used in acupoint injection therapy to treat myofascial pain.

E. As noted above, there are many types of herbs that are used for Dampness.

Dampness is considered the central pathogenic factor in Painful Obstruction (Bi) Syndromes. It is a viscous, substantial, and sticky pathogen, and it attracts and adheres to other Pathogenic Factors. It also attracts and adheres to the body tissues. Bi (and Damp) syndromes are, for these reasons, often said to be difficult to eliminate. In Damp disorders the condition may be predominately Hot, Cold, or mixed. When mixed, the degree of the involved Pathogenic Factors must be understood; therefore, when treating Dampness one must analyze the patient's condition to ascertain if Dampness is predominate, or if, rather Heat in Damp-Heat, Wind in Wind-Damp, Yang/ Spleen/Kidney-deficiency in Cold-Damp, Qi-deficiency or stagnation in Damp-accumulation predominates. Another aspect that needs to be considered is the location of Dampness and whether it is of endogenous or exogenous origin. When treating Damp syndromes, complex treatment strategies may thus be warranted. Often herbs that are sweet-bland can be combined with other herbs that address any of the above-discussed pathologies. However, since most of these herbs have diuretic effects and are therefore downward moving, attention must be paid to Spleen-deficiency as it is the Spleen's upward movement that is in charge of transporting Fluids and inhibiting Dampness and Fluid pathogens. The root of Dampness, which is either exogenous or endogenous, is often said to be Spleen-deficiency (see page 27). Therefore, in patients with Spleen weakness (and even more in patients with internal Dampness), the emphasis is often on herbs that raise Yang and assist Spleen-transportation.

Other common causes of Dampness are Kidney-Yang-deficiency (the source of Spleen-Yang), failure of the Lungs to regulate Qi and move the Fluids down, and the excessive intake of sweet and rich foods, which weaken the Spleen/pancreas. Addressing the Spleen/pancreas or other causative factors is thus often needed.

In musculoskeletal disorders:

- In patients with Damp-Heat with symptoms of swollen, hot joints and/or other symptoms or signs of Damp-Heat, Cortex Phellodendri (Huang Bai), Radix Scutellariae Baicalensis (Huang Qin) and Caulis Hyptis Capitatae (Mo Gu Xiao) are used to drain, dry and clear Damp-Heat. They are used also as "balancing" herbs in Spicy and Warm formulas to protect Yin/Fluids.

Cortex Phellodendri (Huang Bai) enters the Kidney and Bladder channels. This herb is mostly used in disorders of the lower body/extremities both in Full or Empty-Heat. Together with other herbs, it is often used in inflammatory arthritis. Because it is bitter and cold, this herb should be used with caution in patients with weak digestion or Exterior-Cold and it may cause hidden-Heat.[24] It is often used topically to treat traumatic injuries.

Radix Scutellariae Baicalensis (Huang Qin) enters the Gall Bladder, Large Intestine, Lung, and Stomach channels. This herb is sometimes used in disorders of the upper body/extremities, usually with Full-Heat. Pain that

---

22. Long cooking is needed even though this herb is prepared prior to distribution. To counteract its hot and spicy properties Gypsum (Shi Gao) and/or Rehmanniae (Sheng Di) are commonly used in musculoskeletal practice.

23. Overdose can result in involuntary salivation, nausea, vomiting, diarrhea, dizziness, blurred vision, dry mouth, numbness of the body and extremities, slowed pulse, difficulty breathing, twitching limbs, convulsions, disorientation, urinary and fecal incontinence, hypotension, hypothermia, heart rhythm disorders, and possibly death. To treat toxicity, Rou Gui can be used in early stages (within four to six hours of ingestion). Other herbs such as Gan Cao, Gan or Sheng Jiao, Lu Dou, Huang Lian, Ren Shen, and Huang Qi can also be used.

24. Any cold-bitter herb or formula is said to be capable of trapping pathogenic Cold resulting in Hidden/Latent Heat or complex Heat Cold syndrome. For hidden-muscle-Heat or for muscle pain from Spring-Warm and/or Summer-Heat the use of modified Ten Spirit Decoction (Shi Shen Tang) may be helpful: Notopteryggi (Qiang Huo), Radix Puerariae (Ge Gen), Radix Ligustici (Chuan Xiong), Radix Angelica (Bai Zhi), Radix Paeoniae (Chi Shao), Folium Perillae (Zi Su), Pericarpium Citri (Chen Pi), Rhizoma (Cimicifugae (Sheng Ma), Rhizoma Cypri (Xiang Fu), Bombys (Jiang Can), and Radix Glycyrrhizae (Gan Gao).

responds to this herb usually involves the Liver or Gall Bladder channels. Because it is bitter and cold, this herb should be used with caution in patients with weak digestion or Exterior-Cold, as this can result in hidden pathogenic Heat.

Caulis Hyptis Captitatae (Mo Gu Xiao) enters the Kidney and Liver channels. This herb is cold and bland so that it drains Dampness and Heat. It can be used to treat arthralgias, neuritis and sciatica.

- To *dispel Dampness via the surface*, spicy Exterior releasing herbs such as: Ramulus Cinnamomi Cassiae (Gui Zhi), Radix Ledebouriella (Fang Feng), Rhizoma et Radix Notopterygii (Qiang Huo), and Herba cum Radix Asari (Xi Xin) are used especially in Exterior Cold-Damp syndromes.

  Fructus Viticis (Man Jing Zi) and Radix Puerariae (Ge Gen) are used in Exterior Heat-Damp syndromes.

- *Purgative herbs such as*: Rhizoma Rhei (Da Huang) and Herba Aloes (Lu Hui) are sometimes used when constipation is a factor.

- *Dampness bland draining/precipitating* herbs such as: Poriae Cocos (Fu Ling), Polypori Umbellati (Zhu Ling), Semen Coicis Lachrma-jobi (Yi Yi Ren), Semen Plantaginis (Che Qian Zi), Rhizoma Dioscoreae Hypoglaucae (Bei [Bi] Xie), Rhizoma Alismatis Orientalitis (Ze Xie), Radix Stephaniae Tetrandrae (Han Fang Ji) and Medulla Tetrapanacis (Tong Cao) are used to drain Dampness and Heat via urination, especially in patients with lower extremity edema and/or swelling.

  Poriae Cocos (Fu Ling) enters the Heart, Spleen, Stomach, Lung, and Kidney channels. This is a mild diuretic that can be used in both Damp-Heat and Damp-Cold syndromes. It can be used in most cases because it is mild and neutral. This herb can be used to treat edema and swelling due both to accumulation of pathogenic water secondary to local blockage and from the Spleen failing to metabolize and move Fluids. This herb can tonify the Spleen without being cloy and thus is usually free of side effects. It also has a mild sedative effect.

  Polypori Umbellati (Zhu Ling) enters the Kidney and Bladder channels. This herb has a stronger diuretic effect than Poriae Cocos (Fu Ling) and is mostly used for edema and swelling. It does not strengthen the Spleen.

  Coicis Lachrma-jobi (Yi Yi Ren) enters the Spleen, Lung, and Kidney channels. This herb is used more commonly in musculoskeletal disorders, as it can promote urination to leach out Dampness, dispel Wind-Dampness, and clear Heat. It is said to sooth the sinews and increase the flexibility of tendons and joints. Although slightly cold, this herb can be used in most cases without side effects but is usually more appropriate in Hot Painful Obstruction (Bi) syndromes. It is used most often in chronic cases to treat swollen and stiff joints, crampy/spasm pains, and heaviness and numbness of the limbs. Because it enters the Spleen, it can be used to treat Dampness in the muscles and flesh with or without weakness or atrophy (Wei syndromes). When powdered this herb is said to absorb pathogenic-Dampness when used externally.

  Semen Plantaginis (Che Qian Zi) enters the Bladder, Kidney, Liver, and Lung channels. This herb is cold in nature and is therefore mostly used for Damp-Heat type edema and pain. This herb also has mild effects on joint swelling. It can be used in patients with Yin-deficiency as it does not injure Fluids. The extracts of the herb can be used as an injectable proliferent in the treatment of joint and ligament laxity.

  Rhizoma Dioscoreae Hypoglaucae (Bie Xie or Bi Xie) enters the Urinary Bladder, Liver, and Stomach. This herb is neutral and can treat turbidity, separate Heat from Dampness, and treat Wind-Dampness. Because this herb is neutral and is said to relax the sinews and treat Wind-Dampness, it is often used in patients with generalized muscle aches. It can be used to treat Painful Obstruction due to Deficiency or Excess such as: Cold-Dampness with symptoms aggravated on cold and rainy days; Heat-Dampness with symptoms aggravated on hot days; or in Kidney-deficiency with weakness and soreness of the low back and knees (or limbs).

  Rhizoma Alismatis Orientalitis (Ze Xie) enters the Kidney and Bladder channels. This herb is also a mild diuretic with a cold nature. It is used mostly to treat Damp-Heat in the lower body and to clear Empty-Heat. It can be added to tonic formulas to prevent the formation of pathogenic Heat and rising of Kidney-Fire.

  Radix Stephaniae Tetrandrae (Han Fang Ji) enters the Bladder, Spleen, and Kidney channels. This herb is cold and very bitter and is used mainly to treat Damp-Heat in the lower extremities. It can also eliminate Wind and therefore is often used in Wind-Damp-Heat Painful Obstruction (Bi) syndromes, with painful and heavy extremities and/or swollen and inflamed joints. This herb should be used with caution in weak patients or patients with kidney disease, as it may be nephrotoxic.[25]

  Radix Coculi (Mu Fang Ji) promotes the circulation of water, eliminates water accumulation, and can treat all forms of neuralgias.

  Medula Tetrapanadis (Tong Cao) enters the Heart, Lung, and Small Intestine channels. This herb promotes urination, clears Heat, and cools the Blood. Although it does not enter the Spleen channel, this herb can be useful in the treatment of muscle soreness.

- *Wind-Dampness-dispelling herbs*: In general there are two main methods of dispelling Wind-Dampness Bi syndromes. The first is via the surface, using spicy herbs. This is used mainly for Exterior syndromes of short dura-

---

25. Han Fang Ji should not be confused with Radix Aristolochia Fangchi (Guang Fang Ji), a toxic herb that contains Aristolochic acid, which is highly toxic to the liver, kidneys, and adrenal glands. Mu Fang Ji should not be confused with Han Fang Ji as well.

tion (often called Exterior-Damp). The second method is used to treat exogenous or endogenous Wind-Dampness which lodges more deeply (i.e., in the sinews, bones, and collaterals/network-vessels) and therefore is used for acute or chronic disorders. Herbs that promote the flow of Qi and Blood, move Yang, and possibly tonify Spleen, Liver, Kidney, Qi and Blood are often used at the same time. Many of the herbs in the category of Wind-Damp-dispelling enter the Liver channel and can be used in musculoskeletal disorders. Formulas often include a large number of them in small doses. Warm and hot herbs are often used together with cool and cold herbs.

For Cold conditions, Radix Angelicae Pubescenis (Du Huo), Radix Clematidis (Wei Ling Xian), Excrementum Bombycis Mori (Can Sha), Cortex Acanthopanacis (Wu Jia Pi), Agkistrodon seu Bungarus (Bai Hua She), Ramus Piperis Wallichii (Hai Feng Teng), Herba Lycopodii Claviati cum Radice (Shen Jin Cao), Herba Speranskiae seu Impatients (Tou Gu Cao), Lignum Pini Nodi (Song Jie), Fructus Chaenomelis (Mu Gua) and Radix Achefflerae (Qi Ye Lian) are commonly used.

For Hot conditions, Radix Gentianae (Qin Jiao) [both hot and cold conditions], Ramus Lonicerae Japonicae (Ren Dong Teng) Ramulus Mori Albae (Sang Zhi) [both hot and cold conditions], Herba Siegesbeckiae (Xi Xian Cao), Folium Clerodendri Trichotomi (Chou Wu Tong), Caulis Trachelospermi (Luo Shi Teng), Ramus Tinosporae Sinensis (Kuan Jin Teng), Herba Solidaginis (Liu Zhi Huang), Rhizoma Doscoreae Nippnicae (Chuan Shan Long), and Radix Tripterygii Wilfordii (Lei Gong Teng) are used.

) Cortex Erythrinae (Hai Tong Pi), Zaocys Dhumnades (Wu Shao She), Exuviae Serpentis (She Tui) and Caulis Sinomenii (Qing Feng Teng) are neutral.

To moisten Yin and tonify the Kidneys, Herba Pyrolae (Lu Xian Cao) and Ramulus Loranthus (Sang Ji Sheng) are used often. Yang tonics are also used to treat Wind-Dampness (see below).

Radix Angelicae Pubescenis (Du Huo) enters the Kidney and Bladder channels. Although this herb is pungent and warm, it is not too harsh, has a mild moistening effect, and can be used in weak patients and chronic disorders. It treats Wind-Damp-Cold Painful Obstruction (Bi) syndrome of mainly the tissues controlled by the Kidneys; the bones, the back, and lower extremities. The pain is characterized by heaviness, stiffness, and numbness. It can also enter the peripheral channels and collaterals to dispel pathogens. It therefore can be used for both acute and chronic aches and pains of the muscles and joints.[26]

Radix Clematidis (Wei Ling Xian) enters the Bladder (or all twelve) channels. This herb is said to open all the channels and network-vessels/collaterals, strongly promoting the movement of Qi and eliminating Phlegm and accumulations. It treats Wind-Dampness, especially when Wind predominates. It can be used in arthritic disorders anywhere in the body, especially when symptoms of numbness and tingling (Wind) are seen. It is most effective for lumbar and lower extremity pain. Because it enters the collaterals, it is said to be capable of treating stagnated Blood and Qi. Clinically, it is often used for musculoskeletal disorders with muscle cramping and spasms, stiffness of joints, difficulties in both flexion and extension, and for numbness. The extract of the herb can be injected for the treatment of hypertrophic spondylitis. This herb should be used with caution in weak patients and should not be used to treat stiffness and pain due to Blood or Yin deficiency.

Excrementum Bombycis Mori (Can Sha) enters the Liver, Spleen, and Stomach channels. This substance treats Wind-Dampness, and, because it enters the Spleen and Stomach, it is used to treat muscle pains and spasms, especially of the calves. It can be helpful when the patient experiences numbness or itching with the pain.

Cortex Acanthopanacis (Wu Jia Pi) enters the Liver and Kidney channels. This herb can both expel Wind-Dampness and strengthen the Liver and Kidneys (sinews and bones). It is therefore used in chronic Painful Obstruction (Bi) syndrome with weakness of the sinews and bones, and for muscular atrophy. It can also be used for muscles spasms and cramps due to Excess or Deficiency. This herb is especially useful for elderly and weak patients. Because it has a mild diuretic effect, it can be used to treat mild edema and joint swelling as well. This herb has both anti-inflammatory and analgesic effects and can quicken Blood circulation.

Agkistrodon seu Bungarus (Bai Hua She) enters the Liver and Spleen. This substance (a snake), like many other animal medicinals, is said to be capable of penetrating deeply, reaching all tissues and channels. It is said to be capable of seeking out pathogenic Wind, no matter how long it has been retained. This medicinal is therefore used for many chronic conditions characterized by stiffness, cramping/spasms, numbness, tingling, and moving pains. Extracts of the snake can be used for injection therapy.

Herba Lycopodii Claviati cum Radice (Shen Jin Cao) enters the Liver channel and has a mild moistening nature. This herb treats Wind-Dampness, opens and clears the channels and collaterals/network vessels, increases circulation, and "relaxes" the sinews. It is considered to be especially important when treating tendons. This herb is commonly used in chronic Painful Obstruction (Bi) syndromes with symptoms of stiffness, contracted soft tissues, soreness of joints and muscles, and numbness. It is also used in acute traumatic injuries of soft tissues.

Herba Speranskiae seu Impatients (Tou Gu Cao) enters the Liver and Kidney channels. This herb is mainly used to treat bones and is said to eliminate Wind-Damp-Cold from deep tissues and bones. It is used mostly in chronic

---

26. Some sources warn against using Du Huo in patients with Yin/Blood-deficiency, even though the herb has moistening qualities.

cases when Wind-Dampness lingers and affects the bones and joints, with stiffness being predominate. It can also be used to treat traumatic injuries as it can vitalize Blood circulation and break-up stasis. This herb is said to promote the generation of tissues. It may be used to treat bone spurs, especially when the affected area is "steamed," or rapped with this herb cooked in vinegar.[27]

Lignum Pini Nodi (Song Jie) enters the Liver channel. This herb primarily treats Wind-Cold and pain due to acute injury. It is also used for chronic and difficult joint pains (including rheumatoid arthritis), and for hypertonicity of muscles and sinews and stiffness of joints.

Ramus Piperis Wallichii (Hai Feng Teng) enters the Liver channel. This herb is only slightly warm and is therefore gentle. It treats Wind-Dampness-Cold in both muscles and joints, which become worse during damp weather. Symptoms are usually characterized by achy pains, cramping, heaviness, numbness, and stiffness of joints. It can be used for pain due to trauma, as well.

Fructus Chaenomelis (Mu Gua) enters the Liver and Spleen channels. This herb relaxes the sinews and opens the channels and collaterals. While warm, this herb is mild, not drying, and therefore can be used for most patients. It is commonly used to treat musculoskeletal disorders characterized by muscle cramps, spasms, and stiffness and is best for the lower extremities. Mu Gua is the papaya fruit, and, therefore, some of the above effects may be due to digestive enzymes found within this fruit.

Radix Schefflerae (Qi Ye Lian) enters the Liver channel. This herb is mainly used for its analgesic properties. It can be used for both acute (traumatic) and chronic pains with swelling. It can also be used to treat headaches, tension, or migraines. It is also said to be helpful in the treatment of neuropathies. The herb can be used as injectable to treat muscular pain and trigger points.

Radix Gentianae (Qin Jiao) enters the Gall Bladder, Liver, and Stomach channels. This herb is slightly cold and also has a mild moistening property. It can therefore be used in all types of painful Wind-Damp disorders, including Hot, Cold, Deficient or Excess (although it is best for Hot type pains and for pains aggravated by weather changes). It relaxes the sinews and opens channels and collaterals and thus is used especially for painful extremities. It also guides other herbs to the spine and lumbar areas. Because of this herb's moistening quality, it is also used to balance the dry hot nature of other herbs that treat Wind-Dampness and to prevent constipation.

Ramus Lonicerae Japonicae (Ren Dong Teng) enters the Large Intestines, Lung, Stomach, and Liver channels, as well as the collaterals/network-vessels. This herb primarily treats Wind-Damp-Heat and is used most often in inflammatory arthritis. Since it enters the collaterals, it can be used to clear Heat from the collaterals/network-vessels and to treat muscle aches.

Ramulus Mori Albae (Sang Zhi) enters the Liver channel. This herb is neutral (or slightly cold) with an affinity for the upper extremities, particularly the hands. It is mainly used to treat Wind transforming to Heat of the hands, but can also be used for all other joints. It is also used for Wind-Dampness. Clinically, it is used for muscle aches, cramping and pain. It is commonly used to treat tendinosis/tendinitis.

Herba Siegesbeckiae (Xi Xian Cao) enters the Liver and Kidney channels. This herb treats weakness in the muscles and sinews due to Wind-Damp-Heat. It strengthens the Liver and Kidneys, and, because it is slightly moistening, it can treat Liver-Yang rising. It is used often for back and leg pain and weakness and/or paralysis when Dampness is severe. It is useful in treating secondary paralysis or muscle weakness due to neuritis.

Folium Clerodendri Trichotomi (Chou Wu Tong) enters the Liver channel and is mainly used to treat numbness in the extremities.

Caulis Trachelospermi (Luo Shi Teng) enters the Liver and Heart channels. This herb is mainly used to treat pain and spasms due to inflammatory conditions as it can also cool the Blood. It is used also when Wind-Dampness transforms into Heat (transformation/congested-Heat) and there is pain and tension in the sinews and joints. It is useful in the treatment of neuritis in its primary stage or sequelae with muscle weakness and/or atrophy.

Herba Solidaginis (Liu Zhi Huang) enters the Lung, Liver, and Kidney channels. This herb opens the channels and collaterals/network-vessels and therefore is used to treat pain and inflammation. It can be used to treat trauma-related pain or tightness of tendons.

Rhizoma Dioscoreae Nipponicae (Chuan Shan Long) enters the Liver and Lung channels. Because this herb can dispel Wind-Dampness, invigorate the Blood, and open the channels and collaterals/network-vessels it is used to treat painful joints with numbness and stiffness. It can also be used to treat pain from traumatic injuries.

Radix Tripterygii Wilfordii (Lei Gong Teng) enters the Liver channel. It is used to relieve pain and swelling in patients with inflammatory disorders. This herb can suppress the immune system and therefore is used in many autoimmune disorders such as rheumatoid arthritis. psoriatic arthritis, lupus, etc. It has also been recommended for discogenic disorders. Although toxic, this herb can be used safely and can be quite effective for these disorders.[28]

Ramus Tinosporae Sinensis (Kuan Jin Teng) enters the Liver channel. This herb is mainly used to treat pain and spasms due to inflammatory conditions. It is also used to treat inflammation secondary to trauma.

Cortex Erythrinae (Hai Tong Pi) enters the Liver, Spleen, and Kidney channels. This herb is neutral and can be used in most patients. It is mostly used to treat Wind-

---

27. Vinegar is often used to "soften" bones, treat spurs, and increase absorption of topical herbal applications. Soaking the feet in vinegar is said to be helpful in treating all the Sinew channels.

Damp numbness, pain, or cramping in the lower extremities, and waist muscles or sinews. It is also important when treating traumatic swelling. Its analgesic properties are relatively pronounced. It can also relax striated muscles. Large doses should not be used as it can be cardiotoxic.

Zaocys Dhumnades (Wu Shao She) enters the Liver and Spleen channels. This medicinal snake is used in similar ways to Agkistrodon seu Bungarus (Bai Hua She) except that it is milder and not toxic. An extract made from this snake can be used for injection therapy as an anti-inflammatory and analgesic.

Caulis Sinomenii (Qing Feng Teng) enters the Liver channel and is neutral. It dispels Wind-Dampness and relieves pain. It is mainly used for patients that experience tightness, swelling, and painful joints. This herb has significant anti-inflammatory and analgesic effects.

Herba Pyrolae (Lu Xian Cao) also called (Lu Han Cao) enters the Liver and Kidney channels and is both capable of treating Wind-Dampness and of replenishing Kidney-Yin/Essence. This herb can be used in arthritic, bony, and sinew disorders, as it is said to be capable of strengthening the sinews and bones. It is also used to treat bone spurs. Its nourishing quality can be used to balance the dryness of other herbs in this category.

Ramulus Loranthus (Sang Ji Sheng) enters the Kidney and Liver channels. This herb is neutral and can be used in most patients. It tonifies the Liver and Kidney, strengthens the sinews and bones, and expels Wind-Dampness. Some texts list it under the category of tonifying Yin herbs. It is used most often in chronic arthritic disorders that involve the lower back, knees, and lower extremities. However, it can be used in other joint disorders characterized by weakness, with or without Wind-Dampness. The extract of the herb can be used as an injectable for poliomyelitis.

- *Aromatically transforming Dampness herbs*: Herba Eupatorii Fortunei (Pei Lan), Rhizoma Atractylodis (Cang Zhu), and Fructus Amomi (Sha Ren) are used mainly for Dampness at the Exterior, middle warmer (digestive symptoms), and in edema.

---

28. Lei Gong Teng is a highly toxic herb which can cause bleeding in the stomach, intestines, liver, and lungs. It can also cause irregular menstruation. Signs of toxicity include: dizziness, dry mouth, palpitations, headaches, fatigue, vomiting, chills, fever, abdominal pain, diarrhea with black stools, generalized aches and pains, tachycardia, irregular heart rhythms, frequent urination and urgency. Most of these side-effects occur within two to three hours after ingestion. Within two to three days, some patients complain of low back pain, hair loss, facial edema, and decreased or increased urinary output. Some patients also develop hypotension, hypothermia, altered consciousness, convulsion, respiratory depression, and hypoxia. There have been several deaths attributed to this herb. With chronic use some patients have developed decreased white blood cell and platelet counts due to bone marrow suppression. A periodic CBC should therefore be ordered. Vitamin B12 and B6 have been advocated to prevent some of the side-effects. Acute toxicity is treated by emetic methods or gastric lavage. Herba Pteris (Feng Wei Cao) or Radix Notoginseng (San Qi) can be given to address systemic reactions and to stop bleeding.

Herba Eupatorii Fortunei (Pei Lan) enters the Spleen and Stomach. This herb is neutral and mild and can be used with little worry of damaging Yin. It is mostly used to treat heaviness from Dampness.

Rhizoma Atractylodis (Cang Zhu) enters the Spleen and Stomach channels. This herb is important in treating Dampness, as it can both strongly transform Dampness and strengthen the Spleen. It is often used in Damp-Cold or Damp-Heat arthralgias, especially of lower extremities with swelling and soreness. Its spicy character can induce slight "perspiration," dispelling Dampness via the surface.

Fructus Amomi (Sha Ren) enters the Spleen and Stomach and is used mostly to balance cloy tonic herbs.[29]

- *Phlegm transforming*: Bulbus Fritillariae Thunbergii (Zhe Bei Mu), Radix Trichosanthis Kirilowii (Tian Hua Fen), Succus Bambusae (Zhu Li), Succus Biticis Negundi (Jing Li), Succus Zingiberis (Jiang Zhi), and Thallus Algae (Kun Bu) are used sometimes to treat Hot-Phlegm swellings with nodular tissues in muscles and/or joints such as seen in fibromyocitis, cysts and spurs.

Rhizoma Pinelliae Ternatae (Ban Xia), Rhizoma Arisaematis (Tian Nan Xing), Rhizoma Typhonii Gigaantei (Bai Fu Zi), Semen Sinapis (Bai Jie Zi), and Spina Gleditsiae (Zao Jiao Ci) are sometimes used for Cold-Damp/Phlegm swelling with nodular and *tight* muscles and/or joints. Some of these herbs are poisonous and should be used with care.[30] Although not a "Phlegm" herb, Semen Arecae Catechu (Bing Lang) can break up Phlegm due to its bitter and pungent quality. It is used for pain and swelling of the feet.

Bulbus Fritillariae Thunbergii (Zhe Bei Mu) enters the Lung, Triple Warmer, Stomach, and Liver channels. Like other herbs in this category, which are salty, it can "soften" and dissipate nodules and is sometimes used to treat bony and soft tissue nodules.

Radix Trichosanthis Kirilowii (Tian Hua Fen) enters the Lung and Stomach and is used in ways similar to Bulbus Fritillariae Thunbergii (Zhe Bei Mu), especially if the patient is thirsty or suffers from dry mouth. It is often used to treat traumatic swelling. It can be used to treat bone spurs and to moisten tissues without being cloy.

Succus Bambusae (Zhu Li) enters the Heart, Lung, Spleen and Stomach channel and is said to be capable of reaching the whole body. It is used mostly to treat Phlegm-Heat with symptoms of numbness, tingling or cramping of the limbs.

Thallus Algae (Kun Bu) enters Spleen, Stomach, Lung and (Kidney) channels. This herb can soften and dissipate

---

29. Sha Ren is automatically added to premade formulas containing Shu Di Huang (or Di Huang which has been cooked with Sha Ren is used) at Guangzhou municipal hospital (unless specifically deleted by the doctor).

30. There are many traditional methods of processing poisonous herbs that reduce their potential dangers.

nodules and is sometimes used to treat bony and soft tissue nodules, edema, and leg obstruction (beriberi like disorders).

Rhizoma Pinelliae Ternatae (Ban Xia) enters the Spleen and Stomach channels and is a very important herb in treating Dampness and Phlegm. This herb is used mostly in treating systemic Dampness and Phlegm nodules, and to balance cloy tonic herbs.

Rhizoma Arisaematis (Tian Nan Xing) enters the Liver, Lung and Spleen channels and collaterals/network-vessels. This herb is powerful and poisonous, and therefore should be used with care. The processed varieties (Zhi Nan Xing and Dan Nan Xing) are less toxic. It is used to treat Phlegm in the channels and collaterals with symptoms of numbness, spasms/cramps (because it dispels Wind), paralysis, swelling, and arthritis/arthrosis. It is often used in facial disorders and traumatic swelling.[31]

Rhizoma Typhonii Gigaantei (Bai Fu Zi) enters the Liver and Stomach channels. It is used in ways similar to Rhizoma Arisaematis (Tian Nan Xing), especially in facial disorders with convulsions, clenched jaws, tremors, paralysis, and deviation of mouth and eyes. It is often used to treat headaches and migraines as well as to eliminate toxins and dissipate nodules. Extracts of the herb can be used for acupoint injection to treat facial neuritis.

Semen Sinapis (Bai Jie Zi) enters the Lung channel. This herb can regulate-Qi, dissipate nodules, open the channels and collaterals/network-vessels to relieve pain. It is used to treat Phlegm obstruction causing pain, numbness and pain, especially around the waist and back. This herb can be used to treat acute low back sprains when fried until yellow, powdered, and administered with rice wine. Its spicy nature is used to penetrate and scatter Phlegm-nodules (cysts).

Spina Gleditsiae (Zao Jiao Ci) enters the Liver and Stomach channels. This herb can eliminate toxicity, drain pus, activate Blood circulation, and reduce swelling. It can be used to treat cysts, nodules, and bone spurs.

- *Yang lifting herbs*: Low dosage of Rhizoma Cimicifugae (Sheng Ma), Radix Bupleuri (Chai Hu), Radix Puerariae (Ge Gen), Rhizoma et Radix Notopterygii (Qiang Huo), Radix Ligustici Sinensis (Gao Ben) and Radix Ledebouriellae Sesloidis (Fang Feng) can be added to formulas in patients with weakness of Spleen and Yang-Qi, with endogenous or exogenous Dampness.

Rhizoma Cimicifugae (Sheng Ma) enters the Spleen, Stomach, Large Intestine and Lung channels. This herb can be used to treat pain in the forehead and to aid lift Clear-Yang.

- *Strengthening Yang to transform Dampness herbs*: To treat Cold-Damp, Phlegm, accumulated Fluids or edema, or when Cold predominates over Dampness with more symptoms of chills and general aches that become worse by cold exposure/weather, herbs such as Cortex Cinnamomi Cassiae (Rou Gui), Aconiti Carmichaeli Praeparata (Fu Zi) Radix Aconiti Carmichaeli (Chuan Wu), Radix Aconiti Kusnezoffii (Cao Wu) are used together with bland draining/precipitating herbs such as Poriae Cocos (Fu Ling), Polypori Umbellati (Zhu Ling), and Semen Coicis Lachrma (Yi Yi Ren).[32]

Yang tonification, especially of the Kidneys and Liver, is often used in conditions in which the sinews and bones are "weak." There is waist (low back) and lower extremity pain and weakness. They are used frequently in the elderly. Rhizoma Curculiginis Orchioidis (Xian Mao), Radix Morindae (Ba Ji Tian), Herba Epimedii (Yin Yang Huo), Cortex Eucommiae Ulmoidis (Du Zhong), Radix Dipsaci Asperi (Xu Duan), Rhizoma Cibotii Barmometz (Gou Ji), Cornu Cervu Parvum (Lu Rong), Rhizoma Gusuibu (Gu Sui Bu), Fructus Psoraleae Chinesis (Bu Gu Zhi), Semen Cuscutae (Tu Si Zi), and Herba Cistanshes (Rou Cang Rong) are often used.

Rhizoma Curculiginis Orchioidis (Xian Mao) enters the Kidney and Liver channels. This herb is very pungent and can expel Coldness, but only slightly strengthens the Kidneys. Because its nature is very pungent, this herb can easily injure Yin and is therefore used for short durations in chronic and obstinate Cold-Damp Painful Obstruction. Clinically, this herb is used in patients that suffer from cold limbs, intolerance and aggravation of pain by cold, weakness, and pain in the low back and knees.

Radix Morindae (Ba Ji Tian) enters the Liver and Kidneys. It is only slightly warm and is therefore mild and can be used on most patients. This herb is used in very similar cases as Rhizoma Curculiginis Orchioidis (Xian Mao), but it is stronger in tonifying Kidney-Yang. It is often used in chronic cases with weakness and pain in the low back (waist) and knees, and in chronic Painful Obstruction (Bi) syndromes.

Herba Epimedii (Yin Yang Huo, also called Xian Ling Pi) enters the Liver and Kidney channels. This herb has characteristics similar to the above Yang tonic herbs but is most useful in expelling Wind-Dampness. It can tonify both Yin and Yang and steady (pull-down) rising-Liver-Yang with symptoms of dizziness and/or headaches. This herb is therefore used in chronic and acute cases of Painful Obstruction and Kidney and Liver weakness.

Cortex Eucommiae Ulmoidis (Du Zhong) enters the Liver and Kidney channels. This herb is gentle and beside tonifying Yang it can smooth/regulate the flow of Qi and

---

31. Overdose can result in numbness of the tongue and mouth, swelling and pain in the tongue and mouth, headache, dizziness, palpitations, nausea, vomiting, slurred speech, hoarse voice, convulsions, and respiratory depression. Treatment may include a large dosage of Sheng Jiang, Fang Feng, and Gan Cao.

32. For Cold-Dampness in somatic tissues (muscles and sinews) Rhizoma Zingiberis (Gan Jiang), Radix Aconiti (Fu Zhi), Cortex Cinnamomi (Rou Gui) and Flos Caryophylli (Ding Xiang) can be used with or without Dampness herbs.

Blood. It is often used in chronic cases of Kidney-deficiency, with symptoms of painful and weak low back and knees. Because it can regulate Blood flow, it is also used to aid the healing of sinews and bones in both acute and chronic injuries. It is especially important for low back pain and can be used in all types of lumbar pain.

Radix Dipsaci Asperi (Xu Duan) enters the Liver and Kidney channels. This herb, like Cortex Eucommiae Ulmoidis (Du Zhong), is gentle and can promote Blood flow. It is often used in the treatment of weak and painful sinews and bones, in both acute and chronic conditions. It can aid in healing fractures and in repairing tendons and ligaments. It is often combined with Cortex Eucommiae Ulmoidis (Du Zhong) for chronic or acute low back pain.

Rhizoma Cibotii Barmometz (Gou Ji) enters the Liver and Kidney channels. Like the above two herbs, this herb can regulate Blood flow. However, it is warmer and more pungent and is not as mild. It is used to expel Wind-Damp Painful Obstruction in patients with chronic stiffness of the joints and crampy, shortened muscles. It is used also to treat edema and swelling resulting as an aftermath of illness. It is also said to have an affinity for the spine.

Cornu Cervu Parvum (Lu Rong) enters the Liver and Kidney channels but can also tonify the Governing channel. This substance is used to benefit Essence and Blood as well as to tonify Kidney-Yang. It is therefore used in developmental disorders, skeletal deformities, and soreness of the waist (low back) and knees. It is particularly useful in aiding to heal bone fractures.

Rhizoma Gusuibu (Gu Sui Bu) enters the Kidney and Liver channels. This herb can move Blood, stop bleeding, and supplement the Kidneys, sinews, and bones. It is particularly useful in treating ligamentous, tendinous and bony injuries. It aids in mending these tissues in both chronic and subacute injuries.

Semen Cuscutae (Tu Si Zi) enters the Liver and Kidney channels. This herb is mild and is not cloy and therefore can be used in most cases. It tonifies the Kidney, Liver, Yin and Yang, and benefits the Essence. It is used mostly in chronic disorders, in patients with weakness of the back and knees, or with constitutional weakness.

Fructus Psoraleae (Bu Gu Zhi) enters the Kidney and Spleen channels. This herb tonifies the Kidney and fortifies Yang. It also consolidates Essence and retains urine. It is therefore used to treat degenerative joint diseases (especially effecting bone) and can be used for sequelae of S4 nerve root lesions with loss of urinary and bowl control.

Herba Cistanshes (Rou Cang Rong) enters the Kidney and Large Intestine channels. This herb is moistening, mild, and can nourish Essence. It can invigorate the Yang and warm the Kidneys without drying. It is therefore used to balance other Yang tonics that have a drying effect and to treat weakness of sinews and bones.[33]

- *Qi regulating herbs*: Pericarpium Citri Reticulatae (Chen Pi), Pericarpium Citri Reticulatae Viride (Qing Pi), Rhizoma Cyperi Rotundi (Xiang Fu), Semen Arechae Catechu (Bing Lang) and the Blood-moving Radix Ligustici Wallichii (Chuan Xiang) are often used to push Fluids by moving Qi and Blood, especially in the middle-Burner or extremities.

Pericarpium Citri Reticulatae (Chen Pi) enters the Stomach and Spleen channels. Because it is aromatic, it can transform Damp-Phlegm. It is used mainly to motivate and regulate Qi and to help digest cloy herbs, countering the sticky "staying" effects of many tonifying herbs.

Pericarpium Citri Reticulatae Viride (Qing Pi) enters the Liver and Gall Bladder channels. It has a stronger function of regulating Qi than Pericarpium Citri Reticulatae (Chen Pi). It is used mainly for pain in a Liver or Gall Bladder channel distribution (chest, subcostal, and trunk) caused by Phlegm accumulations.

Cyperi Rotundi (Xiang Fu) enters the Liver and Triple Warmer channels and is an important herb for regulating Liver-Qi. It can be used without fear of damaging Yin or Blood.[34] Because it enters the Triple Warmer, it can be used to treat Qi-stagnation anywhere in the body and to spread Qi throughout the body.

Semen Arechae Catechu (Bing Lang) enters the Large Intestine and Stomach channel. This herb has a descending property and can be used to lead other herbs to the lower extremities. Because it is bitter, pungent, and warm, it treats water accumulation and swelling especially in the feet. It can be used with other herbs to treat tight lumpy muscles. It can also eliminate parasites.

There are many other herbs that may be used in the treatment of musculoskeletal disorders, but in general they are less important. Table 7-1 summarizes the most important aspects of commonly used herbs (including some that have not been covered), Table 7-2 on page 401 summarizes herbs used for Extra channels, Table 7-3 on page 402 summarizes herbs used to conduct formulas to channels, Table 7-4 on page 402 summarizes herbs and point used to treat pain be region, Table 7-5 on page 403 summarizes herbs and point by pathology, Table 7-6 on page 404 summarizes commonly used prepared formulas, Table 7-7 on page 406 summarizes herbal combination used by pathologies and regions, Table 7-8 on page 417 summarized the pharmacological effects of herbs, and Table 7-9 on page 419 summarizes TCM contraidications.

---

33. Other non-drying Kidney-Yang tonics are Herba Cynomorii (Suo Yang) and Semen Juglandis (Hu Tao Ren).

34. There are differing opinions as to how mild this herb is, and some practitioners consider it to be capable of damaging Yin and Blood.

Table 7-1: Highlights Of The Most Commonly Used Herbs In Musculoskeletal Disorders

Category	Herbs
Spicy Warm Exterior Releasing [A]	**Ephedrae (Ma Huang):** Used as vasoconstricter, warms channels to relieve pain mostly in upper extremity but also knees. Used for Excess type Cold pains. **Cinnamomi (Gui Zhi):** Used for warming and vasodialating effects. Treats many conditions with cold extremities such as Raynaud's disease. Often added to colder formulas. Can be used for Deficient or Excess type pains. Often used topically. **Ledeboriella** [Siler or Saposhnikovia] **(Fang Feng):** Used to expel pathogens from the flesh/muscles and subcutaneous regions. Also for muscle spasms, cramps, tetanus, trembling of hands and feet, and for seizures. Also used in moving arthritis/pains. **Schizonepetae (Jing Jie):** Used sometimes in Painful Obstruction and muscle spasms. **Perillae (Zi Su Ye or Zi Su Gen):** Used for its Liver and Qi moving effects mostly in sensitive patients or when the patient also has digestive symptoms. **Zingiberis (Sheng Jiang):** Used for warming as well as analgesic and anti-inflammatory effect. Often used in patients that also have digestive issues. **Notopterygi (Qiang Huo):** Used to treat pain in the back of the neck and head (occipital) and for pain in the upper extremities. **Ligustici (Gao Ben):** Used mostly to treat vertex headaches. **Angelicae (Bai Zhi):** Used for painful disorders in the upper-frontal body areas, especially forehead pain. Also used to treat ganglion cysts, especially when found on the thumb or index finger tendons. It has anti-inflammatory and analgesic effects. Often used topically. **Asari (Xi Xin):** Very important in the treatment of pain. Penetrates deeply and is useful for bone and sinew/soft tissue pains. Often used for arthritic pains, chronic and Deficient (especially Kidney) disorders, acute Painful Obstruction, and to treat headaches. Small amounts are often added to cold formulas. Often used topically.
Spicy Cool Exterior Releasing	**Arctii (Niu Bang Zi):** Used in high doses for discogenic pain. **Chrysanthemi (Ju Hua):** Used to treat headaches and Liver-Heat. A mild herb that can be used to treat weak patients with Liver-Heat. **Puerariae (Ge Gen):** Used for Pathogenic Factors in the subcutaneous and muscle layers. For muscular weakness and wasting, and for "dryness" in the flesh. Often used for pain in the back of the neck and shoulder. Also used topically. **Bupleuri (Chi Hu):** Used to harmonize the Shao-Yang and to raise Qi. It can also "open" the Liver and treat Liver-congestion. **Sojae (Dan Dou Chi):** Used to treat irritability and insomnia in post viral pain syndromes.
Clear Heat and Purge Fire [B]	**Gypsum (Shi Gao):** Important herb in treating inflammatory joint diseases. Can be combined within warming formulas. Often used for Yang-Ming (body front) pains. Often used topically. **Anemarrhenae (Zhi Mu):** Used to both clear Heat and to moisten. Often used to treat inflammatory joint diseases. Can be used for both Deficiency and Excess type disorders. **Gardeniae (Zhi Zi):** Used to treat Triple Warmer Damp-Heat and irritability. **Prunellae (Xia Ku Cao):** Sometimes used to treat bony spurs and cysts. It can also treat headaches from Liver-Fire especially eyeball pain.
Clear Heat and Toxin	**Caulis Loncerae (Ren Dong Teng):** Used in inflammatory arthritis. Also treats muscle aches. **Tracaxaci (Pu Gong Ying):** Sometimes used for inflammatory or infectious joint diseases. **Abri (Ji Gu Cao):** Sometimes used for Heat type Painful Obstruction.
Clear Heat Dry Dampness	**Scutellarae (Huang Qin):** Used for upper body Damp-Heat. Can also be used to balance spicy, warm dry herbs. Used often in post viral pain syndromes. **Coptidis (Huang Lian):** Used for middle Warmer Damp-Heat. Often used to treat Heart-Fire when the patient has a red-tipped tongue. Can be added to warm formulas in patients with red-tipped tongue. Used often in post viral pain syndromes. **Phellodendri (Huang Bai):** Used for lower Warmer Damp-Heat. Can be used for both Excess and Deficiency type syndromes. Often used to treat inflammation in the lower extremities. Often used topically. **Centellae (Long Dan Cao):** Used to treat Liver-type headaches. Helpful for acute discogenic pain. **Sophorae (Ku Shen):** Used for post viral pain syndromes.

Table 7-1: Highlights Of The Most Commonly Used Herbs In Musculoskeletal Disorders (Continued)

CATEGORY	HERBS
CLEAR HEAT AND COOL BLOOD	**Rehmanniae (Sheng Di Huang)**: Used in both Empty-Heat and Full-Heat disorders. Can stop bleeding. Used frequently for inflammatory disorders and to calm the spirit when the patient suffers from irritability and thirst. Can treat acute or chronic diseases. Also used to balance Yang-tonics. **Scrophulariae (Xuan Shen)**: Used to treat soft swellings and clear Blood-Heat. Used for many inflammatory type disorders. Can be used to balance spicy and hot formulas. **Mountan (Mu Dan Pi)**: Used to both move and cool the Blood. Mostly for deep-Heat with lack of perspiration. Can treat swelling and acute injuries. Can treat both Empty-Heat and Full-Heat. Also used to balance Yang-tonics, preventing side-effects. **Lycii (Di Gu Pi)**: Used for deep Heat with perspiration. Sometimes used for inflammatory joint diseases. Mostly for Deficiency type syndromes. Can be used to balance spicy-hot and Yang-tonic herbs.
PURGATIVE	**Rhei (Da Huang)**: Used to treat Blood-stasis and circulate Blood. It clears Heat and constipation. Mostly used in Excess type syndromes but can be combined with other herbs for Deficiency syndromes. Often used topically.

Table 7-1: Highlights Of The Most Commonly Used Herbs In Musculoskeletal Disorders (Continued)

CATEGORY	HERBS
ELIMINATE WIND-DAMPNESS[c]	**Angelicae (Du Huo)**: Used in weak patients and chronic disorders. Treats Painful Obstruction of bones, the back and lower extremities. Characterized by heaviness, stiffness and numbness. Used for both acute and chronic aches and pains of the muscles and joints. Not too harsh, has a mild moistening effect. **Clematidis (Wei Ling Xian)**: Used in arthritic disorders anywhere in the body, especially when symptoms of numbness and tingling (Wind) are seen. Most effective for lumbar and lower extremity pain. Used often for musculoskeletal disorders with muscle cramping (spasms), stiffness of joints and difficulties in both flexion and extension, and for numbness. Often used topically. **Bombycis (Can Sha)**: Used to treat muscle pains and spasms, especially of the calves. Can be helpful when the patient experiences itching with the pain. **Acanthopanacis (Wu Jia Pi)**: Used in chronic Painful Obstruction with weakness of the sinews and bones, and for muscular atrophy. Also used for muscles spasms and cramps due to Excess or Deficiency. Especially useful for the elderly and weak patients. Can be used to treat mild edema and joint swelling. Has both anti-inflammatory and analgesic effects. It can also quicken Blood circulation. **Agkistrodon (Bai Hua She)**: Used to penetrate deeply and treat all tissues and channels. Used for many chronic conditions characterized by stiffness, cramping/spasms, numbness, tingling and moving pains. **Zaocys (Wu Shao She)**: Used in similar ways as Bai Hua She except that it is milder and is not toxic. **Lycopodii (Shen Jin Cao)**: Used to "relax" the sinews. Especially important when treating tendons. Commonly used in chronic Painful Obstruction with symptoms of stiffness, contracted soft tissues, soreness of joints and muscles and numbness. It is also used in acute traumatic injuries of soft tissues. **Speranskiae (Tou Gu Cao)**: Used to treat bones, mostly in chronic cases with stiffness being predominant. Can also be used to treat traumatic injuries. Said to promote the generation of tissues. May be used to treat bone spurs, especially when the affected area is "steamed," or wrapped with this herb cooked in vinegar. **Pini (Song Jie)**: Used for pain due to acute injury. Also used for chronic and difficult joint pains (including rheumatoid arthritis), and for hypertonicity of muscles and sinews and stiffness of joints. **Piperis (Hai Feng Teng)**: Used for pain in muscles and joints which become worse during damp weather. Characterized by achy pains, cramping, heaviness, numbness, and stiffness of joints. It can be used for pain due to trauma. **Chaenomelis (Mu Gua)**: Used to relaxes the sinews. Treats musculoskeletal disorders characterized by muscle cramps, spasms, and stiffness. Best for the lower extremities. **Schefflerae (Qi Ye Lian)**: Used for its analgesic properties. Can be used for both acute (traumatic) and chronic pains with swelling. Can treat headaches, tension, or migraines. Helpful in the treatment of neuropathies. **Gentianae (Qin Jiao)**: Used in all types of Painful Obstructions, including Hot, Cold, Deficient or Excess (although best for Hot type pains and for pains aggravated by weather changes). Relaxes the sinews especially for painful stiff extremities. Guides other herbs to the spine and lumbar areas. Also used to balance the dry hot nature of other herbs and to prevent constipation. **Mori (Sang Zhi)**: Used for the upper extremities, particularly the hands, but can also be used for all other joints. Used often for muscle aches, cramping, and pain. It is commonly used to treat tendinitis. **Siegesbeckiae (Xi Xian Cao)**: Used to treat weakness in the muscles and sinews due to Wind-Damp-Heat. Used often for back and leg pain and weakness and/or paralysis when Dampness is severe. It is useful in treating secondary paralysis or muscle weakness due to neuritis. **Clerodendri (Chou Wu Tong)**: Used to treat numbness in the extremities. **Trachelospermi (Luo Shi Teng)**: Used to treat pain and spasms due to inflammatory conditions. Used for transformative/congested-Heat with pain and tension in the sinews and joints. Useful in the treatment of neuritis in its primary stage or sequelae with muscle weakness and/or atrophy. **Solidaginis (Liu Zhi Huang)**: Used to treat pain and inflammation. Can be used to treat trauma-related pain or tightness of tendons. **Dioscoreae (Chuan Shan Long)**: Used to treat painful joints with numbness and stiffness. Also used to treat pain from traumatic injuries. **Tripteryggi (Lei Gong Teng)**: Used to relieve pain and swelling in patients with inflammatory disorders. Suppresses the immune system and therefore is used in many autoimmune disorders such as rheumatoid arthritis, psoriatic arthritis, lupus, etc. Also recommended for discogenic disorders. **Tinosporae (Kuan Jin Teng)**: Used to treat pain and spasms due to inflammatory conditions. Also used to treat inflammation secondary to trauma. **Erythrinae (Hai Tong Pi)**: Used to treat pain, or cramping in the lower extremities, and waist muscles or sinews. Also important when treating traumatic swelling. Its analgesic properties are relatively pronounced. Can also relax striated muscles. **Sinomenii (Qing Feng Teng)**: Used for patients that experiences tightness, swelling and painful joints. This herb has significant anti-inflammatory and analgesic effects.

Table 7-1: Highlights Of The Most Commonly Used Herbs In Musculoskeletal Disorders (Continued)

CATEGORY	HERBS
ELIMINATE WIND-DAMPNESS NOURISH YIN	**Pyrolae (Lu Xian Cao or Lu Han Cao)**: Used in arthritic, bony and sinew disorders, said to strengthen the sinews and bones. Also used to treat bone spurs. Can be used to balance dryness of other herbs. **Loranthus (Sang Ji Sheng)**: Used to strengthen the sinews and bones in chronic arthritic disorders that involve the lower back, knees, and lower extremities. Also for other joint disorders characterized by weakness, with or without Wind-Dampness.
ELIMINATE WIND-DAMPNESS TONIFY YANG	**Curculiginis (Xian Mao)**: Used to expel Coldness, but only slightly strengthens the Kidneys. Used for short duration in chronic and obstinate Cold-Damp Painful Obstruction. Treats cold limbs, intolerance and aggravation of pain by cold, weakness, and pain in the low back and knees. **Epimedii (Yin Yang Huo or Xian Ling Pi)**: Used to tonify both Yin and Yang and steady (pull-down) rising-Liver-Yang with symptoms of dizziness and/or headaches. Often used in chronic or acute cases of Painful Obstruction with Kidney and Liver weakness. **Cibotii (Gou Ji)**: Used to treat Painful Obstruction in patients with chronic stiffness of the joints and crampy, shortened muscles. Also used to treat edema and swelling resulting as an aftermath of illness. Said to have an affinity with the spine.
TONIFY YANG STRENGTHEN SINEWS AND BONES (SOME ALSO VITALIZE BLOOD)	**Radix Morindae (Ba Ji Tian)**: Used in chronic cases with weakness and pain in the low back (waist) and knees, and in chronic Painful Obstruction (Bi) syndromes. **Eucommiae (Du Zhong)**: Used in chronic cases of Kidney-deficiency, with symptoms of painful and weak low back and knees. Also aids healing of sinews and bones in both acute and chronic injuries. Especially important for low back pain and can be used in all types of lumbar pains. **Dipsaci (Xu Duan)**: Used to treat weak and painful sinews and bones, in both acute and chronic condition. Aids in healing fractures and in repairing tendons and ligaments. **Cistanshes (Rou Cang Rong)**: Used to moisten and nourish Essence and to balance other Yang tonics that have a drying effect and to treat weakness of sinews and bones. **Cuscutae (Tu Si Zi)**: Used in chronic disorders, in patients with weakness of the back and knees, or with constitutional Essence weakness. **Cervu (Lu Rong)**: Used in developmental disorders, skeletal deformities, and soreness of the waist (low back) and knees. Particularly useful in aiding to heal bone fractures. **Drynaria (Gu Sui Bu)**: Used to stop bleeding and supplement the Kidneys, sinews, and bones. Particularly useful in treating ligamentous, tendinous, and bony injuries. Aids in mending tissues in both chronic and subacute injuries. **Psoraleae (Bu Gu Zhi)**: Used to treat degenerative joint diseases (especially affecting bone) and can be used for sequelae of S4 nerve root lesions with loss of urinary and bowl control.
FRAGRANT DAMP DISSOLVING	**Atractylodis (Cang Zhu)**: Used to treat joint swelling, cysts, and nodules. **Amomi (Sha Ren)**: Used to balance cloy and greasy herbs. **Agastache (Huo Xiang)**: Used to treat post viral pain syndromes. **Eupatorii (Pei Lan)**: Used to treat post viral pain syndromes.
WATER REGULATING DAMPNESS PERMEATING[D]	**Poriae (Fu Ling)**: Used to treat edema and swelling, due both to accumulation of pathogenic water secondary to local blockage and from the Spleen failing to metabolize and move Fluids. Also has a mild sedative effect. **Polypori (Zhu Ling)**: Used for edema and swelling. **Coicis (Yi Yi Ren)**: Used in musculoskeletal disorders to leach out Dampness. Sooths the sinews and increase flexibility of tendons and joints. More appropriate in Hot Painful Obstruction (Bi) syndromes. Used most often in chronic cases to treat swollen and stiff joints, crampy/spasm pains, heaviness and numbness of the limbs. Also used to treat Dampness in the muscles and flesh with or without weakness or atrophy (Wei syndromes). **Plantaginis (Che Qian Zi)**: Used for Damp-Heat type edema and pain. Has mild effects on joint swelling. **Dioscoreae (Bie Xie or Bi Xie)**: Used to treat turbidity and relax the sinews. Treats patients with generalized muscle aches. Can treat Painful Obstruction due to Deficiency or Excess such as: Cold-Dampness with symptoms aggravated in cold and rainy days; Heat-Dampness with symptoms aggravated in hot days; or in Kidney-deficiency with weakness and soreness of the low back and knees (or limbs). **Alismatis (Ze Xie)**: Used to treat Damp-Heat in the lower body and to clear Empty-Heat. Can be added to tonic formulas to prevent the formation or pathogenic Heat and rising of Kidney-Fire. **Stephaniae (Han Fang Ji)**: Used to treat Damp-Heat in the lower extremities with painful and heavy extremities, and/or swollen and inflamed joints. **Coculi (Mu Fang Ji)**: Used to treat all forms of neuralgia. **Tetrapanadis (Tong Cao)**: Useful in the treatment of muscle soreness.

Table 7-1: Highlights Of The Most Commonly Used Herbs In Musculoskeletal Disorders (Continued)

CATEGORY	HERBS
WARM INTERIOR AND ELIMINATE COLD	**Aconiti (Fu Zi)**: Used for Painful Obstruction when Cold is predominant with symptoms of severe pain, stiffness, cramping of the muscles and sinews, all of which are aggravated by cold weather. Also helpful in treating atrophy with spasms and contractures; inability to walk and cyanotic or dark complexion of the limbs or face. **Aconiti (Chuan Wu)** and **(Cao Wu)**: Used in treatment of Painful Obstruction with symptoms of severe pain, generalized pain, numbness, stiffness, cramping, and spasms. Both can be used for acute or chronic pain; however, for short periods only. Beside pain both herbs can be used to reduce swelling and treat abscesses (Yin-abscesses). Often used topically. **Cinnamomi (Rou Gui)**: Used mostly for patients with low back pain, weakness of waist and knees, and difficulty walking due to Kidney-deficiency. Also to treat floating-Yang that is due to Mingman-deficiency (Cold and/or false Heat). Can treat edema and generate flesh. **Zingiberis (Gan Jiang)**: Use as an anti-inflammatory and can treat joint pains, especially of the low back and lower extremities. Used with aconiti to both strengthen the effects and to counteract toxicity.
REGULATING QI[E]	**Pericarpium (Chen Pi)**: Used to balance cloy and tonic herbs. **Pericarpium (Qing Pi)**: Used for palpable masses from Phlegm and Qi-stagnation. **Aurantii (Zhi Shi)**: Used for extremity cold pains from Qi-stagnation. **Aurantii (Zhi Ke)**: Used for painful chest from Qi-stagnation. Also used for pain accompanied with itching. **Auckadiae/Saussureae (Mu Xiang)**: Used to balance cloy and greasy herbs. **Cyperi (Xiang Fu)**: Used for pain due to Liver-congestion Qi-stagnation. Pain changing characteristics. **Toosendan (Chuan Lian Zi)**: Used for pain due to Liver-related disorders with Heat. **Linderae (Wu Yao)**: Used for referred groin and abdominal pain. **Rosae (Mei Gui Hua)**: Sometimes added to formulas that treat Blood-stasis secondary to trauma and when treating females with concomitant menstrual disorders.
HEMOSTATICS	**Radix Pseudoginseng (San Qi)**: Used to stop bleeding (when used as a raw powder) and at the same time unblock the channels and network-vessels and to purge congealed-Blood. Treats traumatic bleeding, swelling and chronic arthritis with swelling. Important in the treatment of pain. Used topically to stop bleeding. **Pollen Typhae (Pu Huang)**: Used mostly as weak a anti-inflammatory effect and to treat traumatic swelling. **Lignum Sappan (Su Mu)**: Used in acute injuries to stops bleeding, invigorates the Blood, reduces swelling, and alleviates pain. Also used in some chronic disorders.

Table 7-1: Highlights Of The Most Commonly Used Herbs In Musculoskeletal Disorders (Continued)

Category	Herbs
Vitalizing Blood[F]	**Ligustici (Chuan Xiong)**: Used to treat headaches, neuralgias, traumas and/or arthritis. Also used for crampy (cold) pain in any part of the body. Can be used for Excess, Deficiency, Cold, or Hot condition. **Salvia (Dan Shen)**: Used in most musculoskeletal pains to promote circulation, remove congealed-Blood and reduce pain. Aids deposit calcium at a bone fracture zone. Often used to treat arthritis or traumatic injuries, especially with swelling and pain due to Heat-type stasis. **Millettiae (Ji Xue Teng)**: Used to treat chronic conditions such as chronic arthritis, neuropathic pain, numbness, stiffness and cramping pain in the limbs. Often used in elderly patients. **Corydalis (Yan Hu Suo)**: Used to treat pain. It can be used for somatic or visceral pains. **Curcumae (Yu Jin)**: Can treat pain, mostly in patients with Liver-Qi-stagnation and Blood-stasis or with Heart-Heat. **Lycopi (Ze Lan)**: Used to treat edema and joint swelling. Can be used to treat back or other joint pains from traumatic injuries. Also used for chronic arthritic pains with swelling. **Paeoniae (Chi Shao)**: Used treat inflammation, swelling, and pain from traumatic or other origins. **Persicae (Tao Ren)**: Used in a wide variety of Blood-stasis patterns, especially with palpable masses. **Carthami (Hong Hua)**: Used in a wide variety of Blood-stasis patterns both in the Interior or Exterior. It is especially helpful for pain in the extremities. Used to treat trauma, reduce swelling, stasis and pain. Often used topically to treat pain. **Zedoriae (E Zhu)**: Used to treat substantial Blood-stasis masses. Can be used to treat bone hypertrophy. **Sparganii (San Leng)**: Used to treat substantial Blood-stasis masses. Can be used to treat bone hypertrophy. **Olibanum (Ru Xiang)**: Used to "relax" the sinews for stiff, swollen and painful joints or soft tissues. Used for traumatic sprains, strains and fractures, because it is analgesic and can disperse swelling and aid in healing. Often used topically. **Myrrha (Mo Yao)**: Used to treat pain. Has anti-inflammatory effects. Often used topically. **Achyranthis (Niu Xi)**: Used to treat lower body pain especially low back and knees as it can tonify the Liver and Kidney. Treat chronic disorders with low back ache, weakness of waist and knees, and difficulty walking. **Sanguis (Xue Jie)**: Used to treat sprains, strains, contusions, and fractures. Used topically to stop bleeding due to external injury. **Lignum (Su Mu)**: Used for traumatic pain. **Trogopterorum (Wu Ling Zhi)**: Used in chronic pain patients, both in muscular and articular disorders. Also transforms stasis and stops bleeding. Useful in treating swelling. **Lycopodii Serrati (Jin Bu Huan)**: Used to treat sinew and bone pains. It can stop bleeding. **Hirudo (Shui Zhi)**: Used to penetrate masses and break up and drive out Blood-stasis. Sometimes used in acute traumas. **Eupolypaga (Tu Bie Chong)**: Used to penetrate masses and break up and drive out Blood-stasis. Aids in healing of sinews and bones. Often used in trauma and acute lumbar sprain. **Cyathulae (Chuan Niu Xi)**: Used for lower extremity or lower back pains. Pulls Blood downward and clears Heat and therefore used to treat dizziness. **Manis (Chuan Shan Jia)**: Used to treat swelling, stiffness, numbness and tingling or spasms of the limbs. Often added to formulas that treat chronic arthritic pains.
Tonify Qi[G]	**Ginseng (Ren Shen)**: Used in chronic cases specially after hemorrhaging. Helpful when pain becomes worse after (not during) activity. Used to treat underlying Qi deficiency. **Astragali (Huang Qi)**: Used for patients with Qi-deficiency (pain getting worse after activity). Also important in patients with muscular weakness, as this herb is said to be capable of increasing the strength of the muscles. Treats numbness and pain due to insufficient nourishment and circulation of Qi and Blood. **Codonopsis (Dang Shen)**: Used to treat underlying Qi deficiency. **Pseudostellariae (Tai Zi Shen)**: Used to treat underlying Qi-deficiency and Dryness. Can be used for post neuritic weakness. **Dioscoreae (Shan Yao)**: Used to treat underlying Qi and Yin deficiency. **Atractylodis (Bai Zhu)**: Used to treat underlying Qi and Spleen deficiency and to treat Dampness. **Ziziphi (Da Zao)**: Used to harmonize the formula and to nourish Heart and Qi. **Glycyrrhizae (Gan Cao)**: Used to harmonize the formula and to reduce toxicity of other herbs. Used in inflammatory disorders. **Polygonati (Huang Jing)**: Used to treat underlying Qi, Yin and Essence deficiency. Often used as a substitute for Shu Di in patients with Spleen-deficiency or with Dampness.

Table 7-1: Highlights Of The Most Commonly Used Herbs In Musculoskeletal Disorders (Continued)

CATEGORY	HERBS
TONIFY BLOOD	**Rehmanniae (Shu Di):** Used to treat underlying Blood, Yin and Kidney weakness. **Polygoni (He Shou Wu):** Used to treat underlying Blood, Essence, Yin, Kidney and Liver weakness. **Angelicae (Dang Gui):** Used to treat underlying Blood-deficiency or Blood-stasis. Has analgesic effects and can be used for both acute and chronic disorders. **Paeoniae (Bai Shao):** Used to treat underlying Blood and Liver deficiency. Also important in treating pain especially spasmodic pains. Used in both acute and chronic disorders. **Lycii (Gou Qi Zi):** Used to treat underlying Blood, Yin and Essence deficiency. Especially helpful for Liver-Blood and Yin deficiency. **Mori (Sang Shen Zi):** Used to treat underlying Blood and Yin and deficiency. Especially helpful for sensitive patients that cannot tolerate other Blood tonics (i.e., mild approach).
TONIFY YIN	**Glehniae (Bei Sha Shen):** Sometimes used for post neuritic weakness and atrophy. Or in underlying Yin-deficiency especially in Stomach and Lungs. **Ophiopogonis (Mai Men Dong):** Sometimes used for post neuritic weakness and atrophy. Or in underlying Yin-deficiency especially in Stomach. **Asparagi (Tian Men Dong):** Sometimes used for post neuritic weakness and atrophy. Or in underlying Yin-deficiency especially in Lungs and Kidney. **Dendrobii (Shi Hu):** Sometimes used for post neuritic weakness and atrophy. Or in underlying Yin-deficiency especially in Stomach and Kidney with Empty-Heat. Said to strengthen the Back, sinews and bones. **Polygonati (Yu Zhu):** Sometimes used for post neuritic weakness and atrophy. Or in underlying Yin-deficiency especially of Stomach and Lung and for Qi and Yin deficiency. **Lilii (Bai He):** Sometimes used for post neuritic weakness and atrophy. Or in underlying Yin-deficiency especially in Heart and Lung. **Ecliptae (Han Lian Cao):** Used to treat underlying Yin-deficiency with Empty-Heat. Can stop bleeding. **Ligustri (Nu Zhen Zi):** Used to treat underlying Liver and Kidney Yin-deficiency. **Testudinis (Gui Ban):** Used to treat underlying Yin-deficiency with rising Yang. Said to strengthen bones and sinews.
ASTRINGENT[H]	**Schisandrae (Wu Wei Zi):** Sometimes used to treat post neuritic weakness and atrophy. Also used for sequelae of S4 nerve root lesions. **Myristicae (Rou Dou Kou):** Sometimes used to treat sequelae of S4 nerve root lesions. **Corni (Shan Zhu Yu):** Used to treat underlying Liver and Kidney deficiency. Sometimes used to treat post neuritic weakness and atrophy. Also used for sequelae of S4 nerve root lesions. **Rosae (Jin Ying Zi):** Sometimes used to treat post neuritic weakness and atrophy. Also used for sequelae of S4 nerve root lesions. **Mantidis (Sang Piao Xiao):** Sometimes used to treat underlying Kidney and Essence deficiency and for sequelae of S4 nerve root lesions. **Nelumbinis (Lian Zi):** Used to treat sensitive patients with Spleen and Kidney deficiency. **Stamen (Lian Xu):** Used to consolidate Kidney Essence preventing further loss.
DISSOLVING PHLEGM	**Pinellia (Ban Xia):** Used in treatment of systemic Dampness and Phlegm nodules, and to balance cloy tonic herbs. **Arisaematis (Tian or Dan Nan Xing):** Used to treat numbness, spasms/cramps (because it dispels Wind), paralysis, swelling, and arthritis/arthrosis. Used in facial disorders and traumatic swelling. **Typhonii (Bai Fu Zi):** Used in facial disorders with convulsions, clenched jaws, tremors, paralysis and deviation of mouth and eyes. Also used to treat headaches and migraines as well as to eliminate toxins and dissipate nodules. **Sinapis (Bai Jie Zi):** Used for numbness and pain, especially around the waist and back. For acute low back sprains fry herb until yellow, powder, and administer with rice wine. Also used to penetrate and scatter Phlegm-nodules (cysts). **Gleditsiae (Zao Jiao Ci):** Used to eliminate toxicity, drain pus, activate Blood circulation, and reduce swelling. Used to treat cysts, nodules and bone spurs. **Laminariae (Kun Bu):** Used to soften and dissipate nodules. Sometimes used to treat bony and soft tissue nodules, edema, and leg obstruction (beriberi like disorders). **Fritillaria (Zhe Bei Mu):** Used to soften and dissipate nodules and is sometimes used to treat bony and soft tissue nodules. **Trichonsanthis (Tian Hua Fen):** Used to soften and dissipate nodules especially if the patient is thirsty or suffers from dry mouth. Often used to treat traumatic swelling. Also used for bone spurs and to moisten tissues without being cloy.

Table 7-1: Highlights Of The Most Commonly Used Herbs In Musculoskeletal Disorders (Continued)

CATEGORY	HERBS
PACIFY SPIRIT	**Draconis (Long Gu):** Used to calm patients and to promote healing of wounds. Said to be helpful in patients with Qi-wild pulses (Shen-Hammer style). **Succinum (Hu Po):** Used to calm patients and to reduce swelling and promote healing of wounds. **Ostreae (Mu Li):** Used to calm patients and soften nodules. Sometimes used to treat bone-spurs. Said to be helpful in patients with Qi-wild pulses (Shen-Hammer style).
NURTURE HEART AND PACIFY SPIRIT	**Zizyphi (Suan Zao Ren):** Used to calm patients with insomina due to Liver and Empty-Heat. **Polygalae (Yuan Zhi):** Used to calm patients by nourishing Heart and to dispel Phlegm. **Albiziae (He Huan Pi):** Used to nourish Heart and calming patients. Can open channels and collaterals and treat swelling, invigorate the Blood, and to facilitate healing of soft tissues and bone. **Polygoni (Ye Jiao Teng):** Used to calm patients and also to treat soreness and pain in the limbs from Blood-deficiency. Can open channels and collaterals and treat Painful Obstruction.[i] **Valerianae (Xie Cao):** Used to calm patients and to relieve cramps, spasms and pain due to Liver-congestion-Qi-stagnation.
EXTINGUISH WIND RELIEVE SPASMS [j]	**Uncariae (Gou Teng):** Used mostly for its sedative effect and to treat spasms. **Gastrodiae (Tian Ma):** Used for both internal and external Wind. Moistening nature and used in both Excess or Deficient-Yin/Blood Wind disorders. Symptoms of muscle twitching, cramping, spasm, tonic-clonic convulsions, stiffness, numbness, tingling, or headache. Commonly used to treat headaches including migraines and arthritic problems characterized by pain, numbness, and decreased agility. **Lumbricus (Di Long):** Used to "dig-in" and "penetrate," to break up obstructions. Treats Wind with convulsions, seizures, mania, and fever. Often used for Painful Obstruction with symptoms of stiffness, weakness, numbness, and pain in the limbs (mostly lower limbs). Used also in chronic arthritic disorders characterized by Heat with redness, warmth and swollen joints, and/or pains increasing with exposure to heat. Or for arthritic disorders characterized by coldness, numbness, stiffness, and pain that increases by exposure to cold. Also treats bone fractures with swelling and pain. **Buthus (Quan Xie):** Used for acute or chronic spasms, tremors, or convulsions from Liver-Wind and Heat. Useful for chronic and stubborn headaches, especially frontal, temporal and migraines. Also treats arthritic disorders with severe pain, numbness, decreased mobility, or paralysis. May inhibit joint destruction and stiffness. **Scolopendra (Wu Gong):** Used in similar ways as Quan Xie but better for Cold conditions. Commonly used for pain of the sinews and muscles with numbness and stiffness. For joint pains characterized by pain that moves from one joint to another. It is also used for chronic and stubborn headaches. **Batryticatus (Jiang Can):** Used in similar ways as Di Long, but stronger effect on Dampness/Phlegm. Used for fascial (and facial) pain, spasm, numbness and paralysis in the extremities. Most commonly for head and face pain, and for Wind-Damp arthritis/arthrosis. **Vespae (Lu Feng Fang):** Used for intractable Painful Obstruction, often with Heat-Toxin symptoms.

a. Herbs that treat Cold are pungent and warm and are capable of activating Qi, opening the pores and subcutaneous layers, and some can out-thrust Pathogenic Factors to the Exterior, connect the Interior with the Exterior and harmonize the Nutritive and Defensive -Qi. They may be chosen from the pungent warm Exterior, or pungent warm Interior category. All these herbs may injure Qi, Yin, Fluids, or Blood and thus should be used with care.
b. Herbs that clear Heat are often cold and may be bitter and thus can easily injure the digestive system. Their bitter quality however can dry Dampness and thus may aid the Spleen.
c. Herbs that treat Wind-Dampness are usually used to treat Painful Obstruction (Bi) syndromes and by enlarge are divided to those that mainly treat Wind, Cold, Heat, or Dampness. Many are pungent, warm, and bitter so that they may harm Yin/Fluids and thus should be taken with care. Almost all enter the Liver, Spleen, and Kidney channels. Those that enter the Liver tend to treat the sinews, those that enter the Spleen tend to treat the muscles and flesh, and those that enter the Kidney tend to treat the bones.
d. Herbs that treat Dampness may be chosen from several categories. Some are bland and promote urination, some are bitter and can dry-Dampness, some are pungent and can transform-Dampness, some are warm and can steam-Dampness, some promote movement of Qi thus dispersing Dampness, and some treat the Spleen, Kidneys, Lungs, and Triple Warmer as they can lead to Dampness.
e. Herbs that treat Qi-stagnation are often pungent and warm and therefore may injure Qi, Yin, Fluids, or Blood. Other herbs that have pungent flavour may also be used to move-Qi.
f. Herbs that move-Blood are often analgesic and are used often in the treatment of pain. Some of these herbs are warm and should be used with care in patients who bleed. Some, however, can both move and stop bleeding.
g. Most tonic herbs, and especially Yin and Blood tonics, are difficult to digest, are cloy, and, therefore, tend to "stick" (not move) or promote pathogenic-Dampness. They are therefore likely to cause digestive side-effects or may lead to retained Pathogenic Factors. Herbs that regulate Qi should be used at the same time.
h. Astringent herbs are sometimes used topically to treat swellings.
i. The first four herbs are often used to treat Painful Obstruction in sensitive patients (i.e., mild approach).

j. Herbs that treat Wind may be chosen from warm or cold Exterior category, or from those that subdue Interior-Wind. Animal herbs are said capable of digging into the body, searching-out Pathogenic Factors.

There are eighteen (or nineteen) incompatibilities between herbs. There are also some incompatibilities between foods and herbs. Salvia (Dan Shen) and Poria (Fu Ling) are said to interact negatively with vinegar. All Blood tonics are said to interact negatively with strong tea (especially black tea). Rehmanniae (Shu and Sheng Di) and Polygoni (He Shou Wu) are said to interact negatively with onions, garlic, and radishes. Rehmanniae (Shu Di) is said to also be incompatible with animal blood. Also, Smilacis (Tu Fu Ling) and Quisqualis (Shi Jun Zi) with tea and Dichroae (Chang Shan) with onions. Radix Glycyrrhizae (Gan Cao), Coptidis (Huang Lian), Platycodi (Jie Geng), Radix et Rhizoma Rhei (Da Huang) and Mume (Wu Mei) with pork. Fructus Psoraleae (Bu Gu Zhi) with pork blood. Rhizoma Atractylodis (Cang Zhu) with black carp, peach, plum and Chinese cabbage. Rhizoma Acrori Graminei (Shi Chang Pu) with meat, lamb blood and maltose. Radix Aconiti (Fu Zi) with soy sauce and millet. Rhizoma Zingiberis (Sheng Jiang) with horse meat. Perillae (Zi Su Ye and Zi Su Geng), Os Draconis (Long Gu) with carp. Rhizoma Pinelliae (Ban Xia) is said to be incompatible with lamb and sheep blood and maltose.

Radix Glycyrrhizae (Gan Cao) is said to interact with Herba Sargassii (Hai Cao) and Radix Euphorbiae (Da Ji). Radix Aconiti (Wu Tou) is used often to treat pain and is said to have bad interactions with Bulbus Fritillareiae Cirrhosae (Bei Mu), Fructus Trichonsanthis (Gua Lou), Rhizoma Pinelliae (Ban Xia) and Rhizoma Bletillae (Bai Ji). Radix Ginseng (Ren Shen) interacts with Excrementum Trogopterori (Wu Ling Zhi). Cortex Cinnamomi (Rou Gui), Halloysitum (Chi Shi Zhi), Flos Caryophylli (Ding Xiang) and Tuber Curcumae (Yu Jin) are all said to reduce each other's function. Fructus Zizyphi (Da Zao) interacts with Herba Sargassii (Hai Zao) and some of the harsh diuretics. There are a other interactions however they are not commonly used in orthopedic patients.

It is also said however that Radix Aconiti (Wu Tou) can restrain any toxic effect of Cornu Rhinoceri (Xi Jiao). Radix Ginseng (Ren Shen) restrains toxicity of Excrementum Trogopterori (Wu Ling Zhi). And Cortex Cinnamomi (Rou Gui) restrains Radix Paeonia Rubra (Chi Shao).

Table 7-2: Herbs for Extra Channels/Vessels

CHANNEL	HERBS
GOVERNING (DU)	Cervi (Lu Rong) and its preparations (Lu Jiao, Lu Shuang), Aconiti (Fu Zi), Cinnamomi (Rou Gui and Gui Zhi), Asari (Xi Xin), Zanthoxyli (Chuan Jiao), Ligustici (Gao Ben), Zingiberis (Gan Jiang). Soups made with bones/vertebrae, and sinews. Fructus Xanthii (Cang Er Zi), Plastrum Testudinis (Gao Ben), Fructus Lycii (Gou Qi Zi), Radix Astragali (Huang Qi).
CONCEPTION (REN)	Rehmanniae (Di Huang), Lycii (Gou Qi Zi), Testudinis (Gui Ban), Amydae (Bie Jia), Placenta (Zi He Che), Flouritum (Zi Shi Ying), Salviae (Dan Shen), Codonopsis (Dang Shen), and Morindae (Ba Ji Tian). Scrophulariae (Xuan Shen), Anemarrhenae (Zhi Mu), Phellodendri (Huang Bo) and Scrophulariae (Xuan Shen)
Girdle (Dai)	Schisandrea (Wu Wei Zi), Euryales (Qian Shi), Nelumbinis (Lian Zi), Flouritum (Zi Shi Ying). Mantidis (Sang Piao Xiao), Os (Long Gu), Concha (Mu Li), Astragali (Sha Yuan Zi), Os Sepiae (Wu Zei Gu), Rosae (Jing Ying Zi), Rubi (Fu Pen Zi), Dioscoreae (San Yao), Paeoniae (Bai Shao), Rehmanniae (Shu Di), Lycii (Gou Qi Zi), Angelicae (Dang Gui), Dipsaci (Xu Duan), Artemisiae (Ai Ye), and Cimicifugae (Sheng Ma).[a]
YANG LINKING (WEI)	Cinnamomi (Gui Zhi), Paeonia (Bai Shao) and Astragali (Huang Qi).
YIN LINKING (WEI)	Angelicae (Dang Gui), Biotae (Bai Zi Ren), and Ligustici (Chuan Xiong).
HERBS THAT TREAT *BOTH* YIN AND YANG (WEI) LINKING CHANNELS	Cinnamomi (Rou Gui), Stephaniae (Fang Ji), Manitis (Chuan Shan Jie), Os (Hu Gu) Paeoniae (Bai Shao), Corni (Shan Zhu Yu), Rehmanniae (Shu Di), Testudinis (Gui Ban), Tritici (Huai Xiao Mai), Zizyphi (Da Zao), Glycrrhizae (Gan Cao), Schisandrae (Wu Wei Zi).
YANG (QIAO) MOTILITY	Sileris (Fang Feng), Ephedrae (Ma Huang), Stephaniae (Fang Ji), Atracylodis (Cang Zhu), Testudinis (Gui Ban), Rehmanniae, (Shu Di), Phellodendri (Huang Bai), Poriae (Fu Ling), Corni (Shan Zhu Yu), Schisandrae (Wu Wei Zi), and Polygalae Tenuifoliae (Yuan Zhi).
YIN (QIAO) MOTILITY	Corydalis (Yan Hu Sou), Pinellae (Ban Xia), Arisaemae (Dan Nan Xing), Polygalae (Yuan Zhi), Ziziphi (Suan Zao Ren), Acori (Shi Chang Pu), Anemarrhenae (Zhi Mu), Phelodendri (Huang Bai). Paeoniae (Bai Shao), Corni (Shan Zhu Yu), Hallyositum (Bai Shi Ying), Tritici (Huai Xiao Mai), Zizyphi (Da Zao), Radix Glycyrrhizae (Gan Cao).
PENETRATING (CHONG)	Flouritum (Zi Shi Ying), Haemitium (Dai Zhe Shi), Astragali (Sha Yuan Zi), Rehmanniae (Shu Di), Lycii (Gou Qi Zi), Biotae (Bai Zi Ren), Testudinis (Gui Ban), Amydae (Bei Jia), Juglandis (Hu Tao Ren), Phellodendri (Huang Bai), Cistanchis (Rou Cong Rong), Eucommiae (Du Zhong), Morindae (Ba Ji Tian), Dioscoreae (Shan Yao), Angelicae (Dang Gui), Ligustici (Chuan Xiong), Corydalis (Yan Hu Suo), Persicae (Tao Ren), Salviae (Dan Shen), Meliae (Chuan Lian Zhi), Poriae (Fu Ling), Curcumae (Yu Jin), Cyperi (Xiang Fu), Citri (Qing Pi), Pinelliae (Ban Xia), Magnoliae (Hou Po), Evodiae (Wu Zhu Yu), Atractylodis (Cang Zhu), Leonuri Heterophylli (Yi Mu Cao), Lignum (Jiang Xiang), and Foeniculi (Xiao Hui Xiang).
HERBS THAT ENTER THE LIVER, KIDNEY, AND ALL EIGHT EXTRA CHANNELS (YANG 2002)	Lycii (Gou Qi Zi), Amomi (Sha Ren), Eucommiae (Du Zhong), Achyranthis (Niu Xi), Dipsaci (Xu Duan), Rehmanniae (Sheng Di Huang), Sesame (Zi Ma), Mori (Sang Shen), Cuscutae (Tu Si Zi), Croni (Shan Zhu Yu), Ligustri (Nu Zhen Zi), (Hao Ren Zao), Cynomorri (Suo Yang), Rubi (Fu Pen Zi), Magnetitum (Ci Shi), and Os (Long Gu).

a. Although many of these herbs are traditionally used to treat discharges associated with the Dai channel. They can also hold and conserve Essence (Jing) and thus are used also to protect the Kidneys and help *stabilize* Essence.

Table 7-3: Herbs that Conduct Formulas to a Particular Channel

Channel	Herbs
Tai-Yang	*Urinary channel*: Notopterygii (Qiang Huo), Puerariae (Ge Gen), Ledebouriellae (Fang Feng). *Small Intestine channel*: Ligustici (Gao Ben), Akebiae (Mu Tong), Phellodendri (Huang Bai).
Yang-Ming	*Large Intestine channel*: Cimicifugae (Cheng Ma), Angelica (Bai Zhi), Gypsum (Shi Gao), Rhei (Da Huang). *Stomach channel*: Puerariae (Ge Gen), Angelica (Bai Zhi), Gypsum (Shi Gao).
Shao-Yang	*Gall Bladder channel*: Bupleuri (Chi Hu), Citri (Qing Pi). *Triple Warmer channel*: Viticis (Man Jing Zi), Gardeniae (Zhi Zi), Cinnamomi (Gui Zhi), Lycii (Di Gu Pi), Citri (Qing Pi), Aconiti (Fu Zi).
Tai-Yin	*Lung channel*: Platycodi (Jie Geng), Atractylodes (Cang Zhu), Cimicifugae (Sheng Ma), Angelica (Bai Zhi). *Spleen channel*: Atractylodes (Bai Zhu), Angelica (Bai Zhi), Atractylodes (Cang Zhu), Cimicifugae (Sheng Ma), Paeoniae (Bai Shao).
Shao-Yin	*Heart channel*: Asari (Xi Xin), Coptidis (Huang Llian). *Kidney channel*: Angelicae (Du Huo), Asari (Xi Xin), Cinnamomi (Rou Gui), Anemarrhenae (Zhi Mu).
Jue-Yin	*Pericadium channel*: Bupleuri (Chi Hu), Mountan (Mu Dan Pi). *Liver channel*: Ligusticum (Chuan Xiong), Citri (Qing Pi), Bupleuri (Chi Hu), Evodiae (Wu Zhu Yu).

Table 7-4: Basic Herbs and Points by Pathology

Type of Pain	Herbs	Acupoints
Cold	Ephedra (Ma Huang), Cinnamon (Gui Zhi), Radix Angelicae (Bai Zhi), Asari (Xi Xin) Ginger (Sheng Jiang), Aconiti (Fu Zi).	Moxa-GV-14, GV-4, CV-4.
Heat	Puerariae (Ge Gen), Gardeniae (Zhi Zi), Fel Bovus (Niu Dan), Moutan (Dan Pi), Caulis Lycii (Di Gu Teng).	LI-11, Sp-10, Liv-2, GV-14.
Wind	Ledebouriellae (Fang Feng), Notopterygium (Qiang Huo), Piperis (Hai Feng Teng), Lycii (Gou Qi Gan), Uncariae Cum Uncis (Gou Teng), Gastrodia (Tian Ma), Lumbricus (Di Long), Buthus Martensi (Quan Xie), Scolopendra (Wu Gong).	GB-20, GB-21, GB-31, UB-12.
Qi-stagnation	Cyprus (Xiang Fu), Saussurea (Mu Xiang), Lindera (Wu Yao), Corydalis (Yan Hu Suo), Curcuma (Yu Jin), Bupleurum (Chai Hu), Rosa (Mei Gui Hua).	Liv-3, Liv-14, UB-18, CV-17, Cv-6.
Blood-stasis	Corydalis (Yan Hu Suo), Red Paeoniae (Chi Shao), Salvia (Dan Shen), Safflower (Hong Hua), Ligusticum (Chuan Xiong), Turmeric (Jiang Huang), Achyranthes (Niu Xi), Millettia (Ji Xue Teng).	UB-17, Sp-10, LI-4, LI-11, Liv-3, Liv-4, St-36.
Damp	Poria (Fu Ling), Coicis (Yi Yi Ren), Alismatis (Ze Xie), Atractylodes (Cang Zhu), Stephaniae (Fang Ji).	St-40, Sp-9, CV-9, UB-20, UB-21.
Wind-Damp-Heat	Gentianae (Qin Jiao), Erythrinae (Hai Tong Pi), Mori (Sang Zhi).	Combination of above points.
Wind-Damp-Cold	Angelica pubescens (Du Huo), Clemetisis (Wei Ling Xian), Erythrinae (Hai Tong Pi), Chaenomelis (Mu Gua), Acanthopanacis (Wu Jia Pi), Caulis Piperis (Hai Feng Teng).	Combination of above points.
Deficiency	**Qi**—Condonopsis, (Dang Shen), Astragalus (Huang Qi), Atractylodes (Bai Zhu), Poria (Fu Ling). **Blood**—Angelica (Dang Gui), Prepared Rehmannia (Shu Di), Paeoniae (Bai Shao), Ligusticum (Chuan Xiong), Lyceum (Gou Qi Zi), Mulberry (Sang Shen).	CV-6, CV-4, St-36, LI-11, LI-4, Sp-6. Lu-7, UB-17, UB-18, Sp-10.

Table 7-5: Basic Herbs and Points by Region

LOCATION	HERBS	ACUPOINTS
HEAD/ FACE	**General**—Ligusticum (Chuan Xiong).	Beside Three Miles.
	Supraorbital, Forehead—Angelica (Bai Zhi), Gypsum (Shi Gao) or Cimicifuga (Sheng Ma).	GV-23, UB-2, LI-4, St-36 1/2 (deep insertion), St-44.
	Orbital/Temporal, Zygomatic—Vitalizes (Man Jing Zi), Ligustici (Gao Ben).	TW-5, GB-41.
	Temporal or Bilateral— Bupleurum (Chai Hu), Scutellaria (Huang Qin), Cassia (Cao Jue Ming).	GB-20, Taiyang (M-HN-9), GB-38, GB-43, UB-62, TW-3.
	Vertex— Ligustici (Gao Ben), Asari (Xi Xin), Ledebouriellae (Fang Feng), Evodia (Wu Zhu Yu).	GV-20, GB-20, UB-7, Liv-3, 2, K-1.
	Occipital—Notopterygium (Qiang Huo), Puerariae (Ge Gen), Ephedra (Ma Huang).	GB-20, GV-20, 19, UB-10, TW-5, GB-41, UB-60, 65, SI-3.
	Left-sided—Schizonepetae (Jing Jie), Menthae (Bo He).	Right side, TW-5, GB-41, 38.
	Right-sided—Atracylodis (Cang Zhu), Pinelliae (Ban Xia).	Left side, St-40, 37 (deep).
	Radiating to gums or facial spasms — Cicadae (Chun Tui), Gypsium (Shi Gao).	LI-4, St-4, 44, TW-2, GV-27.
	Sinus/Eye— Magnolia (San Yi Hua), Asari (Xi Xin), Centipedae (E Bu Shi Cao), Angelicae (Bai Zhi).	UB-5, 9, 2, GB-14 Sp-3,4, UB-59, 64, 65.
	Distending, boring, stabbing, or trauma— Salviae (Dan Shen), Persicae (Tao Ren), Carthami (Hong Hua).	GB-44, UB-17, 18, Sp-10, LI-11.
	Pounding pain—Achyranthis Bidentatae (Niu Xi), Haematitum (Dai Zhe Shi).	LI-5. GV-22, LI-4, St-8, TW-5, UB-62, K-1.
	Chronic Headaches/Migraine—Buthus Martensi (Quan Xie), Scolopendra (Wu Gong).	GB-20, Sishencong (M-HN-1), LI-4, Lu-7, SI-3, UB-62, 65, TW-5, GB-41.
	Dizziness, irritability, pain—Uncariae (Gou Teng).	UB-56, TW-1, GB-44.
	Severe lateral, facial pain, migraine—Rhizoma Typhonii Gigantei (Bai Fu Zi).	Beside Three Miles, bleed local triggers.
NECK	Puerariae (Ge Gen), Notopterygium (Qiang Huo).	GB-20, GB-21, UB-10, SI-15, GV-14, Hua tuo jia ji points Correct tendons, GB-39, UB-60, TW-5, SI-3.
SHOULDER	Turmeric (Jiang Huang).	LI-15, TW-14, SI-9 St-38, St-39, Beside Three Miles, Sp-9 1/2.
UPPER LIMBS	Turmeric (Jiang Huang), Mori (Sang Zhi), Notopterygium (Qiang Huo), Ledebouriellae (Fang Feng), Cinnamon (Gui Zhi), Clematis (Wei Ling Xian).	LI-15, LI-11, LI-4, TW-5, SI-6 GB-30, GB-34, GB-39, St-39, St-36.
LOWER LIMBS	Achyranthes (Niu Xi), Gentianae (Qing Jiao), Chaenomelis (Mu Gua), Angelicae (Du Hou), Stephaniae (Fang Ji), Bombyx Batryticatus (Jiang Can).	GB-30, GB-34, GB-39, St-36 LI-15, Shoulder Center Middle (44.06), SI-6, UB-43 (bleed).
LOWER BACK	Ciboti (Gou Ji), Eucommia (Du Zhong), Dipsacus (Chuan Duan), Loranthus (Sang Ji Sheng).	UB-23, UB-52, UB-25, GV-4 Huatuojiaji points, Tender points GV-26, UB-7, GV-20, State H20.
FOOT/ HEEL	Eucommia (Du Zhong), Dipsacus (Chuan Duan), Loranthus (Sang Ji Sheng), Deer Horn (Lu Rong), Arecae (Bing Lang).	K-3, K6, UB-60, Correct tendons, P-7, P-7-1/2, UB-43 (bleed).

Table 7-6: Commonly Used Prepared Medicines for Musculoskeletal Pain Syndromes

MEDICINE	USE	DISEASE APPLICATION
Feng Shi Xiao Tong Wan Wind-Wet Reduce Pain Pills	Wind-Damp (Bi syndrome).	Fibromyalgia, weakness, pain, rheumatism, myofascial pain syndromes, leg cramps.
Shi Wei Cuo San Astragalus and Aconite Formula	Cold-Wind-Damp.	Weakness and stiffness; severe cold-sensitive arthralgia.
San Bi Tang Three-Painful Obstruction Decoction	Wind-Damp-Cold, deficient Qi and Blood.	Fibromyalgia, rheumatism, myofascial pain syndromes, leg cramps.
Fang Feng Tang Ledenouriella Decoction (Siler Combination)	Wind-Damp (Wind).	Arthritis with symptoms that vary considerably in intensity and site.
Shu Feng Liu Shi Yin Clematis and Chin-chiu Combination.	Wind-Damp (more Dampness), Blood-stasis.	Dampness accumulation; numbness.
Mu Gua Wan Chaenomeles Pill	Dampness, Blood-stasis.	Numbness and pain in the lower body.
Qing Huang San Schizonepeta and Ma-huang Formula	Dampness-Wind (Dampness).	Upper body and arms Dampness pain.
Xiao Juo Luo Dan Pill Minor Invigorate Collaterals Special Pill	Wind-Cold accumulation, Wind-Damp accumulation, Blood-stasis.	Joint pain and stiffness (especially lower body), pain, numbness, paresthesias.
Jiu Wei Qiang Huo Tong Nine Herb Tea with Notoptrygium	Wind-Cold-Damp.	Fibromyalgia, URI, acute lower back sprain, fever and chills without perspiring, headache or stiff neck, generalized aches/pains.
Yi Yi Ren Tang Coicis Decoction (Coix Combination)	Dampness (Wind-Damp).	Rheumatic disorder dominated by Dampness.
Shu Jing Hou Xue Tang Relax the Channels and Invigorate the Blood Decoction (Clematis and Stephania Combination)	Blood-stasis, Wind-Damp.	Lower limb arthralgia, lumbago and sciatica.
Da Qin Jiao Tang Major Gentiana Qinjiao Decoction (Major Chin-chiu Combination)	Wind-Damp with Blood-deficiency.	Joint pain with muscle contraction and stiffness.
Da Fang Feng Tang Major Ledebouriella Decoction (Major Siler Combination)	Wind-Damp, Blood and Qi stagnation, Cold-deficiency.	Pain and weakness in the legs due to downward flow of cold Fluid; knee swelling; atrophy.
Shu Jing Lian San Clematis and Carthamus Formula	Wind, Blood-stasis (deficiency).	Recalcitrant arthritis producing severe pain.
Juan Bi Tang Remove Painful Obstruction Decoction (Chiang-huo and Turmeric Combination)	Wind-Damp, Qi and Blood obstruction.	Early-stage painful obstruction (joint of soft tissue pain); mostly in the neck, shoulder, and upper back. Osteoarthritis, rheumatoid arthritis, gouty arthritis, bursitis, post viral myofascial pain.
Ping Wei San Calm the Stomach Powder	Dampness, distention fullness, loss of appetite, fatigue, digestive symptoms.	Post-viral myofascial pain, fibromyalgia, abdominal distention.
Lian Po Yin Coptis and Magnolia Bark Tea	Damp-Heat.	Post-viral myofascial pain, fibromyalgia, sudden turmoil (vomiting and diarrhea), abdominal distention.
Chu Shi Wei Ling Tang Eliminate Damp Calm Stomach with Poria Tea	Damp-Heat.	Post-viral myofascial pain, fibromyalgia, especially lower body, distention fullness, edema, loss of appetite, fatigue.
Dang Gui Nian Tong Tang Tang-kuei and Anemarrhena Combination	Dampness, Damp-Heat.	Dampness accumulation in the lower body, swelling and pain.
Jia Wei Er Miao San Augmented Two-Marvel Pill	Damp-Heat.	Rheumatoid arthritis, gouty arthritis, gonococcal arthritis, UTI, post-viral myofascial pain, scanty yellow urine, atrophy of lower extremities, painful area feels hot (worse in rainy or hot weather), fidgetiness, thirst with no desire to drink.

Table 7-6: Commonly Used Prepared Medicines for Musculoskeletal Pain Syndromes (Continued)

MEDICINE	USE	DISEASE APPLICATION
Gui Zhi Shao Yao Zhi Mu Tang Cinnamon twig, Peony, and Anemarrhena Decoction (Cinnamon and Anemarrhena Combination).	Recurrent Wind-Cold-Damp stagnated with transformation-Heat.	Swollen stiff joint(s), warm to the touch, worse at night.
Yunnan Bai Yao Yunnan White Medicine	Bleeding, pain, stasis.	Sprains, strains, trauma.
Shu Feng Hou Xue Tang Disperse Wind Invigorate Blood Decoction (Stephania and Carthamus Combination).	Blood-stasis, Wind-Damp.	Excess syndrome, red and swollen joints, muscle aches, radiating leg pains, numbness.
Fu Yuan Huo Xue Tang Revive Health By Invigorating the Blood Decoction (Tang Kuei and Persicae Tea)	Blood-stasis.	Acute injuries, costochondritis, chest and/or flank pain.
Tao Hong Si Wu Tong Four Substances Tea plus Tao Ren (Persicae) and Hong Hua (Carthamus)	Blood-deficiency with Blood-stasis.	Neurogenic headache, fibromyalgia, often used for women, lusterless complexion, generalized muscle tension and menstrual dysfunction.
Gu Zhe Cuo Shang San Broken Bones and Bruise Powder	Blood-stasis.	Fractures, lacerations, trauma, aids regeneration of bone and soft tissues, fixed stabbing pain.
Qi li San Seven Pinches Powder	Blood-stasis.	Trauma, sprains, strains, fixed stabbing pain.
Shen Tong Zhu Yu Tang Drive Out Blood Stasis from a Painful Body Decoction (Cnidium and Chiang-huo Combination)	Blood-stasis.	Fixed stabbing pain, trauma, sprains, strains.
Yan Hu Suo Zhi Tong Pian Tetrahydropalmatine 50 mg. (This product is a pharmaceutical formulation)	Strong analgesic, strong sedative.	Severe pain.
Huo Luo Xiao Ling Dan Fantastically Effective Pill to Invigorate the Collaterals	Blood-stasis, Wind-Damp.	Fixed local stabbing pain (especially if increases at night), pain in various locations.
Du Huo Ji Sang Wan Angelica Pubescens and Sangjisheng Decoction/Pill (Angelica Loranthus Pill)	Wind-Damp accumulation, deficiency of Liver, Kidney, Qi and Blood.	Chronic arthritis in elderly.
Jin Gui Shen Qi Wan Kidney Qi Pill	Kidney-Yang-deficiency.	Diabetes, hypothyroid, arthritis, asthma, adrenal insufficiency, ligamentous insufficiency, cold sensation in lower body, edema, asthma, often used in geriatrics, strengthens the sinews.
Yao Tong Pian Back Pain Tablets	Kidney deficiency.	Chronic low back pain with Kidney weakness, nocturia, weak knees, adrenal insufficiency, ligamentous insufficiency.
Jian Bu Hu Qian Wan Healthy Steps Tiger Stealthily Pills	Heat and Deficiency symptoms combined.	Wei syndrome (wasting syndrome), paralysis, sequelae of poliomyelitis, flaccid paralysis, muscular atrophy, congenital weakness.
Kang Gu Zeng Sheng Pian Against Bony Hyperplasia	Liver and Kidney Weakness, Cold-Phlegm.	Proliferated Bi syndrome, bony hyperplasia, spurs, chronic spinal joint pains.
Zuo Gui Yin Restore the Left (Kidney) decoction	Deficient Kidney-Yin.	Chronic weakness, chronic low back pain.
You Gui Wan Restore the Right (Kidney) Pill	Deficient Kidney-Yang.	Chronic weakness, chronic low back pain.

Table 7-7: Herb Combinations for Commonly Seen Musculoskeletal Disorders

RHEUMATIC DISEASE PAINFUL OBSTRUCTION (BI)	*Fundamental formula for pain due to Painful Obstruction (can be used for inflammatory Damp-Heat type as well):* Arisaematis (Nan Xing), Clematidis (Wei Ling Xian), Angelicae (Bai Zhi), Phellodendri (Huang Bai), Atractylodis (Cang Zhu), Ligustici (Chuan Xiong), Persicae (Tao Ren), Gentianae (Long Dan Cao), Massa (Shen Qu), Stephaniae (Fang Ji), Cinnamomi (Gui Zhi), Carthami (Hong Hua), Notopterygii (Qiang Huo). *Soft tissues and/or joints general pain, Pathogenic Factors, fundamental combination:* Cinnamomi (Gui Zhi), Angelicae (Du Huo), Notopterygii (Qiang Huo), Ledebouriellae (Fang Feng), Clematis (Wei Ling Xian), Carthami (Hong Hua), Aconiti (Fu Zhi), Anemarrhenae (Zi Mu), Coicis (Yi Ren), Pini (Song Jie). *Wind-Damp, chronic, difficult:* Speranskiae (Tou Gu Cao), Aconiti (Chuan Wu), Lycopodii (Shen Jin Cao). *Predominance of Wind, wandering, moving pain and swelling:* Cinnamomi (Gui Zhi), Angelicae (Du Huo), Notopterygii (Qiang Huo), Ledebouriellae (Fang Feng), Clematis (Wei Ling Xian), Spatholobi (Ji Xue Teng), Carthami (Hong Hua), Gastrodia (Tian Ma), Peoneae (Chi Shao), Vaccariae (Wang Bu Liu Xiang), Manitis (Chuan Shan Jia). *Wind-Damp and Blood-deficiency:* Cinnamomi (Gui Zhi), Angelicae (Du Huo), Notopterygii (Qiang Huo), Ledebouriellae (Fang Feng), Clematis (Wei Ling Xian), Carthami (Hong Hua), Aconiti (Fu Zhi), Anemarrhenae (Zhi Mu), Coicis (Yi Ren), Pini (Song Jie), Angelica (Dang Gui), Ligustici (Chuan Xiong). *Wind-Damp-Heat:* Cinnamomi (Gui Zhi), Ledebouriellae (Fang Feng), Clematis (Wei Ling Xian), Carthami (Hong Hua), Anemarrhenae (Zhi Mu), Coicis (Yi Ren), Pini (Song Jie), Salviae (Dan Shen), Moutan (Dan Pi), Gypsum (Shi Gao). *Wind-Damp-Cold, swelling:* Notopterygii (Qiang Huo), Ledebouriellae (Fang Feng), Clematis (Wei Ling Xian), Angelica (Dang Gui), Coicis (Yi Ren), Lycopodii (Shen Jin Cao), Spatholobi (Ji Hue Teng). *Wind-Damp-Cold, stiff and hypertonic:* Notopterygii (Qiang Huo), Ledebouriellae (Fang Feng), Clematis (Wei Ling Xian), Angelicae (Du Huo), Angelica (Dang Gui), Coicis (Yi Ren), Mori (Sang Zhi), Aconiti (Fu Zhi). ***Or:*** Notopterygii (Qiang Huo), Ledebouriellae (Fang Feng), Clematis (Wei Ling Xian), Angelicae (Du Huo), Angelica (Dang Gui), Coicis (Yi Ren), Mori (Sang Zhi), Ligustici (Chuan Xiong), Angelicae (Dang Gui), Myrrha (Mo Yao), Carthami (Hong Hua), Lumbricus (Di Long). *Wind-Damp-Cold, stiff and hypertonic, chronic and difficult:* Notopterygii (Qiang Huo), Clematis (Wei Ling Xian), Angelicae (Du Huo), Carthami (Hong Hua), Pini (Song Jie), Cinnamomi (Gui Zhi), Asari (Xi Xin), Lycopodii (Shen Jin Cao), Speranskiae (Tou Gu Cao), Chaenomelis (Mu Gua), Stephaniae (Fang Ji), Manitis (Chuan San Jia). *Wind-Damp, pain and weakness of legs:* Siegesbeckiae (Xi Xian Cao), Taxilli (Sheng Ji Sheng), Angelicae (Du Huo), Dipsaci (Xu Duan), Acanthopanacis (Wu Jia Pi), Achyranthis (Niu Xi), Clematidis (Wei Ling Xian), Coicis (Yi Ren), Stephaniae (Fang Ji). *Blood-stasis due to Wind-Damp-Cold, with numbness:* Codonopsis (Dang Shen), Astragali (Huang Qi), Ligustici (Chuan Xiong), Paeoniae (Bai Shao), Angelicae (Dang Gui), Rehmanniae (Sheng Di), Eucommiae (Du Zhong), Achyranthis (Niu Xi), Cinnamomi (Rou Gui), Asari (Xi Xin), Gentianae (Qin Jiao), Angelicae (Du Huo), Ledebouriellae (Fang Feng). *Transformation/congested/binding-Heat, flare-ups:* Trachelospermi (Luo Shi Teng), Ledebouriellae (Fang Feng), Mori (Sang Zhi), Peoneae (Chi Shao), Lonicerae (Ren Dong Teng), Ligustici (Chuan Xiong), Angelicae (Dang Gui), Myrrha (Mo Yao), Carthami (Hong Hua), Siegesbeckiae (Xi Xian Cao), Lycopodii (Shen Jin Cao). *Chronic, spasmatic contractions, weakness, Yin-deficiency:* Asparagi (Tiang Dong), Ophiopogonis (Mai Dong), Polygonati (Yu Zhu), Dendrobii (Shi Ju), Angelicae (Dang Gui), Gentianae (Qin Jiao), Chaenomelis (Mu Gua), Lycii (Gou Qi Zi), Mori (Shang Ren), Coicis (Yi Ren), Trachelospermi (Luo Shi Teng), Lycopodii (Shen Jin Cao), Achyranthis (Huai Niu Xi), Paeoniae (Bai Shao), Rehmanniae (Sheng Di), Glycyrrhizae (Gan Cao), Mori (Sang Zhi).

Table 7-7: Herb Combinations for Commonly Seen Musculoskeletal Disorders (Continued)

ARTHRITIS (ACTIVE/HOT)	*General, fundamental combination*: Cinnamomi (Gui Zhi), Gypsum (Shi Gao), Peoneae (Chi Shao), Anemarrhenae (Zhi Mu), Coicis (Yi Ren), Pini (Song Jie), Salviae (Dan Shen), Moutan (Dan Pi), Lonicerae (Ren Dong Teng). *Acute*: Lonicerae (Ren Dong Teng), Gypsum (Shi Gao), Clematidis (Wei Ling Xian), Gentianae (Qin Jiao), Angelicae (Du Huo), Notopterygii (Qiang Huo), Phellodendri (Huang Bai), Atractylodis (Cang Zhu), Stephaniae (Fang Ji), Chaenomelis (Mu Gua), Speranskiae (Tou Gu Cao), Paeoniae (Chi Shao), Carthami (Hong Hua). *Acute/subacute Wind-Heat*: Cinnamomi (Gui Zhi), Paeoniae (Chi Shao and Bai Shao), Anemarrhenae (Zi Mu), Gypsum (Shi Gao), Poria (Fu Ling), Ephedrae (Ma Huang), Astragali (Huang Qi), Pollen (Pu Huang), Spatholobi (Ji Xue Teng), Ligustici (Chuan Xiong), Erythrinae (Hai Tong Pi), Clematis (Wei Ling Xian). *Acute/subacute Blood-Heat, Lupus/RA*: Rehmanniae (Sheng Di), Scrophulariae (Xuan Shen), Paeoniae (Bai Shao), Gypsum (Shi Gao), Lonicerae (Jin Yin Hua), Arctii (Niu Bang Zi), Schizonepetae (Jing Jie), Ledebouriellae (Feng Fang), Imperatae (Bai Mao Gen), Anemarrhenae (Zhi Mu), Glycyrrhizae (Gan Cao), Angelicae (Dang Gui), Carthami (Hong Hua). *Subacute-active with Yin-deficiency, Lupus/RA*: Ophiopogonis (Mai Men Dong), Ligustri (Nu Zhen Zhi), Mountan (Mu Dan Pi), Anemarrhenae (Zhi Mu), Corni (Shan Zhu Yu), Tripterygium (Lei Gong Teng), Sargentodoxae (Hong Teng), Alismatis (Ze Xie), Glycyrrhizae (Gan Cao). *Acute or Subacute, Transformation/congested/binding-Heat, flare-up*: Salviae (Dan Shen), Lonicerae (Ren Dong Teng), Gentianae (Qin Jiao), Coicis (Yi Ren), Clematis (Wei Ling Xian), Phellodendri (Huang Bai), Peoneae (Chi Shao), Carthami (Hong Hua), Angelicae (Du Huo), Notopterygii (Qiang Huo), Mori (Sang Zhi), Bombycis (Can Sha). *Yin-deficiency, Network-vessels Obstruction, RA*: Siegesbeckiae (Xi Xian Cao), Sinomenii (Qing Feng Teng), Trachelospermi (Luo Shi Teng), Lonicerae (Ren Dong Teng), Milletiae (Ji Xue Teng), Sambucidis (Lu Ying), Mori (Sang Zhi), Paeoniae (Chi Shao), Angelicae (Dang Gui Wei), Chaenomelis (Mu Gua), Dipsaci (Xu Duan), Buthus (Quan Xie), Glycyrrhizae (Gan Cao). *Wind-Dampness, RA*: Siegesbeckiae (Xi Xian Cao), [very large dose100g], Angelicae (Dang Gui) [also large dose 30g]. *Chronic RA or OA with deformed joints, Wind and Blood-deficiency, a mild approach for sensitive patients*: Gentianae (Qin Jiao) Ledebouriellae (Fang Feng), Uncariae (Gou Teng), Paeoniae (Bai Shao), Cassiae (Cao Jue Ming), Ziziphi (Suan Zao Ren), Chrysanthemi (Ju Hua), Hordei (Mai Ya), Biotae (Bai Zi Ren), Clematidis (Wei Ling Xian), Glycyrrhizae (Gan Cao).
GOUT	*Acute general*: Atractylodis (Cang Zhu), Phellodendri (Huang Bai), Achyranthis (Huai Niu Xi), Akebiae (Mu Tong), Stephaniae (Han Fang Ji), Liquidambaris (Lu Lu Tong), Coicis (Yi Yi Ren), Lonicerae (Ren Dong Teng), Rehmanniae (Sheng Di), Smilacis (Tu Fu Ling), Fraxini (Qin Pi), Glycyrrhizae (Gan Cao). *Subacute, chronic, Kidney-deficiency*: Gypsum (Shi Gao), Oldenlandiae (Bai Hua She She Cao), Mori (Sang Zhi), Stephaniae (Fang Ji), Alismatis (Ze Xie), Plantaginis (Che Qian Zi), Rhei (Da Huang), Phellodendri (Huang Bai), Poriae (Fu Ling), Pyrolae (Lu Han Cao), Corni (Shan Zhu You), Dioscoreae (Shan Yao), Cuscutae (Tu Si Zi), Fraxini (Qin Pi), Glycyrrhizae (Gan Cao). *Chronic, multi-system, Wind-Damp-Heat*: Phellodendri (Huang Bai), Atractylodis (Cang Zhu), Arisaematis (Zhi Nan Xing), Clematidis (Wei Ling Xian), Cinnamomi Cassiae (Gui Zhi), Stephaniae (Fang Ji), Pruni (Tao Ren), Carthami (Hong Hua), Gentianae (Long Dan Cao), Ligustici (Chuan Xiong), Angelicae (Zhi Bai Zhi), Notopterygii (Qiang Huo), Massa (Shen Qu). *Chronic, multi-system, Blood-stasis*: Ephedrae (Ma Huang), Cinnamomi (Gui Zhi), Carthami (Hong Hua), Angelicae (Bai Zhi), Puerariae (Ge Gen), Aconiti (Chuan Wu), Antelopis (Ling Yang Jiao Fen), Astragali (Huang Qi), Ledebouriellae (Fang Feng), Stephaniae (Han Fang Ji), Notopterygii (Qiang Huo), Anemarrhenae (Zhi Mu), Gypsum (Shi Gao), Moutan (Mu Dan Pi), Paeoniae (Chi Shao), Rubiae (Qian Cao Gen), Eupolyphagia (Tu Bie Chong), Zaocys (Wu Shao She). *External use*: Persicae (Tao Ren), Armeniacae (Xing Ren), Methae (Bo He), Schizonepetae (Jing Jie), Gardeniae (Zhi Zi), Wine. **Or**: Rhei (Da Huang), Phellodendri (Huang Bai), Curcumae (Jiang Huang), Angelicae (Bai Zhi), Arisaematis (Tian Nan Xing), Citri (Chen Pi), Atractylosis (Cang Zhu), Magnoliae (Hou Po), Glycyrrhizae (Gan Cao), Trichosanthis (Tian Hua Fen), Wine.

Table 7-7: Herb Combinations for Commonly Seen Musculoskeletal Disorders (Continued)

PSORIATIC ARTHRITIS	*Damp-Heat subacute, chronic*: Peoneae (Chi Shao), Dictamni (Bai Xian Pi), Phellodendri (Huang Bai), Coicis (Yi Ren), Atractylodis (Cang Zhu), Stephaniae (Fang Ji), Chaenomelis (Mu Gua), Pini (Song Jie), Ledebouriellae (Fang Feng), Clematis (Wei Ling Xian).
	Or: Atractylodis (Cang Zhu), Phellodendri (Huang Bai), Gentianae (Qin Jiao), Dictamni (Bai Xian Pi), Sophorae (Ku Shen), Coicis (Yi Ren), Smilax (Tu Fu Ling), Notopterygii (Qiang Huo), Carthami (Hong Hua), Persicae (Tao Ren), Olibanum (Ru Xiang), Polyporus (Zhu Ling), Cyathulae (Chuan Niu Xi).
	Chronic, subacute, acute, Wind-Cold: Astragali (Huang Qi), Cinnamomi (Gui Zhi), Notopterygii (Qiang Huo), Angelica (Dang Gui), Carthami (Hong Hua), Persicae (Tao Ren), Gentianae (Qin Jiao), Olibanum (Ru Xiang), Glycyrrhizae (Zhi Gan Cao), Kochiae (Di Fu Zi), Zaocys (Wu Shao She).
	Chronic, subacute, acute, Wind-Heat: Lonicerae (Jin Yin Hua), Tripterygium (Lei Gong Teng), Rehmanniae (Sheng Di), Anemarrhenae (Zhi Mu), Glycyrrhizae (Gan Cao), Serpentis (She Tui), Dendrobii (Shi Hu), Gypsum (Shi Gao), Peoneae (Chi Shao), Salviae (Dan Shen), Moutan (Dan Pi), Kochiae (Di Fu Zi).
	Acute or chronic Heat-toxin: Lonicerae (Jin Yin Hua), Traxaci (Pu Gong Ying), Isatis (Ban Lan Gen), Rehmanniae (Sheng Di), Anemarrhenae (Zhi Mu), Glycyrrhizae (Gan Cao), Dendrobii (Shi Hu), Gypsum (Shi Gao), Peoneae (Chi Shao), Salviae (Dan Shen), Moutan (Dan Pi), Bubali (Shui Niu Jiao).
	Chronic, Liver and Kidney deficiency: Rehmanniae (Sheng and Shu Di), Angelicae (Dang Gui), Eucommia (Du Zhong), Corni (Shan Zhu Yu), Lycii (Gou Qi Zi), Gentianae (Qin Jiao), Notopterygii (Qiang Huo), Carthami (Hong Hua), Persicae (Tao Ren), Olibanum (Ru Xiang), Ligustici (Chuan Xiong).
ARTHROSIS DEGENERATIVE JOINT DISEASE	*General joint pain, fundamental combination*: Spatholobi (Ji Xue Teng), Trogopteri (Wu Ling Zhi), Cinnamomi (Gui Zhi), Mori (Sang Zhi), Clematidis (Wei Ling Xian), Angelica (Du Huo), Notopterygii (Qiang Huo), Angelica (Dang Gui), Carthami (Hong Hua), Manitis (Chuan Shan Jia), Aconiti (Fu Zhi), Lycopi (Ze Lan).
	Cold painful: Cinnamomi (Gui Zhi), Angelicae (Du Huo), Notopterygii (Qiang Huo), Ledebouriellae (Fang Feng),[a] Clematis (Wei Ling Xian), Angelica (Dang Gui), Aconiti (Fu Zhi).
	Chronic, severe, with joint deformity, Cold: Cinnamomi (Gui Zhi), Angelicae (Du Huo), Notopterygii (Qiang Huo), Ledebouriellae (Fang Feng), Clematis (Wei Ling Xian), Angelica (Dang Gui), Aconiti (Fu Zhi), Coicis (Yi Ren), Mori (Sang Zhi), Lycopodii (Shen Jin Cao), Psoraleae (Bu Gu Zhi), Dipsaci (Xu Duan), Manitis (Chuan San Jia), Carthami (Hong Hua), Chaenomelis (Mu Gua).
	Progressive with weakness (back, knee, feet): Taxilli (Sang Ji Sheng), Angelicae (Du Huo), Cinnamomi (Rou Gui), Morindae (Ba Ji Tian), Aconiti (Fu Zhi), Dipsaci (Xu Duan), Chaenomelis (Mu Gua), Angelicae (Dang Gui), Condonopsis (Dang Shen), Astragali (Huang Qi).
	Chronic-enduring, joint deformity: Epimedii (Yin Yang Huo), Curculiginis (Xian Mao), Lycii (Gou Qi Zi), Placenta (Zi He Che), Glycyrrhizae (Gan Cao).
	Spurs and nodules: Gleditsiae (Zao Jiao Ci), Sargassum (Hai Cao), Laminariae (Kun Bu), Eupolyphaga (Tu Bie Chong), Scorpio (Quan Xie).

Table 7-7: Herb Combinations for Commonly Seen Musculoskeletal Disorders (Continued)

AUTO IMMUNE	*Active Ankylosing Spondylitis*: Cibotii (Gou Ji), Cuscutae (Tu Si Zi), Dipsacii (Xu Duan), Drynariae (Gu Sui Bu), Rehmanniae (Shu Di), Paeoniae (Bai Shao and Chi Shao), Angelica (Dang Gui), Manitis (Chuan Shan Jia), Gleditsiae (Zao Jiao Ci), Olibanum (Ru Xiang), Myrrhae (Mo Yao), Agkistrodon (Bai Hua She), Sinapis (Bai Jie Zi), Hirudo (Shui Zhi), Scolopendra (Wu Gong), Cervi (Lu Jiao), Testudinis (Gui Ban Jiao). *Active RA, lupus, Heat in Blood/Nutritive*: Bubali (Shui Niu Jiao), Rehmanniae (Sheng Di), Moutan (Dan Pi), Paeoniae (Chi Shao), Anemarrhenae (Zhi Mu), Gypsum (Shi Gao), Scrophulariae (Xuan Shen), Gardeniae (Zhi Zi), Forsythiae (Lian Qiao), Lonicerae (Ren Dong Teng), Lophatheri (Zhu Ye), Rhapntici (Lou Lu). *Subacute RA, chronic, Qi and Yin deficiency*: Lycii (Di Gu Pi), Amydae (Bie Jia), Macrophyllae (Qin Jiao), Artemisiae (Qing Hao), Mume (Wu Mei), Scrophulariae (Xuan Shen), Dendrobii (Shi Hu), Angelicae (Dang Gui), Astragali (Huang Qi), Tripterygii (Lei Gong Teng). Zaocys (Wu Shao She). *Chronic RA, Liver and Kidney Yin-deficiency*: Reumanniae (Sheng and Shu Di), Mountan (Dan Pi), Corni (Shan Zhu Yu), Lycii (Gou Qi Zi), Ligustri (Nu Zhen Zi), Gentianae (Qin Jiao), Paeoniae (Bai and Chi Shao), Salviae (Dan Shen), Zaocys (Wu Shao She), Speranskiae (Tou Gu Cao), Phlellodendri (Huang Bai), Lonicerae (Ren Dong Teng). *Chronic RA, Yin and Yang deficiency*: Epimedii (Yin Yang Huo), Curculiginis (Xian Mao), Salvia (Dan Shen), Cistanchis (Rou Cang Rong), Reumanniae (Sheng Di), Anemarrhenae (Zhi Mu), Glycyrrhizae (Zhi Gan Cao), Coicis (Yi Ren), Dioscoreae (Shan Yao), Lycii (Gou Qi Zi). *Chronic RA, deficient, mild approach for sensitive patients*: Ziziphi (Suan Zao Ren), Poria (Fu Ling), Dolichoris (Bian Dou Hua), Perilla (Su Geng), Capillaris (Mian Yin Chen), Scutellariae (Huang Qin), Trichonsanthis (Tian Hua Fen), Glycyrrhizae (Zhi Gan Cao), Hordei (Mai Ya), Uncariae (Gao Teng), Anemarrhenae (Zhi Mu), Beninacasae (Dong Gua Ren), Cassia (Jue Ming Zi), Aurantii (Zhi Ke), Taxilli (Ji Sheng), Corydalis (Yan Hu Suo). *Mixed connective tissue disease, chronic, Kidney-deficiency with Blood-stasis*: Leonuri (Yi Mu Cao), Cinnamomi (Gui Zhi), Curenliginis (Xian Mao), Epimedii (Yin Yang Huo), Psoraleae (Bu Gu Zhi), Ligustici (Chuan Xiong), Cistanches (Rou Cang Rong), Phellodendri (Huang Bai), Tripterygium (Lei Gong Teng), Spatholobi (Ji Xue Teng), Glycyrrhizae (Gan Cao).

Table 7-7: Herb Combinations for Commonly Seen Musculoskeletal Disorders (Continued)

LIMB(S)	*Cold, painful and stiff, fundamental formula*: Cinnamomi (Gui Zhi), Carthami (Hong Hua), Peoneae (Chi Shao), Lycopodii (Shen Jin Cao). *Painful, stabbing, fixed limb(s) pain (Blood-stasis)*: Persicae (Tao Ren), Carthami (Hong Hua), Ligustici (Chuan Xiong), Angelicae (Dang Gui), Gentianae (Qin Jiao), Notopterygii (Qiang Huo), Myrrhae (Mo Yao), Trogopterorum (Wu Ling Zhi), Cyperi (Xiang Fu), Glycyrrhizae (Gan Cao). *Upper limb(s) pain, fundamental formula*: Cinnamomi (Gui Zhi), Notopterygii (Qiang Huo), Curcumae (Jiang Huang), Corydalis (Yan Hu Suo), Mori (Sang Zhi). *Upper limb(s) Wind-Damp, general ache or pain:* Notopterygii (Qiang Huo), Gentianae (Qin Jiao), Angelicae (Dang Gui Wei), Cinnamomi (Gui Zhi), Curcumae (Jiang Huang), Carthami (Hong Hua), Ledebouriellae (Fang Feng). *Lower limb(s) pain, fundamental formula*: Dipsacii (Xu Duan), Angelicae (Du Huo), Loranthi (Shang Ji Sheng), Corydalis (Yan Hu Suo), Achyranthes (Niu Xi). *Hypertonic and achy limb(s)*: Xanthii (Cang Er Zi), Notopterygii (Qiang Huo), Coicis (Yi Ren), Speranskiae (Tou Gu Cao). *Painful swelling lower limb(s), Damp-Heat*: (Fang Ji), Coicis (Yi Ren), Lumbricus (Di Long), Achyranthis (Niu Xi), Poria (Fu Ling), Arecae (Bing Lang); Or: Anemarrhenae (Zhi Mu), Gypsum (Shi Gao), Cinnamomi (Gui Zhi), Atractylodis (Cang Zhu), Phelodendri (Huang Bai), Stephaniae (Han Feng Ji), Mori (Sang Zhi), Achyranthis (Niu Xi), Glycyrrhizae (Gan Cao). *Painful swelling lower limb(s), Cold-Damp (more Damp)*: Coicis (Yi Ren), Atractylodis (Cang Zhu), Notopterygii (Qiang Huo), Angelicae (Du Huo), Ledebouriellae (Fang Feng), Aconiti (Chuan Wu), Ephedrae (Ma Huang), Cinnamomi (Gui Zhi), Angelicae (Dang Gui), Ligustici (Chuan Xiong), Zingiberis (Gan Jiang), Glycyrrhizae (Gan Cao). *Painful achy lower limb(s) Wind-Damp (more Wind)*: Ledebouriellae (Fang Feng), Ephedrae (Ma Huang), Angelicae (Dang Gui), Achyranthis (Niu Xi), Gentianae (Qin Jiao), Cinnamomi (Rou Gui), Poria (Fu Ling), Zingiberis (Sheng Jiang), Zizipus (Da Zao), Glycyrrhizae (Gan Cao). *Painful achy lower limb(s) Wind-Damp-Cold (more Cold):* Aconiti (Chuan Wu), Ephedrae (Ma Huang), Paeoniae (Bai Shao), Glycyrrhizae (Gan Cao), Astragali (Huang Qi). *Weak and limp lower limb(s)*: Angelicae (Du Huo), Achyranthes (Niu Xi), Atractylodes (Cang Zhu), Lumbricus (Di Long), Acanthopanacis (Wu Jia Pi), Dipsaci (Xu Duan). *Progressive weakness and atrophy (Wei syndrome)*: Eucommiae (Du Zhong), Drynariae (Gu Sui Bu), Dipsaci (Xu Duan), Cistanches (Rou Cang Rong), Lycii (Gou Qi Zi), Angelicae (Dang Gui), Trachelospermi (Luo Shi Teng), Cyathulae (Chuan Niu Xi), Carthami (Hong Hua) Eupolyphaga (Di Bie Chong). *Progressive weakness and atrophy from damaged Essence by Damp-Heat*: Rehmanniae (Shu Di), Dioscoreae (Shan Yao), Corni (Shan Zu Yu), Poria (Fu Ling), Eucommiae (Du Zhong), Schisandrae (Wu Wei Zi), Morindae (Ba Ji Tian), Foeniculi (Xiao Hui Xiang), Cistanches (Rou Cang Rong), Polygalae (Yuan Zhi), Acori (Shi Chang Pu), Lycii (Gou Qi Zi), Jujubae (Dao Zao).
LIMB(S) NUMBNESS	*General formula, Qi Blood deficiency and stagnation*: Angelica (Dang Gui), Astragali (Huang Qi), Ligustici (Chuan Xiong), Carthami (Hong Hua), Pinelliae (Ban Xia), Ledebouriellae (Fang Feng), Cinnamomi (Gui Zhi), Peoneae (Bai Shao), Rehmanniae (Shu Di Huang), Manitis (Chuan Shan Jia). *Phlegm-Wind in channels and collaterals, numbness*: Arisaematis (Tian Nan Xing), Inulae (Xuan Fu Hua), Lumbricus (Di Long). *Malnourishment of sinews*: Loranthi (Shang Ji Sheng), Mori (Sang Zhi). *Wind-Damp, aching*: Clematidis (Wei Ling Xian), Angelicae (Du Huo), Xanthii (Cang Er Zi), Epimedii (Yin Yang Huo), Aconiti (Fu Zi), Ligustici (Chuan Xiong), Dipsaci (Xu Duan). *Qi and Blood deficiency*: Angelica (Dang Gui), Astragali (Huang Qi).

Table 7-7: Herb Combinations for Commonly Seen Musculoskeletal Disorders (Continued)

ANKLE SPRAIN	*Acute stage*: Carthami (Hong Hua), Olibani (Ru Xiang), Resina Myrrhae (Mo Yao), Dragon's Blood (Xue Jie), Acacia (Er Cha), Ligusticum (Chuan Xiong), Angelica (Dang Gui), Persicae (Tao Ren), Rhubarb (Da Huang), Corydalis (Yan Hu Suo), Aurantii (Zhi Qiao). *Chronic stage*: Aconite (Zhi Chuan Wu), Carthami (Hong Hua), Olibani (Ru Xiang), Myrrhae (Mo Yao), Salviae (Dan Shen), Paeoniae (Bai Shao, Chi Shao), Angelica (Dang Gui), Lumbricus (Di Long), Angelicae (Du Huo), Notopterygium (Qiang Hou), Lycopodii (Shen Jin Cao), Cinnamomi (Rou Gui), Psoralea (Bu Gu Zhi), Chaenomelis (Mu Gua), Loranthus (Sang Ji Sheng), Gentianae (Qin Jiao), Glycyrrhizae (Gan Cao).
FEET	*Painful and cold, fundamental formula*: Ephedrae (Ma Huang), Rehmannia (Shu Di), Cinnamomi (Gui Zhi), Carthami (Hong Hua), Sinapis (Bai Jie Zi), Zingiberis (Pao Jiang), Mantis (Zhi Shan Jia). *Swollen numb*: Lumbricus (Di Long), Chaenomelis (Mu Gua), Stephaniae (Fang Ji), Evodiae (Wu Zhu Yu), Arecae (Bing Lang), Perillae (Zi Su Gen). *Chronic pain, deficiency of Liver, Kidney and Essence*: Reumanniae (Shu Di), Corni (Shan Zhu Yu), Dioscoreae (Shan Yao), Poria (Fu Ling), Alismatis (Xe Xie), Angelicae (Dang Gui), Ligustici (Chuan Xiong), Eucommiae (Du Zhong), Dipsaci (Xu Duan), Achyranthis (Niu Xi), Loranthi (Sang Ji Sheng), Eupolyphaga (Di Bie Chong), Glycyrrhizae (Gan Cao). *Heel pain (chronic planter fasciitis)*: Carthami (Hong Hua), Persicae (Tao Ren), Mantitis (Chuan Shan Jia), Gleditsiae (Zao Jiao Ci), Eucommiae (Du Zhong), Dipsaci (Xu Duan), Phellodendri (Huang Bai), Alismatis (Xe Xie), Rehmannia praeparata (Shu Di), Sebastan (Po Bu Zi Ye), Trichonsanthis (Tian Hua Fen), Cyathulae (Chuan Niu Xi), Gummi (Ru Xiang), Myrrha (Mo Yao). *Bunions, painful*: Astragali (Huang Qi), Angelicae (Bai Zhi) Codonopsis (Dang Shen), Angelica (Dang Gui), Salvia (Dan Shen), Achyranthes (Niu Xi), Paeoniae (Chi Shao, Bai Shao), Cinnamomi (Gui Zhi), Chaenomelis (Mu Gua), Ophiopogonis (Mai Dong), Loranthus (Shang Ji Sheng), Morindae (Ba Ji Tian), Lycii (Gao Qi Zi), Rehmannia praeparata (Shu Di), Mori (Sang Zhi), Glycyrrhizae (Gan Cao).
SHOULDER	*Cold pain*: Cinnamomi (Gui Zhi), Curcumae (Jiang Huang), Ledebouriellae (Fang Feng). *Arthrosis, "periarthritis," general formula*: Notopterygii (Qiang Huo), Gentianae (Qin Jiao), Angelicae (Dang Gui Wei), Clematidis (Wei Ling Xian), Mori (Sang Zhi), Cinnamomi (Gui Zhi), Tripterygii (Lei Gong Teng), Spatholobi (Ji Xue Teng), Curcumae (Jiang Huang). *Or*: Curcumae (Jiang Huang), Salviae (Dan Shen), Notopterygium (Qiang Hou), Clematidis (Wei Ling Xian), Angelica (Dang Gui), Peoneae (Chi Shao), Ledebouriellae (Fang Feng), Schizonepeta (Jing Jie), Cinnamomi (Gui Zhi), Zingiberis (Sheng Jiang), Astragali (Huang Qi), Glycyrrhizae (Gan Cao), Scolopendra (Wu Gong), Lumbricus (Di Long). *Active inflammation*: Angelica (Dang Gui), Mori (Sang Zhi), Impatiens (Tou Gu Cao), Notopterygium (Qiang Hou), Rehmanniae (Sheng Di Huang), Cyperi (Xiang Fu), Olibani (Ru Xiang), Myrrhae (Mo Yao), Gentianae (Qin Jiao), Scolopendra (Wu Gong), Rhei (Da Huang), Tripterygium (Lei Gong Teng). *Acute traumatic arthritis (capsular pattern, night pain, possibly numbness), Cold, Deficient*: Astragali (Huang Qi), Cinnamomi (Gui Zhi), Paeoniae (Bai Shao), Zingiberis (Sheng Jiang), Red Date (Hong Zao), Curcumae (Jiang Huang), Notopterygii (Qiang Huo), Aconiti (Fu Zi), Coicis (Yi Ren), Bombycis (Can Sha). *Bursitis (can be used for elbow)*: Notopterygium (Qiang Hou), Asari (Xi Xin), Curcumae (Jiang Huang), Salviae (Dan Shen), Ligusticum (Chuan Xiong), Glycyrrhizae (Gan Cao), Ledebouriellae (Fang Feng), Atractylodes (Cang Zhu), Atractylodes (Bai Zhu), Poria Cocus (Fu Ling), Radix Stephaniae Tetrandrae (Fang Ji), Alismatis (Ze Xie), Coicis (Yi Yi Ren), Tripterygium (Lei Gong Teng), Moschus (She Xiang).

Table 7-7: Herb Combinations for Commonly Seen Musculoskeletal Disorders (Continued)

ELBOW	*Epicondylitis (tennis or golfer elbow), chronic*: Rehmanniae (Shu Di), Angelicae (Dang Gui), Ligustici (Chuan Xiong), Curcumae (Jiang Huang), Cinnamomi (Gui Zhi), Angelica (Bai Zhi), Paeoniae (Chi and Bai Shao), Persicae (Tao Ren), Carthami (Hong Hua), Gentianae (Qin Jiu), Gleditsiae (Zao Jiao Ci).
	Epicondylitis (tennis or golfer elbow), acute: Millettia (Ji Xue Teng), Salviae (Dan Shen), Moriae (Sang Zhi), Carthami (Hong Hua), Ligustici (Chuan Xiong), Gentianae (Qin Jiu), Clematidis (Wei Ling Xian), Angelica (Bai Zhi), Notopterygii (Qiang Huo), Paeoniae (Chi and Bai Shao), Manitis (Chuan Shan Jia), Gleditsiae (Zao Jiao Ci).
	Epicondylitis (tennis or golfer elbow), chronic or acute, tendinosis: Mori (Sang Zhi), Spatholobi (Ji Xue Teng), Clematidis (Wei Ling Xian), Angelicae (Dang Gui), Notopterygii (Qiang Huo), Cinnamomi (Gui Zhi), Paeoniae (Bai Shao), Curcumae (Jiang Huang), Ledebouriellae (Fang Feng), Asari (Xi Xin).
	Arthrosis, general formula: Notopterygii (Qiang Huo), Ligustici (Chuan Xiong), Gentianae (Qin Jiao), Angelicae (Dang Gui Wei), Clematidis (Wei Ling Xian), Mori (Sang Zhi), Cinnamomi (Gui Zhi), Lycopodii (Shen Jin Cao), Curcumae (Jiang Huang). Reumanniae (Shu Di), Dipsaci (Xu Duan), Loranthi (Sang Ji Sheng), Eupolyphaga (Di Bie Chong), Astragalus (Huang Qi), Glycyrrhizae (Gan Cao).
	Active inflammation: Angelica (Dang Gui), Mori (Sang Zhi), Notopterygium (Qiang Hou), Rehmanniae (Sheng Di Huang), Cyperi (Xiang Fu), Olibani (Ru Xiang), Myrrha (Mo Yao), Gentianae (Qin Jiao), Scolopendra (Wu Gong), Rhei (Da Huang), Tripterygium (Lei Gong Teng), Curcumae (Jiang Huang).
HAND AND FINGERS	*Arthrosis, Cold-Damp*: Astragalus (Huang Qi), Cinnamomi (Gui Zhi), Paeoniae (Qi Shao), Peoneae (Bai Shao), Ginger (Gan Jiang), Lumbricus (Di Long), Tumeric (Jiang Huang), Millettiae (Ji Xue Teng), Carthami (Hong Hua), Aconiti (Fu Zi), Glycyrrhizae (Gan Cao).
	Inflammatory arthritis: Loncerae (Jin Yin Hua), Chrysanthemum (Ye Ju Hua), Phellodendri (Huang Bai), Angelica (Dang Gui), Salviae (Dun Shen), Olibani (Ru Xiang), Myrrhae (Mo Yao), Scutellariae (Huang Qin), Rehmanniae (Sheng Di), Glycyrrhizae (Gan Cao), Tripterygium (Lei Gong Teng).
LOW BACK PAIN	*Damp-Cold*: Angelicae (Du Huo), Loranthi (Sang Ji Sheng), Cinnamomi (Gui Zhi), Atractylodes (Cang Zhu), Zingiberis (Gan Jiang), Cyathulae (Chuan Niu Xi).
	Damp-Heat: Phellodendri (Huang Bai), Atractylodis (Cang Zhu), Achyranthis (Niu Xi), Coicis (Yi Ren), Stephaniae (Feng Ji), Bombycis (Can Sha), Dioscoreae (Bei Xie).
	Blood-stasis: Angelicae (Dang Gui), Achyranthis (Niu Xi), Eupolyphaga (Tu Bie Chong), Carthami (Hong Hua), Persicae (Tao Ren), Manitis (Chuan Shan Jia), Myrrhae (Mo Yao).
	Kidney-Yang-deficiency: Rehmanniae (Shu Di), Cibotii (Gou Ji), Lycii (Gou Qi Zi), Dipsaci (Xu Duan), Eucommiae (Du Zhong), Psoraleae (Bu Gu Zhi), Juglandis (Hu Tao Ren), Cervi (Lu Jiao Pian).
	Kidney-Yin-deficiency: Rehmanniae (Shu Di), Plastrum (Gui Ban), Ligustri (Nu Zhen Zi), Cibotii (Gou Ji), Lycii (Gou Qi Zi), Dipsaci (Xu Duan), Eucommiae (Du Zhong), Juglandis (Hu Tao Ren).
LOW BACK AND KNEES PAIN	*Of any type*: Eucommiae (Du Zhong), Dispaci (Xu Duan).
	With Damp-Cold add: Cinnamomi (Gui Zhi), Angelicae (Du Huo), Notopterygii (Qiang Huo).
	With Damp-Heat add: Phellodendri (Huang Bai), Atractylodes (Cang Zhu), Achyranthis (Niu Xi), Coicis (Yi Ren).
	With Static-Blood add: Achyranthis (Niu Xi), Lycopi (Ze Lan).
LOW BACK ACUTE SPRAIN/STRAIN	General: Sinapis (Bai Jie Zi)
	Qi-stagnation: Aristolochiae (Qing Mu Xiang), Cypri (Xiang Fu), Lycopi (Ze Lan), Corydalis (Yan Hu Suo), Olibani (Ru Xiang), Myrrhae (Mo Yao), Loranthi (Sang Ji Sheng), Carthami (Hong Hua), Glycyrrhizae (Gan Cao).
	Blood-stasis: Angelica (Dang Gui), Lycopi (Ze Lan), Cyathulae (Chuan Niu Xi), Trachelospermi (Luo Shi Teng), Carthami (Xu Duan), Ciboti (Gou Ji), Salviae (Dan Shen).
	Muscle strain from twisting or contusion: Foeniculi (Hui Xiang), Sinapis (Bai Jie Zi), Ligustici (Chuan Xiong), Cinnamomi (Gui Zhi), Amomi (Sha Ren), Citri (Zhi Ke), Lycopi (Ze Lan), Myrrhae (Mo Yao).

Table 7-7: Herb Combinations for Commonly Seen Musculoskeletal Disorders (Continued)

HERNIATED LUMBAR DISC	*General formula (also for cervical)*: Radix Angelicae (Dang Gui), Lycopi (Ze Lan), Cyathulae (Chuan Niu Xi), Angelicae (Du Huo), Chaenomelis (Mu Gua), Acanthopanacis (Wu Jia Pi), Loranthi (Sang Ji Sheng), Tripterygii (Lei Gong Teng), Carthami (Hong Hua), Lignum (Jiang Xiang), Poriae (Fu Ling). *General herbs*: Arctii (Niu Bang Zhi), Eucommiae (Du Zhong), Dipsaci (Xu Duan), Achyranthis (Niu Xi). *Weak spine, Kidney-Essence deficiency, Blood-stasis*: Arctii (Niu Bang Zhi), Bombyx (Bai Jiang Can), Angelicae (Du Huo), Notopterygii (Qiang Huo), Eucommiae (Du Zhong), Dipsaci (Xu Duan), Cibotii (Gou Ji), Persicae (Tao Ren), Carthami (Hong Hua), Lumbricus (Di Long), Rehmannia (Shu Di), Drynariae (Gu Sui Bu), Angelicae (Dang Gui). *General formula, Pathogenic Factors, Cold*: Lumbricus (Di Long), Ephedrae (Zhi Ma Huang), Cinnamomi (Rou Gui), Asari (Xi Xin), Angelicae (Dang Gui), Carthami (Hong Hua), Phellodendri (Huang Bai), Morindae (Ba Ji Tian), Sappan (Su Mu), Glycyrrhizae (Gan Cao), Cervu (Lu Jiao), Persicae (Tao Ren). *General formula, Pathogenic Factors (also for cervical), swelling*: Arctii (Niu Bang Zhi), Sinapis (Bai Jie Zi), Lumbricus (Di Long), Lycopi (Ze Lan), Achyranthis (Niu Xi), Clematidis (Wei Ling Xian), Arisaematis (Dan Nan Xing), Glycyrrhizae (Gan Cao), Salviae (Dan Shen), Angelicae (Dang Gui).
SEQUELAE TO S4 DISC LESION (CAUDA EQUINA SYNDROME);[B]	*Weakness of limbs, loss of control of urine or bowl*: Eucommiae (Du Zhong), Dipsaci (Xu Duan), Rehmanniae (Shu Di Huang), Epimedii (Yin Yang Huo), Cistanches (Rou Cang Rong), Mantidis (Sang Piao Xiao), Achyranthis (Niu Xi), Dioscorea (Shan Yao), Corni (Shan Zhu Yu), Aconiti (Fu Zhi).
KNEES	*Pain, Cold-Damp, nodular, Craine's knee*: Rehmanniae (Shu Di), Ephedrae (Ma Huang), Cervi (Lu Jiao), Cinnamomi (Rou Gui), Zingiberis (Pao Jiang), Sinapis (Bai Jie Zi), Glycyrrhizae (Gan Cao). *Pain, inflammation, nodular, Craine's knee, Deficiency and Excess*: Rehmannia (Shu Di), Achyranthes (Niu Xi), Angelica (Dang Gui), Angelica (Du Hou), Tripterygium (Lei Gong Teng), Corni (Shan Zhu Yu), Lycii (Gou Qi Zi), Poria (Fu ling), Eucommiae (Du Zhong), Ligustricum (Chuan Xiong), Psoraleae (Bu Gu Zhi), Loranthus (Sang Ji Sheng), Glycyrrhizae (Gan Cao). *Pain, inflammation, nodular, Craine's knee, Hot and Cold, flare-up*: Lonicera (Ren Dong Teng), Atractylodes (Cang Zhu), Coix (Yi Ren), Phellodendron (Huang Bai), Zingiberis (Sheng Jiang), Cinnamomi (Gui Zhi), Anemarrhenae (Zhi Mu), Atractylodes (Bai Zhu), Ledebouriellae (Fang Feng), Paeoniae (Bai Shao), Ephedrae (Ma Huang), Glycyrrhizae (Gan Cao), Aconite (Fu Zhi). *Pain, Cold-Damp*: Pini (Song Jie), Chaenomelis (Mu Gua), Erythrinae (Hai Tong Pi). *Arthritis active, inflammation, flare-up*: Phellodendri (Huang Bai), Atractylodes (Cang Zhu), Tripterygium Wilfordii (Lei Gong Teng), Angelica (Dang Gui), Stephaniae (Fang Ji), Achyranthes (Niu Xi), Dioscorea (Bei Xie), Loncerae (Ren Dong Teng), Scutellariae (Huang Qin), Mountan (Dan Pi), Paeoniae (Chi Shao), Rehmanniae (Sheng Di), Clematis (Wei Ling Xian). *Sprained meniscus*: Bletillae (Bai Ji), Paeoniae (Bai Shao), Melo (Hu Gua Zi), Albizziae (He Huan Pi), Homalomenae (Qian Nian Jian), Eupolyphagae (Tu Bie Chong), Dioscoreae (Bi Xie), Angelicae (Bai Zhi), Dipsaci (Xu Duan), Polygalae (Yuan Zhi), Glycyrrhizae (Gan Cao), Egg White.

Table 7-7: Herb Combinations for Commonly Seen Musculoskeletal Disorders (Continued)

NECK AND HEAD	*Pain, acute sprain*: Cinnamomi (Gui Zhi), Isatidis (Ban Lan Gen), Paeoniae (Chi Shao), Puerariae (Ge Gen), Ledebouriellae (Fang Feng), Notopterygii (Qiang Huo), Glycyrrhizae (Gan Cao). *Subacute pain with pre-existing disease*: Notopterygii (Qiang Huo), Chaenomelis (Mu Gua), Lycopodii (Sang Ji Sheng), Drynariae (Gu Sui Bu), Angelica (Dang Gui), Loranthi (Sang Ji Sheng), Acanthopanacis (Wu Jia Pi), Citri (Chen Pi). *Chronic arthropathy (DDD, DJD), general formula*: Puerariae (Ge Gen), Cinnamomi (Gui Zhi), Ledebouriellae (Fang Feng), Paeoniae (Bai Shao), Angelicae (Du Huo), Gentianae (Qin Jiao), Uncariae (Gou Teng), Gastrodia (Tian Ma), Carthami (Hong Hua), Trachelospermi (Luo Shi Teng). *Arthropathy with numbness, Blood-deficiency and stasis*: Puerariae (Ge Gen), Codonopsis (Dang Shen), Astragali (Huang Qi), Angelicae (Dang Gui), Cinnamomi (Gui Zhi), Ligustici (Chuan Xiong), Cimicifugae (Sheng Ma), Carthami (Hong Hua), Salviae (Dan Shen), Paeoniae (Chi Shao), Spatholobi (Ji Xue Teng), Curcumae (Jiang Huang). *Dizziness or vertigo from vertebral artery and/or arthrosis*: Gastrodia (Tian Ma), Bupleuri (Chi Hu), Cyperi (Xiang Fu), Ligustici (Chuan Xiong), Salviae (Dan Shen), Haliotidis (Shi Jue Ming), Scolopendra (Wu Gong), Uncariae (Gao Teng), Lycii (Gou Qi Zi), Schisandrae (Wu Wei Zi), Citri (Fo Shou Gen), Lignum (Jiang Xiang). *Tension headache, general*: Bupleuri (Chai Hu), Gardeniae (Zhi Zi), Corni (Shan Zhu Yu), Dioscoreae (Shan Yao), Angelicae (Dang Gui), Ligustici (Chuan Xiong), Paeoniae (Bai Shao), Rehmanniae (Sheng Di, Shu Di), Menthae (Bo He) Glycyrrhizae (Gan Cao), Moutan (Dan Pi), Poriae (Fu Ling), Alismatis (Ze Xie). *Chronic headache of any kind with/without neck pain*: Ligustici (Chuan Xiong), Puerariae (Ge Gen), Angelica Dahuricae (Bai Chi), Cyperi (Xiang Fu), Glycyrrhizae (Gan Cao), Cinnamomi (Gui Zhi), Uncariae (Gao Teng), Schizonepeta (Jing Jie), Gypsum (Shi Gao), Lumbricus (Di Long), Bombyx (Bai Jiang Can), Scorpio (Quan Xie), Carthami (Hong Hua), Persicae (Tao Ren), Paeoniae (Bai Shao), Trichosanthis (Tian Hua Fen). *Post traumatic (whiplash) pain and confusion*: Bupleurum (Chi Hu), Auranthii (Zhi Shi), Paeoniae (Bai Shao), Glycyrrhizae (Gan Cao), Salviae (Dan Shen), Trogopterori (Wu Ling Zhi).
CHEST AND RIB CAGE	*Trauma, sprain, Blood-stasis*: Angelica (Dang Gui), Paeoniae (Chi Shao), Luffae (Si Gua Luo), Salviae (Dan Shen), Curcumae (Yu Jin), Corydalis (Yan Hu Suo), Citri (Qing Pi), Aurantii (Zhi Ke), Olibani (Ru Xiang), Myrrhae (Mo Yao). *Trauma, sprain, Qi-stagnation*: Cyperi (Xiang Fu), Corydalis (Yan Hu Suo), Aristolochia (Qing Mu Xiang), Ligustici (Chuan Xiong), Aurantii (Zhi Ke), Linderae (Wu Yao), Curcumae (Yu Jin), Glycyrrhizae (Gan Cao). *Trauma, sprain, Qi and Blood stagnation*: Aconiti (Cao Wu), Angelicae (Dang Shen), Salviae (Dan Shen), Sparganii (San Leng), Citri (Xiang Yuan Pi), Citri (Fo Shou Gen), Lignum (Jiang Xiang). *Ribs, chest or trunk pain, Qi and Blood stagnation*: Aurantii (Zhi Ke), Curcumae (Jiang Huang), Platycodi (Jie Geng), Toosendan (Chuan Lian Zi), Cyperi (Xiang Fu), Corydalis (Yan Hu Suo), Cinnamomi (Gui Pi, and Gui Zhi), Luffae (Si Gua Luo). *Fracture, injury early stage*: Bupleuri (Chai Hu), Meliae (Chuan Lian Zi), Lumbricus (Di Long), Angelicae (Dang Gui), Rhei (Da Huang), Carthami (Hong Hua), Persicae (Tao Ren), Trichosanthis (Tian Hua Fen), Gentianae (Qin Jiao), Astragali (Huang Qi), Pseudoginseng (San Qi powdered), 3g, Asari (Xi Xin), Glycyrrhizae (Gan Cao). *Fracture, injury late stage*: Dipsaci (Xu Duan), Drynariae (Gu Sui Bu), Pyritum (Zi Ran Tong), Paeoniae (Chi Shao), Curcumae (Jiang Huang).
PAIN	*Fixed, Blood-stasis*: Ligustici (Chuan Xiang), Carthami (Hong Hua), Persicae (Tao Ren), Trogopteri (Wu Ling Zhi), Olibanum (Ru Xiang), Myrrha (Mo Yao). *Musculoskeletal of any type*: Ligustici (Chuan Xiang), Pseudoginseng (San Qi), Myrrhae (Mo Yao), Olibani (Ru Xiang), Corydalis (Yan Hu Suo), Typhae (Pu Huang), Trogopterori (Wu Ling Zhi), Moschus (She Xiang). *Intractable with difficulty walking*: Aconiti (Cao Wu Tou), Loranthi (Sang Ji Sheng), Angelicae (Du Huo), Dipsaci (Xu Duan), Eucommiae (Du Zhong), Achyranthis (Niu Xi), Olibanum (Ru Xiang), Myrrha (Mo Yao), Aconiti (Fu Zhi), Clematidis (Wei Ling Xian), Drynari (Gu Sui Bu), Lycopodii (Shen Jin Cao), Homalomenae (Qian Nian Jian).

Table 7-7: Herb Combinations for Commonly Seen Musculoskeletal Disorders (Continued)

Muscles	*Spasm, cramps, or tension*: Peoneae (Bai Shao), Glycyrrhizae (Gan Cao), Chaenomelis (Mu Gua), Erythrinae (Hai Tong Pi). *Whole body myalgia*: Erythrinae (Hai Tong Pi), Gentianae (Qin Jiao). *Weakness*: Astragali (Huang Qi).
Sinews/Muscles	*Rupture, strain/sprain*: Angelicae (Dang Gui), Carthami (Hong Hua), Sappan (Su Mu), Persicae (Tao Ten), Pyritum (Zi Ran Tong), Dynariae (Gu Sui Bu), Dipsaci (Xu Duan), Piperis (Hai Feng Teng) Eupolyphaga (Tu Bie Chong), Pseudoginseng (San Qi), Olibanum (Ru Xiang), Myrrha (Mo Yao). *Hypertonicity*: Chaenomelis (Mu Gua), Paeoniae (Bai Shao), Lycopodii (Shen Jin Cao), Manitis (Chuan San Jia), Gentianae (Qin Jiao). *Tendon muscle spasm (hypertonicity/"hardness") and pain*: Angelica (Dang Gui), Scrophulariae (Xuan Shen), Rehmanniae (Sheng Di), Coicis (Yi Ren), Bupleuri (Chi Hu).
Weakness Atrophy of Muscles, Sinews and Bones Deficiency of Liver and Kidneys	*Fundamental formula*: Ginseng (Ren Shen), Astragali (Huang Qi), Angelicae (Dang Gui), Achyranthis (Niu Xi), Cistanchis (Rou Cang Rong), Rehmanniae (Shu Di), Ligustici (Chuan Xiong), Eucommiae (Du Zhong), Chaenomelis (Mu Gua), Os (Hu Gu), Poriae (Fu Ling), Phlellodendri (Huang Bai), Ophiopogonis (Mai Dong), Schisandrae (Wu Wei Zi). *General formula*: Plastrum (Gui Ban), Dendrobii (Shi Hu), Achyranthis (Niu Xi), Dioscorea (Shan Yao), Corni (Shan Zhu Yu), Psoraleae (Bu Gu Zhi), Juglandis (Hu Tao Rou), Eucommiae (Du Zhong), Dipsaci (Xu Duan), Rehmannia (Shu Di Huang). *If also numbness*: Achyranthis (Niu Xi), Dendrobii (Shi Hu), Phellodendri (Huang Bai), Dioscorea (Shan Yao), Eucommiae (Du Zhong), Dipsaci (Xu Duan), Rehmannia (Shu Di Huang), Coicis (Yi Ren), Chaenomelis (Mu Gua), Os (Gu).[c] *For elderly*: Rehmanniae (Shu Di), Angelicae (Dang Gui), Lycii (Gou Qi Zi), Homalomenae (Qian Nian Jian), Acanthopanacis (Wu Jia Pi), Dipsaci (Xu Duan), Cinnamomi (Ru Gui), Angelicae (Du Huo), Notopterygii (Qiang Huo), Dioscoreae (San Yao), Atractylodis (Bai Zhu), Corni (Shan Zhu Yu), Ligustici (Chuan Xiong).

Table 7-7: Herb Combinations for Commonly Seen Musculoskeletal Disorders (Continued)

BONES	*Fracture general*: Angelicae (Dang Gui), Carthami (Hong Hua), Sappan (Su Mu), Persicae (Tao Ten), Pritum (Zi Ran Tong), Dynariae (Gu Sui Bu), Dipsaci (Xu Duan), Eupolyphaga (Tu Bie Chong), Pseudoginseng (San Qi), Olibanum (Ru Xiang), Myrrha (Mo Yao). *Early-stage fracture*: Angelicae (Dang Gui), Rehmanniae (Shu Di Huang), Paeoniae (Bai Shao), Ligustici (Chuan Xiang), Olibanum (Ru Xiang), Myrrhae (Mo Yao), Lycopodii (Shen Jin Cao), Liquidambaris (Lu Lu Tong), Plantaginis (Che Qian Zi), Loncerae (Jin Yin Hua), Chrysanthemi (Ju Hua), Paridis (Zao Xiu). *Mid-stage fracture (bone union stage)*: Sanguis (Xue Jie), Eupolyphaga (Tu Bie Chong), Manitis (Chuan Shan Jia), Pyritum (Zi Ran Tong), Strychnotis (Ma Qian Zi), Drynari (Gu Sui Bu), Pyrolaceae (Lu Xian Cao), Ephedra (Ma Huang), Os (Gu). *Late-stage fracture with stiffness and pain*: Angelica (Dang Gui), Spatholobi (Ji Xue Teng), Salviae (Dan Shen), Mori (Sang Zhi), Carthami (Hong Hua), Dynariae (Gu Sui Bu), Ligustici (Chuan Xiong), Gentianae (Qin Jiu), Clematidis (Wei Ling Xian), Curcumae (Jiang Huang). *Late-stage bone pain, bone spur pain*: Aconiti (Chuan Wu and Cao Wu), Asari (Xi Xin), Angelicae (Bai Zhi), Angelicae (Dang Gui), Dioscoreae (Bie Xie), Carthami (Hong Hua). *Wilting atrophy*: Plastrum (Gui Ban), Achyranthis (Niu Xi), Dioscorea (Shan Yao), Corni (Shan Zhu Yu), Psoraleae (Bu Gu Zhi), Juglandis (Hu Tao Rou), Eucommiae (Du Zhong), Dipsaci (Xu Duan), Rehmannia (Shu Di Huang), Achyranthis (Niu Xi), Dendrobii (Shi Hu), Phellodendri (Huang Bai), Dioscorea (Shan Yao), Eucommiae (Du Zhong), Dipsaci (Xu Duan), Drynariae (Gu Sui Bu), Chaenomelis (Mu Gua), Os (Gu). *Spurs and nodules*: Gleditsiae (Zao Jiao Ci), Sargassum (Hai Cao), Laminariae (Kun Bu), Eupolyphaga (Tu Bie Chong), Scorpio (Quan Xie), Sebastan (Po Bu Zi Ye). *Pain or weakness from overuse*: Psoralea (Bu Gu Zhi), Beef Marrow (Niu Gu Sui), Dear Horn (Lu Rong), Drynaria (Gu Sui Bu) and Os Tiger [or any bone] (Hu Gu).
SINEW AND BONE	*Weakness due to Wind-Damp*: Atractylodes (Cang Zhu), Coicis (Yi Ren), Acanthopanacis (Wu Jia Pi), Dioscoreae (Bi Xie), Achyranthis (Niu Xi), Chaenomelis (Mu Gua), Angelica (Du Huo), Notopterygii (Qiang Huo).
SCAR TISSUE	*Topical*: Galla (Wu Bei Zi), Evodiae (Wu Zhu Yi), Schefflera (Qi Ye Lian), Speranskiae (Tou Gu Cao), Homalomenae (Qian Nian Jian), Angelica (Dang Gui), Paeoniae (Chi Shao), Olibanum (Ru Xiang), Myrrhae (Mo Yao), Carthami (Hong Hua), Vinegar.

a. Fang Feng can be used to reduce the toxicity of Aconiti (Fu Zhi) as large doses of Aconiti are often needed in the treatment of musculoskeletal disorders.
b. Cauda Equina syndrome (S4) is a medical emergency which must be treated surgically to avoid sequelae.
c. Traditionally tiger bone (Hu Gu) is used, but any bone may be substituted.

Table 7-8: Pharmacology of Commonly Used Herbs

Function	Herbs
Activate Pituitary-Adrenocortical System	Bai Hua Se She Cao, Di Huang, Du Zhong, Gan Cao, Qin Jiao, Ren Shen, Xuan Shen, Yan Hu Suo, Zhi Mu.
Adrenergic	Ma Huang, Xi Xin, She Xiang.
Analgesics	Bai Fu Zhi, Bai Shao, Bai Zhi, Bing Pian, Cao Wu, Chi Hu, Chan Su, Chun Tui, Chi Shao, Chou Wu Tang, Chuan Wu, Dang Gui, Dan Shen, Ding Xiang, Due Huo, Du Zhong, Fang Feng, Fen Fang Ji, Fu Zhi, Gan Cao, Gan Jiang, Gao Ben, Gui Zhi, Han Fang Ji, Hong Hua, Hua Jiao, Jiao Gu Lan, Jing Jie, Ling Zhi, Man Jing Zi, Mu Dan Pi, Mu Zei, Mu Tong, Niu Xi, Qing Hao, Qi Jiao, Qi Ye Lian, Qing Feng Teng, Quan Xie, Ren Shen, Rou Gui, San Qi, San Zhi Zi, Sang Bai Pi, She Xiang, Sheng Jiang, Sheng Ma, Shui Chang Pu, Suan Zao Ren, Tian Ma, Tian Nan Xing, Tian Zhu Huang, Wei Ling Xiang, Wu Zhu Yu, Xi Xin, Xian He Cao, Xiang Fu, Xiao Hui Xiang, Xu Chang Qing, Xu Yang Jin, Xun Gu Feng, Yan Hu Suo, Yi Yi Ren, Ying Su Ke, Zao Xiu.
Anesthetics	Chan Su, Chuan Wu, Da Suan, Huan Jiao, She Chuang Zi, Xi Xin, Xiang Fu, Xin Yi Hua.
Antiadrenergics	Du Huo, Ge Gen, Huang Lian.
Antiallergics	Ai Ye, Bai He, Bi Cheng Qie, Chen Pi, Chuan Tui, Chen Xiang, Dao Zao, Di Long, E Bu Shi Cao, Fang Feng, Fen Fang Ji, Gan Cao, Gui Zhi, Han Fang Ji, Huang Qin, Jing Jie, Lian Qiao, Ling Zhi, Ma Huang, Qiang Huo, Qin Jiao, Qin Pi, She Xiang, Tao Ren, Wu Mei, Wu Yao, Xi Xin, Xin Yi Hua, Xu Chang Qing, Yu Xing Cao, Zhi Shi, Zhu Dan.
Anticholinesterase	Bo Lou Hui, Gang Liu Pi, Huang Lian.
Anticonvulsants	Chan Tui, Chi Shao, Dang Shen, Di Long, Ding Xiang, Fang Feng, Fo Shao, Gan Cao, Gou Teng, Gui Zhi, Hu Jiao, Jiang Can, Ju Ye San Qi, Ling Yang Jiao, Ling Zhi, Long Chi, Long Dan Cao, Long Gu, Lu Rong, Mu Dan Pi, Niu Huang, Peng Sha, Qi Ye Lian, Qin Pi, Quan Xie, Ren Shen, Sang Bai Pi, Sang Jiang, Sheng Ma, Shi Chang Pu, Suan Zao Ren, Tian Ma, Tian Nan Xing, Wu Gong, Xi Yang Shen, Xiang Mao, Xie Cao, Xuan Shen, Yuan Zhi, Zao Xiu, Zhu Dan, Zhu Sha.
Antihistamine	Chan Tui, Chen Pi, Fang Feng.
Anti-Inflammatory	Ba Ji Tian, Bai Shao, Bai Zhi, Bing Pian, Cang Er Zi, Cao Wu, Chai Hu, Chan Su, Che Qian Cao, Chi Shao, Chau Wu Teng, Chuan Wu, Chuan Xin Lian, Ci Wu Jia, Da Huang, Da Qing Ye, Da Qing Ye, Dan Shen, Dang Gui, Di Huang, Di Yu, Dong Ling Cao, Du Huo, Du Zhong, Fang Feng, Fen Fang Ji, Fu Zhi, Gan Cao, Gan Jiang, Gao Ben, Ge Jie, Gu Sui Bu, Guang Jin Qian Cao, Hai Ge Fen, Han Fang Ji, Hei Zhi Ma, Hong Hua, Hu Zhang, Huai Hua, Huang Jing, Huang Lian, Huang Qi, Huang Qin, Jiang Huang, Jie Geng, Jin Jie, Jin Qiao, Jin Yin Hua, Ku Shen, Lai Fu Zhi, Lei Gong Teng, Lian Qiao, Long Dan Cao, Lu Lu Teng, Lui Huang, Ma Bian Cao, Ma Dou Ling, Ma Huang, Man Jing Zi, Mao Dong Qing, Mu Dan Pi, Mu Tong, Niu Huang, Niu Xi, Nu Zhen Zi, Pi Pa Ye, Pu Huang, Qin Jiao, Qing Feng Teng, Ren Dong Teng, Ren Shen, San Qi, Sang Bai Pi, Sha Yuan Zi, Shan Dou Gen, Shang Lu, She Gan, She Tui, She Xiang, Sheng Jiang, Sheng Ma, Su Mu, Tao Ren, Tian Ma, Wu Jia Pi, Xi Xiang Cao, Xi Xin, Xia Ku Cao, Xian Mao, Xiang Fu, Xiang Fu Zi, Xian He Cao, Xi Xian Cao, Xi Xin, Xiao Ji, Xu Chang Qing, Xuan Shen, Xue Yu Tan, Ye Ju Hua, Yin Yang Huo, Yu Xing Cao, Ze Xia, Zhi Zi, Zi Cao Gen, Zhu Dan.
General Stimulants	Ban Bian Lian, Chan Su, Du Huo, Huang Lian, Jin Yin Hua, Kuan Dong Hua, Ma Huang, Ma Qian Zi, Qin Jiao, Ren Shen, Wu Wei Zi, Wu Zhu Yu, Xi Xin.
Cholinergics	Bing Lang, Chuan Wu, Gou Qi Zi, Huang Lian.
Coagulants and Hemostatics	Ai Ye, Bai Ji, Bai Mao Gen, Bu Gu Zhi, Ce Bai Ye, Chen Pi, Da Huang, Da Ji, Di Huang, Di Jin Cao, Di Yu, Fang Feng, Fu Ling, Guang Zhong, Han Liang Cao, Hu Zhong, Hua Rui Shi, Huai Hua, Jin Yin Hua, Jing Tian San Qi, Liang Fang, Long Qi, Long Gu, Ma Mian Cao, Pu Huang, Qian Cao Gen, Qu Jie, San Qi, Shen Ma, Shi Liu Pi, Su Mu, Xi Yang Shen, Xian He Cao, Xiao Ji, Xue Yu Tan, Yin Yang Huo, Wu Yao, Zi Cao Gen, Zi Zhu, Ziang He Cao, Zong Lu Zi.
Diuretics	Bai Mao Gen, Bai Zhu, Ban Bian Lian, Bian Xu, Cang Zhu, Chan Su, Che Qian Cao, Che Qian Zhi, Chuan Mu Tong, Da Huang, Dang Gui, Dan Zhu Ye, Di Fu Zhi, Di Huang, Du Zhong, Fang Feng, Fu Ling, Guan Mu Tong, Gui Zhi, Hai Jin Sha, Huang Qi, Huang Qin, Jie Geng, Jin Qian Cao, Ku Shen, Lian Qiao, Long Dan Cao, Lu Rong, Ma Huang, Ma Ti Jin, Mu Dan Pi, Mu Tong, Niu Xi, Qu Mai, Sang Bai Pi, Sang Ji Sheng, San Qi, Shi Hu, Ting Ling Zi, Wu Zhu Yu, Yin Chen, Yu Xing Cao, Ze Xie, Zhi Ke, Zhu Ling.
Enhancers of Tolerance to Hypoxia	Chuan Shan Long, Dan Shen, Di Huang, Fo Shou, Gua Lou, Hong Hua, Jin Qian Cao, Ju Hua, Ku Shen, Ling Zhi, Mai Dong, Pu Huang, San Qi, Yin Yang Huo, Yu Zhu.
External Wound Healing	Di Yu, Gu Sui Bu, Lu Hui, Lu Lu Tong, Shan Yao.
Fracture-Healing Promotors	Hu Gu, Jiu Jie Feng, Lu Rong.
Immunosuppressants (Modulators)	Bei Sha Shen, Chai Hu, Chan Tui, Chuan Shan Long, Chuan Wu, Chuan Xin Lian, Dong Ling Cao, Gan Cao, Gan Sui, Hong Hua, Huang Qin, Jin Jie Feng, Ku Shen, Lei Gong Teng, Long Dan Cao, Shan Dou Gen, She Chuang Zi, Shu Di Huang, Tian Jua Fen, Tian Men Dong, Wu Jia Pi, Wu Wei Zi, Xia Ku Cao, Ze Xie.

Table 7-8: Pharmacology of Commonly Used Herbs (Continued)

Function	Herbs
Peripheral Vasodilators	Bai Zhu, Can Wu, Chuan Shan Long, Chuan Wu, Chuan Xiong, Ci Wu Jia, Dan Shen, Dang Gui, Da Qing Ye, Du Zhong, Fu Zi, Ge Gen, Gua Lou Shi, Gui Zhi, Hai Feng Teng, Hong Hua, Huang Lian, Huang Qi, Lei Gong Teng, Luo Bu Ma, Lu Xian Cao, Mu Zei, Pu Huang, Ren Shen, Sang Bai Pi, Sang Ji Sheng, Shui Cang Pu, Tao Ren, Tian Ma, Wu Wei Zi, Xi Xian Cao, Xie Cao, Xin Yi Hua, Suan Shen, Yang Jin Hua, Yin Guo Ye.
Sedatives and Hypnotics	Ai Ye, Bai He, Bai Jiang, Bai Shao, Ce Bai Ye, Chai Hu, Chan Su, Chan Tui, Chi Shao, Cho Wu Tong, Ci Wu Jia, Dang Gui, Dan Shen, Di Huang, Di Long, Dang Chog Xia Cao, Du Huo, Du Zhong, Fang Feng, Fo Shou, Fu Ling, Gou Teng, Gan Song, Gui Ban, Gui Zhi, He Huan Hua, Hong Huan, Hou Po, Huang Lian, Huang Qin, Jiang Can, Ju Hua, Ling Zhi, Long Chi, Long Dan Cao, Mu Dan Pi, Mu Tong, Mu Zei, Niu Huang, Qing Feng Teng, Qin Jiao, Qi Ye Lian, Ren Shen, Sang Bai Pi, San Zhi Zi, Shan Zha, Sheng Jiang, Sheng Ma, Shi Cang Pu, Shui Cang Pu, Suan Zao Ren, Tian Ma, Tian Nan Xing, Wu Wei Zi, Xi Xin, Xiang Fu, Xian Mao, Xuan Shen, Yan Hu Suo, Yi Yi Ren, Yu Mi Xu, Yuan Zhi, Zao Xiu, Zhu Dan, Zhu Sha.
Striated Muscle Relaxants	Ba Jio Feng, Bei Dou Gen, Han Fang Ji, Hou Po, Long Dan Cao, Ren Shen, Xin Yi, Xi Sheng Teng, Yan Hu Suo.
Tranquilizers	Luo Fu Mu, Qing Feng Teng, Ren Shen, Sang Bai Pi, Shi Cang Pu, Shui Chang Pu, Suan Za Ren, Yan Hu Suo.

Table 7-9: TCM Contraindications for Commonly Used Herbs in Musculoskeletal Disorders

Herb	Contraindication
Artemisiae (Ai Ye)	Yin-deficiency, Blood-Heat.
Morindae (Ba Ji Tian)	Yin-deficiency, Fire-effulgence, Insufficiency of Fluids and Humors, Difficult urination, Damp-Heat.
Amomi (Bai Dau Kou)	Yin-deficiency, Blood agitation without Dampness and Cold.
Patriniae (Bai Jiang Cao)	Blood-stasis with Qi-stagnation without Excess-Heat.
Sinapis (Bai Jie Zi)	Lung-deficiency with enduring cough, Yin-deficiency, Fire-blazing, Stomach-Fire.
Paeoniae (Bai Shao)	Weak confirmation with abdominal pain, diarrhea.
Dictamni (Bai Xian Pi)	Weak and Cold confirmation.
Angelicae (Bai Zhi)	Yin-deficiency, Blood-Heat.
Atractylodis (Bai Zhu)	Yin-deficiency, Internal Heat or Fluids and humors damage with thirst.
Pinelliae (Ban Xia)	Blood diseases, Yin-deficiency, Dry cough, Fluid damage, thirst.
Scutellariae (Ban Zhi Lian)	Edema due to Deficiency.
Fritillariae (Bei Mu)	Spleen and Stomach Deficiency and Cold, Damp-Phlegm.
Glehniae (Bei Sha Shen)	Wind-Cold cough, Lung and Stomach Deficiency, Cold.
Piperis (Bi Bo)	Excess-Heat, Yin-deficiency-Fire.
Dioscoreae (Bi Xie)	Yin-deficiency, Fire-blazing.
Trionycis (Bie Jia)	Spleen/Stomach Deficiency and Cold, Poor appetite and loose stools, Pregnancy.
Arecae (Bing Lang)	Spleen-deficiency, loose stools.
Borneolum (Bing Pian)	Yin-deficiency, Yang-Excess, Fright in children, Diarrhea and vomiting due to Spleen-deficiency, Eye diseases due to Liver and Kidney Deficiency, Pregnancy.
Methae (Bo He)	Exterior-deficiency with spontaneous sweating.
Psoraleae (Bu Gu Zhi)	Yin-deficiency, Fire-blazing, constipation.
Atractylodis (Cang Zhu)	Yin-deficiency with internal-Heat, Qi-deficiency with perspiration.
Aconiti (Cao Wu)	Yin-deficiency, Pregnancy, Excess-Fire.
Bupleuri (Chi Hu)	Yin-deficiency, Fluid damage, Hyperactive Liver and Intestines.
Plantaginis (Che Qian Zi)	Essence and Qi Deficiency.
Paeoniae (Chi Shao)	Blood-deficiency.
Toosendan (Chuan Lian Zi)	Weakness of Spleen and Stomach.
Manitis (Chuan Shan Jia)	Insufficiency of Blood and Qi, Open carbuncles, Pregnancy.
Ligustici (Chuan Xiong)	Yin-deficiency, Fire-blazing, Headache due to hyperactive Liver and Intestines, Excessive Mensis.
Rhei (Da Huang)	Qi and Blood Deficiency, Spleen and Stomach Deficiency Cold, Absence of true Heat, Pregnancy and Lactation.
Salviae (Dan Shen)	Hemorrhagic disease.
Angelicae (Dang Gui)	Dampness and stagnation causing fullness of abdomen, Loose stools or diarrhea.
Condonopsis (Dang Shen)	Excess pathogens in middle burner, Qi and Fire Excess and effulgent.
Lycii (Di Gu Pi)	Exterior contraction, Wind, Cold with fever, Spleen-deficiency, Loose stools.
Angelicae (Du Huo)	High fever not resolving Cold, Yin-deficiency with Heat.
Eucommiae (Du Zhong)	Yin-deficiency, Fire-blazing, Dry stools or constipation.
Curcumae (E Zhu)	Qi and Blood Deficiency, Spleen and Stomach weakness without stasis and stagnancy, Excessive menstruation.
Ledbouriellae/Siler (Fang Feng)	Blood-deficiency, Yin-deficiency leading to Wind, Fire-blazing.
Stephaniae (Fang Ji)	Yin-deficiency without Dampness, Heat.
Poria	Deficiency-Cold, Immature emission or deficient-Qi downward-surging.
Aconiti (Fu Zhi)	Yin-deficiency, Yang Excess (false Cold), True Heat, Yin-deficiency with internal-Heat, Pregnancy.
Glycyrrhizae (Gan Cao)	Dampness with fullness and choking feeling in chest and abdomen, Edema, Retching.

Table 7-9: TCM Contraindications for Commonly Used Herbs in Musculoskeletal Disorders (Continued)

Herb	Contraindication
Ligustici (Gao Ben)	Blood-deficiency with headache, Hot confirmation.
Puerariae (Ge Gen)	Cold perspiration in hot weather.
Cibotii (Gou Ji)	Yin-deficiency with fever, short urination with dark color.
Lycii (Gou Qi Zi)	Excess Heat of surface, Spleen-deficiency, Dampness and stagnation, Sensitive intestines with diarrhea.
Dynoariae (Gu Sui Bu)	Yin-deficiency with Heat.
Testudinis (Gui Ban)	Yang-deficiency, Spleen and Stomach-deficiency-Cold, Exterior pathogens, Pregnancy.
Cinnamomi (Gui Zhi)	Heart disease with Yin-deficiency, Yang-excess, Blood-Heat, Excessive mensis, Pregnancy.
Erythrinae (Hai Tong Pi)	Blood-deficiency.
Ecliptae (Han Lian Cao)	Excess pathogens without Deficiency.
Polygoni (He Shou Wu)	Loose stools or diarrhea, Sever Dampness, Phlegm.
Phellodendri (Huang Bai)	Spleen-deficiency with diarrhea, Weak Stomach, Poor appetite.
Polygonati (Huang Jing)	Spleen-deficiency with Damp stagnation, Cough with lots of Phlegm.
Coptidis (Huang Lian)	Yin-deficiency with Heat-palpitations, Vomit due to Stomach Cold, Spleen-deficiency with diarrhea.
Astragali (Huang Qi)	Excess external pathogens, Qi-stagnation, Damp-plug, Food-stagnation, Yin-deficiency, Yang-excess, Beginning of carbuncle with Heat-poison.
Scutellariae (Huang Qin)	Spleen and Stomach Deficiency Cold, Poor appetite, Loose stools.
Spatholobi (Ji Xue Teng)	Excessive mensis, Pregnancy.
Bombyx (Jiang Chan)	Blood-deficiency, Averse Wind.
Lonicerae (Jin Yin Hua)	Spleen and Stomach Deficient Cold, Qi-deficiency, Carbuncles with clear discharge.
Schizonepetae (Jing Jie)	Spontaneous perspiration, Yin-deficiency headache.
Cervi (Lu Jiao)	Yin-deficiency, Hyperactive-Yang.
Cervi (Lu Rong)	Yin-deficiency, Hyperactive-Yang, Blood-Heat, Stomach-Fire, Phlegm, Heat.
Trachelospermi (Luo Shi Teng)	Fear of Cold, Frequent diarrhea.
Ephedrae (Ma Huang)	Spontaneous perspiration due to Exterior-deficiency, cough or short breath due to Qi-deficiency, Spleen-deficiency with edema.
Ophiopogonis (Mai Men Dong)	Mild cold flu, Phlegm retention cough, Spleen and Stomach Deficiency Cold with diarrhea.
Viticis (Man Jing Zi)	Headache and dizziness due to Blood-deficiency with Fire, Weak Stomach.
Moutan (Mu Dan Pi)	Blood-deficiency with Cold, Pregnancy, Excessive mensis without Blood-Heat.
Chaenomelis (Mu Gua)	Deficiency of Essence and Blood, True-Qi-Yin-deficiency.
Arctii (Niu Bang Zi)	Qi-deficiency, Loose stools, Open carbuncles with clear discharge.
Ligustri (Nu Zhen Zi)	Spleen and Stomach Deficiency Cold, Diarrhea, Yang-deficiency.
Typhae (Pu Huang)	Pregnancy.
Notopterygii (Qiang Huo)	Blood-deficiency.
Gentianae (Qin Jiao)	Enduring pain becoming deficiency, Weakness, Frequent urination, Loose stools.
Scorpio (Quan Xie)	Blood-deficiency, Heat.
Ginseng (Ren Shen)	External pathogens, Extreme internal-Heat, Damp-carbuncles, Food-stagnation with abdominal distension, constipation or diarrhea.
Cistanches (Rou Cang Rong)	Kidney-deficiency with Fire-blazing, Spleen-deficiency, Loose stools.
Cinnamomi (Rou Gui)	Yin-deficiency-Fire, Fluid damage from Heat, True Heat false Cold.
Sparganii (San Ling)	Qi-deficiency, Weakness, Menorrhagia, Pregnancy.
Notoginseng (San Qi)	Bleeding due to Yin-deficiency, Thirst, Pregnancy.
Dioscoreae (Shan Yao)	Spleen-deficiency with Excess-Dampness, Abdominal or chest fullness and distress.
Corni (San Zhu Yu)	Hyperactive-Liver and Intestines, Contraction of Damp-Heat, Difficult urination.
Musk (She Xiang)	Deficiency of Yin-Yang-Qi-Blood, Pregnancy.

Table 7-9: TCM Contraindications for Commonly Used Herbs in Musculoskeletal Disorders (Continued)

HERB	CONTRAINDICATION
REHMANNIAE (SHENG DI HUANG)	Spleen-deficiency with diarrhea, Weak Stomach, Poor appetite, Phlegm.
CIMICIFUGAE (SHENG MA)	Yin-deficiency, Yang-floating, Excess dyspnea or counter-flow, Eczema at ripe stage.
REHMANNIAE (SHU DI HUANG)	Spleen and Stomach Deficiency and Weakness, Dampness, Chest oppression, Loose stools.
ZIZIPHI (SUAN ZAO REN)	Excess-Fire, Loose stools or diarrhea.
CYNOMORII (SUO YANG)	Yin-deficiency-Fire, Spleen-deficiency with diarrhea, Excess-Heat constipation.
TRICHOSANTHIS (TIAN HUA FEN)	Spleen and Stomach Deficiency Cold, Loose stools.
GASTRODIAE (TIAN MA)	Blood-deficiency, Yin damage.
ARISAEMATIS (TIAN NAN XING)	Yin-deficiency, Sticky Phlegm, Pregnancy.
SMILACIS (TU FU LING)	Liver and Kidney Yin-detriment.
CUSCUTAE (TU SI ZI)	Yin-deficiency-Fire, Dry stools with constipation, Short dark urination.
CLEMATIDIS (WEI LING XIAN)	Qi-deficiency, Blood-deficiency, Absence of Wind-Cold.
ACANTHOPANACIS (WU JIA PI)	Blood-Heat, Liver and Intestines hyperactivity and uprising.
SCHISANDRAE (WU WEI ZI)	External pathogens not resolved or Excess-Heat, Early cough, Measles, Eczema.
ACANTHOPANACIS (WU JIA PI)	Blood-Heat, Liver and Intestine hyperactive counterflow.
LINDERAE (WU YAO)	Qi-deficiency, Interior-Heat.
EVODIAE (WU ZHU YU)	Yin-deficiency, Fire Blazing.
ASARI (XI XIN)	Yang-hyperactive headache, Yin-deficiency cough due to Lung-Heat.
PRUNELLAE (XIA KU CAO)	Spleen-deficiency, Weak Stomach, Pregnancy.
CYPRI (XIANG FU)	Exterior-deficiency with perspiration.
DRACONIS (XUE JIE)	Lack of Blood-stasis.
LEONURI (YI MU CAO)	Yin and Blood Deficiency.
ALPINIAE (YI ZHI REN)	Yin-deficiency-Fire, Nocturnal emission, enuresis and metrorrhagia due to internal-Heat.
ARTEMISIAE (YIN CHEN HAO)	Jaundice without Damp-Heat and Cold-Dampness.
EPIMEDII (YIN YANG HUO)	Ministerial-Fire unrooted, Spontaneous erections.
CURCUMAE (YU JIN)	Yin-deficiency, Loss of Blood with Qi-stagnation and Blood-stasis, Pregnancy.
POLYGONATI (YU ZHU)	Spleen-deficiency with Phlegm.
POLYGALAE (YUAN ZHI)	Excess-Heat, Toxic-Heat, Yang-excess, Spleen and Stomach weakness.
GLEDITSIAE (ZAO JIAO)	Pregnancy, Weak confirmation with Bloody cough.
ALISMATIS (ZE XIE)	Kidney weakness, Spermatorrhea.
ACONITI (ZHI CHUNG WU)	Yin-deficiency, Yang-Excess, Pains of Heat type, Pregnancy.
ANEMARRHENAE (ZHI MU)	Spleen and Stomach Deficiency Cold, Loose stool or diarrhea.
AURANTII (ZHI QIAO)	Spleen-deficiency, Stomach weakness, Pregnancy.
AURANTII (ZHI SHI)	Spleen-deficiency, Stomach weakness, Pregnancy.
GARDENIAE (ZHI ZI)	Spleen-deficiency diarrhea.
POLYPORUS (ZHI LING)	Lack of water retention and Dampness.
VIOLA (ZHI HUA DI DING)	Deficiency Cold.
PERILLAE (ZI SU YE)	Febrile disease, Qi-deficiency and Exterior-deficiency.
BAMBUSAE (ZU RU)	Stomach Cold vomit.

8

FOUNDATION FOR INTEGRATIVE ELECTROTHERAPUTICS

This chapter covers electrotheraputics and related techniques. These have been integrated into OM/TCM as well as into related Western therapies.

Bioenergetic Field Therapy

Ideas from the "bioenergetic" field of medicine are increasingly being integrated into modern OM. Bioelectromagnetics (BEM) is the emerging science that studies how living organisms interact with electromagnetic (EM) fields. Electrical phenomena are found in all living organisms. Moreover, electrical currents exist in the body that are capable of producing magnetic fields that extend outside the body. Consequently, they can be influenced by external magnetic and EM fields as well. Changes in the body's natural fields may produce physical and behavioral changes. All of the known frequencies of EM waves or fields are represented in the EM spectrum, ranging from DC (zero frequency) to the highest frequencies, such as gamma and cosmic rays. The EM spectrum includes x-rays, visible light, microwaves, and television and radio frequencies, among many others. Moreover, all EM fields are force fields that carry energy through space and are capable of producing an effect at a distance. These fields have characteristics of both *waves* and *particles*. Depending on what types of experiments one performs to investigate light, radio waves, or any other part of the EM spectrum, one will find either waves or particles called "photons." A photon is a tiny packet of energy (a discrete particle of quantum electromagnetic energy) that has no measurable mass and is the packet carrying the energy of every frequency in the electromagnetic spectrum. A photon is generated when an electron makes a transition from an upper to a lower energy level (state). The greater the energy of the photon, the greater the frequency associated with its waveform (Rubik et al *ibid*).

To understand how these field effects may occur, it is first useful to discuss some basic phenomena associated with EM fields. This involves understanding the electrical nature of the cells of the body and how this affects our health. It is obvious that the biological molecules within our bodies are not just resting. They are constantly on the move to maintain homeostasis and hence our health. The very fact that negative and positive ions in the form of biological molecules are constantly moving means that they are conducting electric energy. While they are moving, as with electrical theory, they are also generating an electromagnetic field and placing varying strengths of electrical forces on neighboring molecules. This undoubtedly facilitates communication and is probably one of the ways the TCM channel systems communicate. A good example of a moving charge and hence an electrochemical magnetic field is that of nerve impulses during muscle contraction and relaxation. Proprioceptors respond to a change in the environment and send nerve impulses to the central nervous system (CNS). Here's our first produced field as biological ions move along the neural pathway to alert the CNS that a response is required to a particular situation. The CNS will then decide on an appropriate response, and, via the endocrine or sympathetic nerve pathways, send signals to effect a reaction to the change in environment. When this response is directed to the muscles, nerve impulses at neuromuscular junctions break down the resting 70mV membrane potential, and muscle contraction occurs. The cells within the muscle tissue then react in a number of ways to establish equilibrium again (thereby re-establishing the balanced membrane potential). Once this is achieved, muscle relaxation will occur. The physiological mechanisms are not limited to the negative feedback systems such as the nervous and endocrine systems. These changes will affect all systems and tissues, and, more specifically, neurotransmitters in the brain and adrenal functions. (Tume 2004).

(OM: Electromagnetic and electroacupuncture stimulators can be used to influence the TCM channels systems, specific tissues, and other biological fields. When discussing the channel systems in TCM, we usually speak of trajectories of communication systems that manifest and are described by Yin Yang polarities. Potential differences within channels are traditionally described as rivers and reservoir with differential potentials (Yin and Yang) of stored or moving Qi (Transport points). There is, therefore, some overlap between electrical theories and cell biology with gradient potentials and the channel systems. (The ideas of positive and negative potential extremes of Yin and Yang, i.e., the communication systems of Qi, and electrical, electrochemical and other biological informations systems that relay on potential gradients are therefore quite similar).

Aristotle (400 BC) was probably the first person in Western history to talk about the therapeutic use of magnetism, or as he called it, the "White Magnet." The ancient use of magnetism is also seen in China, Egypt, India, and within the Arab and Hebrew worlds.[1] Up until the middle of the 20th century, the use of magnetism in healing was limited to what today are called permanent or static magnets. Modern research into static magnetic therapy didn't begin until the mid-nineteen thirties when Albert Roy Davis, with the help of Walter C. Rawls Jr., initiated basic research into the use of the two poles of a magnet on living systems. Davis continued to investigate this until his death, and this research still continues today. Kyoichi Nakagawa MD proposed the theory of "Magnetic Field Deficiency Syndrome" in the mid-nineteen fifties. He postulated that due to the reduction of the earth's magnetic field over time, the connection of the human body to magnetic field effects, and support by his clinical findings, that the idea of a "magnetic deficiency" in humans is viable. The symptoms of the "Magnetic Field Deficiency Syndrome" are said to include: stiff shoulders, stiff upper back, chest pains for no reason, dizziness and insomnia for no apparent reason, general lassitude, and, habitual constipation amongst many others. The key factor to the theory was that there was no obvious medical reason for the conditions seen and that the application of magnetic therapy in a majority of cases alleviated the symptoms described. In 1819 Hans Christian Oersted, having cited the first theories of electromagnetism, combined electricity and magnetism under a single concept. Up until this time, electricity and magnetism had been seen as separate phenomena. Bjorn Nordenström discovered a circulatory system that is based on spontaneously occurring electrical potentials. Potential gradients have long been known to develop in normal organs as a result of metabolism and in injured or diseased tissue as a result of hemorrhage or necrosis. His work has shown these potentials to be more than just a source of error in bioelectric measurements, they drive electric current through what he calls a *biologically closed electric circuits* (BCEC). BCEC works in part via ionic media, such as blood plasma and interstitial fluid, that are capable of conducting current. Blood vessel walls and the cells and membranes that surround interstitial spaces may function to insulate these conducting media from their surroundings. Plasma and interstitial fluid are electrically joined across capillary membranes. Thus, blood vessels and interstitial spaces function as insulated electric cables that carry current and transport charged particles over short and long distances. Other BCEC probably also exist. Nordenström's work (described in his book, *Biologically Closed Electric Circuits*) examines this particular circuit in detail, documenting its existence and function with a series of experiments using physical analogs of biologic organs and organ systems, animal models, and tumor and tissue specimens obtained at autopsy or surgical resection. The resultant hypotheses are tested in a series of careful and humane diagnostic experiments and therapeutic trials performed on consenting human volunteers with malignant diseases (Glickman 1984). Nordenström suggests that the forces flowing in BCEC's may be thought of as Qi, with positive and negative charges that are comparable to Yin and Yang in OM. In his text he offers other analogies with OM concepts of how the Qi in nature can affect human health, performance, and possibly aging. He also relates the concepts of aptosis and apoptosis of the repetitive cycle of death and rebirth to the Generation and Control cycles of the Five-Phases theory.

Naturopathic thought, modern "Bioenergetic Philosophy," and the philosophic position of "Vitalism" all share the ida of "Vital Force" or energy. Within Bioenergetic Therapies currently emerging, we see a system of electrical states and potentials in the body, which respond to the application of subtle electrical and electromagnetic emissions that can aid in rebalancing the body's homeostatic resonance. By understanding the basic theories of electricity, we can be in a better position to understand the mechanisms of electrical potentials within the body and how they may be affected bioenergetically to restore a natural physiological homeostatic balance. Energy takes on many forms in life within both the internal and external environments. The forms of energy are electrical, thermal, light, chemical, magnetic, electromagnetic, and radioactive. While the effects and uses of radioactive energy are well known, it is the uses of electrical, chemical, magnetic, and electromagnetic that are most related to Bioenergetic Therapies (Tume *ibid*).

Nonionizing electromagnetic medical applications may be classified according to whether they are thermal (producing heat in biologic tissue) or nonthermal. Thermal applications of nonionizing radiation (i.e., the application of heat) include radio-frequency (RF) hyperthermia, laser and RF surgery, and RF diathermy. The most important electromagnetic (EM) modalities in alternative medicine are the nonthermal applications of nonionizing radiation. For example, microwave resonance therapy, which is used primarily in Russia, employs nonthermal, low-intensity (either continuous or pulse-modulated) sinusoidal microwave radiation to treat a variety of conditions, including arthritis, ulcers, esophagitis, hypertension, chronic pain, cerebral palsy, neurological disorders, and the side effects of cancer chemotherapy. Thousands of people in Russia also have been treated by specific frequencies of extremely low-level microwaves applied at certain *acupuncture points* (Rubik et al *ibid*).

Foundations of Electricity and Biomagnetic Therapy

Electricity is an invisible force that can be made to produce heat, light, motion, and many other physical effects. While the force of electricity is said to be achieved by attraction or repulsion between electrical charges (electrons and protons),

---

1. Both the Egyptian (2500 BC) and the Greek physician Hippocrates (400 BC) used electric fish to treat pain. Iron ore may have been used for healing in Africa as far back as 100,000 years ago (Oschman 2000).

Table 8-1: Nomenclature

DATE	NAME	UNIT	SYMBOL	NAMING BODY
1867	FARAD	Electrical capacitance	F	British Association Committee (London)
1881	VOLT	Electric potential	V	1st International Electrical Congress (Paris)
1881	COULOMB	Electric charge	C	1st International Electrical Congress (Paris)
1881	AMPERE	Electric current	A	1st International Electrical Congress (Paris)
1889	WATT	Power, radiant flux	W	2nd International Electrical Congress (Paris)
1891	GAUSS	Magnetic field density	B	3rd International Electrical Congress (Frankfort)
1891	WEBER	Magnetic flux	Φ	3rd International Electrical Congress (Frankfort)
1893	HENRY	Inductance	H	4th International Electrical Congress (Chicago)
1894	GILBERT	Magnetomotive force	mmf	AIEE Standards Committee (Chicago)
1894	OERSTED	Magnetic reluctance	r	AIEE Standards Committee (Chicago)
1900	MAXWELL	Magnetic flux	Φ	5th International Electrical Congress (Paris)
1930	OERSTED	Magnetic field strength	Oe	IEC Technical Committee (Paris)
1932	HERTZ	Frequency	Hz	IEC Technical Committee (Paris)
1932	WEBER	Magnetic flux	Wb	IEC Technical Committee (Paris)
1932	SIEMENS	Electrical conductance	S	IEC Technical Committee (Paris)
1956	TESLA	Magnetic flux density	T	IEC Technical Committee (Munich)

Robert Beck B.E., D.Sc., states that he does not know what electricity is and neither anybody else. Atoms consist of a nucleus, protons and electrons. Neutrons have no electrical charge, protons have a positive electrical charge, and electrons have a negative electrical charge. Generally, atoms have no net electrical charge as they have an equal number of electrons and protons. During atomic bonding however, an atom loses or gains electrons; we see a change in the net electrical charge. This process of bonding is known as *ionic bonding*. If for example, an atom gains electrons during bonding, it then has a higher number of electrons and therefore a greater negative electrical charge. This is known as a *negative ion*. If on the other hand an atom loses electrons during bonding, it then has a greater number of protons and therefore a greater positive electrical charge. This is known as a *positive ion*. Magnetic fields are produced by moving electrical currents. For example, when an electrical current flows in a wire, the movement of the electrons through the wire produces a magnetic field in the space around the wire. Therefore electroacupuncture is also a type of electromagnetic field therapy.

Electrical conduction is usually described as one of three types: metallic conduction, ionic conduction and semi-conduction. Metallic conduction is said to occur only in metal wires (although, when non-metallic materials are formed to make tensegrity tubes, they can become conductive as well). Ionic conduction occurs through cell membranes and travels minute distances. Semi-conduction is possible within the body (via crystalline-like protein structures, such as perineural glial cells), or other crystalline structures (e.g., electronic transistors), and is capable of conducting small currents (and hence information) over long distances.

Piezo-electricity is the tendency of a crystalline structure to release electrical charges when deformed or struck. Movements within the body are said to constantly release and trigger piezo-electric activity. The main points to remember when talking about electrical current flow are:

- Insulators are substances that are poor or non-conductive such as glass, plastic, rubber and wood.
- A resting static charge flows through conductors as electrical current and then resumes its static nature after it stops flowing.
- Electrical current flows from a region of high charge or "potential" to a region of low charge or potential.

- When a current is flowing through a conductor (for instance a wire), it creates a magnetic field around it.

An electric circuit (a closed circuit) must have a source of potential difference (the volts or power supply), and a complete path for the current to flow from one side of the applied voltage source, through the circuit, and return to the other side of the voltage source. More specifically, electricity can be explained in terms of charges, currents, voltage and resistance. The corresponding electrical units are the coulomb (C) for measuring charge (Q), the ampere (A) for current (I), the volt (V), for potential difference (PD), and the ohm (Ω) for resistance (R). These properties of electricity are combined in Ohm's Law, which states that the current (I) is equal to the applied voltage (V) divided by the resistance (R). Coulomb's law states that *like charges repel and unlike charges attract*. Table 8-1 summarizes the nomenclature used in magnetic and electro-therapeutics. The following terms are often used to describe electric circuits and are also used in Bioenergetic field of health care:

- Coulomb: The coulomb is a unit of charge. One Coulomb (C) is equal to a charge of 6.25 times 10^{18} electrons. It can describe any charge, even static electricity, in which the electrons or protons are not in motion (not connected to a circuit).
- Volt: The volt is a unit of potential differences. When one charge is different from the other, there is a difference of potential between them (a Yin/Yang gradient). The Volt (V) is a measure of the work needed to move an electric charge across the differential. The potential difference of 1V equals the work required to move 1C of electrons between two points, each with its own charge. In general, hi volt therapy is considered to be greater than 100-150V. Low volt therapy is less than 100-150V.
- Ampere: The ampere is a unit of current or charge in motion. To produce a current the charge must be moved by a potential difference (V). The current is a continuous flow of electrons. Only the electrons move, not the potential difference. The number of free electrons that can be forced to drift through the wire (body) to produce the moving charge depends on the amount of potential difference across the wire. One ampere (A) of current is when the charge moves at the rate of 1C electrons flowing past a given point per second.

  Average Current (also called Root Mean Square) describes the "average" intensity. This will depend on the pulse amplitude, pulse duration, and wave form. DC will have more net charge over time and therefore has higher thermal effects. AC current will have a zero net charge.

  Current Density describes the amount of charge per unit area. With surface stimulation (TENS) this is usually relative to the size of the electrode; the density increases with a small electrode, but the small electrode also offers more resistance. The farther the two electrodes are placed from each other, the deeper the electrical penetration and lower the density.

- Ohm. The ohm is a unit of resistance in opposition to current. In any medium that conducts electricity there is always "opposition," which limits the amount of current that can be produced by a given voltage. This is called "resistance" (R). Metal conductors have very little resistance, insulators have a large amount of resistance. Resistance is measured as ohms (Ω). The greater the length through which electricity has to travel the greater the resistance. The hotter the material the greater the resistance as well. Superconductors which offer almost no resistance must be kept at a temperature close to absolute zero.
- Amplitude: The amplitude is used to describe the total power (height) of stimulation and is a product of all the above (although sometimes refers just to A or V).
- Direct Current (DC): The current in a closed circuit that flows in one direction with a DC voltage source which has a fixed polarity, as produced by a regular battery, whether this is steadily or in pulses.
- Alternating Current (AC): The current in a closed circuit that periodically reverses its direction, resulting from an alternating voltage source, such as a wall outlet. The wave form will be replicated on both sides of the isoelectric line (with symmetrical waves). Related to AC (sine wave) currents is the square wave. Unlike the sine wave (which is found in nature), the square wave is produced by specific equipment known as *function generators*. Function generators can produce a wide variety of wave shapes, but within Bioenergetics, sine and square waves (and variations of the square wave) are the most predominantly used wave shapes.[2]
- Frequency (f): The number of cycles per seconds (frequency) is measured in hertz (Hz). One should not assume that lower frequencies mean longer pulse duration.
- Period (T): The amount of time for one cycle to complete is the period. With a frequency of 60Hz the time for one cycle is 1/60 seconds.

---

2. By definition the square wave has an infinite number of odd harmonics, and there might be bad waves in that mix, as well as good. One can't tell what the mix is by looking at the wave using an oscilloscope which is a time domain display. It will show the wave forms (some of waves) and the frequency of the pulse repetition rate, but it cannot show what the harmonics of those wave forms are actually producing in the way of frequencies. What is needed is a spectrum analyzer, and most of the companies the build electrotheraputic devices probably don't own one (because of the high expense). Many engineers confuse pulse repetition rate with frequency. They are two entirely different things. For example, the number of taxi cabs that are going by a specific corner per hour would be the repetition rate of taxis passing. But knowing the rate does not tell you what's inside these taxicabs until you look inside. In electrotherapy this means looking at the wave on a spectrum analyzer. A spectrum analyzer is a frequency domain display, an entirely different thing from time domain. Many of the devices being sold as electro-medical stimulators, either cranial electro-stimulators or generic TENS devices have got the wrong frequency spectra (Beck interview from: Megabrain Report, Vol. 1 No.1 edited by Michael Hutchison).

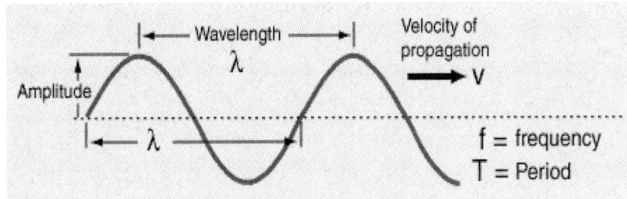

Figure 8-1: Sine wave of AC current (Tume 2004 with permission).

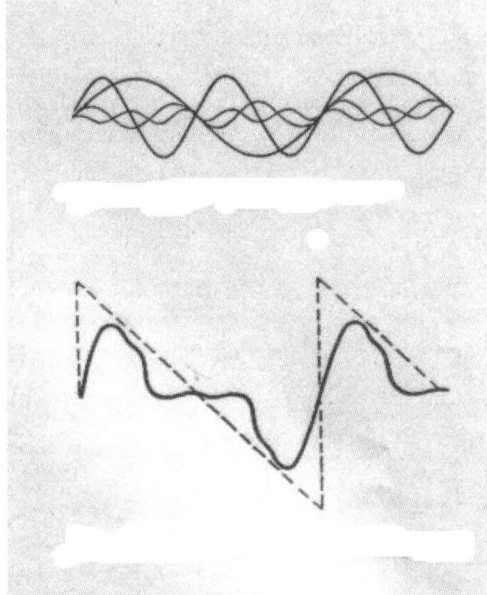

Figure 8-2: Harmonics and their Complex Vibration. Sawtooth illustrated with doted line is used in many therapeutic stimulators in order to simulate harmonics found in nature (with permission Tume *ibid*).

- Wavelength (λ): The periodic variation with respect to distance in one cycle or wave.
- Duty Cycle: The duty cycle is the on-off time. It may also be called the inter-pulses. The more rest of "off" time, the less muscle fatigue will occur: 1:1 ratio fatigues muscles rapidly; 1:5 ratio is less fatiguing to muscles; and 1:7 ratio will not fatigue a muscle.
- Waveforms: The basic wave forms are nonalternating (monophasic) or DC current, and Sinusoidal AC waveforms (alternating). Non-sinusoidal AC waveforms such as sawtooth wave, symmetrical square wave, unsymmetrical rectangular wave, etc. are used often in electroacupuncture.

  The greater the amplitude and wavelength of a wave shape, the greater penetration and distance that wavelength has. This is important when dealing with penetration depths in human tissues.
- Pulses: A pulse is a sudden increase or decrease in current flow. It allows a large amount of energy or current to be used in a very short amount of time to produce work, or large amounts of energy to be transmitted. Pulses can also be used effectively within Bioenergetic fields.
- Pulse rise time: The time to peak intensity of the pulse (ramp) is known as the pulse rise time. Rapid rising pulses tend to cause nerve depolarization, Slow rise time tend to result in nerve accommodation.
- Signal: A periodic waveform that conveys information. Signals are mostly related to radio station signals that convey voice and sound information. The process that generates signals is known as "Modulation." *Modulation* is a very important term used within the Bioenergetic fields, as certain basic pieces of equipment such as a laser or a magnetic therapy unit can be modulated with another frequency, e.g., different information.
- Open circuit: When a part of the path for electrical flow is broken it is said to be an open circuit (as when a light switch is not turned on). There is no current or flow, only potential differences.
- Short circuit: When there is no resistance between the two poles of the potential difference (across the source of electricity) there would be an "infinite" current, which often results in heat and usually burns a fuse, which is a safety found in most instruments. Short circuits can also burn wires and electronic components as well as flesh.
- Noise: Noise relates to randomly generated, unwanted currents that can be sometimes generated by electronic devices and circuits. Noise can also enter electronic equipment and circuits by way of electromagnetic waves generated by other large electronic devices, lightning, electric motors, and the like. If noise interference is substantial enough, it can interfere with the normal operation of some electrical systems.

Up to this point, we have discussed conductors, insulators, resistance, voltage, types of current flow and various wave shapes. There are however, a few more terms to cover that are relevant to Bioenergetic Therapies. These are: Capacitance, Inductance, and Resonance.

- Capacitance is the ability to store electrons. Electronic capacitors store electrons within electronic circuits for when there is a need for a brief large source of current flow (discharge) or when there is a need to receive a gradual, continuing source of current. The higher the capacitance the longer before a response occurs. Body tissues have different capacitance. Nerves have the least and therefore fire first when healthy. Muscle fibers have more and muscle tissues even more. The muscle membrane has 10 times the capacitance of nerve. More intensity (with decrease pulse duration) is needed to stimulate tissues with a higher capacitance. Because large diameter nerves have a lower capacitance they will respond more quickly.
- Inductance is related to the transfer of energy. When we look at current flowing through a coil of wire, as stated

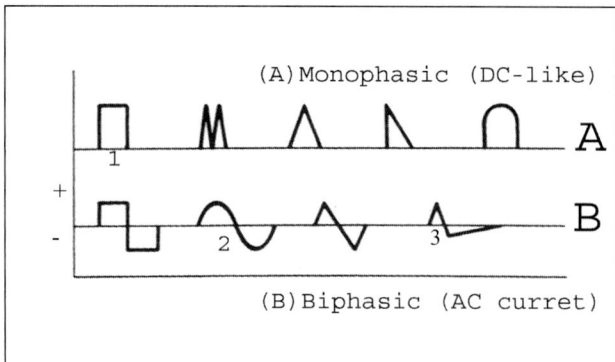

Figure 8-3: Basic wave forms: **1A)** is monophasic square wave. There is no alternation between the - and + poles; there is a net positive polarity. **B2)** is a sine wave. Flow alternates between the + and - poles; no net polarity achieved. **B3)** is an example of an asymmetric biphasic wave form, commonly used with electroacupuncture with differing configurations; no net polarity achieved because of the algorithmic configuration of the wave, i.e., while the positive phase is higher the negative phase is longer which is designed to achieve a 0-net gain (after Alon 1991).

previously, there is a magnetic field generated around the coil itself. When a secondary coil is induced close to the primary coil, the magnetic field can be induced (transferred) to the secondary coil. This transfer of energy will then generate a current within the secondary coil so that it may pass on this current for the production of work. This is one of the most important terms used in electromagnetic therapy. It is by inductance that electromagnetic energy is induced into biological systems to achieve a transferal of energy when the "Vitality" of a person is low.

- **Resonance:** This is another term, related to frequency, that is often used in the field of Bioenergetic health care. The lowest resonant frequency of a vibrating object is called its *fundamental* frequency. Most vibrating objects have more than one resonant frequency, and those used in musical instruments typically vibrate at harmonics of the fundamental. An *harmonic* is defined as an integer (whole number) multiple of the fundamental frequency. If we look at Figure 8-2, the top picture demonstrates a number of waves or harmonics that would make up a complete (total some) frequency with the widest of the sine waves (that is, the sine wave with the longest wavelength) being the fundamental frequency. The overall whole of these harmonics, for a single wave, including the fundamental frequency is known as a "complex vibration" (because it is made of many parts), represented mathematically by "composite curve." The dotted line through this complex vibration represents a sawtooth wave motion, which roughly represents the path of the complex vibration.[3] This is one reason why certain electromagnetic and electroacupuncture therapy outputs have been in a sawtooth wave motion rather than a sine or square wave motion. Resonance in AC circuits is said to imply a special frequency, which is determined by the values of resistance, capacitance, and inductance. (Tume *ibid*).

- **Rate of Current:** How fast electrical energy travels depends on two factors: the voltage (the driving force) and the resistance.

Electromagnetic fields have a wave motion. The wave moves outward at the speed of light (roughly 186,000 miles per second). As a result, it has a wavelength (i.e., the distance between crests of the wave) that is inversely related to its frequency. For example, a 1-Hz frequency has a wavelength of millions of miles, whereas a 1-million-Hz, or 1-megahertz (MHz) frequency has a wavelength of several hundred feet, and a 100-MHz frequency has a wavelength of about 6 feet (Rubik et al *ibid*).

The Electrical Properties of The Body

So that we can fully utilize the bioelectrical knowledge clinically, it is essential to have an understanding of how our bodies act in an electrical manner. This involves understanding the electrical nature of the cells of the body and how this affects our health. Electricity can be defined as the flow of energy caused by change in resting potentials, which by enlarge is expresses as Yin-Yang potentials in OM/TCM.

The electrical potentials of our cells, and hence of our bodies, begin with the chemical reactions within our cells. From the study of anatomy and physiology we learn about the process of cellular nutrition, which allows nutrients to enter the cells and waste products from cellular metabolism to be eliminated.[4] Essentially, cellular nutrition and cellular respiration involve biologically necessary molecules crossing the cell membrane (to feed the biological reactions that sustain life) by processes such as: osmosis, diffusion, facilitated diffusion, and receptor mediated endocytosis. If we look at the structure of the molecules involved in these processes, we will see that they have a certain "polarity." That is, they are charged either positively or negatively depending on their ionic structure and hence their balance of electrons and protons.

During cellular nutrition there are positively and negatively charged molecules moving across the cell membrane. At certain times there are more negative ions inside the cell than outside it and vice versa. This being the case, during these active states, the overall or net charge inside and outside the cell constantly changes. (In terms of OM/TCM we

---

3. The "sawtooth wave" in not an actual wave form, unless generated by a clinical stimulator, but rather it is a schematic approximation of a total some effect.

4. To some extent all disease can be defined as failure in either cellular nutrition or failure of cellular detoxification. In physiologic medicine the practitioner assesses the bodies ability to successful absorb and transport essential substances (as well as keep out what needs to stay out) and the bodies ability to detoxify and excrete what is toxic.

can see that this is a Yin/Yang interplay.) As with all chemical reactions, these states strive to reach equilibrium. In the body, this constitutes the homeostatic balance that sustains life within normal limits. This homeostasis is not total equilibrium. Total equilibrium would probably mean death as all life is characterized by movement. *(OM: Qi can never not be moving)*.

When the cell reaches the appropriate level of equilibrium, that is, when reactions are functioning normally, the cell is said to be in a stable state. The electric "potential" (or the difference in charge between the inside and outside of the cell) in this case is approximately 70mV. We may ask, why is there a 70mV potential rather than a net even charge? This is due to the fact that ionic bonding such as occurs in H_2O will sometimes need more of one element than another to reach its state of equilibrium, so there must be different numbers of negatively and positively charged ions inside and outside the cell to provide the "biological equilibrium" that is the stable homeostatic state of life.

Nernst (a physicist) worked out an equation to calculate the voltage across the cell membrane as: V (across membrane) = K x log concentration of ions inside the membrane times concentration of ions outside the membrane. So we can see that a homeostatic state is a balance of negative and positive polarity depending on ionic bonding and chemical reactions within the cell and the surrounding tissues. These states are related to cellular needs depending on the health of the cells and establishes the existence of polarity within the body, and that, in stable states or states of rest, there will be an electrostatic charge (potential) to the system depending on the balance of ions. When these ions (molecules) move, however, we come back to the principle of electricity *(OM: Yin and Yang potentials, Qi, and channels)*. As can be seen, our whole body is affected by changing electromagnetic fields that are produced electrochemically and continue to react with each other.

It is important to note here that while these fields at a cellular level are quite small, when the cells aggregate into tissue and then into organs and systems, the aggregated magnitude of the fields make the body an electro-magnetic entity of considerable intensity. *(OM: This is not unlike the growth of Qi circulation as it moves proximally to affect larger systems)*.

Becker (*ibid*) found that the human body is positively polarized along the central spinal axis and negatively peripherally. The normal voltage reading is said to be -10 µV (microvolt), however when a fracture occurs, the voltage is decreased toward zero. Jaffe et al (1982) showed that the human skin has a resting potential across its epidermal layer of 2-90mV with the outside of the skin being negative and the inside positive.

Nordenström suggested that any injury to the body creates a voltage that continuously fluctuates between positive and negative (like an AC current) until it finally reaches electrical equilibrium, a state he believes to be associated with healing. He found that the electrical resistance of the walls of the veins and arteries was at least 200 times that of blood. In effect, he states, these vessels act as insulated cables, and the blood flowing within them conduct electricity between tumors (or injured cells) and the surrounding tissues. When an injury occurs, a positive charge builds up in the area of injury, which may then result in a potential gradient acting as a bioelectric battery. Bioelectricity is said to be conducted through five main components that may be found in any vascularized part of the body:

1. Insulating walls of blood vessels.

2. Conducting intravascular plasma.

3. Insulating tissue matrix (possibly including lymph vessels).

4. Conducting interstitial fluid.

5. Transcapillary electrical junctions for redox reactions.

A change in the electrical insulating properties of capillary membranes is said to turn on the "biological battery." As the membranes become less permeable to the flow of ions and more electrically insulated, the flow of intrinsic bioelectricity is forced to take the path of least resistance, which is through the bloodstream to the injured area. The capillary cell membranes act as naturally charged electrodes that allow ions to move through the cells via gates and vesicles. Additional ions flow between the cells through pores. This local ion flow stops when excess electrons cross enzyme bridges in the capillary walls, closing the pores and gates and thereby closing the local circuit. This occurrence creates a long distance bioelectrical circuit in which the ions flow. The capillary cell membranes, therefore appear to be the key component in switching from local ion flow across the capillary membranes to long distance ion flow down the capillary walls. When Nordenström applied a positive electric current to the blood vessels, white blood cells, which are said to curry negative charges on their surface, were attracted to the positive electrode. Blood clots, too, would form in the vessels in response to the current which may be used to treat tumors. If the polarity is switched the clots would dissolve (Nordenström *ibid*, Becker *ibid*). Polar effects can be used to treat musculoskeletal disorders (see below).

From this viewpoint we can then establish that if miniature magnetic fields within the body act on each other in varying degrees, then it is possible that electromagnetic radiation from our external environment, when at a high enough density, can affect these internal fields both beneficially and detrimentally. Whether or not electromagnetic radiation is hazardous to human health (and all biological systems) has been debated for years. Generally speaking, the mainstream line is that electromagnetic pollution is not hazardous to human health except in certain circumstances (Tume *ibid*).

HAZARDOUS TO HUMAN HEALTH. In radiation biophysics, an EM field is classified as ionizing if its energy is high enough to dislodge electrons from an atom or molecule. High-energy, high-frequency forms of EM radiation, such as gamma rays and x-rays, are strongly ionizing in biological matter. For this reason, prolonged exposure to such rays is harmful. Radiation in the middle portion of the frequency and energy spectrum—such as visible or even ultraviolet light—is weakly ionizing (i.e., it can be ionizing or not, depending on the target molecules; Rubik et al *ibid*).

The fact that the World Health Organization (WHO), National Health and Medical Research Council (NHMRC), Australian Radiation Protection and Nuclear Safety Agency (ARPANSA), Environmental Protection Agency (EPA) and many more agencies have specific branches dedicated to research into the health effects of electromagnetic radiation pollution say that there is obviously something worth researching here. Most branches of these agencies concentrate on non–ionizing radiation. The National Radiation Protection Board (NRPB) in the UK defines non–ionizing radiation as follows: "Non-ionizing radiation (NIR) is the term given to the part of the electromagnetic spectrum where there is insufficient quantum energy to cause ionizations in living matter. It includes static and power frequency fields, radiofrequencies, microwaves, infrared, visible, and ultraviolet radiation." The South Australian EPA states that, unlike natural fields, commercial fields expose us to 50 Hz EMR (this 50 Hz frequency is more commonly known as "Mains Hum," in the US, it is 60 Hz) by: small and large power lines, wiring in homes and office buildings and, all domestic and industrial appliances that use electricity which *may* be harmful. The Australian EPA also states that there is generally *no sound evidence* of ill health effects of EMR but do say that the risk of leukemia in children can be increased especially when exposed to prolonged EMR at 0.3 to 0.4 micro Tesla. Furthermore, in 1996, the WHO established the International Electromagnetic Fields (EMF) Project. This was done to research the accuracy of statements from some members of the scientific community that there are possible health hazards associated with EMF. One partner of the WHO's International EMF Project: The International Commission on Non–Ionizing Radiation (ICNIRP), has even developed international guidelines on exposure limits for all EMF's although these are only limited to acute short term exposure. This is because the ICNIRP considers the potential carcinogenicity of extremely low frequency (ELF) fields (ELF fields having been classified by the International Agency for Research on Cancer (IRAC) as possibly carcinogenic) as having insufficient evidence to establish similar limits on exposure (Tume *ibid*).

CLINICAL IMPLICATIONS: The use of electromagnetic diagnostics is well-known: the diagnostic procedures of electroencephalography (EEG) and electrocardiography (ECG) are based on the detection of endogenous EM fields produced in the central nervous system and heart muscle, respectively. Taking the observations in these two systems a step further, current biological EM research is exploring the possibility that weak EM fields associated with nerve activity in other tissues and organs might also carry information of diagnostic value. New technologies for constructing extremely sensitive EM transducers (e.g., magnetometers and electrometers) and for signal processing recently have made this line of research feasible (Rubik et al *ibid*). Clinically, as far back as 1935, Burr described the detection of ovulation by monitoring changes in voltage during the ovulatory cycle. According to Oschman (2000), measurement of acupuncture point conductance and skin surface electrical potentials have been shown to detect organ degeneration and inflammation, tuberculosis, cirrhosis, lung disease, and tumors.

Several studies have found evidence for the presence and influence of electricity and magnetism in connective tissue function and injury (Nordenström 1983; Becker *ibid;* Oschman *ibid;* Hunt 1995). According to Hunt (1995) various body tissues omit differing electromagnetic currents within acupuncture-like meridians. Denser tissues like bone and cartilage exhibit slower moving, lower frequencies that were associated more with direct current (DC). Lighter tissues like nerves and glands were associated with higher frequencies and alternating currents (AC). Dr. Hunt associated healing with a local injury "switching" from predominately electrical to becoming predominately magnetic, and Nordenström with switching from primarily DC (not oscillating) to AC (oscillating). Slow waves of electrical depolarization are set up across the skin in response to injury which are important in triggering tissue repair (Oschman *ibid*). The discovery that tissues and systems are polarized may be used in clinical practice, for example, by the use of DC electrostimulation to attract white blood cells to an injured area. If a silver electrode (needle) is used this will increase the bodies ability to fight infection (as silver ions are antibiotic). The addition of electromagnetic stimulation to acupuncture may therefore influence *intrinsic* repair.

The Russian scientist Pressman summed-up three main effects for bioelctromagnetic fields: they allow living things to sense information about the environment; they facilitate organization and control within the organism; and they are used for communication between living things (Presman 1970). These are all applicable in Bioenergetic medicine. At the same time, however, the state of clinical evidence for "bioenergetic medicine" is mixed and more high quality studies are needed.

Introduction to Electromagnetic and Electrical Stimulation Therapy

Electricity creates magnetism and magnetism can produce electricity. Electromagnetism is a combination of the two which allows, by the use of clinical instruments, for magnetism to be turned on and off at will (that is: pulsed). An iron bar with a coil of wire around it through which a current flows can be turned into a temporary magnet. A magnetic field always surrounds an electric current when it is flowing but disappears when the current stops. This magnetic field has a specific direction and spin, either North or South, similar to any other magnetic field. Early inventors discovered that electricity could be created whenever any electrical conductor travelled across the lines of force of a magnetic field. (This is why when an electromagnetic field source is placed near acupuncture needles, the needles become magnetic.) Magnetic resonance imaging machines enable a scan to be made of the body, particularly its soft tissues and fluids, to detect what is happening deep within the body. As the patient lies in a huge magnetic field, computer pictures are made from the returning signals it receives.

Coils of wire through which an electric current is flowing are called *solenoids*. Solenoids fitted with an iron core are called *electromagnets*. A *magnetic* field is produced when electric currents pass through the solenoid. When an iron core is added to the solenoid, the magnetic field becomes stronger and the iron becomes magnetized for as long as the current keeps flowing.

The therapeutic uses of electromagnetic systems are the same as for static magnetic therapy; however, they present an extra benefit in that the power of the magnetic field can be increased, and the penetration of the magnetic energy can in this way be deeper and hence more beneficial for the patient, while still being a non-invasive form of therapeutic application. It also allows for the use of specific frequencies for specific conditions.

Essentially, the benefit of EM therapy is that, as stated above, the magnetic field can be pulsed at different frequencies. This allows beneficial frequencies to be transmitted to the body by the EM field. According to Sanserverino (1992) 11 year study on 3014 patients, interrupted stimulation (pulsed) is more effective than continuos one since sensitive receptors and excitable membranes are usually stimulated by energy variations. Specific changes in the field configuration and exposure pattern of low-level EM fields can produce highly specific biological responses. More intriguing, some specific frequencies have highly specific effects on tissues in the body, just as drugs have their specific effects on target tissues. The actual mechanism by which EM fields produce biological effects is under study. Evidence so far suggests that the cell membrane may be one of the primary locations where applied EM fields act on the cell. EM forces at the membrane's outer surface could modify ligand-receptor interactions (e.g., the binding of messenger chemicals such as hormones and growth factors to specialized cell membrane molecules called receptors), which in turn would alter the state of large membrane molecules that play a role in controlling the cell's internal processes. Experiments to establish the full details of a mechanistic chain of events such as this, however, are just beginning (Rubik et al *ibid*).

CLINICAL EVIDENCE. Pulsed electromagnetic therapy is being used for a variety of muculoskeletal disorders as well as wound and fracture healing. For example, Thuile and Walzl (2002) have shown in two prospective, randomized studies in patients with either lumbar radiculopathy in segments L5/S1 or whiplash syndrome, that magnetic field applied twice a day for a period of two weeks has a considerable and statistically significant potential for reducing pain. Acupuncture needles in a magnetic field have been shown to stimulate the immobilization of blood vessels which may be used to decrease blood supply to tumors, facilitating tumor necrosis (Rotariu et al 2004). Musaev, Guseinova and Imamverdieva (2003) studied pulsed electromagnetic fields with complex modulation (PEMF-CM) in the treatment of patients with diabetic polyneuropathy (DPN). PEMF-CM at 10 Hz was found to have therapeutic efficacy, especially in the initial stages of DPN and in patients with diabetes mellitus for up to ten years. Usichenko, Ivashkivsky, and Gizhko (2003) studied the efficacy and safety of electromagnetic millimeter waves (MW) applied to acupuncture points in patients with rheumatoid arthritis (RA) and showed significant pain relief and reduced joint stiffness during and after the course of therapy. Lappin et al (2003) reported on the effects pulsed electromagnetic therapy has on multiple sclerosis fatigue and quality of life in a multi-site, double-blind, placebo controlled, crossover trial. Each subject received four weeks of the active and placebo treatments separated by a two-week washout period. This trial was consistent with results from smaller studies suggesting that exposure to pulsing, weak electromagnetic fields can alleviate symptoms of MS. The clinical effects were small, however, and need to be replicated. Woldanska-Okonska and Czernicki (2003) have shown that pulsating magnetic field used in magnet therapy and magnet stimulation can alter cortisol levels in patients with chronic low back pain by as much as 100%. Nicolakis et al (2002) reported on pulsed magnetic field therapy (PMF) for osteoarthritis of the knee in a double-blind sham-controlled trial. They found PMF treatment can reduce impairment in activities of daily life and improve knee function. Transcranial magnetic cortical stimulation has been used to treat central pain (Canavero et al 2002). Mark et al (1995) reported on the usefulness of Transcranial Magnetic Stimulation on mood in depression. Sandyk et al (1992) reported on the use of magnetic fields in the treatment of Parkinson's disease. Foley-Nolan et al (1990) has shown electromagnetic therapy to be useful in persistent neck pain. Binder et al (1984) reported on the use of electromagnetic therapy in persistent rotator cuff tendinitis. Kuz'menko (1982) reported positive effects in 240 amputees for limb stump pain. Finally, a review article by Rubnic et al (1992) reported on the useful uses of electromagnetic therapy in: bone and cartilage repair, soft tissue and wound healing, neural tissue growth and regeneration, behavioral problems, acupuncture-style pain reduction, modifications in the pineal gland's production of melatonin, immune system effects, arthritis treatment, and cellular and subcellular effects on tumors.

Electrical Stimulation

Electrical stimulation is used frequently in treatments of musculoskeletal disorders, either by surface application or via acupuncture needles. Electrical stimulation has three

Table 8-2: Electrode Effects

ANODE (+)	EFFECTS	CATHODE (-)	EFFECTS
Nerve excitability	decrease	Nerve excitability	increase
Acidity	increase	Alkalinity	increase
Fluid	decrease	Fluid	increase
Red blood cells	decrease	Red blood cells	increase
White blood cells	increase	White blood cells	decrease
Skin hardness	increase	Skin hardness	decrease
Used more in acute injuries		Used more in chronic injuries	

basic biological effects: electrothermal, electrochemical, and electrophysical. These effects can be seen locally (on a tissue/cellular level), systemically, and segmentally. Sisken and Walker (1995) have reviewed research employing electric and magnetic fields on soft tissues. Low energy and frequency fields may be emanated by the hands of practitioners of therapeutic touch and related methods (Oschman *ibid*).

LOCAL EFFECTS. Locally, electrical stimulation can cause peripheral nerve excitation, alteration of enzymatic activity, and alteration of protein synthesis (Owens and Malone 1983; Stanish, Valiant, and Bonen et al 1982). Local contraction of muscles and an increase in venous blood and lymph circulation (a segmental effect) may: slow atrophy that has occurred due to denervated muscles; reduce swelling; and facilitate the healing process (Weiss, Kirsner and Eaglstein 1990; Bettany, Fish and Mendel 1988). Electrical stimulation has been shown to have analgesic and other effects, both systemic and segmental. Loss of presynaptic inhibition, such as occurs with Type I mechanoreceptors on Type IV nociceptors, facilitates the noxious input at the dorsal horn, allowing more pain signals to register in the brain (see chapter 2). Electrotherapy (including spinal stimulators) are a common therapeutic choice.

Electrical stimulation may (Bourguignon and Bourguignon 1978; Owoeye, Spielholx and Fetto et al 1987; Akai, Oda, Shiraski and Tateishi 1988; Brighton and Pollack 1986, Sisken and Walker 1995, Oschman *ibid*):

- Diminish pain;
- Influence the migratory, proliferative, functional capacity of fibroblasts;
- Enhance capillary formation;
- Reduce swelling;
- Speed repair of tendons, muscles, and ligaments and improve their tensile strength;
- Reduce muscle loss after ligament surgery;
- Accelerate functional recovery after injuries;
- Influence bone regeneration;
- Accelerate nerve regeneration and functional recovery;
- Bring about gel-to-sol state of ground substance and release "toxins."

Because of these effects, electrostimulation and/or electroacupuncture is commonly used to: stimulate Type I inhibitory receptors and A-δ fibers to activate the "gate control" and other analgesic mechanisms such as stimulating endogenous polypeptides and catecholamine-mediated analgesia (although the slow onset may preclude the gate theory); affect joint mobility due to muscle group contraction; possibly modulate internal organ activity due to somatovisceral reflexes; help repair and prevent scars in minor muscular tears; forestall atrophy of muscles in root palsy; and stimulate the proliferation of cells for soft-tissue or bone-growth and repair.

EFFECTS IN THE VICINITY OF THE ELECTRODES. Direct (DC or monophasic) electrical stimulation has several effects in the immediate vicinity of the electrodes (Table 8-2), (Shriber 1974, *ibid*). In general with DC electrostimulation, proton gradients are formed across the mitochondrial membrane. The current produces a gradient when electrons at the cathode react with water to form hydroxyl-ions while producing protons at the anode side (+). This results in voltage gradient across the tissues between the electrodes. The influence of the electrical field and the proton concentration difference produce a *proton-current* that moves from anode (+) to cathode (-). Electrons move from the cathode (-) to the anode (+). As the migrating protons cross the mitochondrial membrane-bound-H+ATPase, ATP is formed. The increased ATP production stimulates amino acid transport, and these two factors contribute to increased protein synthesis (Cheng et al 1982, *ibid*).

The body's attempt to restore pH balance results in increased local circulation. Electrophoresis (interchange of ions between the two poles, also called iontophoresis) can be used to deliver medication through the skin (Figure 8-4). This increased circulation and the interchange of ions may contribute to reported acceleration of bone healing and the regeneration of other tissues by electrical stimulation.

Research evidence on microcurrent stimulation supports negative (cathode) microcurrents as being more effective with bone and nerve repair and regeneration, while positive (anodal) microamp stimulation may be more effective in healing skin lesions. Contradictions appear in literature regarding optimal polarity with tendon injuries (Oweye, Speilholtz et al 1987; Stanish 1988). Stanish and Gunlaughson (1988) in a summery article of research into tendon healing acceleration, including human injuries of the anterior cruciate ligament and the Achilles tendons, stated that while the results are subjective, the individuals in both treated groups appear to have returned to usual activities more quickly, and have greater mobility, than people treated conventionally. Nessler and Mass (1987) showed that in vitro a 1.4 volt direct current (DC) connected through a 150 kOhm resistor at a current of about 7 uA is useful in repairing tendons. It was found that currents any higher than this caused

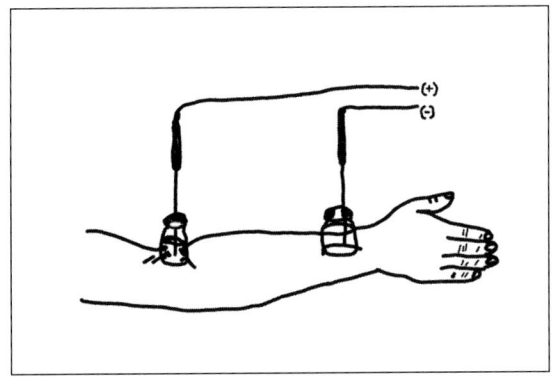

Figure 8-4: Combined electroacupuncture and iontophoresis.

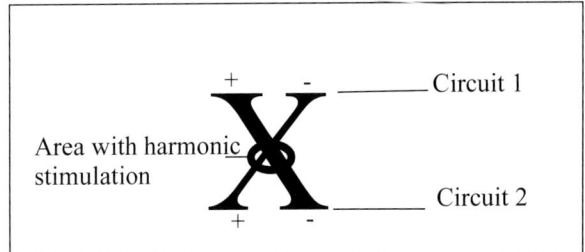

Figure 8-5: Quadra pole two circuit asynchronous (cross) configuration.

"discoloration" of the tendons. Healing was measured by proline uptake and bridging of the repair site by the epitendon. Continuous direct current was shown to increased tendon cell activity within seven days and the increased activity may persist as long as 42 days. Oweye et al (1987) showed greater healing strength in injured Achilles tendon in rats stimulated with 75 microamps, at 10 Hz. with the group treated with anodal current (+) withstanding significantly greater loads than either the group which healed normally (i.e., without stimulation) or the group treated with cathodal currents.

In general, more studies suggest that local anodal (+) stimulation result in greater *tendon strength* than cathodal (-) stimulation or no stimulation (Owoeye, Spielholx and Fetto et al 1987), although according to Nuccitelli (1984) and McCaig (1987) in most cases there is enhanced cell growth toward the cathode (-) and reduced cell growth toward the anode (+), in electric fields of physiological strength (not just microamp). High-volt cathode (-) galvanic stimulation has been said to be sclerolytic or tissue-softening, and anode (+) stimulation is said to be tissue-hardening, possibly associated with dehydration, and therefore to have some effects similar as prolotherapy. Clinical use of biphasic (AC like current, or any of the biphasic waves), nonpolarized stimulation has been shown to cause collagen formation and osteogenesis as well (Brodsky and Khalil 1988; *ibid*).

Nordenström suggests using direct mircocurrent stimulation of cancer tumors to control cancer pain. He suggest placing the anode (positive) pole in the tumor and the cathode (negative) pole at a distance which is said to reduce oxygen supply to the tumor by attracting white blood cells and rejecting (and possibly by creating blood-clots) red blood cell at the anode (Nordenström 1989). He also reports curing patients with lung cancer.

According to Dr. Liss, the manufacturer of the LISS Cranial Stimulator,[5] blood circulation can increase at the cathode (-), and blood can be mobilized from areas where the anode (+) is placed towards the cathode (-). He also states that no effects on blood circulation are seen with a bipolar version of the LISS stimulator. Therefore a monopolar device is advocated, if there is a clinical need to reduce pain through the increase of blood in a given body area as in diabetic neuropathy, Raynud's disease, multiple sclerosis, or in the head as in migraine headaches. To treat orthopedic disorders, placement of the cathode (-) at the injured (painful) site and the anode (+) proximally (over the trunk or spine) is often recommended. If there is a need to reduce pain by altering the level of neurobiochemicals (including reduction of stress hormones) such as in chronic back and other musculoskeletal pain, facial pain, or neuropathic pain such as reflex sympathetic dystrophy, a bipolar device may be used as a cranial stimulator (Figure 8-6).

QUADRIPOLE STIMULATION. It is possible to use two separate circuits (i.e., four electrodes) positioned in a cross (X) configuration to create harmonics and the greatest amplitude-frequency-modulated biologic interference effects (Figure 8-5). This configuration may be particularly helpful when treating peripheral joints. The current delivered to the tissues from the first circuit intersects and blends with the current delivered to the tissues in the opposite direction from the second circuit. Harmonics occur when the two circuits are slightly out of sink with each other. The two waves slightly out of phase would collide and form a single wave with progressively increasing and decreasing amplitude. Asynchronous stimulation to muscles can result in motor unit contraction and relaxation at different rates. This results in a smoothly graded muscle contraction that requires less energy and is therefore less fatiguing than would be the case if motor units were recruited synchronously (*ibid*).

In order for the two waves to not have "destructive interference" they should not be half a wavelength (of any multiple) from each other.

IONTOPHORESIS AND GALVANIC STIMULATION. Continuous, unidirectional (galvanic) current (DC) is the current of choice for iontophoresis. Other current forms, such as con-

---

5. The LISS Cranial Stimulator is used as a TENS unit and can treat pain by stimulating both "brain" activity and chemicals, placing the pads on the head. It can also treat the extremities by placing the pads there.

Table 8-3: Clinical Iontophoresis (Cummings 1991)

ION	SOURCE	POLARITY	INDICATION
Acetate	Acetic Acid	Negative	Calcium deposits
Chloride	Sodium chloride	Negative	Scars and adhesions
Copper	Copper sulfate	Positive	Fungus infections
Dexamethasone	Decadron (brand name)	Negative	Inflammation
Hyoluronidase	Wyadase	Positive	Edema
Magnesium	Mag sulfate (Epsom salts)	Positive	Muscle spasm
Salicylate	Sodium salicylate	Positive	Edema
Tap water		Alternating polarity	Hyperhydrosis
Xylocaine	Xylocaine/Lidocaine	Positive	Pain
Zinc	Zinc oxide	Positive	Dermal wounds

ventional pulsed high-voltage, sine wave, asymmetrical biphasic, and interferential currents are not effective in iontophoresis. Galvanic stimulation is usually characterized by high voltage pulsed stimulation and is used primarily to treat local edema. Edema is often comprised of negatively charged plasma proteins, which leak into the interstitial spaces. Galvanic stimulation is thought to work by having the negative electrode placed over the edematous area which may repel the charged plasma toward the positive electrode (Lenz's law), which is placed at a distant site (proximally). Due to the risks of electrical burns from DC currents, the stimulation is usually kept under 1 mA/cm^2. Also, because the caustic effects from alkalinity under the cathode (-) pole is greater than the acidic reaction under the anode (+) pole, the practitioner reduces the current under the cathode by increasing the cathode (-) electrode size—it should be at least twice the size of the anode. The practitioner should also keep in mind that DC currents have anesthetic effects on the skin, and, therefore, the patient may not be aware of ensuing burns (Cummings 1991, *ibid*). In iontophoresis low volt stimulators are usually used. Low voltage direct current is also used to stimulate denervated muscles where peripheral nerve injuries have occurred. Table 8-3 summarizes common substances used in (biomedical) iontophoresis.

When combining acupuncture and iontophoresis, a medicinal ampule can be cut at the bottom and the glass smoothed. An herbal extract, usually containing herbs that clear Wind, Cold, and promote Qi and Blood circulation are placed in the ampule filling about a third of it. The ampule is placed on the skin and a syringe is used to draw out the air, creating the needed suction. Then an acupuncture needle is inserted through the rubber stop, which can either penetrate the skin or just contact it. A monopolar stimulator is then connected to the needle handle (only if the polarity of the medicines are known). Stimulation lasts fifteen to forty-five minutes and is repeated daily or every other day (Figure 8-4). Because the polarity of herbal formulation is usually not known, the solution can be placed at both ends and a monopolar wave form used (this however may not result in iontophoresis and no penetration studies are available).

TRANSCUTANEOUS STIMULATION (TENS). Transcutaneous stimulation is often used to treat pain. TENS can be prescribed for home use and therefore can be a cost-effective method of treating pain. TENS can be used for acute and chronic pain, but clinical efficacy evidence is mixed. There are currently four major TENS modes used in clinical practice (Walsh 1997). *Conventional TENS* is a high-frequency, low intensity TENS and is the most commonly used. Typically, the frequency is around 100 Hz and pulse duration is usually short (50-80 microseconds, [ms]). The effect is usually of quick onset and short-lasting analgesia. The pads are usually placed over the painful area. *Acupuncture-like-TENS* is a low-frequency (1-4 Hz), high- intensity TENS, which primarily stimulates type III and IV nociceptors and small motor fibers. The pulse duration tends to be long—about 200 ms. This type of stimulation can result in muscle contractions. These contractions are thought to be important. The pads are placed over the myotome related to the painful area. *Burst train (sequential) TENS* is a combination of conventional TENS and acupuncture-like-TENS, in which a low-frequency baseline stimulation is delivered and which contains high-frequency trains (also called dense disperse). Typically, the baseline frequency is 1-4 Hz with internal frequency trains of around 100 Hz (such as the Han frequency). The pads can be used locally, over related myotomes, or both. *Brief, intense TENS* uses a high-frequency (100-150 Hz), long pulse duration (150-240 ms) and highest tolerable intensity for a short time (< 15 min). This type of stimulation is often recommended for procedural pain such as skin debridement. The pads can be placed locally or on related dermatomes.

Other TENS methods are available as well. DC-TENS can be used to treat a variety of painful disorders as it can functionally interrupt the pathways running in certain nerves (Jenkner 2002). The small anode (+), which is placed directly over the nerve transmitting the pain, "focusses" dense electric field lines along that nerve—which can be a peripheral or sympathetic nerve. The larger cathode (-) can be placed over the opposite surface of the trunk or extremity, or it can be placed at the contralateral appropriate spinal level, over a back Shu point or related segment.

Forty minutes of stimulation seems to be the optimal treatment duration of TENS treatment of knee pain (Cheing et al 2003). The treatment can be repeated several times per day; however, in animal studies the repeated administration of low- and high-frequency TENS leads to a development of opioid tolerance. Clinically, it may be inferred that a treatment schedule of repeated daily TENS administration should be avoided to possibly obviate the induction of tolerance (Chandran and Sluka 2003).

Microamp TENS delivers a below-sensory-level stimulation and is said to encourage healing. It is less frequently used in the treatment of pain. Data collection by Lynn and Wallace (1990) showed microcurrent therapy to be affective in reducing pain during the first treatment in 94% of 1531 patients. A popular and well-studied device, Alpha-Stim[R] uses a random, biphasic stimulation (10-600 microamps continuously adjustable, 0.5, 1.5 or 100 Hz, bipolar asymmetrical rectangular wave, and 50% duty cycle) and has been used in the treatment of pain as well as psychiatric disorders. "Transcranial" stimulation is achieved by connecting the Alpha-Stim to the earlobes. The LISS stimulator has also been used to treat psychiatric and pain disorders. It uses a modulated waveform with a carrier wave of 15,000 Hz and a first modulated wave of 15 Hz and a second of 500 Hz transmitted simultaneously. (This causes an harmonic.) The current is usually in the micro-to-miliamp range. The LISS stimulator can also be used to stimulate acupoints. A high-frequency "carrier" wave (either in micro- or miliamp stimulation) referred to as interferential stimulation is used.

True *interferential stimulation* uses two biphasic medium-frequency currents simultaneously (four electrodes). Higher frequencies lower tissue resistance eliciting a stronger response with a lower current intensity. This allows for stronger stimulation since these frequencies decrease sensory perception between the electrodes and more current can be handled. The two currents are superimposed when the electrodes are placed diagonally across the area of treatment. Through constructive interference, the perceived stimulation is concentrated in the target area, providing a tingling and massaging sensation (Boniquit et al 2002). A carrier wave is not need when doing electroacupuncture.

The type of TENS to be used may depend on previous patient and practitioner experience. Most of the time, conventional TENS is tried first, as most patients find the light tingling associated with high-frequency stimulation soothing and less painful or frightening than acupuncture-like-TENS. The intensity and duration of stimulation should be increased slowly, and the patient should understand that more is not necessarily better. The first session may last thirty minuets or so. After the initial session, the duration may be increased to one hour, and the intensity may be experimented with. It is advisable to stop stimulation for a while every hour or so to prevent adaptation and loss of efficacy. It is best to have a unit that allows for adjustments of frequency, intensity, and

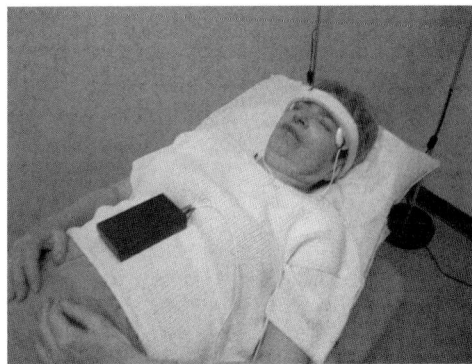

Figure 8-6: Patient treated with LISS stimulator.

pulse duration, as all of these parameters may need to be adjusted to any individual patient or changed when one setting stops to be effective. Pad placement may be experimented with as well. In general, pads are placed at the painful area, the related peripheral nerve (related channel), the related spinal segment (back-Shu-point), or at specific points such as motor points, trigger points, or acupuncture points. The use of superficial electrodes instead of needles using acupuncture-like-TENS (pulse width 0.3 ms; frequency of 2 and 100 Hz) can produce the same analgesic effects achieved by electroacupuncture (Han *ibid*).

While the type of TENS to be used often needs to be chosen based on trial and error, in general, when treating an acute soft tissue injury, a low-frequency, high-intensity TENS (or electroacupuncture) may not be appropriate, as this may cause increased pain from muscle contractions. Low frequency (acupuncture-like-TENS) is more appropriate over muscular tissues as muscle contraction pulses are thought to be an important component of the therapy. (The muscle should be placed in a shortened position to avoid strain.) Therefore, when treating bony and joint capsules directly, acupuncture-like-TENS may not be the best type of stimulation. During the subacute stage of soft tissue injury, however, using acupuncture-like-TENS (or electroacupuncture) with the effected muscle in a shortened position can result in mild and comfortable contraction and may prevent adhesion formation.

Frequency and Intensity

Many neurotransmitters and physiologic mediators have been implicated in the many electrostimulation, electromagnatism, and electroacupuncture effects. Most studies show normal bodily biomagnetic and bioelectromagnetic fields to vary between 2-30 Hz (although some state that the basic bodily friquency is 72Hz). The frequency of *electrical stimulation* used in treatment appears to have specific effects summarized in Table 8-7. When speaking of frequency and pulse repetition Becker (*ibid*) thinks that when a pulse is composed of a number of other individual pulses of a higher frequency,

Table 8-4: Healing Effects of Specific Frequencies

Frequency (Hz)	Effects
2	Nerve regeneration
7, 15	Bone growth
10	Ligament healing
15, 20, and 75	Stimulation of capillary formation and fibroblast proliferation
25 and 50	Synergistic effects with nerve growth factor

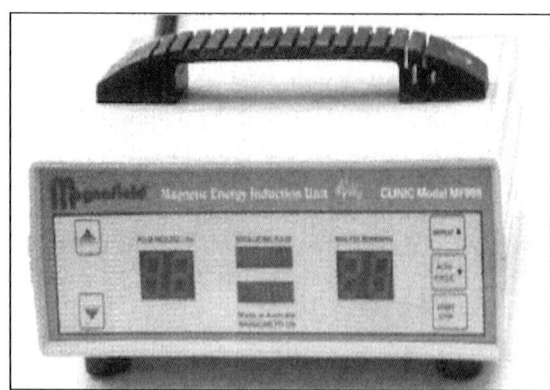

Figure 8-7: Magnafield.

the effects are going to depend upon the relationship between these parameters, as to which one the body is most likely to "see." When a fairly low frequency, like 15 Hz is modulated with a couple of hundred Hz, or even higher frequency in the individual pulses within each pulse burst, Becker thinks there would not be much of an effect from the high frequency but the effect will be due to the body "rectifying" the whole wave and looking at it as a 15 Hz signal which is closer to normal body frequencies. (15 Hz is often used in bone-growth stimulators.) This is an opinion and is not backed up with data.

At the same time high frequency stimulation can be used to induce numbness or neural blockade (Woessner 2002) and may be more appropriate for neuropathic pain (although Han emphasizes low frequency with shorter duration of high frequency stimulation when using electroacupuncture to treat neuropathic pain). It seems that the effects of high frequency (80 Hz and above) are mediated more by catecholamine than opioid mechanisms. Muscle spasms may respond better to 100 Hz versus 2 Hz. 2-Hz electrical stimulation seems to effect the reticular formation, resulting in nonsegmental analgesia (Browsher 1975), and a decrease in sympathetic tone for >10 hours. 3-Hz results in even longer effects on sympathetics (Andersson *ibid*). Healing effects of specific frequencies have been described by Sisken and Walker (*ibid*) and summarized in Table 8-4.

The most accepted effects of electomagnetic frequencies within *electromagnetic* therapy circles are summarized in Table 8-5. Other specific effects for electromagnetic frequencies are summarized in Table 8-6 (Tume *ibid*).

As can be seen from the above tables, there are a number of frequencies that cover a wide range of clinical uses. It generally comes down to practitioner preference and experience as to which frequencies to use. While electromagnetic fields are used to transmit a specific frequency into biological tissue, they are also transmitting an electromagnetic filed with a gauss rating. Depending on the number of coils of wire in magnetic pads, you will get a different gauss rating. Generally these are only small (in the range of 500 to 1000 gauss), but they will still have an underlying beneficial affect, which is synergistic with the modulated frequency that is used. Although some clinical evidence has been put forth to support the above parameters, additional high quality controlled studies are still greatly needed.

Equipment. Electromagnetic therapy can be delivered via electroacupuncture (electrical pulses delivered to needles or to fixed magnets) or by instruments designs to deliver an electomagnetic field. The Diapulse (electromagnetic stimulator) emits 27 MHz (25 million pulses per second) and is said to reduce swelling, accelerate wound healing, stimulate nerve regeneration, reduce pain, and hasten functional recovery (Sisken and Walker *ibid*). The Curaton PC has preprogramed frequencies and time-settings to treat various conditions. Most of the programs use varying frequencies and intensities to "prevent adaptation." The Magnafield is another instrument which is commonly used clinically. It has a preset treatment time of twenty minutes, but this does not mean that one needs to use the full twenty minutes for every patient. For example, when treating young children and in certain cases elderly people, one can use shorter treatment times, as these groups will respond to treatment quicker than most. However, for the average-aged patient, the full twenty minutes can be used quite comfortably. In most cases, treatment every second day is sufficient, and adjunctive therapies such as acupuncture, laser, and static magnetic therapy can be used. When integrating other therapies, one should remember, however, that laser therapy and electromagnetic therapy should not be used at the same time, as the field produced by electromagnetic machines can interfere with the laser diode and possibly cause it to malfunction.

In most cases, one starts to see results within the first week or so, but this is dependant on many factors, such as the stage of the ailment (acute or chronic), the systems of the body affected, age of the patient, the general health of the patient, diet, and lifestyle. Therefore, it is important to take into account all of these factors, and in certain cases suggest

Bioenergetic Field Therapy

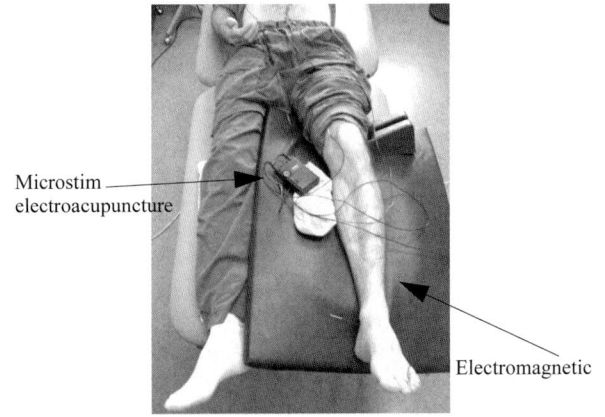

Figure 8-8: Patient with medial collateral ligament strain treated with combined electroacupuncture (P-6 and K-3) and electro magnetic therapy. A wedge is used to reduce physical stress. (Potentially a magnetic field may interfere with the electronics of the microstim however the measured output was not effects)

dietary and lifestyle changes to help the patient recover from the condition and lead a healthier life from that point on.

Table 8-5: Most Accepted Frequencies In Electromagnetic Therapy

Frequency (Hz)	Effect
8 and below	Causes vaso-dilation.
12 and above	Causes vaso-constriction.
0.87 - 3	For tendons, muscles, nervous system in harmony with blood and lymph.
2	Used where there is inflammation or infection.
3 - 8	For central and peripheral nervous system.
1 - 4	Used to fight infections by stimulation of phagocytes and the immune system in general.
4	Used to counteract muscular and nervous spasm and is found to be sedating.
4 - 8	Used for its sedative effect to help counteract muscular spasm.
8	Used as an analgesic tonic and is seen to be stabilizing; stabilization helps to stop pain.
5 - 13	Alpha to Theta range of Brain waves.

Table 8-6: Additional Frequencies used in Electromagnetic Therapy

Frequency (Hz)	Effects
8 - 16	Used for its analgesic tonic and stabilizing effects.
15	Commonly used to treat bone fracture nonunion.
16	Specific for rheumatic complaints (more specifically in chronic cases).
16 - 32	Used for its generally stimulating effects.
32	Stimulating and tonifying.
1 - 32	Generally used for acute pain syndromes or compulsive disorders.
3 - 4 (Delta Waves)	Related to deep sleep and certain brain disorders.
4 - 7 (Theta Waves)	Related to various stages of sleep and during emotional stress.
8 - 14 (Alpha Waves)	Related to a normal and alert state of mind.
14 - 50 (Beta Waves)	Related to the frontal portion of the brain during intense mental activity.

Generally speaking, in the clinical setting, after taking the case history, one can apply an electromagnetic treatment. Then one can safely use button magnets for the patient between visits to continue the treatment away from the clinic. In this way, the practitioner can continue the treatment without the need for the patient to keep coming to the clinic on a daily basis, even though the latter is preferable although impractical for most patients. Laser can also be used after the electromagnetic treatment and before applying button magnets to help accelerate healing in most cases. As these are all non-invasive forms of therapy, they are quite safe to use in this fashion (Tume *ibid*). For information on electroacupuncture instrumentation see below.

INTENSITY OF STIMULATION. In general, *mild stimulation* (both in manual and electroacupuncture, and in electrotherapy) of large nerve fibers will have mainly segmental effects. *Moderate stimulation* of large fibers would have mixed effects but still mainly segmental, and *strong stimulation* has more general (nonsegmental) and possibly anti-inflammatory effects (Han *ibid*, Stux and Pomeranz *ibid*). However, lower-intensity electroacupuncture stimulation of 2mA (or < 1mA) seems to be better than higher intensity stimulation (2-3mA) for the treatment of *chronic pain* from *inflammation* and when the pain is of *neuropathic* origin (Han 1998, *ibid*). Other authors, however, found that high-intensity electroacupuncture stimulation is more effective than low-intensity in *chronic* pain patients (Mao et al 1980).

High-level electroacupuncture or via TENS stimulation is likely to be accompanied by visible muscular contractions which may be important therapeutically (and may further stimulate bata-endorphins and mechanoreceptors). Increasing the level of electroacupuncture stimulation to above pain threshold can result in additional analgesia (Han *ibid*). High-intensity electroacupuncture may be most appropriate for acute pain states, especially C-fiber responses. The effects however are also dependent on the frequency with low-frequency-high-intensity electroacupuncture (2-5 Hz, 5-6 mA) producing the strongest analgesia. The inhibition of C-responses induced by weak electroacupuncture tend to increase progressively with increased frequency, highest at 50 Hz (Han *ibid,* You et al 1999).

Microcurrent TENS stimulation and electroacupuncture have been advocated because their closeness to the body's "natural currents" that seem to be in the microcurrent range (10 to 30 µA; Backer *ibid*). Microcurrent stimulation has been shown to stimulate adenosine triphosphate (ATP) production, and this may aid in tissue-healing. Stimulation at a miliamp current rage seems to decrease ATP production (Cheng et al 1982). Cheng also found that aminoisobutyric acid uptake increased dramatically beginning at 10 microamps and inhibitory effects began at 750 microamps. Uptake of aminoisobutyric acid is essential for protein synthesis and membrane transport, and showed an increase of 30 - 40% with microstimulation. Slandish (1984) has stated that implanted electrodes delivering 10-20 µA of current hastened the recovery of injured athletes suffering from ruptured ligaments and tendons. Most microcurrent devices with low voltage (MENS) use a longer duty cycle that results in as much as 50% increase in stimulation time regardless of the frequency selected. This may make these devices less suitable for electroacupuncture, as they may be more apt to cause electrolysis of the needles (but they are not problematic with disposable needles and due to the low current used in microstim probably do not cause any harm). An interrupted pulse can be used which allows the tissues to discharge (i.e., tissue capacitance). A modified square wave in a monopolar setting may act as DC stimulation. A TENS device such as MIRCO-Plus™ can be adapted for acupuncture use (Figure 8-8). The use of microcurrents allows for the use of longer bursts in which *resonance* is possible (when using square waves as achieved with the Alpha-Stim). This would be more difficult when using mA currents because it may cause burning. The majority of electroacupuncture research, however, has been undertaken with stimulation in the mA range. When using microcurrent to treat a fast twitch muscle a higher frequency may be required than when treating a slow twitch muscle.

More research is needed to demonstrate the efficacy (and advantages) of microcurrent, as both positive and negative studies have been published. Many wave forms and intensities such as H-wave, modulated, ramped, multi-channel random, etc., have been tried, but no clear advantages have emerged.[6]

Electroacupuncture

The use of electricity to augment the therapeutic effects of acupuncture has a long history. In 1765, a Japanese acupuncturist, Gennai Hiaga, reported the use of electrical stimulation on acupuncture needles. In 1825, the French physician, Chevalier Sarlandiere, described the application of an electric current applied to acupuncture needles to treat rheumatic conditions (Ulett 1992). In 1921, Dr. Goulden reported on the successful treatment of neuritis with electroacupuncture in the *British Journal of Medicine*. Since the 1950s, practitioners in the Orient have been using and researching the use of electroacupuncture extensively. (The first electroacupuncture device produced in China was in 1934.)

Jaffe et al (1982) showed that the human skin has a resting potential across its epidermal layer of 2-90mV with the outside of the skin being negative and the inside positive. It is possible that acupuncture needles "short circuit" this "endogenous battery" and result in electrotheraputic messages, including the initiation of the so-called "current of injury" and the facilitation of intrinsic repairs. If acupuncture points are a low-resistance (low-impedance) pathway in the skin, they could provide a path of least resistance for currents driven by the natural 2-90mV resting potential over the skin. This would be consistent with the 5mV higher readings found in acupoints compared to surrounding skin (Pomeranz *ibid*). Electroacupuncture devices may aid to influence such electrical phenomenon.

Early in the field of electroacupuncture, the German physician Reinhold Voll developed an instrument that is said to be capable of both diagnosis and treatment, as did Nakatani with the Ryodoraku instrument.[7] According to Starwyn, a six-second mircrostimulation in patients with pathologies results in a consistent increase of skin electrical conductivity as compared to "healthy" controls which he measures with the positive electrode proximal and negative distal. Voll also measures the point's "response" to stimulation and says that a great indicator drop after an initial high measurement is probably the most important and safest diagnostic sign of a pathological change in the measured organ and should be taken as an alarm signal (Leonhardt 1980). Strarwynn claims

---

6. H-wave stimulation is a form of electrical stimulation that differs from other forms of electrical stimulation, such as TENS, in terms of its waveform. H-wave stimulation has been used for the treatment of pain related to a variety of etiologies, such as diabetic neuropathy, muscle sprain's, temporomandibular joint dysfunctions or reflex sympathetic dystrophy. H-wave stimulation has also been used to accelerate healing of wounds, such as diabetic ulcers. H-wave is said to emulate the H waveform found in nerve signals (Hoffman reflex) and may penetrate the body with lower frequencies and currents as compared to other stimulators. H-wave is a bipolar exponentially decaying wave of 2, 16, and 50 Hz. All the frequency are delivered together and therefore the wave allows the therapist to apply two "treatments" at the same time— low frequency muscle stimulation and high frequency deep analgesic pain control.

7. Unfortunately, little validation has been provided for either (as well as other instruments such as the Vaga) with *high quality* controlled studies.

Table 8-7: Effects of Electrical Frequencies in Electroacupuncture/stimulation

SOURCE	FREQUENCY	INTENSITY	RESPONSE
Le Bars et al. 1979	Low	High	Activation of A delta and C fibers
Cheng, Pomeranz 1979	Low (2-6 Hz)	High	Tends to activate high threshold A-delta (IIIb) fibers Like strong manual stimulation Opioid systems[a] Slow-onset (20-30 minutes), long-lasting, cumulative analgesia General analgesia, nonsegmental
Melzack, Wall 1965 Cheng, Pomeranz 1979	High (200 Hz)	Low	Activation of thick A-beta and delta (II and IIIa) fibers Like mild manual stimulation Fast onset, short-lasting, non-cumulative analgesia (mostly only during stimulation) Serotonin mediated[b] and may be best for neuropathic pain. Segmental analgesia
Han *ibid*, Stuz and Pomeranz *ibid*.[c]	Low (2 Hz)		Activation of Beta-endorphins, sympathetic inhibition
	Medium (15 Hz)		Activation of Methionin-enkephalin, Leucin-enkephalin and A, B dynorphin[d]
	High (100)		Activation of dynorphin A and B, segmental analgesia, for some types of neural pain
	(Medium 30 Hz)		(All three opioid receptors)
Shanghai Inst. of Physiology	Low (2 Hz) High (90 Hz)		General, distal analgesia Segmental analgesia
Woessner 2002	High (1000-20,000 Hz)		Prevent nerves from repolarizing Conveys more energy to neurons effecting cAMP depletion Results in a nerve block
Lin, Chen and Han 1991 Han ibid.	High 2000 Hz High 5000 Hz High 9100 Hz in human and rat, and 30 Hz in rabbit		Opioid mediated analgesia Nonopioid mediated analgesia Accelerating the release of dynorphin in the spinal cord
Shen et al 1996	Low (2 Hz) Low (4 Hz) Medium to High (8-100 Hz)		Moderate decrease of spinal substance P[e] No change in spinal substance P Marked increase of spinal substance P. 15 Hz increased the most

a. Blocked by naloxone, an opioid blocker.
b. Blocked by chlorophenylalanine, a serotonin synthesis inhibitor.
c. Han states that 2 Hz and 15 Hz release two different kind of opioid peptides.
d. !5 Hz has also been shown to stimulate endomorphin, β-endorphin, enkephalin and dynorphin (Han *ibid*).
e. This may be the best frequency for fibromyalgia patients as they have high levels of substance P in the spinal cord.

that a change in reading is needed for successful treatment of pain and restricted range of motion. Voll also studied the effects of various frequencies extensivly.

Electroacupuncture and manual acupuncture seem to stimulate different regions in the brain. In studying the effects of both on LI-4, Kong et al (2002) found that electroacupuncture mainly produced fMRI signal increase in the precentral gyrus, the postcentral gyrus/inferior parietal lobule, and the putamen/insula; in contrast, manual needle manipulation produced prominent decreases of fMRI signals in the posterior cingulate, the superior temporal gyrus, and the putamen/insula.

Electroacupuncture is usually applied to acupuncture needles using a pulsating electrical current as a means of stimulating the acupoints. Most electroacupuncture devices are designed to deliver variable amplitudes and frequencies. Their waveforms and pulse widths are usually fixed, and the duration of the positive pulse is usually between 0.2-0.4 milliseconds (ms; Figure 8-9). This duration of stimulation minimizes the activation of unmyelinated C-fibers (i.e., naked

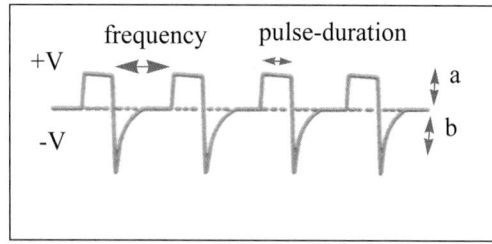

Figure 8-9: The modified saw-tooth (square) wave is the most commonly used with acupuncture stimulators. a) shows the positive (or polarization) phase of stimulation. b) shows the negative (or depolarization) phase of the stimulation (i.e., nerve depolarization or stimulation).

pain fibers which can get activated when the pulse width/duration is above 0.6ms). Usually the current used is between 0-16 milliampere (mA) with an upper limit of about 40 mA, usually via TENS. (Most commonly 2-10 mA is used for electroacupuncture, and 8-15 mA for a stamp-sized skin are via TENS). 3-8 mA is usually the sensory threshold, and double sensory threshold is often recommended for the treatment of pain; this however can lead to muscle contractions and may be uncomfortable especially with high frequencies. Some newer acupuncture stimulators are said to deliver currents in the microamp range; however, if turned up, the current is often within the patient's sensory range and probably more likely to be in the mA range. When using the so-called dense disperse (high and low) rates/frequency a good solution would be to increase the pulse width to 0.6ms during the low frequency cycle and decrease it to 0.2ms during the high frequency cycle. However as stated earlier most electroacupuncture devices use a fixed pulse width. Because it is the negative pulse that stimulates nerve tissues symmetrical biphasic wave forms have been advocated (Pomeranz ibid).[8] This may be due to the emphasis on neural paradighm in electroacupuncture research and ignore the possible safe uses of monophasic stimulation and their biological effects.[9]

---

8. The WQ-6F stimulator shown on Figure 8-12 does modulate the pulse width between the X10 frequency setting and the X1 setting. Circuit B X10 setting is set at pulse width of 0.2-0.3ms while in circuit one this setting is 0.4-0.6ms. In both circuit one and two the pulse width in the X1 setting is 0.6-0.8.

9. Even if a "net-DC" would occur the tissues stimulated would probably act as capacitors discharging most of the current absorbed during rest periods (rest periods between pulses and will depend on the duration of the rest period between pulses). This has been shown in a rabbit bone none-union study comparing pulsed and non-pulsed currents (Richez, Chamay and Biele 1972). A newly published study used implanted electrode devices in paralyzed shoulder muscle of post stoke patients. The muscles were stimulated with a monopolar wave form for at least one hour per day without any negative effects. The patients shoulder instabilities improved dramatically.

When using a wave form which has a "net-DC" effect some advocate the placement of the cathode (-), which excites (depolarize) the nerve, proximally to the anode (+). This is said to allow impulse transmission to the CNS to be "unimpeded." This is recommended with the neural gate theory in mind, i.e., activating large fibers in the direction of the CNS. This however is contra to others which advice the use of opposite placement, which is said to be the normal polarity of the body.

The common range of voltage is about 0-24V with an upper limit at 60V (usually not used with needles). The range of frequency is usually from 1-300Hz, but some instruments can go up as high as 10,000Hz.

Most electroacupuncture devises administer variations of alternating current (AC): square wave, modified square wave or sawtooth wave, and may be symmetric biphasic, alternating or asymmetrical biphasic, of varying configurations. Therefore, most electroacupuncture instruments do not have a true polarity (i.e., positive and negative leads regardless of wire color code). Some devices use direct current (DC), but the use of these has been discouraged as it can cause a local burn and can ionize the needles, which may make the needle brittle. Ionazation also increases resistance and may therefore result in decreased stimulation. Some devises have a modified wave which stimulates one pole (or direction, called monopolar square wave) and then stop before stimulating the same pole again and therefore have a polar bias. These can be considered as having a polar effect.[10] The rest period, if long enough, allows the tissues to discharge. Because the size of the two electrodes (i.e., the needles) are the same, when using DC-like electroacupuncture the current should be kept low to avoid burning (unless it is the desired effect such as in "electroacupuncture-prolotherapy"). When using silver needles to increase the antibiotic effects of electroacupuncture (inducing sliver ions), a low current is sufficient.

THE PHYSICS OF POWER IN ASYMMETRIC WAVE FORMS. Some manufactures of acupuncture electrostimulators state that only *symmetrical* biphasic wave forms do not have polar effects, and do not produce a so-called net-DC effect, which may cause ionazation which occur with asymmetrical electroacupuncture wave forms. This however is not always true as asymmetrical bipolar waves may be designed to achieve a net-0 effect; it will depend on the algorithmic design of the wave (i.e., how much current is allowed to move in the positive and negative phase of the wave, called the effective current). An oscillating voltage wave form applied to a device is able to produce instantaneous power equal to the square of the current times the resistance of the circuit where the power is expended ($P=I^2 R$). Based on this, it can be derived that the average power (P_{av}) expended in a circuit for a sine wave (alternating current; Figure 8-10 [a]) is the sum of all incremental ordinates squared time the resistance (the same applies to voltage V since $V= I R$, and R is a constant). By means of mathematical calculus, the result can be demonstrated to be: $P_{av} = 1/2\, R\, I_m^2$ (R= resistance of circuit, I_m = maximum ordinate of the sine wave). Assume now that the same resistance is calculated in a Direct Current (DC) circuit

---

10. While some modified saw-tooth acupuncture stimulators may result, at times, in one pole of the device showing local bleeding as compared to the other lead, this may be due to a "pulsed current" effect (i.e., short duration high intensity stimulation usually at the negative pole) and not due to a polar effect. Asymmetrical biphasic stimulation does not work for iontophoresis which relies on polar effects showing little if any polar effects.

Bioenergetic Field Therapy

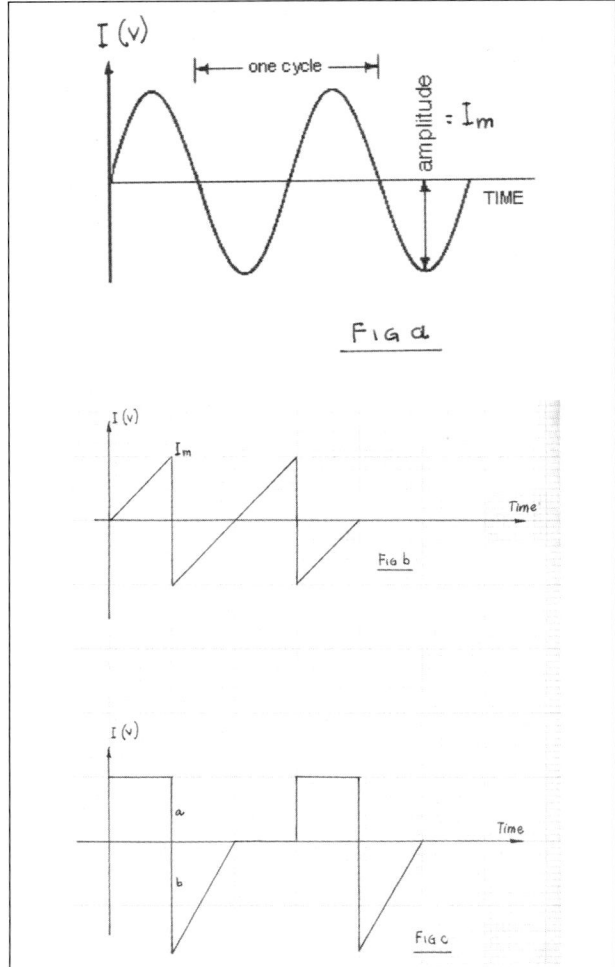

Figure 8-10: Effective currents with differing wave forms. Figure c shows an asymmetrical biphasic wave form with 0 "net-DC" effect.

until the power dissipated is equal to that dissipated by the resistance in an AC circuit. We can explain this as $RI^2=1/2\ RI^2_m$ or $I=1$ divided by square root of 2 times I_m; or $0.707\ I_m$. This is called the effective current. Following the same method for a triangle wave (Figure 8-10, b) it can be demonstrated that $I_{eff}=1$ divided by square root of 3 times I_m; or $I_{eff}=0.578\ I_m$. Now if we have an alternating wave as shown in Figure 8-10 (c) (approximation of real output curves of acupuncture simulators) in which a=0.578 b, the effective value of the triangular side of the wave will be equal to that of the square side (equivalent to DC input). The DC voltage equivalent of the alternating wave shown (asymmetric biphasic square wave) will be zero. The energy produced (power during a lapse of time) will be the sum of the one produced by the square wave, plus the one produced by the triangular wave.

PRACTICAL CLINICAL USE. In China (in general), the needles are first stimulated manually to attain the De Qi (needle sensation), then the needles are connected to the electrostimulator. The electrical stimulation then substitutes for frequent or prolonged manual stimulation and allows for a stronger stimulation if needed. Electroacupuncture is often used to treat neurological diseases, including acute and chronic pain, "spasms," and paralysis and is also used in surgical anaesthesia/analgesia. Strong stimulation is often used in cases of paralysis and neuralgia (although some advocate weak stimulation for neuralgias). It should also be mentioned that some studies have shown negative effects with strong muscle electrostimulation to paralyzed muscles. Since muscle atrophy and damage may take a long time to develop, it may be unwise to use strong stimulation on muscles with a recent onset of paralysis. Nerves grow at rate of about one inch per month, so innervation to the muscle may reestablish itself before any permanent damage results in muscular tissues. The addition of electrical simulation (via surface pads) has not shown clear positive effects in such cases.

Electrical frequency and intensity can be controlled and may have specific effects. During treatment, the patient may become adapted to the stimulus (lose sensation), especially when using constant (non-alternating) pulse stimulation (or if needle ionazation occurs). The intensity may be increased (or frequency changed) to resume sensation. Variable frequency output can be used to circumvent adaptation (so-called "dense disperse pulse waves" which usually only mean two pulse rates not a change in true frequencies; Figure 8-11). Another possibility is to use constant current devices. Constant current devises however are not readily available.

For analgesic effects, Han recommends an alternating stimulation switching between 2Hz, (15Hz), and 100Hz every three seconds. This is said to stimulate all four types of endogenous opioids and catecholamines—the so-called "Han frequency," and is also said to be better than having two devices, one set at 2Hz and the other at 100Hz.[11] Repeated "Han-stimulation" is said to induce the expression of the opioid peptides and the enzyme-coding genes involved in monoamine (catecholamine, neurotransmitters) synthesis, which results in a prolonged and *cumulative* therapeutic effect.

Electrosimulating acupuncture devices should not be turned on until the needles are in place and the electrodes connected. All changes in intensity or frequency should be carried out gradually to avoid sudden pain, excessive spasm (especially with dense-disperse) or twitching of the muscles. The proper amount of stimulation is dependent on patient tolerance and the condition for which he/she is being treated. In general, it should be in the range between just sensing the electrical effect and being uncomfortable. High intensity with high frequency is said to be "sedating," while low intensity and low frequency are more "tonifying." (However no real criteria or proof have been provided for these beliefs,

---

11. Han recommends using local/segmental points as well as LI-4 for maximum release of endogenous opioid peptides and catecholamines (neurotransmitters). The use of St-36 will increase the effects. This can be done as acupuncture-like-TENS as well which would be more comfortable to the patient.

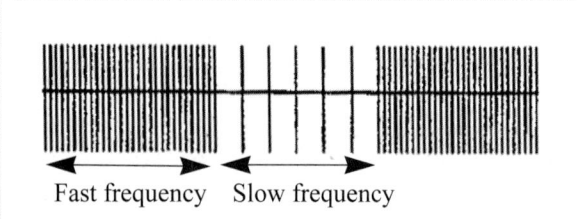

Figure 8-11: Dense-disperse pulse rate.

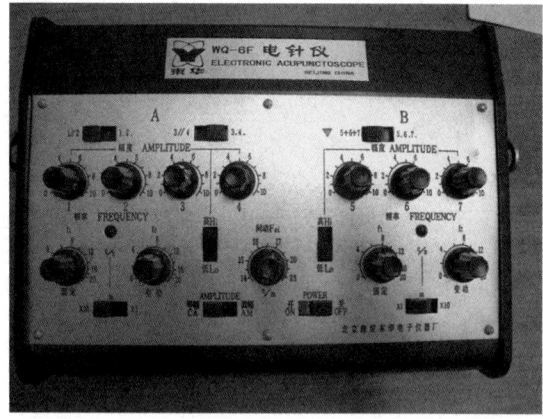

Figure 8-12: Typical electroacupuncture instrument. This one has two separate circuits, continuos amplitude (CA) or ramped amplitude (AM), and two setting for frequencies that can achieve different combinations. The two circuits can be used out of phase to create additive fields and harmonics. There are 8 variations of waveforms with differing pulse frequencies that can be achieved with combinations of the various settings: continuos, intermittent, dense- disperse, rise- fall (modulation), normal sawtooth, inverse sawtooth, rise dense- fall disperse, and fall dense- rise disperse. When the resistance between the two needles is 250 Ohm, the peak current is 40 mA at 10V.

they are usually surmised from comparison with traditional manual needle manipulation). Clinically, therefore it is often recommended that the practitioner use stronger stimulation when trying to sedate a "spasmed" muscle (in order to fatigue the muscle) or when treating pain. For spasms, Han recommends using 100Hz in a ratio of 2:1 with 2Hz stimulation to emphasize dynorphins stimulation. Milder stimulation is often recommended to strengthen a point, channel, or muscle, although as, stated earlier, in China it is common to use very strong stimulation when treating paralysis. High intensity stimulation can produce dorsal root potentials that can result in multi-segmental (generalized) effects (Han *ibid*). For neuropathic pain, Han recommends low frequency and low intensity stimulation. His devise, however, still incorporates 100Hz bursts, but less frequently than slow waves of electrical depolarization when used for regular analgesia. It is recommended that one use electrical stimulation only on experienced acupuncture patients, as electroacupuncture is more likely to cause vaso-vagal reactions. (The patient should be lying down to prevent a fall.)

In musculoskeletal practice a device capable of delivering mono-polar stimulation or DC current may be useful. Electroacupuncture can then be used with the appropriate electrode placed at the points that activate the applicable channel system or tissues. In general, the cathode (-) pole/lead is considered to have a "tonifying" (stimulating) effect (Kenyon 1983), although the anode (+) shows greater proliferative effects on soft tissues in *some* studies and therefore may be considered tonifying. Other studies show a higher proliferation of cells near the cathode pole.[12] Nerves grown in cell cultures under a weak DC electrical field show maximal growth to be near the cathode (-) pole (Baker *ibid*).[13]

"Holes" made by needling are said to cause a negativity at the site of injury due to the current of the injury (Pomeranz *ibid*). Often for pain *channel treatments,* the cathode (-) pole may be used at the distal areas and the anode (+) pole at proximal areas (mostly for peripheral joint pain), to move/activate Qi proximally in the direction of the Sinew channels (which is also said to be the "polarity of the body"). Electrical stimulation may be used to facilitate (tonify) circulation, or inhibit (sedate) circulation within the channel. To promote circulation, the cathode (-) pole may be used close to the origin of the channel (points with lower numbers) and the anode (+) pole down stream.[14] To sedate, the electrodes are switched and the anode (+) pole is used close to the origin of the channel. Electrical stimulation is used together with local or special function points to channel the Qi/energy to and through the lesion.

The polar effects can be also used to influence blood circulation, tissue proliferation, nerve excitation, therapeutic ions, change tissue pH, treat edema, etc.

While electroacupuncture is reported to be safe, it is generally recommended that one avoid placing the elec-

---

12. There is controversy regarding which pole is "tonifying" and which is "sedating" or if there is such effects at all.

13. In electroacupuncture field of medicine, polar effects are often viewed as having negative and/or damaging effects and as stated earlier this may be so because of the neural doctrine which dominates electroacupuncture research (only the negative phase stimulates nerves so that some state that both electrode should be stimulated alternating a negative pulse). However, many studies on humans as well as animals show that DC stimulation can be used safely and may have advantages in some circumstances.

14. It should be remembered however, that the direction of Qi flow within the channels is inconsistent between classic literature. A study by Ionescu-Tirgoviste and Pruna using an electroacupunctureogram that can measure the electrical potential as well as polarity of points (and is said to not significantly stimulate the points on its own) showed that extremity points, for example, can have positive or negative charges in relation to ground. They also state that blockage in the "normal" flow of these currents leads to a high concentration of positive or negative electrical charges that may cause pain and other symptoms of different diseases.

trodes near or across the heart, especially if the patient is using a pace-maker. Whether one should cross the spinal cord is controversial (i.e., treating both sides of Hua Tuo or UB channel points), but the author does not know of any reported problem regarding this, and does so often.

In conclusion, there are still many unanswered questions related to the use of electric stimulators in electroacupuncture and electrotheraputics in general. For example, is micro or miliamp stimulation better? If it is better then for what conditions? Does miliamp stimulation really "fry" the point or tissues as some proponent of microstimulation state? If it does, why were most positive studies on electroacupuncture, or TENS devices, undertaken with miliamp stimulators? What are the best frequencies and intensity settings? What effects can be attributed to polarity or wave forms and do they have clinical advantages? Do asymmetrical wave forms have harmful effects? If yes, does the type of needle (metal) used make a difference? The electronic acupuncture market is replete with instruments for sale and claims about them. While the above discussion did not answer these questions, available information has been reviewed. There is still a great need for high quality studies in the field of electroacupuncture.

Static Magnetic Therapy

When using Static Magnetic Therapy, it is essential to understand the following (Tume *ibid*):

- What Magnets are;
- the Properties of magnets;
- polarity and Poles of magnets;
- effects of Magnets on living tissues.

A magnet can be described basically as a metal having the properties of attracting iron or other ferrous substances, and pointing in a North and South direction (i.e. it acts as a compass). We use magnets and magnetic materials every day, e.g. door catches, fridge magnets, magnetic audio, video, and computer tapes and disks. Magnets are also used in industry and in medicine, e.g., MRI. A "magnet", usually referred to as a "static" or "permanent" magnet, has the most orderly focus of what we may call "matter polarity," whereas a crystal represents the most orderly focus of the "spirit polarity."

A magnet has a *North* and a *South* pole, and, if it is broken into pieces, each piece also has a North and South pole. Magnets have "domains," which are groups of magnetic atoms combining to form miniature magnets. Magnets have "vectors," referred to as "vector potentials" that produce electromotive energy from moving electrons in the magnetic field. An iron bar, if stroked with a magnet, in one direction, will line up these domains, and the iron bar will become a magnet itself.

While permanent magnets are usually not thought of as capable of creating a pulsed field, which is often associated with biological effects, the interaction between the wearer's movements and the static/permanent magnet may actually cause such pulsations. That is the interaction between the magnet and nervous tissues may result in moving electric charges (as shown by Faraday's research of electromagnetic fields). The predominant effects of induced magnetic energy fields in living tissue are as follows:

1. ionic change, shift or balance;
2. stimulation of peripheral circulation;
3. transfer of energy by the electron activity;
4. balancing pH by correct applications;
5. balancing cell wall membrane voltage;
6. correcting calcium and other nutrient transfer.

Magnetic fields are all around us and can be measured, captured for use, or changed. The earth's magnetic field is the most commonly recognized magnetic field, and a compass will indicate the energy flow from the South to the North pole.[15] The magnetic field of a permanent (static) magnet can be determined by instruments such as a compass (Figure 8-13). The lines of a magnetic field from a bar magnet are closed. By convention, the field direction is taken to be outward from the North pole and in toward the South pole of the magnet. Permanent magnets can be made from ferromagnetic materials.

Electric sources are inherently "monopole" or point-charge sources. Magnetic sources are inherently dipole sources: you can't isolate North or South "monopoles." In reference to biological molecules and their dipole status, a dipole is a state which atoms and molecules attain because of their electron charges. It affects the electric and hence the magnetic field when these molecules are in motion. When there is separation of the positive and negative charges within a molecule, the molecule is said to be dipolar. In other words, the molecule looks a little like a miniature magnet (Figure 8-14), having a positive and negative end, or technically a North and a South pole. When dipolar molecules are in this state, they are said to be "polarized," which essentially means that they have polarity or a negative charge at one end and a positive charge at the other. This is the antithesis of a "non-polarized" molecule, which has a disorganized mixture of polarities within the molecule. Body tissue will conduct electricity, so a current will flow through the tissue in the pattern of the electric field through the tissue created by the dipole.

The orbital motion of electrons creates tiny atomic current loops which produce magnetic fields. When an external magnetic field is applied to a material, these current loops

---

15. The earth's magnetic field is known to be weakening and to have changed its polarity several times throughout history. Mice placed in a magnetically insulated cage die showing that magnetic fields are essential for life. The weakening of the earth's magnetic fields therefore may have significant health effects.

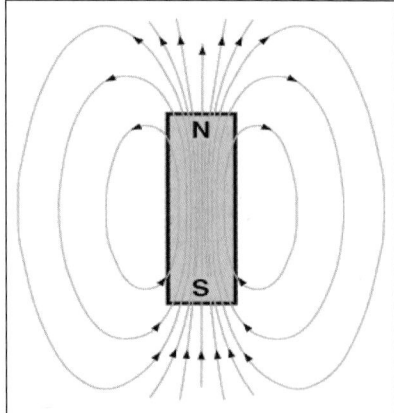

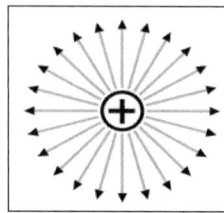

Figure 8-13: Magnetic field of a permanent (static) magnet (with permission Tume *ibid*).

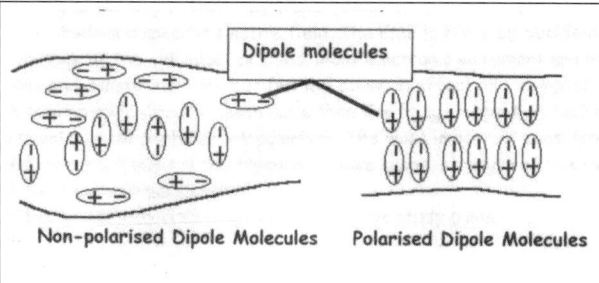

Figure 8-14: Dipole molecule (courtesy of Tume *ibid*).

will tend to align in such a way that they oppose the applied field. This may be viewed as an atomic version of Lenz's law: induced magnetic fields tend to oppose the change which created them. Materials in which this effect is the only magnetic response are called "diamagnetic." All materials are inherently diamagnetic, but if the atoms have some net magnetic moment as in paramagnetic materials, or if there is a long-range ordering of atomic magnetic moments as in ferromagnetic materials, these stronger effects are always dominant. Diamagnetism is the residual magnetic behavior when materials are neither paramagnetic nor ferromagnetic. Any conductor will show a strong diamagnetic effect in the presence of changing magnetic fields, because circulating currents will be generated in the conductor to oppose the magnetic field changes. A superconductor will be a perfect diamagnet since there is no resistance to the forming of the current loops (Tume *ibid*).

Pole Polarity

It is generally accepted that the South-seeking pole of a magnet, hence the *North pole, is the negative polarity*, and the North-seeking pole of a magnet, hence the *South pole, is the positive polarity*. It is important to remember these definitions, as the two polarities are said to have very different effects on biological tissues. Noel Norris describes the different effects of North and South polarities as follows: The North-seeking pole (the South pole of magnet) with Positive polarity effects may (Tume *ibid*):

- increase positive ions and decrease oxygen in cells;
- act to increase the pain of chronic ailments;
- act as a stimulant on the body;
- promote bacterial growth (infections);
- have a negative effect on healing and tissue repair;
- act to increase acidity;
- increase depression;
- tonify acupuncture points;
- improve hypo conditions of major organs;
- decrease fluid retention;
- result in mental hyper-activity and increase symptoms of stress;
- act to increase fat build-up;
- assist in treatment of bruising or inflammation of soft tissue not associated with infection;
- act to contract muscle tissue.

The South-seeking pole (North pole of the magnet) with Negative polarity effects may:

- increase negative ions and increase oxygen in cells;
- act to relieve, inhibit, and control pain of chronic ailments;
- promote restful sleep;
- improve athletic performance;
- fight and counter infection;
- assists fat burning;
- immediately and continuously encourage healing and repair of tissue;
- act to increase alkalinity;
- act to relieve stress symptoms by sedating and calming;
- encourage general well being and contentment;
- disperse acupuncture points;
- improve hyper conditions of major organs;
- increase and enhance mental alertness and function;
- act to relax muscle tissue;
- act on pineal gland to increase melatonin and growth hormone secretion.

As can be seen from the above examples, static magnetic therapy may be useful in a large variety of conditions. While the North and South poles of magnets are specifically used in the above ways, there are also Bi-polar magnets on the market. These are generally accepted as having similar effects to the North pole of a magnet. There is a wide range of magnetic products on the market today. The most commonly used magnetics in the clinic are products made of neodymium and ceramic materials such as:

- Magnetic buttons: commonly in the size range of 2.5 x 2 mm up to 50 x 12.5 mm. These magnets generally range from approximately 500 to 3000 gauss.
- Magnetic Bars: these exist up to 75 x 15 x 10 mm in size and can have slightly larger gauss ratings than the button magnets.
- Magnetic Blocks: up to 50 x 50 x 12.5 mm in size and, again, having a higher rating generally than the accessible button magnets.

Depending on where one purchases these products you may find other ranges of therapeutic magnets such as flexible plastiform strips and other shapes and sizes and gauss ratings. On the other hand, there is a wide range of cosmetic jewelry such as bracelets, rings and necklaces, bed underlays and joint supports and many other products. While some of these may be helpful in a general way, they are not strictly produced for a specific clinical application. That is, for example, an elbow support may provide some relief, but the specific positioning of button magnets on tender points (Ah Shi points) related to an elbow injury may provide more specific energy at the soft tissue and joint structure involved with the injury.

One important point that should be taken into consideration when purchasing any clinical magnet is the gauss rating. It is generally accepted that the higher the gauss rating, the better the therapeutic effect. While this may be true, one needs to be aware that with therapeutic magnets there are actually two gauss ratings. The first is *remnant gauss rating*. This relates to the gauss rating of the magnet at its core. As this energy radiates towards the surface of the magnet, it will reduce in intensity until there is a consistent rating at the surface. This is the *surface gauss rating*. Depending on the material used to produce therapeutic magnets, the reduction between the two ratings can be as high as 50 or 60%. For example, one may have a magnet rated at 3000 gauss; however, a remnant gauss rating of 3000 gauss could be as low as 500 or 600 gauss active surface rating.

Safety of Permanent Magnetic Therapy

Most of the literature suggests that permanent magnetic (or electromagnetic) therapy is safe. Magnetic resonance imaging (MRI) machines expose patients to magnetic fields as high as 15,000 gauss without apparent harm. Some areas in Norway and Sweden have high levels of lodestone and thus high background magnetic fields. People living in these areas do not show any ill effects. A study commissioned by the World Health Organization in 1987 stated that permanent magnetic therapy has never been implicated in any mutagenic process. However, a study by Ardito et al (1984) suggests that exposure of human lymphocyte cultures to a magnetic field of 740 gauss causes a slight increase in chromosome aberration. The applicability to a clinical setting is unknown.

Clinical Evidence

Control studies of magnetic therapy is difficult to design as usually it takes a few days of use to see clinical effects and the difference between a magnetized and non magnetized piece of metal is easy enough to detect. There is mixed evidence for static magnetic therapy with both positive and negative controlled studies. For example, Brown et al (2002) reported that static magnetic field therapy significantly improves disability and may reduce pelvic pain. Active magnets were worn continuously for four weeks over abdominal trigger points in patients with chronic pelvic pain. Blinding in the study however was compromised. Hinman, Ford, and Heyl (2002) reported on the effects of static magnets in patients with chronic knee pain and loss of physical function in a double-blind study. They concluded that the application of static magnets over painful knee joints appears to reduce pain and enhance functional movement. Man, Man and Plosker (1999) reported that permanent magnetic field therapy enhanced wound healing in suction lipectomy (postoperative wounds) patients in a double-blind study. A static magnetic field from a permanent magnet may accelerate and stimulate bone grafting in surgically repaired patients (Rogachefsky 1997). According to Takesshige and Sato (1996) magnetic therapy is as effective in the treatment of pain as is acupuncture. Prince (1983) reported that low strength magnets placed on EAV points is effective in reducing injection pain during surgical interventions. Baron et al (1983) reported that magnets may be effective in treating vertigo secondary to whiplash and head injuries.

On the other hand, Winemiller et al (2003) reported in JAMA that cushioned insoles, with either active bipolar magnets or sham magnets, which were worn daily by the participants for eight weeks showed no difference between sham and active treatment. Martel, Andrews, and Roseboom (2002) compared static and placebo magnets on resting forearm blood flow in young healthy men. Static magnets placed for up to thirty minutes showed no significant alterations in resting blood flow. Alfano et al (2001) reported mixed results in the treatment of fibromyalgia in a randomized controlled trial, although the functional pad groups showed improvements in functional status, pain intensity level, tender point count, and tender point intensity after six months of treatment. With the exception of pain intensity level, these improvements did not differ significantly from changes in the Sham group or in the usual care group.

Principles of Static Magnetic Therapy

To completely understand the nature of why one would use static magnetic therapy for any condition, it is beneficial to understand the body and its magnetic properties and how these might affect the health of a person (Tume *ibid*).

The body is said to be essentially comprised of two magnetic characteristics. The first is *paramagnetic*. Paramagnetism (as discussed in bioenergetic philosophy) is the ability of a substance to retain a magnetic stimulus on a temporary basis. The second is *permanent* magnetism. The body has a number of structures that can be considered to have permanent magnetic characteristics. These structures (organs) contain magnetite crystals (possibly related to calcifications and, in the case of the pineal gland, known as "Brain Sand.") These crystals allow the organs to retain a permanent magnetic field. These structures include:

- the pineal gland;
- neurons;
- bones;
- the ethmoid organ at the back of the nose.

All other structures within the body such as blood, muscles, and other organs are considered to be paramagnetic. That is, when stimulated by a magnetic influence, they will become temporarily magnetized until that stimulus is taken away. This brings us to the effects of local vs. systemic treatment.

Local treatment using magnetic therapy may bring about a temporary magnetism of the tissues in the area where the magnetic field is applied. If this field is applied for long enough, this temporary magnetism may be held by tissues and fluid and may be carried by the blood to other parts of the body. This allows for certain local treatments to bring about a minor systemic response, which may be beneficial for the body. With time and experience one may learn how to affect different areas of the body with localized and distal treatments.

POLARITY OF THE BODY: It is important to be aware of the differences in polarity in the body so that one can better utilize the correct placement of static magnets for beneficial effects. While Philpott states that the brain and spinal cord are positive in nature, and the tissues peripheral to the CNS are negative, Rawls and Davis state that the anterior right side of the body is positive, the anterior left side of the body is negative, the posterior right side of the body is negative and the posterior left side of the body is positive. While both may be right to a certain degree (and further research is needed), it is the concepts that the body is electromagnetically balanced, has polarities, and when disturbed may cause dis-ease, that is important to remember.

It is also important to remember that injuries and the pathophysiology of disease bring about an electro-positive states in biological systems. The application (in most cases) of negative magnetic energy (the North [south-seeking] pole of a magnet) will help the body to neutralize and reduce the positive polar nature of pathogenic conditions (Tume *ibid*).

REVISION OF MAGNETIC EFFECTS: It may be important to understand the different effects that can be achieved by applying different polarities of magnetic energy to the body. By understanding the effects that magnetic polarity is said to produce, one may be better able to specifically treat different conditions with beneficial effects. Philpott lists the effects of *Negative Magnetic Energy*. Some of these are: Increasing cellular oxygen, pulling fluids and gasses, reducing fluid retention, reducing inflammation, relieving or stopping pain, supporting biological healing, and reducing symptoms. *Positive Magnetic Energy* on the other hand will have the opposite effect such as: decreasing cellular oxygen, pushing fluids and gasses, inhibiting healing, increasing pain and inflammation, and intensifying symptoms. Basically, these effects are said to allow one to affect the physiology of each condition in a very specific way, and explain why it is important that one have a firm grasp of anatomy, physiology, pathophysiology and the body's ability to heal itself (Tume *ibid*).

SIDE EFFECTS AND CONTRA-INDICATIONS: While there have been no observed adverse affects from the use of static magnets,[16] there are a number of considerations that must be kept in mind. Firstly, if pain or symptoms are affected adversely, there are a couple of things that can be done. It is important to note here that one must be completely sure that the magnets used are correctly marked. It is essential to use the correct polarity for the indicated condition. Different suppliers will have their magnets marked in different ways. For example, some manufacturers mark the North pole (south-seeking) with a dimple, while others will not mark the magnets in any way. Other manufacturers of block magnets will mark positive in red and negative in green. Therefore when encountering symptomatic aggravation, if there is no indicated reason as to why the condition is aggravated, it is best to remove the magnet or reverse the polarity. If the correct polarity is being used, simply moving the magnet away from the spot slightly may help to reduce these affects.

One other precaution is to be aware of the effects that a magnetic underlay may have on people that are taking medications. There is however little information available and clinical observation may be the only guide.

As with any other modality, there are certain contra-indications the professional Bioenergetic practitioner must be aware of:

- Do not use magnets on the abdomen during pregnancy.
- Do not use magnets over the thoracic area on patients with pacemakers or defibrillators.
- Magnetic underlays should not be used twenty-four hours a day. This can affect adrenal function. Use of magnetic

---

16. Including in the neonatal unit (Moran personal communication).

underlays overnight are acceptable (keeping in mind the precautions relating to those people who are on medication).

- Magnetic therapy should not be used over the abdomen until 1.5 hours after meals. This can affect the process of peristalsis.
- Positive magnetic energy should be applied only under medical supervision.

TYPE OF MAGNETS TO USE: There are many variables that will be encountered when deciding on which types of static magnets to use. Blechman et al (2002) has shown that over-the-counter magnets studied showed the actual field flux density measurements to be significantly lower than the values claimed by suppliers. This can have significant implications in clinical practice. Variables can be as follows:

- Button magnets: These are the most common magnets used for sports injuries and for very specific point treatments such as magnetic acupuncture point stimulation or treatment of specific muscles and ligaments. These are generally cost-effective and very easy for any one to use.
- Plastiform magnets: These can be used for larger treatment areas such as large muscle tears or joint problems.
- Block Magnets: These are generally used in a clinical setting for initial practitioner treatments. They can be a bit too expensive for patients to buy and treat themselves with. Generally, practitioners might treat a condition with block magnets in the clinic and provide button magnets for ongoing treatments outside of the clinic.
- Other forms of magnetic products available are the joint straps and braces that have button magnets strategically positioned within the brace. These are generally alright but will not necessarily provide specific relief for everyone. These types of products generally come down to practitioner preference regarding whether they are used or not.

PLACEMENT OF MAGNETS: Obviously the placement of magnets will vary according to the different conditions seen in the clinic. Essentially, static magnetic therapy involves the application of static magnets directly over the injury or condition. In certain cases (such as sprains or strains of large muscle groups) certain distal placements will also benefit the condition being treated. However, to put it simply, most conditions will respond to the direct application of negative magnetic energy. Obviously, apart from the contra-indications, conditions such as wounds, ulcers, and the like will not allow direct application of magnets. In these cases, one can place the magnets as close as is practical to the lesion and still achieve the desired results. As has been stated previously, one must be aware of certain limitations that one has as a Bioenergetic practitioner. For most other applications however, direct application over the site of injury or afflicted area is the most advisable protocol. For example, for muscle strains and strains, direct application over the area which has swelling or bruising and over the insertion or origin points of ligaments and tendons will bring about the most effective results.

Patients that don't have a good diet and exercise balance may have sluggish lymphatic drainage. By assisting lymphatic drainage, the practitioner may help the body rid itself of the toxins as well as reduce the severity of symptoms. Also, in chronic cases, placement of button magnets over the lymph nodes may help the body clear out the lymphatic system and aid in the elimination of infection or cellular debris.

In cases of neuritis, and more so in chronic neuritis, it is important not to simply treat the affected area but to treat along the nerve pathways and dermatomes (those areas of skin affected by the nerve in question). In cases of chronic neuritis, the nerve involved will be affected along the nerve due to hypersensitivity. By treating along the nerve pathway, magnetic therapy may be able to promote healing of the whole nerve and not just the affected area.

When treating conditions such as headaches, shoulder tension, and other repetitive strain injuries, it is important to consider topics such as occupation, posture, stress, and lifestyle. While Magnetic and other Bioenergetic therapies will assist in reducing the severity of symptoms, if the causes of of strain are not removed, the patients' symptoms will continue to occur as an ongoing trend. Again, it is about treating the whole and not simply a portion of the body.

Laser and Photonic Therapy

Lasers and Light Photonic Therapy are increasingly being used in the treatment of musculoskeletal disorders. In recent years, Low Level Laser Therapy (LLLT) has become widely publicized in a variety of medical and/or "alternative" areas. However, the current state of evidence is not clear and many conflicting studies have been published. Baldry (1998) states that the controlled trials and a recently conducted meta-analysis leave considerable doubt as to whether any pain relief obtained with LLLT is greater than that obtained with a placebo. Brosseau et al (2003) also found mixed results. Conflicting results may reflect differences in equipment, wavelengths, power, and differing protocols.

Recent bioelectromagnetic (BEM) research has uncovered a form of endogenous electromagnetic (EM) radiation in the visible region of the spectrum that is emitted by most living organisms, ranging from plant seeds to humans. Some evidence indicates that this extremely low level light, known as *biophoton emission*, may be important in bioregulation, membrane transport, and gene expression. It is possible that the effects (both beneficial and harmful) of exogenous fields may be mediated by alterations in endogenous fields. Thus, externally applied EM fields (and laser light) from medical devices may act to correct abnormalities in endogenous EM fields characteristic of disease states. Furthermore, the energy of the biophotons and processes involving their emission as well as other endogenous fields of the body may prove to be involved in energetic therapies, such as healer interactions.

Light energy is generally described as photonic. The electrons stimulated to produce additional photons in a laser do so because the photons are partially "trapped" in an optical cavity to build the optical wave through positive feedback (Liu 2002). The human eye detects only a narrow band of frequencies within the EM spectrum: light between 400 and 800nM (an nM is one billionth of a meter). Ultraviolet is below 400nM and infrared above 800nM. A photon gives up its energy to the retina in the back of the eye, which converts it into an electrical signal in the nervous system that produces the sensation of light (Rubik et al *ibid*). Laser light may exist in the visual range or not.

"Laser" is an acronym for "light amplification (via) stimulated emission (of) radiation." The term "radiation" should not be confused with the alpha, beta, and gamma rays of nuclear radiation. Laser devices produce a highly monochromatic (single colored) light, typically visible red or near the infrared spectrum (630-950 nanometer or nM). Lasers, therefore produce radiation that is coherent, as apposed to regular light that radiates in all direction, i.e., lasers produce parallel rays that are sequential or "in step" over both distance and time. However, even laser light disperses when directed into human tissues.

Some photonic infrared stimulators produce a range of wavelengths (i.e., not monochromatic) which are also not coherent and therefore are not considered as lasers. According to some clinicians these may be more effective clinically especially in neuropathic pain.

The effects of low-energy laser stimulation has been reviewed by Sasford (1989) and are thought to be harmless (except if directed at the eyes). LLLT does not result in a rise of bodily tissue temperature above 36.5-37° C, i.e., normal body temperature (although a slight increase of 0.3-0.62° C has been reported, compared with 5° C achieved with modalities such as diathermy, ultrasound, and hot packs).[17]

The active medium in which to produce laser light can be solid (Ruby laser), a liquid (Dye laser), gas (Helium Neon, Argon, Rypton, etc.), or semiconductor (diode lasers). In LLLT, the two most commonly used are the Helium Neon lasers which produce visible red laser and diode lasers emitting in the visible or near non-visible infrared range. The Helium Neon unit is usually limited to from 1-10 milliwatts (mW) at 632nM, while diode units can vary from 1mW to 500mW (or as high as 1000mW, usually as a cluster of several beams totaling 1000mW of energy), and at wavelengths of 630-904nM. A Diode laser usually has a divergent bream (12-15°) and needs a collimating lens system to deliver a narrow beam. However, because of the infrared wavelength range (780-904nM) of the usually invisible beam of a diode laser, it is best used with some divergence for the sake of eye safety. Diode lasers also have a small range of wavelengths

---

17. The output of lasers used in surgery is around 10W/cm^2 (1 W=1000 mW).

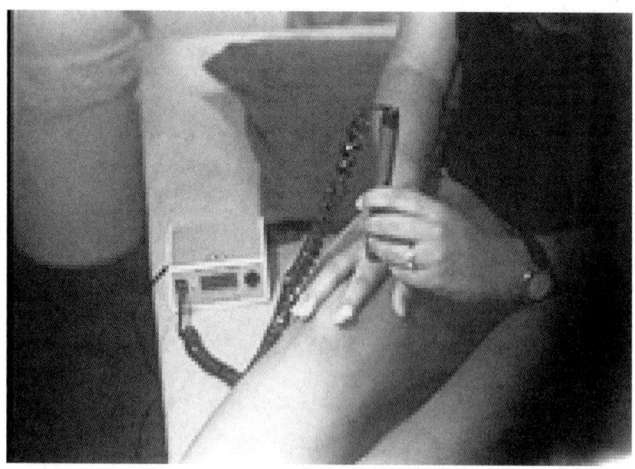

Figure 8-15: Patient self-treating with a laser.

and therefore are not truly monochromatic. Five mW (or higher) visible lasers may be used; however, their *active* energy penetration is shallow, and exposure time needs to be fairly long, about three minutes per one joule (J) of energy (for the 5mW). The joule is a unit of energy. One joule is equal to radiant power (W) times time in seconds. Each point is usually stimulated with 1-15 (but can be much higher with some patients needing as much as 3000J per treatment; Saputo personal communication) joules per site (Naeser *ibid*). Joules should be calculated based on cm^2. Visible red lasers are said to be more effective in the treatment of skin disorders.

Tissue Penetration

Laser light does not penetrate tissue to a greater degree than any other form of light. It has been estimated that an infrared laser beam will loose half of its energy for every 1mm of tissue in people with light colored skin. It would loose even more in dark-colored people (Seichert 1991). That would make the energy available at a depth of 1cm 1/1000 of the surface strength. Some manufacturers use a pulsed device and claim that it has a deeper penetration (and power); however, this is difficult to explan unless a higher output is used with each pulsed output (as by definition each time one uses a pulsed light the total on time is reduced as compared to a constant stimulation).

General Effects and Clinical Studies

Low-energy laser stimulation has been shown to stimulate collagen formation, protein synthesis, cell granulation, neurotransmitter release, phagocytosis, prostaglandin and ATP synthesis, among other effects (Basford 1989).

Many musculoskeletal disorders including neck pain, low back pain, joint pain, generalized muscle pain, and acceleration of wound healing have been reported to respond to LLLT (Martin 2003). Burke (2001) has shown LLLT to increase sensation in diabetic neuropathy patients from 20 grams to 2 grams using Semmes-Weinstein monofiliament test. In psoriatic arthritis, sacroileitis, tenosynovitis and bursitis, Hegyi (1999) has shown a decrease in medication use in 60% of patients and discontinuation in 30%. Gur (2002) has shown significant decrease in pain, stiffness, tender point numbers in fibromyalgia patients, and Simunovic (1996) 60-70% reduction in pain in patients with myofascial trigger point and in acute and chronic pain. Bjordal et al (2001) published a review paper on LLLT therapy for tendinopathy. Their conclusion was that the mean effect over placebo was 32%. A clinical comparative study of microcurrent electrical stimulation, mid-laser and placebo for the treatment of degenerative joint disease of the temporomandibular joint showed laser to be superior to placebo and microcurrent therapy (Bertolucci and Grey 1995). According to Tume (*ibid*) there have been 254 studies in 37 countries and 94% of them have been positive.

However, not all studies have been positive, for example, while some studies have shown lasers to be effective in the treatment of carpal tunnel syndrome (Chen 1990; Naeser 1996); Ysla and McAuley (1985) found laser treatment to be no better than placebo in the treatment of median nerve compression. Another study that compared conventional acupuncture and laser acupuncture found conventional acupuncture to be more effective in the treatment of lateral epicondylagia (Baxter 1997). While LLLT has been shown to be helpful in rheumatoid arthritis (Bliddal et al 1987; Colov et al 1987; Oyamada and Izu 1985), controlled studies on osteoarthritic knee pain (Jensen, Harreby and Ker 1987; McAuley and Ysla 1985) and osteoarthritic thumb pain showed no subjective or objective benefit (Basford et al 1987). At the same time a review by Bjordal et al (2003) of 11 studies including 565 patients showed that appropriately used LLLT can result in significant reduction in pain and improvement in health status in chronic joint disorders including osteoarthritis.

According to Martin (2003) LLLT has been shown to be effective in three major categories: inflammation reduction, pain reduction, and accelerated tissue healing.

Inflammation is reduced by the stabilization of cellular membranes; ATP production and synthesis (by stimulation of Cytochrome c Oxidase); vasodilation stimulation by increase of serotonin (although others found no effects on serotonin) and nitric oxide (NO); increased prostaglandin synthesis, particularly conversion of the prostaglandins PGG2 and PGH2, which have vasodilating and anti-inflammatory actions with some attributes similar to COX-1 and COX-2 inhibitors; reduction in interleukin 1 which is proinflammatory; enhanced lymphocyte response and activity; increased angiogenesis which results in improved circulation and profusion as well as increase in NO and growth factors; temperature modulation; enhanced superoxide dismutase (SOD) levels, which helps terminate the inflammatory process; and decreased C-reactive protein and neopterin levels, which are inflammatory markers (particularly in rheumatoid arthritis patients).

Pain reduction is achieved by increase in β-endorphins; blocking depolarization of C-fiber afferent nerves; increased NO production, which has both direct and indirect impact of on sensation and circulation (NO can relax blood vessels); axonal sprouting and nerve cell regeneration of damaged nerves; decreasing bradykinin levels (bradykinin is an inflammatory mediator that can both stimulate and sensitize pain fibers); increased release of acetylcholine, which helps normalize nerve signal transmission in autonomic, somatic, and sensory neural pathways; and ion channel normalization.

Tissue healing is increased by impacting all the phases of inflammation and repair by enhanced leukocyte infiltration; increased macrophage activity; increased neovascularization; increased fibroblast proliferation; keratinocyte proliferation; early epithelialization; enhanced cell proliferation and differentiations; and greater healed wound tensile strength. According to Dyson and Young (1986), a frequency of 700 Hz enhances healing, while 1200 Hz inhibits healing.

Because lasers are senstionless, they are particularly useful for the treatment of children or nervous patients, for patients with communicable blood diseases, for patients who are very sensitive such as those with neuropathic pain and for sensitive points such as the Well/Jing/Ting acupoints and in for auricular therapy (Figure 8-15).

Clinical Parameters

The total dosage used to treat *a new* patient should probably not exceed 100J (although it is common to use much larger doses especially with photonic stimulation). This can be delivered as 1J at 100 points or 10J at 10 points, etc. For acupuncture-laser, 1-3J is said to tonify and 4-5J to sedate. Most patients will experience some dosage reaction, which can range from an immediate improvement (usually in acute conditions) to an increase in pain (most often limited to chronic or neuropathic conditions when over stimulated), both of which can vary considerably in different patients. A slight flare is harmless, but the possibility should be explained to the patient. By reducing the dose, such a reaction can usually be minimized or avoided. Overdose is said to be capable of causing muscle spasms, mild fatigue, mild nausea, headache, and increase in the severity of symptoms. These reactions can occur during treatment, or more often, some hours after treatment, and may last from two to twenty-four hours (Tume 2003). However, as stated earlier some patients require much higher dosages with as much as 3000J per treatment. In general, the more sensitive the patient is the lower should be the first treatment dosage. For example, many fibromyalgia patients are overly sensitive in general, often they can not tolerated pharmaceutical medications except in lower doses, they are intolerant of heavy bodywork, etc. Such patients should be treated with a much lower dose at the beginning than robust patients that can tolerate

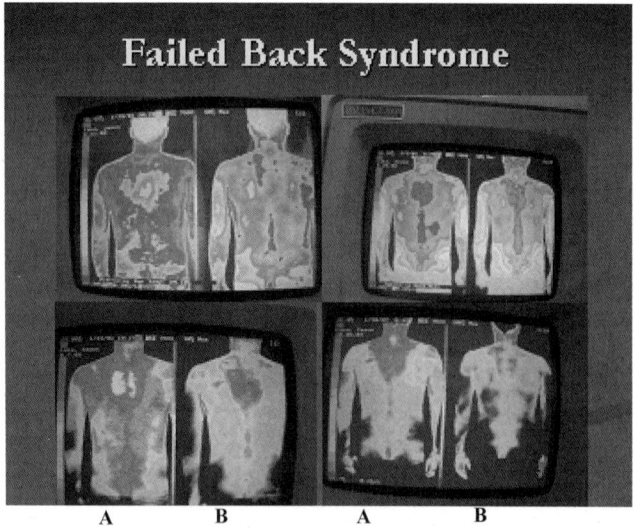

Figure 8-16: Thermogram done during infrared photonic light therapy on a failed back syndrome patient. Left side upper and lower (A) are baseline images at start of therapy. Left side upper and lower (B) are images at the end of first visit. A and B images on right side are baseline and end of treatment images several months into treatment. Note the dark areas indicating heat at baseline compared to end of treatment (courtesy of Saputo).

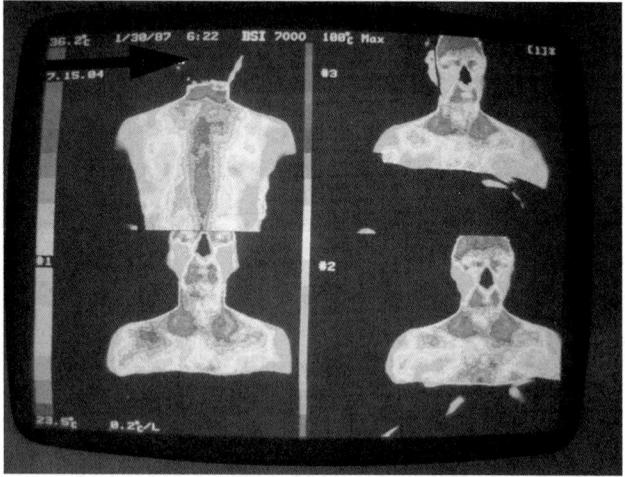

Figure 8-17: Thermogram done during infrared photonic light therapy for a patient with left sided shoulder capsulitis of five week duration. Scans on the left side are pretreatment. Note that her symptomatic shoulder is colder (lighter color) than the well shoulder despite inflammation. Right lower scan shows the shoulders after light therapy to the left St-38 acupoint area. Note the more equal heat distribution post treatment. At the end of stimulation the patient was able to rase her arm with glenohumeral abduction at 90° (normal). She still had pain on full internal rotation at the scapular area. The upper right scan shows the patient after light therapy to left SI-6 area. Note the further equalization of the temperature between left and right. The patient's pain improved as well. Three days after this treatment the patient's range of motion did not show improvement but her pain, including night pain improved significantly.

pharmaceuticals, etc. Also in general, fair skinned and blue eyed individuals are said to be more sensitive to the effects of laser and photonic stimulation.

Thermography can be used to guide treatment parameters determining both dosage and areas to be stimulated. Normalization of skin temperature can usually be demonstrated during treatment. According to Dr. Saputo clinical impressions,[18] 90-95% of patients suffering from diabetic neuropathy get relief from pain ranging from 70-100%, and restoration of sensation and proprioception ranging in 50-90% recovery of nerve function. This is achieved after only 5 daily treatments and in most patients is lasting. In his experience about 90% of patients with failed backs are helped with symptom relief ranging from 25-100% (with the bulk of patients having around 75% reduction in pain; Figure 8-16). He has also seen good response in patients suffering from plantar fasciitis, sprains and strains, carpal tunnel (with almost all of the patients being able to avoid surgery), and pressure sores. In general, neuropathic conditions respond better than orthopedic conditions (Saputo personal communication).

Lasers are best held at a right angle to the tissue to be treated and applied with firm contact pressure, although other methods such as scanning, a technique of moving the hand piece backwards and forwards over the selected area can be used.

---

18. Len Saputo MD is the medical director of the Health Medicine Institute and has been using thermography guided photonic stimulation for a verity of medical and pain syndromes. A formal study is currently underway studying the effects of photonic stimulation on diabetic neuropathy.

A typical treatment regime is to treat two to three times a week for up to three to four weeks, or until satisfactory relief is observed by the patient. Based on a Spanish study, the following dosages are recommended as a starting point for general LLLT therapy:

- Analgesic effects: Muscular pain 2-4J/cm^2
  — Joint pain 4-8J/cm2.
- Anti-inflammatory effect: Acute 1-6J/cm^2
  — Chronic 4-8J/cm^2.
- Circulatory effect: 1-3J/cm^2.

The manufacture of the Tume Clini-Laser recommends the following routines as general guide lines in the treatment of musculoskeletal disorders:

MUSCLE PROBLEMS: Always treat the origin and insertion points of the affected muscle. Choose two or three points at each location, and treat each point with at least 4Jcm^2. If the muscle belly is tender, treat two or three points around the motor points with 2-3J/cm^2 at each point. The bulk of the muscle (if tender) can also be treated with four to six points of 2-3J per point. Following this palpate for myofascial trigger points (TPs), and, where found, treat with firm pressure and deliver 4-6J to the TP. Test for easing of symptoms, treat with further dosages of 2-4J/cm^2 per point, and again palpate the TPs, if still present, then treat the TPs again with at least 4J/cm^2.

LIGAMENTS AND TENDONS: Treat all ligament/tendons at 10mm points along their length. Treat with 4-6J/cm^2 per point. These points can be directed over the ligament/tendon, and along both sides.

WOUNDS: Wounds can be treated with either of two methods. First, a grid pattern of 4-5mm is selected over the wound bed. (A grid is a figure of imaginary intersecting lines over the selected area. The tip of the laser is applied at each intersecting point on the grid.) This grid is treated with 4-6J/cm^2 per intersecting point. The healthy tissue immediately around the wound is treated at 5mm points with 1-2J/cm^2 per point. The second treatment method is to treat the wound bed by "scanning" back and forth. This method must allow for the size of the area, and thus the dosage setting. A wound of, lets say, 25mm in diameter would need an initial dosage setting of at least 15-20J/cm^2. Again the surrounding healthy tissue is treated as in the first method.

FRACTURES: To promote healing, at least eight points surrounding the fracture are chosen, and each is treated with 4-6J/cm^2. Additionally, four to six points on each side of the fracture site approximately 30mm away are treated with 2-3J/cm^2 per point.

DIABETIC NEUROPATHY. Diabetic neuropathy can be treated by first stimulating segmental levels associated with peripheral innervation of the feet (L5-S1; using segmental points on the Urinary Bladder and Governing (GV) channels), Kidney/kidney and adrenal related acupoints are stimulated for 4-15J/cm^2. Then the femoral artery at the inguinal area is stimulated (to treat sympathetic nerves). St-36, Sp-9, Sp-6, Sp-4, K-1, Liv-3 and GB-34 are then stimulated with about 1-30J per point. The foot is then scanned stimulating with between 20J-150J for the entire bottom and sides of the foot.

Supplantation with 500mg of GLA from evening primrose oil, 50mg of DHA from fish oil or other sources, 400-800mg of alpha lipoic acid, 8mg of biotin, 200-600mcg of chromium and 50mg of vanadyl sulfate can greatly enhance the treatment. Some patient will initially feel increased pain as nerves are healing. If the patient is very sensitive a much lower dosages should be started with.[19]

---

19. This therapy in not a Tume protocol.

9

INTEGRATIVE MANUAL THERAPIES, REHABILITATION, AND ORTHOSIS THERAPY

The following section covers both TCM and non-TCM treatment methods. *Golden Book for Original Medicine* ("Important Notes on Orthopedics" section) tells us that manual therapy (Shou Fa) is the main TCM method of treating musculoskeletal disorders. Manual therapy is also what partially distinguishes Orthopaedic Medicine form traditional allopathic orthopedics. Rehabilitation empowers patients and is imperative to maintaining the therapeutic effects achieved in an office setting. While there are many effective TCM-styles of manual therapies, this chapter focuses mainly on Osteopathic and Orthopaedic techniques. TCM manual therapy often demands great strength by the practitioner and is often non-specific. It is the author's belief that modern Osteopathic methods of manual therapy are better tolerated by patients than TCM styles and are also more clinically effective. Orthosis are often needed to address foot and other structural problems that can lead to musculoskeletal pain syndromes.

Massage/Manipulation

TCM manual therapy includes massage therapies such as Tui-Na (push and grab), medicinal massage, bone setting/bone-connecting-manipulation (for fractures and dislocations), and spinal manipulation (Zheng Ji). The Chinese characters that make up the words "Tui-Na" and the ones that represent manual medicine are composed of the character for hand together with the characters for vertebra and unify. The Chinese characters that represent the words for massage are composed of the character for hand together with the characters for safe and numbness. Hence, the art of manual medicine (Shou Fa) incorporates high-velocity manipulations and nonthrust techniques. Table 9-2 introduces TCM manual techniques for treating sinew disorders, some are shown in Figure 9-1.

Massage and many types of manipulation have been used in the treatment of musculoskeletal disorders since the beginning of time. Techniques are often similar in different schools; however, since the theories explaining pathophysiology vary considerably, the descriptions of similar techniques vary also. Massage might be beneficial for patients with subacute and chronic nonspecific low back pain (and other musculoskeletal disorders), especially when combined with exercise and education. Some evidence suggests that *acupuncture-massage* (acupressure) is more effective than "classic massage" (Furlan, Brosseau, Imamura and Irvin 2002). According to the *Classic of Internal Medicine,* massage and manipulation should not be performed in the winter, i.e., when the patient is cold.

Massage/Mobilizations without Impulse

Massage is widely used in the treatment of musculoskeletal disorders and may have both palliative and curative effects. Massage techniques can also be used to prepare the tissues for additional specific joint thrust manipulation. Used in both the acute and chronic stages of injuries, massage has circulatory, mechanical, and neurological effects. Massage can:

1. reduce swelling;
2. inhibit spasms;
3. circulate blood;
4. soften adhesions;
5. flush out extravasated blood and damaged cells;
6. restore correct placement of tissues;
7. increase local metabolism;
8. reduce pain;
9. induce piezoelectric stimulation in connective tissues;
10. transform tissues from a gel to a sol (more liquid) state.

Schools of massage therapy have many similarities and, while the descriptions in the following bullets describe Osteopathic techniques (Kuchera and Kuchera *ibid*), their utilization and description are similar to those seen in other systems, including TCM:

- *Deep friction* or deep pressure is used to relax deep short muscles such as the rotators and multifidi of the spine. Application with the thumb, fingers, knuckles, or elbow requires short amplitude with deep strokes.
- *Pertrissage* is a good soft tissue technique for chronic fibrotic areas, especially when they occur between the deep and superficial fascial layers. It may be used over

Table 9-1: General Considerations for TCM Regulating Sinew Techniques

ACUTE CONDITIONS	Use light (not necessarily superficial) manipulative techniques that reach dysfunctional tissues. For chronic condition, one may use stronger manipulative techniques, but they must be measured.
SLIGHT JOINT DISLOCATIONS, DEVIATION OF SINEWS, TURNED OVER SINEWS (CONTRACTIONS)	To relax and relocate displaced tissues safely; flex, extend, and rotate the joint to its physiological ROM. Use Pushing methods to restore correct tissue location. High-velocity manipulation to gap joints restore correct location/function.
ACUTE SOFT TISSUE INJURY WITH SWELLING AND INTERNAL BLEEDING	Use pressing method, by thumbs or by palm of hand. • Helps stop further bleeding. • Helps reduce swelling.

Table 9-2: TCM Massage-Manipulation Techniques

PRESSING	• Inhibitory or stimulatory. • Used mostly on local and distal channel points and tissues. • Stops bleeding, analgesic.
ROLLING CIRCULAR RUBBING	• Warming and vitalizing. • Used in large areas or locally to mobilize Qi and Blood.
PUSHING	• Inhibitory. • Used locally on affected tissues. • Rearranges soft tissues. • Stops bleeding.
GRASPING	• Dispersing. • Usually used locally, but also can be used distally. • Analgesic, Blood vitalizing.
AUXILIARY METHODS	• Kneading. • Splitting. • Rubbing. • Rolling. • Rotation. • Traction. • Lifting. • Tapping, clopping, hammering etc. • Shaking. • Moving. • Tugging (pulling) 　—promotes Blood circulation; 　—disperses Blood stagnation; 　—reduces swelling; 　—relaxes and activate Sinews; 　—loosens or breaks adhesions; 　—softens scars; 　—reduces pain; 　—restores normal location to displaced tissues/bones.

healed scars to which there are adhesions that are believed to be causing subjective complaints. It is also used in cellulosis. It involves pinching or tweaking one layer and lifting and/or twisting it away from the deeper layers. Skin-rolling and cupping achieves the same effects. Initially, these techniques are often uncomfortable.

• *Tapotement* is used to break adhesions or move bronchial secretions. It involves the hammering, clopping, beating, squashing of tissues. These actions are commonly used in TCM.

- *Effleurage* is performed on subcutaneous tissues by softly stroking them to move fluids along the lymphatic vessels. The motion is toward the heart in most cases. It is soothing and decongests subcutaneous tissues. To be most effective, fascial pathway restrictions must first be removed. This technique is used often in patients with tendinosis, by stroking from the periosteal attachments towards the muscle belly. Repeated strokes ("milking") are used to drain the tendon from accumulated fluids.

In general, most TCM massage techniques fall within the following three categories:

Opening Obstruction, Separating Adhesions, Breaking Scars, Invigorating Muscles and Sinews

These methods are used for both acute and chronic soft tissue injuries. The tissue is rubbed perpendicularly to the course of the fibers, which encourages muscle fibers to broaden, breaking microscopic adhesions that may be binding them together. Similar techniques are known as *deep transverse friction* in Orthopaedic Medicine. The technique is useful for mobilizing scars and other tissues such as tendons and ligaments. It also has analgesic effects. When used in TCM, the technique is often *less* specific and is used over large areas (an entire sinew channel, for example), as opposed to a small local specific lesion. Techniques such as rolling, kneading, grasping, and pinching are TCM methods included in this category.

Cross-fiber massage can be used to prepare tissues for thrust manipulation, especially when used to rupture adhesions. It is effective in capsular and ligamentous adhesions, and in many cases of tendinitis and in some patients with tendinosis. Cross-fiber massage can also be used as a *prophylactic* treatment in patients with recurrent strains or tendinitis/tendinosis. Most overuse tendinitis can be treated by cross-fiber massage, except (Ombregt et al *ibid*) the tenoperiosteal origin of the extensor carpi radialis bravis (type II tennis elbow).[1] In general, in Orthopaedic Medicine, the technique is applied for ten to twenty minutes and repeated three times a week for six to twelve sessions. In some cases this has to be done for up to six weeks before full effect takes place. If tenderness persists after two days, the pressure used during treatment should *not* be diminished, but the interval between sessions should be increased. When performed in Orthopaedic Medicine, it is vital that the massage be applied only at the site of the lesion, since the effects are very local. Unless the finger pressure is applied to the exact site and friction given in the right direction, relief cannot be expected; therefore, a very accurate diagnosis is mandatory. No movement is ever allowed between the practitioner's finger and the patient's skin as a blister can form. A cotton can be placed between the practitioner's finger and the patient's skin to prevent skin irritation. The skin must be dry; therefore no oil or lotion should be used.

In minor muscular tears, cross-fiber massage is usually followed by active movement; in ligamentous tears by passive movement; and in tendinous lesions by *avoidance* of any painful activity until full resolution has been achieved. Friction (cross-fiber) massage to a muscle belly should always be given with the muscle relaxed. It can be used in contusions—lesions due to repeated overuse in myosynovitis and after a minor tear. Tendons with a sheath and ligaments are treated with the tissues in tension. Tenosynovitis usually responds well to this treatment. The musculotendinous junctions often respond only to this type of treatment (Ombregt et al *ibid*).

During the acute phase of sprain/strain injuries, cross-fiber massage can be used gently—beginning with one to two minutes and building up to fifteen minutes—on a daily basis, to prevent scar formation. For more information see page 537.

The following conditions are said to be curable only by cross-fiber massage (Ombregt et al *ibid*):

- Muscle belly disorders of:
  — Subclavius, brachialis, supinator, adductors of the thumb, interosseous of hand, intercostal, abdominal oblique, interosseous of foot.
- Tendinitis of:
  — Tendon body of long head of biceps in the sulcus, pectoralis major at the humeral insertion, interosseous of hand, quadriceps expansion of the patella.
- Ligametous lesions of:
  — Posterior carpal of wrist, coronary of knee, posterior tibial, anterior tibiotalar.

Contraindications

Contraindications to cross-fiber massage are: Ossification and calcification of soft tissues (not described as contraindication in TCM), bacterial and rheumatoid-type tendinitis (also described as contraindication in TCM for Damp-Heat and Toxic-Heat), skin problems such as ulcers, psoriasis or blisters, neighboring bacterial infection, bursitis, disorders of nerve structures, and large haematomas.

Rearranging Displaced Tissue and Restoring Their Normal Function

To rearrange displaced tissues and restore their normal functions, force is applied along the fibers in a longitudinal direction. This type of technique (as used in effleurage, stretching, bone setting) can be used to relax muscles and disperse edema and extravasated blood. Therapeutic passive movements also fall within this category, as well as many of

---

1. Type II tennis elbow is the most common type. Often it is better first to use effleurage massage. Cross-fiber massage can be helpful when used within an integrative approach that combines herbs, acupuncture, laser, and electromagnetic therapy. Cross-fiber massage is very effective in treating type II tennis elbow within the first two weeks of acute onset.

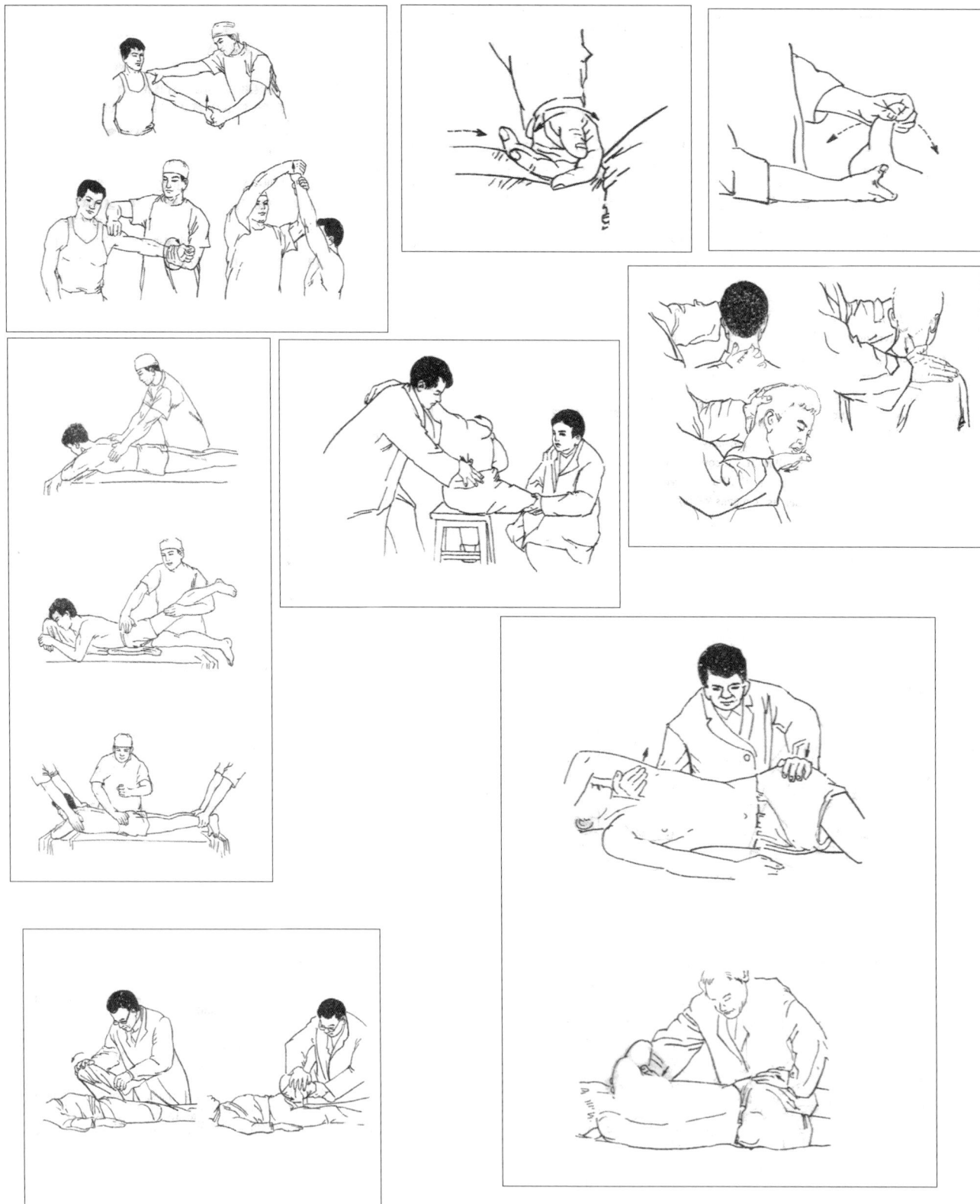

Figure 9-1: Examples of Traditional Chinese manual therapy techniques. These include soft tissue massage, stretching, traction, mobilization, and high velocity low amplitude techniques.

Massage/Manipulation

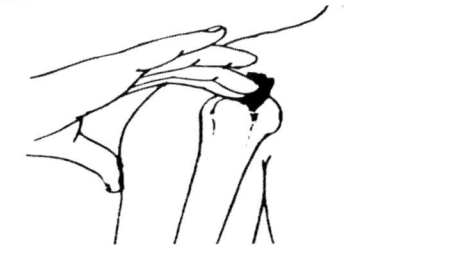
Cross-fiber massage of supraspinatus tendon. The patient's arm is positioned behind his/her back.

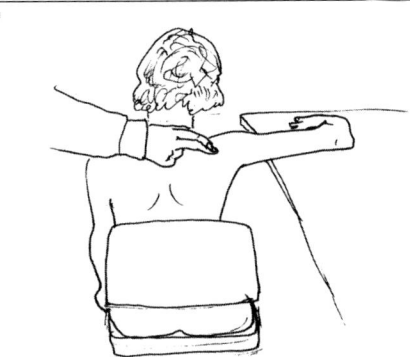
Proper position for cross fiber massage of the supraspinatus musculotendinous junction.

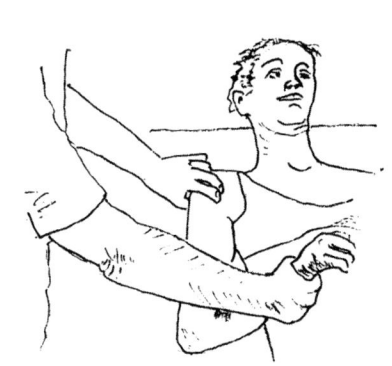
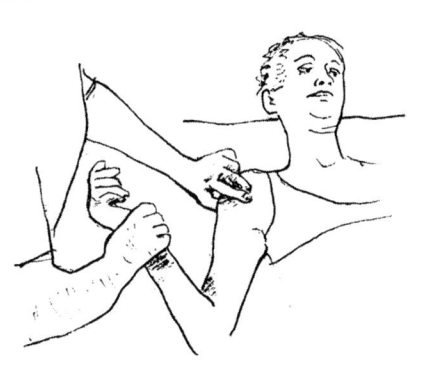
Cross-fiber massage technique for the biceps tendon. Here the finger pressure remains constant while the arm is moved from internal rotation to external rotation.

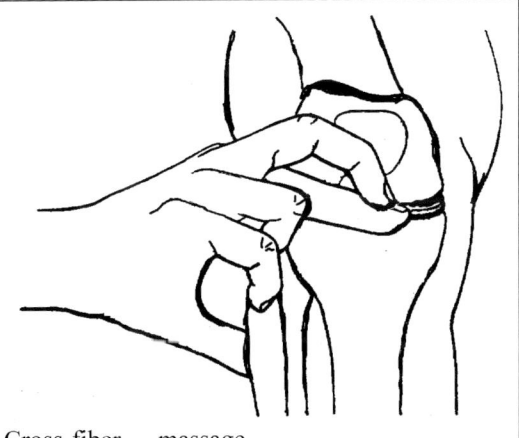
Cross-fiber massage technique for the coronary ligament of the knee.

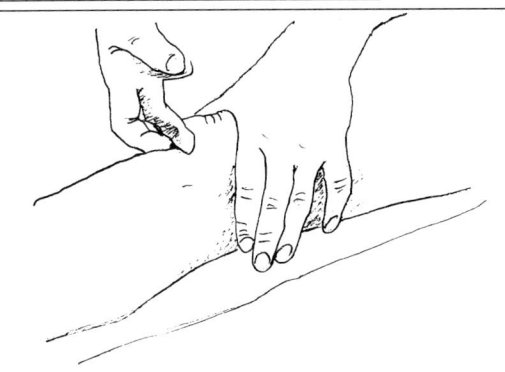
Cross-fiber massage technique for infrapatellar tendinitis.

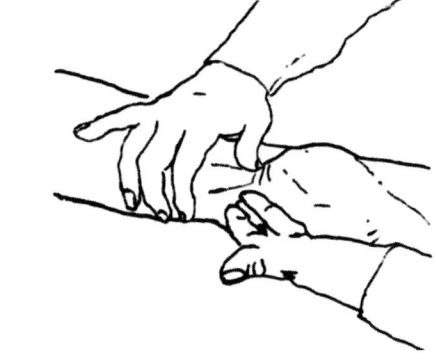
Cross-fiber technique for a lesion at the anterior aspect of the Achilles tendon. The thumb exposes the lesion while the other fingers role over the lesion with pressure.

Figure 9-2: Examples of specific cross-fiber massage techniques.

the thrust manipulations used in TCM. Both thrust and passive mobilization techniques used in TCM can be performed in the direction of restriction (called direct techniques in Osteopathic medicine) or direction of pain, or away from restriction (called indirect techniques in Osteopathic medicine) or the direction of pain. Rotation and shaking methods also fall under this category.

Inhibitory and Stimulatory Techniques

Inhibitory techniques are performed by deep, steady pressure to acupuncture, Ashi (painful) points, muscle insertions, and origins, etc. Inhibitory techniques are used mostly at the beginning or end of treatment for their analgesic effect, or as preparation for other techniques. *Stimulatory* techniques, which are more vigorous, with quicker motions and pressures, are used mostly in chronic cases to improve circulation and activate the channels (they are often said to be sedating). The direction in which such techniques progress also have "tonifying" or "sedating" effects. Some of these techniques are similar to the *Articulatory techniques* described in Osteopathic medicine, i.e., the springing of joints into their restricted barriers. The pressing and pushing methods fall under this category

TCM describes many other techniques that fall within the above three categories such as rubbing, tweaking, flicking, knocking, patting, hammering, treading, holding, and supporting. Table 9-1 lists general precautions to exercise when using these methods.

Commonly Used TCM Tuina Techniques

Tuina is used extensively in the treatment of musculoskeletal as well as internal medical disorders. The following are descriptions of the most important Tuina methods and techniques (Cusick 2003).

Rolling Method (Gun Fa)

Rolling is a modern Tuina technique introduced in the twentieth century. It is one of the most commonly used manipulations in clinical practice. The rolling method is somewhat difficult to master but once skill is achieved it is an effective technique. Rolling is a a good technique with which to begin a massage therapy. One can roll through broad areas of the body to warm and circulate Qi and Blood, open the channels, relax tendons and muscles, and lubricate the joints. It has a deep, gentle, warming and penetrating effect. It produces micro movements in the tissues and a rhythmic movement throughout the patient's body.

APPLICATION: The practitioner begins with the knife-edge of his/her hand which is kept in contact with the area to be treated. The hand is rolled in a diagonal fashion across the back of the hand. The contact begins at the base of the ulnar wrist around the SI-4, 5 acupoints. The slightly cupped hand roles forward toward SI-3 and across the dorsum of the hand towards the MCP (knuckle) joint of the index finger. The fifth MCP will stay in contact at all times.

Movement is initiated by supination and pronation of the arm. The hand rolls but does not rub, chafe or push. Movement begins slowly and builds to increasing speed. With practice 100-160 roles per minute is easily attained. Important points for the practitioner to remember are:

- The technique is deep but not forceful;
- Make sure that both patient and you are comfortable and adapt a grounded stances;
- Keep your shoulder and elbow relaxed. They should drop naturally;
- The wrist also remains supple. (this may take some practice;)
- Be consistent in speed and pressure. Avoid jerky motions;
- Stay relaxed and rounded in your body. Keep upright and avoid hunching over;
- Keep your anchor hand gently resting on the patient. This hand can also introduce a gentle swaying motion. Keep a space underneath both of your armpits. This keeps your frame rounded and energy expansive.

Kneading Method (Rou Fa)

Kneading in a simple technique to learn and can be applied in lots of ways. Kneading "tools" include fingers, thumb, whole palm, heel of palm, and elbow. The most commonly used are the palm, palm-heel, and knife hand methods.

APPLICATION: The technique begins with the heel of the palm, whole palm, or "small fish belly" pressed against the skin. Kneading is achieved with a rotating motion, slowly increasing and varying downward pressure. The hand is relaxed. As the palm moves from place to place it does not drag the skin; or it is slightly lifted from the skin. The skill lies in the frequency of rotations, fluidity of movement, and moving the hand while remaining in contact but without producing too much friction. The rate of frequency is generally 50-60 times per minute. Important points for the practitioner to remember are:

- Always engage the muscle tissue, do not skim over the skin;
- Engage the muscle but do not aim to compress it too deeply, the tissue must twist and turn on itself. Kneading should be deep yet pliable;
- The practitioner's movement should begin in the feet, transfer to the hips, and express via his/her arms.

Chafing Method (Ca Fa)

Chafing strokes look similar to kneading but here the object is to produce heat through friction. The force used depends upon the reaction of the patient's skin. The purpose is to reach as deep as the skin and subcutaneous tissue and no farther. This is a good technique for applying therapeutic oils or liniments.

Rubbing Method (Cuo Fa)

Rubbing is similar to chafing except that it is lighter. The purpose is to produce a gentle heating and dispersing action. It is a "harmonizing" technique.

Pressing Method (An Fa)

This is the oldest and simplest Tuina technique. It can be relaxing and comforting or it can be intense. Knowing how and when to apply what pressure is the main clinical issue. The thumb, palm, fingers, or elbow can be used. Pressure is always applied slowly and with sensitivity. Pressure can be continues, for a comparatively long period of time, or intermittent, at a fixed rate. Pressure can be deep or shallow. Important points for the practitioner to remember are:

- Use your weight not your strength;
- Listen with your hands, if the tissue strongly resists, back off;
- Relax. Allow yourself to find a way through the tissue: do not force your way in.

Pushing Method (Tui Fa)

Pushing is simple technique that can be developed into a sophisticated tool. The pad of the thumb, heel of palm, or the thumb-in-palm (two-handed) methods are very effective. In its simplest use, the pushing method involves pushing in a straight line from one place to another, often along a channel or muscle group. One pushes forward and then gently drags backwards. A more advanced method involves pushing obliquely across muscle fibers, using small strokes and affecting a swaying rhythm throughout the muscle. This technique has a soft feeling like rolling.

For thumb-in-palm pushing the thumb of one hand is in contact with the patient and the palm of the other hand overlies the thumb. The thumb and palm are *completely relaxed*. The palm heel of the upper hand delivers the force of the body to the thumb. The result is a focused yet relaxed pressure which is not injurious to the practitioner's hands.

Grasping Method (Na Fa)

Grasping can be applied with the pads of the thumb and fingers or with the whole hand. One or both hands can be involved.

APPLICATION: The practitioner simply grasps the selected tissue, gripping and gently squeezing, then lifting it way from the bone. Then the tissues are released and the technique is repeated. Twisting or shearing motions can be added to lifting. Important points for the practitioner to remember are:

- Use the pads of your fingers, not fingertips, use care not to get your fingernails involved;
- Keep an even rhythm;
- Stay gentle, think about softening the tissues not pulling them;
- The patient may feel soreness during this technique but not pain.

Pinching Method (Nie Ha)

The pinch method employs the fingers to squeeze and pinch muscle and fascial tissues. The flesh is squeezed with the thumb on top and the rest of the fingers below. The fingers below become a fulcrum and the thumb with the entire arm is the lever delivering force through the thumb. The practitioner rolls the thumb and treated fibers over one another while moving forward, following the outline of the muscle or a channel. Important points for the practitioner to remember are:

- Avoid using hand power for squeezing. This will easily tire your hand and can lead to tendinitis of the thumb;
- Use your whole body to transfer pressure through the thumb;

One Finger Meditation Method (Yi Zhi Chuan Fa)

This technique takes lots of practice but is essential when stimulating individual acupoints. Here the thumbs are used like an acupuncture needle. The hand is cupped gently, the thumb is straight but loose. The shoulder is relaxed while the elbow and wrist are raised. The wrist remains supple as the elbow rhythmically swings the forearm inward and outward. The frequency should be 100-150 times per minute. To tonify a gentle technique is used, to sedate a more vigorous pressure is used:

It is important to remember that the thumbs are often the first joint injured in bodyworkers. This technique, if done properly, will not damage but strengthen the thumbs. Important points for the practitioner to remember are:

- Practice is a must but must be increased slowly;
- Practice starts by 2-3 minutes each day with each thumb;
- Work up to twenty minutes per day;
- Bilateral proficiency is a must.

Rotation Method (Yao Fa)

Rotation method is a very simple and very important technique in which smooth rotation can be introduced to any joint in the body from the neck to the toes. This method relaxes the tissues, trains the patient to release holding patterns, lubricates the joint and often restores motion to a joint. With skill, forces can be applied to rupture adhesions. Important points for the practitioner to remember are:

- Caution must be exercised to not over stretch a joint;

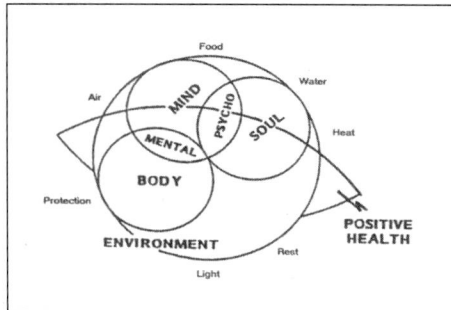

Figure 9-3: Osteopathic philosophy (From Kuchera WA and Kuchera ML, Osteopathic Principles in Practice, KCOM press 1993, with permission).

- Correct body mechanics are necessary to ensure practitioner safety;
- Vary amplitude, direction and speed;.
- Do not let the patient "help you," coach him/her to surrender.

Shaking Method (Dou Fa)

This is only used on the legs and arms but with skill the whole body can be harmonically affected. Important points for the practitioner to remember are:

- Vary shaking speed;
- Vary shaking amplitudes;
- Vary amount of traction;
- Be mindful not to cuff the skin in such a way as to produce a "skin burn."

Stretching Methods (Yin Shen Fa)

Stretching methods are commonly used and with skill can be applied to any joint in the body including the spine and pelvis. When a high speed overpressure is added at the end of a slow stretch this method becomes a high velocity manipulation.

Western Manual Therapies

Western Osteopathic techniques are often effective and frequently better tolerated by patients then TCM or Orthopaedic Medicine manipulations. In general, Osteopathic techniques tend to be joint *specific* or directed toward specific tissue restrictions.[2] Many of these techniques can be adapted and used in less specific ways when integrated with acupuncture with great benefit to patients.[3]

Table 9-3: Classic Osteopathic Philosophy (*ibid*)

HEALTH	• Health is a natural state of harmony. • The human body is a perfect machine created for health and activity. • A healthy state exists as long as there is normal flow of body fluids and nerve activity
DISEASE	• Disease is an effect of underlying, often multifactorial causes. • Illness is often caused by mechanical impediments to normal flow of body fluids and nerve activity. • Environmental, social, mental, and behavioral factors contribute to the etiology of disease and illness.
PATIENT CARE	• The human body provides all the chemicals necessary for the needs of its tissues and organs. • Removal of mechanical impediments allows optimal body fluid flow, nerve function, and restoration of health. • Environmental, cultural, social, mental, and behavioral factors need to be addressed as part of any management plan. • Any management plan should realistically meet the needs of the individual patient.

Osteopathic Medicine

Osteopathy originated with the work of Andrew Tylor Still (1828-1917), a Medical Doctor. Osteopathic philosophy is similar in many ways to principles found in Chinese Medicine.[4] Osteopathic philosophy acts as a unifying set of ideas for the organization of scientific knowledge in relation to all phases of physical, mental, emotional, and spiritual health, along with distinctive patient management principles. In the 21st century, this viewpoint is particularly useful, as practitioners from a wide variety of disciplines confront increasingly complex physical, psychosocial, and spiritual problems affecting individuals, families, and populations from a wide variety of cultures and backgrounds. Dr. Still believed that life exists as a unification of vital forces and matter. Since the body is controlled by the mind to exhibit purposeful motion in attaining the needs and goals of the organism, Dr.

---

2. The question of clinical accuracy and the consistency between practitioners using Osteopathic and other manual diagnosis techniques is controversial. Data is quite mixed with many negative and positive studies. While cross-fiber massage used in Orthopaedic Medicine is very tissue specific, high velocity manipulations are not. Manipulations and massage techniques used in TCM are usually not joint or tissue specific.

3. They do however work best when used to treat an identified restriction and applied accurately to the area/vertebra/joint of greatest restriction.

4. The author heard but cannot verify that Still's first clinic was rented from a Chinese laundry owner, the implications of which can only be speculated on. Littlejohn finds the foundation of Osteopathy in Greek and Roman medicine. Hulett and Downing trace the origins of various Osteopathic concepts to the philosophy and practice of medicine found in other ancient writings, such as those of the Ptolemies, Brahmins, Chinese. and Hebrews (Seffinger et al *ibid*).

Osteopathic Medicine

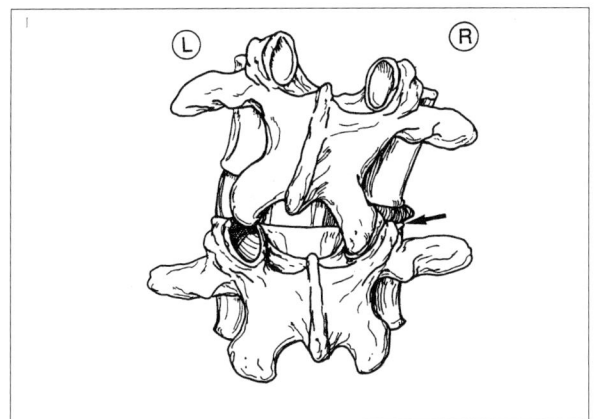

Figure 9-4: Arrow pointing to the facet that remains closed during flexion. This results in fixation in extension, rotation and sidebending to the right, when the spine is forward bent (i.e., in flexion; courtesy of Dorman and Ravin).

Still stated that, "Osteopathy...is the law of mind, matter and motion...Life is matter in motion. Each tissue, organ, and structure is designed for motion...All diseases are mere effects, the cause being a partial or complete failure of the nerves to properly conduct the fluids of life." *(OM: Qi can never not be moving).* Even in infectious diseases, Dr. Still (as in TCM) saw germs (or Pathogenic Factors) as opportunists in relation to decreased host function *(OM: Zheng or Righteous Qi weakness),* not as primary agents in themselves. Osteopathic medicine, in contrast to TCM, is firmly rooted in the in-depth study of modern (biomedical) anatomy and physiology. As in TCM, in Osteopathic medicine the body is seen as a whole. This interdependence of body components is mediated by the communication systems *(OM: channels and vessels)* of the body: exchange of substances via circulating blood and other body fluids and exchange of nerve impulses and neurotransmitters through the nervous system. The circulatory and nervous systems also mediate the regulation and coordination of cellular, tissue, and organ functions and thus the maintenance of the integrity of the body as a whole. The patient must be viewed in the context of the environment in which all the body parts live and function and in which the mind finds expression (as is in TCM/OM). Everything about the patient: genetics, history (from conception to the present moment), nutrition, use and abuse of body and mind, parental and school conditioning, physical and sociocultural environment must be considered. Another important tenant of Osteopathic medicine is that *structure determines function, structure and function are reciprocally interrelated* (Seffinger et al 2003).

Because the musculoskeletal system is the largest system in the body, it is the largest consumer in the "body economy." To meet this demand, all other bodily systems such as the cardiovascular, respiratory, digestive, renal, and other visceral systems must participate for normal and efficient function. Impairment or failure in the musculoskeletal or its related systems can therefore have extensive implications upon health.

Comprehensive Osteopathic treatments include patient education strategies with emphasis on moderation (as is in TCM). These includes advice for removing noxious or toxic substances from the diet and environment, and behavioral adjustments such as adding exercises and stopping smoking, drug and alcohol abuse. Dr. Still emphasized manual therapy (body work) to restore normal motion, but continued to use surgery and medical interventions. He also described the importance of giving hope to patients and, at the same time, providing them with a realistic approach to managing their clinical condition. Each patient is treated as a unique individual, not as a disease entity (Seffinger et al *ibid*). Table 9-3 summarizes classic Osteopathic philosophy.

Joint Dysfunctions and Manual Medicine Models

While this discussion uses Osteopathic and orthopedic language, it must be emphasized that many of the same general ideas can be found in TCM literature, except for the *specificity* of modern Osteopathic medicine.

Coupled Movement, Fryette Rules of Motion

Coupled movements of the spine have been described by Fryette and divided into three basic patterns. These three patterns are used to diagnose and treat spinal joint dysfunctions using Osteopathic techniques. Although it is difficult to demonstrate the validity of the first two "patterns," some radiographic evidence has shown support. As a model for analysis of vertebral joint dysfunction, there is no other theory with the predictive power of Fryette's formulation (Mitchell *ibid*). Table 9-4 describes the three types of coupled movements (also see Radiology in Chapter 4).

Vertebral, pelvic, and other joint (somatic) dysfunctions can be divided into subluxation, neutral and non-neutral, vertebral, sacroiliac, and iliosacral dysfunctions. The distinction between sacroiliac and iliosacral dysfunctions (which occur in the same joint) is as follows: sacroiliac dysfunction pertains to the behavior of the sacrum between the ilia during spinal movements; iliosacral dysfunction pertains to iliosacral motions in response to lower limb movements.

Subluxations

Subluxations are non-physiologic dysfunctions resulting from, or showing as movement greater than normal joint motions. They are fairly common in the pelvic joints and occasionally may be detected at the costovertebral joints. Subluxations in the lumbar spine, although described in older chiropractic literature, are very rare, unless they are part of spondylolisthesis. The Chiropractic "subluxation" theory is not supported by evidence (Lewit 1999). Pelvic shears, if not treated, can last indefinitely and often are very painful. Bizarre displacements of bony landmarks are seen often and can be quite confusing when analyzing for somatic dysfunction (Mitchell 1993).

Table 9-4: Coupling of Vertebral Movement, Fryette Rules

Dysfunction	Descriptions
Neutral Type I	Bending of spine to one side is coupled with rotation to the opposite side. —Found in lumbar and thoracic spine. —Not found in the cervical spine except in occipital atlantal joint.[a] —Occurs only when normal spinal curvature is maintained, i.e. without flexion or extension that engage the facet joints. —Often lost with dysfunction. —Often seen as rotoscoliosis due to compensation to nonneutral dysfunctions or unlevel sacral base or short leg syndrome. In "neutral" mechanics the spine is relatively stable and injuries occur less frequently.
Nonneutral Type II	Refers to vertebral motions when the spine is flexed or extended which engages the facets. Side bending coupled with rotation to same side. —Results in less stability than neutral spine mechanics. —Found in cervical, thoracic, and lumbar spine. —Results in increased injury risk.
Restrictive	Movement in one direction reduces motion in all other directions. —Used for localizing manipulation techniques and diagnosis screening.

a. Not all authors/practitioners agree with this, and some find pathological neutral behavior in the cervical spine as well.

True subluxation must be treated with manual techniques (manipulation), except possibly in cases of pubic shears that can, at times, respond to acupuncture.

Vertebral Dysfunctions

In the lumbar, thoracic, and cervical spine, the practitioner can find restrictions of flexion and extension that often are due to *nonneutral* (Type II) *dysfunctions* called FRS and ERS. FRS is a *positional* term that describes a segment as "stuck," flexed, rotated, and sidebent to one side—possibly because the facet on one side is not closing with extension movement. The F represent flexed, R represents rotated and S sidebent. The side to which the segment is rotated and sidebent is marked in parentheses. For example, if a dysfunction of a motion segment (a pair of vertebra) is diagnosed as FRS(rt), it is *stuck:* flexed, rotated, and sidebent to the right. The restricted motions and often the provocation of pain are in the opposite directions, i.e. extension, rotation, and sidebending to the left. Usually (Bourdillon and Day 1992) the

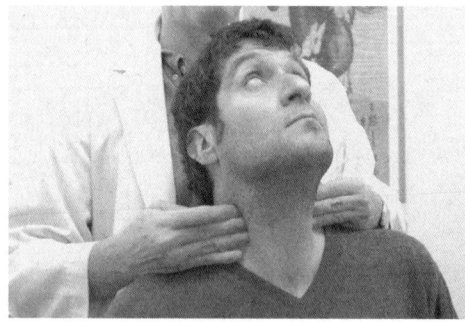

Figure 9-5: Patient being assessed for extension restriction (FRS) at the cervical spine. Note rotation present when the patient extends the neck. The practitioner's fingers are used to assess the anterior aspect of the vertebra. As the patient extends the neck both the right and left side of the vertebra should move posteriorly. If one does not, this shows the facet at that side to be "stuck" open.

total range of extension and flexion (in the sagittal plane) will be reduced.

The opposite is true for ERS(rt). The segment *positional diagnosis* is extended (E), rotated (R) and sidebent (S) to the right (rt). Restricted motions and often the provocation of pain would be to the opposite side, i.e, are flexion, rotation, and sidebending to the left. The spinous process and the supraspinous ligament are tender. Often the transverse processes (TrPrs) and/or the articular capsule are very tender (Bourdillon and Day *ibid*). Flexion restriction may be due to a facet joint not opening on one side during flexion movement.[5] Figure 9-4 shows a segment with flexion and left sidebending rotation restriction. (The right facet is stuck closed). Figure 9-5 shows an evaluation technique used in the cervical spine. Figure 9-6 shows findings associated with Non-neutral dysfunctions. Figure 9-8 shows several other methods used to assess vertebral dysfunctions.

In the lumbar and thoracic spines, the practitioner often finds *neutral group* (Type I) *dysfunction*. Neutral *group* dysfunction is usually a compensatory reaction to a nonneutral dysfunction elsewhere in the spine, or to a dysfunction of the lower extremity (Greenman *ibid*). Described as "NR(side)," the N represents neutral, and the R represents rotation, with the direction written in parentheses. Sidebending is always to the opposite side of rotation. Motion is restricted toward the convex side of the group, and rotation is restricted in the opposite direction. The total range of flexion and extension (in the sagittal plane) usually is reduced (Bourdillon and Day *ibid*). Neutral group dysfunctions (Mitchell *ibid*) are maintained by multiarticular muscles that span several joints and are seen with scoliosis.

In the cervical spine, occiptioatlantal (CO-C1) restrictions mostly affect flexion and extension, limiting posterior gliding of CO on C1 with flexion, anterior gliding with extension, and to a lesser but important extent, sidebending. C1-C2 restrictions largely involve rotational movements. In

---

5. There are many theories trying to account for restricted vertebral movement and the facet dysfunction being one.

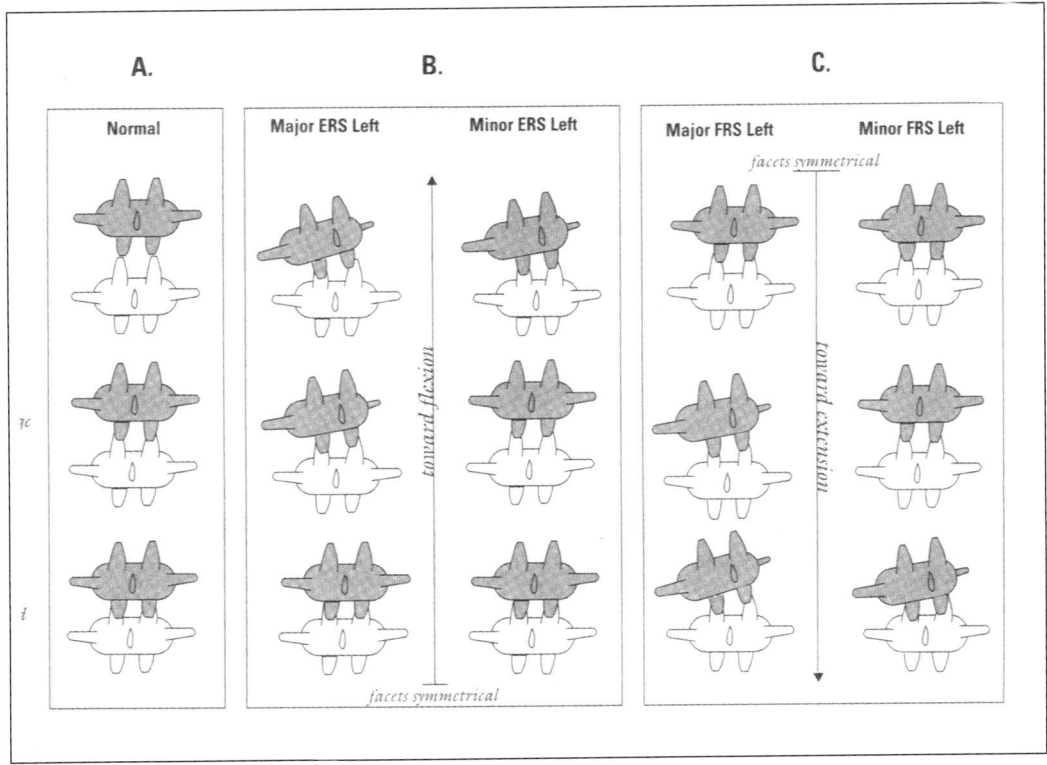

Figure 9-6: Somatic dysfunctions. Normal shows the ability of both facets to open in flexion and in extension. ERS dysfunction shows the ability of both facets to close during extension, but the left facet does not open during flexion. FRS dysfunction shows the ability of both facets to open during flexion, but the right facet does not close in extension (courtesy of Mitchell *ibid*).

the typical (C3-C7) segments, both flexion restrictions (ERS) and extension restrictions (FRS) are common.

Depending on evaluation style, the practitioner may find neutral dysfunction in the cervical spine, usually affecting a single motion segment, and only when using passive evaluations.

The ideas of flexion and extension restrictions, especially as they are explained in the Osteopathic muscle energy model (the Mitchell model), are quite similar to ideas expressed in the TCM *General Treatise on the Causes of Symptoms of Disease*: "When the Yang aspect is damaged, the patient has difficulty flexing (as seen in ERS dysfunctions)...When Yin is damaged, the patient has difficulty extending (as seen in FRS dysfunction).

Pelvic Dysfunctions

Movements of the sacrum between the innominates are described as sacroiliac motions. These are all physiological movements that can become restricted or exaggerated (Greenman *ibid*; Mitchell *ibid*; Bourdillon, Day and Brookhout *ibid*). Figure 9-7 shows the Gillet's Stork test, a method for assessing sacroiliac joint movement.

NUTATION. Nutation is movement of the sacral base anteriorly and inferiorly down the L-shaped track of the joint

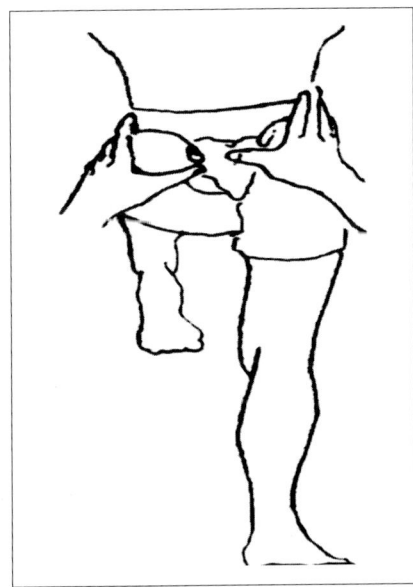

Figure 9-7: Gillet's Stork Test. In assessing SI joint mobility, normally the finger at the PSIS moves downward when the leg is flexed on the same side. Figure shows a negative test for the left SI joint.

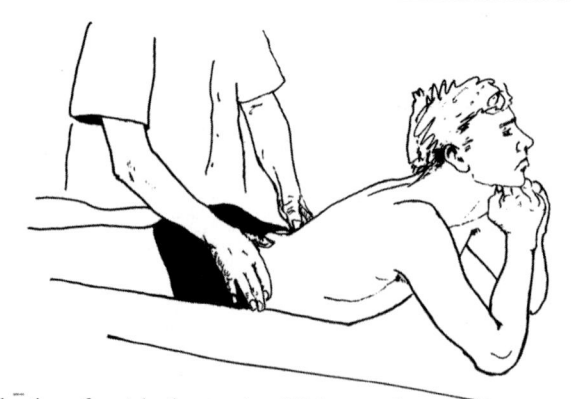

Evaluation of vertebral extension. With normal extension, both facets close and the transverse processes translate posteriorly, equally. One side not showing this movement indicates that the facet on that side is stuck *open* and is not closing. This would cause a rotation of that segment only during extension. In flexion, the transverse processes are equal because both facets can open. There is an FRS dysfunction.

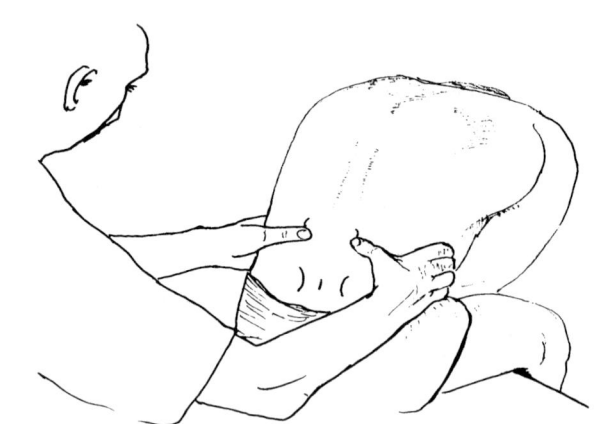

Evaluation of vertebral flexion. Both transverse processes should translate forward equally. If one side does not, the facet on that side is stuck closed. This would result in rotation of this segment during flexion only. In extension, both sides are equal, as both facets can close. There is ERS dysfunction.

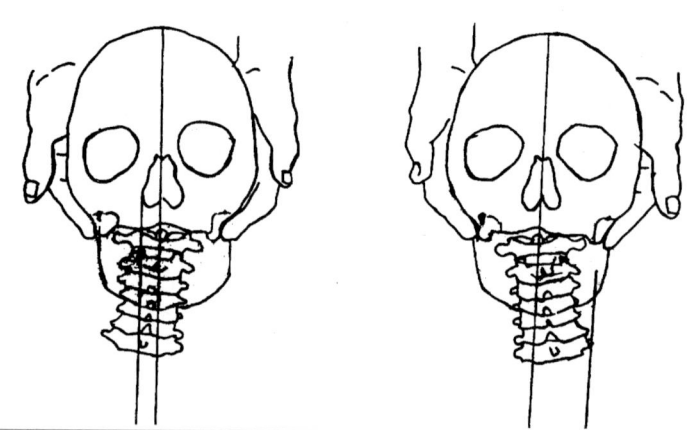

Evaluation of OA function. The fingers are placed at the OA junction and the head is translated from side to side. This is done in slight flexion and extension. Resistance and distance of movement are assessed. While in the rest of the cervical spine sidebending and rotation are said to be restricted always to the same side, at the OA junction rotation and sidebending can become restricted on opposite sides. It is repeated in flexion and extension to see which is more limited (courtesy of Mitchell 1995).

Evaluation of C1-to-C7 function. Here C2-C3 is evaluated by assessing lateral translation. It is done by passively moving the superior vertebra over the one below. Translating the vertebra from left to right creates a left sidebending. If more sidebending exists in one direction than the other, there is restriction. It is repeated in flexion and extension to see if an FRS or ERS dysfunction exists. (courtesy of Mitchell 1995)

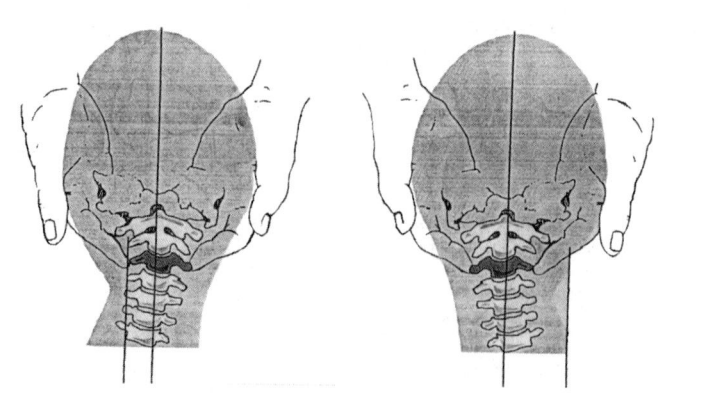

Figure 9-8: Assessment of spinal function.

Osteopathic Medicine

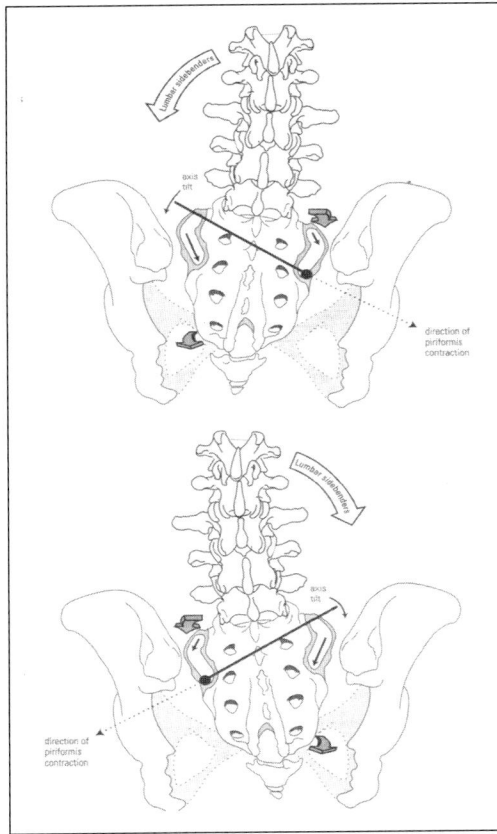

Figure 9-9: Sacral torsions (courtesy of Mitchell *ibid*).

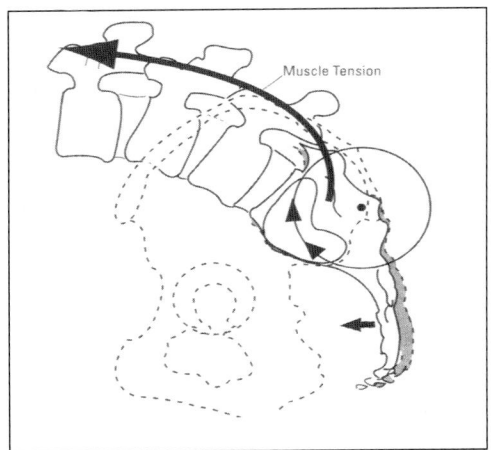

Figure 9-10: Counternutation hypothesis (Mitchell *ibid*).

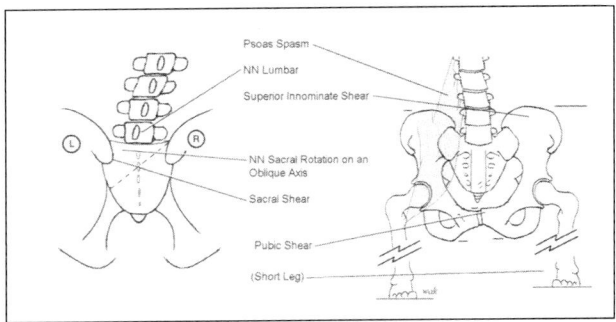

Figure 9-11: Dirty half dozen in failed back syndrome (courtesy of Kuchera and Kuchera 1994).

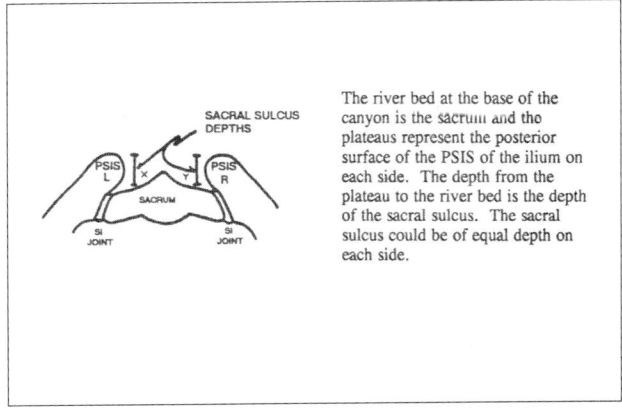

Figure 9-12: Sulcus depths (From Kuchera WA and Kuchera ML, Osteopathic Principles in Practice, KCOM press 1993, with permission).

between the innominates. It involves a rotation of the sacrum about a transverse axis and a translation of the sacrum caudally (inferiorly) within the joint. Sacral nutation is a normal, movement coupled to extension of the lumbar spine. During sacral nutation, the two PSISs approach each other slightly while the pubic symphysis is caudally extended and cranially compressed. The multifidus and erector spinae, which also constrain nutation by pulling the ilia together, are thought to induce nutation. The long dorsal SI ligaments become lax, and the sacrotuberous ligament tightens (Vleeming et al *ibid*). Bilateral restrictions are rare; unilateral restrictions are common (Mitchell *ibid*).

COUNTERNUTATION. Counternutation (posterior nutation) occurs when the sacral base moves posteriorly and superiorly on the innominate bones in the same axis as nutation. The sacral base becomes prominent posteriorly, with the inferior lateral angles (ILAs) less so. Counternutation is a normal reaction to *extreme* lumber flexion in *some* people. With counternutation the dorsal SI ligaments tighten up and become part of a pattern of flattening the lumbar spine. This occurs especially late in pregnancy, when women counterbalance the weight of the fetus (Vleeming et al 1997). When the SI becomes restricted (stuck) in counternutation, con-

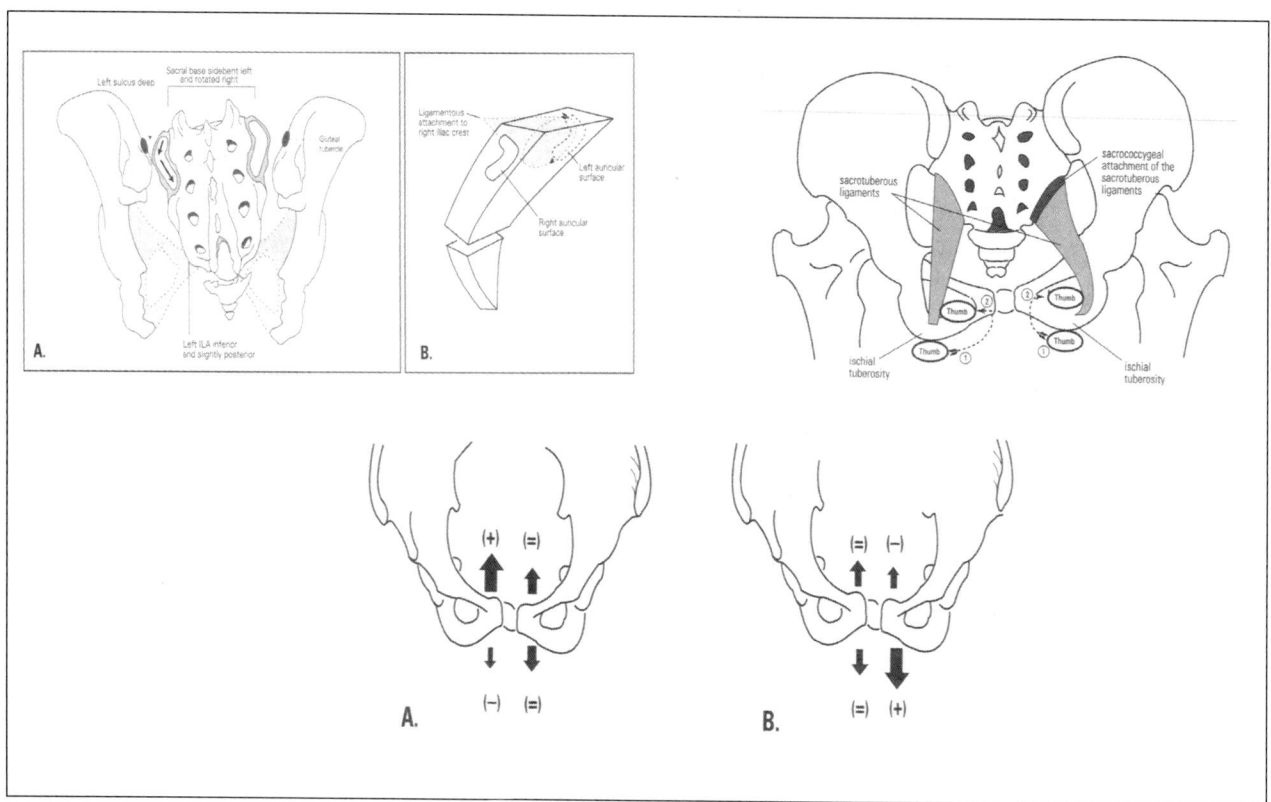

Figure 9-13: Shear dysfunctions. Upper left shows Flexed left sacrum. Upper right shows upslip innominate on the right. Bottom shows pub subluxations (courtesy of Mitchell *ibid*).

stant tension of the dorsal ligaments can lead to sprain and pain. Restrictions (Mitchell *ibid*) can occur both unilaterally and bilaterally.

NUTATIONAL DYSFUNCTIONS. Both forward and backward nutational dysfunctions are probably maintained due to SI ligamentous insufficiency and/or lack of muscle stabilization on the joint.

SHEARS. Sacral "shears" have been described in the literature as non-physiological (i.e., beyond normal range). However, they are part of normal sacral movement during nutation and counternutation (Mitchell *ibid*). True dysfunctional, sacral or innominate shears probably represent ligament insufficiency.

SACRAL TORSIONS. *Anterior/forward torsion* is a normal movement around a theoretical oblique axis that accompanies the counter-rotation of the two innominates and the lateral shifts of the spine in normal walking. During walking, the lumbar sidebending muscles on the swing-leg side contract at mid-stride, elevating the hip to allow the swing leg to pass. The *piriformis* muscle on the non-swing side contracts and stabilizes the sacrum, creating an axis by which the sacrum rotates. This probably creates an oblique axis between the lower and the opposite upper sacroiliac region. The sacrum rotates toward the side of the oblique axis (Mitchell *ibid*).

Posterior/backward torsions occur during lumbar non-neutral mechanics that result in co-contraction of lumbar sidebenders and hip external rotators. This induces a backward torsional movement of the sacral base on an oblique axis. Backward torsional movement is thought to be a normal physiological motion in response to non-neutral lumbar movements.

Backward torsion dysfunctions are maintained principally by the lumbar sidebenders (*quadratus lumborum* and *piriformis*) on the same side (Mitchell *ibid*).

COMMON CLUSTERS: Dysfunction often shows in clusters. In patients with chronic low back pain and posain, i.e., they complain of pain when standing for prolonged periods but the pain improve with movements, the cluster often includes: superior pube on left, unilateral flexed sacrum on left, and a posterior innominate on the left. Often there is also ERS dysfunction at L5. This cluster is often seen in patients with an unstable SI joint. Another common presentation seen in patients with lifting injuries and in which the patient may look like he/she is suffering discogenic pain are: right on left torsion, right anterior innominate, and right inferior pub. This is usually seen with non-neutral dysfunction in the lumbar spine, especially FRS at T12 (Greenman *ibid*).

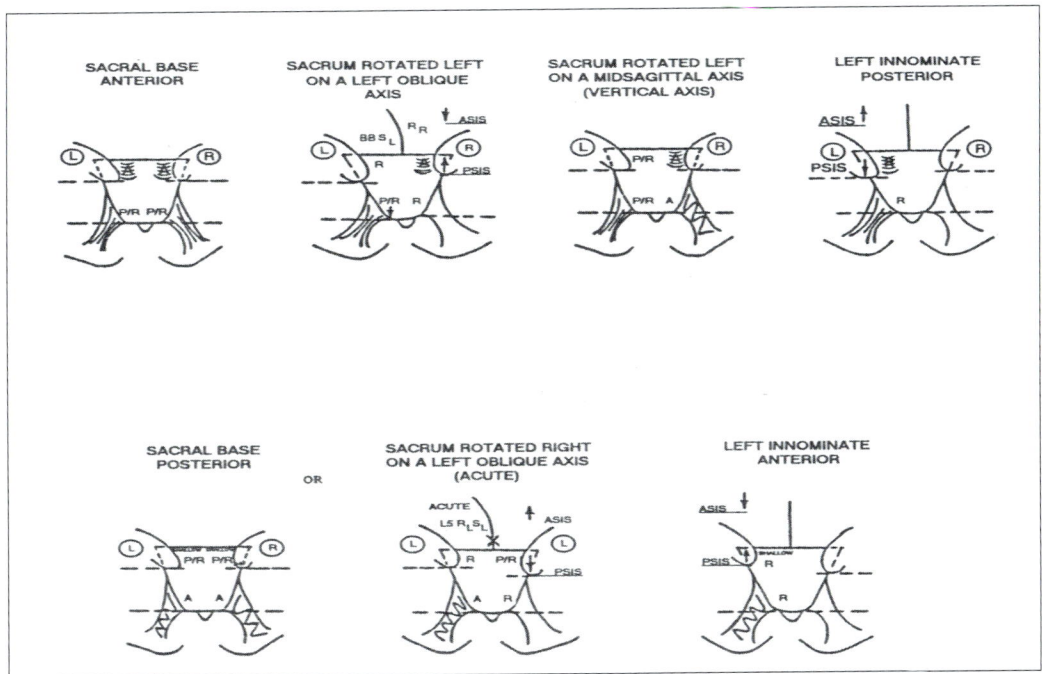

Figure 9-14: Passive palpatory clinical finding in some sacral and innominate dysfunctions (Courtesy fo Kuchera WA and Kuchera ML)

Table 9-5: Osteopathic Vertebral Dysfunctions

AREA AND DYSFUNCTION	FINDINGS AND GENERAL INFORMATION
LUMBAR AND THORACIC SPINE	Restrictions of flexion or extension that often are due to: • Nonneutral (Type II) dysfunctions called "FRS" and "ERS." • Neutral (Type I) dysfunctions called "NR."
NEUTRAL GROUP DYSFUNCTION NR (SIDE)	• Usually a compensatory reaction to a nonneutral dysfunction. • N represents neutral, R represents the rotation, (the direction of the rotation in the parentheses). • Sidebending is to the side opposite of rotation. • Motion is restricted toward the convex side of the group, and rotation is restricted in the opposite direction. • Total range of flexion and extension usually is reduced. • Neutral restriction, i.e., rotation and sidebending to opposite sides, can occur in one motion segment (not a group dysfunction) when passive testing is used for diagnosis.
FRS (SIDE)	Describes a segment as flexed, rotated, and sidebent to one side. (The side is marked in parentheses.): • Often restrictions of movements and provocation of pain are in the opposite directions. • Usually the total range of extension and flexion is reduced.
ERS (SIDE)	Opposite of FRS: • Restricted motions, often the provocation of pain, are in flexion, rotation, and sidebending to the opposite side. • Spinous process and the supraspinous ligament are tender. • Transverse process (TrPs) and/or the articular capsule often are very tender.

Table 9-6: Osteopathic Sacroiliac Dysfunctions (The Mitchell Model)

DYSFUNCTION	GENERAL INFORMATION	FINDINGS
GENERAL RULES	In all torsions, the prominent sacral inferior lateral angle (ILA) and deeper sacral sulcus are on opposite sides. The torsion is toward the prominent ILA side. In flexed sacral dysfunction, the prominent ILA and deeper sacral sulcus are on the same side.	If the ILAs are symmetrical and remain symmetrical for 10 seconds, there is no torsion or unilateral flexion dysfunction. If the sacrum oscillates (large rocking sacral movements back and forth), it indicates a dysfunction in the cranial mechanism, usually in the posterior cranial fossa, or involving the temporal bone. If the asymmetry is predominately posterior, the lesion is probably sacral torsion toward the side of the posterior ILA. If the sacral sulcus of one side is deeper, and the sacral ILA of that same side is more inferior and posterior relative to the opposite ILA, there is unilaterally flexed sacrum on that side.
PUBIC SHEARS	The most common subluxation of the pelvis, especially during pregnancy. Can be inferior or superior. Inferior shears tend to be self-correcting by weightbearing.	Positive, standing flexion (++), seated flexion (+), and Stork tests on the dysfunctional side. Superior or inferior pube on the dysfunctional side ASIS position, with patient supine, as per position of pube.
ANTERIOR TORSIONS	Quite common, often associated with mild symptoms.	

LEFT-ON-LEFT	About 4:1 compared to right on right.	Standing flexion test (+) positive on the right.
		Seated flexion test (++) positive on right.
		Sacral right base loses its function of posterior nutation.
		    —Therefore malposition and dysfunction (and possibly pain) are exaggerated when patient is forward bent.
		• Sacral ILA posterior (++) and inferior (+) on the left.
		• Sacral base is posterior (rotated left) on the left in flexion with deep sacral sulcus on right.
		    —The sacral base becomes level in extension.
		    —The left ILA is also a little inferior, but not as much as in nutation dysfunction (unilaterally flexed sacrum).
		L-5 is rotated to right and lumbar adaptation is convex to right.
		Short leg with patient prone on left (++).

RIGHT-ON-RIGHT		Findings are reversed.

BACKWARD TORSION DYSFUNCTIONS	Less common.
	Prominent ILA and deeper sacral sulcus on the opposite sides.
	Described as right-on-left (or left-on-right) oblique axis.
	    —Associated with lumbar nonneutral dysfunction.
	    —Often with extension restrictions (FRS).
	    —Often are acute and severely painful.
		Normal nutation movement of one side of the sacral base is restricted,
		    —therefore signs, and usually symptoms, are exaggerated by extension of the lumbar spine.

LEFT ON RIGHT	More common than Right on Left.
	    —May be found with dysfunction of FRS(lf) at L5-S1, a combination that is very painful.
	    —L5 should be treated first.
	    —The left sacral base is posterior; rotated left and sidebent right and posteriorly nutated at left base
		Seating flexion test (++) positive on the left.
		Standing flexion test (+) positive left.
		The sacral base and the ILA are posterior (++) on the left in extension, sacral sulcus deep on right.
		    —ILA also slightly inferior (+).
		    —Both are level in flexion.
		Lumbar lordosis and spring are reduced.
		L-5 rotated right.
		Short leg with patient prone on left (++).
		PSIS with patient prone inferior on left (++).
		ASIS with patient supine inferior on right (++).

RIGHT ON LEFT		Findings are reversed.

Table 9-6: Osteopathic Sacroiliac Dysfunctions (The Mitchell Model) (Continued)

UNILATERAL FLEXED SACRUM (LEFT)	Left unilateral flexed sacrum (anterior sacral nutations, inferior shear on left.) Prominent ILA and deeper sacral sulcus on same side. —Are much more common than right-sided dysfunctions (about 9:1). —Must be treated with manual therapy. —Often patient suffers from morning pain. —Often seen in so-called cocktail syndrome with ERS(lf) at L5, left pub dysfunction, and left innominate dysfunction.	Often the seated flexion test is positive on the left (++). Often the standing flexion test positive on the left (+). The base on that side is "stuck" in anterior nutation (flexed) (with loss of counternutation). —Base is found anterior to the iliac crest, especially in spinal flexion, —but slightly less in neutral. —In extension it is only little improved. —Sacrum is sidebent to the left. —ILA is inferior (++) on the same side, about 1 cm, and is slightly posterior (+), but not as much as in torsional dysfunctions. The leg is short with patient prone on right side (++). Lumbar compensation is usually rotation of L-5 to the left. Lumbar spine usually convex on left. With lordosis (-spring).
UNILATERAL EXTENDED SACRUM (RIGHT)[a]	Sacrum loses its nutation function. More common in patients that have had spinal surgery. Findings are more pronounced in lumbar extension. Much more common on the right.	Often the seated flexion test is positive (++) on the right. Often the standing flexion test positive (+) on right. In extension the sacral base is found even more posteriorly on the right, sacral sulcus deep on left. —The ILA are more anterior (+) and superior (++) on right. —in neutral or in flexion they are only little improved. The lumbar lordosis and spring is reduced. Long leg with patient supine on right. Lumbar compensation is usually with L5 rotation to the right.

a. Mitchell claims this dysfunction does not occur, and the diagnosis may be based on erroneous interpretation of the flexion test (personal conversation). Others disagree.

Table 9-7: Osteopathic Iliosacral Disorders

DYSFUNCTION	GENERAL INFORMATION	FINDINGS
ILIOSACRAL DYSFUNCTIONS GENERAL	First treat pelvic subluxation and SI dysfunctions	The standing flexion test is still positive after treatment to SI. The ASISs are still found to be unequal. An iliosacral dysfunction is probable.
UPSLIPPED INNOMINATE	Second most common pelvic "dislocation." More common on right side (questionable).	Seated (++) and standing (++) flexion tests are positive on the upslipped side. The ischial tuberosity, iliac crest, and leg are found superiorly on that side. The sacrotuberous ligament is lax on the subluxed side, unless the innominate is also posteriorly rotated.[a]
POSTERIOR INNOMINATE (LT)	More common on the left side.	The left ASIS will be superior on the side of the positive standing flexion test (++). The leg on that side appears to be shorter.
ANTERIOR INNOMINATE	Anterior innominate is much more common on the right side.	The findings are the reverse of posterior innominate.
ILIAC OUTFLARE (LT)	Found in pathologic joints with reverse relation of convex concave plane of the joint.	Standing flexion test positive (++) on left. ASIS further from midline on left.
ILIAC INFLARE (RT)	Found in pathologic joints with reverse relation of convex concave planes of the joint.	Standing flexion test positive (++) on right. ASIS further from midline on right.

a. The patient may be treated prone if associated with anteriorly rotated innominate and supine if associated with posterior rotation (Lee *ibid*).

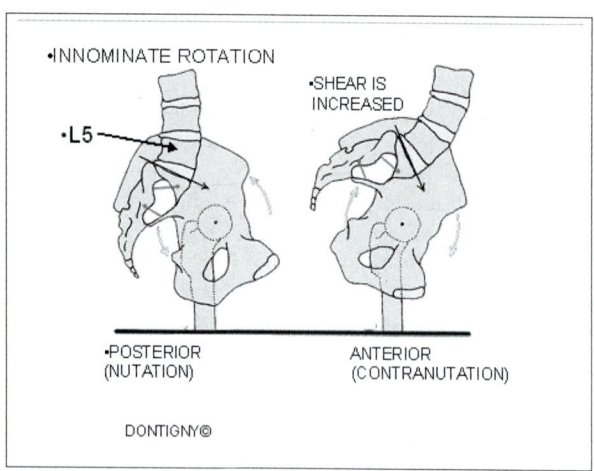

Figure 9-15: Influence of innominate rotation on lumbosacral dynamics (courtesy of Dontigny)

Figure 9-11 illustrate common clusters found in failed low back patients.

SEGMENTAL RELATIONS. Joint dysfunctions often result in predictable secondary dysfunctions due to mechanical and neural phenomena. Neural interconnection from somatic, sympathetic, dermatomal, sclerotomal, myotomal, and visceratomal in the left and right columns can cause a local segmental disorder to spread to its related segments. These are commonly seen as (Brown *ibid*):

- C8/T1/T2 affecting or being affected by C1/C2;
- T2/T3/T4 affecting or being affected by C3/C4;
- T5/T6 affecting or being affected by C5/C6;
- T7/T8/T9 affecting or being affected by C7/C8;
- T10/T11 affecting or being affected by L3/L4;
- T12/L1/L2 affecting or being affected by L5/S1/S2.

When any symptoms present at any of the above segments, the related segment should be assessed and treated if needed, either by manual therapy or acupuncture.

The osteopathic literature describes three main types of indirect methods which will be reviewed later in this chapter (Ward *ibid*):

- Balance and hold;
- Dynamic functional procedures;
- Countertension-positional-release-(Strain-counterstrain™).

And four main types of direct methods:

- Muscle energy;
- Myofascial release;
- High velocity techniques;
- Articulatory techniques.[6]

Functionally Oriented Screen Tests

Screening tests vary according to the system used and personal preferences. It is this author's practice to often pay special attention to the lower kinetic chain as it is the base of posture and can have far reaching effects. However, the screen tests are often made to ascertain which area of the body is most restricted, and, therefore, no preconceived ideas should guide assessment and thereafter treatment. Treatment should always follow what an individual patient's body tells us at any given moment. The musculoskeletal screening can lead the practitioner to areas of dysfunction that are outside of the patient's complaint areas. Often these are primary and must be addressed.

The problems, dysfunctions and compensatory mechanisms that this section has described are multi-layered and complex. Treatment requires accurate diagnosis, which can take time. The practitioner should always perform a full examination, and the treatment approach should always be systematic. Some practitioners suggest that performing the examination before conducting the interview can reduce bias and help identify the root lesion. At times dysfunctions only reveal themselves after treatment. Therefore, one should not be too quick to take credit for successful treatment after previous failure by others.

Osteopathic and Functional Tests

It is the author's practice to screen the entire spine following a protocol taught by Dr. Ed Stiles DO, especially when considering manual therapies. This process is helpful also when using acupuncture. The objective of this screen is to find the area of greatest *restriction*. It is Dr. Stiles belief that one should follow *a treatment sequence* to treat musculoskeletal and other somatic dysfunctions effectively, starting at the area of greatest restriction (like opening a combination lock which requires a particular *sequence* to be opened). After each intervention, the screen is repeated and treatment of the next area of greatest restriction commences. By following this sequence one may avoid the trap of treating secondary compensation or chasing symptoms.

There are several restriction patterns that may indicate: upper extremity, lower extremity, cranial, or rib-cage dysfunction. If one encounters one of these patterns, then that area is screened again to find the area of next greatest restriction (e.g., cranial suture, acromioclavicular joint, etc.). The patterns are as follow:

---

6. There are many variations of such methods including: Fascial-Ligamentous Release Techniques, Balanced Ligamentous Tension Techniques, Neuromuscular Release Techniques, Cranial Techniques, Lymphatic Techniques, Visceral Manipulation Techniques, among others.

Functionally Oriented Screen Tests

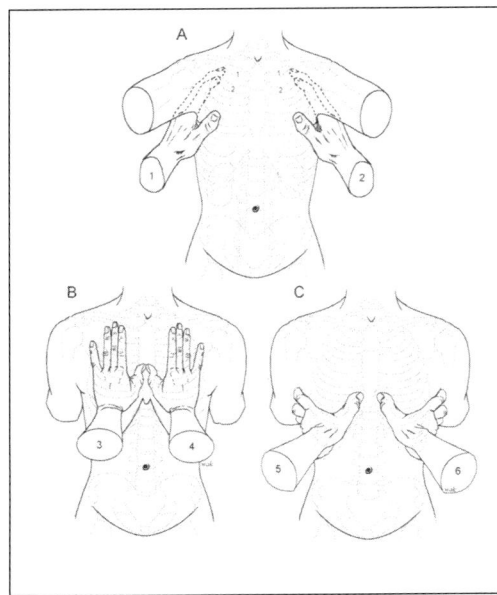

Figure 9-16: Palpation of respiratory rib motions ((From Kuchera WA and Kuchera ML, Osteopathic Principles in Practice, KCOM press 1993, with permission).

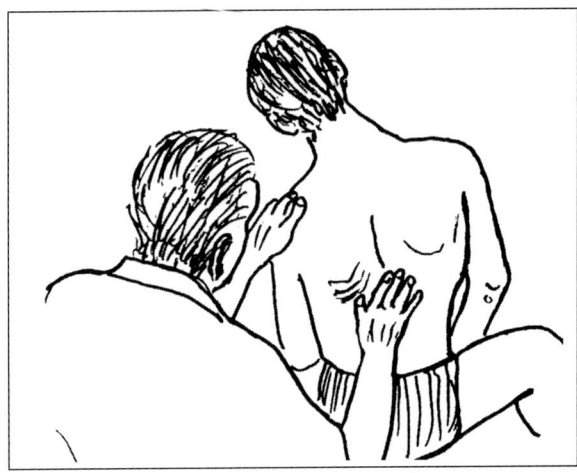

Figure 9-17: Joint play assessed at thoracic spine.

- At the occipital-atlantal joint, if one experiences a hard end-feel without muscle tightening, this can indicate a cranial problem, so the cranial motions are screened and treated (as long as this is the area of greatest restriction in the spine).
- If a group of periscapular joints and muscles are restricted and tight on one side, this can indicate an upper extremity problem. The upper extremity on that side is screened for the area of greatest restriction.
- If one segment at the thoracic spine seems to be the area of greatest restriction, then the rib at that level is evaluated for springing. If the rib feels tighter than the facet at that level, then the entire rib cage is screened for respiratory restrictions. According to Dr. Stiles, when following this process one only needs to treat respiratory rib dysfunction. If the facet (close to spine) is more restricted than the ribs (tested by springing the rib angles), then that joint is assessed for extension and flexion dysfunction and treated.
- If one finds a group of tight facets with a tight quadratus lumborum on one side, then this may indicate a lower extremity problem. The lower extremity is screened.

In a clinical audit of 100 of his low back patients, Dr. Stiles found that in most cases the area of greatest restriction was in the thoracic region and rib cage. He also found that after treating these areas, findings in the pelvis would often change. During the screening the patient either sits or stands with the practitioner standing on the side and slightly behind. The screening is performed as follows:

1. The practitioner places one of his thumbs on one side at the occipital-atlantal area. The other hand is placed on top of patients head. The practitioner then stacks up (i.e., adds) movement into: slight flexion, sidebending, and finally rotation to the thumb side, using the hand on top of the head. He then translates his thumb forward at a 60-degree angle toward the spine while at the same time moving the patient's head toward his thumb with his other hand and tests end-feel. This process is repeated for the entire cervical spine, flexing slightly more each time a lower segment is evaluated.

2. When reaching the thoracic spine the hand that was on the patient's head is moved to his shoulder repeating the same process except that now the movements are into: extension, sidebending and rotation (Figure 9-17),

A variation which the author uses frequently is to induce sidebending to one side of the spine while monitoring the other side with the thumb for non-neutral responses (e.g., if the segment at the apex of the induced curve rotates toward the concavity the monitoring thumb moves forwards). The information is assessed at the beginning of motion before muscle splinting obscures palpatory information (Figure 9-18).

The screen tests described below can be used as well. The practitioner tests active movement with the patient in several positions.

Active Movement, Patient Standing and Sitting Tests.

With the patient standing the practitioner:

1. tests trunk, lumbar and cervical sidebending, extension, rotation, and flexion;

2. observes for asymmetry;

3. observes for increased or decreased AP curves, scoliosis, paravertebral asymmetry, and muscle tone;

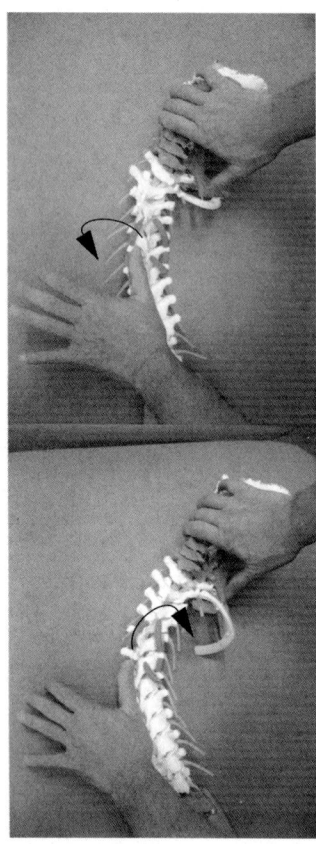

Figure 9-18: Upper shows normal/neutral sidebending coupled with opposite rotation. Lower shows dysfunctional sidebending coupled with rotation to the same side. The rotation is assessed at the beginning of movement as apposed to endfeel.

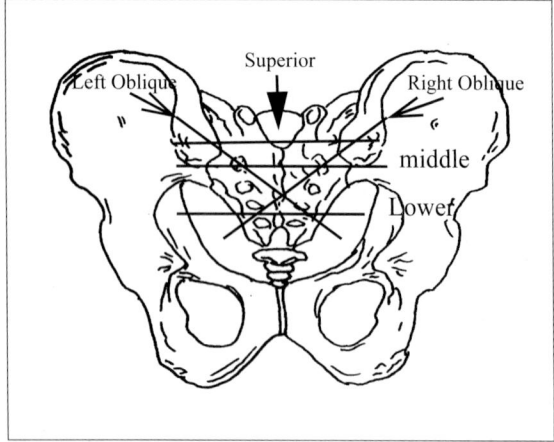

Figure 9-19: Sacral axis. Superior axis reflect cranial motion. mid-axis reflect sacral motions and lower axis innominate motion.

4. performs a standing flexion test;

5. repeats these observations with the patient sitting;

6. tests upper extremity function by having the patient abduct his arm while touching the backs of his hands

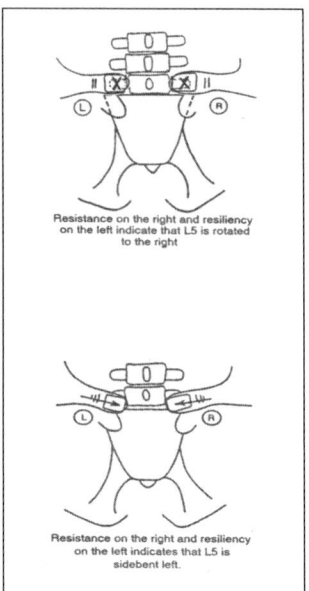

Figure 9-20: Joint function (play) assessment. Superior figure shows passive testing of rotation. Inferior figure shows passive testing of sidebending (From Kuchera WA and Kuchera ML, Osteopathic Principles in Practice, KCOM press 1993, with permission).

above the head. He palpates the clavicle during this movement for the clavicular jump test.

With the patient prone, the practitioner:

1. checks bony symmetry;

2. tests joint play in the spine by pushing on the transverse and spinous processes, springing individual vertebra (Figure 9-20).;

With the patient supine, the practitioner:

1. checks for bony symmetry and resting foot positions;

2. performs the compression (squish) test by anterior pressure on the ASISs. Pressure directed towards the upper (SI) pole reflects cranial axis function; pressure towards the middle (SI) pole reflects the pelvis and SI joints functions; and pressure towards the lower (SI) pole reflects functions of the innominates and lower extremities (Figure 9-19 and Figure 9-28 on page 478);

3. tests respiratory movement of the rib cage for symmetry. Inhalation and exhalation should be equal bilaterally;

4. performs a straight leg raise (SLR), and dural tension test which are part of the general orthopedic evaluation;

5. performs *Patrick's Faber* maneuver to test the hips and SI joints (flexion, abduction and external rotation). The test is also part of the general orthopedic evaluation. Normally the end-feel is leathery and range is equal on both sides

Functionally Oriented Screen Tests

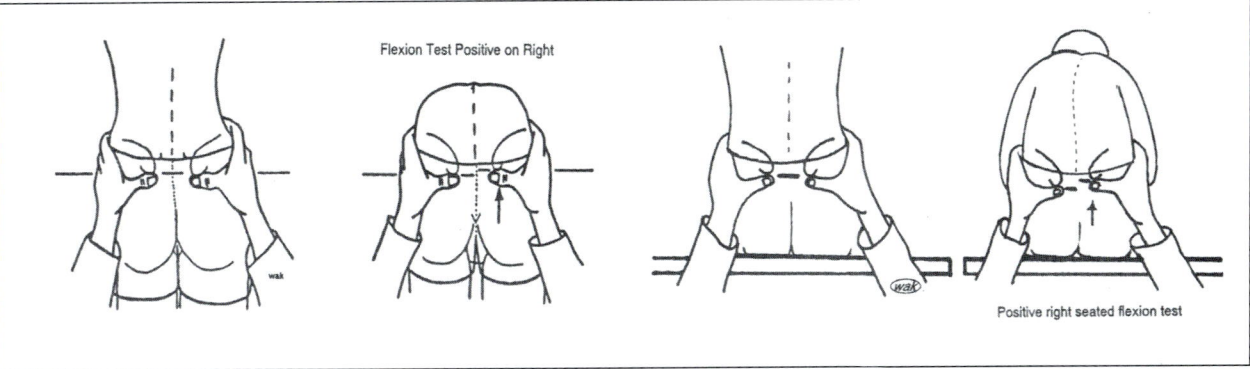

Figure 9-22: Standing and sitting flexion test (From Kuchera WA and Kuchera ML, Osteopathic Principles in Practice, KCOM press 1993, with permission).

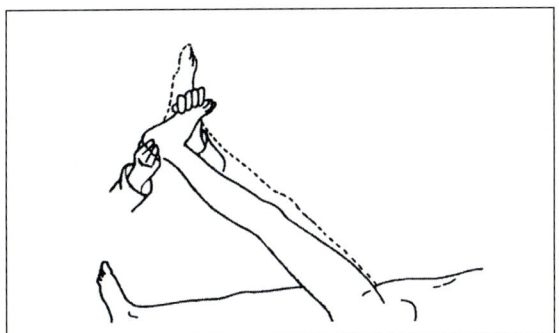

Figure 9-21: Straight leg rase (doted line). Dural tension test solid line.

Standing and Sitting Flexion Tests.

The standing flexion test is used to evaluate iliosacral motion and lower extremity function; the seated flexion test is used to evaluate sacroiliac motion. In the former, the patient is standing with feet hip-width apart. If, before performing the standing flexion test, the ilial crests are not level, the practitioner can place a shim under the leg on the lower side. If, after leveling the ilial crests the PSISs are not level, there may be an iliosacral somatic dysfunction. (Dr. Stiles does not level the hips and prefers to test the patient as he or she is.) Anterior-posterior asymmetry suggests hip rotator imbalance, which would cause the entire pelvis to rotate (Mitchell ibid). The practitioner then places two thumbs just at the inferior slope of the Posterior Superior Iliac Spines (PSISs) (which are found about a cm or more inferior to the dimple of Michaels) or on the gluteal tubercles. The patient is then asked to bend forward and touch the floor, keeping the knees straight. Movements of the PSISs are followed (Figure 9-22).

The upward movement of each PSIS should be equal. If either moves further or earlier, the iliosacral motion at that side is said to be restricted. Special attention is paid to the end of movement as a sudden acceleration is often noted on the positive side. A tight hamstring can cause a false positive. While the patient is flexed, the hamstring can be palpated. One can also perform a reverse test, seeing which PSIS moves first when the patient returns to the upright position. (Mitchell considers this more accurate and reproducible.)

The practitioner repeats the same test with the patient seated (Figure 9-22).

NOTE: Testing the patient seated focuses the tests on the pelvis and spine, eliminating contribution from the lower extremities.

- If abnormal findings are decreased in the seated test, the problem is likely to come from the lower extremities and the iliosacral axis.

- If abnormal findings with the seated test do not change or if they increase, the problem is more likely to originate in the pelvis or spine.

Squat Test

To test the knees, hips, ankles, quadriceps, and calf muscle, the practitioner asks the patient to perform a squat. The test is best performed bare footed with feet parallel, allowing for adaptation if needed, at about hip width apart. Any difficulty may reflect dysfunctions in these areas (Figure 9-23). The practitioner pays special attention to the heels, checking to see if one starts moving first (this often reflects an unstable foot and ankle) or to see if the patient cannot squat without lifting the ankles (testing for heel cord tension). An unstable foot and/or ankle has implications for the entire musculoskeletal system. When this test is positive, especially in patients with low back pain, attention to the foot and ankle are of utmost importance. The practitioner also observes how the knees track in relation to the foot. Poor knee track often result in knee pain and pathology. Does the patient need to shift their weight, or do the heels move medially as the test progresses? If it does this often shows that the patient cannot stabilize the foot due to excessive subtalar pronation or foot ligamentous laxity. This test is often used as part of a basic orthopedic evaluation.

Clavicular Jump Test

This test is used to look for clues in three areas of the body: lumbar spine, thoracic spine, and pelvis (Bear 1999). The patient stands with their arms hanging at their sides. The practitioner:

1. instructs the patient to place the palms of their hands against the sides of their legs;

2. lightly places the pads of his index fingers on the medial ends of the clavicles and evaluates for levelness of the clavicles;

3. instructs the patient to slowly raise their arms over their head without bending the elbows or rotating the arms. This should bring the backs of the hands together;

4. evaluates the new position of the clavicles.
   Findings: If the clavicles were uneven to start with and are now even (level), the problem will be found from T10 inferiorly.
   If the clavicles were even to start with and are now uneven, the problem may be found in the pelvis on the side which is now superior (with the most likely dysfunction being an upslip).
   If the clavicles were uneven to start with and are still uneven but the sides are reversed, the problem may be found above T6.
   This test will not work in a patient who has sustained a fracture of the clavicle or who has limited range in the shoulder due to any pathology. This test in not used as part of a basic orthopedic exam.

Patrick's Faber Test

This test is said to evaluate the hip joint, but it can also compress the sacroiliac (SI) joint. The hip is put in flexion,

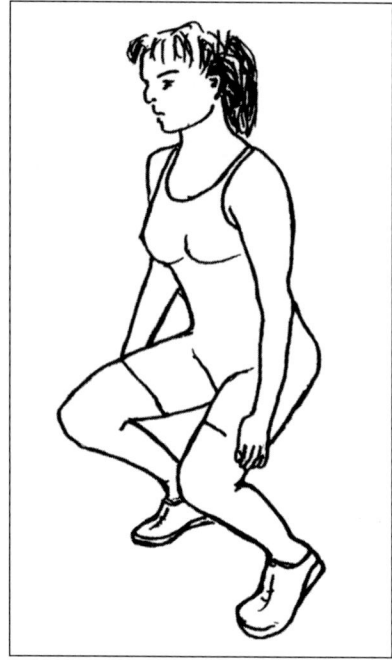

Figure 9-23: Squat test.

abduction, and external rotation (Figure 9-24). After reaching the end of movement, the femur is fixed in relation to the pelvis. The practitioner holds down the anterior superior ilia spine (ASIS) on the opposite side and increases the pressure at the medial side by pressing down on the knee. This stresses the anterior sacroiliac ligaments; in particular, on the side of the abducted leg.

With hip pathology, the patient often complains of anterior or proximal posterior femur pain. With sacroiliac disorders, the patient often complains of pain in the sacroiliac region. In the presence of L4 or L5 disc disease, this test can be markedly restricted.

Forced lateral rotation with the leg held in 90° of flexion and resisted adduction of the thigh exerts a distraction force at the SI joints and indirectly stretches the anterior SI ligaments. Forced medial rotation at the hip joint with the hip and knee held at 90° of flexion and resisted abduction of the thigh pulls the ilium away from the sacrum. In the absence of hip joint pathology, pain experienced over the SI joint is highly suggestive of a SI problem (Ombregt et al *ibid*).

Fascial Asymmetries

Fascial screen tests evaluate for preferences in rotation of body fascial planes. The four primary areas to be tested are the Occipito-Atlanta area (OA), the Cervico-Thoracic area (CT), the Thoraco-Lumbar area (TL), and the Lumbo-Sacral area (LS). Ideally, the fascial planes would have equal rotational ability to the right and left at each of these areas. The

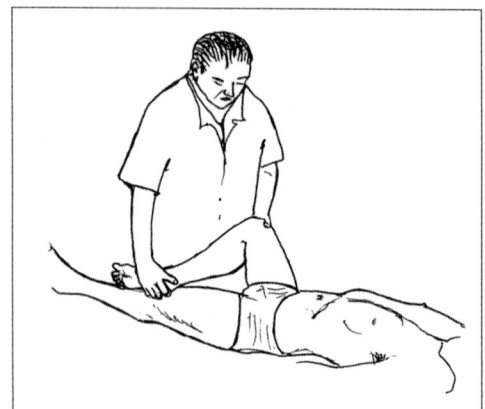

Figure 9-24: Patrick's Faber Test.

tests are performed by placing the practitioner's palm on the patient's area to be assessed, gently pressing down and then rotating (or side-moving) the palm left and right. Commonly areas have sequential rotational preferences which is viewed as proper adoption. For example, if the OA rotates more easily to the right, the CT area will do so to the left. If both the OA and CT areas have similar preferences, this is viewed as poor compensation (Figure 9-25).

To test the sacral area, the practitioner stands on one side facing the head of the supine patient and reaches across to place one hand under the opposite hip and slightly under the gluteal muscle. The other hand is placed over the ASIS closest to the practitioner. The hip is then picked-up and a mild attempt to rotate it toward the practitioner is made two or three times. The hands are then reversed, and the test repeated. When a preference is present (which is so almost universally), one side will lift easily and the other less so (Kuchera and Kuchera *ibid*).

Tissue Congestion and Terminal Lymphatic Drainage

There are six major areas that provide clues to regional congestion on each side of the body (Kuchera and Kuchera *ibid*).

1. Supraclavicular for the head and neck. Palpated by gently compressing the tissues. Fullness or bogginess on either side indicates dysfunction.

2. Posterior axillary folds for the upper extremities. The practitioner's hand is held with the palm up and the index finger placed against the rib cage and posterior to the posterior axillary fold; the lateral side of the thumb is also against the rib cage but anterior to the posterior axillary fold; the straight fingers and the straight thumb are brought together in a compressing clamp-like manner. Pressure is sequentially applied from the top of the region to the bottom—from the second to the eighth rib level. Dysfunction is indicated by tender nodules or areas of fullness.

3. Epigastric area for the abdomen. The area is observed and palpated for puffiness.

4. Inguinal areas for the thigh, leg, and/or feet. The area is palpated with the fingers. Dysfunction is indicated if the region is taut, ticklish, and/or tender.

5. Popliteal areas for legs and/or feet. With the knee slightly flexed, the practitioner palpates each popliteal space for fullness, which indicates dysfunction.

6. Achilles tendons for ankles and feet. The tendon is gently squeezed between the thumb and the index and middle finger. The tendon feels thicker on the side of dysfunction.bv

Fascial asymmetries and tissue congestion are functionally related. When the fascias are not freely moveable they can produce tensions which will not only affect the pathways

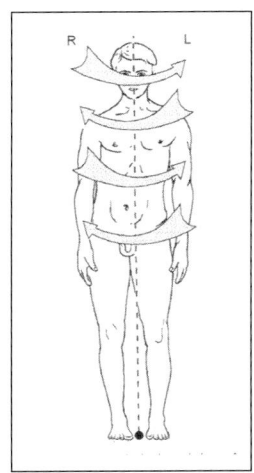

Figure 9-25: Assessment for fascial asymmetries (From Kuchera WA and Kuchera ML, Osteopathic Principles in Practice, KCOM press 1993, with permission).

for veins, lymphatics, and nerves but also the function of the abdominal diaphragm which acts as an extrinsic pump of the lymphatic system.

Joint Play

Mennell describes "joint play" as a motion within a synovial joint, in which the motion is separate from, and cannot be initiated by, voluntary muscle contraction. Joint play consists of fine movement (less than 1/8-inch) in any plane the natural laxity of the joint capsule allows. The play available at each joint is the sum of all passive angular and translatory movements (such as x-y-z planes).

The range of joint play is the same for any given joint of the same kind (the shoulder, the wrist etc.) with that type's characteristic end-feel. Loss of joint play impairs function and is associated with pain.

Restoration of joint play is considered crucial for normal joint function. Familiarity with joint play is essential for the understanding of manual therapy techniques. Proper manipulation therapy is effective for restoring normal movement.

ASSESSING JOINT PLAY. Mennell has proposed nine rules for assessing joint play. The practitioner:

1. Must see that the patient is relaxed. To avoid painful movement, the patient's joint must be supported and protected.

2. Must be relaxed. The practitioner's grip must be comfortable for the patient.

3. The practitioner and patient must isolate and examine one joint at a time (when possible).

4. Test one movement at a time.

5. Hold one aspect of the joint stable while mobilizing the other.

6. Ascertain the extent of normal joint play by examining the unaffected side (if not symptomatic).

7. Stop the movement at any point that pain is elicited.

8. Never use forced or abnormal movement.

9. If the patient presents with obvious inflammation or disease, the practitioner must not perform an examination of movement.

For more joint specific information see the author's book *Musculoskeletal Disorders: Healing Methods from Chinese Medicine, Orthopaedic Medicine and Osteopathy* North Atlantic Books 1998.

Analysis of Findings

Distance Between Patient's Legs, Spine, and Pelvic Sway

The distance between the patient's legs is usually two to four inches. A wider stance can indicate that the patient has a feeling of instability, unsteadiness and poor balance and could be due to brain and spinal cord lesions, peripheral neuropathy, or inner ear disorders. Both stride and step length vary with the patient's age, size, fatigue, dysfunction, and pathology. Stride inequality usually indicates lower limb dysfunction, but it may also be due to pain avoidance from symptoms in the head, neck, or trunk (Hoppenfeld ibid; Mitchell ibid). Elevated ilia with concurrent lowering of the homolateral shoulder may indicate long limb dysfunction. Flexion at the waist during single support phase of gait may indicate functional hallux limitus (FHL; Dananberg *ibid*).

Tilted Shoulders, Arms, Head, Upper Body. Neck and/or Pupillary Line

If the pupillary line or neck lines are not level or straight, this may point to a failure of the cervical spine or occipital-atlantal joint to adapt, since the righting reflex strongly tries to maintain a level visual line. If there is a change between standing and sitting, then the pelvis must be examined (Bear *ibid*).

Tilted shoulders, head, or upper body can be either primary or secondary to lower trunk and limb dysfunctions and/or pathology. Commonly, the shoulder on the dominant side is a little lower with a small tilt of the head to the same side. A raised shoulder often indicates a weak lower trapezius and serratous muscles with hyperactivity of the upper trapezius and levator scapula muscles (Janda *ibid*; Mitchell *ibid*).

An anteriorly protruded head (*forward head posture*) can affect the entire musculoskeletal system and is usually due to weakness of the deep neck flexors and dominance or tightness of the suboccipitals and sternocleidomastoid muscles; the pectoralis major is often tight as well. Tightness of the upper trapezius and levator scapulae can be observed on the neck and shoulder line; the contour may straighten. These findings are collaborated with palpation of the muscles of the OA junction and with OA functional tests (head-nod test).[7] OA muscle tension is tested with the patient standing and seated. The seated position removes influences by pelvis/low extremities. When positive standing and negative seated, the dysfunction (forward head posture) is likely to be due to the lower extremity, innominate, or (Chaitow *ibid*) to forward-downward pelvic rotation and sacroiliac joint hypermobility in flexion—often a unilaterally flexed left (hyper-lordosis is often seen) and anteriorly rotated right innominate. Forward head posture may result from functional hallux limitus.

Excessive head and neck *movements* could suggest impaired mobility in the lower spine or limbs and/or short limb. An unequal distance of the upper arms from the trunk or an asymmetric arm swing can be seen with scoliosis or upper limb dysfunction or pain avoidance (Mitchell *ibid*). One internally rotated arm, may indicate a weak mid-trapezius and hyperactive latissimus dorsi muscles (Janda *ibid*). Lack of shoulder motion during gait, especially if unilateral, often indicates long limb functional accommodation (Dananberg *ibid*).

Scapula

Scapular winging can be seen in C5 palsy or palsy of the long thoracic nerve. It also indicates weakness of the serratus anterior and hyperactivity of the rhomboids, demonstrated with the push-up test (which brings on winging) (Ombregt et al *ibid*). A round shoulder and protracted scapula can indicate weakness in the mid-trapezius and tightness of pectoral muscles (Janda *ibid*).

Lumbar Lordosis

Decreased lumbar lordosis suggests paravertebral muscle spasm (commonly due to backward sacral dysfunction), disc disease or other significantly painful lesions. There is usually extension restrictions at lumbar joints (stuck in flexion). Often there is also a component of an anterior and/or lateral shear of those lumbar vertebrae, which contributes to the loss of lordosis.

Lordosis is increased with "sway back" (weak abdominal and psoas muscles, associated with Janda's pelvic crossed syndrome), spondylolisthesis, and anterior sacral dysfunctions. There is often flexion restriction at the lumbar vertebrae (stuck in extension).

Antalgic Posture

Antalgic postures (typical lumbago list, deviation away from pain) are commonly seen with psoas syndrome, disc lesions,

---

7. The supine patient's head-nod test is performed and observed by having the patient rest his/her head on the table. Then an up and down nodding or the chin (without rasing the head from the table) is assessed. Nodding should result in no sidebending or rotation of the head. If it does an OA dysfunction exists.

Functionally Oriented Screen Tests

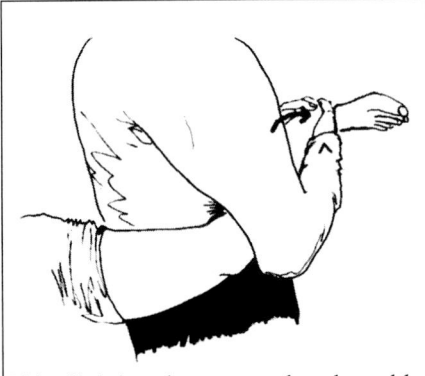
Side tilt joint play assessed at the ankle joint.

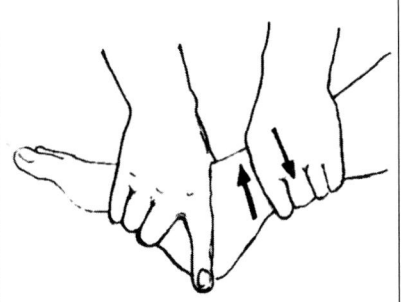
Anteroposterior glide of tibia and fibula on the talus.

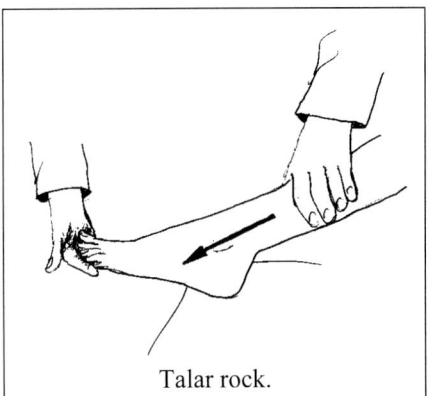
Talar rock.

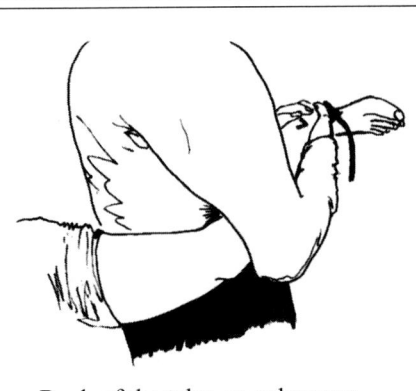
Rock of the talus on calcaneus.

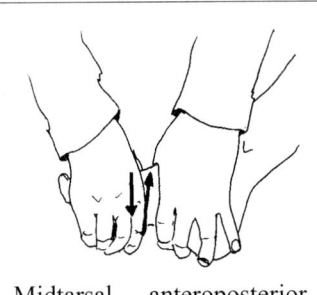
Midtarsal anteroposterior glide.

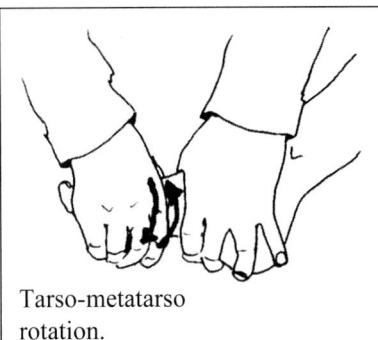
Tarso-metatarso rotation.

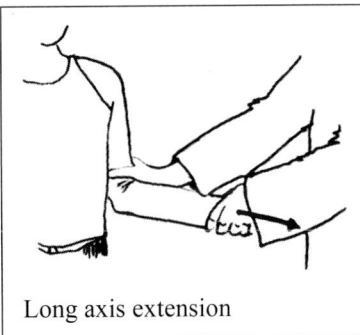
Long axis extension

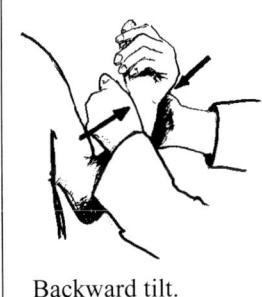
Backward tilt.

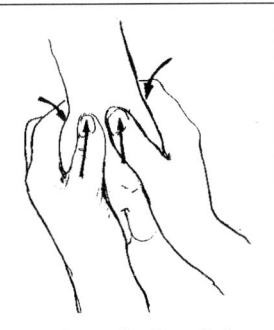
Backward tilt of the scaphoid and lunate upon the radius.

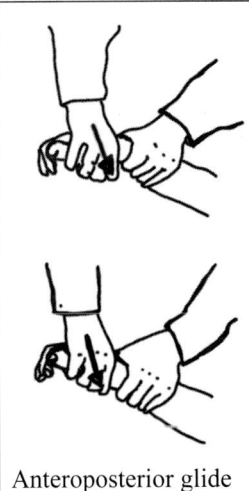
Anteroposterior glide

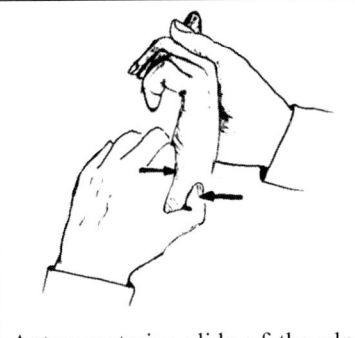
Anteroposterior glide of the ulna on the triquetrum

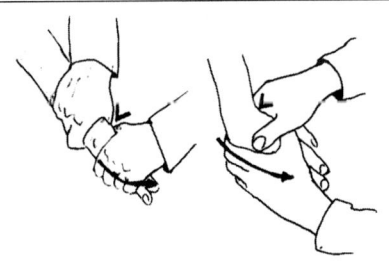
Side tilt of scaphoid on the radius

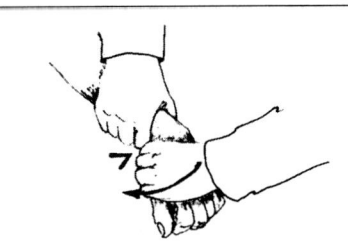
Side tilt of the triquetrum away from the ulna and the meniscus.

Figure 9-26: Example of joint play assessments and treatments.

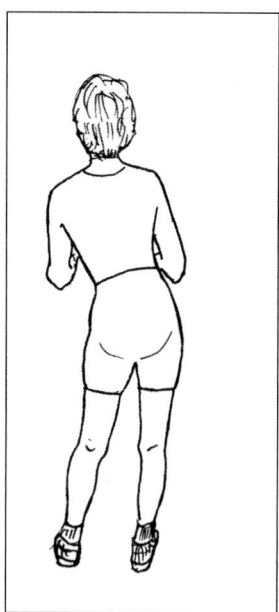

Figure 9-27: Postural list.

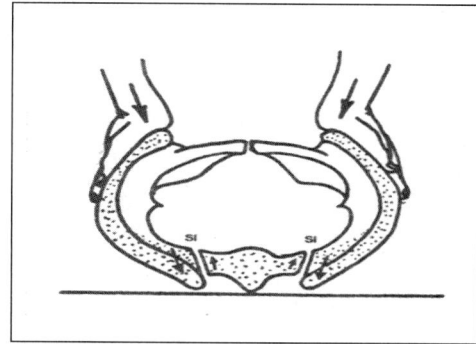

Figure 9-28: Pelvis compression (squish) test to ascertain SI joint restriction. The practitioner presses the ASIS towards the SI joint and feels for restriction. It is also possible to press on one side while feeling response on the other side. A restricted SI joint will result in faster and more significant movement on the opposite side (From Kuchera WA and Kuchera ML, Osteopathic Principles in Practice, KCOM press 1993, with permission).

and backward sacral torsions. They are also seen with extremity pain from the hip, knee, or feet (Figure 9-27).

Passive Rotation and Sidebending

Asymmetrical rotation and sidebending can point to somatic dysfunction at the area involved. Unequal trunk rotation with the patient seated-up-tall can indicate a lower thoracic/ upper lumbar dysfunction which should then be examined more closely. Normally, one is able to rotate ninety degrees to each side (Mitchell *ibid*).

Rib Cage Motions

When rib cage respiratory motions are bilaterally unequal, it is important to ascertain which key rib is restricted. When a group of ribs are restricted on inhalation, the key rib is the most superior of the group. When a group of ribs are restricted on exhalation, it is the bottom rib of the group that is usually the key rib.

Knee Tracking

Failure to keep the knee in line with the foot during the squat test often indicates a problem with the patient's subtalar joint. With over pronation, usually the patella will shift medially. Lack of full knee extension during gait is often seen with functional hallux limitus.

Pelvic Tilt (Oblique Position)

A pelvic tilt due to a shortening of the lower extremity can be detected as a "short leg gait." Here, the patient shows a lateral shift toward the shorter leg and a downward pelvic

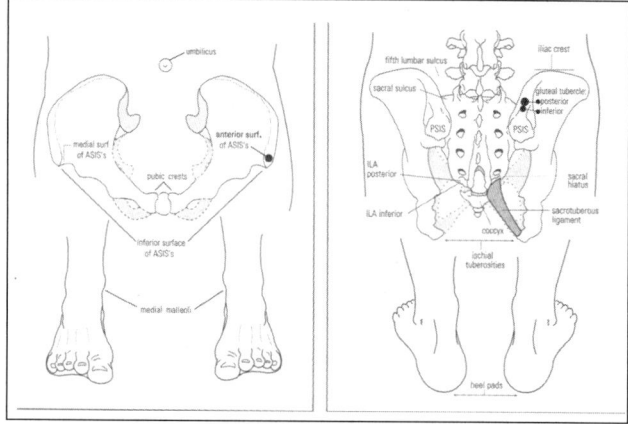

Figure 9-29: Important landmarks for palpation of pelvic obliqueness and dysfunction (courtesy of Mitchell *ibid*).

tilt. These result in a limp-like gait, depending on the discrepancy between leg lengths. Patients may compensate for a short leg by rotating their innominates posteriorly on the long leg side and anteriorly on the short leg side. Such patients do not show a short leg gait; however, on the short leg side, the heel lifts prematurely in mid-stance (Kuchera and Kuchera *ibid*). Often the short leg is externally rotated (Mitchell *ibid*), the foot on the long leg side often pronates.

A pelvic twist is associated often with shortness of the piriformis and/or iliopsoas. Shortness of the thigh adductors and tightness of the quadratus lumborum and of the iliopsoas can lead to a functional short leg. Tightness of the piriformis makes the leg appear longer (Janda 1996). *(OM: while pelvic tilts often reflect a complicated pattern, most patients will also show reactions in the Girdle (Dai) channel).*

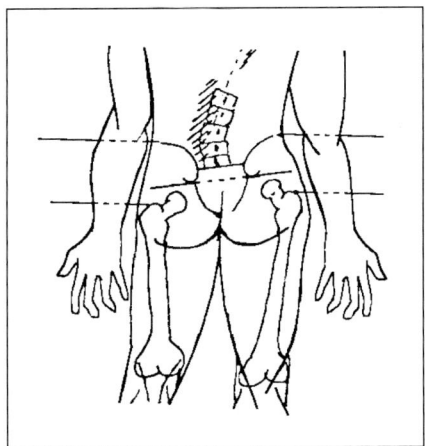

Figure 9-30: Scoliosis due to short leg (From Kuchera WA and Kuchera ML, Osteopathic Principles in Practice 1994, with permission).

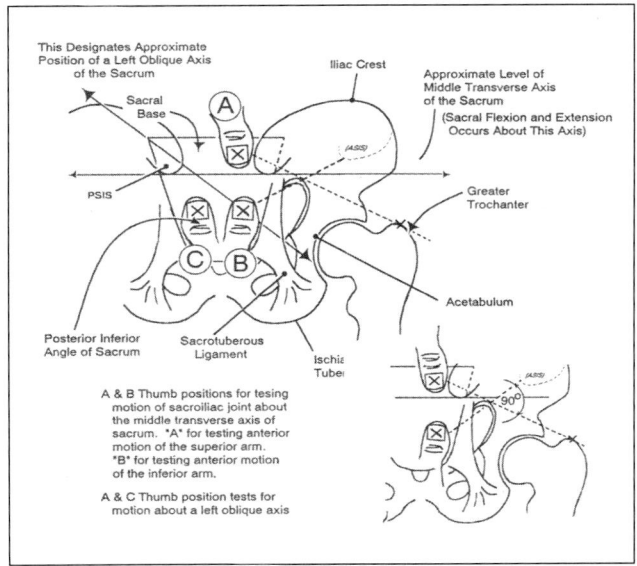

Figure 9-31: Passive motion testing for SI joint motions (From Kuchera WA and Kuchera ML, Osteopathic Principles in Practice, KCOM press 1993, with permission).

Pelvic Lateral and Vertical Movements, Spinal Movements

Pelvic lateral movement (normally one inch or so) is to the weight bearing side. Vertical movement is highest in midstance, usually is about two inches, and may be increased on the side with pathology. A patient walking with a stiff spine but with free pelvic superior shifts and rotational movements is more likely to have a spinal lesion than a pelvic lesion. Irregularities of hip sway suggest anatomic asymmetries of the lumbar and pelvic joints (Hoppenfeld *ibid*; Mitchell *ibid*; Dorman *ibid*).

Scoliosis

Scoliosis can be structural or functional. Abnormally high ilia, hips, unleveling of the sacral base, or inequality in leg length can result in secondary scoliosis. (*OM: scoliosis is most often associated with weakness in the Governing (Du) channel and with marrow and Kidney weakness.*)

Hypertrophy at the thoracolumbar erector spinae, with/or without a scoliotic curve, is due often to lumbosacral instability and poor muscle tone.

Rotated Leg, Feet

Normal gait is with the feet pointed straight ahead. An internally or externally rotated leg is due usually to a rotation imbalance of the hips and frequently are a compensation for pelvis and/or trunk asymmetries (Mitchell *ibid*). A flexed knee and internally rotated foot (Dorman and Ravin *ibid*) may represent either a problem in the affected hip or pain from the posterior superficial sacroiliac ligaments (*OM: Tai Yang Sinew channel, Divergent channel and/or Yin Motility [Qiao] deficiency.*) Bilateral toe-out (slew-foot) usually reflects poor trunk and head/neck posture. Toe-in (pigeon-toe) is commonly seen in athletes and is thought to enhance agility (Mitchell *ibid*) (*OM: Yang Motility (Qiao) deficiency*). Failure to raise the heel during single support phase of gait often indicates functional hallux limitus, or, if unilaterally present, may suggest an unequal leg length (Dananberg *ibid*).

A toed-out (push-off) phase of gait can result as a compensation to over pronated forefoot, hallux valgus with a flattened midtarsal joint, and forefoot and rearfoot varus; functional hallux limitus is seen often in these patients. They often develop buttock pain and a piriformis syndrome. Often the tibialis muscles are weak. (*OM: toe-out is often a result of Shao Yang channel and/or Yang Motility (Qiao) channel excess, Yin Motility (Qiao) deficiency. The Kidney and Bladder Sinew channels are weak*).

The positions of the patellae relative to the position of the feet can call attention to problems of the femur and knee, tibial torsions, and traumatic or degenerative displacements of the patella. (*OM: Altered patellar position is mostly due to Shao Yang and Yang Ming Sinew channels disorders and to degenerative Bi syndromes.*)

Alteration of Weight Transfer and Foot Arch

Aberration of weight transfer across the sole of the foot during gait is commonly due to somatic dysfunction (or ligamentous laxity) in tarsal articulations or rearfoot disorders.

Brisk walking should stimulate the *plantar myotatic reflexes* which are stimulated by a stretch of the plantar fascia and help in keeping the foot arch intact. This reflex involves the tendon of the tibialis posterior, which comes from the medial side of the foot, curves around the navicular bone, and crosses under the sole of the foot to attach to the cuboid, often extending to the head of the fifth metatarsal. It

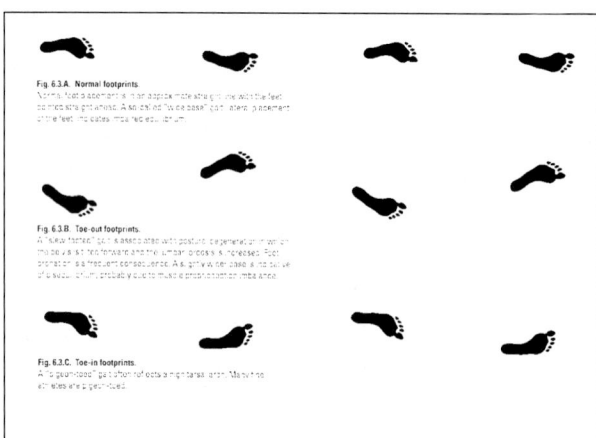

Figure 9-32: Normal gait, toe-in and toe-out gait (courtesy of Mitchell *ibid*).

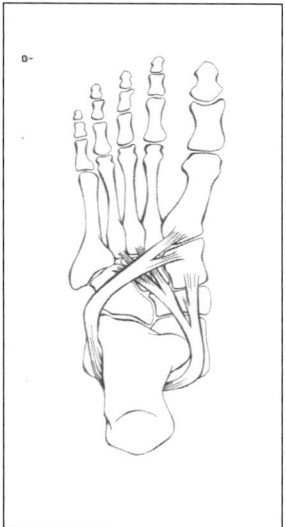

Figure 9-33: Tendinous arrangement that supports the foot (courtesy of Mitchell *ibid*).

also involves the peroneus muscles, the tendon of which come from the lateral side, passing under the cuboid, crossing under the arch, to attach at the first metatarsal head (Figure 9-33). These tendons create a stirrup for the foot. The simultaneous contraction of these muscles is a myotatic reflex response to a sudden stretch of the plantar fascia. When these muscles contract, they pinch the transverse tarsal arch together, rotating the tarsal bones into a close-packed relationship for the transmission of weight through the foot. The reflex is observed at mid-stride of the weight bearing foot. Absence of the reflexes is seen in mild cases of sciatic neuritis, suggesting the possibility of lumbo-pelvic somatic dysfunction. Tarsal or fibular dysfunction may inhibit this reflex (Mitchell *ibid*; Figure 9-34).

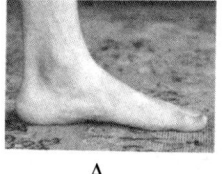 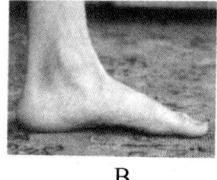

A   B

Figure 9-34: Myotatic reflex, absent in A), normal in B) (courtesy of Mitchell *ibid*.

Foot Callouses and Footwear

Most patients with significant foot problems develop callouses on their feet. Callous under the fifth (little) toe and along the medial side of the first (big) toe often indicates an uncompensated forefoot varus pattern (inverted position of the forefoot relative to the rearfoot at the level of the midtarsal joint).[8] This is the most common problem causing disability found in the foot. A callous pattern in the middle of the foot behind the third (middle) toe indicates a compensated forefoot varus, and does not mean a lack of a problem (Bear *ibid*). This type of callous is found in a "Morton's foot," as well as in subtalar varus (calcaneal varus). A callous under the big toe only is seen often in forefoot valgus and plantarflexed first ray, and in hallux abducto valgus (Valmassy *ibid*)]

Problems of the feet sometimes can be deduced from abnormal wear on the sole of the shoes. With foot varus, the inside of the sole frequently wears more quickly than the outside; with foot valgus, the outside of the sole can wear more quickly than the inside (although many pronators show excessive shoe wear on the inside edge of the heel or sole). (*OM: Yang Motility (Qiao) deficiency, Yin Motility (Qiao) excess. Sinew channel imbalances.*) Some faster wear of the outside rear sole is normal, because at heal strike weightbearing takes place first on the outside and then moves up and across the front at toe-off. A "swirl" pattern (Mitchell *ibid*) may indicate excessive external rotator muscle tightness during the stance phase of the gait. Excessive wear on the lateral heel and medial side of the sole of the patient shoe may be

---

8. Forefoot varus (inversion/supinatus) is due to inadequate frontal plane torsion of the head and neck of the talus occurring during the normal development of the foot. With forefoot varus, the big toe is high (off ground/dorsiflexed first ray). This is usually due to a dorsiflexory force placed on the lateral aspect of forefoot. The foot is assessed by placing it in its subtalar neutral position, and the midtarsal joints are locked via a dorsiflexory force placed on the lateral aspect of the forefoot. Subtalar neutral is at a "peak" where the foot seems to fall off more easily to either side between pronation and supination and is assessed with the non-weight bearing foot (Figure 9-85 on page 532). At this "peak," a minimal amount of dorsiflexion is required to lock the subtalar joint in neutral. An uncompensated forefoot varus is a structural forefoot varus and there is no calcaneal eversion beyond the vertical available. One can not correct the forefoot supinatus by plantar pressure on the first ray, when the foot is in subtalar neutral. With a compensated forefoot varus the patient is often maximally pronated in weight bearing and the force falls medially to the subtalar joint axis of motion (Valmassy *ibid*).

seen with a Morton's foot (Morton *ibid*) and with functional hallux limitus.

Universal Pattern

A common adaptation known as the "universal pattern" usually includes (Greenman 1996; Mitchell 1995):

- A slightly lower right shoulder, with a slight tilt of the head to the right (in right-handed people);
- Minimal scoliosis of the upper thoracic spine (convexity to the left);
- Slight forward rotation of the right innominate, commonly seen with a left-on-left sacral torsion;[9]
- Flattening of the right foot arch, somewhat more than in the left foot;
- Slight external rotation of the right leg.

Poor posture often results in a weak and relaxed abdomen, with a tendency towards a drooped chest, with narrow rib angle, forward shoulders, prominent shoulder blades, a forward position of the head, tight and weak back extensors, and probably pronated feet. When the human system is out of balance, physiological function cannot be perfect, muscles and ligaments are in an abnormal state of tension and strain and consume unnecessary energy. Abnormalities develop, and, since a well-poised body means a machine working perfectly, with the least amount of muscular effort and therefore better health and strength for daily life, poor posture may lead to chronic dysfunctions and fatigue (Chaitow *ibid*).

---

9. A sacrum that is twisted and sidebent to the left.

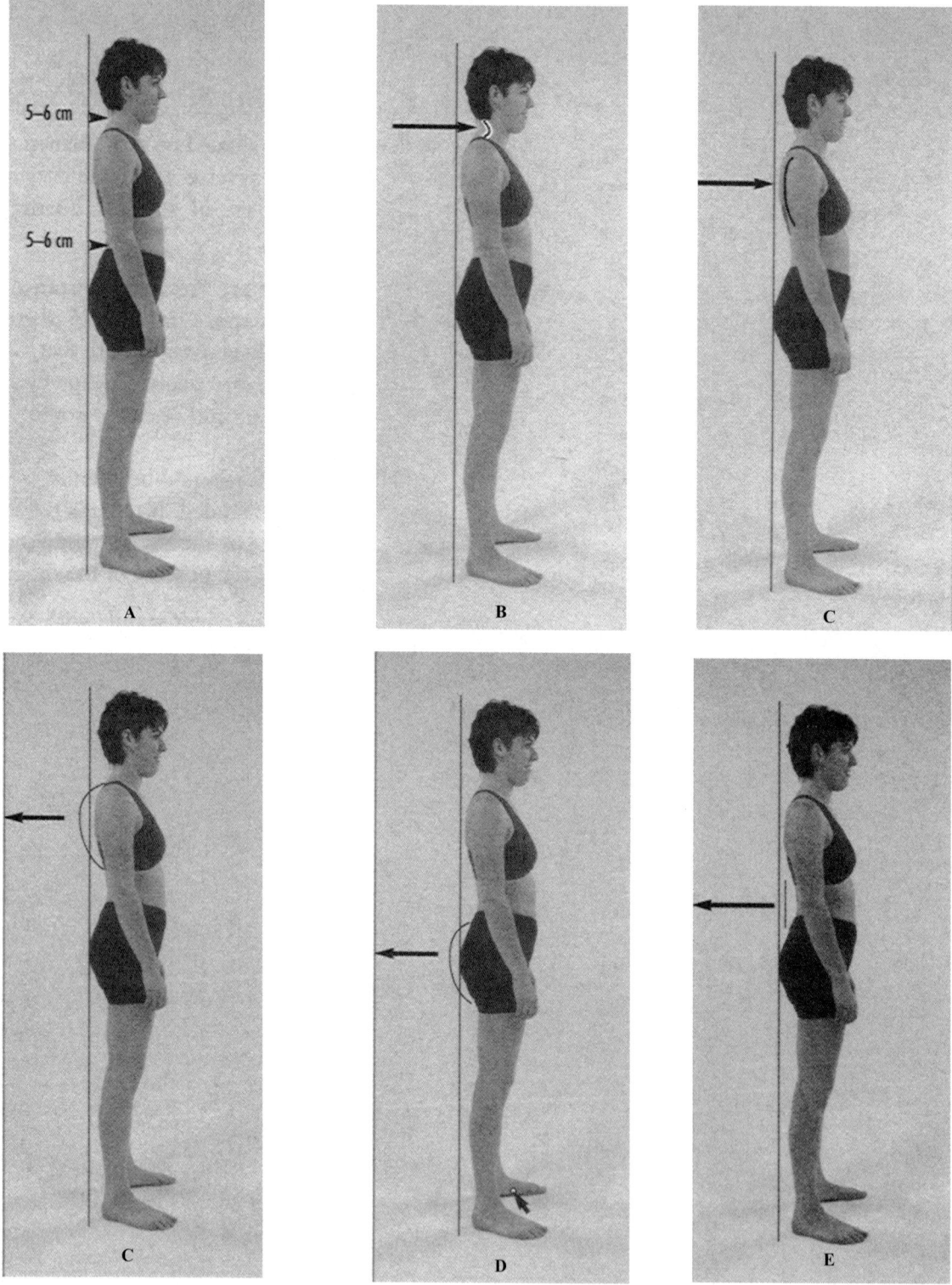

Figure 9-35: **A)** Normal posture with approximately 5-6 cm distance from plumb line. **B)** Forward head and neck posture. One or more vertebrae are usually "stuck" flexed, with anterior and/or lateral shear. **C)** Loss of thoracic kyphosis which is often caused by thoracic vertebrae that are stuck extended or anterior, and/or lateral shear. **C)** Excessive thoracic kyphosis which is often due to vertebrae that are stuck flexed. Often, there is spinal cord and/or nerve root tissue tension as well as ostopenia/osteoporosis in the thoracic spine. Excessive kyphosis may also occur in order to protect internal organs. **D)** Posterior buttocks, which is almost always due to dysfunction in the sacroiliac joints and the lumbosacral junction. There may be the *appearance* of excessive lumbar lordosis. **E)** Loss of lumbar lordosis, which occurs often when vertebrae are stuck flexed. Often there is also a component of an anterior and/or lateral shear of those lumbar vertebrae, which contributes to the loss of lordosis. Also, loss of lordosis is often due to discogenic pain (From Giammatteo and Giammatteo Integrative Manual Therapy for Biomechanics Application of Muscle Energy and Beyond" Technique 2003, with permission).

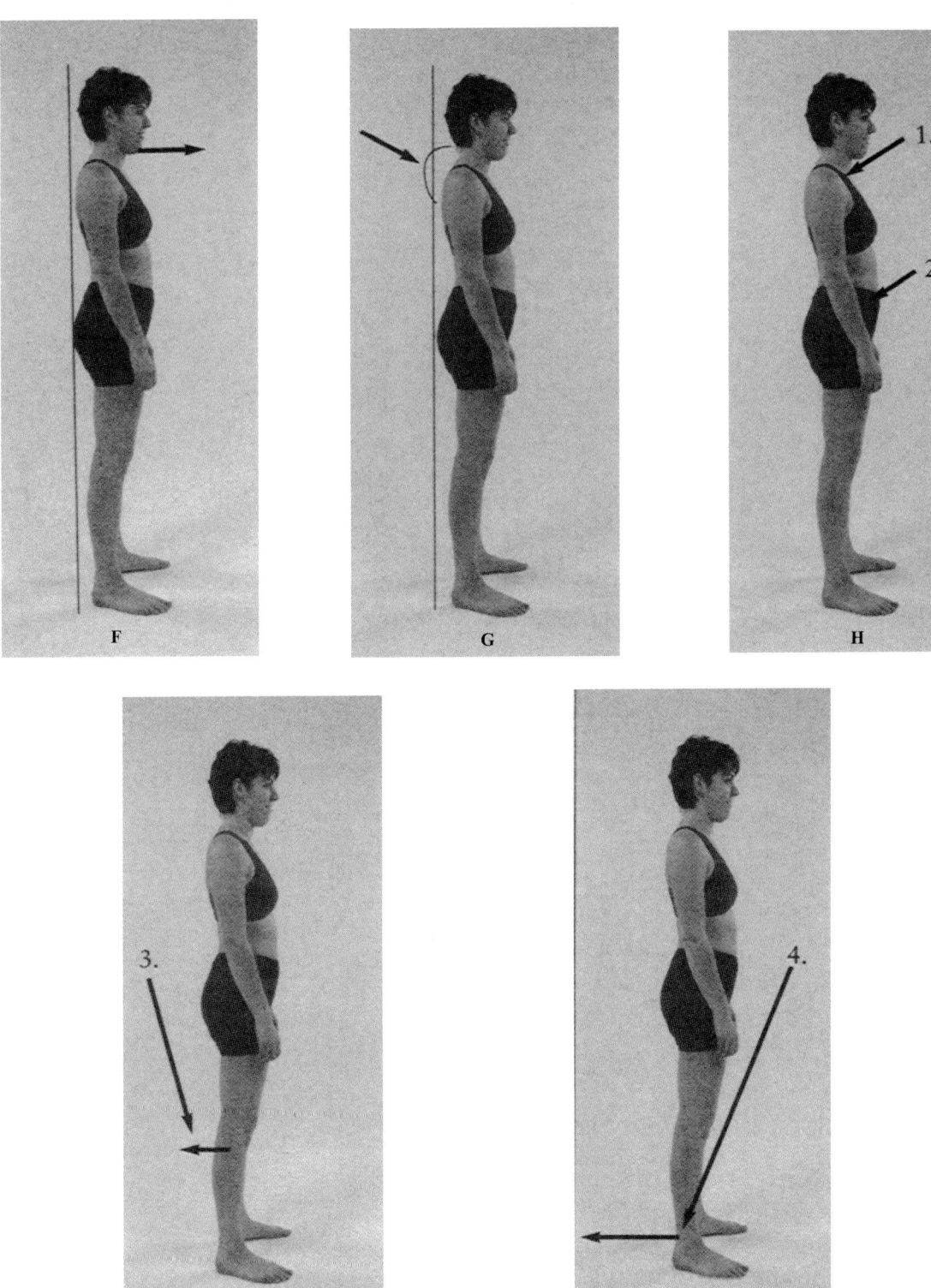

Figure 9-36: **F)** Protruding chin, in which there is often hyperextension of the occiput on the atlas. Often, the subcoccipital tissues become compressed causing tension on the occipital region, inferior brain stem, and other neurovascular tissue. **G)** Dowager's hump, which is usually due to dysfunction of the cervicothoracic junction. Often there is: flexed C7 and/or anterior shear; flexed T1; compressed C7/T1 interspace, with compromise of the C7/T1 disc; nerve root impingement of C7 nerve roots; cervical plexus neural tissue tension; compromise of dural mobility; spinal cord fibrosis at the level of the cericothoracic spine; and biomechanical dysfunction of sacrum. **H) 1.** Anterior shoulders, which most often are caused by short pectoralis minor and subscapularis muscles. **2.** Flexed hip, which is often secondary to sacroiliac joint and lumbosacral dysfunctions. **I)** Recurvarum of knees, which is most often caused by ligamentous laxity as well as muscle shorting of the quadriceps. Gastrocnemius shorting and limited dorsiflexion of the foot is common as well. **J)** Posterior tibial glide commonly seen with limited dorsiflexion. When there is a limitation of dorsiflexion, the tibia is stuck in posterior glide on the talus. (From Giammatteo and Giammatteo Integrative Manual Therapy for Biomechanics Application of Muscle Energy and Beyond" Technique 2003, with permission).

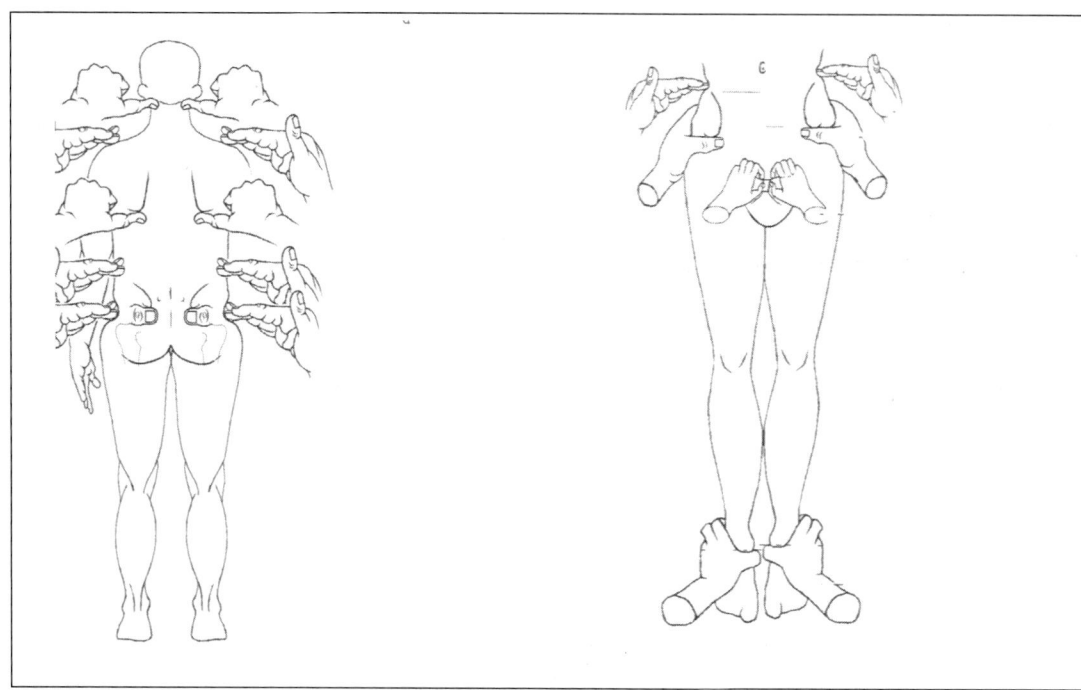

Figure 9-38: Assessment for levelness (From Kuchera WA and Kuchera ML, Osteopathic Principles in Practice, KCOM press 1994, with permission).

Osteopathic Treatment Methods

Many of the following treatment methods can be adopted to TCM/OM practice, or used in conjunction with them. They are often helpful in treating musculoskeletal disordered.

Balance and Hold

With balance and hold, motions at the joint are introduced in seven directions to identify:

- The point of maximal ease within each movement.
- The point of maximal ease within the respiration cycle.

After the practitioner identifies these positions, the patient is asked to hold them for as long as possible. This procedure is repeated as many times as necessary to correct the dysfunction (Greenman *ibid*).

Integration of Balance and Hold Techniques in TCM Practice

Balance and hold techniques can be easily adapted in TCM/OM practice using general palpatory evaluation or by paying attention to Sinew channel distributions. They are also useful integrated with distal or local acupoint stimulation. For example, when treating low back pain, it is often helpful to position the patient on the treatment table in such a way that the dysfunctional area is at maximal ease. This can be done with the assistance of wedges, pillows, or other devices using palpatory guidance as is done in Balance and Hold techniques. The patient can then be needled combining the benefit of balanced positioning and acupuncture.

Dynamic Functional Techniques

As the name implies, the practitioner uses dynamic functional techniques to try to restore normal function by means of motion. The joint or area is guided by applicable movements along a new path of increased "ease" to restore normal motion patterns. This may be performed using either "functional" methods, "facilitated positional release" (Schiowitz 1990), or "Still technique" (Van Buskirk 2001) approaches, which involve the operator's finding a position of maximum ease. A number of variations on the theme of placing the patient or area into ease are available. This (Greenman *ibid*) process may reduce nociceptive and abnormal mechanoreceptive output, allowing the joint to *relearn* a more normal behavior. The technique can be applied based on Osteopathic positional diagnosis, usually starting treatment at the *dysfunctional position* (i.e., at the stuck position). This position is then *slightly exaggerated* and an *activating force* such as compression is introduced, waiting and allowing the joint or tissues to "unwind," or letting "the body do what it wants to do." The practitioner can also move the joint more deliberately to-and-through its restricted barrier while maintaining a slight compression, as is done with the Still technique (Van Buskirk *ibid*).

In general, in functional techniques one uses a "listening hand" which must not move or initiate any movement. Its function is to contact the area under assessment/treatment to

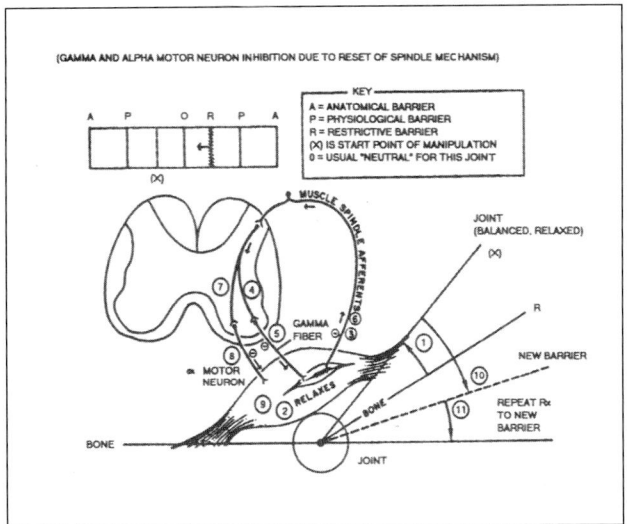

Figure 9-39: Indirect and functional methods (From Kuchera WA and Kuchera ML, Osteopathic Principles in Practice, KCOM press 1993, with permission).

gather information from the tissues, making sure that any movement (inherent or induced) results in increasing "tissue compliance" and softness.

Functional techniques are probably one of the safest techniques, especially for cranial structures, but should be followed through to their inherent "still point" or tissue calmness, at which point the area is done "unwinding."

Johnston (2003) lists six guidelines to help ensure success in the application of indirect functional techniques:

1. The initial introduction of motion in any one elementary direction is small (not range), with minimal forces applied.

2. Motion directions are toward a sense of *immediately* increasing ease.

3. Single elements of rotary and translatory directions are combined, effecting the control of an eventually smooth torsion arc for body movement. The order of introduction of these elements is not important.

4. The final step of the functional procedure involves request for a specific direction of active respiration, whichever direction (inhalation or exhalation) contributes further to the increasing ease. For example, if inhalation, the request is for the subject to take a deep breath slowly and hold it briefly.

5. This respiratory interval, adding to a continuous feedback of decreasing resistance, allows the operator to fine-tune the combination of translatory and rotary directions. The objective is to reach a sense of release of tissue tension at the fingertips, which are continually monitoring response at the dysfunctional segment.

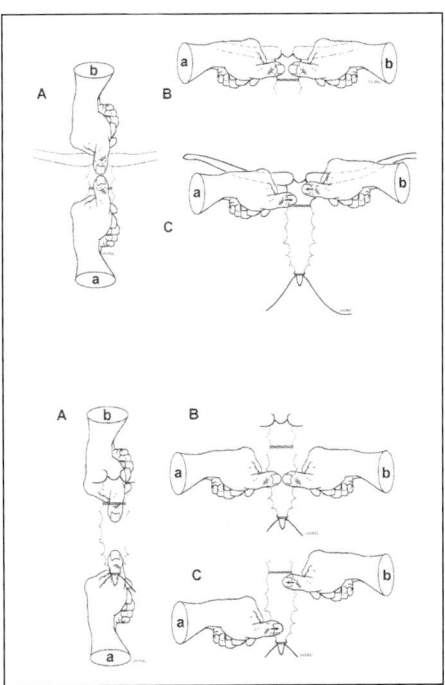

Figure 9-40: Assessment of sternal and manubrial motions. In direct techniques the restrictions are engaged and for indirect techniques increased compliance is engaged (From Kuchera WA and Kuchera ML, Osteopathic Principles in Practice, KCOM press 1993, with permission).

6. The release of restraint in the motor mechanism allows a return to midline resting, unobstructed by any sense of the resistance previously encountered in the return direction.

A successful outcome is signaled by a sensed release of the segmental tissues' holding forces, which then allows a free return to a resting position, and a new tissue tone at rest.

Adaptation Of Functional Techniques In TCM Practice

The *Classic of Internal Medicine* states that when Yin is dysfunctional there is difficulty in extension, when Yang is dysfunctional there is difficulty in flexion. Functional techniques can be used by identifying tightness and then moving the patient's body part towards the tight area, body part, sinew channel, etc., until feeling maximal compliance (relaxation) of the tissue. Once there, a variety of methods may be used. The practitioner may add a compressive, or distractive force and then move the joint, tissues, or channel toward the restricted motion. Another possibility is to wait for inherent tissue release and to flow with it as the body unwinds itself.

Functional type techniques are also very helpful following local acupuncture techniques in which the patient feels increased stiffness and/or pain. The reactive muscles, channel, or joint is identified and its two ends approximated. When maximal relaxation is felt, a compressive or distractive force is added, and the area mobilized towards tightness. For example, if the patients feels tightness or increased pain

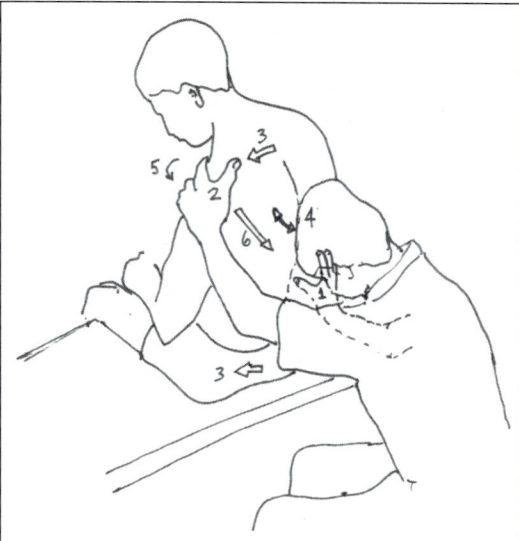

Lumbar Extension Restriction FRS(rt)

1. Palpate locked side (left facet).
2. Contact right trapezius area.
3. Shift (translate) weight to right ischium (side of rotation).
4. Translate (A-P) to get flexion at segment.
5. "Float" (loose-pack) joint with lateral translation/rotation.
6. Fascial load the right shoulder by compression to begin "unwinding;" to right, to still point and into previously restricted area.

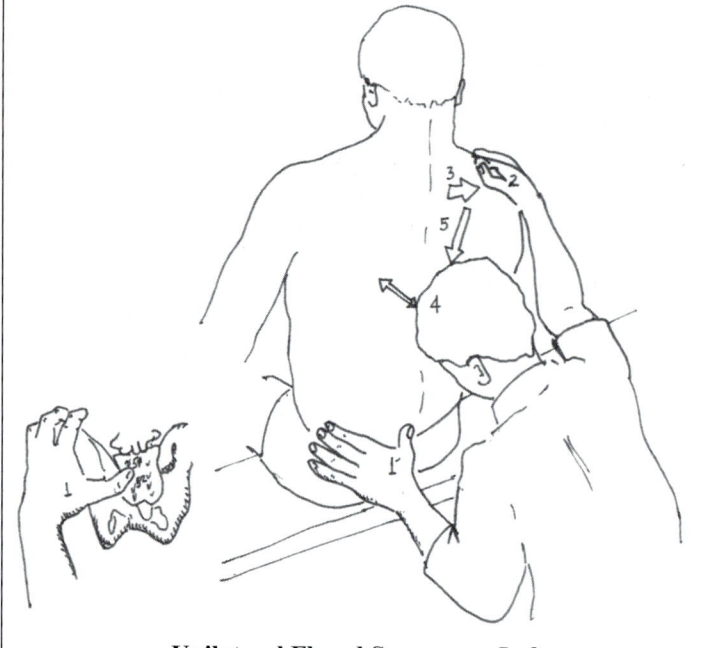

Unilateral Flexed Sacrum on Left

1. Palpate locked side (left sacral base).
2. Contact right trapezius area
3. Shift patient to right ischium (side of rotation).
4. Translate (A-P) to middle transverse sacral axis (S-2).
5. Loose-pack left SI (with right translation) and fascial load right shoulder by compression to begin "unwinding"; to right, to still point and into previously restricted area.

Figure 9-41: Examples of functional techniques as taught by Dr. Stiles

in the low back following local needling of UB or Jia Ji points, assess if flexion or extension is more painful or limited. If flexion results in pain or stiffness, extend, sidebend and rotate the patient until feeling maximum tissue compliance; add compression and slowly mobilize the aria towards flexion, sidebending and rotation to the other side. If needed, repeat technique sidebending and rotating towards the other side.

Another simple adaptation is to have the patient sit on top of a seated practitioner's thighs (with one ischium on each thigh), while, at the same time, holding the patient's pelvis with both hands. Simple small movements and a shifting of weight are explored, paying attention to compliance by the patient's pelvis. The techniques are continued until the practitioner feels a sinking (or a letting go) in the patient's body. This can be very helpful in treating secondary stiffness or pain following acupuncture and dry needling techniques.

A related *needling technique* is to needle fascial layers, usually between muscle groups, while monitoring tension at the affected area. For example, it is often beneficial to needle between the quadratus lumborum (QL) and neighboring muscles (instead of needling the muscle it self). The needle is inserted and moved deeply within the fascial layers (or just subcutaneously). No tissue resistance should be felt, and the needle should slide in easily. The non-needling hand is placed over the QL to monitor tension. Slow rotations, pressures, pressure combined with rotations, or pulling of the needle are then explored in all directions, and only movements that increase muscle relaxation are used. Another application is to thread a thin-gauge needle along a tight muscle band (along its fibers) and then to gently rotate the

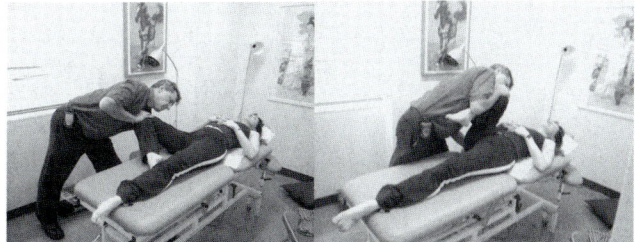

Figure 9-42: Stimulation of distal points with mobilization. This patient suffers from low back and leg pain in L3 and L5 dermatomal distributions. The patient has tenderness at right ASIS which is also anteriorly rotated. GB-41, TW-5, and K-7 on the opposite side are needled while the leg is moved from hip extension, abduction and lateral rotation (left photo) into flexion (right photo), under compression focused at the lower pole (innominate axis) of the SI joint. This addresses the patient's SI and innominate dysfunctions and is synergistic with needle therapy.

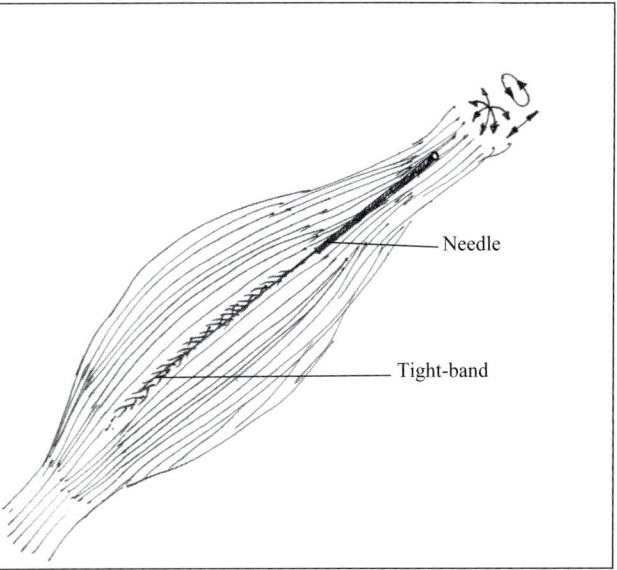

Figure 9-44: Functional needle technique. The needle is inserted into, or just above, a tight-band and manipulated in all direction to find those that result in release and softening.

needle in the direction that relaxes tension. This is often helpful on periscapular muscles (Figure 9-44). Figure 9-42 shows the integration of distal needle therapy and functional treatment to the lower pole of the SI joint.

Release by Countertension-Positioning and Related Techniques

Countertension *positional release* (strain-counterstrain™) was developed by Larry Jones DO., although, apparently, there are Ayurvedic writings from the third or fourth millennium that describe very similar techniques (Rex [Bear] personal communication). Countertension-positional release is effective especially for muscle spasm with an accompanying exquisitely tender point, but can also be used to treat vertebral and joint dysfunctions, as well as cranial (Greenman *ibid*) and visceral autonomics.

In contrast to Jones' technique in which therapy is mainly localized to the main area of symptoms and in which six to eight points might be treated with each position held for ninety seconds, D'Ambrogio and Roth (1997) emphasize a systematic scanning evaluation in which all or most of the tender points are assessed prior to treatment. They recommend treatment to only one to three points. This would take care of many other tender points including points in the dominant or symptomatic area.

The mechanism by which this technique works may be that, by keeping the muscle in a countertension (shortened) position and slightly increasing tension on its antagonist, the sensory (afferent) input from proprioceptors is "shut down," effectively suppressing the local protective cord reflex and inducing muscle relaxation. Thus, countertension positioning is thought to achieve its benefits by means of an automatic resetting of muscle spindles, which helps to dictate the length and tone in the tissues. Studies (Chaitow *ibid*) on cadavers have shown that when a radio-opaque dye is injected into muscles, the dye is more likely to spread into the vessels of the muscle when a "counterstrain" position of ease is adopted than when the muscle is in a neutral position. It is possible, therefore, that a circulatory affect is enhanced when muscles are in a shortened position.

Countertension-positional release is performed by first identifying tender points anywhere in the muscular system (often located at acupuncture or trigger points) or at the prescribed Jones points (Figure 9-43). Jones tender points (Chaitow *ibid*) are usually found in tissues which were in a shortened state at the time of strain (whether acute or chronic), rather than those which were (or are being) at stretch (which often develop trigger points). The patient is then positioned in such a way that discomfort and tenderness at these tender points are greatly reduced. When positioning the body (part) in countertension positioning techniques, a sense of "ease" is noted as the tissues reach the position in which pain vanishes from the palpated point. The patient is then held, by the practitioner if:

1. The monitored-point pain has reduced by at least 70%.

2. There is no additional pain in the symptomatic area.

3. No new or additional pain is created.

This position is maintained for around ninety seconds (according to Jones, but may be shorter or as much as twenty minutes for "fascial responses," according to D'Ambrogio and Roth *ibid*) before slowly and passively being returned to normal position without any patient effort. The patient should be told to avoid strenuous activities for several days and to expect post-treatment soreness. (Figure 9-45 and Figure 9-46 show some examples of countertension techniques.)

Goodheart (1984) suggests using a "functional" evaluation approach to choosing points for positional release (instead of tenderness). He suggests finding a point on mus-

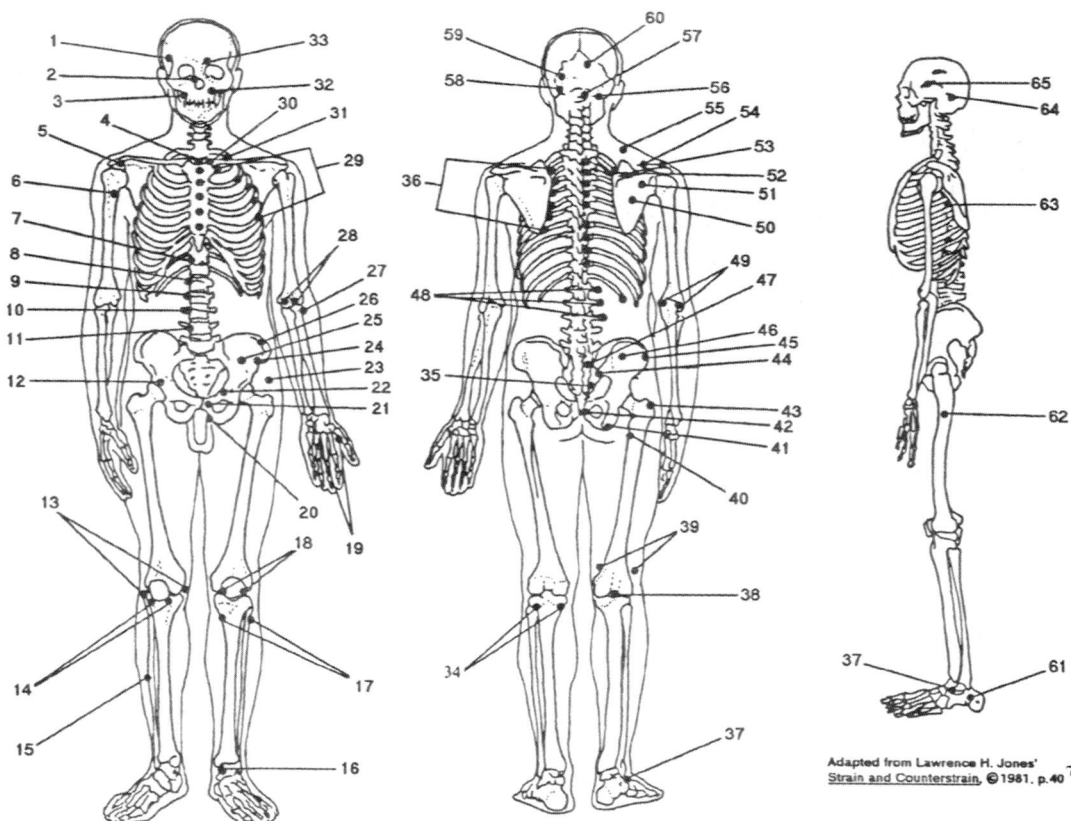

LOCATIONS OF TENDER POINTS

1. Squamosal
2. Nasal
3. Masseter-temporomandibular
4. Anterior first thoracic
5. Anterior acromioclavicular
6. Latissimus dorsi
7. Anterior seventh thoracic
8. Anterior eighth thoracic
9. Anterior ninth thoracic
10. Anterior tenth thoracic
11. Anterior eleventh thoracic
12. Anterior second lumbar
13. Medial and lateral meniscus
14. Medial and lateral extension meniscus
15. Tibialis anticus medial ankle
16. Flexion ankle
17. Medial and lateral hamstrings
18. Medial and lateral patella
19. Thumb and fingers
20. Low-ilium flare-out
21. Anterior fifth lumbar
22. Low ilium
23. Anterior lateral trochanter
24. Anterior first lumbar
25. Iliacus
26. Anterior twelfth thoracic
27. Radial head
28. Medial and lateral coronoid
29. Depressed upper ribs
30. Anterior eighth cervical
31. Anterior seventh cervical
32. Infraorbital nerve
33. Supraorbital nerve
34. Extension ankle (on gastrocnemius)
35. High flare-out sacroiliac
36. Elevated upper ribs (on rib angles)
37. Lateral ankle
38. Posterior cruciate ligament
39. Anterior cruciate ligament
40. Posterior medial trochanter
41. Also posterior medial trochanter
42. Coccyx (for high flare-out sacroiliac)
43. Posterior lateral trochanter
44. Lower-pole fifth lumbar
45. Fourth lumbar
46. Third lumbar
47. Upper-pole fifth lumbar
48. Upper lumbars
49. Medial and lateral olecranon
50. Third thoracic shoulder
51. Lateral second thoracic shoulder
52. Medial second thoracic shoulder
53. Posterior acromioclavicular
54. Supraspinatus
55. Elevated first rib
56. Posterior first cervical
57. Inion
58. Left occipitomastoid
59. Sphenobasilar
60. Right lambdoid
61. Lateral calcaneus
62. Lateral trochanter
63. Subscapularis
64. Posteroauricular
65. Squamosal

Figure 9-43: Jones points (From Kuchera WA and Kuchera ML, Osteopathic Principles in Practice, KCOM press 1993, with permission).

cles that are antagonistic to painful movement, i.e. muscles that are being stretched (and which probably have a trigger point). For example, if abduction of the shoulder is painful, one would look for tender points in adductor muscles. Because a variety of movements may produce pain or restriction in any given dysfunctional joint, a variety of tender points may be identified and treated using this approach. Goodheart also suggests teaching the patient to self-treat using this approach. For more detailed descriptions see the author's book *Musculoskeletal Disorders: Healing Methods from Chinese Medicine, Orthopaedic Medicine, and Osteopathy*, North Atlantic Books 1998.

Adaptation Of Countertension Techniques To TCM Practice

Since countertension techniques basically involve wrapping the body part around a tender point and keeping it there for about ninety seconds, this technique can be easily adapted to TCM practice. Tender channel or Ashi points are identified and monitored for tenderness by the practitioner while at the same time wrapping the area of the body around the tender point. After about ninety seconds the area is slowly stretched.

FACILITATED POSITIONAL RELEASE (FPR): The advantage of FPR is that it can be performed quickly and does not require a ninety-second hold. With this approach, one must first modify the sagittal posture, so that in the spinal area to be treated the curves are slightly reversed to achieve a balance between flexion and extension. With FPR, the practitioner adds to the position of ease a "facilitating" element. This might involve either compression or traction, or a combination of both, inducing an immediate tissue release in terms of hypertonicity or restriction of motion—and thus one does not need to hold for ninety seconds. When treating the cervical spine, for example, a pillow is placed below the head to slightly flex the neck and reverse cervical lordosis before a position of ease is sought (Schiowitz *ibid*).

INTEGRATED NEUROMUSCULAR INHIBITION TECHNIQUE. Integrated neuromuscular inhibition technique (INIT) has been described by Chaitow (*ibid*) and involves using a "position of ease" for tissues housing a tender/pain/trigger point as part of the sequence leading to its deactivation. The sequence begins by the locating tender/pain/trigger point, followed by:

1. Application of ischemic compression, i.e. direct pressure on the point. (This is optional and is avoided if pain is too intense or the patient too fragile or sensitive.)

2. Introduction of positional release positioning.

3. After an appropriate length of time, during which the tissues are held in ease, the patient is asked to introduce an isometric contraction into the affected tissues for seven to ten seconds.

4. After the muscles are relaxed, they are stretched (or they may be stretched at the same time as the contraction, if *fibrotic tissue* calls for such attention).

5. Subsequently, a further position-of-ease period may be instigated, facilitating the activation of the antagonists to the muscles involved, may be introduced.

The following are contraindications and cautions for positional release listed by Chaitow (*ibid*):

- Particular care should be taken in application of strain counter strain (SCS) in cases of malignancy, aneurysm, and acute inflammatory conditions.
- Skin conditions may make application of pressure to the tender point undesirable.
- Protective spasm should not be treated unless the underlying conditions are well considered (osteoporosis, disc herniation, fractures, etc.).
- Recent major trauma or surgery precludes anything other than gentle superficial positional release methods concerning SCS in hospital settings.
- Infectious conditions call for caution and care.
- Any increase in pain during the process of positioning shows that an undesirable direction, movement, or position is being employed. Sensations such as numbness or aching may arise during the holding of the position of ease, and as long as this is moderate and not severe the patient should be encouraged to relax and view the sensation as transient and part of the desirable changes taking place.
- Caution should be exercised when placing the neck into extension. It is important to maintain verbal communication with the patient at all times and to ask them to keep their eyes open so that any signs of nystagmus are observable.

Some TCM techniques use a supporting/stimulating method (treating Yin within Yang) which is somewhat similar to indirect Osteopathic techniques. The joint is moved away from pain or toward the nonpainful barrier and held there while acupuncture points are stimulated (by massage) along the channel that affects the pathological (painful) side of the joint. The joint-channel is then stretched as massage stimulation continues. Mobilization movements with increasing amplitude going from the nonpainful position toward the painful or restricted directions are used as well.

Muscle Energy Techniques

Osteopathic muscle energy technique (MET) was developed by Fred Mitchell Sr. and uses postisometric relaxation,[10] reciprocal inhibition[11], and isotonic contraction to restore

---

10. The relaxation of a muscle after isotonic contraction.

11. The activation of antagonist muscles which then inhibit the agonist muscle or post isometric techniques.

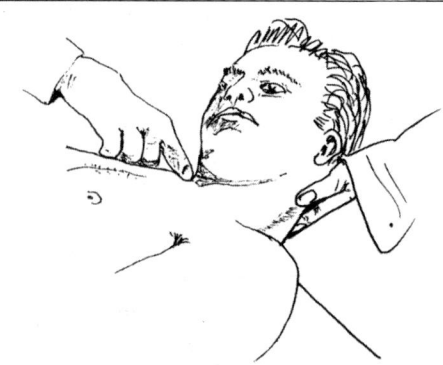

Countertension technique for C7 anterior tender point (or LI-16 area). The practitioner's right index finger monitors the tender point while his right hand flexes, sidebends, and, if needed, rotates the head and neck until tenderness is minimized.

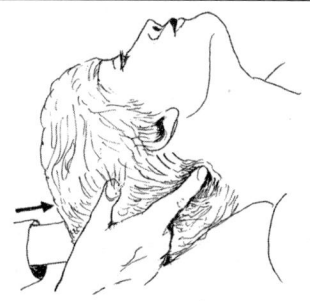

Counter tension technique for posterior C1. The finger monitors the tender point, while the head is positioned so that tenderness is at a minimum. Can be used of GB-20 or UB tender channel points. The practitioner's right index finger is being used to monitor point tenderness, while the left hand extends and compresses the head until point tenderness in minimized.

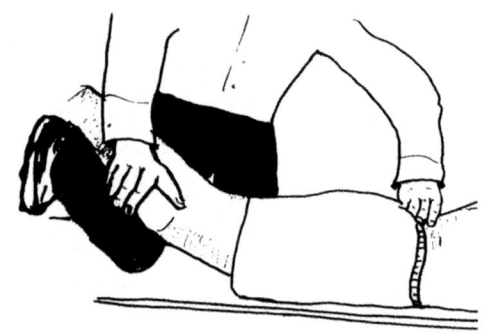

Countertension technique for quadratus lumborum muscle (UB-23-24 or Jia Ji points). The practitioner's left index finger monitors the tender point, while the patient's leg is lifted and abducted or adducted until tenderness is minimized

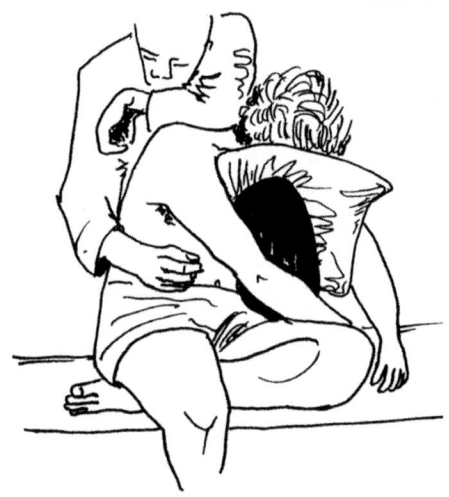

Countertension technique for anterior point tenderness at subcostal or epigastric region. The practitioner's right hand is monitoring the tender point (Liv-14 for example) while using his body to "wrap" the patient's body around the point until tenderness is minimized.

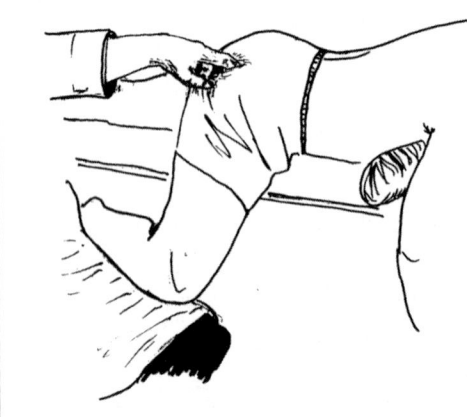

Countertension technique for piriformis muscle (or GB-30). The finger monitors the tender muscle, while the leg is abducted and rotated until tenderness at the muscle is minimized.

Figure 9-45: Examples of Countertension techniques.

Osteopathic Treatment Methods

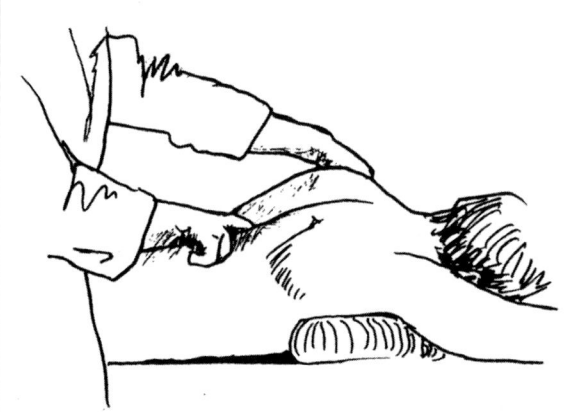

Countertension technique for posterior thoracic tender point with marked deviation of spinous processes. The practitioner's right finger monitors the tender point, while the left hand lifts the left shoulder until tenderness is minimized.

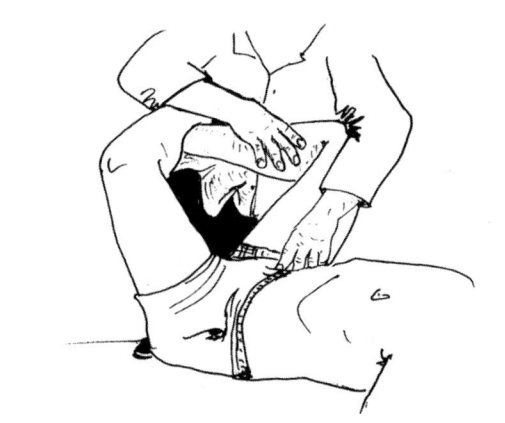

Countertension technique for iliopsoas muscle (St-12, GB-27, Liv-12). The finger monitors the tender points, while the patient's body is wrapped around the point until tenderness at the point is minimized.

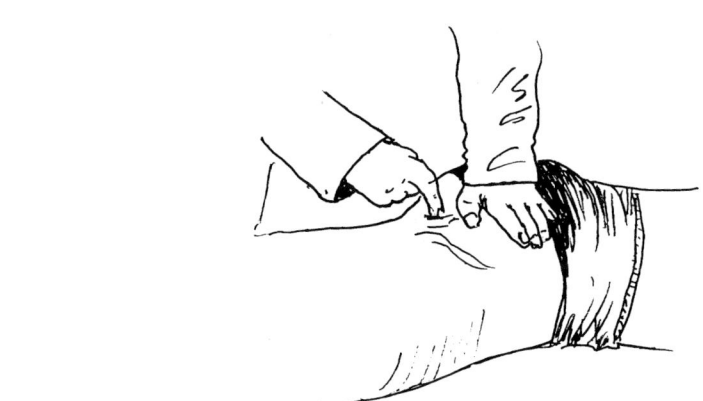

Countertension technique for posterior sacral tender point (or UB-32 area), posterior torsions of the sacrum and levator ani muscle. The practitioner's right index finger monitors the point and the other hand applies downward pressure to the sacral apex in order to extend the sacral base until tenderness is minimize.

Figure 9-46. Examples of Countertension techniques.

mobility to joints. Similar techniques are used by other systems and with different rational. Liebenson (*ibid*) describes three variations of muscle energy techniques that are used by Lewit, Janda, and himself. MET is both passive and active (requiring patient participation) and are therefore a favorite of this author. *(OM: An OM treatment system developed in Japan called So Tai Kan Gen Ho (return the body back to alignment) uses isotonic muscle contractions away from the dysfunctional barriers, integrated with breath activation. Evaluation is made by looking for joint dysfunctions in cross patterns [i.e., right ankle, left knee, right hip, etc.]. The joint is taken to its dysfunctional barrier and then the patient moves the joint against practitioner resistance away from the dysfunctional barrier, isotonically).*

One MET hypothesis is that a light, brief isometric voluntary contraction of the hypertonic muscle externally stretches the nuclear bag fibers of the spindles. The bag annulospirals, after brief excitation, promptly adapt to a lengthened muscle condition, even though the muscle length does not change. With postisometric relaxation, the muscle may actually be lengthened without stimulating myotatic reflexes. The isometric contraction may also press fluid from the spindle lymph space, reducing the postisometric tension in the capsule of the spindle. The slower adapting nuclear chain fibers attached to the capsule of the spindle may, therefore, undergo a change in tension with a reduction of annulospiral stimulation. It is thought that suprasegmental systems, as well as the muscle spindle receptors, are reprogrammed by MET techniques (Mitchell *ibid*).

In the Osteopathic model, which for the most part uses *positional diagnosis*, muscle energy is used most commonly to treat joint (somatic) dysfunctions. Postisometric relaxation and reciprocal inhibition relax the affected muscles (Figure 9-47), resulting in the restoration of normal function (postisometric relaxation is used most often; Mitchell 1985). MET is considered a direct technique, in that it addresses the restrictive barrier of a dysfunctional joint by slow postisometric stretching. For MET to be effective, the joint barriers must be accurately engaged at the feather edge of their dysfunctional limits (i.e., not too far into barriers: joint must remain loose packed), in all three planes.[12] This requires a great degree of palpatory skill by the practitioner. Some common mistakes beginners make are:

1. Overpassing the barrier and loosing joint play, i.e. going beyond the resistance barriers of the joint or muscle treated.

2. Inadequate patient instruction, making the patient tense, resulting in difficulties for the practitioner in moving the joint/muscle into the newly gained barrier passively (with no help from patient).

---

12. Mitchell states that it may not be possible or necessary to engage all three barriers; two may be sufficient.

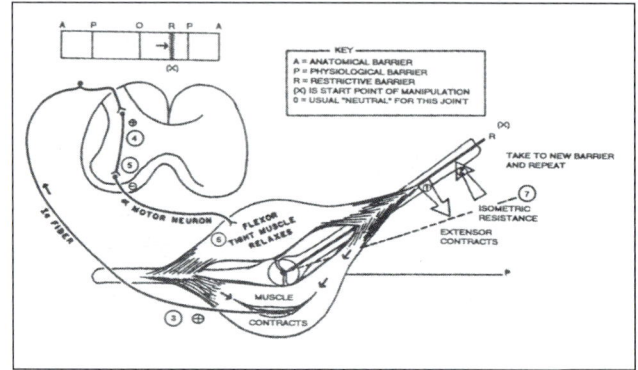

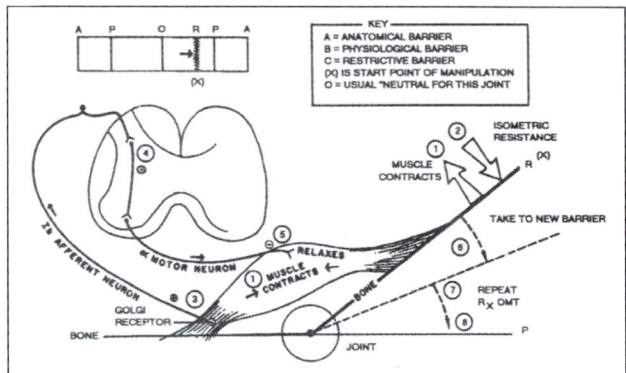

Figure 9-47: Reciprocal inhibition of motor neurons to the opposing muscle (upper); Postisometric relaxation (bottom), (From Kuchera WA and Kuchera ML, Osteopathic Principles in Practice, KCOM press 1993, with permission).

3. Moving the muscle to its newly gained barrier too quickly, not allowing the connective tissues to begin to lengthen (ideally after about ten seconds when primarily treating a muscle).
   — Note: when treating *joints* using osteopathic MET, there is *no* need to hold soft tissues at stretch in order to achieve a lengthening. Once the new barrier is reached, and after the patient has let go from his isometric effort, and after the practitioner has taken up available slack, without force (i.e. without stretching), the next contraction is called-for and the process is repeated.

4. Applying inadequate counterforce to the patient's contraction effort. This results in poor localization, movement, and therefore the muscle effort is not isometric.

5. Using too much or not enough force. (Most often the beginner is likely to use too much force, especially when treating the spine.)

The muscle contraction force made by the patient must be away from the restricted barrier (i.e. activating the shortened muscles). It should be no more than a few ounces when treating short muscle restrictors, as is the case in non-neutral (type II) vertebral dysfunction. The patient/practitioner should apply only moderate force when treating multisegmental muscles as is the case in neutral group (type I) dysfunction; otherwise, muscle recruitment can reduce the effect (Mitchell *ibid*). The contraction is resisted by the practitioner to ensure that the muscular effort is isometric (i.e., no movement of the joint is allowed). This position is held for four to six seconds, after which the patient is instructed to completely let go. The joint is then moved to the edge of the newly-gained restrictive barrier, after which the procedure is repeated three to five times.

Following isometric contraction, whether the agonist or antagonist muscle is being used, there is approximately fifteen seconds during which movement towards the new barrier of a joint or muscle can be easier (due to reduced tone). The barrier (Chaitow *ibid*) used in MET treatment is a "first sign of resistance" barrier, at which the very first indication of the onset of "bind" is noted (i.e. taking up the slack only). This is the place at which further movement would produce the stretching of *some* fibres of the muscle(s) to be treated. It is also where (at the feather edge of tension barrier), in *acute* problems, MET isometric contractions, whether these involve the agonists or antagonists, commence and, short of which, contractions commence in *chronic* problems (when primarily treating shortened multisegmental/joint/large muscles). When treating joint dysfunction, the first sign of movement, *at the joint*, is often used for localization (Mitchell *ibid*).

When treating *shortened* muscles in *chronic* conditions, Chaitow suggests using reciprocal inhibition (i.e., working the antagonist muscle) with a contraction of between ten and twelve seconds, commencing from a *mid-range position* rather then at the tension/resistance barrier. The patient's effort should be more than 20% but not more than 50% of the patient's available strength. After each contraction, a short rest period (between two and three seconds) is allowed before a stretch is introduced to take the tissues to a point *just beyond* the previous barrier of resistance. It is useful to have the patient gently assist in taking the (now) relaxed area towards and through the barrier, thus reducing the danger from the stretch reflex (i.e, preventing a reflex spasm). Each new effort is repeated from *midrange* instead of the newly gained barrier (Chaitow *ibid*).

For *acute* conditions, Chaitow suggests using postisometric relaxation with the muscle *at the stretch barrier* and the patient's effort at no more than 20% of available strength. The contraction is held for seven to ten seconds—the time it is thought necessary for the "load" to the Golgi tendon organs to influence the intrafusal fibres (muscle spindles). This inhibits muscle tone. The muscle (joint) is then taken to a new resting tension/resistance barrier with far less effort, or else it is stretched through the barrier of resistance, if appropriate. The process is repeated to see whether even more release is possible, starting from the *new resistance barrier* to whatever new range is gained following each successive contraction.

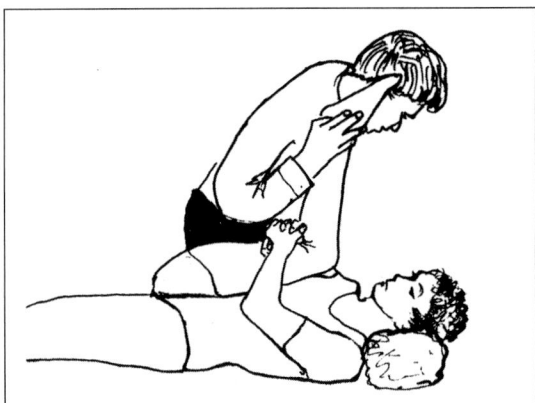

Figure 9-48: Post isometric stretching of tight hamstring muscle.

It is this author's practice, however, to first use reciprocal inhibition technique in *acute condition,* working the antagonists, often with great but not maximal force. This effort may be isometric or isotonic. With isotonic technique having a yielding resistance which allows lengthening of the acutely shortened muscle during the antagonist's (inhibiting) effort. The muscles requiring treatment are placed just short of their resistance/tension barrier at the beginning of each effort. A concentric effort of the shortened muscle may proceed—as illustrated by Mitchell (1995) for acute torticollis (crick in the neck).

Some techniques classified as "muscle energy" use both respiratory assistance and isotonic/concentric and isolytic/eccentric contractions.

Muscle Weakness

Muscle weakness is commonly seen clinically. *Isometric* exercises are especially useful in strengthening weak muscles about an unstable joint. For example, in shoulder instability the scapular stabilizers: lower trapezius, serratus anterior, rhomboids and pectoralis minor are strengthened using isometric training (Ombregt et al *ibid*).

Isokinetic contractions, the progressive resisted exercise at uniform velocity of movement, can be done using an isotonic/concentric (shorting of fibers), isolytic/eccentric (lengthening of fibers) effort, or a combination of both, to strengthen weak muscles.[13] The patient starts with a mild effort which rapidly progresses to a strong effort, while the practitioner moves the muscle/joint through its full ROM. To perform an eccentric muscle training the practitioner effort overcomes the patient's effort stretching the muscle while its fibers are tense. For concentric training the patient's effort overcomes the practitioner's. The above technique should

---

13. *Isolytic* contraction is what happens when the practitioner or load "wins" and overpowers the patient's effort. *Isometric* contraction is what happens when there is equal resistance between the patient and the practitioner or load. *Isotonic* contraction is when the patient overpowers the practitioner's or load effort.

take no more than four seconds at each contraction, in order to achieve maximum benefit with as little fatiguing as possible. The use of isokinetic contraction is reported to be a very effective way of building muscle strength and is superior to high repetition, lower resistance exercises (Blood 1980)—one must be careful not to strain the contractile unit.

A simple form of isotonic *concentric* contraction is to use *isokinetic* contraction (also known as *progressive resisted exercise*). The patient starts with a weak effort but quickly advances to a maximal contraction of the affected muscle(s). This can be performed with exercise equipment or with resistance to the practitioner's effort to mobilize the joint/muscles through a full range of motion (Chaitow *ibid*).

In order (Norris 1999) to tone postural (type 1) muscle fibers which may have lost their endurance potential but are important stabilizers, *eccentric* isotonic exercises, *performed slowly,* are said to be more effective. *Rapid* movement is used in isotonic *concentric* exercises, to treat phasic (type II) muscle fibres.

In Orthopaedic Medicine, isotonic exercises are used in three ways (Ombregt et al *ibid*):

1. In minor muscular tears after the lesion has been prepared by gentle cross fiber massage. Here, the contraction is carried out with the muscle in the shortened position.

2. To strengthen weakened muscles as in arthritis or after local or generalized immobilization.

3. To strengthen muscles so they can protect joints or inert structures from being painfully overstretched.

When treating weakness, it is also important to re-establish proprioception and proper muscular contraction timing to increase joint support. The use of tilting boards, swiss balls, and other unstable surfaces are recommended (Janda *ibid*). Dual channel electromyography biofeedback can be used in the treatment of patellofemoral dysfunction and glenohumeral instability. Eccentric training is also said to re-establish proprioception (Ombregt et al *ibid*).

According to Dr. Goodheart if a specific muscle is weakened by being slightly separated from the bone, a manual procedure of firm, goading pressure on the attachment points of the weak muscles can result in an immediate response "turning on" the muscle. For more information on strength training see "Rehabilitation and Exercise" on page 513.

Muscle Fibrosis and Adhesions

An *isolytic* contraction performed with a *quick* stretch into *eccentric* contraction can be used to treat adhesions within muscles. The practitioner applies a force which is just greater than that being exerted by the patient, thus opening the joint or lengthening the muscle(s) being treated, while the patient maintains muscle contraction. This procedure can be uncomfortable and cause microtrauma (lysis), and the patient should be warned. Limited degrees of effort on the part of the practitioner are therefore called for at the outset of isolytic contractions (Chaitow *ibid*).

Another technique to treat fibrotic, tight muscles is an isolytic contraction performed against a vibratory oscillating counterforce of at three to five Hz., provided by the practitioner (Mitchell *ibid*).

In conclusion, the above techniques have the ability to treat tight, shortened, and weak tissues. The healing will depend, to a large extent, on the subsequent use of the area (exercise, etc.), as well as the nutritive status of the individual. Collagen formation is dependent on adequate vitamin C and on a plentiful supply of amino acids such as proline, hydroxyproline, and arginine. Manual therapies, aimed at the restoration of a degree of normality in connective tissues, should therefore take careful account of nutritional requirements (Chaitow *ibid*). Resistive exercises may be of concern in patients with severely painful arthritic joint or painful neck or back problems. Performed incorrectly they can aggravate symptoms. However, MET and rehabilitation exercises can be used on patients with arthritis and can be modified for osteoporosis with very little risk. Anybody who has a serious heart problem or extremely fragile bones should be handled with care. Patients should avoid holding their breath during the exercises. Breathing out during the resistive strengthening activity is an essential part of the exercise. Weight bearing exercise if performed with sufficient force can stimulate muscles at their attachment to bone and stimulate optimal bone formation (Chaitow *ibid*).

MET can be used as the principal method for treating vertebral, pelvic, and peripheral joint dysfunctions. The patient should be warned of possible increased discomfort for twelve to thirty-six hours after treatment. Drinking plenty of water and applying moist heat and effleurage massage to the area may reduce such discomfort For more detailed descriptions see the author's book *Musculoskeletal Disorders: Healing Methods from Chinese Medicine, Orthopaedic Medicine, and Osteopathy*, North Atlantic Books 1998.

Adaptation of Muscle Energy Techniques To TCM Practice

Post-isometric relaxation can be easily adapted to TCM practice without a specific somatic dysfunction diagnosis. For example, when treating low back pain, the practitioner can follow acupuncture or dry needling techniques with a set of muscle energy positions for the post-isometric relaxation of muscles and to increase functional range of motion. The series can be performed regardless of specific diagnosis and is not harmful in any way, i.e., treating for flexion restriction when the patient actually has extension restriction will not harm the patient. For example, in treatmernt of the spine, after acupuncture or dry needling, the patient is positioned as seen in Figure 9-49 and post-isometric techniques are used to increase range of motion and to decrease post-treatment soreness.

Osteopathic Treatment Methods

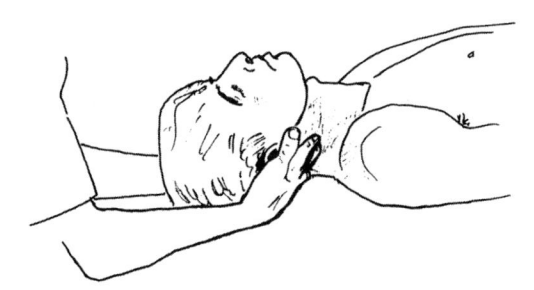

Position for treating FRS(lf) (anterior Yin channel tightness). The joint is extended, rotated, and sidebent to the right and the opposite movements are resisted for muscle energy stretch techniques.

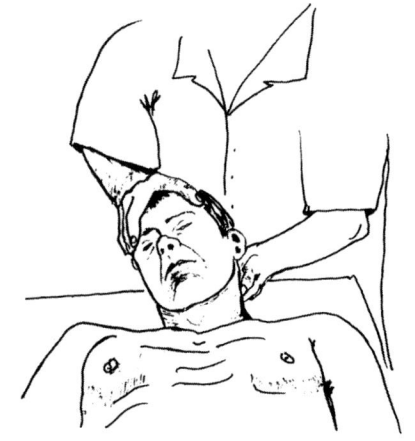

Position for treating ERS(lf) (posterior Yang channel tightness). The joint is flexed, sidebent, and rotated to the right. Movements in the opposite direction are slowly increased using post-isometric muscle energy techniques.

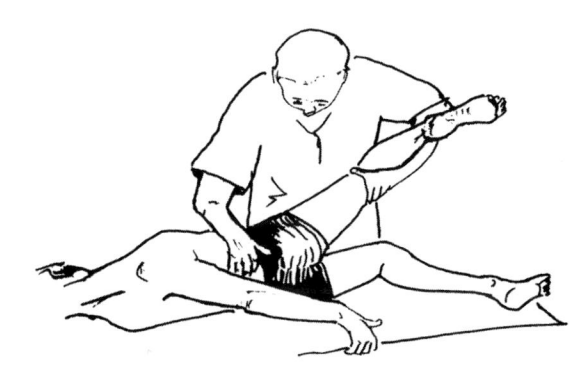

Muscle energy technique for extension restriction— FRS(lt) at lower lumbar, (tightness in anterior Yin channel). The joint is slowly extended, rotated, and sidebent to the right following resisted muscle energy stretch techniques.

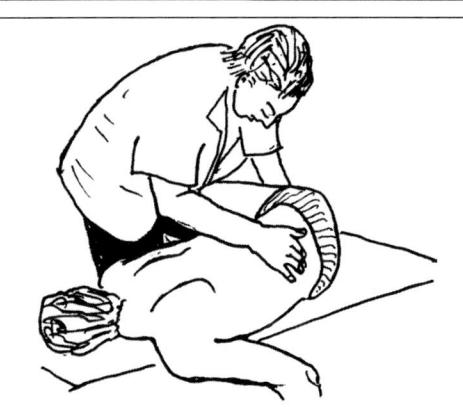

Position for treating ERS(rt) (posterior Yang channel tightness) in lower lumbars. The joint is flexed, sidebent, and rotated to the left. Movements in the opposite direction are resisted for post-isometric muscle energy technique. A similar position can be used to treat forward sacral torsions.

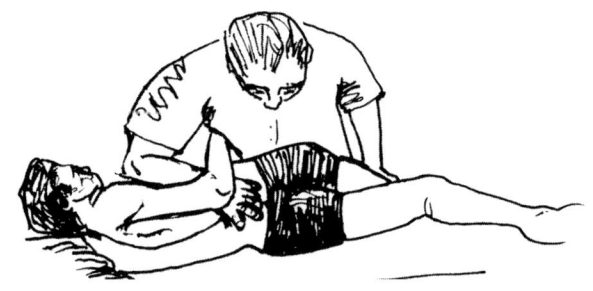

Position for treating backward sacral torsion. The spine is extended until the sacrum begins to move.

Figure 9-49: Examples of a few muscle energy techniques.

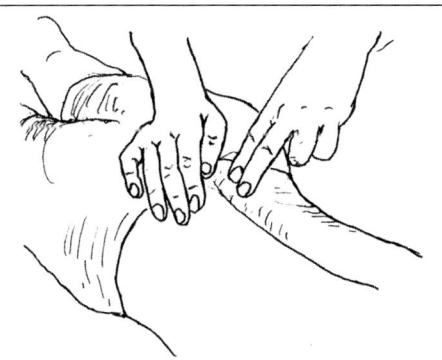

Position for treating left flexed sacrum. With this technique the patient's respiratory effort is used as an activating force.

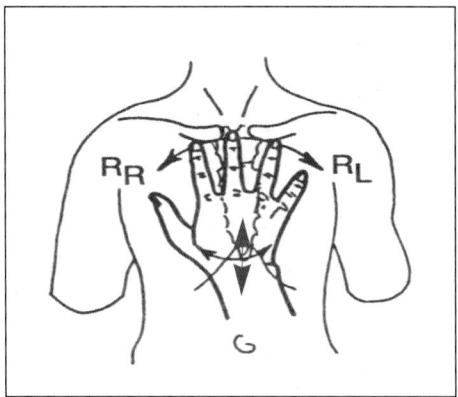

Figure 9-50: Myofascial release assessment or treatment. The practitioner, after engaging the fascia by compression, moves his/her hand in all directions and combinations and stacks up tension. The same principles can be used on joints or any other structure including bone (Kuchera and Kuchera 1994).

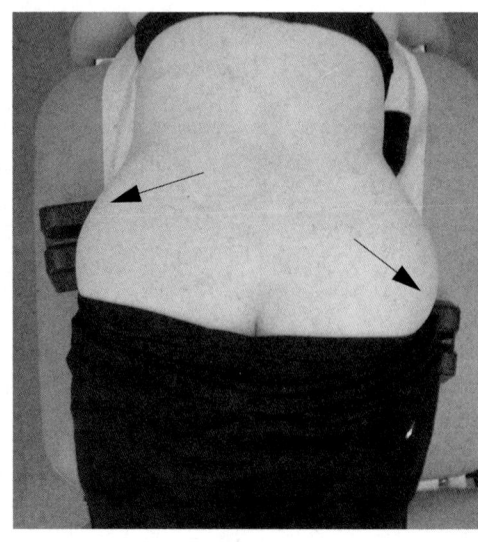

Figure 9-51: Wedges used to align and unload the pelvis during acupuncture treatment.

Myofascial Release Techniques

Myofascial Release (MFR) and Integrated Neuromusculaoskeletal Release techniques are relatively new additions to Osteopathic treatments, although Ward states that the ideas of both have been a part of American Osteopathic thinking from early in the profession's history (Ward 2003). They have also been referred to as isometric and isotonic methods, fascial release, and functional techniques. Various approaches to myofascial release techniques are used by physical therapists as well as other body work professionals.

All tissues exhibit nonlinear, stress-strain responses that are functions of their densities and viscosities. For example, tendons deform at different rates than muscle fibers, ligaments, and bones (Ward *ibid*). Fascia often behaves as if it has a memory, as it is able to maintain tissue deformation for long periods.

In Osteopathic Myofascial Release techniques the practitioner applies pressure on the fascia in a specific direction while an activating force, such as deep breath, is initiated by the patient. This method "re-educates" the fascia back to the normal physiologic state (Greenman *ibid*). Myofascial Release techniques may also combine principles and techniques from MET, other soft tissue techniques, as well as Osteopathic cranial techniques. As both static and dynamic movement barriers are encountered when using these techniques, they are released by sequentially loading areas of tightness using combined compression, traction, and twisting maneuvers (Figure 9-52). A key to their clinical success is the practitioner's ability to identify tethering (restriction) effects that persistently create and maintain pathologic asymmetries. *Tightness suggests tethering, while looseness suggests joint and/or soft tissue laxity with or without neural inhibition* (Ward *ibid*). According to Ward, the integration of a variety of patient-invoked cranial nerve activities such as eye, tongue, jaw, and oropharyngeal isometric and kinetic movements are helpful, especially in patients suffering from cognitive symptoms due to whiplash injury.

With direct techniques the tissues are moved in increasing degrees of tightness, after which the patient is asked either to breath in or out, depending on which further tightens the tissues. The patient is then asked to add other activating movements such as moving fingers, toes, arms, or legs, or to activate cranial nerves by facial and eye movements. Its important to make sure that the patient's skin in not lubricated so that forces are transferred to the fascial layers.

John Barnes advocates the use of *traction* placed on fascial planes and held as long as needed to achieve a release. This may take several minutes. He also advocates the use of wedges to align the pelvis when treating pelvic restrictions. For example, in a prone patient one wedge can be placed under the ASIS (most often on the right, as anterior right innominate is seen in the majority of patients) and a second wedge under the left greater trochanter of the femur to align the two sides of the pelvis (Figure 9-51). It his belief that most pelvic and other bodily asymmetries are due to fascial plane shortening rather then joint and/or muscle dysfunctions. After aligning the pelvis by the use of wedges, traction is applied by the practitioner's hands, using downward pressure on the sacrum with one hand and upwards pressure on the spine with the other. The barrier is gently engaged until a release is felt. To treat the sacroiliac joint, for example, the hands can be placed across the joint and traction applied until a release is sensed. (This is a technique that in fact can be applied across any joint.) For integrated upper or lower extremity technique, the practitioner may engage the restricted fascial barriers gently by moving the limb in varying directions that engage tightness and then applying gentle traction by pulling the limb until a release is felt. The traction is always released slowly.

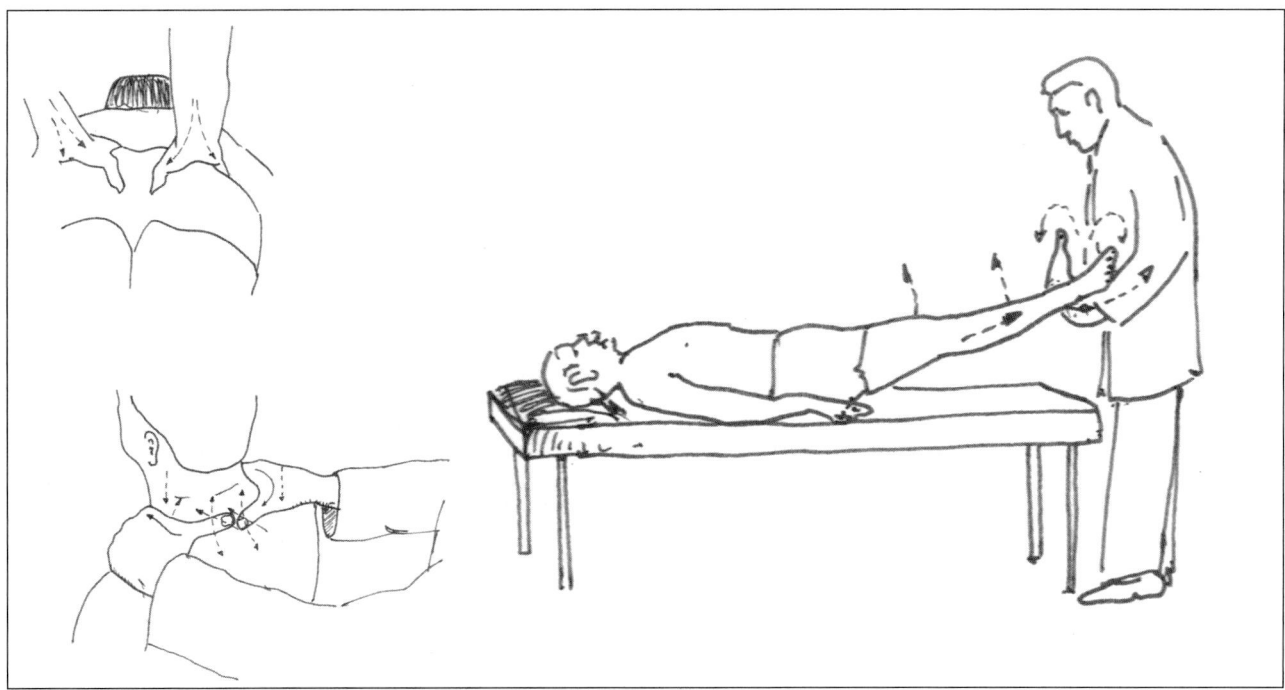

Figure 9-52: Myofascial release techniques. Performed by sequentially loading areas of tightness using combined compression, traction, and twisting maneuvers. This is a direct technique.

Integration of Myofascial Release to TCM Practice

Myofascial release techniques are helpful and can be easily integrated within TCM practice. Normal tissue palpatory, or Sinew channels assessment can be used (i.e., one can visualize the pathways of the Sinew channels as a guide for testing fascial tension). These techniques are also often helpful when used in combination with distal acupoint stimulation. The appropriate Sinew channels or Main channels are needled and proximal tissues are released manually. After needling the appropriate Sinew channel, the limb is moved to its restricted barriers and held until a release is sensed. Wrist-Ankle acupuncture is particularly helpful in facilitating myofascial release technqiues.

Articulatory Techniques

Articulatory techniques (springing techniques) are direct methods that use repetitive and gentile forces applied to parts of the body that are restricted, gently springing against the fixed barriers. These techniques are also known as low-velocity moderate-to high-amplitude, or short-lever techniques. They are especially helpful for simple problems with a single restrictive barrier or complex problems with multiple joint and tissue restrictive barriers. Very young and old patients respond well to this type of treatment (Patriquin and Jones 2003).

An example would be applying slow, gentle, and controlled pressure against a restricted vertebra. This pressure can be applied to the spinous process or transverse process, engaging the restricted barrier and gently encouraging the affected vertebra into movement through the fixation. The pressure is in-line with the facet orientation. Repeated attempts are made until the restricted barriers are fully engaged. The patient is then asked to take a deep breath. This breath further helps to restore proper motion.

Procedure

In general, the patient is placed in a comfortable position that permits the problem area to be mobilized. The affected joint is moved to the limit of all ranges of motion. As the restrictive barrier is reached, slow, firm, gentle, and continuous force against the limit of tissue motion or up to the patient's tolerance of pain or fatigue is applied. After a few seconds, the pressure is slowly released and the joint is allowed to return to its newly gained resting position. The process is repeated several times. Activating forces such as deep breathing or even muscle energy (post-isometric contractions) can be integrated. They often increase the effectiveness of the treatment. At times, it is helpful to release the pressure quickly. This results in a sudden springing of the joint and may facilitate mobility. A quick direct thrust may be tried as well.

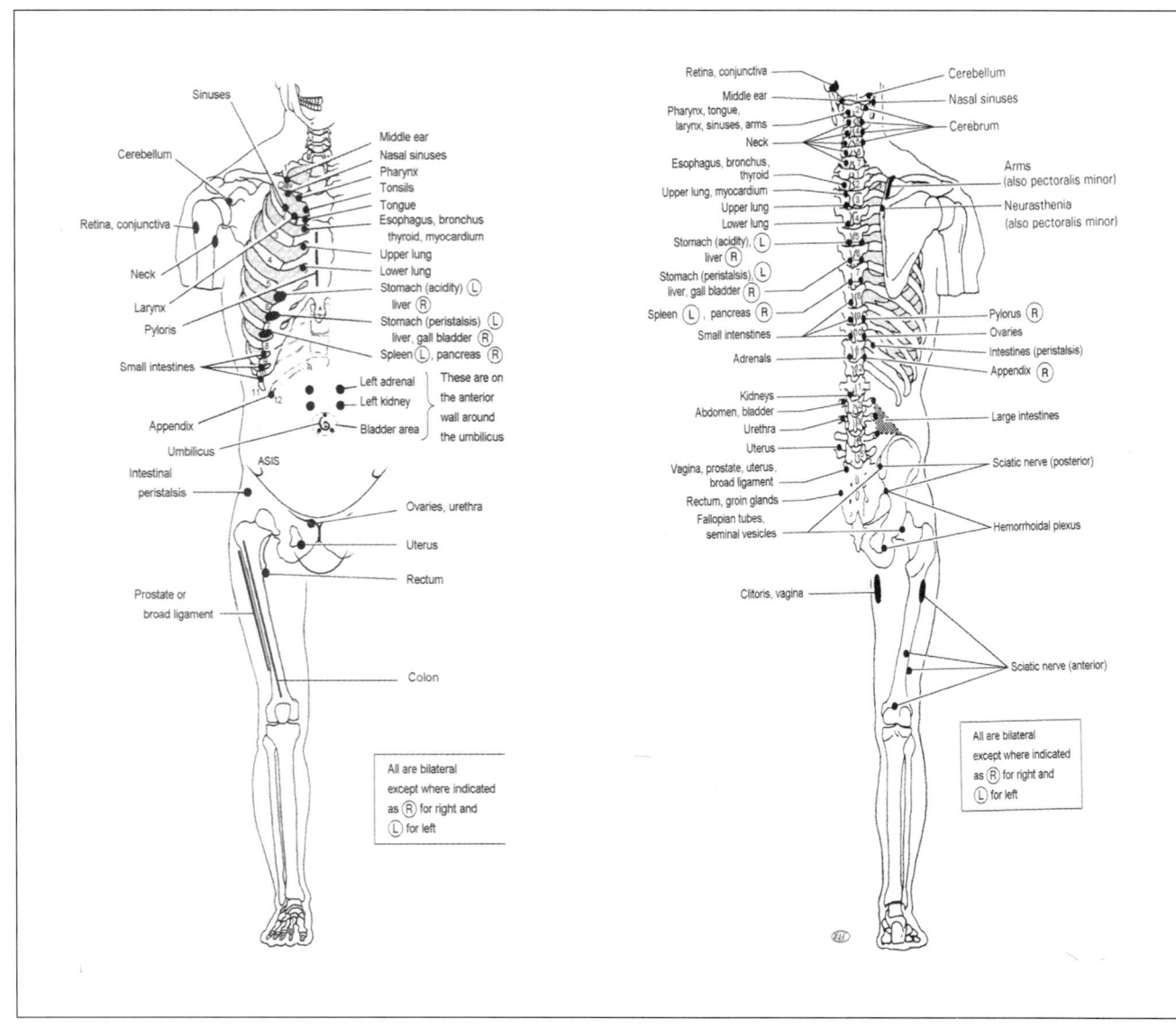

Figure 9-53: Chapman's reflexes (From Kuchera WA and Kuchera ML, Osteopathic Principles in Practice, KCOM press 1993, with permission).

Integration of Articulatory Techniques to TCM Practice

Articulatory techniques are very similar to the stimulatory techniques used in TCM. The difference between TCM and Osteopathic articulatory techniques is the precision and gentleness used when springing the affected joint or area as well as differences in functional assessments. While in TCM springing often involves quick rocking movements, with Osteopathic articulatory techniques movements are usually slow and gentile. The use of breath by the patient to facilitate release is also unique to Osteopathy. Direct pressure articulatory TCM techniques are often based on spinous process positioning, i.e., the position of the vertebra is determined by the position of the spinous process. Articulatory techniques can be very helpfully integrated with acupuncture therapy either following local needling, or when applied at the same time with distal or microsystem needling (for example see page 277).

Chapman Reflexes

Chapman reflexes are areas of particular viscerosomatic reflexes discovered by Dr. Chapman (Patriquin 2003; Kuchera and Kuchera 1994). Chapman's reflexes can be useful when differential diagnosis is needed to ascertain if pain is due to visceral or somatic causes. The reflexes can be used for treatment as well.

These reflexes are areas that develop *tissue changes* and *tenderness* as a result of visceral and other disorders (mostly neurolymphatic). They are found bilaterally. The *anterior* reflexes (points) are used more for diagnosis and the *posterior* reflexes (points) are used more for treatment (although both anterior and posterior points can be used for both). Many of the posterior reflexes (and palpable nodes) are found in the paraspinal areas midway between the tip of transverse process and the spinous process, in the area (level) which corresponds to the anterior reflex points (i.e., fifth anterior intercostal correspond with T5 posterior point). Other posterior reflex areas are found over the scapula, sacrum and ilia, buttock, and posterior thigh. Many of the anterior reflexes (and palpable nodes or points) are located next to the sternum in the intercostal spaces, or in the intercostal spaces next to the costal cartilages. Other points are located over the abdomen, pelvis, and thigh.

On palpation, these areas are located deep to the skin and subcutaneous areolar tissue, most often lying on the deep fascia or periosteum (or within the fatty tissue just under the skin). The nodules are said to feel small, smooth, firm, and discretely palpable, or grouped in irregular patches. If found alone they are said to be approximately 2-3mm in diameter. They can be easily confused with lipomas. Once found, the reflex point is identified and isolated by the practitioner's fingertip. Gentle but firm pressure on it usually causes a deep, disagreeable pain response by the patient. The pain is said to characteristically be pointed, nonradiating, sharp, and exquisitely distressing.

Chapman's reflexes are said to be particularly helpful when signs of lymphatic congestion are seen. Symptoms of lymphatic congestion may include edema, congested or enlarged lymph nodes that may or may not be tender, low resistance in general, infections and poorly healing wounds. These (Frost 2002) reflexes may be useful in treating poor muscular endurance.

Treatment to these points is advocated only after the pelvis has been treated for somatic dysfunctions. Treatment is usually performed by applying uncomfortable pressure to the nodular mass. The finger tip is then slowly moved in a circular fashion, attempting to "flatten" the mass. The technique is performed for ten to thirty seconds.

Adaptation of Chapman's Points to TCM Practice

Chapman's reflexes are obviously similar in many ways, and used in similar ways, to *Mu (Alarm) and back-Shu (or Jia Ji)* circuits in TCM. They can easily be used to supplement somatic palpation in visceral and circulatory diagnosis and treatment. The author has found that Japanese gentle needle techniques using a thin thirty-six to thirty-eight gauge, or even a 00 Serin needle works well. After insertion, the needle is held *loosely* by the practitioner and gently inserted to *pack* the nodule. The needle is held loosely so as to only tease the outer edge of the nodule instead of penetrating it.

Cranial Techniques

Cranial technique was added to the armamentarium of Osteopathic medicine around 1940 through the work of William G. Sutherland (Greenman *ibid*). Dr. Sutherland concluded that the cranial sutures are not fused as was previously thought, but rather allow for motion. The cranial system is closely related to the sacrum via connections of the dural tube. The technique is therefore also known as CranioSacral Therapy. When one places both hands on the skull one can feel a rhythmic sensation of widening and narrowing. This sensation occurs at a rate of about 10-14 times per minute and is of relatively low amplitude. At the same time the sacrum also moves rhythmically at the same rate with the sacral base nodding forward and backwards (around the upper sacral axis at S1). This rhythmic movement is known as the primary respiratory mechanism. When treating spinal pain (low back pain) one can assess movement of the sacrum by placing two hands one on each side of the sacrum (lateral aspects of sacrum). If large rocking, as apposed to normal nodding, movement (unrelated to breathing with slow velocity) is seen this is known as sacral oscillation, and a cranial cause of pain should be considered. Often dysfunctions can be detected at the cranial base and/or temporal bones.

While craniosacral function and treatment is important in the general management of musculoskeletal disorders, it is beyond the scope of this text.

Adaptation of Cranial Techniques to TCM Practice

Cranial evaluation techniques can be used to assess the appropriateness and effectiveness of Scalp acupuncture, as well as guiding the practitioner to scalp aria points. When treating low back pain the practitioner is confronted with endless choices of point selection. One can use local point, distal points on the lower or upper extremity, or points on the scalp. State Waters (1010.25) (two scalp points) is commonly used to treat low back pain in Tong-style acupuncture. The choice of using these two points is often arbitrary and mostly based on having midline low back pain. Bleeding or needling UB-40 is another choice that can treat low back midline pain. Cranial evaluation techniques, or the presence of sacral oscillation can then be used to guide the practitioner to cranial point. When sacral oscillation is seen, the cranial sutures at the cranial base and temporal bones can be palpated for tension. Areas that feel excessively tight are then needles using a horizontal subcontious approach along the suture.

Manipulation with Impulse and Other Western Techniques

Thrust (high-velocity, short-amplitude) techniques are commonly used in many traditional therapies around the world.

Short-Lever Techniques

Short-lever techniques (Figure 9-56) are achieved by the practitioner manipulating his thrust directly on the joint

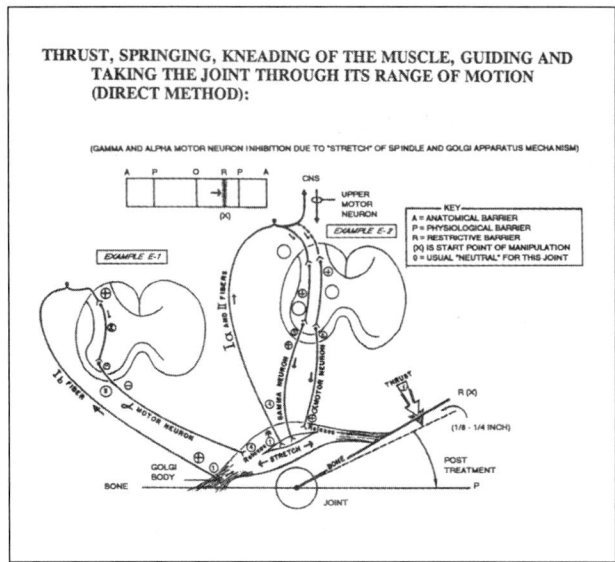

Figure 9-54: Direct methods (From Kuchera WA and Kuchera ML, Osteopathic Principles in Practice, KCOM press 1993, with permission).

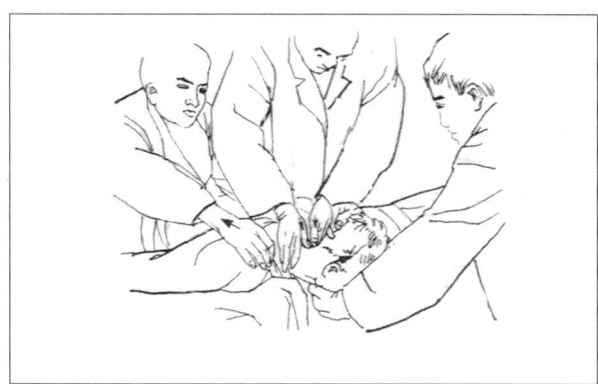

Figure 9-55: Combined long- and short-lever manipulation.

without using a lever arm. Many TCM manipulations are short-lever and require significant physical strength. In TCM, short-lever techniques are sometimes used in combination with long-lever techniques (Figure 9-55). They are used also by other systems such as Orthopaedic, Osteopathic, and Chiropractic, especially on the thoracic spine.

Long-Lever Techniques

TCM, Orthopaedic, Osteopathic and other manual therapy styles commonly use long-lever thrust techniques (Figure 9-56). Parts of the body (leg, arm, hip, shoulder, trunk, and spine) are used as lever arms to transmit the manipulator's force to the desired segment or joint.

These manipulations are performed in order to increase the joint's range of motion, displace any structure blocking a joint, rupture ligamentous or tenoperiosteal adhesions, distract a joint, stretch soft tissues, or restore the normal location and function of a misaligned or dysfunctional joint. The joint is usually placed at its restrictive barrier (or away from pain), and an activation force is delivered via the lever arm. This type of manipulation often gaps the two joint surfaces and allows them to spring back into a more physiologic position.

Joint-specific techniques may be designed to gap or not gap the joint, and usually are directed through the restrictive barrier. Orthopaedic Medicine and some TCM long-lever techniques are less joint-specific as compared to Osteopathic techniques, which usually are also less forceful. TCM, Chiropractic, Osteopathic, and some Orthopaedic techniques combine short-lever together with long-lever techniques. These combinations can increase localization. TCM and Orthopaedic Medicine also commonly use manipulation techniques under traction.

Many theories attempt to explain the therapeutic action of high-velocity, short-amplitude manipulation (thrust techniques), not all of which consider the direct "mechanical/positional" action of the thrust. For example, high-velocity, short-amplitude manipulation forcefully stretches hypertonic muscles against their muscle spindles, leading to a barrage of afferent impulses to the CNS. This may then, by reflex inhibition of gamma and alpha motor neurons, lead to re-adjustment of muscle tone and relaxation. Stimulation of mechanoreceptors may in turn shut down the "gate" by inhibiting small-caliber nociceptors and may also result in reciprocal inhibition. Although this can easily explain the short-term effects of manipulation, it does not explain long-term effects. The main hypotheses for the effects of high-velocity, short-amplitude manipulation are: the release of entrapped synovial folds or plica, relaxation of hypertonic muscle by sudden stretching, disruption of articular or peri-articular adhesions, and unbuckling of motion segments that have undergone disproportionate displacements.

Manipulation can be performed in the pain-free direction, as determined by provocation tests. Or the practitioner can use motion restriction rather than pain as a guide. Slack is taken up in the spinal segments adjacent to the dysfunctional joint. Localization of movements should be painless. The thrust must be sufficient to gap and move the restricted joint in the desired direction, or to stimulate the antagonist muscle to release the joint (via reciprocal inhibition). This is achieved by a quick thrust of low amplitude (distance).

Dangers of High-Velocity Thrust Manipulations

The dangers of *cervical* thrust manipulation have been greatly exaggerated. The inherent risk of thrust techniques and non-thrust procedures in which the head and neck are rotated, (especially if extended at the same time) must however, be kept in mind. Weintraub and Khoury (1995), have documented by magnetic resonance angiographic analysis,

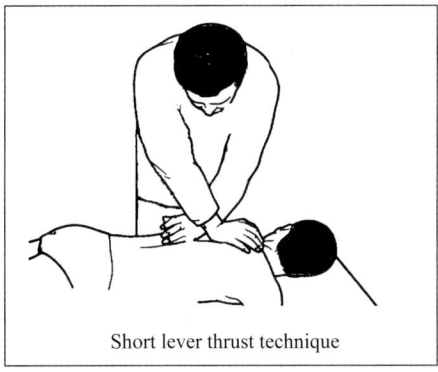
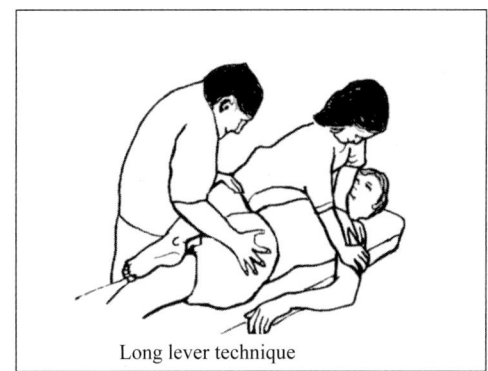
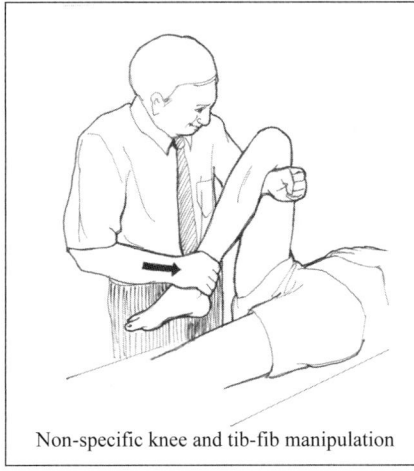
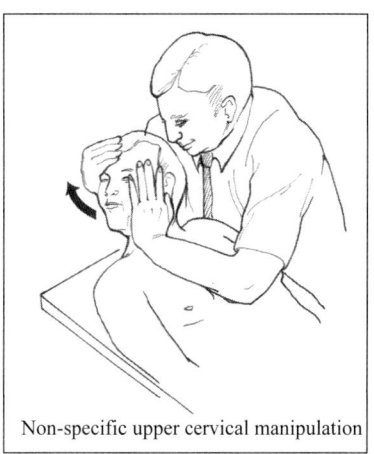

Figure 9-56: Example of high velocity low amplitude manipulations.

and others (Ombregt et al *ibid*) by other techniques, that neck and head positions of rotation and hyperextension can result in abnormalities of perfusion at the atlantoaxial and atlantooccipital junction and in the distal vertebral artery.

- Rotation slightly decreases blood flow in the ipsilateral vertebral artery and significantly decreases blood flow in the contralateral artery.
- Sidebending slightly decreases flow in the ipsilateral artery and has no effect on blood flow in the contralateral artery.
- Pure flexion or extension do not effect blood flow at all.
— However, flexion combined with rotation significantly reduces flow bilaterally, and flexion combined with sidebending and contralateral rotation slightly decreases flow in the contralateral artery, while complete cessation of flow is seen in the ipsilateral artery.
- Patients with degenerative joint disease are at increased risk.

A 1993 estimate states that one in 17,000 manipulations results in *mild* complications, most commonly a *transient* disturbance of consciousness or radicular signs (Dvorák, Baumgartne, Antinnes 1993). More serious complications have been reported. Kunnasmaa (1993) reviewed all European journal reports and found 139 cases of cerebrovascular accidents (CVA). Kunnasmaa reported thirty-one deaths and twenty-nine severe residual neurological deficits following cervical manipulation. Considering that at least several million manipulations are performed each year and that so few reports of complications are published, the procedure can be regarded as safe when performed appropriately. Estimates for CVA range from one-per-million to three-per-million manipulations (Middleeditch 1991; Carey 1993). In a review of malpractice data from the Canadian Chiropractic Protective Association evaluating all claims of stroke following chiropractic care over a ten-year period between 1988 and 1997, approximately 134.5 million cervical manipulations were performed by chiropractors over this time period. There were forty-three cases of neurological symptoms fol-

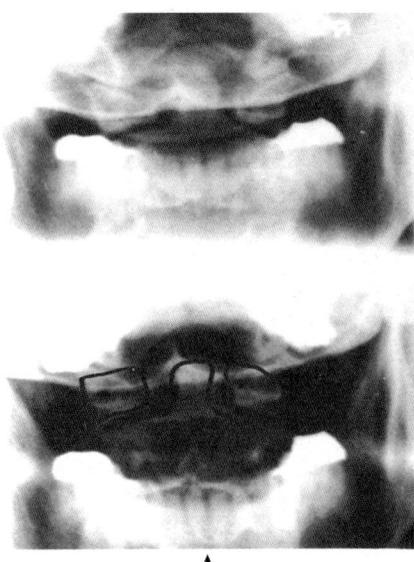
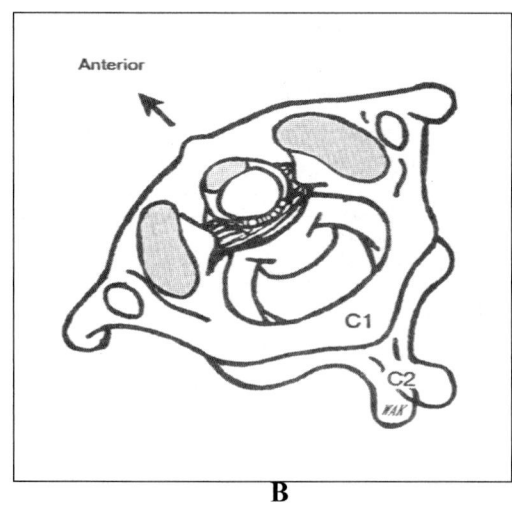

Figure 9-57: (A) Open mouth x-ray to assess upper cervical instability. (B) Possible movement of upper cervical vertebra when supporting ligaments are injured. Seen post-traumatic or in patients with inflammatory diseases ([B] (From Kuchera WA and Kuchera ML, Osteopathic Principles in Practice, KCOM press 1994, with permission).

lowing cervical manipulation over this ten-year period. Twenty were minor and were not diagnosed as a stroke by neurologists. Twenty-three cases of stroke or vertebral artery dissection following cervical manipulations were noted. With over 4,500 licensed chiropractors in Canada, the likelihood that a chiropractor would be made aware of an arterial dissection following cervical manipulation is approximately 1:8.06 million office visits, 1:5.85 million cervical manipulations, 1:1,430 chiropractic practice years, and 1:48 chiropractic practice careers. This is significantly less than the estimates of 1:500,000-1,000,000 cervical manipulations that have been calculated by surveys of neurologists. Characteristics of the twenty-three patients who developed vertebral artery dissections following cervical manipulations were: median age of 42.5 years, 26% male and 74% female, 17.4% with hypertension, 4.3% used oral contraceptives, 17.4% with migraine headache and 22% who smoked (Haldeman, Carey, Townsend, Papadopoulos 2001).

In comparison, nonsteroidal anti-inflammatory (NSAIDs) medications result in 2,000 (or upto 20,000) *deaths* and cost $200,000,000 for treatment of side effects per years in the US, alone. It is estimated that 8% of the world adult population is prescribed an NSAID for a variety of conditions (Simon 1997, *ibid*).

Contraindications to Spinal Thrust Manipulations

Manipulations with impulse should not be used in patients with:

- Bleeding disorders or anticoagulant medications.
  —May cause disastrous complications from bleeding. This is only a relative contraindication.
- Rheumatoid disease, Reiter's syndrome, and psoriatic arthritis.
  —May result in ligamentous laxity and instability, especially in the cervical spine were the transverse ligament is affected often. These are only relative contraindications.
- Spinal cord compression is absolutely contraindicated to manipulation.
- Radicular pain with/without sensory, reflex and motor signs.
  —Such patients rarely benefit from thrust techniques and often are made worse; thrust techniques are probably better avoided.
- Susceptibility to fractures from infections, osteoporosis, neoplastic disease etc.
- Hypermobility unless mild.
  — Is a relative contraindication.
- Evidence of upper motor neuron lesion (cord signs and symptoms).
- Adherent dura.
- Basilar ischemia.
- Drop attacks.
- Catalepsy.
- Infection and active inflammation, including ankylosing spodylitis.

Other relative contraindications to thrust manipulation are:

- Weakness and pain associated with pain on contralateral sidebending (may be a sign of a tumor).

Table 9-8: Sample Considerations for Thrust Manipulation

PRESENTATION	CONSIDERATION
Articular Signs	If the patient has articular signs, limitation of movement in some directions, no clear root signs, and at least three directions of free movement, manipulation therapy can be tried.
Acute Facet Sprain	If the patient has an acute facet sprain with hemarthrosis, thrust techniques often are painful and unhelpful.
Nervousness or Muscle Guarding	If the patient is nervous or has severe muscle guarding, the practitioner applies acupuncture, massage, and indirect techniques first.
Root Signs	In the presence of root signs (such as positive compression test with arm pain), thrust manipulation often fails—especially if a nucleus protrusion has occurred—and even might aggravate symptoms. In these cases, the practitioner applies traction first.

- Instability of the spine (can be caused by rheumatoid arthritis, by trauma, or may be congenital).
- Disc protrusions and radial tears that pass from the annulus into the nucleus.
- Hyper-sensitivity.

Thrust manipulation should follow the findings of the examination, as described in the examples in Table 9-8.

Joint Crack

In 1995, Reggars and Pollard reported that in fifty patients, a relationship between the side of head of the rotation and the side of joint crack during the "diversified" rotatory manipulation of the cervical spine was found. When they analyzed the "joint crack" sound by wave analysis of digital audio tape recordings, 94% exhibited cracking on the ipsilateral side to head rotation; one subject exhibited joint cracking on the contralateral side only; and two subjects exhibited bilateral joint crack sounds. Statistically, the rate of exclusively ipsilateral joint cracking in subjects who had a history of neck trauma was significantly lower. The joint crack sound is thought to result from joint space enlargement. The fluid within the joint may transform from a liquid to a gases state (as when opening a champagne bottle) resulting in the popping sound.

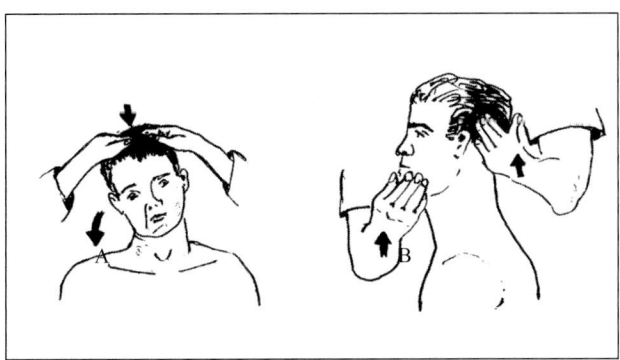

Figure 9-58: A: Foraminal compression test, positive if pain increases. B: Distraction test for assessment of root pain, positive if reduces pain.

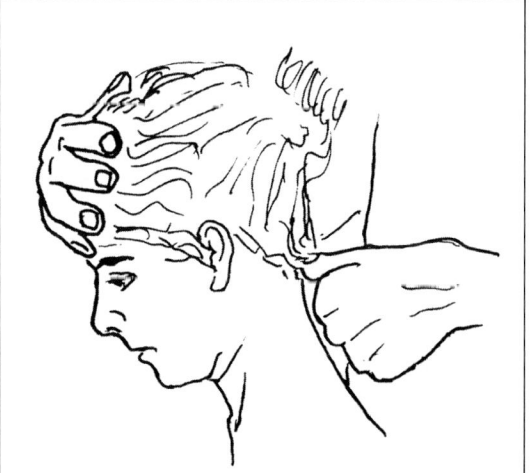

Figure 9-59: Sharp-Purser test for upper cervical instability. The head is pushed posteriorly gently against the practitioner's thumb which is on the spinous process of the axis. The test is positive if a sense of gliding movement or a sound is heard as the atlas and the skull subluxate forward and backward.

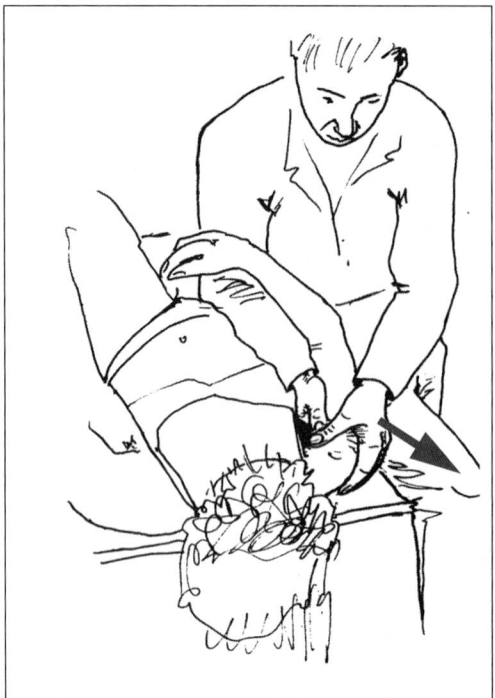

Figure 9-60: Distraction technique for shoulder capsulitis. The practitioner gently lifts (superiorly) and pulls laterally the humeral head, gently holding it until a sense of relaxation is sensed.

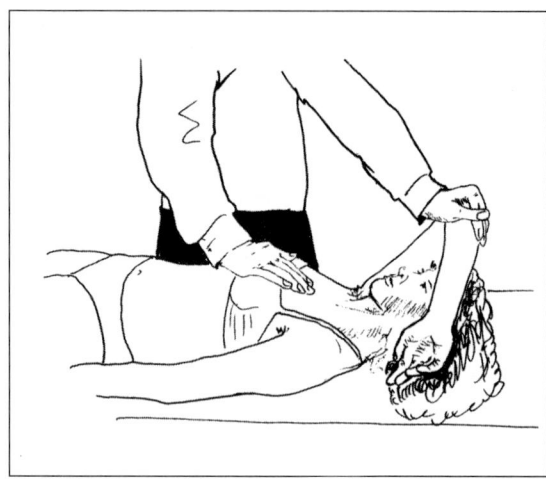

Figure 9-62: Shoulder capsule stretch.

Additional Commonly Used Techniques

Traction and Distraction

Traction/distraction can be used both therapeutically and diagnostically. When traction reduces pain from spinal origin, the pain is likely to be of a discogenic origin as traction can distract the intervertebral disc space, widen the intervertebral foraminae, but can also pull on the facets and thus influence pain coming from the hypophyseal (facet) joints as well (Figure 9-63). In the spine, traction can be used for nuclear disc protrusion. Traction can cause a negative intradiscal pressure with centripetal "suction" on the protrusion. The posterior longitudinal ligament is tightened which may help reduce a displaced fragment. For *nuclear* protrusions a continuous twenty-four hours traction is recommended which allows the traction to be of a low degree of pull. In outpatients, *sustained* traction may be required, in which stronger steady traction is applied daily for about half an hour. *Intermittent* (manual) traction is not recommend as it takes time for the muscles to relax, but it can be used for *radial* disc pains (Ombregt et al *ibid*).

Traction/distraction can be used also to treat peripheral joints. For example, in acute shoulder arthritis distraction can be used as an alternative to steroid injections (Figure 9-60). Traction is often combined with therapeutic manipulations to treat joint derangement (e.g. meniscus, loose bodies etc.), (Figure 9-61).

Stretching Techniques

Stretching can be used to treat shortened muscles or joint capsules. Capsular stretching is required often in early stage arthrosis and in some cases of early arthritis, as long as the end-feel is still "stretchable," i.e. not too hard/bony (Figure 9-62). When stretching a tight capsule it is helpful to first

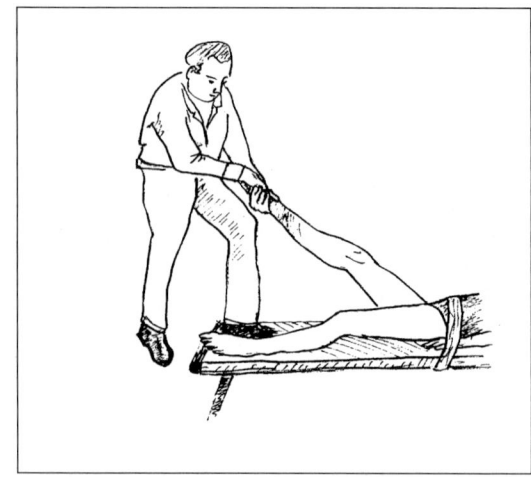

Figure 9-61: First manipulative technique for a loose body of hip under traction.

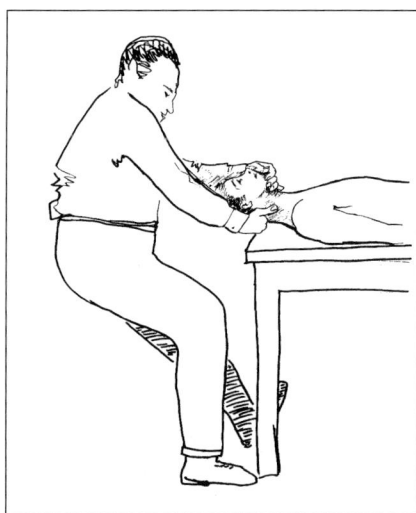

Figure 9-63: Manual traction treatment of cervical spine.

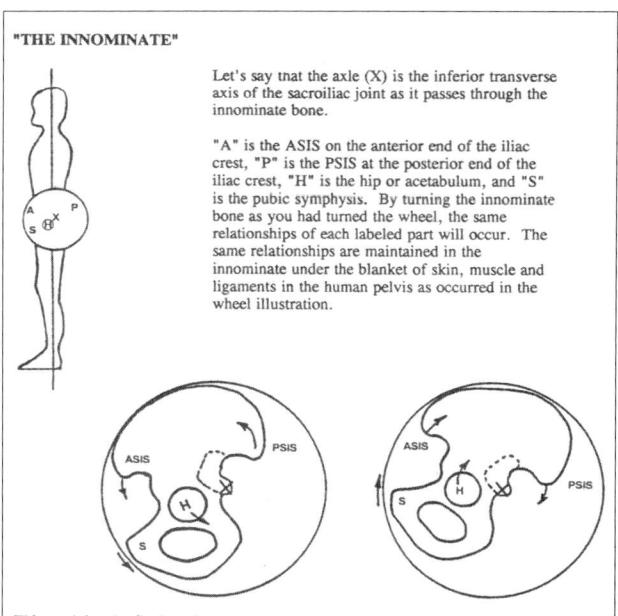

Figure 9-64: Innominate rotations (From Kuchera WA and Kuchera ML, Osteopathic Principles in Practice, KCOM press 1993, with permission).

treat myofascial triggers with light acupuncture stimulation and to warm the joint just prior to stretching. Capsular stretching is done by applying a steady pressure for about thirty seconds to one minute, with as much force as is reasonable for the patient to bear. Tension is then slightly reduced for a few seconds, and then again increased. From time to time the pressure is completely released and the patient rests. Some pain may be felt when tension is released and, therefore, it may be wise to bring the limb back to neutral position under *traction*. Normally, capsular stretching is given for fifteen to twenty minutes, three times a week. The therapeutic effect is slow. If the patient feels increased pain after a stretching session for more than a day, then the technique is too forceful or is inappropriate for the joint (Ombregt et al *ibid*).

Muscles may be stretched by sustained stretching force, preferably for ninety seconds, and/or after a post-isometric effort. To prevent rebound-tightness, it is often better to stretch only the tight muscle fibers (if they contain a tight band), leaving the uninvolved muscle fibers slack. The stretch sensation should then be felt in the muscle belly only, *not* at the tendons. *Stretch-and-spray* may be used, and the spray sweeps should be applied in one direction only, covering first the full length of the muscle and then covering the complete pain reference zone, if one exists. Only the skin should be cooled, not the muscle. Tight muscles may be treated by other methods, such as positional release for example.

Paralyzed muscles may lead to a loss of normal ROM of related joints. Stretching these as well as joint capsules may help prevent such complications and should be started as soon as possible to prevent contractures.

The Dontigny Model

There are many models that can be used to design manual therapy interventions. Many are complex, especially when dealing with the pelvic girdle. Dontigny PT proposes a simple model for SI joint dysfunction (SIJD) based on the loss of self-bracing from innominate rotation. He advocates a simple treatment and exercise routine which is said to be appropriate in all SIJD and effective 85% of the time. According to him, *all* SIJD are due to anterior innominate rotation, regardless if present as posterior or anterior (Osteopathic) dysfunctions (Dontigny 2003).

The Biomechanics of the Pelvis

Vleeming et al (*ibid*) have shown that anterior pelvic rotation *loosens* the sacrotuberous ligament and increases the lumbosacral angle, the lordotic posture, as well as shear forces at L5-S1. Weight bearing on the sacrum increases the ventral inclination of the sacrum and tightens the sacrotuberous ligament. The origins and insertions of the sacrospinalis and multifidus are approximated and may undergo a positional inhibition with atrophy. When moving from standing with a loaded sacrum to supine, the sacrotuberous ligaments unload allowing the S3-sacral segment to move somewhat anteriorly on S3-ilial. Simultaneously, the posterior interosseous ligaments are unloaded, allowing S1-sacral to move somewhat posteriorly on S1-ilial and causing the sacrum to incline dorsally. When moving from a supine to an erect posture, the posterior interosseous ligaments are loaded first, causing the S1-sacral segment to move anteriorly. The sacrum inclines ventrally causing a simultaneous secondary loading on the sacrotuberous ligaments.

When the line of gravity is posterior to the acetabula the innominate bones rotate posteriorly on an acetabular axis (Figure 9-64). Posterior rotation of the innominate bones

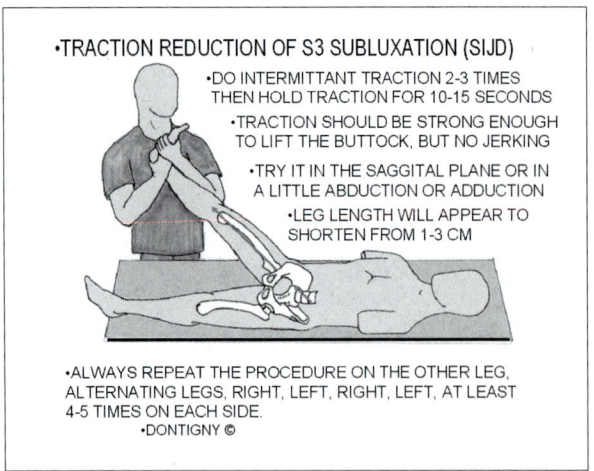
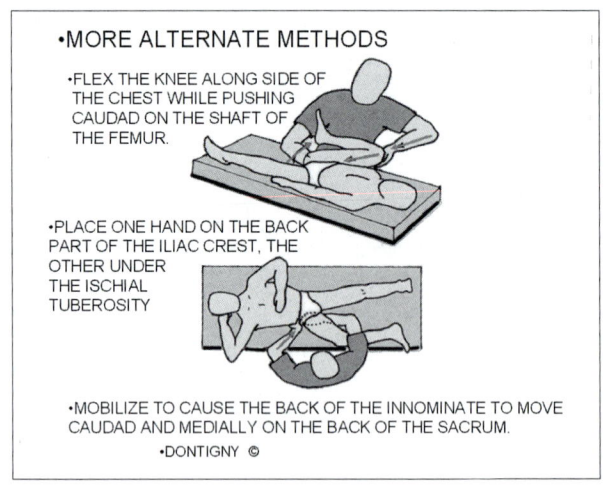
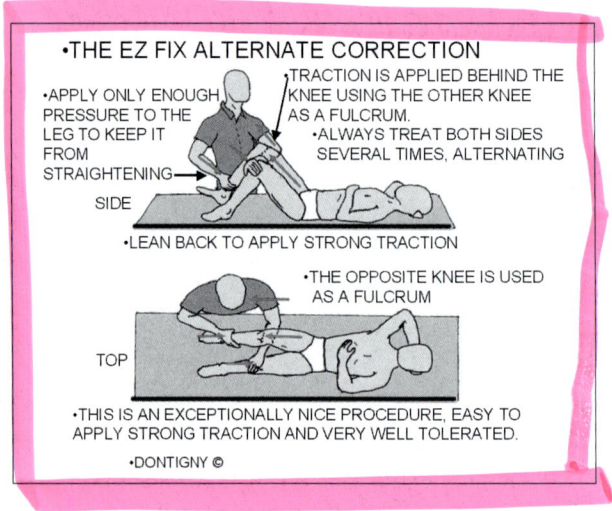

Figure 9-65: Treatment methods using Dontigny techniques (courtesy of Dontigny).

tightens the sacrotuberous ligament. Experiments by Vleeming et al (*ibid*) have shown that tightening the sacrotuberous ligament increases friction, and enhances the self-bracing and stability of the SIJs. Once the SIJ is self-braced, loading may be increased without causing further movement in the SIJ. 15Kg of pressure to the apex of the sacrum caused sacral deformation of 0.5-1.0 cm with no movement of the SIJ (Dontigny *ibid*).

Mechanisms

According to Dontigny, anterior innominate rotation may result in failure of the "force couple" and will cause a pathological release of self-bracing. The resulting "subluxation" is at the S3 segment of the sacroiliac joint. This may cause a broad range of effects on nearly all of the tissues and structures in and around the pelvis. Loss of muscular or ligamentous force-closure may cause slow or a sudden pathological release of self-bracing forcing the innominate bones to rotate anteriorly on the sacrum, on an acetabular axis. When one leans forward to perform any task, their line of gravity moves anteriorly to the acetabula. The anterior aspect of the innominate then tends to rotate down, and the posterior aspect tends to rotate up on the sacrum on an acetabular axis. This anterior rotation tends to loosen the sacrotuberous ligament and may cause a loss of friction and stability. An insidious onset of SIJD may result from excess weight being deposited on the anterior pelvis in people who are overweight, hyperlordotic, flat-footed, or in women during pregnancy. This may result in a slow onset of low back pain.

In summary, forward bending and the situp position may result in anterior rotation of the pelvis on an acetabular axis resulting in a loss of anterior pelvic support, which, in turn, decreases the secondary loading. Friction at the joint is then lost; this results in a loss of force coupling, since force coupling is dependent on SIJ axis. Loading is increased on the posterior interosseous ligaments. A sudden pathological

Additional Commonly Used Techniques

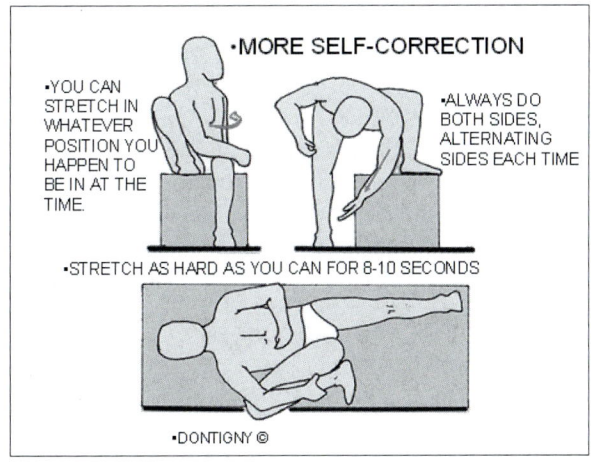
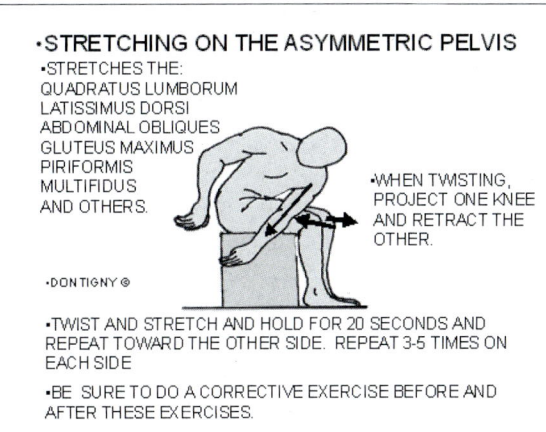
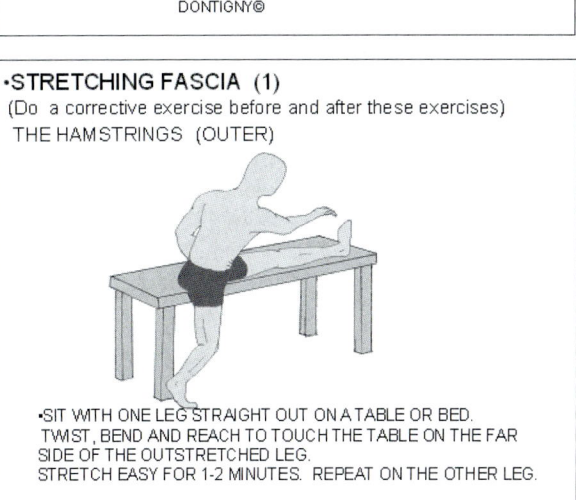
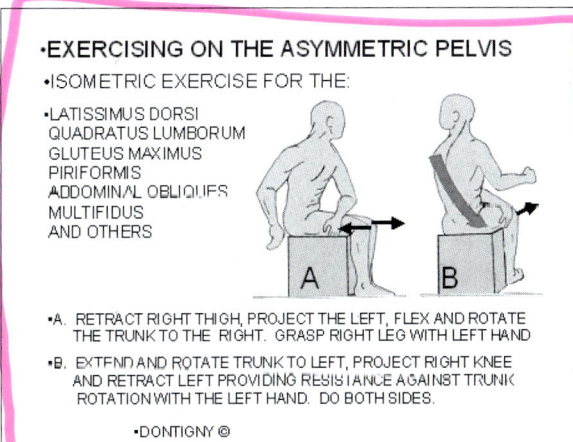
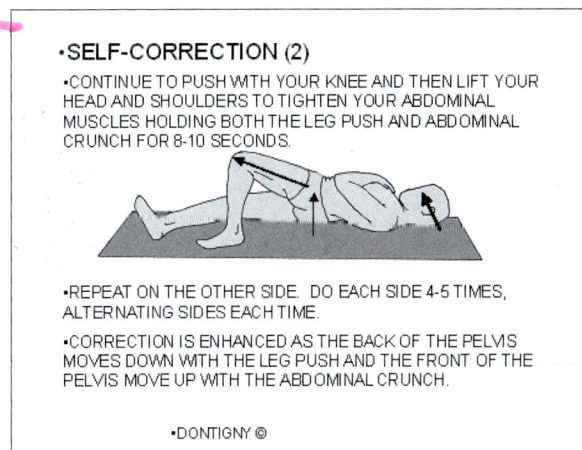

Figure 9-66: Self-correction and exercise methods (courtesy of Dontigny).

release of self-bracing may then increase the tension on the hamstring muscles, which may, in turn, rotate the innominates on the sacrum on an acetabular axis and subluxate at the S3 segment of the SIJ. As the innominate bones tend to spread and separate the SIJs with this subluxation, any increase in intra-abdominal pressure such as is caused by a sudden cough or the straining that occurs with a bowel movement will tend to further increase this spreading and thus increase the pain. The piriformis muscle, which passes immediately caudad to this subluxation and has a secondary bony origin on the ilium at the superior margin of the greater sciatic notch may be affected. Any shearing at that point can separate the dual origins of the piriformis muscle with a resultant muscle separation. Left uncorrected, subluxation at the SIJ may cause a visco-elastic failure of the collagen in stressed ligaments, inflammatory and arthritic changes, and changes in gait. These degenerative processes may result in rents in the SIJ capsule, which may leak synovial fluid into the lumbosacral plexus, the root of the fifth lumbar nerve, and into the body of the psoas and cause neurological symptoms. This may mimic symptoms of a herniated intervertebral disc.

Dysfunctions

Dontigny sees all SIJD as having an essentially pathological release of self-bracing with a subluxation of the innominates cephalad and laterally on the sacrum at the S3 segment. There are four basic manifestations, which may vary in severity and variations of impairment:

1. Bilateral symmetrical.
2. Bilateral oblique (asymmetrical).
3. Unilateral oblique.
4. Bilateral with a secondary caudad movement at the S1 segment.

BILATERAL SYMMETRICAL LESION: The innominates are rotated anteriorly, increasing the lumbar lordosis and the lumbosacral angle. The sacrotuberous ligaments are loosened. The superincumbent weight increases the ventral tilt of the pelvis within the limits of the loosened sacrotuberous ligaments. The origins and insertions of the multifidus and sacrospinalis muscles are approximated and may result in a positional inhibition with atrophy. Both SIJs move cephalad and anteriorly relative to the acetabula increasing the height of the iliac crests and the apparent length of both legs. Posteriorly, the innominate bones move cephalad, laterally and anteriorly on the sacrum on the S3 segment. Anteriorly, the ASISs and the pubes, with the innominates, move forward and down on the S1 sacral segment.

BILATERAL OBLIQUE SUBLUXATION: Asymmetric pelvic loading at the time of subluxation may cause the SIJs to sublux bilaterally, anteriorly, and obliquely, one side more than the other. The oblique bilateral subluxation will cause an asymmetrical pelvis. Both legs will appear to lengthen, one more than the other. This is similar to a unilateral SIJD, which is also asymmetrical, but far less common.

UNILATERAL OBLIQUE PELVIS: With a unilateral SIJD, the sacrum moves above the acetabulum on one side, making the crest and PSIS higher on that side when standing. The sacral base tilts away from the painful side. When supine, the sacral base is level and the leg on the painful side appears longer. This is less common than the bilateral SIJD, which can be symmetrical or asymmetrical.

OBLIQUE PELVIS WITH SECONDARY CAUDAD SLIP: After a bilateral anterior subluxation, on one side gravity may cause the S1 sacral segment to slip caudad on the S1 ilial segment, compromising the original lesion. The crest is lower on the more painful side when standing and the leg appears shorter on that side when supine. The points of pain are the same and the treatment is the same as for bilateral SIJD. This secondary movement only occurs with and after the bilateral subluxation at S3 and because of the variation in the angulations in the S1 and S3 segments. It may give the impression of an anterior dysfunction on one side and a posterior dysfunction on the other, or an "upslip" on one side, or an outflare on one side and an inflare on the other. It is corrected in the same manner as a bilateral anterior subluxation.

In conclusion, it does not matter if one leg is longer or shorter than the other, or if one pubis is higher or lower, or if the sacrum is canted or rotated, or if one iliac crest is higher or lower than the other. All of these things are merely minor variations of the primary subluxation at the S3 segment. They will all be corrected and pelvic symmetry restored and pain relieved with the manual correction of both of the innominate bones to the self-bracing position on the sacrum (Dontigny *ibid*).

Treatment of SIJD using Dontigny Techniques

Assessment for S3 subluxation can begin by reviewing the appropriate history to exclude other causes of pain. The primary indication of SIJD is pain and tenderness at the posterior inferior iliac spine (PIIS), and at points medial and caudal to the posterior superior iliac spine (PSIS). The strait leg raise may be painful contralaterally because of the resulting anterior rotation of the innominate.

Treatment is simply restoring the SIJs to the self-bracing position by rotating the back of the innominates caudad and medially on the sacrum to correct the subluxations at S3. With each maneuver the legs will appear to shorten, presumably correcting the subluxation and restoring the self-bracing position. The corrective procedure is not a vertebral manipulation. No high or low speed manipulative thrust is necessary or indicated. No jerking or popping or twisting is necessary or desirable. Correction is achieved by specifically applied traction on the properly positioned joint or by a precise manual rotation of the innominates posteriorly on the sacrum. Any of several similar methods can be used. For example,

Additional Commonly Used Techniques

Table 9-9: Correspondences of Channels, Muscles and Organs/Glands (Frost 2002)

Channel	Muscle	Organ/Gland
Central	Supraspinatus.	Brain.
Governing/Du	Teres major.	Spine.
Stomach	Pectoralis major and minor. SCM.	Stomach. Stomach.
Spleen	Latissimus dorsi. Trapezius (middle and lower).	Pancreas. Spleen.
Heart	Subscapularis. Subclavius (Dewe).	Heart. Heart.
Small Intestine	Rectus femoris. Rectus abdominis.	Small Intestine. Small Intestine.
Urinary Bladder	Peroneus muscles. Sacrospinalis.	Urinary Bladder. Urinary Bladder.
Conception (Ren)	Gluteus medius. Adductors. Gluteus maximus. Piriformis. Sartorius (& Triple Warmer).	Reproductive organs and glands (ovaries). Reproductive organs and glands. Reproductive organs and glands. Reproductive organs and glands (prostate). Adrenals (esp. the medulla portion).
Triple Warmer	Teres minor. Infraspinatus.	Thyroid. Thymus.
Gall Bladder	Popliteus.	Gallbladder.
Liver	Pectoralis major. Rhomboid major and minor.	Liver. Liver/stomach.
Lung	Serratus anticus. Deltoids.	Lung. Lung.
Large Intestine	Tensor fascia lata. Hamstrings.	Large intestine. Rectum.

direct posterior rotation can be achieved by either bringing the patient's knee to axilla or simply by grasping the innominate bone and rotating it posteriorly. Post isometric muscle energy techniques can be used to achieve added rotation. If there is no history of a congenital leg length difference, polio, or serious leg fracture, the legs will appear to be of equal length after correction.

The patient is then taught correction techniques as well as stretching and rehabilitation maneuvers so that he/she will not be dependent on-going care. Figure 9-65 on page 506 illustrates SIJD correction methods and Figure 9-66 on page 507 illustrates patient self-corrections and exercises for SIJD.[14]

Applied Kinesiology

Applied Kinesiology (AK) was developed by a the Chiropractic practitioner, George Goodheart, and incorporates manually resisted muscle testing, muscle length (tension) testing, with therapeutic stimulation of reflex neural mechanisms. Dr. Goodheart also incorporated Chapman's reflexes, relating them to specific muscles which he tested for weakness or tightness. The manipulation of muscle proprioceptors was then used to manually adjust muscle length, tension, and strength. The goal was the restoration of balance in the muscular system and therefore in the somatic frame. Good muscular balance is also said to maximize normal visceral, neural, circulatory, lymphatic, and endocrine functions.

Depending on the cause of the muscular dysfunction, the spindle cells, Golgi tendon organ, or tendinous insertions can be stimulated to achieve the desired effect. The effects from applying pressure in different direction to spindle cells and Golgi tendon organs seems to have opposite effects. To *decrease* tension in muscle fibers, both sides of the spindles (at the muscle belly) are *pushed toward* each other. If

---

14. While this methods is very simple and often useful, the author finds that posterior torsions and unilateral extended dysfunctions do not respond satisfactory to this method.

510 Chapter 9: Foundations for Integrative Manual Therapies, Rehabilitation and Orthotic Therapy

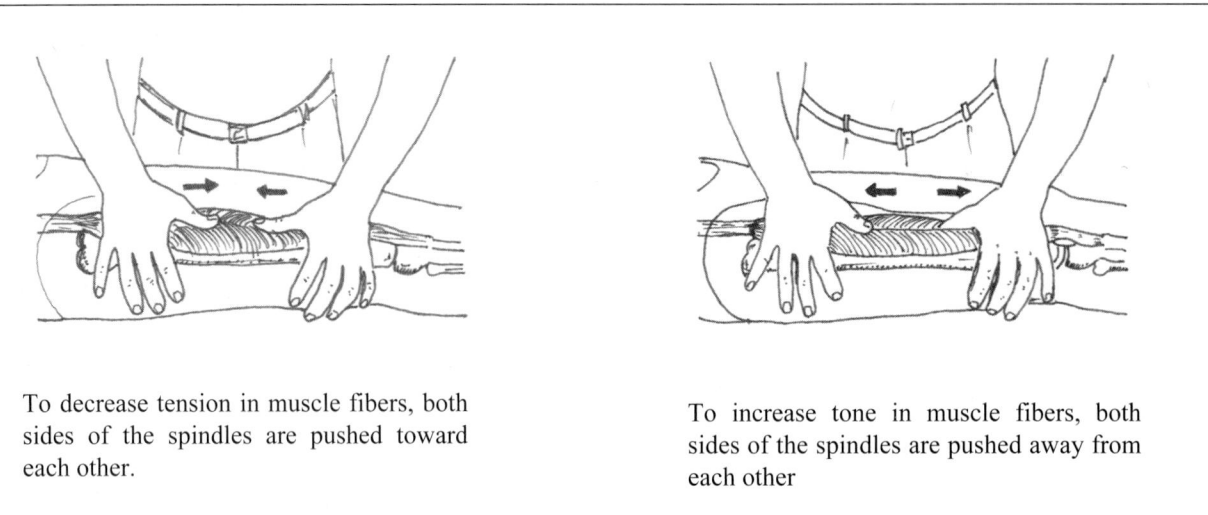

To decrease tension in muscle fibers, both sides of the spindles are pushed toward each other.

To increase tone in muscle fibers, both sides of the spindles are pushed away from each other

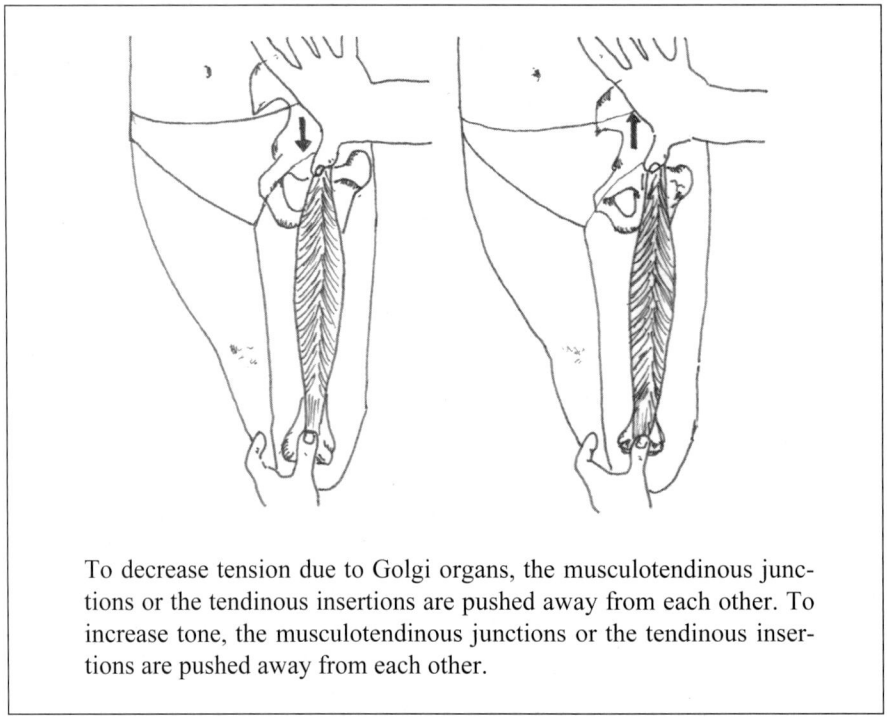

To decrease tension due to Golgi organs, the musculotendinous junctions or the tendinous insertions are pushed away from each other. To increase tone, the musculotendinous junctions or the tendinous insertions are pushed away from each other.

Figure 9-67: Effects of pressure to Golgi and Spindle mechanisms.

increased muscle tension is due to the Golgi organs, the musculotendinous junctions or the tendinous insertions are *pushed away* from each other. The opposite is true if the practitioner is trying to *increase* tension in muscle fibers. The spindles are pushed away from each other and the Golgi organs toward each other (Figure 9-67). The author has found that, at times, this also applies to the direction of needle stimulation.

To determine if muscular problems are arising from spindle cells or the Golgi organ, Applied Kinesiology tests the dysfunctional muscle while pressing the muscle belly (spindles) or the musculotendinous junction (Golgi organ). The pressure is said to over-ride their output and restore normal strength to the muscle. If pressure over the muscle belly restores strength, then the spindles are used for treatment. If pressure over the tendinous insertions or the musculotendinous junction restores strength then the Golgi organs are used for treatment. The pressure needed to treat the muscle is between 1-7 kg (Frost *ibid*).

This type of muscle testing is also said to be helpful in deciding if a muscle is primarily tight or primarily weak. An important clinical decision needs to be made when a muscular imbalance is found that is thought to cause musculoskeletal dysfunction and pain. For example, in chronic low back pain patients, it is common to find tightness in the posterior postural muscles and weakness in abdominal muscles (possibly from reciprocal inhibition). While Janda (*ibid*) often emphasizes the inhibition of the abdominals by tight spinal postural muscles (which is usually how reciprocal inhibition works), it is also possible that the lack of tone in the abdominals results in excessive tightness in back muscles, which are then called on to compensate for changes in posture from loss of abdominal bracing. The patient usually has a forward tilt of the pelvis and increased lordosis (curve) in the lumbar spine from tightness in the spinal muscles. Applied Kinesiology tests are said to be helpful in deciding which is primary in each patient.

Specific acupuncture points are said to sedate (reduce tone in) muscles. A normotonic muscle is said to become weak when the sedation points are needled, palpated, tapped, or simply touched (Figure 9-68 on page 512; Frost *ibid*):

- H-7: Subclavius and subscapularis.
- SI-8: Rectus abdominis and rectus femoris.
- P-7: Gluteus maximus & medius, adductors, piriformis and sartorius.
- TW-10: Teres minor and infraspinatus.
- Sp-5: Latissimus dorsi, middle and lower trapezius.
- St-45: Pectoralis major; clavicularis & sternalis, pectoralis minor and SCM
- Lu-5: Serratus anterior, and anterior, middle, and posterior deltoid.
- LI-2: Tensor fascia lata and hamstrings.
- K-1: Iliopsoas and upper trapezius.
- UB-65: Peroneus tertius, longus & brevis and Sacrospinalis.
- Liv-3 (2): Pectoralis major sternalis and rhomboids.
- GB-38: Popliteus.

Table 9-9 on page 509 summarizes AK correspondences of channels/meridians, muscles and organs/glands. According to Frost, AK can be used to diagnose channel/meridian imbalances as well as their related muscles, organs/Organs, and glands. The channels are said to manifest muscle weakness to AK testing before organic or other symptoms appear. The organs and glands associated with the channels in TCM are said to "fit like a glove" with AK's previously established system of correspondences. If a channel is "deficient," some or all of its associated muscles are said to test weak. Stroking a channel against its flow is said to weaken its muscles for ten seconds. If this does not occur, the muscle is said to be in a hypertonic state.

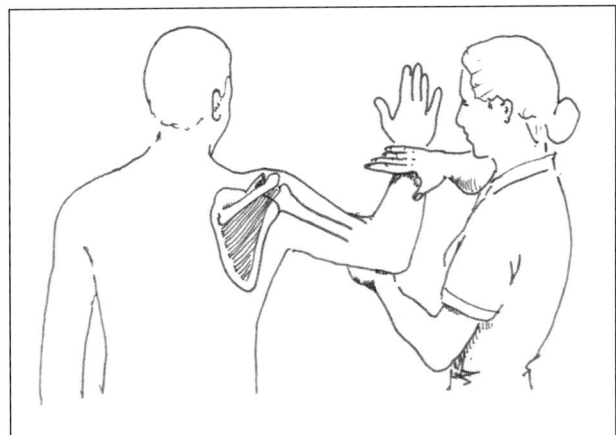

Figure 9-69: Resisted shoulder external rotation muscle testing in Applied Kinesiology. Note that the muscle is tested in a shortened position as apposed to being in neutral as is done in Orthopaedic Medicine.

Applied Kinesiology Muscle Testing in Orthopedics[15]

Muscle testing in Applied Kinesiology (AK) is said to evaluate the muscle's ability to appropriately respond to a challenge by the practitioner, and to evaluate all the regulatory mechanisms that affect muscle tone and strength. The muscle to be tested is placed so that its fibers are partially shortened (i.e., the joint(s) or origin and insertion of the muscle are approximated toward each other, as opposed to being in neutral as it is in Orthopedic Medicine). The test is initiated in a way similar to the way it is described in chapter 4, but in AK, at the end of the patient's maximal effort (which is resisted by the practitioner to create an isometric contraction), an extra load of 2-5% is placed on the muscle by the practitioner. The ability of the muscle to "lock" is therefore assessed (Figure 9-69).

Muscles are said to be weak if the patient is unable to lock the muscle and resist the extra load. If the muscle is strong, i.e., if the patient is able to lock the muscle and resist the extra load, the muscle is said to be strong. Strong muscles can then be further tested to see if they can become appropriately weak when an inhibiting stimulation is used. An inhibiting stimulation is provoked by manipulating the muscle spindles or Golgi organs, pressing sedation points, or by having the patient touch dysfunctional areas or reflex points. A normal (normotonic) muscle is said to respond to inhibition by becoming temporarily weak. Somatic dysfunctions (and joint dysfunctions) are said to be areas capable of stimulating inhibition of muscles. For example, a normotonic muscle is used to test joints (including cranial) to see if dysfunction is present. When the patient touches a dysfunctional joint or area, the normotonic muscle should become

---

15. Applied Kinesiology is said to be used also to assess for medical conditions by muscle testing but is not part of what is discussed here.

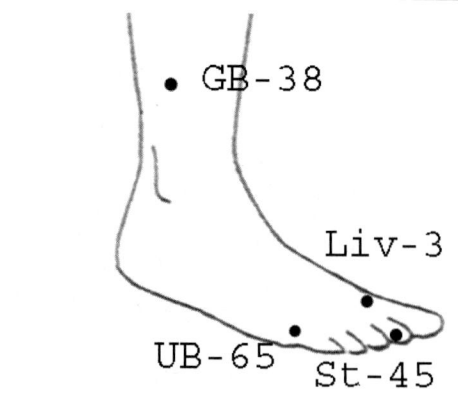

GB-38: Popliteus

UB-65: Peroneus muscles, sacrospinalis

St-45: Pectoralis muscles, clavicularis, sternalis and SCM

Liv-3 (2): Pectoralis major, sternalis, rhomboids

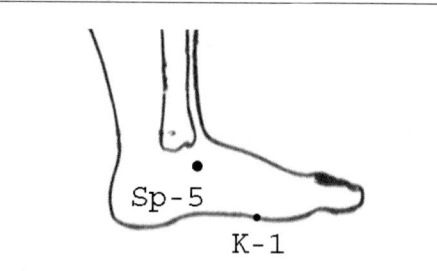

Sp-5: Latissimus dorsi, middle and lower trapezius

K-1: Iliopsoas, upper trapezius

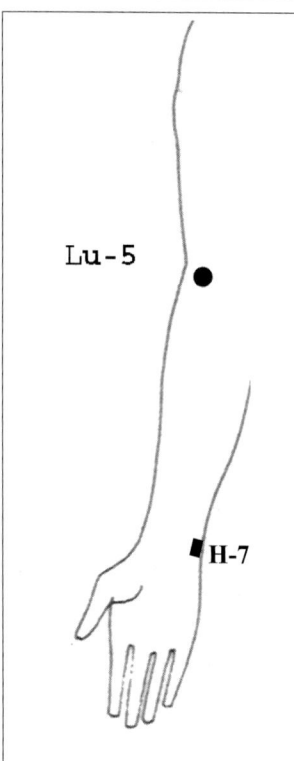

Lu-5: Serratus anterior, deltoids

H-7: Subclavious and subscapularis

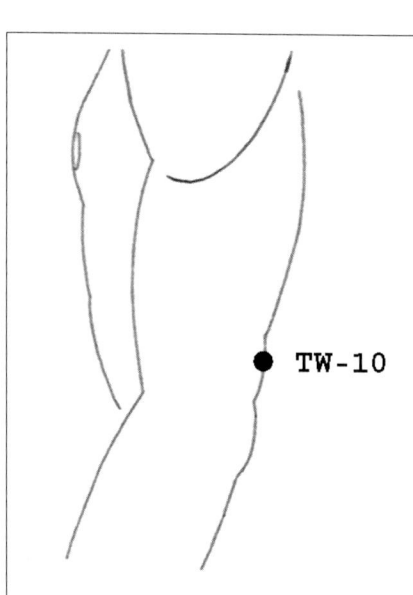

TW-10: Teres minor, infraspinatus

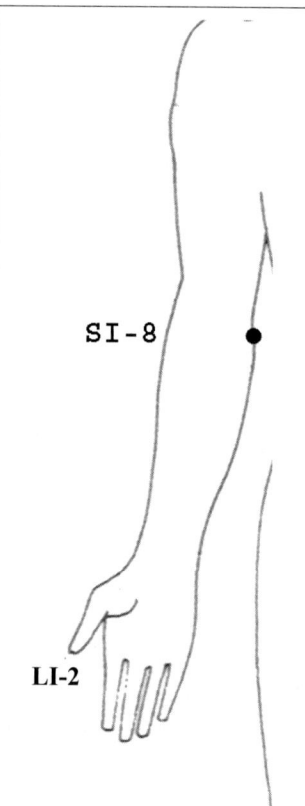

SI-8: Rectus abdominus, rectus femoris

LI-2: Fascia latta, hemstrings

Figure 9-68: AK muscle sedation points.

weak. (Any normotonic muscle can be chosen, and the muscle does not have to be related or connected to the joint.) The practitioner can then move the joint to see which direction (or manipulation technique) will be effective for treatment by retesting the indicator muscle. (For example, the practitioner will push the joint in one direction and retest the muscle, and then push the other way and test the muscle.)

Dysfunction in muscle is said to be caused by mechanical causes (subluxations, fixations, etc.), organ systems (viscera, endocrine, neural, etc.), emotional causes, chemical, dehydration, and nutritional causes.

Integration of Acupuncture With Manual Therapies

Acupuncture can be integrated with all the above techniques in which muscle length and tension are treated. Often this can enhances their effects, allowing for better localization and relaxation. The spinal levels responsible for innervation of the muscle(s) or joint(s) can be needled or moxaed before manual techniques are used. A motor or active trigger can be treated at the involved area and its antagonists. When functional muscle groups are involved, the Sinew channels can be treated, generally at active points (usually one of the first three or four points on the channel) or at the extremities. These can be needled, moxaed, or quickly stroked with an incense stick. It is often a good idea to treat the entire (i.e., lower and upper) related channels (e.g., Yang-Ming, Stomach, and Large Intestines). One can also use contralateral points to facilitate pain relief, joint and muscle relaxation thus allowing for increased accessibility to other manual therapies.

Rehabilitation and Exercise

Rehabilitation exercises are often used within the TCM/OM armamentarium to treat both musculoskeletal and internal disorders. There are exercises that use breath and movement (Tai Chi and Qi Gong) as well as specific rehabilitation and stretching techniques such as Dao Yin. Exercise is also said to be crucial for the practitioner. *Spiritual Axis* states: "Slow joints and pliable muscles, with the Heart and Mind harmonized and in tune, are responsible for guiding and leading the movement of Qi (Qi Gong)."[16]

It is essential for the patient to understand that pain does not always equal harm. Unfortunately, patients with chronic pain tend to refrain from moving a painful body part because the movement itself is painful. This reluctance to move can actually result in increased pain, dysfunction, and disability. This pain, however, does not mean that the movement is harmful. A gradual conditioning program is important for breaking what has been termed the "vicious cycle of chronic pain." Studies have shown that within a matter of days, mus-

---

16. Also see "Muscle Energy Techniques" on page 489.

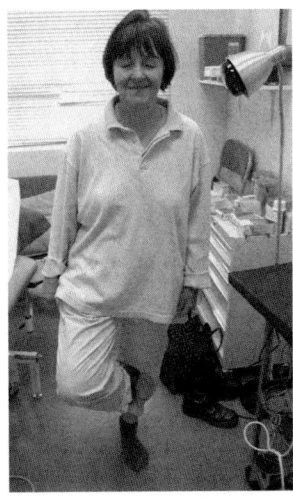

Figure 9-70: Assessment of trunk stability with one leg standing.

culoskeletal gains are lost if athletes stop training. When chronic pain patients are caught in the cycle of pain, their bodies weaken and physical disability develops.

Exercise is essential to maintaining clinical improvements achieved by manual therapies or acupuncture. When possible, a simple and time-efficient exercise program should be carefully taught to the patient. While there is disagreement in the literature as to which and what type exercise programs are best, treatment should probably begin by carefully stretching tight areas without aggravating instability. Weakness is then addressed, being careful not to overly aggravate the pain as many patients see this as evidence of injury. To ensure long-term success, it is also essential to prescribe proprioception training such as one-leg standing activities. A simple evaluation technique to gauge trunk stability, abdominal and gluteus strength, as well as acuity of proprioception, is to have the patient stand on one leg with eyes closed for fifteen to thirty seconds. The patient's failure to be able to do so indicates a need to balance muscle systems and train proprioception (Figure 9-70).

Tai-Chi exercises are particularly helpful in increasing proprioception, even though the pelvic tilt associated with Tai-Chi can easily aggravate discogenic pain, and, for this reason, modification of the Tai-Chi "form" may be needed. Treatments of perpetuating factors are complex and involve both medical intervention and patient education (with participation). Much of the stress our bodies suffer is a consequence of gravity. Therefore, postural re-education is often called for.

Muscle Tension/Length Testing

Many of the problems of the musculoskeletal system seem to involve pain related to aspects of muscle shortening (Lewit 1999). Muscle weakness is often found in patients with muscularskeletal disorders as well. However, before prescribing strengthening exercises, it is important to evaluate muscle tension and length, as often the antagonists to the "weak" muscles are hypertonic and/or shortened, reciprocally inhibiting their tone, resulting in weakness.

It is Janda's (*ibid*) and others' opinion that prior to any effort to strengthen weak muscles, shortened muscles should be dealt with by proper therapies (including treatment of joint dysfunctions). Often after tight muscles are treated, spontaneous toning occurs in the previously "weak" muscles. If muscle tone remains inadequate, then, and only then, should exercise and/or isotonic maneuvers be initiated. This is not universally accepted, and many physical therapists prefer to work on weak structures first. Attention to weak structures may reduce tightness in antagonists; however, such treatment methods cannot reverse the fibrotic state of many chronically shortened structures. It is therefor important to evaluate major muscles for tension/length as part of screening examinations.

Janda (*ibid*) suggests that for the reliable evaluation of muscle shortness:

1. The starting position, or method of fixation and direction of movement must be performed carefully observing correct methodologies;
2. The prime mover (the agonist) must not be exposed to external pressure and/or stress;
3. If possible, the force exerted on the tested muscle must not activate two joints;
4. The practitioner should perform a slow, continuos movement that brakes slowly at the end of the range;
5. The practitioner should avoid jerky movements to keep the stretch and the muscle irritability equal;
6. Pressure or pull must act in the required direction of movement only;
7. The practitioner must recognize that muscle shortening can be correctly evaluated only if the joint range is not decreased, as might be the case should an osseous limitation or joint dysfunction/blockage be present.

Screen muscle tension and length may include tests as illustrated in Figure 9-71 and Figure 9-72.

Rehabilitation and Exercise

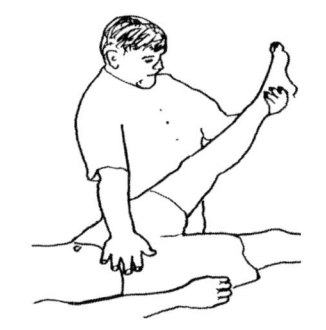

Hamstring tension: monitor opposite ASIS noting how far the leg can be rased before the ASIS begins to move. Tension should be equal on both sides. Leg rasing of less then 45° indicates excess tension.

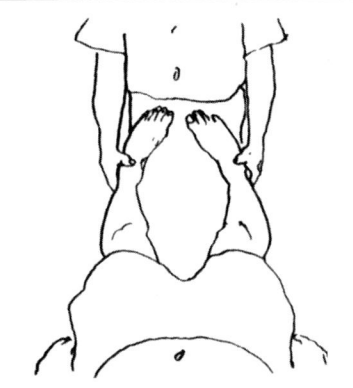

Uncompensated internal rotation at the hip (tension of the external rotators): by rotating the legs internally. The end-feel should be slightly springy and equal on both sides

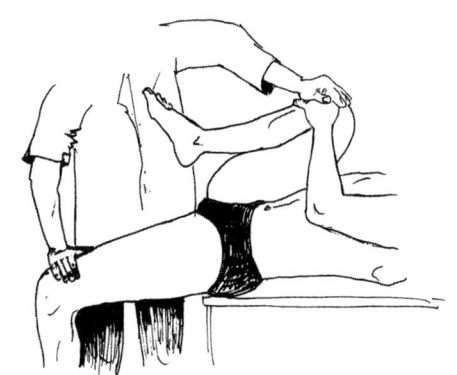

iliopsoas muscle tightness: by having the standing patient bring his thigh to his chest and then leaning backward onto the exam table. Difficulty maintaining hip extension (the patient's lower leg tending to lift off the table) indicates a tight iliopsoas muscle. A tight quadriceps muscle does not allow the knee to flex (while the patient is in this position). When knee flexion is reduced the hips compensate by flexing. The fall of the thigh below the horizontal indicates a hypotonic psoas muscle. The rectus femoris is once again seen to be short, while the relative external rotation of the lower leg (see angle of foot) hints at a probable shortened TFL

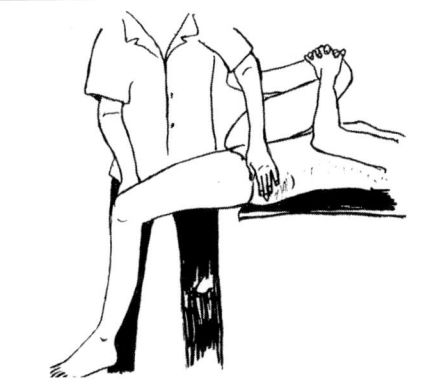

Leg adductor tension: using the same position used in the psoas tension test, but this time the patient's lower leg is abducted. Abduction of less than 25° indicates excessive tension

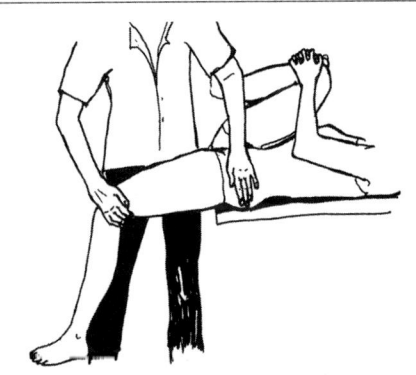

Tensor fascia lata tension: using the same position used in the psoas tension test, but this time the patient's lower leg is adducted. Adduction of less than 15° indicates excessive tension

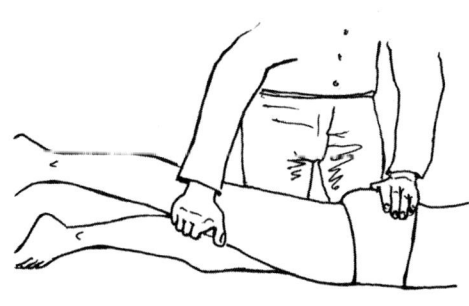

Uncompensated hip extension (psoas major muscle tension): by stabilizing the patient's pelvis and lifting his thigh. Hip extension should be equal on both sides and end-feel should be soft

Figure 9-71: Screening for muscle length and tension.

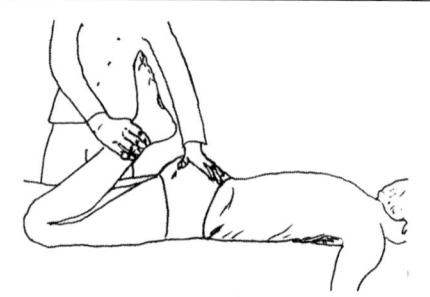

Rectus femoris muscle tightness: by flexing the patient knee. Tightness results in early compensatory lifting of the patient's pelvis on the tested side. Tension should be equal on both sides.

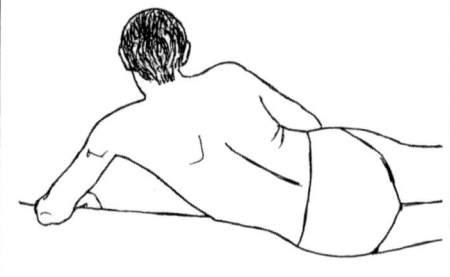

Quadratus lumborum tension: by testing passive trunk sidebending. Normally, tension is equal bilaterally.

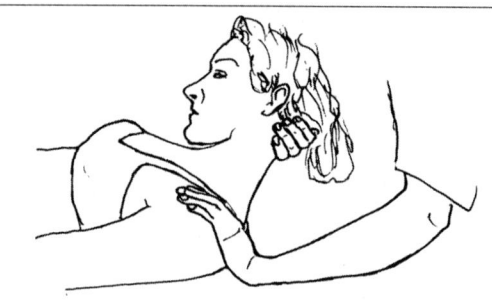

Upper trapezius tension: by flexing and inclining the head contralaterally. Then, from this position, the shoulder girdle is pushed distally. Normally, the end-feel is soft and equal on both sides. Hardness indicates excessive tension.

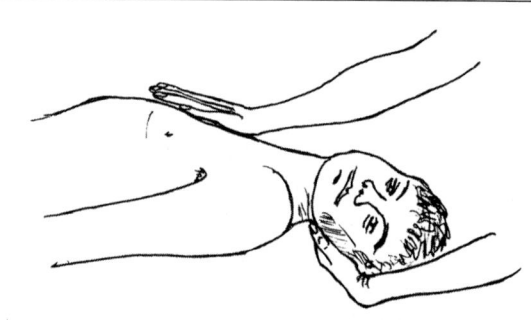

Sternocleidomastoid (SCM) tension: by first flexing the head maximally, then sidebending the neck to the opposite side, and, while rotating the head to the same side, extending the neck. Normally, the end-feel is soft and equal in both sides. Hardness indicates excessive tension

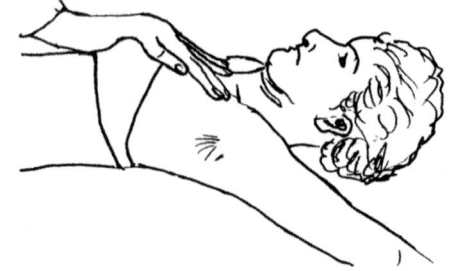

Pectoralis major tension by moving the arm into abduction, making sure the trunk is stable. Normally, the arm should reach the horizontal.

Figure 9-72: Screening for muscle length tension.

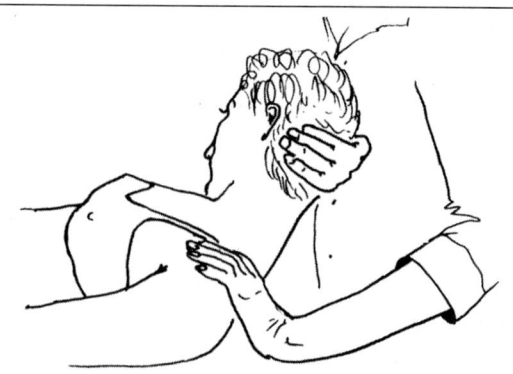

Levator scapulae tension in a similar manner as upper trapezius, but this time the head is also rotated to the contralateral side. The practitioner's hand monitors the medial superior angle of the scapula. Normally, the end-feel is soft and equal on both sides. Hardness indicates excessive tension.

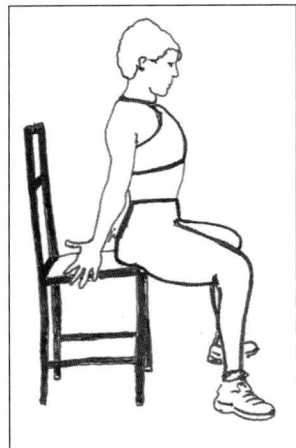

Figure 9-73: Sited posture (Brugger exercise).

Corrective Postural Exercise

The following is Mitchell's recommendation for *exercises to correct postural degeneration.* The instructions for the patient are:

1. *Stand slightly "pigeon-toed,"* (toe-in about ten degrees). Be sure that slightly more than 50% of your weight is on the balls of your feet; in other words, you should raise up on your toes without leaning any further forward. This commences the retraining of your postural control system.

2. *Grip your toes.* Dig your toes into the floor or the soles of your shoes. Keep your feet clenched in that way. This action stimulates the important proprioceptors in the feet, providing data to be integrated into the vestibular, cerebellar, postural control system.

3. *Tilt your pelvis backward.* This is not accomplished by having the abdominal muscles pull the pubic bones up toward the chin but by tucking the tailbone between the legs, dropping the buttocks and flattening the lower back. (The author uses a variation, especially in patients with discogenic pain, where the patient strongly tightens the buttock muscle at this stage of the exercise.)

4. *Make yourself "taller."* Try to move the crown of your head closer to the ceiling. If you are not sure where your crown is, look at an anatomical drawing of the back of the skull and visualize putting your lambda (the junction of the sagittal and lambdoidal sutures) up toward the ceiling. This action diminishes the antero-posterior curvature of the spine. It is sometimes helpful to visualize being hung from the ceiling by a string.

5. *Turn your palms forward.* This action flattens the scapulae against the posterior thorax and reduces the caved-in chest aspect of the postural degeneration.

6. *Turn your kneecaps forward.* This is done by twisting the thighs at the hips until the kneecaps face straight forward. Notice how the foot arches are elevated by this action, making you even taller. Especially notice the sense of tension in the buttock muscles at the hip. Conscious awareness of this tension will be part of gait retraining.

7. *Breath deeply.* The object here is to learn effortless breathing while standing. Breathing should be abdominal; inhalation should distend the abdomen all the way to the pubes. This is counterintuitive in our culture, but the pelvic tilt should be a function of dropping the buttock more than lifting the pubes with the rectus abdominis. If one were to maintain constant abdominal tension, the diaphragm would have to work much harder, increasing intra-abdominal pressure with contraction. This, in itself, is not a bad thing, because it accelerates lymphatic and venous drainage from the lower body, but it is not necessary most of the time. (The author often incorporates a Tibetan exercise with the previously recommended position of tightened buttock muscles: After full *abdominal* and *chest* inhalation, I have the patient exhale forcefully through the mouth, keeping the upper and lower teeth touching. This makes exhalation slower and more difficult. Care must be taken, as fainting may occur.)

This series is additive (and can be repeated as often as possible). The accumulated tensions are sustained for ten seconds at a time. After a few seconds' rest, standing in one place, the series is repeated for as long as the situation allows.

Figure 9-73 shows a seated variation that can be used several times a day to counteract the effects of gravity and flexed (slouched) seated postures. The patient instructions are:

1. Sit at the edge of a chair.

2. Rock your pelvis forward bringing your spine into extension (increase the curve of your low back).

3. Tuck in your chin slightly.

4. With your hands turned forward and elbow straight bring your arm backward and pull your shoulder blades closer to each other.

5. Hold this position for 15 seconds breathing normally.

6. Release and bring your pelvis to a neutral position (do not slouch or flex your spine. Rest for 15 seconds.

7. Repeat the exercise 10-20 times.

8. Repeat as often as possible throughout the day especially when sitting for prolonged periods.

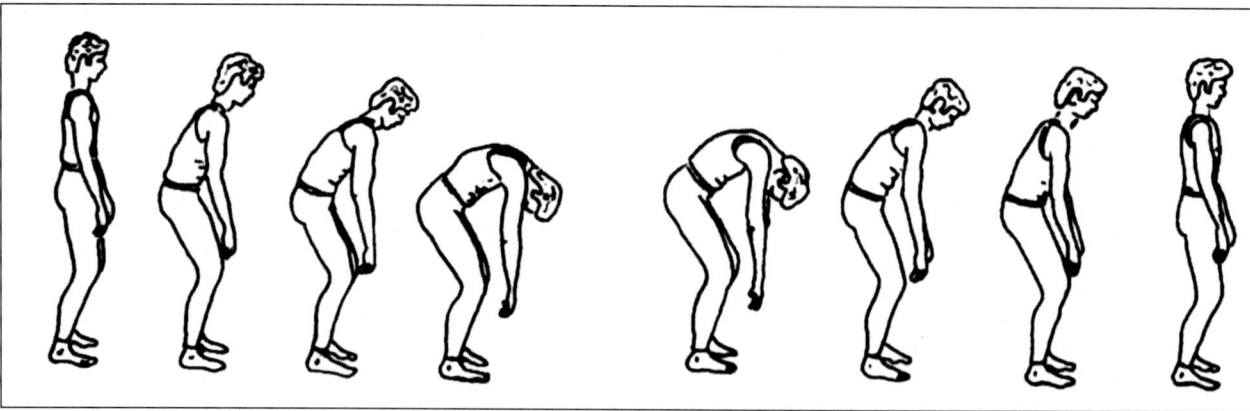

Figure 9-74: Spinal stretch.

Spinal Stretch

Another important exercise that can be used to treat perpetuating postural factors is the *Spinal Stretch*, a Qi-Gong (breath, energy, and movement) exercise that involves a series of flexion/extension movements. Part of a series of exercises in a spinal rehabilitation system, this and other Qi Gong and Tai Chi exercises can be very helpful for chronic pain patients. These movements are performed slowly, first elongating the posterior aspect of the spine with flexion, and then, while maintaining the stretch posteriorly, elongating the anterior aspect during extension.

This exercise is achieved by a "letting go," meditative stretch, rather then a forceful, mechanical stretch. Instructions for the patient are:

1. Stand with knees bent and sacrum slightly tucked under. (note to practitioner, a pelvic tilt achieves a counternutated sacrum with hip flexion, which must be performed carefully in patients with discogenic pain).

2. Starting the exercise from the bottom, relax the lowest vertebra, letting go of any tension, and gradually allowing gravity to flex just this segment. While relaxing the lowest segment hold, the spine above, straight and unyielding, especially the neck and head.

3. When this segment becomes completely relaxed and is flexed as far as it will go, repeat the same process for the next segment.

4. When the last cervical segment has relaxed and is stretched, lower the head while at the same time releasing the joints of the upper extremities.

5. Let the arms hang and try to feel the cranial sutures opening/closing (cranial sacral rhythm).

6. Starting from below, begin relaxing each vertebra and extend segment by segment, opening the front of the vertebral joints.

7. Continue until the last cervical segment has extended; then raise the head while at the same time pushing together the upper extremity joints.

8. Stand in place and feel the new spinal length.

9. Repeat the exercises a maximum of three times (Figure 9-74).

A variation on the spinal stretch can be performed to strengthen and stretch from one to three vertebral segments. The patient performs a series of local small extensions and flexions with the dysfunctional segment at the apex of the exercises. This can be done sitting or standing and is called Bend the Bow and Shoot the Arrow Qi-Gong.

Paradoxical Breathing

Paradoxical breathing is said to be a common source of abuse and overload of the scalene muscles. It is frequently adopted by patients following abdominal surgery and by people who constantly retract a protruding abdomen to improve appearance. According to Simons, Travel, and Simons (*ibid*), people with paradoxical breathing often complain of shortness of breath, a feeling that they are "always out of breath," or that they "run out of breath" even when they perform simple activities like talking on the phone. In paradoxical breathing, the normal expansion of the chest and abdomen during inhalation is lost, and the two movements may even occur in opposition to each other. On inhalation, the chest expands while the abdomen moves in, elevating the diaphragm and thus decreasing lung volume. On exhalation, the reverse occurs. This results in poor efficiency and a condition where the scalene muscles must overwork to exchange sufficient air. The patient should be taught to raise both the chest and abdomen during inhalation, and lower both with exhalation (Figure 9-79). This can be taught to the patient while he/she is supine and seated.

Stabilization Postural Exercises

The following exercises must be performed with care and adjusted to the patient's condition. It is important to train patients in pelvic and trunk stability. Stomach crunches are used first, and the patient is taught to keep the spine in neutral during the entire crunch, both on the way up and the way down. To teach the patient to maintain the pelvis in neutral, first have the patient in the supine position with the knees and hips bent and feet resting comfortably on the floor. (This is known in the physical therapy community as the "hook lying" position). To identify the patient's neutral position, instruct him/her as illustrated in Figure 9-75, additional exercises are illustrated Figure 9-76 through Figure 9-78.

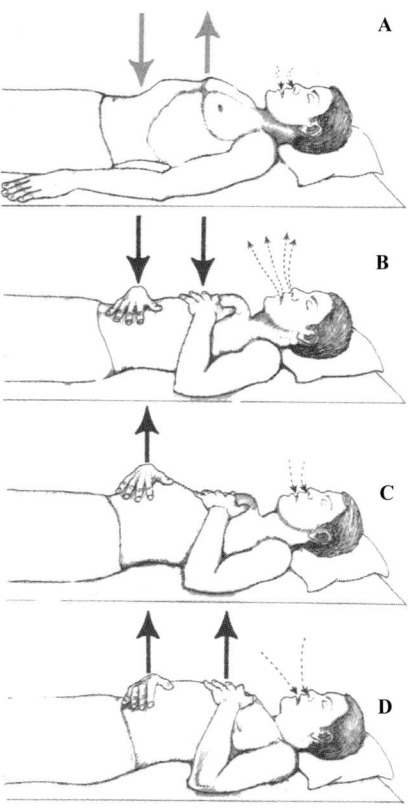

Figure 10-79: Breath training. **A)** Illustrates erroneous, paradoxical breathing, with abdomen in and chest out. **B)** First step in training: complete exhalation. **C)** Next step: inhalation by using the diaphragm only, protruding the abdomen and keeping the chest flat. **D)** Finally, the synchronization of the chest and diaphragm by taking deep breaths while concentrating on moving the chest and abdomen in and out together (after Simons, Travell, and Simons 1999).

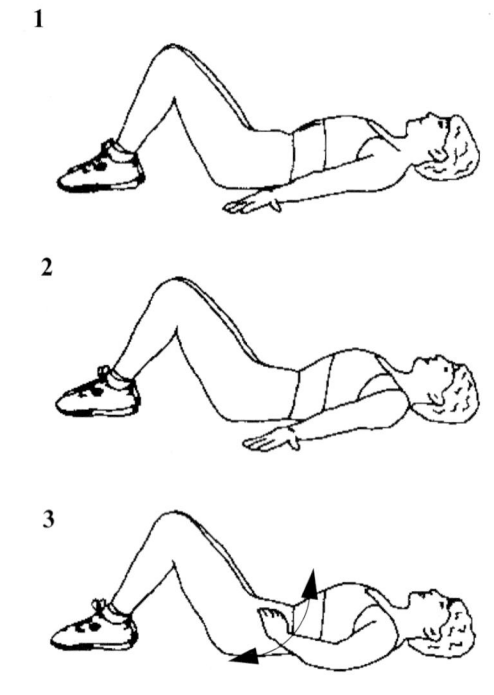

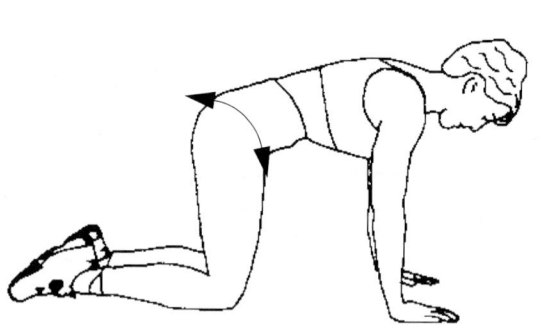

Pelvic Tilt Third Position

1. Turn over on to your hand and knees.
2. Slowly rock your pelvis back and forth.
3. Keep the movements slow and controlled.
4. Explore the entire range and identify the non-painful range.
5. The point of maximal ease is your neutral pelvic position.

Pelvic Tilt First Position

1. Lie on your back with knees and hips bent and feet resting on the floor.
2. Stabilize your shoulder as shown in fig 1 and 2. Press the back of your hand against the floor.
3. Slowly rock your pelvis backward and forwards by pressing your back against the floor and by lifting your tummy, still keeping your rear pressed against the floor.
4. Explore the entire range and identify a point of maximal comfort and ease. This is you neutral position.

Abdominal Tilt Second Position

1. Using the same supine position as above, put your arms at your side with palms facing upwards; push the back of your thumbs into the floor, and keep your fingers spread as far as possible. This will help to stabilize your scapula and upper body during the exercise.
2. Slowly press the small of your back against the floor, moving the pelvis backward.
3. Slowly press your buttock against the floor, moving the pelvis forward.
4. Repeat these movements slowly and try to identify a point somewhere in the middle of the movements in which your back feels the most comfortable. This will probably be your neutral position.

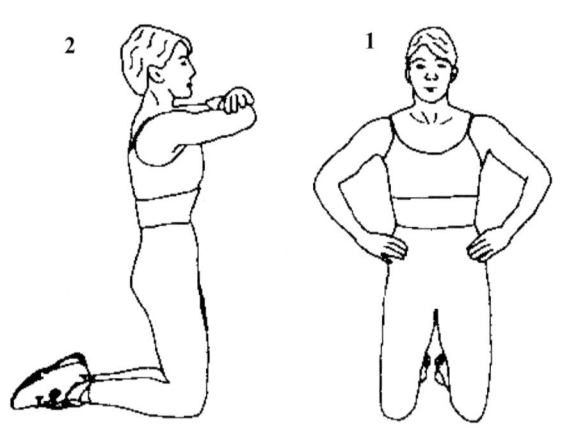

Abdominal Bracing Kneel Position

1. Kneel on your knees and place your hands on your hips then and gently pull your abdomen straight back toward your spine (fig 2). Use your hand to feel your abdominal muscle hardening.
2. While maintaining the abdomen braced raise your arms as shown in fig 2.
3. Hold for a count of 10 and release.

Figure 9-75: Neutral spine training and rehabilitation.

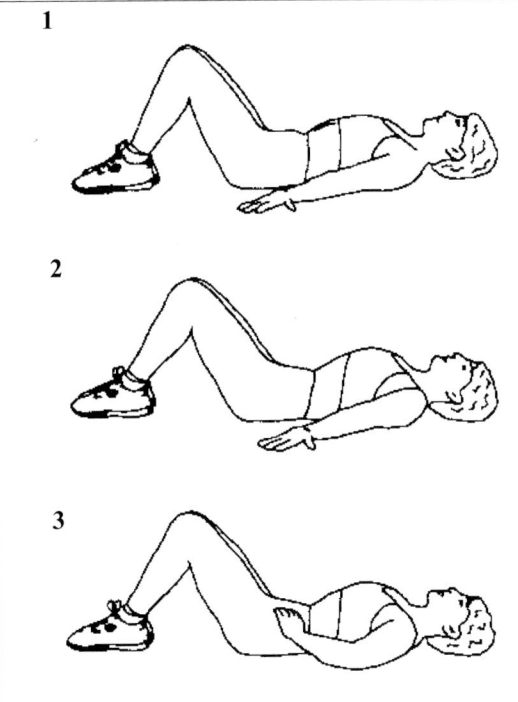

Abdominal Bracing Supine Position

1. Position yourself in the "hook lying" position (fig 1).
2. Maintaining a neutral spine and pelvis, tighten your abdominal muscles by pulling your abdomen straight back toward your spine. Doing this without flattening the spine may be difficult at first, but by remaining relaxed it can be done.
3. Hold for ten seconds and relax.
4. Repeat three to fifteen times.

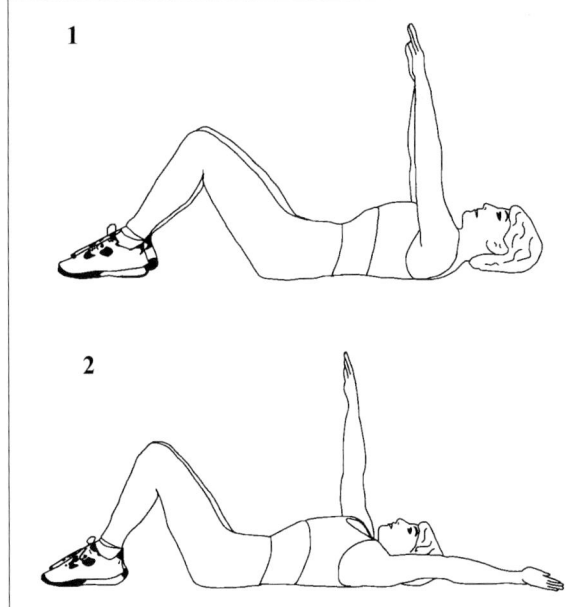

Abdominal Bracing Arm Raise Supine

1. Position yourself in the hook lying position.
2. Keep the abdomen braced to stabilize your spine. Make sure your back is *not* arched but in neutral position.
3. Raise your arms pointing the fingers straight up (fig 1).
4. Lower one arm slowly and then the other.
5. Repeat three to fifteen times.

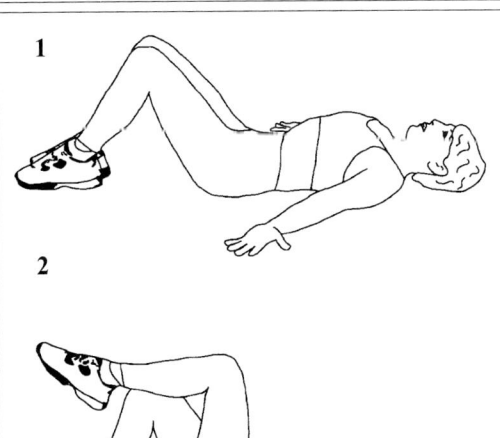

Abdominal Bracing Leg Raise Supine

1. Position yourself in the hook lying position.
2. Keep the abdomen braced to stabilize your spine. Make sure that your back is *not* arched but in neutral position.
3. Slowly raise your leg until your hip is bent to 90° (fig 2).
4. Repeat the movement on the other side.
5. Repeat three to fifteen times.

Figure 9-76: Neutral spine training and rehabilitation.

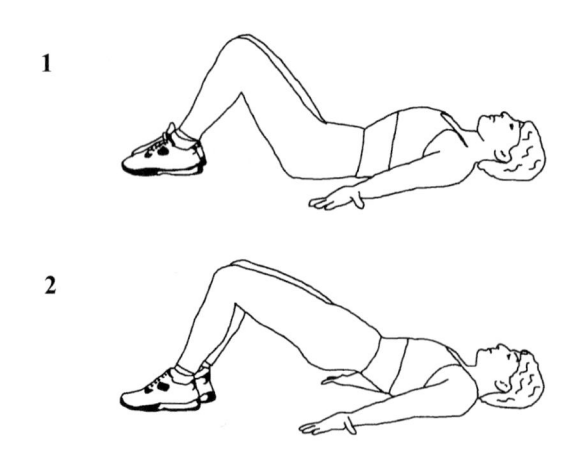

Abdominal Bracing, Bridge Position

1. Position yourself in the hook lying position.
2. Keep the abdomen braced to stabilizes your spine. Make sure your back is *not* arched but remains in neutral position (fig 1).
3. Slowly raise your pelvis of the floor into the bridge position, making sure not to arch or flatten out the spine during any part of the exercise (fig 2).
4. Hold for six seconds and slowly lower your pelvis to the starting position.
5. Repeat three to fifteen times.

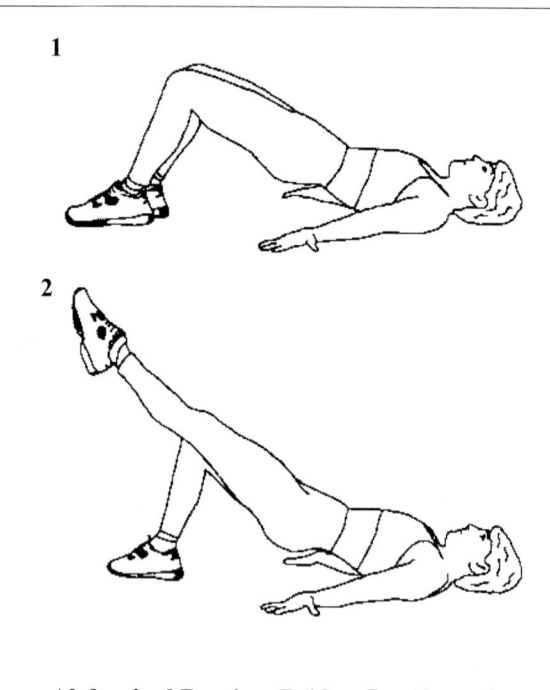

Abdominal Bracing, Bridge, Leg Extension

1. Repeat stabilization instruction from the last exercise (fig 1).
2. Slowly lift your leg and then extend it straight (fig 2).
3. Repeat on other leg.
4. Repeat three to fifteen times.

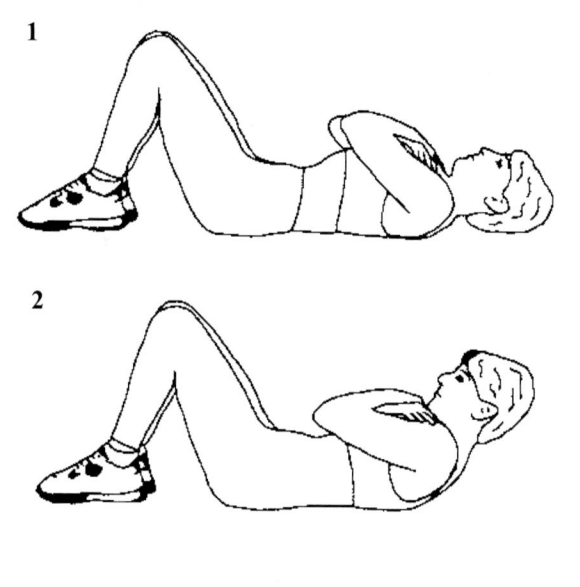

Curl Ups (Abdominal Crunches)

1. Make sure to keep abdominal bracing and neutral spine position throughout the exercise.
2. Cross your arms in front of your chest (fig 1).
3. Keeping your chin slightly tucked, slowly raise your chest off the floor (fig 2).
4. Slowly lower yourself down to the floor, making sure not to extend you lower back.
5. Repeat three to 30 times.

Figure 9-77: Neutral spine training and rehabilitation.

Rehabilitation and Exercise

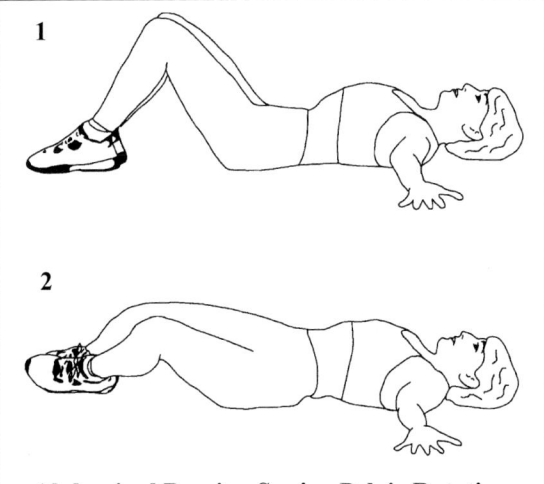

Abdominal Bracing Supine Pelvic Rotation

1. Position yourself in the hook lying position.
2. Keep the abdomen braced to stabilize your spine. Make sure your back is *not* arched but remains in neutral position.
3. Slowly rotate your pelvis until your knees are about halfway to the floor (fig 2).
4. Straighten up and repeat on the other side.
5. Repeat three to fifteen times.

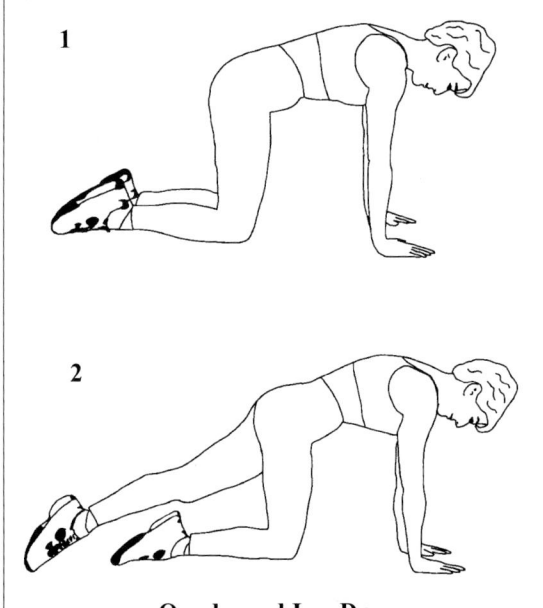

Quadruped Leg Drag

1. Place yourself in the hands and knees position. Keeping your spine stable and in neutral position align your head with the rest of the spine (fig 1).
2. Avoid arching your back or poking your chin, extend your leg back while dragging your foot on the floor (fig 2).
3. Return leg and repeat on other side.
4. Repeat three to fifteen times.

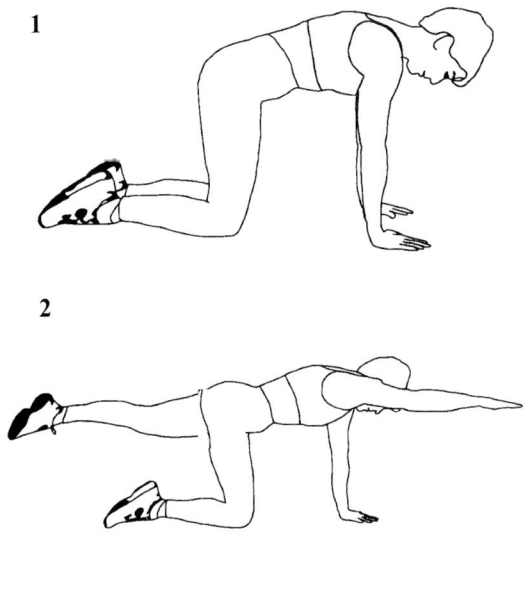

Quadruped Single Leg Raise and Cross-Crawl

1. Place yourself in the hands and knees position. Keeping your spine stable and in neutral position align your head with the rest of the spine during the entire exercise (fig 1).
2. Avoiding any chin poking, raise and extend one leg out behind you.
3. Return to starting position and repeat with the other leg.
4. Repeat three to fifteen times.

Part Two

5. Raise one arm out infront of you while at the same time extend the opposite leg behind your. Make sure to only move your arm and leg, keeping the spine in neutral and abdomen braced (fig 2).
6. Return your arm and leg, and repeat on the other side.
7. Repeat three to fifteen times.

Figure 9-77: Neutral spine training and rehabilitation.

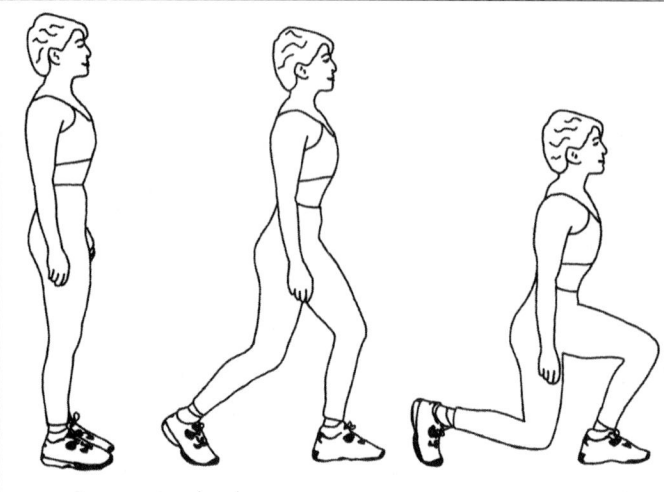

Lunges

1. Stand with your arms at your side (fig 1).
2. Maintain abdominal bracing, and slowly step forward approximately a half stride (fig 2).
3. Slowly lower yourself until your knee slightly touches the floor (fig 3).
4. Slowly raise up and return to the starting position and repeat on the other leg.
5. Repeat three to fifteen times.

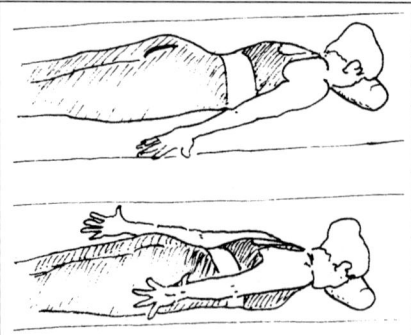

Shoulder Girdle Stabilization 1

1. Lie on front of body with forehead on a small pillow or a rolled towel.
2. Place your arms with palm down and fingers spread. Gently reach towards the feet.
3. Lift the front of the shoulders down and back by gently pulling your shoulder blades together.
4. Hold for 5 seconds.
5. Repeat three to fifteen times.

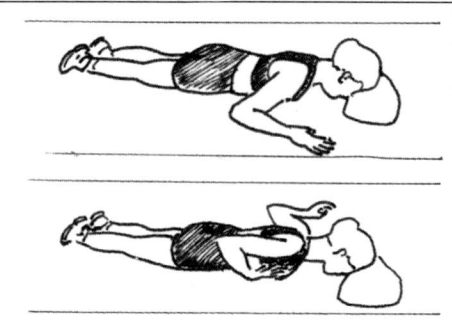

Shoulder Girdle Stabilization 2

1. Continue as per previous exercise but now bring the arms up with palms next to your head and facing down.
2. Lift the front of the shoulders down and back by gently pulling your shoulder blades together.
3. Hold for 5 seconds.
4. Repeat three to fifteen times.

Figure 9-78: Neutral spine training and rehabilitation and Shoulder girdle stabilization which is very important for cervical and shoulder girdle disorders.

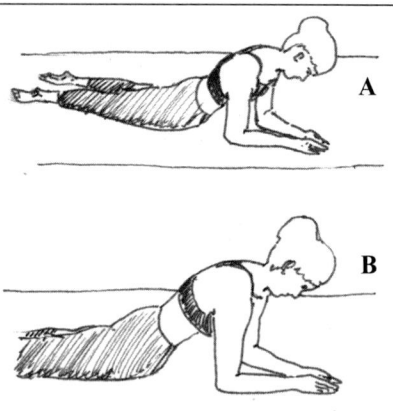

Shoulder Girdle Stabilization 3

1. Make sure your elbows are directly under the shoulders.
2. Maintain a neutral neck alignment.
3. Press chest away from floor (B).
4. Hold for 5 seconds.
5. Repeat three to fifteen times.

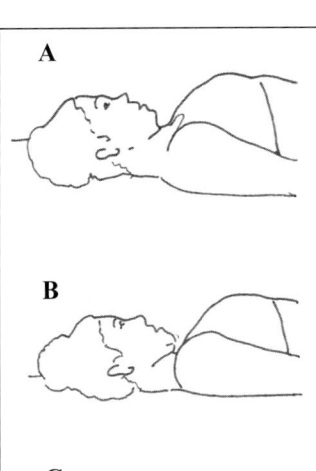

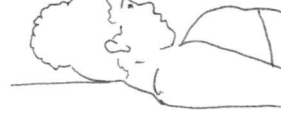

Neutral Cervical Flexion

1. Lie face up on the floor or bedop (A).
2. Slowly tuck your chin down towards the chest without lifting your head (B).
3. Make sure to maintain the chin tucked and slowly lift your head one inch off the floor (C).
4. Hold this position for 5 seconds.
5. Repeat three to fifteen times.

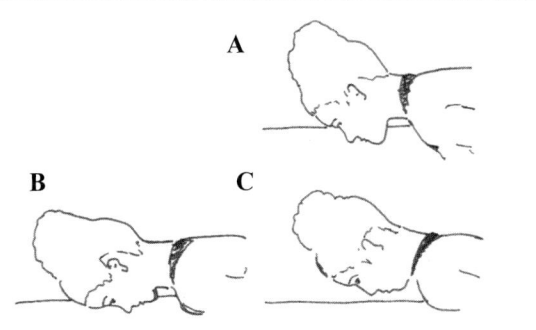

Neutral Cervical Extension

1. Lie face down on the floor or bed (A).
2. Slowly tuck your chin down towards the chest without lifting your head (B).
3. Make sure to maintain the chin tucked and slowly lift your head one inch off the floor (C).
4. Hold for five seconds.
5. Repeat three to fifteen times.

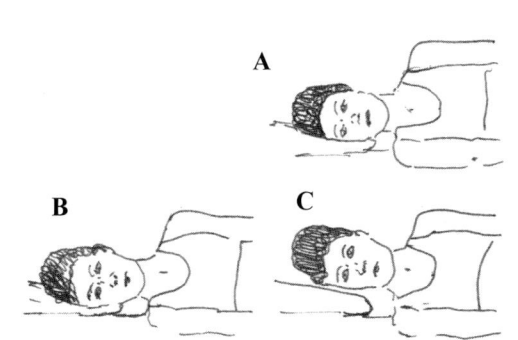

Neutral Cervical Sidebending

1. Lie on your side with a pillow under your head (A).
2. Tuck your chin down towards the chest (B).
3. Make sure to maintain chin tucking and slowly lift your head one inch off the floor (C).
4. Hold for five seconds.
5. Repeat three to fifteen times
6. Turn over and repeat on the other side.

Figure 9-78: Cervical spine stabilization exercises. It is important to make sure that shoulder girdle and lumbar spine exercises be incorporated at the same time.

The McKenzie System

The McKenzie system uses loading strategies to evaluate and treat spinal disorders. Understanding the principles of this system can be very helpful and can enhance rehabilitation as well as acupuncture outcomes. The same principles are used in positioning the patient on the table during acupuncture treatments.

Treatment with McKenzie System

McKenzie has developed a treatment system for disc derangements and other spinal disorders based on the patient's response to load strategies that either increase or decrease the patient's pain. He has originated the "centralization phenomenon," based on the idea that pain often originates from tears within the annulus (McKenzie 1981; Donelson, Silva, Murphy 1990). The goal of the exercise is to centralize the pain; i.e., to concentrate it from peripheral (leg or arm) to central (low back and neck). By controlling posture and avoiding detrimental positions, the patient can promote a return of the nuclear material to the center of the disc (as long the as the disc material is still contained).

In the McKenzie system, spinal disorders are divided into *a postural syndrome, a dysfunction syndrome*, and *a derangement syndrome*. Each of the syndromes responds differently to loading (Jacob and McKenzie 1995).

1. The postural syndrome tends to exhibit a *delayed onset* of symptoms (i.e. it takes some time for symptoms to start) in response to *sustained static loading* at end-range. Symptoms can last for extended periods after loading is terminated.
   The treatment approach is to avoid postures and loading strategies that bring the joints to end range. Stabilization exercises are helpful.

2. The dysfunction syndrome tends to exhibit *immediate onset of symptoms* and mechanical responses at the restricted end-range of the joint. Symptoms are reduced quickly when loading is terminated (e.g., a painful biting sensation when extending or flexing the spine that stops as soon as the movement is terminated).
   The treatment approach is frequent static or dynamic loading at or to the restricted end-range.

3. The derangement syndrome may exhibit *immediate* or *delayed* onset of symptoms following loading at the *obstructed end-range, at mechanically unimpeded end-ranges, during motion*, or *with midrange static loading*. Symptoms persist often, and peripheralization increases when loading is terminated (i.e., seen in a sensitive patient who can easily suffer increased symptoms from many type of movements).
   The treatment strategy involves pursuing and avoiding certain loading tactics (postures and exercises), as well as paying special attention to the order in which each is accomplished. Only movements and postures that result

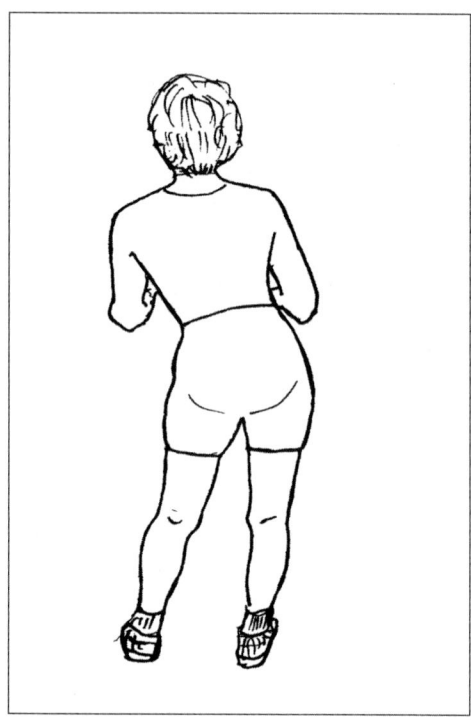

Figure 9-80: Typical posture of a patient who has a posterior-lateral deviation.

in centralization are used (i.e. that bring the symptoms closer to the spine).

Disc derangements have been divided by McKenzie into posterior, anterior, and lateral deviations.

Posterior Deviations

Experiments on cadaverous lumbar motion segments have shown that lordotic postures create a concentration of vertical compressive stresses within the posterior annulus. These stresses can be particularly high following sustained "creep" loading, or following damage to an adjacent vertebra (Adems 1995), probably resulting in posterior deviations. Repetitive loading in a lordotic posture can lead to "hairpin bend" deformations of the lamellae within the posterior annulus, leading to a posterior bulge of the disc (Adams, Dolan and Hutton 1988), leading to posterior deviations.

In posterior deviations of the most common type, the nucleus is shifted backward. Pain peripheralization from posterior deviations increases with flexion and sitting. It decreases with extension and standing (as long as the disc is contained). A newly published study showed that 83% of patients with low back pain with/without leg pain have extension directional preference (i.e., posterior deviation; (Wetzel and Donelson 2003).

Examination for posterior deviation is positive when, after the patient flexes his/her spine ten or more times, there is increased *peripheral* pain, and when subsequent extension movements immediately decrease and *centralize* the pain. The evaluation is performed weightbearing and nonweightbearing.

Anterior Deviations

Anterior deviations are rare (seen in about 7-10% of patients with low back symptoms; (Wetzel and Donelson *ibid*) and are usually characterized by pain and peripheralization on extension and when standing, with reduction of pain and peripheralization when sitting. Anterior deviations are symptomatically very similar to facet syndromes.

Examination is positive for anterior deviations when repeated extension of the spine results in peripheralization and increase of pain, and when subsequent repeated flexion immediately centralizes and reduces the pain.

An increase in pain on extension is common, however, when the disc is desiccated and/or extruded/herniated. Patients with these conditions may not tolerate repeated extension exercises (and would usually feel worse with flexion exercises as well).

Lateral Deviations

Lateral deviation is usually combined either with posterior or anterior deviations. With the addition of lateral deviation, the patient has a side bending component and often presents with a postural list (Figure 9-80). In a newly published study in patients with low back pain with/without leg pain, lateral directional preference was seen in 10% of patients (Wetzel and Donelson *ibid*).

Examination is positive for lateral deviation when lateral gliding to one side *peripheralizes* the pain, while gliding to the other side *centralizes* the pain. A flexion or extension component may be added for anterior or posterior deviations (Figure 9-81).

The Validity of the McKenzie System

The concepts of the McKenzie system have been evaluated by Aprill et al (1995). Remarkably, the McKenzie evaluation showed an 83% agreement on the level of disc associated with pain provocation with magnetic resonance imaging (MRI) and computed tomograpy (CT) discography, a 93% agreement on localization of painful tears within the disc, and an 85% agreement in regard to identifying whether the affected disc was contained or extruded, with drawings drawn by the therapist looking like findings from MRI and discography. In a newly published study, Donelson et al have shown that patients randomly matched to preform direction-appropriate McKenzie exercises report decrease in pain, increase in functional capacity and decrease in medication use, while patients that are mismatched actually suffer increased pain and functional limitations. Figure 9-81 through Figure 9-82 on page 529 illustrate commonly-used movements for evaluation and treatment with the McKenzie system.

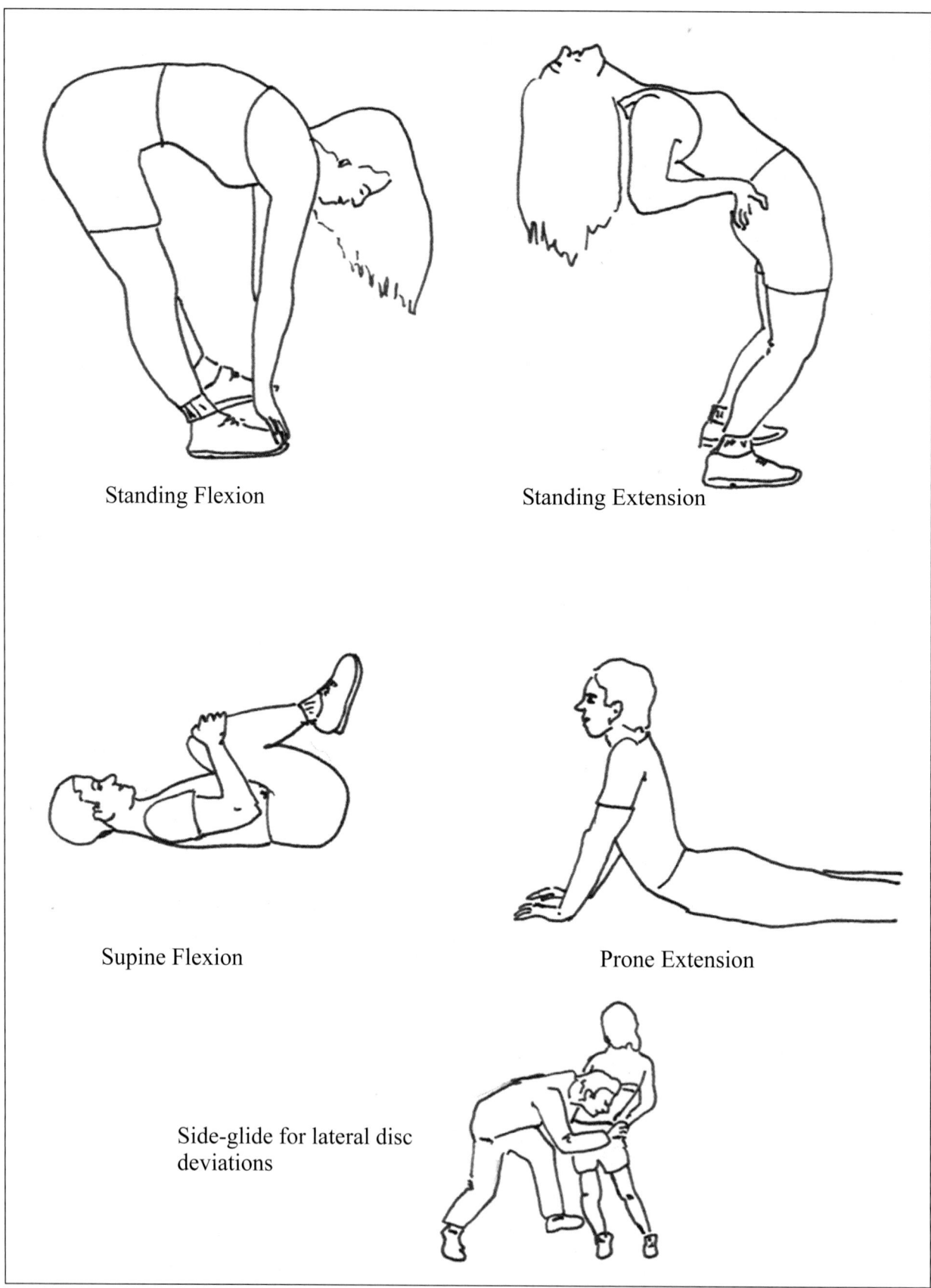

Figure 9-81: Basic McKenzie low back maneuvers.

The McKenzie System

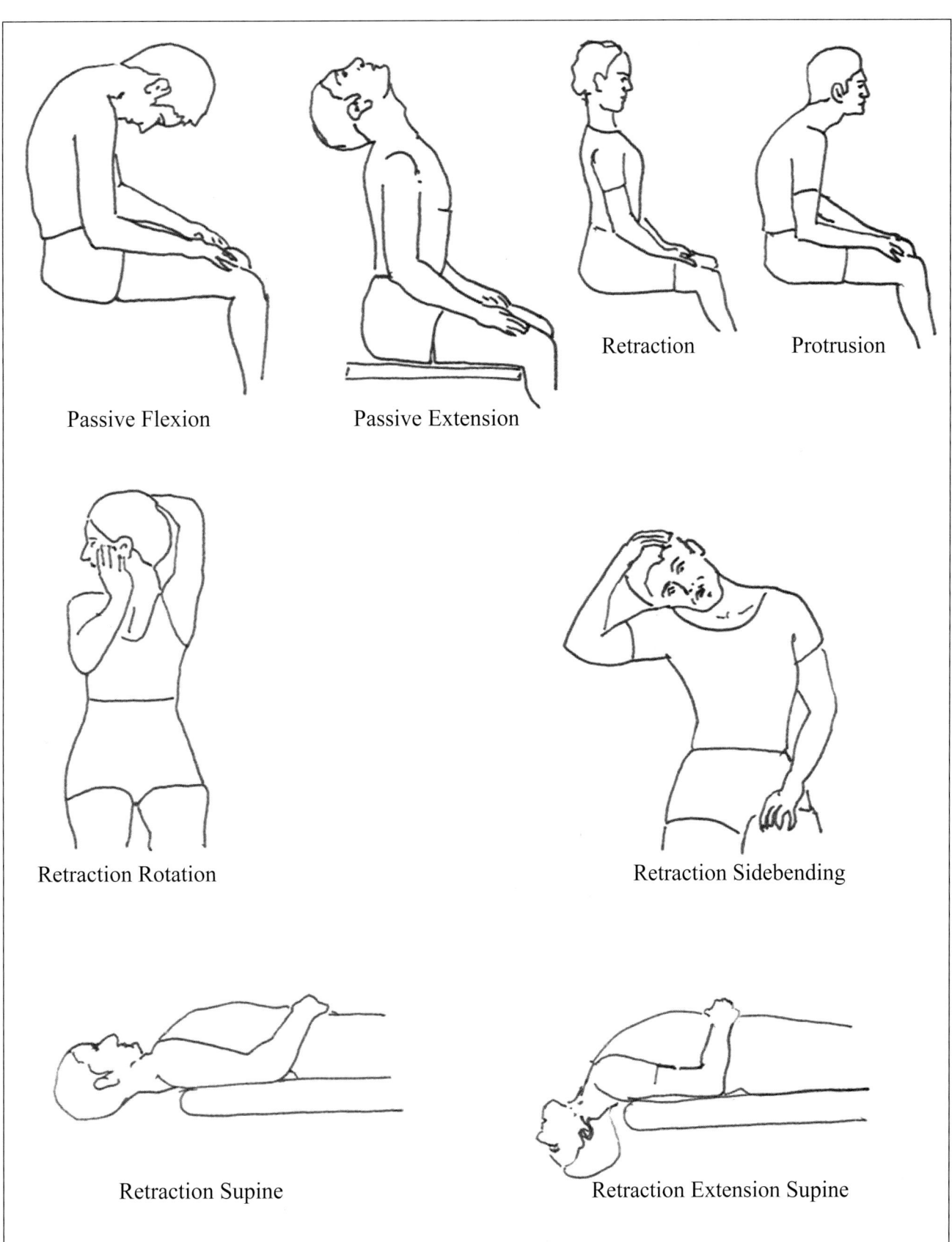

Figure 9-82: Basic McKenzie neck maneuvers

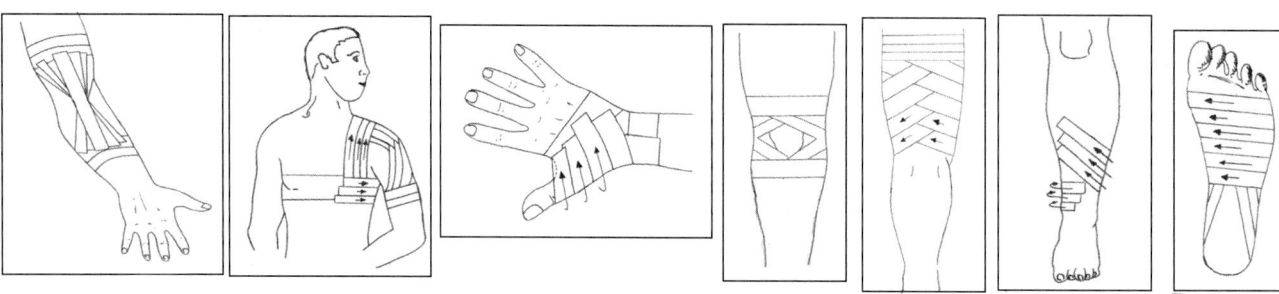

Figure 9-83: Common joints and tissues taped (after Kennedy and Berry 1991).

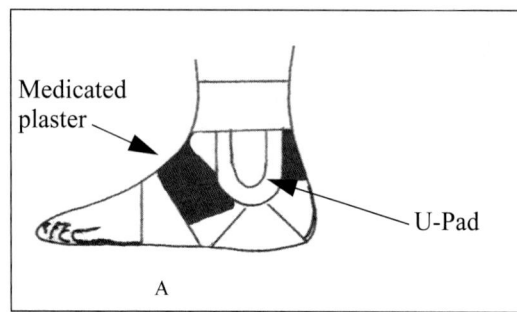
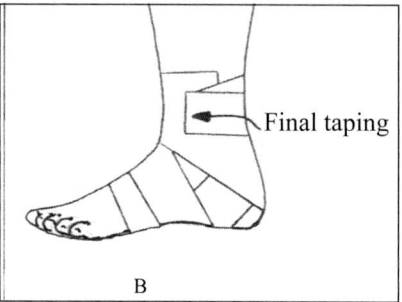

Figure 9-84: Ankle sprain taping. **A)** illustrates the placement of a U-pad and medicated plaster. **B)** illustrates final tape placed on top of the U-pad and medicated plaster (after Kennedy and Berry 1991).

Orthotics and Restraints

Traditionally, in TCM, orthotics and restraints are mostly used in the treatment of trauma and fractures. *Secret Formula of God for Management of Trauma and Fracture* states:

> Sprains and fractures of the hands and feet are treated by topical application of ointment wrapped with cloth, fixation with bamboo, and with intermittent exercise.

In modern times, premade devices are often used in TCM as well as biomedical treatment of musculoskeletal disorders. Foot orthotics, while not used as part of OM, can be very important to control biomechanical dysfunctions, maximize the therapeutic effects and to prevent recurrences.

Taping

According to Dylan Morrissey (2002), taping can be used in a number of ways to reduce movement-associated pain. It can be used as a useful treatment approach in itself, or as a means of maintaining treatment effects. Taping can be used to provide a physical effect on the tissues that lasts for hours, or even days, supplementing the relatively brief practitioner–patient contact. It can be used to affect pain directly by *offloading* irritable myofascial and/or neural tissues. Taping can also be indirectly used to alter the pain associated with identified faulty movement patterns. These affects are essentially proprioceptively mediated. Taping is commonly used in the management of tennis elbow (lateral epicondylitis) and excessive extension at the elbow joint, shoulder instability or impingement syndromes, wrist and thumb joint sprains, patello-femoral pain due to poor patellar traction, hamstring strains, shin splints, and disorders of the feet (Figure 9-83).

Morrissey divides taping techniques into:

- direct and indirect techniques that are proprioceptively mediated;
- longitudinal offload that is used for the inhibition of overactive movement synergists and antagonists;
- transverse offload used for facilitation of underactive movement synergists; promotion of optimal inter joint coordination; direct optimization of joint alignment during static postures or movement.

Longitudinal offloading is useful for painful tissues that are held in tension either because of the unrelieved influence of gravity or because of chronically increased background muscle tone, e.g. due to habitual postures. These conditions are often helped by taping the tissue so that it is passively supported in a shortened position. This type of taping is particularly useful when addressing symptoms associated with adverse neural dynamics.

A transverse offload is used particularly for myofascial tissues that may be mediated either by means similar to that described above or by a more mechanical affect. Transverse offloading of muscle structures effectively lengthens the muscle being used and may be inhibitory.

General Considerations with Elastic and Taping Wraps

Elastic wraps are commonly used to either support an injured joint or to address swelling. Elastic wraps, compression pads, and taping can be very helpful as first-aid in the treatment of musculoskeletal injury and have been shown to reduce rehabilitation time. When used to reduce swelling, the wrap must start below the injury and work upwards to force fluids out and toward the heart. It is often helpful to have the distal part of the warp tighter than the proximal. The warp should be tight but not so tight that it compromises circulation. Pressure provided by the tape or elastic wrap should be transferred to the injured site (the lesion) and not obstruct unaffected areas. To achieve this, pads are often used. For example, a U-shaped pad is needed under the lateral malleolus of the ankle when wrapping an ankle for inversion sprain. This raises the surface contact to a level above the protruding bone (the malleolus) which otherwise prevents the pressure of the wrap from being delivered directly to the injured ligaments (Figure 9-84).

When used to support injured joints and to prevent a joint from entering a painful range, it is necessary to first test the joint and ascertain its non-painful ranges. The joint should remain moveable within the non-painful range after taping or wrapping. This is true when taping as a first-aid or to prevent injury (Kennedy and Berry 1991).

Skin Preparation, Padding, and Clinical Taping

Skin preparation is important to prevent irritation and to maximize the therapeutic effect when using tape. The taped area can be sprayed with Tuff-skin™ or some other adhesive spray. (Skin-prep™ is hypo allergenic.) This helps the tape to stay on longer. The area can also be covered with Pro-wrap™ or some other cover that protects the skin. All areas subject to friction should be lubricated and covered with a piece of gauze or other appropriate pad. For example, when taping over nail beds, a small band-aid can be helpful to prevent irritation from the tape. When taping the ankle, a lubricated heel-and-lace pad or small piece of gauze can be used to cover the achilles tendon. Self-adherent wraps are useful and can provide uniform compression as it secures, and, by being self-adherent, the wrap is stable and does not slip.

When taping or when using elastic wraps it is important to have patient cooperation in maintaining the area in a functional position. It is also important to continually communicate with the patient and to palpate pulses, making sure that circulation is not affected. After skin preparation, usually anchor tapes are placed. These are then used as foundations for the remainder of the taping. When applying the tape, the limb contour is followed and tension is placed on the roll of tape to prevent wrinkles. The strips of tape should overlap by at least one half the width of the tape. When taping over muscles or tendons, the practitioner should have the patient contract the muscle involved, making sure that joint functions are not disturbed (Kennedy and Berry *ibid*).

Pathology-Specific Foot Orthotics

While foot orthotics should always be prescribe on an individual basis, some general rules can be followed. The main purpose of foot orthotics is to correct biomechanical dysfunctions of the foot and ankle. Orthotics can also be used to level the sacral base and to treat leg-length discrepancy (see page 669).

It cannot be overemphasized how critical a quality negative cast is to clinical outcome when prescribing foot orthotics. For orthotic therapy to be effective, the patient's foot should be casted in subtalar neutral (except for specific pathologies in which the foot may be casted other than in neutral). The midtarsal joints should be "lucked" when making the negative cast, by dorsiflexing the ankle until the subtalar joint *starts* to pronate. It is essential that the soft tissue supinatus position of the forefoot (when seen) be removed during the neutral casting. This can be accomplished by pulling plantarly on the medial column at the medial cuneiform and slightly dorsiflexing the hallux. The entire plantar aspect of the foot should be in contact with the plaster. In patients with ankle equinus deformities, however, the first ray should not be plantarflexed during casting. The following are some important points to remember when casting the patient's feet (Huppin and Scherer 2004):

1. The practitioner's "thumb impression" of the plaster cast from holding the foot in the proper position during casting should only be under the 4th and 5th toes. It should not cause any dorsiflexion of the 3ed and 2ed MP joints, nor should it cause a 4th and 5th MP joint dorsiflexion.

   Dorsiflexion of the 4th and 5th toes plantarflexes the 4th and 5th metatarsals. This falsely increases the forefoot varus or decreases the forefoot valgus. Dorsiflexion of the 3ed and 2ed MP joints tightens the plantar fascia and doesn't allow you to fully pronate the oblique midtarsal joint. This produces a higher arched orthotic than the patient can tolerate and can cause medial arch pain.

2. The heel impression should be symmetrical from medial to lateral.

   Pronation of the subtalar joint shifts the fat pad of the heel laterally and makes the plantar aspect flat and shallow. This results in orthotic "bitting" of the medial edge of the heel with loss of foot motion control.

   When the subtalar joint is casted supinated it leads to curved "straight lateral border," (adducted). The oblique midtarsal joint cures the foot and the orthotic will sit with the lateral edge under the foot instead of against the outside border of the shoe. This can lead to pain under the cuboid bone.

3. The highest point of the lateral side of the cast should be under the CC joint.

   Holding the subtalar joint too supinated or not dorsiflexing the forefoot on the rearfoot until the ankle locks, exaggerates the lateral arch (and creates a false forefoot

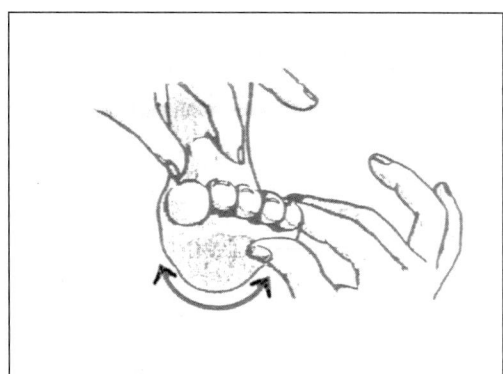

Figure 9-85: Palpation for subtalar neutral. This is the point in which the foot is between supination and pronation. Subtalar neutral is at a "peak" where the foot seems to fall off more easily to either side between pronation and supination and is assessed with the non-weight bearing foot.

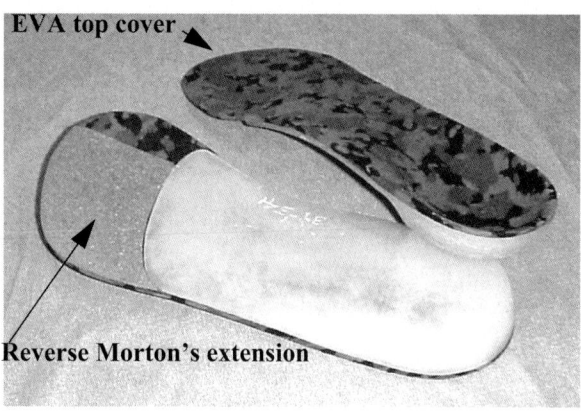

Figure 9-86: Hallux limitus device. Note, this is a CD device, so the heel post is part of the shell itself.

varus). This results in pain (or a rock) in the middle of the orthotic. While this results in a comfortable orthotic it can also result in painful plantar fascia and unsuccessful treatment.

If the foot is casted with the subtalar joint pronated this exaggerates the forefoot valgus in the cast. Exaggerated forefoot valgus creates medial arch pain from the orthotic.

4. The forefoot should not be allowed to invert on the rearfoot (supinatus).

    Some patients, because of the eversion of their heel, invert their forefoot at the midtasal joint causing a supinatus (soft tissue varus). This false inversion of the forefoot persists during casting and produces an invalid cast fatigue (and orthotic fatigue) and fascial pain from the orthotic.

    If you see forefoot varus in more than 1% of your negative casts, you are not seeing forefoot varus—it is likely supinatus. Structural forefoot varus is rare and thus it should be rare to see a negative cast that shows forefoot varus. If you leave this false forefoot varus in the negative cast the results will be little control, painful plantar fascia and unsuccessful treatment.

5. The first met head impression must be symmetrical and concave. The hallux should be dorsiflexed, never plantarflexed. There should be no plaster wrinkle proximal to the head.

    If the patient contracts their tibialis anterior muscle during casting the first ray will be captured dorsiflexed. The shape of the orthotic will hold the first ray dorsiflexed. This will limit the range of motion of the big toe joint, jam the 1st MP joint, will not control midstance and cause pain under the distal arch.

6. Finally, the cast must match the foot and the foot must be measured.

Measure the soft tissue spread at the heel when the patient is standing. If the heel spread is not taken into account this can result in too narrow heel cup.

The following are recommendations made by ProLab orthotics USA (Scherer 2001):

Achilles Tendinitis

The recommended prescription for achilles tendinitis is a milled (CD), rigid wide polypropylene device with: minimum cast fill, normal heel cup depth (14mm), 4mm medial heel skive (in a patient that over pronates), 0/0 polypropylene rearfoot post, EVA top cover to toes, and a 4-5mm heel lift.[17] The heel lift shortens the calf muscles and reduces tension and stress on the Achilles tendon. It should be removed once symptoms are under control. Note, the foot must be fully dorsiflexed when casting to remove all motion from the midtarsal joints. This is the key to good outcome.

Hallux Limitus or Rigidus

The recommended prescription for hallux limitus or rigidus is a semi-flexible CD (or vacuum formed) wide device with: standard cast fill, normal heel cup (however, patients often have an unstable rearfoot and thus a deep heel cup [18-22mm] is often used), 2mm medial skive, 2° cast inversion (both the skive and cast inversion are used on a patient that over pronates), 4/4 poly post (EVA post if shock absorption is needed), EVA topcover to sulcus (or toes) glued posterior only, and reverse Morton's extension. The reverse Morton's extension allows the first toe to drop during the toe-off phase of the gait (see page 196, Figure 9-86). Langer Inc. offers a patented device called a Kinetic Wedge™, which is a fairly accommodating device with a modified reverse Morton's extension. Note, the negative cast should be a neutral suspension cast with the foot fully dorsiflexed and the first ray fully plantarflexed (taking out supinatus). The first ray position is easily accomplished by dorsiflexing the hallux to resistance or pushing down on the medial column.

While most patients with FHL tend to pronate, this dysfunction can be seen also in patients with ankle equinus deformities. In such patients the casting is done without plantar flexing the first ray because this can cause an orthotic that may produce pain or a sense that the orthosis is too high and/or too hard. This occurs because equinus at midstance seeks sagittal plane motion and gets it by lowering the base of the first metatarsal. Flexing the first ray when casting raises the base of the first metatarsal and can result in the arch of the orthotic trying to rase an immovable object.

Shoe recommendations include a wide forefoot and deep toe box if possible. For dress shoes as a second pair of orthotics, a narrow holethotic device with the reverse Morton's extension works well (Figure 9-88).

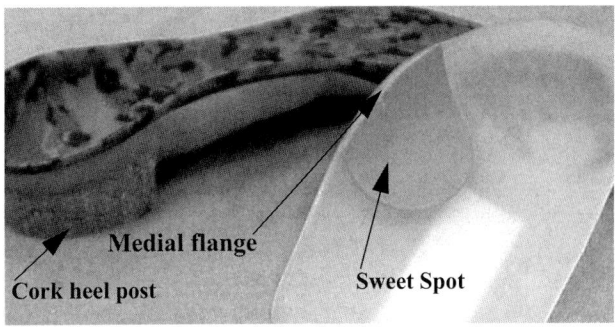

Figure 9-87: Posterior tibialis dysfunction device. Note, this is a vacuum formed device, so the heel post is made of other materials and is not part of the shell itself.

Lateral Ankle Instability and/or Peroneal Tendinitis

The recommended prescription for lateral ankle instability and/or peroneal tendinitis is a wide CD device with: normal heel cup, standard cast fill, 0/0 poly rearfoot post without a lateral bevel, EVA topcover to toes glued posterior only, and 3° valgus extension.

Metatarsalgia

The recommended prescription for metatarsalgia is a wide DC device with: normal heel cup, minimum cast fill, 2°

---

17. A CD device is directly milled out of polypropylene (plastic) after a computer scans the negative cast mailed to the lab by the practitioner. It is an automated system which is computer-controlled. The rearfoot poly post in CD devices is part of the actual device and therefore hard with minimal shock absorption (but it lasts a long time). A vacuum formed device is made by melting the polypropylene over a positive cast made from the negative cast mailed to the lab. With a vacuum formed device, different materials can be used as rearfoot posts which may add shock absorption. The rearfoot post needs to be refurbished once a year or so. It is also possible to make "sweet spots" or strategic holes built into vacuum-formed devices which are used in cases were pressure to a specific point needs to be reduced.

The rigidity of the device is determined by the patient's weight. A medial heel skive or Kirby skive is used to control over-pronation. It inverts the heel.

Inverting the cast is a way of controlling over-pronation and can be used with or without a medial heel skive. It also functions to invert the calcaneus. It is usually used only in patients with flexible flatfoot deformities.

The amount of cast fill done by the lab will determine how close the orthotic will be to the foot (i.e. how high the arch is in the orthotic). A minimal cast fill results in higher arch on the device and more arch support. It may be more difficult to tolerate by some patients.

Rearfoot posts control movement of the orthosis (and therefore the foot) in the shoe. There is some controversy over whether having different angles built into them actually enables them to function differently. A 0/0 post is supposed to minimize rearfoot motion and is often used in cases of arthritis or arthrosis. A 4/4 post is used in most other cases and allows 4° of inversion. A 4/0 post is often used for ski boots.

The wider the device, the more support it will offer. Shoe choices may be limited (i.e., the device may be too wide for the shoe).

A forefoot valgus extension is made with the lateral edge of the extension being thicker than the medial edge.

When the top cover is glued posteriorly only, it allows for modifications to be made and while still keeping the original top cover.

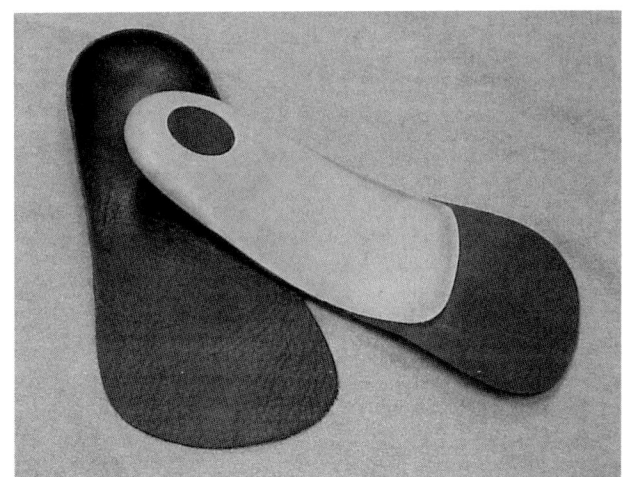

Figure 9-88: Holethotic device.

inversion, 4/4 poly rearfoot post, EVA cover to sulcus glued posterior only, 1/16" Poron forefoot extension, and Poron metatarsal pad.

Neuroma

The recommended prescription for neuroma is a wide CD device with: deep heel cup (18-22mm), minimum cast fill, 2° inversion, 4/4 poly rearfoot post, EVA topcover to sulcus glued posterior only, 1/16" Poron forefoot extension, and Poron metatarsal pad.

Pediatric Flatfoot

The recommended prescription for pediatric flatfoot is a CD device with: deep heel cup, minimum cast fill, 6mm medial skive, 5° inversion, 4/4 poly rearfoot post, and no cover.

Posterior Tibialis Dysfunction

The recommended prescription for posterior tibialis dysfunction (acquired flat foot) is a vacuum formed rigid polypropylene device with: medial flange (increased size support under the medial arch that makes the device extra wide), 20mm heel cup, standard cast fill (although often minimum cast fill may be indicated), 4mm medial heal skive, Birko cork 0/0 rearfoot post, and EVA topcover to sulcus glued at the heel only (Figure 9-87). Note, there may be a need to gently manipulate the foot before casting since in progressive cases the foot may have become accommodated to the abnormal position. During casting, the forefoot should be everted as much as possible while the rearfoot is held in neutral since the weakness has forced the forefoot into inversion (taking out all the soft tissue supinatus).

Sesmoditis

The recommended prescription for sesmoditis is a wide CD device with: normal heel cup, minimum cast fill, 2mm medial heel skive, 3° inversion, 4/4 poly rearfoot post, EVA cover to sulcus glued posterior only, reverse Morton's extension, and Poron metatarsal bar.

Heel Pain, Plantar Fasciitis

The recommended prescription for heal pain and.or plantar fasciitis is a semi-rigid or flexible vacuum formed polypropylene normal width device (or often wide device) with: minimal cast fill (or normal cast fill), 2-4mm medial heel skive, 3° inversion, 4/4 EVA post, heel pad, possible heel lift (if tight heel cord), and cover to sulcus, or toes, glued posteriorly. Note, it is essential that the supinatus position of the foot be removed during the neutral suspension casting. If the patient has a prominent plantar fascia, it can be marked with lipstick before casting. This will leave a mark on the negative cast showing the exact position of the fasciae. A plantar fascia groove (a type of sweet spot) can then be ordered which will reduce local pressure to the plantar fascia.

While most patient's with heel pain or plantar fasciitis over pronate (and then the above orthotic prescription is appropriate), in some patients the rearfoot is stable and not everted on stance. The heel pain is then likely to be caused by dorsiflexion of the first ray due to a flexible forefoot valgus or plantarflexed first ray, both of which increase the force under the forefoot. In these patients the first ray must be plantarflexed during casting. There would be no need for medial heel skive and the heel cup can be of normal depth. A 2° cast inversion will raise the base of the first met and enhance plantarflexion.

Tarsal Coalition

The recommended prescription for tarsal coalition is a wide rigid CD poly device with: 14 mm heel cup, 0/0 (flat) poly post, EVA top cover to toes, and 5mm heel rase (following operative fusion). Note, for tarsal coalition the patient is casted in *maximal pronation* and not in subtalar neutral.

Tarsal Tunnel Syndrome

The recommended prescription for tarsal tunnel syndrome is wide semi-rigid CD or vacuum formed poly device with: normal heel cup, minimum cast fill, 4mm heel skive, 10° inversion (will accentuate the pressure intended to invert the calcaneus), EVA post, sweet spot at the porta pedis (avoids irritation at this spot on the foot), and 4mm heel rase. Note, an accurate negative cast of the foot in the neutral position with forefoot fully dorsiflexed on the rearfoot is essential for a good clinical outcome.

Chondromalcia Patella or Patellow Femoral Pain Syndrome

The recommended prescription for chondramalcia patella or patellow femoral pain syndrome is a wide semi-rigid CD or vacuum formed poly device with: normal heel cup, minimum cast fill, 2mm heel skive, 10° inversion (if the patient has an everted calcaneus in stance), Birko cork post, and EVA top cover to toes. Note, the negative casting must be accomplished with the midtarsal joint "fully loaded." The foot must be completely dorsiflexed until the subtalar joint *starts* to pronate.

Patients with significant ankle arthrosis/arthritis may need a stabilizing device called an Ankle-Foot Orthosis (AFO). There are also many prefab devices that can be quite helpful for such patients.

Proper Shoes

It is important to educate the patient on the choice of proper shoes. This is important whether or not the patient will be using a functional orthotic. Good shoes should function to both support the foot and provide shock absorption. When one is shopping for shoes, to avoid painful foot problems, it is especially important to purchase shoes that fit well. Shoes with a very high heel and a narrow toe box constrict the foot and can cause pain and deformity. They should only be worn for short periods. A good shoe should not be overly flexible. The heel box should offer stiff support. The sole should bend only at the distal third of the shoe when flexed. There should be stiff resistance when trying to twist (torsion) the shoe. Good athletic or walking shoes are ideal when using orthotics. When purchasing a shoe it is best to:

- Have the shoe fitted at the end of the day, when the feet are largest (as they swell during the day). If this is not possible, the foot can be traced on a piece of paper and the width compared to the shoe in the store.
- The patient should be standing while being fitted, since this is when the foot is widest.

- Sizes vary among shoe brands and styles. The shoe should be picked on the basis of how it actually fits the foot, not by the size marked inside.

- The shoe should conform to the shape of the forefoot as closely as possible. There should be one finger's breadth, about 1\2 inch, between the longest toe and the front of the shoe. For greatest comfort, the shoe should be no more that 1\4 inch narrower than the width of the foot. The ball of the foot should fit snugly into the widest part of the shoe, without being overly tight, even if this means that the heel is slightly loose.

While in the store walk around and make sure that the fit feels correct.

10

THE MANAGEMENT OF SPRAINS, STRAINS AND TRAUMA

Sprain, strains, and other traumatic injuries should be treated as early as possible to prevent the development of complications. When treating sprains/strains and many other musculoskeletal disorders, attention to Blood and circulation is of utmost importance. This is true especially for extracellular bleeding and Blood-stasis. In chronic disorders, disturbed Blood/blood circulation, and inadequate nourishment from Blood are often underlying causes of tissue degeneration. Obstacles to circulation may arise from any of the Pathogenic Factors and dysfunction in any of the systems that affect the Blood (Lungs, Spleen, Liver, vessels etc.). Table 10-1 on page 545 through Table 10-6 summarize contemporary TCM classifications and treatment of sprains and strains.

Ligamentous Sprain

Sprains are injuries to ligaments. Sprains characteristically are due to some sort of extrinsic force placed on the joint that moves the joint beyond the limits of the physiologic barrier. They can also be due to fatigue failure and *hysteresis*. When a sprain occurs, some degree of "subluxation" can result. Overall failure of ligaments (and tendons) is usually sudden and is preceded by the microfailure of the attachments between collagen fibers within the tissue and loss of the ability of the ligament (and tendon) to recover its length. It is important to distinguish between an eventual failure due to a sustained load (creep failure, hysteresis) and sustained cyclic loading and unloading (fatigue failure), from acute overload in excess of physiological tolerances. Treatment of subluxations and ligamentous congruity and strength is necessary if the joint is to regain full function.

Grading of Sprains

Sprains, like strains, are graded from mild to severe.

- Mild or Grade I Sprains result in no detectable lengthening of the ligament and therefore no obvious abnormal laxity of the joint. However, the joint is dysfunctional and joint play is often abnormal.
- Moderate or Grade II Sprains are distinguished by lengthening or partial tearing of the ligaments, and almost

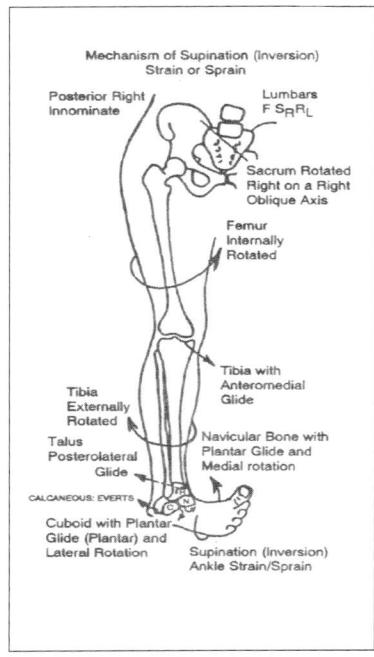

Figure 10-1: Far reaching effects of ankle sprain (From Kuchera WA and Kuchera ML, Osteopathic Principles in Practice, KCOM press 1993, with permission).

always are associated with some degree of subluxation. The joint may be hypermobile, but joint stability is retained mostly.

- Severe or Grade III Sprains result in a complete loss of joint stability. The distinguishing factor on examination is the end-feel, which lacks the normal capsular or leathery end-feel and increased range (unless limited by edema). Usually there is no or only a little pain, and the patient has fears of "giving way."

It is also helpful to grade strains/sprains as: *acute* (first 48 hours), *subacute* (48 hours to 6 weeks) and *chronic* (more than six weeks), each of which grades is related to a different stage of the inflammatory cascade.

This classification is rather arbitrary, and the difference between grades I and II is always subjective. Evaluation of a patient should be done as soon as possible after the injury (especially in mild and moderate sprains), since swelling and pain may make accurate examination more difficult. Tenderness and localized edema indicate the anatomical site of the tear in most instances (Ombregt et al *ibid*).

With sprains the patient is often aware of the injury as soon as it occurs. However, since symptoms are delayed often, the patient may continue with his activities and miss the opportunity to minimize bleeding and swelling. Pain (Garrick and Ebb *ibid*) from severe (grade III) sprains may disappear within minutes and be disproportionately mild. Mild sprains often remain painful for a long time, especially when left untreated.

Muscle Strain

The term *muscle strain* is used to describe injuries to the musculotendinous unit, also called the "contractile unit." Strains can occur anywhere within the contractile unit: In the tendon body, the tenoperiosteal junction, at the musculotendinous junction, or at the muscle belly. Strains can also initiate reflex contraction of the extrafusal fibers (spindles) with resulting viscous cycle of spasm, inhibition, and pain.

Causes of Muscle Strain

Strains usually occur due to intrinsic tension within the musculotendinous unit, most commonly when tension is suddenly and actively increased. This can occur with excessive muscle effort, such as in weight lifting. Strains may be due to overstretching, as well. Increase in tension can result from abrupt contraction of antagonistic (during eccentric contraction) muscles and tendons, causing muscle fibers to fail before the muscle lengthens. Tension in the contractile unit is greatest during deceleration (eccentric action), requiring the muscle to have some ability to lengthen at the same time as it maintains the contraction. Muscle stiffness, with decreased ability to lengthen during deceleration, is a common cause of strain. Another cause, which in part may also depend on muscle flexibility, is a sudden interruption of motion during activity. This occurs frequently during sport activities (Garric and Ebb *ibid*). Muscles that cross two joints, such as the hamstrings, biceps, and gastrocnemii are particularly at risk at their musculotendinous junction (Ombregt et al *ibid*).

The position of a muscle at a point of strain can change the way in which the afferent (sensory) nerves are changed. If the muscle is in a lengthened (eccentric) position, the afferent stimuli generated immediately after will be decreased, whereas if the muscle is in a shortened (concentric) position, the subsequent afferent will be increased (Donaldson et al 2001).

TENDON AVULSION is a strain-type fracture that results from a tendon and its bony attachment tearing loose from the surrounding bone. Such fractures vary in size from a small flake that is barely visible (as is occasionally seen with "tennis elbow") to the large avulsions (many centimeters in length) seen when the hamstring origin avulses a portion of the ischial tuberosity (Garric and Ebb *ibid*).

GRADING OF STRAINS. Strains are graded in severity as mild, moderate, or severe.

- Mild / grade I strains are generally viewed as microscopic disruptions resulting in no defect in the unit on examination.
- Moderate / grade II strains involve significant but not complete disruptions of the musculotendinous unit.
- Severe / grade III strains are complete ruptures of the contractile unit.

It is also helpful to grade strains as: *acute* (first forty-eight hours), *subacute* (forty-eight hours to six weeks) and *chronic* (more than six weeks), each of which is related to a different phase in the inflammatory cascade.

MUSCLE CONTUSIONS. Muscle contusions result from a direct impact to the muscle belly. This results in bleeding and swelling. Intramuscular bleeding (as opposed to intermuscular) can result in severe pain that may last for a long time, as it may be difficult for the body to disperse the blood. If possible, the blood should be aspirated within three days to minimize the chance of myositis ossificans development (Brown *ibid*).[1] After the blood is aspirated, a pressure wrap should be applied. The next day, active contractions with the muscle in a fully shortened position are helpful to prevent the formation of adhesions (Ombregt et al *ibid*). Trauma may be followed by deformation of the sarcomeres in the longitudinal and, more rarely, transverse direction. This may impact the ability of the actine and myosin filaments to slide by each other and cause the muscle to shorten. This can lead to abnormal stimuli and abnormal muscle tension. Such deformations may slightly change the axis of muscular contraction and distort the mobility and motility of a part of the body. Regions of hyperdensity may be formed at the beginning of trauma, edema, and fluid stasis. Some scarring processes may begin, as well (Barral and Croibier 1999). For more information on treatment see chapter 6.

MYOSITIS OSSIFICANS. Myositis ossificans is a benign condition that often results from trauma to muscle tissue. It can also be inherited. The condition is characterized by heterotopic bone formation, which occurs after injury to muscle fibers, connective tissue, blood vessels, and underlying periosteum (Gilmer and Anderson 1959). It occurs most often in males fifteen to thirty years old and the muscles at most risk are the *brachialis* and *quadriceps*. This condition is sometimes found in the hip adductors and pectoralis major and the bony deposit (in the muscle) is often connected to the underlying bone. The patient usually suffers from pain at the

---

1. The TCM technique of surface bleeding and cupping is not helpful in this situation and may result in increased hardening of surface tissues. Aspiration must be done using a large bore needle. Topical and oral herbs are helpful.

affected muscle: The muscle is shortened and resists stretching and often a firm mass is palpable. Often the range of movement in the neighboring joint becomes restricted. Radiographic changes are only evident two to four weeks following trauma. This condition does not respond to conservative treatment, although the administration of diphosphonates may prevent the deposits of bone. Traumatic myositis ossificans may resolve on its own in the course of one to two years (Ombregt et al *ibid*).

Treatment of Acute Sprain/Strain

Treatments of acute injuries follow four steps that address bodily responses to trauma (Kunnus *ibid*). Treating the area with PRICE: **p**rotection, **r**est, **i**ce, **c**ompression, **e**levation, and support is recommended early on.

1. Immediately after injury ice and compression are used to minimize bleeding and swelling (mostly during first seventy-two hours).

2. During the first one to three weeks after injury (depending on severity), protection by immobilization or just rest of the injured tissue/area usually allows healing without extensive scarring. Elevation helps drain edema and clear injured cells.

3. When soft-tissue regeneration begins, controlled mobilization and stretching of muscles and tendons stimulate healing.

4. Later at six to eight weeks post-injury, the rehabilitative goal is full return to pre-injury level of activity.

It must be stated, however, that, though the first step involves immobilization, most experimental and clinical studies demonstrate that early controlled mobilization is superior to immobilization for the primary treatment of acute soft-tissue injuries. Care should be taken not to bring the fibers under longitudinal stress in order not to disrupt the healing breach. Therapeutic movements are of short duration and amplitude, but repeated frequently (Ombregt et al *ibid*). PRICE is therefore used with flexibility.

The following treatment principles are the most important aspects in the treatment of sprains, strains, and contusions.

Treatment Principles

The treatment of acute injury should be directed toward minimizing bleeding, edema, and protection from further injury.

MINIMIZE BLEEDING. Most injuries involve the rupture of small blood vessels. Microscopic capillary bleeding in deep neck muscles, for instance, has been shown to persist for up to five days after motor vehicle collision injuries (Aidman 1987). At the beginning of treatment, preventing or arresting hemorrhaging is the primary concern. The extraversion of blood will produce far more disability than, say, the loss of a few fibers of muscle, tendon, or ligament (Garrick and Ebb

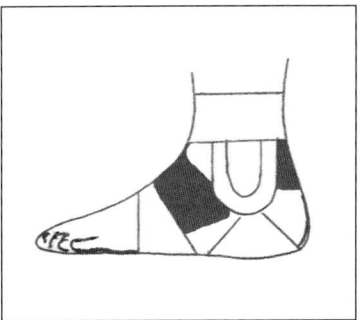

Figure 10-2: An herbal plaster and the U-shape pad that serves to transfer the tapes or elastic wrap pressure to the ligaments.

ibid).

Most sprains and strains are mild or moderate (1st or 2ed degree). Therefore, by definition, the injured structure retains anatomic continuity and ability to function. The accompanying bleeding, however, may distort normal anatomical relationships, resulting in pain and loss of motion/function. Bleeding and inflammation are in fact essential for proper healing. However, it is best to prevent the blood from seeping into unaffected tissues that then suffer unnecessary inflammation and stasis which will further inhibit circulation and drainage of the affected tissues. Also, inflammatory responses are often excessive and may be out of proportion to the severity of the injury and may lead to excessive scarring.

COMPRESSION. Compression is the most effective means of stopping bleeding, but to *be* effective, compression must be selective. Compression must be directed toward, and be in contact with, the bleeding site. For example, tissues injured around the ankle joint are deep to the bony surfaces. They lie in a depression under the malleoluses, where a pressure wrap or tape may be applied. Therefore, to effectively transfer compression to the tissues, a U-shaped pad should be used, or else compressive force will probably only redistribute the swelling to areas where it will do more harm (Figure 10-2). Manual pressure should be applied as soon as possible: within minutes of the injury.

CRYOTHERAPY, LOCAL ANAESTHESIA, AND ANTI-INFLAMMATORY MEDICATIONS. Cold application is helpful, but not as important as immediate compression. The efficacy of cold therapy has been studied on ankle sprains, showing an average of fifteen days reduction in the time of recovery (Knight et al 1980). Cryotherapy has several effects, including reduction of cell metabolism and oxygen consumption. These reductions can prevent secondary hypoxic injuries in uninjured tissues (Knight 1978). Cold also has an analgesic effect by acting as a counter irritant and decreasing inflammatory responses (Cailliet 1991). At the same time, cold/cryotherapy has been criticized, as it can cause edema, especially in the acute phase of an injury and, therefore, may lead to the inhibition of the healing process (Leduc et al 1979). Many TCM physicians are biased against cold therapy and state that it leads to the development of arthritis and scarring. Others use cold therapy during the first twenty-four hours.

Cold packs or ice should be combined with compression early on. Crushed ice or frozen gel capable of contouring around the anatomy should be applied for a minimum of twenty minutes, repeating every two to four hours. Icing of the spine, however, to treat deep-seated lesions is ineffective, and in fact may be detrimental by causing muscle cooling and spasm. In sprains of the sacroiliac (SI) joint, ice is often helpful but should be applied over the SI only, avoiding the lumbar muscles. Icing is helpful for interspinous ligamentous injuries, costotransverse and costosternal sprains, hyperextension/flexion injuries (whiplash) in the neck, tendinitis (acute and chronic), and in the early stage of muscular strain. Cryotherapy is especially helpful in peripheral joint sprains and musculotendinous injuries.

The application of heat in acute injuries has been shown to be detrimental in the early stages (Hohl 1975). Heat is helpful in the chronic stage. In TCM, however, heat is recommended by some physicians in the acute phase (also see page 369).

The immediate induction of *local anaesthesia* at the site of the lesion effectively blocks the nociceptive impulses which are responsible for muscle spasm. This may prevent changes within the nervous system that lead to sensitization. Cryotherapy may work in the same way, since it has local anaesthetic effects. The use of topical Toad venom (Can Su) is effective in some superficial lesions. Hua Tuo's Powder Containing Venenum Bufonis (Doing Su San) may be used as an anaesthetic (taken with a little wine) or used topically. Iontophoresis, ultrasound, or DMSO may be used to increase penetration.[2] Here is the formula for Hua Tuo's Powder:

Venenum Bufonis (Can Su) 3g
Rhizoma Pinelliae (Ban Xia) 2g
Radix Aconitii (Chuan Wu) 6g
Radix Rhododendri Mollis (Yang Zhi Zhu) 2g
Fructus Piperis Nigri (Hu Jiao) 6g
Fructus Piperis Longi (Bi Ba) 6g
Pericarpium Zanthoxyli (Chuan Jiao) 6g

In general, effective analgesia is said to be capable of preventing the onset of complex regional pain (or RSD), or other pathogenic changes in the nervous system. Thus the use of narcotic medications should always be considered if the patient is in severe pain.

Steroids injected within the first forty-eight hours of *ligamentous* sprains can reduce traumatic inflammation and prevent most structural and reflex changes. Pain also disappears, enabling the patient to move the joint in a normal way. Steroids injected during the granulation and repair stage, however, lead to *fewer* fibroblasts, diminished collagen fiber formation, and result in a *weaker* repair. Thus, in acute/early stages of ligamentous sprain, steroids have a beneficial influence, while they may have a harmful one in the later stage. Steroids seem to have larger negative effects on tendons. They are safe intra-articularly in most stages of *traumatic* arthritis (Ombregt et al *ibid*).

ELEVATION. Elevation, or at least avoidance of weight bearing, is another element in the initial treatment of an acute injury. Painful movements should be avoided, but other movements should be encouraged in order to prevent the development of weakness and adhesions from disuse. If the injury is severe, however, a period of rest and immobilization may be needed.

THERAPEUTIC MOVEMENTS AND EXERCISE. Immediately after the injury, one may need to protect and rest the injured area. Strapping the joint to protect it from unwanted movements may be needed. Premature and *intensive* mobilization leads to enhanced type-3 collagen production and weaker tissues than those produced during an optimal immobilization/rest period (Kanus *ibid*). Some acute inflammatory processes may last up to three weeks. Depending on severity, the patient may need to remain immobile or rest for that length of time. This is true especially if sprains are of the 2nd and 3rd degree (i.e., involve clearly torn tissues). However, some movement of tissues by cross-fiber massage and passive motions may be indicated to prevent adhesions and encourage collagen deposition to align in the direction of stress. Movement also stimulates proteoglycan synthesis and tissue repair (*ibid*).

Passive movements in the direct or indirect direction (limited/painful or nonlimited/nonpainful) should be within the allowable joint play and/or soft tissue range, and should be *painless*. They should start as soon as possible, especially in mild to moderate sprains/strains. After three weeks or so, a controlled mobilization in *increasing* magnitude should be started, even in severe sprains.

For *muscle* tears, mobilization should start after three to five days of immobility. This limits the size of the connective tissue area formed within the injury site, reducing scarring and inflammation (Kanus *ibid*). Stretching and resisted movements should be avoided. Ombregt et al (*ibid*), however, advocate light cross-fiber massage and active or electrically induced contractions, with the muscle in a *fully shortened* position to be started on the second day post-injury. They warn against using strong passive stretching or resisted movements. Return to sport activity can be allowed when the strength of the injured limb has been restored to within 10% of that of the unaffected limb (three to six weeks).

For *tendinous* lesions, a gentle passive tissue mobilization by cross-fiber massage together with passive movements are used to orient the randomly distributed collagen. They are performed for no more than a minute or two, starting on the day after injury (Ombregt et al *ibid*).

For *ligamentous* lesions, a gentle passive mobilization in the *non-painful range* together with cross-fiber massage are used, as well. Active movements can be used as long as *no*

---

2. This formula is said to have been used by Hua Tuo as an anaesthetic for surgery. When using DMSO, the herbs are applied topically about twenty minutes following the application of DMSO.

pain is elicited. There should be no attempt to increase this range in the acute or subacute stage (Ombregt et al *ibid*).

For *traumatic arthritis,* it is essential to restore full range of movement as soon as possible. This is true especially in middle-aged and elderly people, as post-traumatic adhesions are apt to form. Movements should be performed to the point of discomfort, but not pain. All possible movements should be attempted, one by one, and a small but definite increase in range should be achieved each day. If this fails, intra-articular steroid injections may be needed (Ombregt et al *ibid*). Other treatments such as functional techniques, muscle energy (MET), joint distraction, acupuncture, and herbs are useful as well, for both the acute and chronic stages.

MASSAGE. Starting on the second day post injury, cross-fiber massage can be used, gently, for a minute or two, and may help prevent adhesions. Effleurage can diminish swelling and pain and encourage restoration of normal movement. Effleurage strokes should always be directed towards the heart.

BLOOD LETTING AND ACUPUNCTURE. Blood letting of visibly congested *blood vessels* (a TCM technique) in the area and Well/Jing/Ting points is helpful to reduce local pressure and encourage circulation, often leading to immediate reduction of pain and throbbing sensations (Figure 10-3). The Sinew channel(s) is activated by needling or bleeding one fen proximal to the Well/Jing/Ting point on the affected channel's side. The Well/Jing/Ting point on the other side is moxaed; then superficial local needles are inserted to surround the area that shows stasis and swelling. No strong or deep stimulation should be attempted at local areas, as this often only increases inflammation and pain. The appropriate Connecting channel is used often. This also helps in dispersing congestion and stasis.

LASER THERAPY: Laser therapy has been reported to both prevent and treat edema and to be generally useful when used early in the treatment of sprains and strains.

MEDICINAL HERBS. Medicinal herbs are prescribed according to the stage of the injury (see below).

SURGERY. Although surgery may be necessary at times, several studies have shown that, for example, non-operative management and early mobilization of medial collateral ligament ruptures of the knee have as good an outcome as surgery. However, if the knee is very unstable and both the medial collateral and ACL are torn, exercise may have an adverse effect. Comparable outcomes have been shown for surgical and non-operative management of acromioclavicular (AC) joint separation, partial Achilles tendon tears, patellar dislocations and complete ruptures of ankle ligaments (Kunnus *ibid*).

Subacute Stage

Treatment is again predicated on severity. The subacute stage starts about thirty-six to seventy-two hours post-injury,

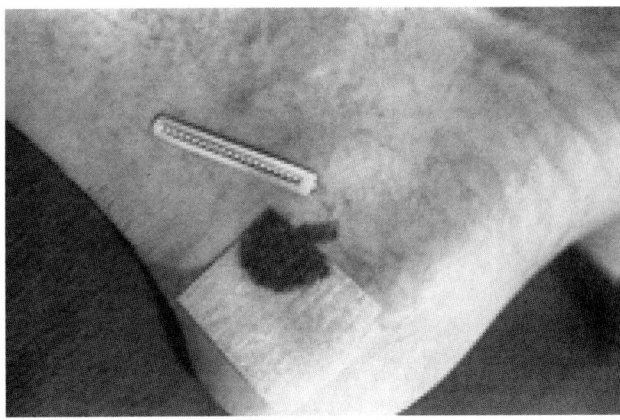

Figure 10-3: Bleeding congested vessels around the ankle.

approximately when edema has stabilized. The practitioner is advised to treat swelling as quickly after the injury as possible, because, once established, edema becomes harder to manage. When patients present at the office a day or two post-injury, the treatment principles remain the same, first arresting all swelling, then eliminating edema, and then restoring function.

1. *Electrogalvanic Stimulation.* Once swelling is stabilized, the addition of high-intensity electrogalvanic or interferential stimulation with the muscle in the shortened position can help eliminate swelling and prevent adhesions from forming. This, however, should not be started too early. *Active* muscle contraction with the muscle in the shortened position may prevent adhesions as well.

2. *Blood Letting and Acupuncture.* Techniques as described for the acute stage are still used.

3. *Topical Herbal Soaks.* Topical herbal soaks and plasters with or without massage are helpful.

4. *Contrast Therapy.* Contrast therapy (alternating hot and cold baths) should start at this time, first soaking the affected area in warm water, or herbal decoction (at 100° F) for about four minutes, followed by one minute of cold icy water bath.

    Heat can increase blood flow, reduce pain and muscle spasm, and relax joints. Encouraging active movement during the heat treatment is very important, as this will facilitate lymphatic and other fluid movements and drainage.

    Thermotherapy. At one time, thermotherapy was seen mainly as a component of the post-cryotherapy rehabilitative process (contrast therapy). However, recently new information has emerged demonstrating that thermotherapy (heat) allows the patient to attain pain relief through the effects understood in the well-known gate-control theory, a concept now known as "thermal analgesia." When muscles and tissues are tight,

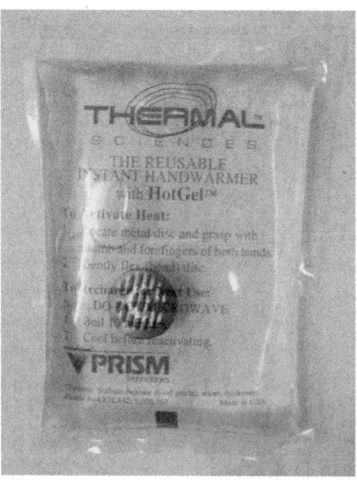

Figure 10-4: Zap Pac.

circulation to the area is restricted, resulting in progressive ischemia and increasing pain. Properly applied heat allows muscular tissue to relax, facilitating increased circulation and relieving pain by allowing metabolic toxins to be removed from the area and increasing tissue oxygenation. While hot water bottles conform well to various body surfaces, they cannot be easily secured to the body. Further, the water in them cools quickly, requiring the patient to continually refill them. Heating pads are usually a safe source of heat. However, the FDA and Consumer Product Safety Commission have logged many cases of injury and death with their use, estimating a total of 1,600 new burns and eight fatalities each year. A patient who wishes to work or carry out sports activities while receiving heat cannot use a heating pad, since it is dependent on an electrical source. Prism technologies manufacture a small plastic bag containing a solution of sodium acetate and a small metal disc. This "Heat Solution" (also known as Zap Pac[R]) is activated by grasping the metal disc inside the bag and clicking it once (Figure 10-4). This action forms a nucleate crystal, which initiates a cascade of exothermic crystalline precipitation. The heat produced may last as long as one hour. The bag can be indefinitely recharged by placing it in boiling water or a microwave oven. Another alternative for heat therapy is the ThermaCare[R] which only begins to heat after the package is opened, and reaches its target temperature of 104°F in about thirty minutes. It provides a consistent heat over an eight-hour period. Two versions are available for musculoskeletal use: a back wrap for low back pain, and a neck-to-arm wrap that treats the neck, shoulders, arms, and wrists. These heat wraps conform to body contours and are fully portable, allowing the patient to carry out normal activities while wearing them.

Heat therapy is mostly suitable for late-stages and chronic disorders. A recent study has shown that heat is superior to icing (or other modalities) in the treatment of chronic low back pain (Mooney 2004).

5. *Exercise and Mobilization Therapy.* Mobilization therapy within the nonpainful range is for the most part passively started. Passive motion should be applied first in the indirect direction (toward the nonrestricted barrier) and initiated within the allowable and comfortable joint-play and soft-tissue range. These measures may prevent the formation of troublesome adhesions, establish appropriate proprioception, and reduce noxious nervous stimulation. Direct movement into the restricted barriers is carried out as tolerated and with care (i.e., without causing any pain or discomfort). Stretching and resisted movement should be avoided at this stage. It may be necessary to immobilize the affected tissues for up to three weeks in some severely injured patients.

Patients usually respond to pain with guarding and avoidance of painful movements. The resulting prolonged disuse leads to muscle weakness. Furthermore, because movements become uncomfortable, the muscles responsible for such movements become less active, and the joint loses the stability normally afforded by these muscles. This increases the likelihood of a recurrent injury. Strengthening exercises at the subacute phase should not be started too soon (especially if a tendon/ligament is involved) before the tissue has had a chance to form a breaching scar. Active exercises are started about two to three weeks after the injury. Light isometric muscle contractions are usually safe. They will not aggravate the condition unless a tendon or fracture is involved, and they should be gauged appropriately. Recently, even fracture care has been changing, and early mobilization, which has been the practice in TCM for a long time, is increasingly being applied. The patient is taught particular exercises and instructed to perform about five repetitions hourly while awake. Vigorous activity should only be resumed after normal function has been restored. Otherwise, immature fibrous healing may rupture and maintain the disability. Also, the body will try to compensate for the dysfunction and establish abnormal patterns that may place unfamiliar stresses on numerous muscles and joints. This will cause a cascading increase in symptoms that may be much more difficult to deal with than those directly resulting from the original injury (Brown *ibid*).

Late and Chronic Stages

The same treatment approach can be used in the chronic stage, with more aggressive techniques. However, in tendinitis or muscular strains, excessive strain from exercise can be detrimental. Often muscle length must be restored first. With instability, strength and length are addressed at the same time. A Rupturing of the adhesion may be needed. For traumatic *arthritis* in the late stage (Ombregt et al *ibid*), stretching out the capsule requires many repetitions of long steady pushes maintained for a minute or so, as long as the patient

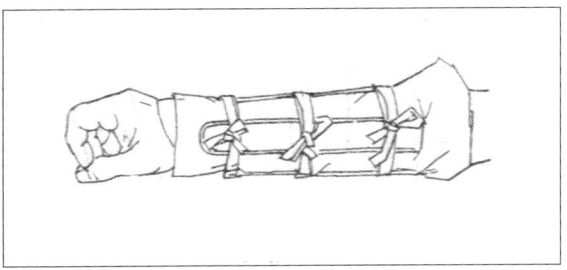

Figure 10-5: Fracture care using splints and herbal rap.

can bear it. No increase in range can be expected for several visits, and persistence is required. Heating the joint prior to treatment is helpful.

A recent multi-site, randomized, actively-controlled, investigator-blinded study compared heatwrap to oral ibuprofen (400 mg TID) and acetaminophen (1,000 mg QID) for lower back pain. Topical heat-wrap therapy was superior to acetaminophen and/or ibuprofen in pain relief, lateral trunk flexibility, decreased muscle stiffness, and disability reduction. Further, investigators discovered that the improvements persisted for over forty-eight hours after removal of the heat wrap, far longer than the duration experienced with nonprescription oral analgesics (Pray 2003).

Many Osteopathic (or TCM) manual therapy techniques can be used in the management of sprain and strains. See "Osteopathic Treatment Methods" on page 484.

TCM Stabilization and Exercise

Management of activity is part of the TCM treatment approach to acute injuries. This approach was also advocated in the West by Hippocrates more than 2400 years ago. Stabilization and restriction of movement with simultaneous exercise was described in the TCM medical book *Secret Formula of God for Management of Trauma and Fracture*:

> Sprains and fractures of the hands and feet are treated by a topical application of ointment wrapped with cloth, fixation with bamboo, and with intermittent exercise. The applicable exercises should be individualized, and the patient must neither overexercise nor under exercise.

For injuries to soft tissues, in order to promote Qi and Blood circulation, prevent stasis and adhesion, and promote healing, the practitioner must create a balance between the need for immobility, stabilization, and mobility. In the acute and middle stages, movement must be soft and fluid to avoid aggravating the condition. In the late and chronic stages, the patient can also use strengthening exercises. Commonly used, especially in acute disorders, are Tai Chi- and Qi Gong-derived techniques. More specific muscle strengthening, stretching, and coordination training is used in middle and chronic stages. Plaster casts are commonly used in the fixation of fractures. Since plaster often contains gypsum (Shi Gao), a stone that is considered to have a cold nature in TCM, patients may develop a Cold syndrome after fixation by a cast (such as stiffness and pain). TCM management of fractures commonly involves early movement and a use of removable bamboo splints.

Herbal Management

In the early and middle stages of acute soft tissue injury, the treatment principles are to activate the Blood, stop bleeding, open the channels and, often, to clear Heat. Representative formulas are Seven-Thousandths of a Tael Powder (Qi Li San) and Trauma Pill (Die Da Wan), which is a warming formula. These formulas facilitate the elimination of Blood-stasis, swelling, bleeding, and pain. The following are basic formulas that can be used in the treatment of soft-tissue sprain and strains. Appropriate modifications are made based on symptoms, signs, and region.

A *guiding* oral and topical herbal formula for early stage sprains and/or strains is:

> Radix Angelicae Sinensis (Dang Gui) 6g
> Radix Notoginseng (San Qi) 15g
> Radix Rehmanniae (Sheng Di Huang) 9g
> Radix Paeoniae Alba (Bai Shao) 9g
> Radix Paeoniae Rubra (Chi Shao) 9g
> Rhizoma Ligustici Wallichii (Chuan Xiang) 6g
> Gummi Olibanum (Ru Xiang) 3g
> Resina Myrrhae (Mo Yao) 3g
> Herba Lycopodii (Shen Jin Cao) 12g
> Fructus Liquidambaris (Lu Lu Tong) 6g
> Semen Plantaginis (Che Qian Zi) 12g
> Flos Loncerae (Jin Yin Hua) 9g
> Flos Chrysanthemi (Ju Hua) 9g
> Rhizoma Paridis (Zao Xiu) 6g
> Radix et Rhizoma Rhei (Da Huang) 6g[3]

If swelling is already prominent:

> Radix Bupleuri (Chai Hu) 9g
> Poriae Cocos (Fu Ling) 20g
> Flos Carthami (Hong Hua) 15g[4]
> Radix Paeonia Rubra (Chi Shao) 12g
> Semen Persicae (Tao Ren) 6g
> Sanguis Draconis (Xue Jie) 9g
> Squama Manitis (Chuan Shan Jie) 12g
> Semen Trichonsanthis (Gua Lou Ren) 9g
> Radix et Rhizoma Rhei (cooked) (Shu Da Huang) 9g
> Resina Myrrhae (Mo Yao) 3g
> Gummi Olibanum (Ru Xiang) 3g
> Radix Notoginseng (San Qi) 12g
> Semen Plantaginis (Che Qian Zi) 15g
> Semen Coicis Lachryma jobi (Yi Yi Ren) 30g
> Rhizoma Dioscoreae Hypoglaucae (Bi Xie) 12g
> Nidus Vespae (Feng Fang) 9g
> Spina Gleditsiae (Zao Jiao Ci) 6g
> Radix Glycyrrhizae (Gan Cao) 3g
> Mirablilitum Depuratum (Mang Xiao) *topically only*

For trauma with stasis, restlessness or complex fracture:

> Pollen Typhae (Pu Huang) 30g
> Rhizoma Corydalis (Yan Hu Suo) 30g
> Radix Paeoniae Rubra (Chi Shao) 30g
> Myrrha (Mo Yao) 30g
> Radix et Rhizoma Rhei (Da Huang) 30g
> Radix Aconiti (Fu Zi) 30g
> Fructus Perillae Frutescentis (Su Zi) 30g
> (Yun Tai Zi) 30g

---

3. For low back strain, add Semen Sinapis Albae (Bai Jie Zi).

4. Care must be paid to bleeding. This herb may be used only if there is no bleeding, or only used in a small dose.

Radix Angelicae Sinensis (Dang Gui) 9g
Cortex Cinnamomi Cassiae (Gui Xin) 9g
Rhizoma Ligustici Wallichii (Chuan Xiong) 9g
An Lu Zi 9g

Grind into powder and take 3g QID with warm wine.

For simple bone fracture, modifications of Join Bone Powder (Jie Gu San) can be used both topically and orally. Vinegar is mixed in when used topically:

Myrrha (Mo Yao) 12g
Gummi Olibanum (Ru Xiang) 12g
Pyritum (Zi Ran Tong) 6g
Os Draconis (Long Gu) 30g
Talcum (Hua Shi) 30g
Hallyositum Rubrum (Chi Shi Zhi) 12g
Sanguis Draconis (Xue Jie) 9g
Lignum Sappan (Su Mu) 9g
Secreto Moschi Moschiferi (She Xiang) 0.1g

During the subacute and chronic stages of bone fracture, the following herbs are added:

Radix Dipsaci Asperi (Xu Duan) 15g
Ramulus Loranthus Sangjisheng (Sang Ji Sheng) 30g
Cortex Eucommiae Ulmoidis (Du Zhong) 15g
Rhizoma Drynari (Gu Sui Bu) 12g
Cornu Cervu Parvum (Lu Rong) 3g

In the subacute stage, when bleeding and inflammation have stabilized, the main treatment principles are to prevent secondary Wind-Dampness and malnourishment of sinews and bones. The following *guiding* formula can be used:

Radix Angelicae Sinensis (Dang Gui) 9g
Gummi Olibanum (Ru Xiang) 3g
Resina Myrrhae (Mo Yao) 3g
Herba Lycopodii (Shen Jin Cao) 12g
Radix et Rhizoma Rhei (Shu Da Huang) 6g
Radix Paeoniae Alba (Bai Shao) 9g
Radix Paeoniae Rubra (Chi Shao) 9g
Radix Notoginseng (San Qi) 9g
Nidus Vespae (Feng Fang) 9g
Radix Ledebouriellae (Fang Feng) 9g
Radix Angelicae Dahuricae (Bai Zhi) 6g
Lignum Sappan (Su Mu) 9g

In the acute late stage and in chronic soft tissue injury, the main pathogenic processes are disharmony between the sinews, channels, and network-vessels. This manifests as pain and the fatigability of the affected tissues. Treatment often consists of nourishing the Blood, re harmonizing the collaterals, and warming the channels to stop the pain and to strengthen the tissues. Representative formulas are Revive Health by Invigorating Blood Decoction (Fu Yuan Huo Xue Tang) and Fixed Bi Empirical Formula (Zhuo Bi Yan Fang).

A *guiding* oral or topical formula for the late stage with stiffness and pain is:

Ramulus Loranthus Sangjisheng (Sang Ji Sheng) 30g
Radix Angelica Sinensis (Dang Gui) 12g
Radix Paeoniae Rubra (Chi Shao) 12g
Caulis Spatholobi (Ji Xue Teng) 12g
Squama Manitis (Chuan Shan Jie) 12g
Radix Salviae Miltiorrhizae (Dan Shen) 12g
Ramulus Mori Albae (Sang Zhi) 9g
Flos Carthami (Hong Hua) 6g
Myrrha (Mo Yao) 9g
Gummi Olibanum (Ru Xiang) 9g
Rhizoma Ligustici Wallichii (Chuan Xiong) 6g
Radix Gentianae Macrophyllae (Qin Jiu) 12g
Radix Clematidis (Wei Ling Xian) 9g
Rhizoma Curcumae Longae (Jiang Huang) 12g
Rhizoma seu Radix Notopterygii (Qiang Huo) 9g

Fructus Psoraleae (Bu Gu Zhi) 9g
Rhizoma Drynari (Gu Sui Bu) 9g
Radix Aconiti Carmichaeli Praeparata (Zhi Chuan Wu) 9g
Herba Asari Cum Radice (Xi Xin) 3g
Secreto Moschi Moschiferi (She Xiang) 0.1g
Scorpio (Quan Xie) 3g
Borneolum (Bing Pian) 0.2g oral use; 3g topical use

A strategy based on modified Pueraria Decoction (Ge Gen Tang) for treating traumatic injury to flash and bone is:[5]

Radix Puerariae (Ge Gen) 30g
Herba Ephedrae (Ma Huang) 9g
Ramulus Cinnamomi Cassiae (Gui Zhi) 10g
Fructus Forsythiae Suspensae (Lian Qiao) 10g
Rhizoma Zingiberis (Sheng Jiang) 3 slices
mix-fried Radix Glycyrrhizae (Zhi Gan Cao) 6g
Radix Paeoniae Lactiflorae (Bai Shao) 15g
Fructus Zizyphi Jujube (Da Zao)12 pieces

Topical soak of Radix Puerariae (Ge Gen) 100g.

For upper extremity add: Rhizoma Curcumae Longae (Jiang Huang) and Ramulus Mori Albi (Sang Zhi).

For lower extremity or the lumbar region add: Radix Achyranthis Bidentatae (Niu Xi).

For severe pain, swelling, and distension add: Rhizoma Cyperi Rotundi (Xiang Fu), Resina Olibani (Ru Xiang) and Resina Myrrhae (Mo Yao).

For traumatic injury and multiple abscesses (i.e., secondary infection)[6] due to Blood-stasis, Removing Blood-stasis Pueraria Decoction (San Xue Ge Gen Tang) can be added to antibiotic therapy:

Radix Puerariae (Ge Gen) 2.5-12g
Rhizoma Pinelliae (Ban Xia) 2.5-9g
Rhizoma (Chuan Xiong) 2.5g-6
Radix Ledebouriellae (Fang Feng) 2.5-9
Rhizoma seu Radix Notopterygii (Qiang Huo) 2.5-9g
Rhizoma Cimicifugae (Sheng Ma) 2.5g-4g
Radix Platycodi (Jie Geng) 2.5-9g
Radix Angelicae Dahuricae (Bai Zhi) 1.5-6g
Radix Glycyrrhizae (Gan Cao) 1.5-3g
Herba Asari (Xi Xin) 1.5g
Folium Perillae (Su Ye) 1.5g-6g
Rhizoma Cypri (Xiang Fu) 1.5-6g

---

5. Ge Gen Tang can relax the muscles and sooth the sinews. When Pueraria is used in large doses, it relaxes the muscles and soothes and softens the sinew channels. Ephedra can "crack patterns of hardness and accumulation," promoting free flow and dissipating. It is used to warm and free the flow of the blood vessels, quicken the Blood, free the flow of the network-vessels, dispel stasis, and stop pain. It frees the flow of the muscles and skin on the Exterior and resolves accumulations of Phlegm and congelations of Blood in the Interior. Cinnamon frees the flow of the Yang. It assists Ephedra in promoting the free flow and circulation of Qi and Blood. Peony assists Pueraria in softening the sinews, relaxing cramping, and stopping pain, as well as mediating the excessively acrid and dissipating properties of Cinnamon and Ephedra. Forsythia is ascending, floating, diffusing, and dissipating, functioning to vigorously course the Qi and Blood. It treats congelation of Blood and accumulation of Qi in the twelve channels. Moreover, Forsythia regulates and soothes the pathways, allowing it to guide the other medicinals to the illness. Ginger and Red Dates harmonize the Constructive (Nutritive) Qi and defensive Qi. An Mo massage, in conjunction with the application of the prescription as a hot soak, promotes the circulation of Blood in the injured area and enhances the therapeutic effect (Chace 2000).

6. Articular infection must be treated with modern antibiotic medications. This formula can be added.

Flos Carthami (Hong Hua) 1.5-6g

For late-stage *weakness* from traumatic injury and bleeding, use Disperse Wind and Nourish Blood Decoction (Shu Feng Yang Xue Tang):

> Herba Schizonepetae (Jing Jie) 6g
> Rhizoma et Radix Notopterugii (Qiang Hou) 9g
> Radix Ledebouriellae/Siler (Fang Feng) 9g
> Rhizoma Ligustici (Chuan Xiang) 9g
> Radix Trichosanthis (Tiang Hua Fen) 15g
> Radix Paeoniae (Bai Shao) 12g
> Radix Gentianae Macrophyllae (Qin Jiu) 12g
> Herba Menthae (Bo He) 5g
> Radix Angelicae Sinensis (Dang Gui) 12g
> Flos Carthami (Hong Hua) 6g

Table 10-5 summarizes the basic treatment principles and classical external formulas used in the treatment of acute injuries. Table 10-6 summarizes commonly used classical formulas for external application in chronic or late stages. Table 10-4 summarizes commonly used classical formulas for oral intake in all stages.

Other Natural Therapies for Sprains and Strains

Proteolytic enzymes have anti-inflammatory, edema-reducing properties and analgesic effects. The analgesic effects are probably due to inhibition of inflammation as well as direct influences on nociceptors. In recent years a significant reduction of pain in various rheumatic diseases including periarthritis of the shoulder, osteoarthritis of the knee, and painful vertebral syndromes have shown effects equivalent to non-steroidal anti-inflammatory agents (NSAIDs) in pain scores (Klein and Kullich 1999). Serratia peptidase (SP) is an anti-inflammatory in wide clinical use throughout Europe and Asia as a viable alternative to salicylates, ibuprofen, and the more potent NSAIDs. Unlike the NSAIDs, SP has no inhibitory effects on prostaglandins and is devoid of gastrointestinal side effects. It is an anti-inflammatory proteolytic enzyme isolated from the microorganism, Serratia E 15. This enzyme is naturally present in the *silk worm* (Bombyx Batryticatus, Jiang Can) intestine and is processed commercially through fermentation. SP is a metalloprotein with a molecular weight of 50,000. Each molecule contains one zinc atom. This immunologically active enzyme is completely bound to the alpha 2 macroglobulin in biological fluids. Histologic studies reveal powerful anti-inflammatory effects of this naturally occurring enzyme.

SP has been introduced and admitted as a standard treatment in Germany and other European countries for treatment of inflammatory and traumatic swellings. In one double-blind study conducted by Esch et al, sixty-six patients with fresh rupture of the lateral ligament treated surgically, were divided into three randomized groups. In the group receiving the SP, the swelling had decreased by 50% on the third postoperative day. In the other two control groups (elevation of the leg, and bed rest, with or without the application of ice), no reduction in swelling had occurred. The difference was of major statistical significance. Decreasing pain correlated for the most part with the reduction in swelling. The patients receiving SP became pain-free more rapidly than the control groups. By the tenth day all patients in the SP treated group were free of pain. The therapeutic daily dose has been reported at one or two tablets (5 mg) three times daily. Serraflazyme, a preparation available in the United States, contains 5mg SP formulated as an enteric coated tablet (Dorman, personal communication). Bromelain, three or four capsules three times per day on an empty stomach, and other proteolytic enzymes may be helpful, as well.

Table 10-1: Soft Tissue Damage

LACERATION OF BONE FRAGMENT	Caused by physical force exerted on tendon-periosteal junction. Palpability and symptoms depend on location.
DAMAGE TO CHANNELS (NERVES AND THEIR ENERVATED STRUCTURES)	Identified by analyzing: • joint movements • loss of sensation • presence of marked muscle contraction. Modern neurological knowledge is useful in this evaluation.
CONGEALED (MIXED) PHLEGM AND BLOOD (OSSIFICATION)	Nontreatment of traumatic injury and/or chronic Phlegm and Blood-stasis can lead to: • channel blockage and formation of "hard nodules" • insufficiency of tissue nourishment. Tissues can react by hardening, resulting in dysfunction, pain aggravation, and formation of osseous lesions.
CONGEALED DAMP BI (INTER-ARTICULAR FREE BODY)	Chronic Obstruction Bi syndrome accompanied by damage due to injury can lead to hardening which becomes interarticular free bodies.
PROLIFERATED BI SYNDROMES (OSSEOUS ARTHRITIS)	Inflamed tissue (where chronic Fire and/or Cold congeals Phlegm and Blood) may transform into "hardness" spurs that attach to joint surface. (Spurs usually develop along stress lines and Sharpey's fibers.)

Table 10-2: Stages of Soft Tissue Damage

Early Stage	Middle Stage	Late Stage	Chronic Stage
First 2-3 days.	Begins 4-14 days after mild-to-moderate or severe injury.	Begins about 2 weeks after injury. Usually results from severe trauma and/or weakness.	Atypical. Usually due to secondary factors, e.g., improper treatment, continuing weakness/deficiency.
Characterized by: severe pain, local Blood-stasis, reddish-purplish color, swelling, dysfunction, local warmth, very noticeable dysfunction	Characterized by: partly reduced swelling, some absorption of Blood-stasis, greenish-purplish color, slightly warm skin, pain reduced greatly, still noticeable dysfunction	Characterized by: change of ecchymotic color to yellow-brown, symptoms reduced greatly, dysfunctions may not be noticeable	(Usually) Characterized by: persistent, mild swelling, development of adhesions and scars, dull pain (ache), sluggish movement of affected parts, painful end-feels
Mild to moderate types may recover. Usually goes to middle stage.	Recovery usually with mild-to-moderate types. Treated correctly, should heal 1-2 weeks.	Recovery expected within 5 weeks of injury, if did not heal by second week of treatment. May progress to chronic	Recovery variable. Good in Mild-Moderate types. Similar to middle stage.
Severe	Severe	Severe	Severe
Goes to middle stage, but middle stage is more prolonged.	By day 14, patient should be improved noticeably, with partial recovery of functions.	May be prolonged. Symptoms may vary greatly by location.	May be prolonged. Symptoms may vary greatly by location.

Table 10-3: Contemporary TCM Classification of Soft Tissue Damage

Cause and Location	Pathology of Damaged Tissue	Stage
Strain/Sprain		
Injury due to indirect (intrinsic) forces such as: • sudden movement. • heavy lifting. Occurs mostly in sinews: • periarticular fascia. • ligaments. • muscles. • tendons.	Blood-stasis. Mild impairment of collateral circulation within: • fascia. • tendons. • muscles. Includes mild lacerations of tissues that do not lead to joint pathology.	Acute stage 1-10th day. Middle stage 4th-14th day.L Late stage 2ed-4 weeks. *Chronic* Constitutionally strong patient with effective treatment, unlikely to progress to chronic stage. With severe injury, tissue severed, or when patient's Righteous is weak its likely to progress to chronic stage, characterized by: • muscular rigidity/flaccidity. • local skin paleness/redness. • swelling and/or tissue hyperplasia or atrophy.
Contusion		
Injury from extrinsic force (trauma). Characterized by damage directly under injuring force to sinews and/or bones: • subcutaneous tissue. • muscles. • tendons. • ligaments. • bones.	Altered Position from Torn Tissue. Malpositioned tissues accompanied by obvious Blood-stasis, swelling, loss of normal function. Affected tissues may include: • muscles. • tendons. • ligaments. • joints. • bones.	*Chronic* Constitutionally strong patient with effective treatment, unlikely to progress to chronic stage. Severe injury, tissue severed, or patient's. Original Qi weak likely to progress to chronic stage, characterized by: • muscular rigidity/flaccidity. • local skin paleness. • swelling and/or tissue hyperplasia or atrophy.

Table 10-4: Internal Herbal Medication: Acute Soft Tissue Injuries

INTERNAL HERBAL APPLICATIONS: ACUTE SOFT TISSUE INJURIES	
Pathologic Processes	• Blockage of Qi. • Blockage of Blood circulation. • Bleeding. • Severe pain due to stasis and ecchymosis.
Treatment Principles	• Activate the Blood. • Dissolve stasis. • Stop bleeding. • Regulate Qi. • Clear Heat.
Injury with Bi Syndrome (Wind-Damp/rheumatism)	• Eliminate Wind-Damp. • Harmonize the collaterals.
Weak Muscles/Tendons	• Supplement Spleen, Liver and Kidney with above principles.
Early Stage Treatment Principles	• Dissolve stasis, activate Blood, stop pain, stop bleeding.
Common Formula	• Stop pain powder (Zhi Tong San). • Yunnan white powder (Yunnan Baha'i).
Middle Stage Treatment Principles	Swelling and Pain Reduced Gradually and Noticeably. • Relax the sinews. • Activate the Blood. • Reduce swelling.
Common Formulas	• Relaxing tendon pill (Shu Jin Wan). • Relaxing sinew and activating Blood Tea (Shu Jin Huo Xue Teng). • Supplementing sinew pill (Bu Jin Wan).
Late Stage, Chronic Stage Treatment Principles	Often accompanied by Wind-Damp, manifest as local swelling, fatigue, muscle contractions, loss of normal function, pain (may be aggravated by weather changes). • Nourish and vitalize the Blood. • Harmonize the Collaterals. • Disperse Wind. • Eliminate Dampness. • Stop Pain.
Common Formulas	• All-Inclusive Great Tonifying Tea (Shi Quan Da Bu Tang). • Minor Invigorate the Collaterals Special Pill (Xiao Luo Luo Dan). • Fantastically Effective Pill to Invigorate the Collaterals (Huo Luo Xiao Ling Dun). • Major Invigorate the Collaterals Special Pill (Da Huo Luo Dan). • Remove Painful Obstruction Tea (Juan Bi Tong).
Elderly Weak patients Treatment Principles	• Supplement Liver, Kidney, Blood. • Eliminate Pathogenic Factors and Blood-stasis.
Common Formulas	• Bushen Zengjin Tong (Tonify Kidney Strengthen Sinews Tea). • Bushen Huoxue Tong (Tonify Kidney Invigorate Blood Tea). • Major Invigorate the Collaterals Special Pill (Da Hou Luo Dan).

Table 10-5: Injury: Basic Treatment Principles, External Applications, and Formulas: Acute Stage

Treatment Principles	• Activate Blood. • Dissolve Stasis. • Eliminate Swelling. • Regulate Qi to Stop Pain.
Common Formulas	• Three Colors Herbal Ointment (Sanshe Gao). • Dissolving Blood-stasis Plaster (Huaxue Zhi Gao). • Stopping Pain Ointment (Zhitong Gao). • Regulate Qi to Stop Pain Plaster (Liqi Zhitong Gao).
Local Heat/Redness	If the injury has local heat and redness, in order to: • Dissolve Blood-stasis. • Clear Heat. • Eliminate Toxin. • Reduce Swelling. • Stop Bleeding. Use • Activating Blood Ointment (Huoxue Gao). • Clearing Ying Ointment (Qing Ying Gao). • Four-Yellow Paste (Sihuang Gao). • Gold-yellow Paste (Jinhuang Gao).
Minor Injuries	For minor injuries, in order to: • Relax Sinews. • Activate the Blood. Use • Thousand Flower Oil (Wanhua Yao). • Fr. Foeniculi Oil (Xue Xiang oil).

Table 10-6: Injury: Basic Treatment Principles External Applications Formulas: Late Stage

Late Stage, Certain Chronic Stages	Pain prolonged. Tissues impaired functionally.
Treatment Principles	• Activate the Blood. • Stop bleeding. • Dispel stasis. • Stop pain.
Common Formulas	• Thousands of responses ointment (Wan Fu Zi Gao). • Pearl ointment (Zhen Zhu Gao). • Transforming channels plaster (Huajian Gao).
Chronic Stages	Skin over lesion cold, somewhat white. Muscles and tendons hardened, swollen, spasmodic.
Treatment Principles	• Warm the channels. • Stop pain. • Facilitate joint movement.
Possible Formulas	• Herbal hydrotherapy. • (Ba Xian Shao Yao Tang, Hai Tong Pi Tang). • Topical spirits.[a] • Huoxue Jiu (activate Blood spirit).
Chronic Pain with Wind-Damp Bi (rheumatism)	
Treatment Principles	• Warm the channels. • Eliminate Wind-Damp. • Stop pain.
Possible Formulas	• External application of steamed herbs. • Teng Yao, Tang Feng Shan. • Plaster: 　—Dog skin plaster (Goupi Gao). 　—Transform channels plaster (Juajian Gao). • Oils/Spirits.

a. A nice combination that can yield a warming effect is to first use Zheng Gu Shui followed by Po Sum On, the area is then wrapped and the patient mobilizes the affected joint.

11

MUSCULOSKELETAL DISORDERS: INTEGRATIVE PRACTICE

The literature is replete with texts that focus on particular aspects of musculoskeletal medicine, often to the exclusion of other (and often conflicting) ways of thinking. Whether the mechanism of the patient's complaint is due to dysfunctions that can be *accurately* understood and described within the lexicon of OM/TCM, or are better understood using biomechanical or biomedical descriptions, it is the purpose of this chapter to review a more holistic/integrated way of thinking about musculoskeletal disorders. In TCM most musculoskeletal conditions, unless due to *direct* forces (trauma), are caused (or allowed) by internal and Deficiency factors. In Painful Obstruction (Bi) syndrome theory, either Deficiency allows exogenous Pathogenic Factors to invade the body, or an internal disharmony reduces flow and leads to blockage that gives rise to Excess-type pain. Another etiology that can result in musculoskeletal pain is malnourishment of sinews and bones with symptoms of fatigue, weakness, susceptibility to injury, and tissue damage. This can lead to Deficiency or mixed type pains. Therefore, in TCM most types of musculoskeletal pain, unless due to trauma, are secondary to a so-called root problem (which may be constitutional, functional, behavioral, or, to a lesser extent, environmental). Emphasis is on the systemic rather than the *anatomical* source of pain.[1] While this approach is especially helpful in regard to metabolic and physiologic processes, it is less developed for disorders that are mainly due to postural and mechanical imbalances.

Soft tissue disorders fall mostly within the domain of OM Painful Obstruction (Bi) and Hit (martial art, bone setting, traumatology) medicine, but internal medicine is almost always an important element (describing root causes). TCM traumatology, or *Exterior-damage,* refers to broken bones, damage to sinews, and wounds. *Interior-damage* refers to musculoskeletal pain resulting from pathological change in the Organ systems or to dysfunctions in Qi/Blood/Essence/Yin/Yang which result in pain or to damage to the above body milieu as a result of trauma which then give rise to Exterior and Interior dysfunctions.

For example, it is said: "If there is wrenching and contusions the Qi counterflows which makes it difficult to bend. Detriment and damage due to carrying heavy loads and taxation leads to congealed Blood. Kidney-deficiency gives a constant, mild pain."

In *Orthopaedic Medicine,* disorders can be grossly categorized as follows (Ombregt et al *ibid*):

- *Traumatic*: Injury resulting either from one single trauma or from multiple small traumas, i.e., the overuse or repetitive use injuries.
- *Inflammatory*: Rheumatoid, poly-or monoarticular, infectious; traumatic.
- *Degenerative*: Arthrosis, tendinosis, etc.
- *Internal derangement*: Loose bodies and displaced menisci in peripheral joints and spine.
- *Functional disorders*: Instability, weakness, proprioceptive disturbances.
- *Psychogenic pain*: There is no existing functional or anatomical explanation for the pain.

This chapter reviews integrative therapies of musculoskeletal disorders.

Inflammation

Inflammation is the means by which the body deals with insult and injury. Insult may be caused: mechanically (e.g., by pressure or foreign bodies), chemically (e.g., by toxins, acidity, alkalinity), physically (e.g., by temperature), by internal processes (e.g., uremia), and by mircoorganisms (e.g., bacteria, virus, parasites). Inflammation is a complicated and not fully understood communication between cellular and humoral elements.[2] Inflammation rids the body of foreign matter and disposes of damaged cells, and initiates wound healing. Inflammation is controlled by mast cells that are in close proximity to autonomic nerves. Mast cells are a constituents of connective tissues containing large granules that contain heparin,[3] serotonin, bradykinin,[4] and histamine.

---

1. Attention to local tissues is still used; however, the development of functional tests and differential of affected tissues is quite rudimentary.

2. Humoral response is one of the two forms of immune response to antigens such as bacteria and foreign tissue. It is mediated by B-cell lymphocytes marked by antibodies. Cellular immunity is dominated by T-cell lymphocytes. It is involved in resistance to infectious diseases, delayed hypersensitivity, resistance to cancer, autoimmune diseases, graft rejection, and allergies.

3. Heparin is an antithrombin factor that prevents intravascular clotting.

These substances are released from the mast cell in response to injury and infection, and, by their degranulation, they control most of the processes of inflammation. Mast cells are responsive to other controls, for example, under the influence of progesterone they release serotonin, and under the influence of estrogen they release histamine. Another important pathway is known as the *arachidonic acid cascade* which is largely controlled by *eicosanoids*.[5] Eicosanoids are local "hormones" made from 20-carbon essential fatty acids (AA, DGLA, EFA), they are short-lived and can affect many aspects of physiological function at the cellular level. Eicosanoids include all the prostaglandins, thromboxanes, and leukotrienes. Depending on genetic as well as other factors eicosanoids transform or control prostaglandins, thromboxanes, and leukotrienes all of which are inflammatory mediators. Eicosanoids can initiate, regulate, and terminate all local inflammatory responses.[6] When inflammation affects a joint (such as in rheumatoid arthritis), the cartilage can be damaged by neutrophils[7] and lysosomal enzymes[8] that enter the area. This leads to a vicious cycle of repeated injury and persistent inflammation.

Inflammation may also lead to mental depression which is commonly seen in chronic pain patients. Indolamine 2.3 dioxygenase (IDO) is a rate-limiting enzyme in the degradation of tryptophan and is induced during inflammation by the cytokines interferon-gamma (IFN-gamma), interferon-alpha (ITN-alpha) and tumor necrosis factor-alpha (TNF-alpha) in a broad variety of cells. Elevated IDO can therefore enhance tryptophan degradation and subsequent serotonin depletion which may cause depression (Wichers and Maes 2004).

Anti-inflammatory drugs such as aspirin and other NSAIDs inhibit prostaglandin synthesis, which may affect inflammatory mediator production and cellular processes. Steroid hormones have been postulated to have a multitude of effects. Probably the most significant in this context is the stabilization of lysosomal membranes (Ryan and Majno 1983).[9] Tripterygium Wilfordii (Lei Gong Teng) is a Chinese herb that has been shown to be quite effective in treating inflammation secondary to auto-immune disorders. It is a toxic herb that should be used with caution as it can cause internal bleeding, kidney damage, decrease in blood cell counts, decreased bone mineral density in females with lupus erythematosus (SLE), hair loss, immune system dysfunction, and even death.[10] Symptoms of toxicity include: dizziness, palpitations, weakness, nausea, vomiting, stomach aches, diarrhea, pain in liver and kidney areas, bleeding of digestive tract, and respiratory and circulation exhaustion. Variations of Two-Marvel Powder (Er Miao San), Cinnamon Twig, Peony, and Anemarrhena Decoction (Gui Zhi Shao Yao Zhi Mu Tang), and White Tiger plus Cinnamon Twig Decoction (Bai Hu Jia Gui Zhi Tang) are often used to treat *active* inflammation.

Chronic Inflammation

Chronic inflammation can evolve from acute inflammation or occur without an acute phase. Histologically, chronic inflammation has two main features: The presence of granulation tissue[11] and mononuclear predominance.[12] The combination of new blood vessels, fibroblasts, and extracellular matrix is termed "granulation tissue." Mononuclear predominance can also be seen in the latter part of acute inflammation as mononuclear phagocytes[13] or macrophages.[14] In comparison to ordinary loose connective tissue, granulation tissue is more cellular and contains neutrophils, inflammatory cells, and fibroblasts.[15] Granulation tissue is more vascular and has "leaky" capillaries. The formation of granulation tissue is the response of connective tissue and vessels to irritation.

In some forms of chronic inflammation, other cell types appear. This suggests the development of immunologic reactions that may include lymphocytes,[16] eosinophils, and plasma cells.[17] In other forms, where no immune response is present, the mononuclear cells are almost entirely macrophages. When inflammation is chronic, the vascular component, vasodilation, and exudation is minimal, and, therefore, manifests clinically with little (possibly no) redness and heat (Ryan and Majno 1983).

Most chronic inflammation without bacterial invasion is pointless and may even prove to be harmful. For example,

---

4. Bradykinin is a peptide of nonprotien origin containing nine amino acid residues and acts as a vasodilator.

5. Arachidonic acid is an essential fatty acid that is a component of lecithin (esterified phospholipid) and a basic material for the biosynthesis of some prostaglandins.

6. Fatty acids are hydrocarbons of varying length with a carboxyl group (-COOH) at one end and a methyl group (-CH3) at the other. Fatty acids are often classified by two types: 1) the saturation (saturated, monounsaturated, polyunsaturated, and trans fats), and by 2) the families of fats, based on physical structure (omega-3, omega-6, omega-9, etc.). Polyunsaturated fats are very susceptible to oxidative damage, and most saturated fats raise serum cholesterol levels. Omega-3 fatty acids make cell membranes more fluid and therefore more permeable. Of the two parent essential fatty acids, both are polyunsaturated. Linoleic acid (LA) is an omega-6 (n-6) oil, and linolenic acid (ALA) is an omega-3 (n-3) oil. Both LA and ALA are transformed by the body into longer and even more polyunsaturated fatty acids using the same cellular enzyme (delta 6 desaturase; which therefore can transform to both pro-inflammatory and anti-inflammatory depending on the amount of substrate from diet and genetic conditions). Many disorders as well as dietary influences can affect the enzyme delta 6 desaturase and thus change fatty acid balance. Three of the metabolites of the enzyme have 20 carbons and have important functions: dihomo gamma linolenic acid (DGLA), arachidonic acid (AA), and eicosapentaenoic acid (EPA).

    Eicosanoids are made by the body via enzymic conversion: Prostaglandins are made by cyclooxygenase enzyme (COX), and leukotrienes and made by lipoxygenase enzymes. EPA can be further desaturate to produce docsahexaenoic acid (DHA, 22:6 n-3; the longest of the fatty acids). DHA is a critical fatty acid that increases membrane fluidity and permeability which allows for proper cell receptor function as well as regulation of nutrients and waste product flow into and out of the cell. Omega 3 fatty acids (fish oils, containing EPA and DHA) are considered anti-inflammatory. However, the omega 6 fatty acid gamma linoletic acid (GLA) may be more appropriate for diabetic patients. The most common causes of fatty acid imbalance is a diet high in omega 6 (animal fat and shell fish), altered delta-6 desaturase activity, vitamin B-3, B-6, biotin, Ca, Zn, and Mg deficiency, and insulin dysregulation.

edema raises tissue tension and causes pain, impeding movements that are important for normal joint function and homeostasis. Pressure from edema to vascular tissues can result in poor drainage of toxins (*ibid*).

SELF-PERPETUATING INFLAMMATION. Self-perpetuating inflammation can result after trauma, especially with minor injuries to tendons and ligaments. Trauma leads to tissue destruction and the release of enzymes that then lead to→inflammation→growth of fibroblasts→formation of fibrils→rest→chaotically formed adherent scar→normal movement→re-injury/irritation→*self-perpetuating inflammation*. Treatment then may be needed to disinflame the scar, or to get rid of the chaotically formed scar, by deep cross-fiber massage or manipulative rupture (Ombregt et al *ibid*).[18] Many conditions that have been labeled as inflammatory, such as chronic tennis-elbow, are not inflammatory.

NEUROGENIC INFLAMMATION. Recent research using immune-histochemical techniques suggests that when ligaments and other connective tissues in the spine (and other areas) that receive a supply of small-diameter fibers become irritated, an initiation of neurogenic inflammation occurs and commonly affects pain and sympathetic receptors. Neurogenic inflammation results from release of neuropeptides that interact with fibroblasts, mast cells, and immune cells in the surrounding connective tissues (Levine et al 1993). When irritated, some of the small-diameter sensory axons can secrete substance-P, which is a proinflammatory, vasodilatory neruropeptide, into the surrounding tissue. This release of an inflammatory agent from a peripheral nerve terminal is involved in initiating the processes of neurogenic inflammation and edema, and results in degranulation of mast cells. Neurogenic inflammation is thought to be a major factor in degenerative diseases and back pain chronicity (Willard *ibid*).

It must be remembered that inflammation anywhere in the body can result in musculoskeletal-like pain, and may be caused by bacteria, viruses, parasites, fungi, spirochetes, and cardiovascular or autoimmune diseases. Septic arthritis should be treated with complete rest and aggressive IV antibiotic therapy.

Wound Healing

Bioelectrical phenomena may initiate and regulate inflammatory process and repair (Oschman *ibid*). Becker (*ibid*) has shown the human body to be polarized. The central spinal axis is said to be positively charged and the periphery is said to be negatively charged. The normal voltage reading is said to be -10 µV; however, when a fracture occurs, the voltage decreases toward zero. Five days after the injury, the voltage is said to move toward normal, and by the fifteenth day, the voltage reading is within normal limits of -10 µV. It is possible that this polarity gradient is a electromotive force driving, in part, the current of injury and the inflammatory cascade that leads to healing. Nordenström has suggested that when an injury occurs, a positive charge builds up in the area of injury, which may then result in a potential gradient acting as a bioelectric battery. A change in the electrical insulating properties of capillary membranes is said to turn on the "biological battery." As the membranes become less permeable to the flow of ions and more electrically insulated, the flow of intrinsic bioelectricity is forced to take the path of least resistance, which is through the bloodstream to the injured area.

When injury occurs, sensory information rapidly alerts the brain and begins the complex sequence of events to reinstate homeostasis. Cytokines[19] are released within seconds after an injury. These substances, such as gamma-interferon, interleukins 1 and 6, and tumor necrosis factor, enter the blood stream in one to four minutes, and travel to the brain. The cytokines, therefore, are able to activate fibers that send messages to the brain and, concurrently, to breach the blood-brain barrier at specific sites and have an immediate affect on the hypothalamic cells. The cytokines, together with eval-

---

7. Neutrophils are the circulating white blood cells essential for phagocytosis and proteolysis by which bacteria, cellular debris, and solid particles are removed and destroyed.

8. Enzymes with hydrolytic actions that function in intracellular digestive processes.

9. Cytoplasmic membrane-bound vesicle measuring 5-8 nm (primary lysosome) and containing a wide variety of glycoprotein hydrolytic enzymes.

10. Vitamin B-12 and B-6 as well as Glycinae Pericarpium (Lu Dou Yi) can be added to minimize the risks.

11. Granulation tissue is any soft, pink, fleshy projection that forms during the healing process in a wound. It consists of capillaries surrounded by fibrous collagen.

12. Mononuclear cells are cells such as leukocytes, lymphocytes and monocytes, with round or oval nuclei.

13. A phagocyte is a cell that is able to surround, engulf, and digest microorganisms and cellular debris.

14. A macrophage is any phagocytic cell of the reticuloendothelial system including histocyte in loose connective tissue. Macrophages probably digest proteins and supply amino acids to the fibroblast.

15. A fibroblast is an undifferentiated cell in the connective tissue that gives rise to various precursor cells, such as the chondroblast, collagenoblast, and osteoblast, that form the fibrous, binding, and supporting tissue of the body.

---

16. A lymphocyte is a type of white blood cell that increases in number in response to infection. Lymphocyte increase permeability and help to activate the phagocytosis of damaged cells.

17. An eosinophil is a granulocytic, bilobed leukocyte (white blood cell) that increases in number in response to allergy and in some parasitic infections.

18. Since most degenerative tendinopathies are non-inflammatory and steroid injection does not result in lasting effects in relation to them, treatments that stimulate cell growth may be needed.

19. Cytokine is a generic term for nonantibody proteins released by one cell population (e.g., primed T lymphocyes) on contact with a specific antigen, which acts as intercellular mediators, as in the generation of an immune response.

uative information from the brain, rapidly begin a sequence of activities aimed at the release and utilization of glucose for necessary actions, such as the removal of debris, the repair of tissues, and, sometimes, the raising of a fever to destroy bacteria and other foreign substances (Melzack *ibid*). Therefore, the sequences that result in wound healing and inflammation integrate both peripheral and brain functions.

Wound healing, regardless of the site of injury or degree of inflammation, occurs in three *overlapping phases* (Banks 1991). The first phase has three major affects: early wound / healing strength secondary to crosslinking, removal of damaged tissue, and recruitment of fibroblasts. The tissues regenerate largely due to inflammatory cells, vascular and lymphatic endothelial cells, and fibroblasts (Ombregt et al *ibid*).

- **First phase**. The first phase, *the inflammatory phase*, is characterized by ischemia, metabolic disturbance, and cell-membrane damage. It is time-dependent and is mediated by vascular, cellular, and chemical events, culminating in tissue repair and sometimes scar (adhesion) formation (Kannus 2000). The inflammatory phase can be divided into early and late stages.
— *Early Inflammatory Stage*. The first reaction is vasoconstriction of small local arterioles that last about five to ten minutes. It is followed by active vasodilatation and increased blood flow for one to three days, during which time, cellular debris and humoral factors attract the initial influx of granulocytes. The first to appear are platelets[20] that secrete many chemical mediators of inflammation, resulting in the arachidonic acid cascade and the release of growth factors such as platelet-derived growth factor (PDGF), platelet factor 4, insulin-like growth factor (IGF-1), and transforming growth factors.
— *Late (Second) Stage*. In the second stage, the monocytes and macrophages release polypeptide growth factors, which activate the fibroblasts. The second stage of the first inflammatory phase lasts about ten days.
- **Second Phase**. The second phase is *the granulation tissue formation* (proliferation) stage. It begins about two days after injury (overlapping with the first phase) and can last up to six to eight weeks. It is controlled by monocytes, which are pluripotential cells capable of essentially directing the complete sequence of events in this proliferative phase.[21]
— Monocytes begin to form, mobilizing a soupy mixture of granulocytes and macrophages with infiltrating fibroblasts from granulation tissue. This is characteristic of a healing wound. Macrophages are capable of releasing numerous growth factors, chemotactants, and proteolytic enzymes. They can activate fibroblasts for tendon and ligament repair.
- **Third phase**. The third phase is *the matrix formation or remodeling maturation* aspect. It is characterized by a trend toward decreased cellularity, decreased synthetic activity, increased organization of extracellular matrix, and a more normal biochemical profile. Type 1 collagen starts to assume a normal orientation and replaces type 3 collagen. Increased chemical cross-linking results in increased strength.
— Fibroblasts remain to build a strong matrix of collagen. In tendon injury, there is intrinsic healing as a result of endotendon fibroblastic response.
— Matrix formation lasts about six months, at which point the tensile strength of the repaired tissue reaches about 50%.[22] Full strength is only reached after one to three years. Collagen maturation and functional linear realignment are usually seen in about two months. Cellular response after tendon laceration can be extrinsic or intrinsic. The extrinsic response is a proliferation and bridging of the injury by epithelial cells. Intrinsic healing is the result of an endotendon fibroblastic response (Brown *ibid*). During maturation, the scar tissue is reshaped and strengthened by removing, reorganizing, and replacing cells and matrix (Ombregt et al *ibid*).

Movement During the Healing Phase

Movement and activity are of primary importance in preserving homeostasis between collagen degradation and synthesis (Amiel and Woo 1981), and are advocated in TCM (and by Hippocrates) in the management of injuries. Movement encourages collagen to be laid down in the correct anatomical arrangement and helps increase the production of ground substance and intermolecular crosslinking, thereby increasing the strength of the tissue. This occurs by improved vascular remodeling (in a longitudinal orientation), and by causing the orientation of fibroblasts and collagen to be laid in parallel to the fibers (Gelberman et al 1989). Movement can also decrease the formation of abnormal scars and adhesions. The result is a more normal looking tissue rather than scar tissue, especially if it is due to treatment such as dry needling or (Dorman *ibid*) prolotherapy. Movement also prevents the randomness of collagen fibers found in regular scar tissue. Movement during the granulation phase (about the first ten days) should not be very stressful on the healing scar, as this can prevent normal healing. Another advantage of early mobilization is the positive affect on skeletal muscles with increased circulation, muscle

---

20. Platelets are the smallest cells in the blood. They are essential for the coagulation of blood.
21. Some types of chronic inflammatory disorders such as tendinitis may occur due to the prolongation of this stage, which may be do to anti-inflammatory therapy.

22. For more information on acupuncture and dry needling, see Chapter 5.

strength and endurance, and maintenace of proprioceptive reflexes, which ensure the active stability of the joint (Ombregt, Bisschop and ter Veer 2002). Exercise increases production of insulin-like growth factor (IGF-1), which is known to stimulate collagen synthesis and cell replication (Brown *ibid*).

Factors That May Influence Healing

Continued joint inflammation can compromise the capacity of lymphatic drainage. When lymphatic drainage is inadequate, the continued edema and resulting pressure may affect healing. Edema can distort anatomical alignment and lead to joint instability, muscle dysfunctions, and ligamentous laxity. Prolonged inflammation and the resulting congestion (swelling) may result in bathing of tissues with serofibrous exudate with resulting adhesions and inflexibility. With poor circulation, congestion, hypoxia and continued re-injury from use, tissue regrowth takes the form of inferior quality granulation tissues, leading to the decreased organization of the extracellular matrix. Poorly healed tissues may be seen with chronic tendinitis, tendinosis, and inflammation of ligament. Therefore, it is important to pay attention to the progress of the healing and related activity of a recuperating patient Simkin (1990).

Healing can be influenced negatively by smoking, collagen diseases, nutritional deficiency, and some medications (Brown, Orme and Richardson 1986; Battié et al 1991, Lawson1989, Brown *ibid*):

- Smoking can decrease fibrinolytic activity and nutritional supply to tissues including discs. This can lead to increased risk of poor healing and can cause disc pathologies and surgical and fracture nonunions.

- Medications, especially anti-inflammatories, may result in poor healing. High levels of corticosteroids can prevent the migration of macrophages.

- Collagen diseases such as Marfan's syndrome and Ehlers-Danlos syndrome result in enzymic deficiencies that influence healing.

- Nutritional deficiencies such as vitamin C, B1, zinc, sulfur, copper, manganese, boron, and proteins can inhibit healing.

Anti-Inflammatory Drugs

While Non-steroidal anti-inflammatory drugs (NSAIDs) often relieve symptoms, they are far from ideal therapeutic agents. NSAIDs work by inhibiting the production of prostaglandins and thus may interfere with normal tissue repair. They inhibit both helpful and non-helpful prostaglandins; hence they can result in unwanted side effects and *interfere* with healing. For example, a recent report presented at the American Orthopaedic Society for Sports Medicine stated that NSAIDs taken for two weeks inhibit tendon-to-bone healing in rotator cuff repair for eight weeks in rats (Medscape 2004). Indomethasin and Naproxen inhibit GAG synthesis and cell proliferation after tendon injury (*ibid*). Patients who use Piroxicam after knee injuries have increased anterior drawer signs compared to those that do not (Slayter et al *ibid*). At least five studies in both humans and animals have reported that NSAIDs may accelerate joint destruction (Newman and Ling 1985; Shield 1993; Brooks, Potter and Buchaman 1982; Ranningen and Langeland 1980; Brandt 1987). The newer COX-2 inhibitors have been shown to significantly inhibit experimentally-induced tibial fractures healing in mice by inhibiting the process of bone cell differentiation (O'Keefe 2002). Corticosteroids may also interfere with healing and the use of NSAIDs and corticosteroids may prolong inflammation in connective tissues (Viidik and Gottrup 1986). The long-term benefits of corticosteroid injections for lateral epicondylitis were shown *not* to be superior to physiotherapy and very comparable to no therapy at all (Smidt et al 2002). Corticosteroids have been associated with tenon ruptures and accelerated cartilage degeneration when used in weight bearing joint. They have been associated with aseptic necrosis and most patients using them develop some degree of osteoporosis.

NSAIDs can cause other serious side effects including peptic ulcer, and, less commonly, hepatic or renal failure. The use of NSAIDs causes about 2000-3000 *deaths* and cost $200-760 million of treatment of side effects in the U.S., per year. Some estimates of deaths caused by NSAIDs in the U.S., are as high as 10,000-20,000 patients per year (Bjorkman *ibid*). It is estimated that 8% of the world adult population is prescribed an NSAID for a variety of conditions (Simon 1997, Bjorkman 1996). A study published in the Archives of Internal Medicine of NSAIDs taken by >80,000 female nurses over a two-year period has found that those who took NSAIDs for twenty-two days or more per month had an 86% increased rate of developing hypertension. The researchers concluded that a substantial proportion of hypertension in the U.S., might be due to the regular use of analgesics. NSAIDs have also been associated with increased rates of non-Hodgkin's lymphoma.

Not all the effects of NSAIDs are harmful. A newly published study on the cyclooxygenase-2 (COX-2) inhibitor Celecoxib has shown it to "enhance the rate of synthesis of both hyluronan and proteoglycans, and concomitantly reduce the net loss of these two glycosaminoglycans," which may, therefore, have protective effects on osteoarthritic cartilage (Manicourt et al 2003). NSAIDs may also protect against the development of glioblastoma multiforme (brain tumors; Niccole and Sivak-Sears 2004). Long-term use should probably be avoided although benefits such as prevention of fatal heart attacks, TIAs, and Alzheimer, and increased early detection of colon cancer have been suggested. Hence, the harm/benefit ratio between the use or nonuse of anti-inflammatory medications is difficult to judge. Inflammation is important for wound repair, but it can also lead to sensitization of nerves. Therefore, anti-inflammatory medication have both beneficial and harmful affects.[23]

Three Phases of Degeneration

Kirkaldy-Willis and Burton (1992) described three phases to the degenerative process. These are: dysfunction, instability, and stabilization. Many of the treatment principles presented in this text are designed to address the consequences of these degenerative processes.

Dysfunction Phase

The dysfunction phase is seen in patients who usually have transient pain that responds well to manual therapies. Pathological tissue alterations are relatively minor, and, by and large, the patient presents with a joint or soft tissue pain that is difficult to document. These patients may have suffered a minor trauma or strain, often due to a lack of good physical condition.

SYMPTOMS AND SIGNS. The patient presents with acute, subacute, or chronic pain. The pain is usually unilateral but may refer in a myotomal or sclerotomal distribution. Often pain is relieved by rest. Patients usually have a postural component to their pain, that is, their pain is usually felt at end-range. The pain usually comes on only after prolonged loading at end-range, such as after sitting for while. Abnormal motions at the affected joint are detectable but may be significant only during symptomatic periods.

If the muscle joint complex or posture is not corrected, soft tissue stress may result in pathological change, such as anoxia of muscle tissue with fibrotic deformations, joint restriction with consequent immobility and increased stress on the ligaments. This process then leads to the second phase: the instability phase.

Instability Phase

Here the patient presents with similar symptoms; however, chronicity is the rule. Patients respond only temporarily to manual therapies. The prolonged dysfunction, poor physiologic posture, immobility, lack of activity, and genetic and other individualized factors result in both mechanical and cellular stress on ligaments and other tissues. Ligaments loose their elastic character, and joint stability is lost. The discs begin to break down and may rupture. This results in an increasing rate of degeneration at the joint complex.

SYMPTOMS AND SIGNS. Signs of hypermobility and ligamentous pain are becoming more pronounced. Patients are often weak and often report a "giving way" or "catching" of the affected region. Discogenic symptoms are common.

Stabilization Phase

In this phase patients often report that a previous severe condition is becoming less painful and that they feel increasingly stiff. Aging causes the ligaments to shrink. Joints develop other ways to stabilize (often referred to as degenerative spondylosis).

SYMPTOMS AND SIGNS. Patients often report feeling less incapacitated, unless degenerative deformations lead to compression phenomenon or sensitization develops.

TCM and the Degenerative Cascade

The following discussion integrates TCM and modern understanding of the degenerative cascade. The principles delineated here can be used to treat musculoskeletal disorders successfully. There is much overlap between the biomedical concept of the degenerative cascade and TCM's understanding of aging and tissue failure. TCM pattern diagnosis tends to change as the patient moves through the stages of their disease, and as the patient undergoes the aging process. The latter relates mainly to the Kidneys, Yin, Essence, and Blood. These diagnostic variations are reflected in the presentation of signs and symptoms representing Pathogenic Factors, the state of the Righteous-Qi (which indicates general health), and the condition of the Form (structure) of the being as a whole and its organs and tissues. In general, disease stages and the aging process undergo the following variations: stages (and processes) where the Righteous-Qi is strong and the Pathogenic Factors are weak; where the Righteous-Qi is strong but the Pathogenic Factors are even stronger (which means to some extent Righteous is weak if pathogens are strong); where the Righteous-Qi is deficient and the Pathogenic Factors are excessive; and where the Pathogenic Factors are eliminated and the Righteous-Qi is recovering. The degenerative cascade is therefore either related to the damage and breakdown of Form[24] by Pathogenic Factors (which damage the Kidneys, Liver, Spleen, and their related tissues as well as Essence and Blood) or to damage from depleted Essence and inherited or postnatal factors.[25]

TCM disease mechanisms that reflect the progression of pathology in musculoskeletal disorders can be summarized as arising from Exterior, Interior, traumatic, or other miscellaneous origins. Early or abnormal degenerative conditions often involve weak (congenital) or depleted Essence.[26]

---

23. There are 2.2 million adverse drug reaction per year in the US and a minimum of 106,000 deaths per year from *appropriate* use of prescriptions drugs (Starfield 2000). Of the 198 drugs approved by the FDA from 1976-1985, 102 had to withdrawn from the market or their label had to be changed due to side effects (FDA drug review 1990). Of all the drugs in the PDR only about 30% have a known mechanism of action.

24. Form is used here to describe structure, not the Taoist ideas of creation and the duality of "Form" and "No Form."

25. The most important acupuncture points that support Essence and Form are: CV-4, 6, 8 (and abdominal points in general), UB-24, 26, 38, 43, 60, GV-4, GB-39, Lu-9 and the rest of the 12 source points.

26. Not a classical statement however has been described to the author by a teacher which follows the Kidney school.

Exterior Pathways

At first, external Pathogenic Factors penetrate the body through the skin, mouth, or nose. Depending on the patient's general condition, he or she develops a superficial syndrome, or, if the pathogens enter more deeply, they may or may not cause immediate symptoms. External Wind-Cold is said first to penetrate the Tai-Yang (UB) channels, and, unless treated, to continue inward (or manifest) via the six channels/stages. Wind-Heat and Dampness are more likely to penetrate through the mouth and nose and tend to progress quickly in the "four level pattern," from the Exterior-division (superficial) to Blood-division (deep) level, or to progress more slowly via the three Warmers, with Dampness often starting in the middle-Warmer and causing digestive symptoms. These stages usually progress in an orderly manner from one to the next. However, in some cases the condition can progress in a non-orderly manner or even remain at the same stage for some time. The stronger the patient's Righteous-Qi, the more likely he/she is to develop a fever/inflammation and eliminate the pathogens. Weak patients often do not develop strong symptoms and are more likely to develop chronicity and retain hidden pathogens.[27]

These models can be applied broadly; however, patients with musculoskeletal pain, especially when mild and non-traumatic, often do not, clinically, fit established TCM patterns. One can always "force" a pattern diagnosis by ignoring some signs and projecting others, but the clinical utility of doing this is often not ideal. The interaction of the ideas that follow has occurred when the author has had to confront these issues.

In the *dysfunction/postural phase* of the degenerative cascade, insufficient *circulation* of Qi and Blood is often the cause of symptoms. External Pathogenic Factors may be one cause that interferes with normal Qi and Blood circulation (especially Dampness, as it is said that Dampness causes Qi-stagnation). These various factors cause stagnation/stasis (congestion) to develop and to advance the dysfunctional/postural phase. Symptoms come on when tissues are under stress and in need of extra nourishment. This stress then activates pain receptors (increase stagnation of Qi and Blood). The Pathogenic Factors are usually weak so that the patient feels symptoms only when the tissue is under prolonged loading and in need of extra nourishment. This nourishment is blocked by pathogens, or by *some other functional disturbance*.[28] Stagnation results in trapped Qi and Blood within an area (with signs such as local swelling or, possibly, an "inflated balloon-like pulse"); or the inability of Qi and Blood to enter an area, (with signs such as *flaccid localized tissues* or, possibly, decreased vessel tone and/or a "flat pulse" quality).[29] With time, lack of nourishment from poor circulation (or blocked circulation), or from pathogens damaging the Yin and Blood (because trapped pathogens often damage Yin/Blood/Essence as they easily transform into Heat or by obstructing flow), results in tissue failure and the patient develops *instability*. Eventually, Blood-stasis and pathogenic Dampness coalesce. This results in hard swellings and a proliferation of tissues with ossification/spurs, resulting in the *stabilization phase*. Hidden pathogens are said to lurk Interiorly and damage Yin and Essence, so that tissue nourishment may be affected, eventually leading to the degenerative cascade.[30]

Interior Pathways

Emotions and/or lifestyle stresses result often in dysfunction of the Qi. This often means stagnation of the Qi. Because Qi moves the Blood, stagnant-Qi can result in poor Blood circulation. Many physical activities demand healthy circulation and tissue nourishment for normal joint and sinew renewal, cell division, and function. When these mechanisms are disturbed, tissue failure can follow. Another common complication of stagnant-Qi is that it can transform into Heat or Fire. This *pathogenic-Heat* can consume Yin/Essence and Blood, all of which then fail to nourish the sinews. The progression of TCM patterns usually reflects the stages of the condition as indexed by the three stages of degenerative cascade; often parallels the dysfunction/postural stage, the instability stage and the stabilization stage. These stages usually progress from one to the next. However, in some cases the condition can progress in a non-orderly manner or even remain at the same stage for some time, as mentioned above.

Another common Interior cause that can lead to the degenerative cascade is lack of inherited Essence or natural endowment (constitution), and decreasing normal bodily functions. Lowered normal functions leads to poor nourishment, and degeneration, or a lack of separation of the pure from the impure, leading to turbidity. This in turn can lead to an accumulation of Pathogenic Factors, mostly Dampness with obstructive-malnourishment, leading to the degenerative cascade.

Just like in Exterior pathways, with Interior pathways the *dysfunction/postural phase* is characterized by Qi and Blood stagnation resulting in symptoms when the tissues are under stress and in need of extra nourishment. Or the patient feels pain when staying still which aggravates the stagnation. Physical movements, which move Qi and Blood, reduce the patient's pain. With time, lack of nourishment from poor cir-

---

27. The priority of Exterior influences on musculoskeletal pain in TCM thinking is probably due to the strong influence of Zhang Zhong jing *Discussion on Cold Damage and Miscellaneous Disorders*. The severity of the disease may not be as obvious in Deficient and old patients.

28. Since often the patient does not have clear patterns associated with TCM ideas, except for channel disturbances, guiding ideas from Painful Obstruction (Bi) syndromes can only be theorized on. While herbs that deal with Pathogenic Factors are used in the next sections, their mechanism of action may be more due to their pharmacological effect on blood circulation than elimination of "Pathogens."

29. Lymphatic drainage (or swelling) increases the extent of tissue damage that follows tissue injury.

30. Not classical conclusions and discussions.

culation or Heat damaging the Yin/Blood/Essence or Form, results in tissue failure and *instability develops*. The body's attempt at compensation will result in proliferated disorders (i.e., Yin producing Yang and vice versa). Hard obstructions (or tissues) develop, resulting in the *stabilization phase* (i.e., congealed/joined/mixed Phlegm/Dampness and Blood-stasis). The dysfunction/postural phase is also associated with *Deficient-detriment* (i.e., taxation, often with low back aching) and aching located at specific locations and which becomes worse on marked strain, in the morning on waking, and improves with light exercise.

Miscellaneous Factors

Many life stresses, dietary influences, iatrogenicity, infections, etc., can affect the body's immune systems/anti-pathogenic systems, or can cause direct insult. This can lead to musculoskeletal damage and pain, which appears, or not, as the *degenerative cascade*. Blood is said to be rejuvenated in the Liver during sleep (which may relate to the production of insulin-like growth hormones at night). Blood and Liver are in charge of nourishing and the strength of sinews. Lack of rest and sleep are increasingly part of modern life, both of which may contribute to the degenerative cascade. Yin, Blood, and Essence are necessary for the normal nourishment of the sinews and bones, all of which are dependent, in part, on healthy diet. Use of therapeutic and recreational drugs can damage the Organic/organic systems and bodily milieu needed for sinew and bone nourishment. Infections can lead to primary or secondary damage to the sinews and bones. High stress levels can result in disequilibrium of the adrenal system with high circulating cortisol levels. Cortisol disequilibrium has been related to the Kidneys in TCM. Chronic high levels of cortisol and Kidney dysfunctions may result in muscle, connective tissue, and bone damage, mostly leading to degeneration (*ibid*). Chronic disorders often affect the normal function of the Kidneys which is needed for bone health as well as nourishment and activation of the Liver, which is then in charge of the sinews and movement of Qi and Blood. Finally, lack of physical activity is increasingly a cause of musculoskeletal pain syndromes. Balanced physical activity is also descried in TCM has important for both physical conditioning as well as Organic health. Excessive physical exercise is thought to damage physical Form as well as the Spleen, Liver, and Kidney systems and their related tissues.

Trauma

Trauma can easily disturb local function and result in poor circulation and/or torn sinews and/or soft tissues. Often this means slight bleeding and hyperemia in the capillary beds, congestion of blood in the precapillary arterioles, edema, accumulation of fluid in the tissue spaces, and petechiae/hematoma/ecchymosis. The result is Blood-stasis and Fluid/fluid accumulation symptoms and signs. Blood-stasis irritates the free nerve endings (nociceptors/pain receptors) found in all connective tissues and leads to inflammation/pain, with or without heat. This process has local and generalized effects via the channel (or neural) systems. Channel (or segmental) effects can result in Organ/organ innervation dysfunction and symptoms. Muscle injury tends to affect the Spleen, sinew damage affects the Liver, and bone damage affects the Kidneys. Local inflammation, swelling, lymphatic congestion, and abnormal fibrosis then lead to the *degenerative cascade*. Facilitated segments are commonly seen (e.g., activation of the Shu-Mu circuits).

The Concept of the Degenerative Cascade in TCM practice[31]

Many patients suffering from musculoskeletal pain, especially in the postural/dysfunction stage, do not present with clear symptoms and signs that correspond to TCM patterns (except channel diagnosis). Understanding the degenerative cascade, the pharmacological effects of herbs, and the physical effects of other traditional interventions can be used to successfully treat these patients. By and large, treatment during the *postural/dysfunction stage* involves: manual therapies to correct joint dysfunctions; channel therapies to open circulation and disperse Pathogenic Factors; and herbs that regulate Qi and Blood circulation, disperse and drain edema, and resolve Pathogenic Factors (depending on cause). Exercise instruction is mandatory if the patient is to arrest the progression of the degenerative cascade and for maintaining the effects of office intervention.

The following formulas can be used as *general* and *flexible guides*, and are often helpful when integrated with manual therapy, acupuncture, and exercise. The first guiding formula can be thought of as treating Pathogenic Factors (possibly) blocking circulation and as moving Qi, Blood, and Fluids. It may be used on patients lacking clear TCM symptoms and signs but whose symptoms are suspected (via the evaluation of risk factors) of being due to Pathogenic Factors. The acrid surface herbs given in small dosages as well as Radix et Caulis (Ci Wu Jia) and Caulis Piperis (Hai Feng Teng) act as vasodilators and increase circulation to *assist* manual and needling therapies:[32]

>Herba Schizonepaetae (Jing Jie) 4g
>Fructus Fossythiae (Lian Qiao) 6g
>Fructus Arctii (Niu Bang Zi) 15g
>Herba Lophtheri (Dan Zhu Ye) 4g
>Rhizoma Ligustici Wallichii (Chuan Xiong) 6g
>Radix Paeoniae Alba (Bai Shao) 6g
>Ramulus Cinnamomi (Gui Zhi) 6g
>Radix Puerariae (Ge Gen) 20g
>Faeces Bombycis (Can Sha) 9g
>Flos Chrysanthemi (Ju Hua) 4g
>Rhizoma Anemarrhenae (Zhi Mu) 4g
>Radix et Caulis Acanthopanacis (Ci Wu Jia) 15g
>Caulis Piperis Kadsurae (Hai Feng Teng) 15g

---

31. Not a classical discussion.

32. It is important to understand that all the formulas in this section have been designed to assist manual and needling therapy. They are not intended to be used on their own. Their utility has been demonstrated often in the author's clinic.

For suspected Phlegm (confusing symptoms that come and go) add: Rhizoma Acrori Graminei (Shi Chang Pu) 6g, Rhizoma Gastrodiae Elatae (Tian Ma) 9g, Herba Eupatorii (Pei Lan) 6g.

For Qi and Blood stagnation (and/or beginning of Deficiency) from daily stress or physical exertion as commonly seen in sedentary patients or athletes that over train (often lacking clear TCM patterns of symptoms and signs) use:

> Rhizoma Curcumae Longae (Jiang Huang) 9g
> Tuber Curcumae (Yu Jin) 6g
> Radix Paeoniae Alba (Bai Shao) 9g
> Fructus Arctii (Niu Bang Zi) 15g
> Poria (Fu Ling) 12g
> Fructus Hordei Vulgaris Geminatus (Mai Ya) 15g
> Radix Astragali (Huang Qi) 12g
> Flos Carthami (Hong Hua) 6g
> Radix Angelicae Sinensis (Dang Gui) 9g
> Semen Citri Reticulatae (Ju He) 6g
> Ramulus Mori (Sang Zhi) 12g
> Herba Eupatorii (Pei Lan) 6g
> Cortex Albizziae (He Huan Pi) 15g
> Caulis Polygoni Multiflorum (Ye Jiao Teng) 15
> Radix et Caulis Acanthopanacis (Ci Wu Jia) 15g
> Caulis Piperis Kadsurae (Hai Feng Teng) 15g

For patients with a *tendency* to develop Interior-Heat signs (often detected only via pulse and tongue) use:

> Flos Chrysanthemi (Ju Hua) 6g
> Poria (Fu Ling) 12g
> Flos Puerariae (Ge Hua) 6g
> Rhizoma Anemarrhenae (Zhi Mu) 4g
> Rhizoma Ligustici Wallichii (Chuan Xiong) 3g
> Fructus Hordei Vulgaris Geminatus (Mai Ya) 12g
> Rhizoma Dioscoreae (Shan Yao) 9g
> Semen Cuscutae (Tu Si Zi) 9g
> Semen Ziziphi Spinosae (Suan Zao Ren) 12g
> Radix Glycyrrhizae Uralensis (Gan Cao) 3g

For Qi-Blood-stagnation (fixed pain felt only at rest that improves temporarily with movement and exercise) add: Rhizoma Curcumae Longae (Jiang Huang) 9g, Tuber Curcumae (Yu Jin) 6g, Ramulus Mori (Sang Zhi) 12g.

For patients who suffer from Deficiency-detriment, mostly from an excessive use of physical resources or from a poor constitution, use modified Young Maiden Pill (Qing E Wan) and Seven-Treasure Special Pill for Beautiful Whiskers (Qi Bao Mei Ran Dan).[33]

While by the time a patient enters the instability stage he/she is likely to present with a clearer TCM pattern diagnosis, some patients do not. In general, once the patient enters the *instability stage,* herbs and acupuncture therapy that increase nourishment to the sinews (mostly ligaments), joints, and bones are needed. More Blood-stasis-resolving and tonic herbs are added, and *strong periosteal* acupuncture is emphasized. The Liver is commonly treated. If needed, the patient is treated with prolotherapy. Strengthening exercises are very important but must be used with care and with an understanding of discogenic pain. Many "back" as well as Tai Chi and Qi Gong exercises can increase symptoms in patients with discogenic pain (especially those that emphasize flexion and pelvic tilts). A *guiding* (general) formula that can be integrated with the above therapies to strengthen the sinews and joints is:[34]

> Radix Notoginseng (San Qi) 20g
> Rhizoma Curcumae Longae (Jiang Huang) 9g
> Cortex Acanthopanacis (Wu Jia Pi) 12g
> Radix Paeoniae Alba (Bai Shao) 15g
> Fructus Arctii (Niu Bang Zi) 30g
> Radix Astragali (Huang Qi) 20g
> Flos Carthami (Hong Hua) 12g
> Radix Angelicae Sinensis (Dang Gui) 12g
> Semen Citri Reticulatae (Ju He) 6g
> Caulis Spatholobi (Ji Xue Teng) 15g
> Herba Lycopodii (Shen Jin Cao) 9g
> Herba Cistanches (Rou Cang Rong) 12g
> Cortex Eucommiae (Du Zhong) 12
> Radix Clematidis (Wei Ling Xian) 9g
> Radix Achyranthis Bidentatae (Huai Niu Xi) 12g
> Ramulus Mori (Sang Zhi) 12g
> Herba Eupatorii (Pei Lan) 6g
> Herba Epimedii (Yin Yang Huo) 9g
> Cortex Lycii Radicis (Di Gu Pi) 20g

Modification of Young Maiden Pill (Qing E Wan) and Seven-Treasure Special Pill for Beautiful Whiskers (Qi Bao Mei Ran Dan) are used often as well.

The *stabilization phase* is by definition a chronic and enduring disease. In TCM, chronic disease is said to be mostly due to Deficiency, blockage, stasis, the network-vessels, and the Liver and Kidney Organs. It is this author's experience, however, that emphasis on resolving blockage/restrictions first may be more important than supplementation of the above Organs, especially when using acupuncture and manual techniques. This means that strong acupoint and dry needling stimulation is often needed, even in elderly or "Deficient" patients. Adhesions may be ruptured by strong manipulative techniques, though care and great skill must be used as the elderly can be easily injured.

Let me Emphasize that herbal treatment must be performed carefully and with the skillful application of TCM methods. Even in older patients, since they are often Deficient, the temptation to tonify too early or too forcefully can be strong. The practitioner must pay attention to blockages/restrictions (Excesses), as these often are the cause of pain, and Excesses can weaken the patient further. At the same time it would be a mistake to ignore a Deficient state; therefore, some support for the patient's Kidneys, Liver, Essence, Blood, Qi, Yin, and Yang are often important. A general

---

33. The ingredients of Young Maiden Pill (Qing E Wan) are: Ginger fried Eucommiae (Jiang Zhi Cao Du Zhong), Wine-fried Psoraleae (Jiu Chao Bu Go Zhi), Juglandis (Hu Tao Ren). Seven-Treasure Special Pill for Beautiful Whiskers (Qi Bao Mei Ran Dan) contains: Polygoni steamed in sesame seeds (He Shao Wu), Poria (Fu Ling), Achyranthis (Niu Xi), Angelica (Dang Gui), Lycii (Gou Qi Zi), Cuscutae (Tu Si Zi), Psoraleae fried with sesame seeds (Bu Gu Zhi).

34. While there are several herbs in this formula that are anti-inflammatory, it is the author's clinical impression that the formula as a whole does not interfere with proper healing after induced ligamentous stimulation by prolotherapy or periosteal needling.

guiding formula that addresses common pathologies at this stage is:

> Radix Angelicae Sinesis (Dang Gui) 9g
> Radix Paeoniae Alba (Bai Shao) 9g
> Radix Rehmanniae (Shu Di) 9g
> Caulis Spatholobi (Ji Xue Teng) 9g
> Scorpio (Quan Xie) 3g
> Semen Sinapis Albae (Bai Jie Zi) 5g
> Agkistrodon Acutus (Bai Hua She) 9g
> Nidus Vespae (Feng Fang) 5g
> Radix Salviae Miltiorrhizae (Dan Shen) 9g
> Fructus Chaenomelis Lagenariae (Mu Gua) 9g
> Radix Astragali (Huang Qi) 12-60g
> Wine fried Rhizoma Rhei (Da Huang) 6g
> Radix Angelicae Dahuricae (Bai Zhi) 5g
> Herba Epimedii (Xian Ling Pi) 5g
> Radix Dipsaci (Xu Duan) 9g
> Cortex Lycii Radicis (Di Gu Pi) 30g
> Herba Siegesbeckiae (Xi Xian Cao) 12g
> Radix Aconiti Lateralis (Fu Zi) 6g
> Spina Gleditsiae (Zao Jiao Xi) 12g
> Rhizoma Pleionis (Shan Ci Gu) 6g

For more Yin-deficiency and Heat add: Radix Rehmanniae (Sheng Di) 12g, Radix Sophorae Flavescentis (Ku Shen) 9g, Rhizoma Anemarrhenae (Zhi Mu) 12g, Radix Pseudostellariae (Tai Zi Shen) 12g.

For stenosis and osteophytes add: Rhizoma Curcumae (E Zhu) 12g, Radix Aconiti Lateralis (Fu Zi) 3-30g, Thallus Algae (Kun Bu) 25g, Radix Scrophulariae (Xuan Shen) 20g, Colla Cornu Cervi (Lu Jiao Jiao) 12g, Herba Ephedra (Ma Huang) 3g.

To transform pathogenic accumulations in Deficient patients who cannot tolerate strong tonification, use:

> Radix Notoginseng (San Qi) 12g
> Rhizoma Atractylodis (Cang Zhu) 4g
> Poriae Cocos (Fu Ling) 9g
> Pericarpium Citri Reticulatae (Chen Pi) 3g
> Rhizoma Cypri Rotundi (Xiang Fu) 6g
> Rhizoma Zingiberis Officinalis (Sheng Jiang) 4g
> Bulbus Fritillaria (Zhe Bai Mu) 15g
> Radix Trichonsanthis Kirilowii (Tian Hua Fen) 12g
> Thallus Algae (Kun Bu) 25g
> Fructus Schisandrae Chinensis (Wu Wei Zi) 6g
> Scorpio (Quan Xie) 5g
> Radix Angelicae Sinesis (Dang Gui) 9g
> Caulis Spatholobi (Ji Xue Teng) 12g

In summary, while the above-discussed approach is not wholly "traditional," the author has used it successfully for many years and in numerous cases when TCM pattern diagnosis was difficult to apply.

Joint Disorders

In this book the term *joint dysfunction* (also called somatic dysfunction), commonly occurring in the spine, is used to describe the loss of intrinsic motions, joint play, or function in the joint complex without obvious pathology. This term implies a loss of motion and usually one or more painful movements. Joint play refers to a motion within a synovial joint, in which the motion is separate from, and cannot be initiated by, voluntary muscle contraction (i.e., it can only be appreciated by motions introduced by the practitioner). Joint motion restriction (dysfunction) represents the end result of a process that probably begins as a neuroreflexive muscle contraction response to trauma, faulty movement patterns, faulty body statics, or viscero-somatic reflexes. With the passage of time, cumulative vascular and connective tissue changes occur in the intrinsic joint tissues and the periarticular tissues, accompanied by a process of general organismic adaptation (Mitchell *ibid*). In chronic cases soft tissues are extensively involved and joint dysfunction is likely to reoccur, often due to instability. (*TCM: In TCM most joint dysfunctions are described as limitations of movements and stiffness.*)

Mechanoreceptors found in the joint capsules (more so than tendon or muscle receptors) are slow-adaptive or non-adaptive. Their effects can be long-lasting both in their ability to maintain dysfunction and in maintaining a therapeutic effect (Brown 1996). These subtle dysfunctions can last for a long time unnecessarily (since they respond to treatment), causing pain and disability. Manual therapy can affect these receptors and result in immediate relief of pain—at least temporarily. Relapses can be challenging to the practitioner. Ligamentous insufficiency or compensations are often the cause.

The Classification of Joint Dysfunctions

Joint dysfunctions can be divided into those caused by internal or intrinsic forces and those caused by external or extrinsic forces (traumas).

Intrinsic Joint Disorders

The proper functioning of a joint relies on diverse factors. Pain and dysfunction can result from interactions among many of these. Often, with unguarded movements (a common cause of intrinsic joint disorders), the driving factor is not that the tissues were injured, or that the joint has an underlying pathology. Rather, a lack of some kind of preparatory integration results in muscle guarding and spasm leading to joint dysfunction. This sudden resetting of muscular tension and length can result in the joint losing normal motion and becoming restricted. This often occurs, not when forces are extreme, but when the patient makes a simple movement absentmindedly or moves from a poor postural position and fails to make preparatory integration. In more chronic cases, ligamentous insufficiency or neural facilitation can be an underlying perpetuating factor.

Extrinsic Causes

Extrinsic injuries are due to trauma. With traumatic injury a small, soft tissue tear can influence joint tensegrity.[35] There may be abnormal load distribution, pain, swelling, muscle guarding and shortening with loss of motion. Trauma can

---

35. Tension integrity.

Joint Disorders

Table 11-1: Chain Joint Muscle Reaction

JOINTS	MUSCLES
Co/C1	Suboccipitals, sternocleidomastoid (SCM), upper trapezius, (masticatories, submandibular)
C1/C2	SCM, levator scapulae, upper trapezius
C2/C3	SCM, levator scapulae, upper trapezius
C3/C6	Upper trapezius, cervical erector spinae, (supinator, wrist extensor, biceps)
C6/T3	SCM, upper or middle trapezius, scaleni, (subscapularis)
T3/T10	Pectoralis, thoracic erector spinae, serratus anterior, (subscapularis)
T10/L2	Quadratus lumborum, psoas, abdominals, thoracolumbar erector spinae
L2/L3	Gluteus medius
L4/L5	Piriformis, hamstrings, lumbar erector spinae, adductors
L5/S1	Iliacus, lumbar erector spinae, hamstrings, adductors
SI JOINT	Gluteus maximus, piriformis, iliacus, adductors, hamstrings, contralateral gluteus medius
COCCYX	Levator ani, gluteus maximus, piriformis, (iliacus)
HIP	Adductors

initiate neural, vascular, and mechanical changes that may cause a "facilitated segment" and chronic dysfunction and pain.

Degree of Joint Dysfunction

Joint restrictions occur within the normal physiologic range of the joint or when joint range is increased (dislocation). One or more vectors of motion are reduced. Dysfunctions are usually seen with some limit in range in varying degrees, and with one vector usually remaining normal.

Subluxation

Subluxations (nonphysiologic dysfunction) result in minor structural changes (minor dislocation) to the joint complex. Therefore, they are not a pure dysfunction; by definition subluxations involves some tissue damage. If a subluxation is extreme, a dislocation occurs and is accompanied by significant structural damage, such as traumatic synovitis and capsular rupture (Garrick 1990).

Hypermobile Joints

Hypermobile joints tend to be more susceptible to developing chronic pain due to ligament sprains, recurrent injury, joint effusions, tendinitis, and early osteoarthritis (Wynne-Davis 1971; Beighton Grahame and Brode 1983).

Hypomobile Joints

Hypomobile joints tend to be more susceptible to muscle strains, tendinitis resulting from overuse, and pinched nerve syndromes (Wynne-Davis 1971; Beighton Grahame and Brode 1983).

SPINAL JOINTS. Most joint dysfunctions in the spine are either caused by, or influence, the zygoapophyseal (facet) joints. Involvement of the vertebral facets can alter normal motion and load distribution. Other structures, especially muscles, are probably involved as well. Changes in load distribution also can result from internal derangement due to excessive forces within a disc or facet meniscus. This can alter facet function and ligament tension and may lead to joint dysfunction without obvious signs of pathology (Wynne-Davis 1986). Hypersensitivity of the joint's type III and IV nociceptors can develop with dysfunction (especially with inflammation) causing hypersensitivity to mechanical stimuli (Willard *ibid*).

Lewit (1991, 1987) identified specific relationships between joint dysfunctions and muscular symptoms, which he called *chain reactions* (Table 11-1).

Prolonged Joint Immobilization

Prolonged joint immobilization can lead to capsular adhesions and decreased ligamentous stress tolerance (Binkley and Peat 1986) and even demineralization (CT 1987; Videman et al 1979). Synovial joints exhibit a 30-40% reduction in concentrations of glycosaminoglycans (GAG) and water content. Loss of the water volume increases friction among the microfibrils and increases the potential for abnormal cross-linking or adhesion formation (Akeson, Amie and Woo 1980) and increasing joint compression (Ombregt et al *ibid*). Other effects of immobilization are increased accumulation of metabolic by-products, muscular atrophy with increase in the relative amounts of connective tissue, and neuromuscular discoordination (Brown *ibid*). Recent studies have demonstrated that disuse of a limb in rodent models can cause pathophysiologic changes that are similar to those that follow nerve injury, including alterations in peripheral nerves and structural and functional alterations in the dorsal horn of the spinal cord (Galer and Dworkin 2000).

The insertion sites of ligaments, tendons, and joint capsules have relatively little vascular supply. Stress and normal joint motion are critical in maintaining tissue integrity at the insertion sites (Noyes et al 1974).

By definition, joint dysfunction results in partial joint immobilization (loss of motion) and therefore may lead to some of the pathologies discussed above. Joint dysfunction is often painful. This can result in protective behavior and further immobilization and therefore should be treated.

It is important to explain to patients with chronic pain that pain does not always equal harm. The natural tendency to refrain from moving a painful body part can result in increased pain, dysfunction, and instability.

Aging

Aging has significant affects on the function of joints and musculoskeletal tissues. Chaitow (*ibid*) discusses connective tissue changes related to aging:

> Aging affects the function of connective tissue more obviously than almost any organ system. Collagen fibrils thicken, and the amounts of soluble polymer decrease. The connective tissue cells tend to decline in number and die off. Cartilages become less elastic, and their complement of proteoglycans changes both quantitatively and qualitatively. The interesting question is how many of these processes are normal and yet contribute blindly and automatically, beyond the point at which they are useful? Does prevention of aging in connective tissues simply imply inhibition of crosslinking in collagen fibrils, and a slight stimulation of the production of chondroitin sulphate proteoglycan?

AGING AND MARTIAL ARTS. Tai Chi has shown to increase endurance and strength in the aged population. It is considered one of the secrets of longevity in the East (Lan, Lai, Chen and Wong 2000). Tai Chi has also been shown to reduce age related bone density loss in the lumbar spine, proximal femur and the ultradistal tibia (Qin, Au, Choy et al 2002). Many Tai Chi systems teach one to control joint play by learning how to open and close joint spaces (a "pumping action") by usage of the small intrinsic muscles. Probably this pumping action also promotes joint function and nourishment. Practice of Tae-kwon-do, a "hard" martial art, has been shown to increase the number of push-ups, degree of trunk flexion and balance time on each foot of elderly individuals practicing Tae-kwon-do (Brudnak, Dundero and Van Hecke 2002).

Somatic Dysfunction

Osteopathic medicine is a system that follows the principle that *structure determines function*, i.e., that structure and function are reciprocally interrelated (Korr *ibid*). *Somatic dysfunction* is therefore an osteopathic term that describes impaired or altered function of related components of the somatic system (skeletal, arthodial, and myofascial structures), and related lymphatic, vascular, and neural elements (and Organs). In the past, somatic dysfunction has been called "osteopathic lesion" (H-ICDA. ED. 3, 1978).

Although not a diagnosis in the regular medical sense, somatic dysfunction describes, in a broad sense, the multiple effects of mechanical dysfunctions, such as how joint dysfunction of the spinal column, pelvis, or extremities may limit motion and produce associated muscular involvement and autonomic reactions such as edema, referred symptoms, and pain (Greenman *ibid*). According to Barral and Croibier (*ibid*), joint dysfunctions (the lesions) as defined in Osteopathy, can occur only as an effect of trauma. The muscular and ligamentous levels do not play a significant restrictive role.

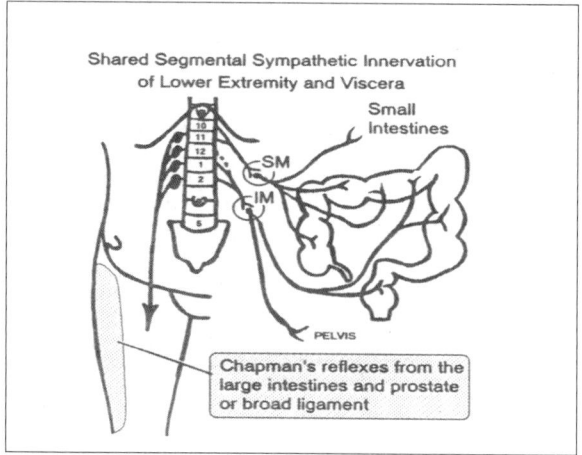

Figure 11-1: Somatovisceral reflexes (From Kuchera WA and Kuchera ML, Osteopathic Principles in Practice, KCOM press 1993, with permission).

Mobility testing reveals a fixed and inelastic barrier in these cases. Barral and Croibier suggest several scenarios:

- Localized drying of the two articular surfaces, modifying the axes of mobility;
- Interruption of the synovial liquid film;
- Indentation and loss of proper alignment of the surfaces;
- Loss of physical capacities (elasticity, plasticity) of the cartilaginous tissue;
- Jamming of bony segments, such as the sacrum between the ilia.

Alone or in combination, these elements are suggested to disrupt articular mechanics through modification of curved surfaces, creation of areas of hypomobility, and changes in axes of mobility. Somatic/joint dysfunction has been classified as (Mitchell *ibid*):

- Acute (short term), characterized by vasodilation, edema, tenderness, and spasm;
- Chronic, characterized by tenderness, fibrosis, paresthesias, and pruritis;
- Secondary, or compensatory, as a result of impairment or pathology in another body part.

Facilitated Segment

Many of the concepts in "somatic dysfunction" came about from work done by the physiologists Sherington, Korr, Denslow and colleagues in the early 1940s and 1950s (Figure 11-2). Through a variety of experiments, including pseudomotor activity as measured by skin resistance, thermography and EMG activity, they studied the osteopathic lesion and showed a complex reaction. Most of this reaction was understood to occur via sympathetic nervous system facilitation. This can develop when a mechanical dysfunction is present (Peterson 1979). As a result of the interconnectedness of the nervous system, when any spinal segment becomes sensi-

Joint Disorders

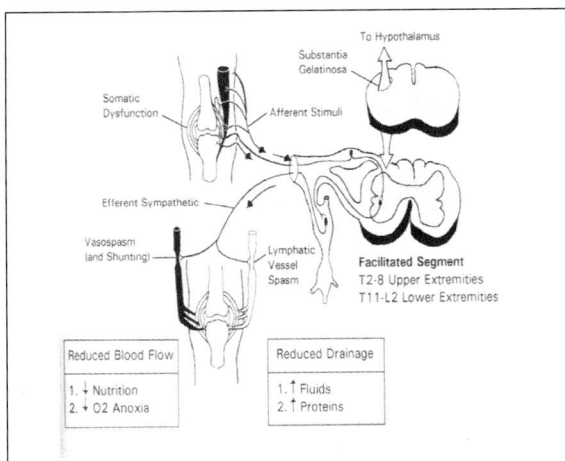

Figure 11-2: Facilitated segment (From Kuchera WA and Kuchera ML, Osteopathic Principles in Practice, KCOM press 1993, with permission).

tized, all of the innervated tissues that are interconnected can become affected and affect each other.

In 1940 Buchthal and Clemmeson noted that a state of enduring muscular excitation in the spinal extensors can be seen in dysfunctional spines. Denslow and colleagues reported that such activity represents chronic segmental facilitation of motor pathways (Denslow, Korr and Krems 1947), which were present mostly in transitional spinal segments (Figure 11-3):

- Occipital-atlanto (OA)
- Cervical- thoracic (CT)
- Thoracic- lumbar (TL)
- Lumbar -sacral (LS).

All of the above are areas where vertebral dysfunctions are found most often. On the average, reflex excitability in response to pressure on the spinous processes is highest in the upper thoracic area and lowest in the midlumbar area. These highly excitable areas are characterized by not only the increased muscular activity in response to pressure on the spinous process, but often by pain and tenderness in the area. In most cases, the individual does not realize that a sensitive area exists. The same pattern of facilitation can occur with psychological stressors. Normal areas remain silent, but low-threshold (facilitated) areas show muscular activity. Although much of our information on the activation of sympathetic afferents (facilitated segments) by skeletal input has come from nociceptive (painful) input, there is evidence that sympathetic output can also be driven independently of nociception by muscle proprioceptors (Patterson and Wurster 2003).

In 1962 Korr, Wright, and Thomas reported that various types of insult, including *disturbed postures* and *injections,* can result in accentuation and increased facilitation of pre-existing facilitated segments. Korr noted that pressure, percussion, other stimulation of the spinous processes of a dys-

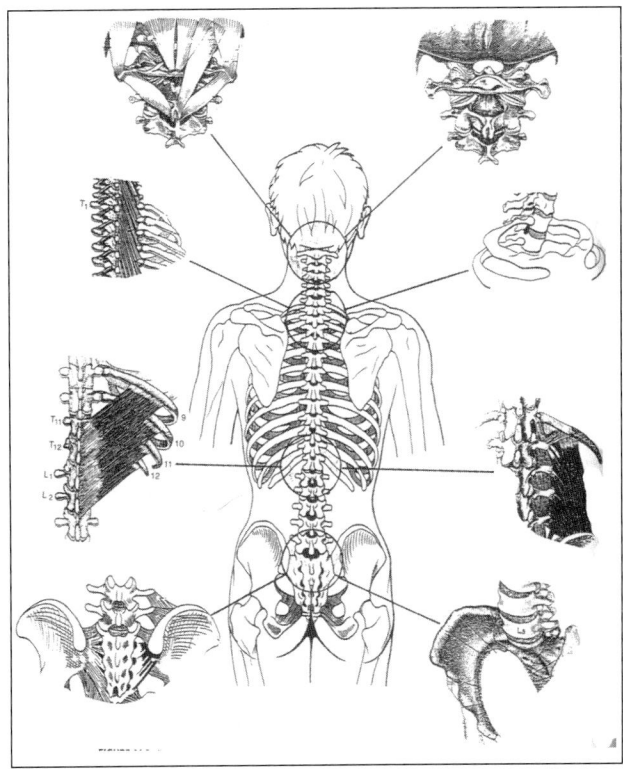

Figure 11-3: Transitional segments. Note the alternating directions of deep myofascial and ligamentous tissues which commonly result in dysfunctions (From Kuchera WA and Kuchera ML, Osteopathic Principles in Practice, KCOM press 1994, with permission).

functional segment, or psychological stress result in the increased electromyographic activity of the corresponding dysfunctional segment. Similar stimulation of the spinous processes of normal segments does not result in such increased activity. However, the stimulation of adjacent "normal" spinal processes may result in increased activity at the dysfunctional segment (referred to as "cross talk"). Percussion of spinous processes is a useful clinical tool for diagnosing somatic dysfunction.

Another important observation by Korr is a relationship between visceral disease and changes of skin resistance. This reduction of skin electro-resistance shows a segmental relationship to the organ involved. Korr reports that in one patient who had been observed for some time, an area of low skin resistance appeared at the appropriate segments three weeks prior to a coronary occlusion. This reinforced the concept of viscerosomatic and somatovisceral reflexes. Changes in spinal cord activity are seen in response to pulmonary afferent stimulation. Electrical stimulation of inflamed tracheobronchial mucosa produces a decrease in electrical skin resistance in the T2-5 dermatomes followed by cutaneous hyperalgesia hours later (Willard *ibid*).

Somatovisceral reflexes demonstrate temporal and spatial summation as indicated by the *windup* phenomenon (sensitization) and the effect of input from different parts of the body. Windup occurs when stimulation is repeated often, and summation occurs when two (or more) different stimuli (from different parts of body, for example) combine to produce a larger response. Windup/winddown is one possible explanation for the additive effects and the need for frequent repetition of therapeutic procedures such as manual therapy (Patterson and Wurster *ibid*) and acupuncture.

Many acupuncture systems and instruments use this phenomenon to diagnose and prescribe treatment for visceral disorders, by evaluating skin impedance at important acupuncture points. According to Dr. Shaw, when *viscerosomatic reflexes* (i.e., lesions originating in internal organs causing somatic symptoms) are responsible for vertebral fixation and somatic symptoms, therapy to the vertebra often results in a very brief change, only one to two hours. Viscerosomatic facilitation should therefore be suspected when patients obtain only short-lasting relief after manipulative therapy. According to Jean Pierre Barral, DO, liver somatic dysfunction is, for example, associated with:

- Restrictions at the thoracic vertebra and rib 7-10;
- Right or bilateral vertebral restriction at C4-C5;
- Right cranial base restriction;
- Glenohumeral periarthritis;
- Sciatica.

Kidney somatic dysfunction is associated with:

- Restrictions of L1-L4;
- Involvement of the knee and foot;
- Lower limb pain due to psoas irritation;
- Glenohumeral periarthritis.

As we can see in Osteopathic medicine, as in TCM, visceral functions are commonly associated with musculoskeletal problems (especially at spine), attention to which may be necessary to resolve pain.

Signs of facilitated segments are often seen as vertebral fixation/dysfunction, tightness and/or weakness and tenderness of the perivertebral muscles adjacent to the dysfunctional vertebra *(OM: or over the Jie Jia and UB acupuncture points)*. Often the deep spinal muscles on one side of the vertebra are hypertonic and those on the other side are hypotonic. Other signs of either denervation or facilitated sympathetics that are often seen are roughness and dryness of the skin over the affected segment (or perivertebral area), and trophic edema at the affected areas or perivertebral area, with sponginess or bogginess of the tissues (Figure 11-4).

Arthritis and Arthrosis

Approximately 40 million Americans suffer from arthritis, costing approximately $54.6 billion annually in medical care and indirect costs. Arthritis is the number one cause of disability in the United States. The number of individuals with arthritis will increase to 59.4 million Americans by the year 2020 (American Arthritis Association).

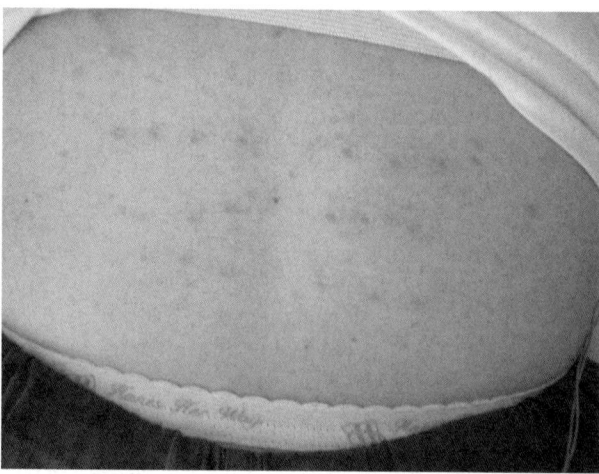

Figure 11-4: Match stick test. The skin is pressed using a dull instrument and the duration of the indentation is compared. The longer and more pronounced the indentations are the more trophic edema is present.

Joint pathology is generally divided into inflammatory and non-inflammatory "arthritis."

Degenerative Joint Disease and Arthritis/Arthrosis

Osteoarthritis (OA), or degenerative joint disease (DJD), is a *non-inflammatory* condition according to radiographic findings. It is characterized by the destruction of articular cartilage, loss of and alterations of subchondral bone, overgrowth of bone with lipping, spur formation, and impaired function. The most common form of arthritis (more appropriately called arthrosis), OA affects more than 40 million Americans. There is a 35% incidence in the knees as early as age 30. Its incidence increases dramatically with age, affecting 80% of persons over the age of 50 (Medical Evidence *ibid*).

OA is usually classified as either primary (idiopathic) or secondary. In the former, no obvious predisposing factor can be identified; in the latter, the arthritis appears to be the result of trauma, repetitive joint use, congenital or developmental defects, metabolic or endocrine disorders, or other factors. Characteristically, the symptoms of OA are use-related joint pain and stiffness after inactivity (posain).[36] According to Alan Gaby, it is estimated that 100,000 people in the United States are unable to walk because of severe OA of the hip or knee. In the past, OA was considered a degenerative disorder, in which the joint gradually "wears out." However, more recent evidence has resulted in a change of thinking concerning the pathogenesis and natural history of OA. It is now known that the joint cartilage of individuals with OA is highly metabolically active, engaging (at least early in the course of the disease) in a process of remodeling and repair of damaged tissue. Arrest or reversal of the disease, once thought to be impossible, has now been shown to

---

36. Positional pain.

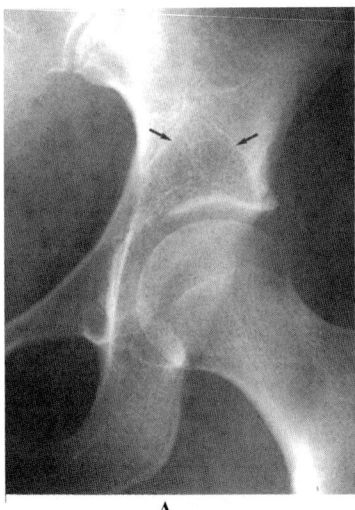 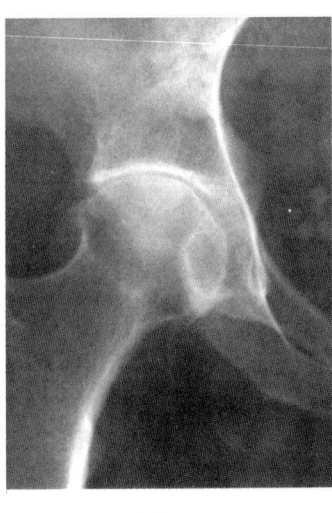 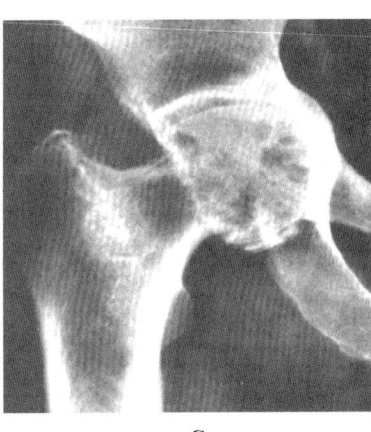

Figure 11-5: X-ray (A) shows a normal hip joint. X-ray (B) shows early degenerative disease. X-ray (C) shows rheumatoid arthritis. Note the uniform loss of joint space as compared to (B). This is the characteristic X-ray finding in rheumatoid arthritis.

occur spontaneously in some individuals with OA (Gaby *ibid*).

Because the environment surrounding the chondrocytes (and cartilage) had been thought to be metabolically inactive, cartilage was thought to "degrade" by being subject to the wear and tear of everyday life. OA and DJD were mostly related to wear and tear of cartilage and old age. However, in recent years a different picture of cartilage metabolism and of the mechanisms involved in damage has emerged. It is now thought to be a disorder of cartilage metabolism or an underlying subchondral bone disorder. The identification of extracellular matrix turnover as a central component of the OA process focused attention on the role of matrix metalloproteinases (MMPs), a family of degenerative enzymes important in the development and normal turnover of all tissues. These enzymes have been shown to be upregulated after joint injury. There is an increase in enzyme activity that parallels the increase in release of collagen and proteoglycan fragments. The finding of increased bone metabolic activity in anatomic association with the involved joint cartilage in OA suggests a close coupling of biologic processes, perhaps both driven by similar mechanisms. A close correlation between positive bone scans and the progression of OA of the knee have been demonstrated. MRI studies have shown that bone marrow edema (actually marrow fibrosis, bone marrow necrosis, and abnormal trabeculae) in patients with knee OA are strong independent predictors of progression of knee OA. Because of the importance of MMP enzymes in cartilage degradation (perhaps affecting bone as well), these enzymes have become a target for potential pharmacological therapy (including the use of glucosamine) to alter the disease process. As MMPs share many structural motifs, it has been possible to develop broad inhibitors of these enzymes, and some of these inhibitors have been tested in humans, including doxycycline (Schnitzer 2004; Spector 2003; Yamada et al 2002; Dodge and Jimenez 2003).

Contrary to popular belief, mild to moderate osteoarthritis often is not painful, as hyaline cartilage and synovium do not contain nerve endings (Wyke 1981). Cartilage is also avascular, and, therefore, damage to cartilage itself is pain-free. The pain associated with OA thus must originate from the surrounding tissues, which are richly innervated by pain endings. Nutrients to the chondrocytes (which are needed for the constant rejuvenation of cartilage) are provided from either the surrounding synovial fluid of the joint or via the underlying bone, which is well vascularities. Degeneration of the joint complex is common with aging, and genetic factors play a major role (Harper and Nuke 1980). If the capsule shrinks and keeps the joint stable, the patient will most likely be pain free and show a capsular pattern of movement limitation with a hard end-feel (Cyriax *ibid*). This condition may be referred to as *osteoarthrosis* (non-inflammatory DJD).

Two phenomena determine the development of arthrosis (Barral and Croibier *ibid*). The first is the gradual degeneration of the cartilage, causing articular incongruence, which modifies in turn the forces of compression and traction exerted on the cartilage. The second is the rapid degeneration of the cartilage during severe contusions or crushing. A simple contusion of cartilage can lead to almost immediate necrosis of the chondrocytes, causing degeneration. Chondrocytes die from loss of proteoglycans, fissure formation, erosion, and eburanation (the disorganization and fragmentation of the superficial layer of cartilage, and the extension of degeneration to a deeper layer).

When arthrosis/osteoarthritis becomes painful, chronic inflammation of the synovium is an important feature in the pathology and pain production. The effects of synovial inflammation probably stimulate pain receptors in the synovial blood vessels, the joint capsule, the fat pads, the collateral ligaments, and the adjacent muscles (Baldry *ibid*).

Osteoarthritis probably is painful only when:

- Active inflammation occurs;
- Nociceptors become oversensitive due to chronic dysfunction and inflammatory mediators (possibly including MDMA receptors within the joint and spinal cord);
- There is an increase of nociceptor rootlets;
- Some mechanoreceptors or sympathetic receptors convert into and function as nociceptors;
- There are bone marrow lesions as seen on MRI (seen as edema);
- There is instability with ligamentous and muscular involvement.

In the advanced stages, when the cartilage is eroded, this condition can become very painful, and joint replacement may be necessary. When degenerative joint disease is accompanied by lax ligaments—a common occurrence—the ligaments may be painful. Proper treatment to them may resolve the pain (Dorman and Ravin *ibid*).

Monoarthritis

Inflammation of a single joint is due most often to injury. Crystalline disease such as gout can also cause a monoarthritis, often first of the big toe. Rheumatoid arthritis can begin in one joint, as well. Other conditions, such as acute exacerbation of degenerative arthritis and, rarely, primary neoplasm of the joint, can present acutely as monoarthritis (Garrick and Ebb 1990).

Oligoarthritis/Polyarthritis

When multiple joints are inflamed (oligoarthritis) and painful, the cause is usually systemic. The leading possibilities are viral (hepatitis, mononucleosis, and rubella) or other infections, autoimmune diseases such as rheumatoid arthritis (RA) and related illnesses. Occasionally a patient may have generalized exacerbation of generalized degenerative arthritis. In rheumatoid type disorders (RA, lupus erythematosus, scleroderma, dermatomyositis), usually the small joints (metacarpophalangeal) are involved first. Reactive type arthritis (e.g., peripheral joint in ankylosing spondylitis, ulcerative colitis, Reither's syndrome, sarcoidosis, or psoriatic arthritis) affects a few large joints (e.g., shoulder, hip, or knee), often asymmetrically. Although both inflammatory and non-inflammatory arthritis can begin at any of the joints, RA most often affects the upper body first (fingers are frequently the first site), while OA/arthrosis most often affects the lower body first (hips and knees). The onset of RA tends to be at a somewhat earlier age than OA, with RA usually starting well before age fifty and OA often starting after age 50. (*OM: Heat often affects the upper body; weakness, Dampness, and degeneration are often worse with age and often affect the lower parts of the body.*) Women are more likely than men to suffer from arthritis of both types (Garrick and Ebb *ibid*; Ombregt et al *ibid*; Brown *ibid*).

CHONDRITIS. Chondritis is the primary response of cartilage to trauma. The thickness and water content of the cartilage markedly increase. This stage, called *edematous chondritis*, is reversible. The next stage, *ulcerative chondritis*, in which the regularity of the surface is disturbed by persistent edema, is partially reversible. If not treated, this leads to chronic ulcerative chondritis, which is irreversible and includes outgrowths on the edges of the articular surface (Barral and Croibier *ibid*).

ALLERGIC SYNOVITIS. Arthritis (mostly the inflammatory types such as rheumatoid arthritis) can sometimes be triggered by certain foods. Food allergy appears to be the mechanism in some patients with synovitis and effusion in joints. In some patients, pain triggered by drinking milk or other foods can occur a few hours after consumption of the offending food. Sometimes arthritis can be triggered by aspirin sensitivity. Leg cramps, swelling, and itching around painful areas may occur due to grass, pollens, house dust, and cat fur (Golding 1990).

FOOD SENSITIVITIES. Food sensitivities are a possible food-related cause of arthralgias, especially in patients with digestive symptoms. Food-related pain is mostly common in inflammatory type arthritis. RAST testing or elimination diet and challenge tests are recommended. Common sensitivities are for milk and dairy products, wheat, eggs, and nuts, although nuts can be therapeutic as well. Food-provoked symptoms may be IgE or IgG mediated. However, many patients do not have evidence of traditional allergies that show with RAST or scratch tests. A leaky gut which may result in large proteins and toxins entering the blood is often the cause.

There are many different ways, known, and unknown, that a food may cause a reaction. The only way to explore this is to perform an elimination and challenge diet. Food reactions may be due to (Hamilton 2001): IgE and IgG-mediated food reactions; possibly, blood-type reactions with specific lectins in foods; metabolic reactions, such as with tyramine-containing foods or monosodium glutamate; reactions that are not immunologically-mediated that occur through the reaction of the white blood cells with a particular food; and finally, transient allergy due to incompletely digested food particles being absorbed by a gut that has increased intestinal permeability.

Whatever the case may be, food elimination, healing the gut mucosa, treating gut pathogens, and using anti-inflammatory nutrients are ways to approach food sensitivity.

THE MAIN JOINTS AFFECTED BY OA INCLUDE:

- Small joints of the hands (mainly the distal interphalangeal joints and thumb base);
- Hips;

- Knees;
- Shoulders and ankles (rarely);
- The facet joints of the lumbar and cervical spine.

The joints affected by OA most often are the knees, hips, spine, and hands.

OSTEOARTHRITIS, BODY MASS, AND ACTIVITY. A study that evaluated physical activity in the presence of knee arthritis has shown an association between activity and knee arthritis. There was a statistically significant positive association between high physical activity and osteoarthritis in women, especially between the ages of fifty-five and sixty-four. A similar trend was seen for men, but it was not significant. Another study involving 166 women and 90 men with knee osteoarthritis found that current body mass index, total body weight, and body mass index at ages twenty-five and forty-five were age-independent predictors of knee osteoarthritis for both males and females. Obesity measured by body mass index increased the risk to osteoarthritis in a "dose-dependent" relationship. This data supports the mechanical etiology for knee osteoarthritis. A metabolic hypothesis cannot be disregarded, however (Orange 1993).

STRESS AND PERSONALITY. In evaluating 128 rheumatoid arthritis (RA) patients and 79 osteoarthritic (OA) patients for the relationship between stress, personality, and disease, it was found that RA patients had more stress at their disease onset than did OA patients. There appeared to be a high stress at onset subgroup of RA patients who had a worse disease prognosis and who corresponded to a personality frequency subgroup (Latman and Walls 1996).

Regeneration of cartilage in rabbits with electrical stimulation has been reported (Beker and Selden 1985). However, the author is not aware of any such evidence in humans. Because of some clinical success, anecdotal observations have suggested that prolotherapy can cause regeneration of cartilage. To date, no study has proven this claim.[37] Recently, surgical scraping and drilling into cartilage have been used to try to regenerate cartilage with variable success. Tissue grafting has been used in early OA, as well. It has also been suggested that glucosamine sulfate can help produce cartilage regeneration, but human studies are scarce. Intra-articular ("purified") hyaluronic acid injections are an FDA approved treatment for knee OA. The injection of 25% dextrose, hyaluronic acid, glucosamine, procaine, B12 and cetamine may work better (Brown personal communication).

Arthritis: TCM Therapy

In 1975 Gaw et al published a study in the *New England Journal of Medicine* on the efficacy of acupuncture on osteoarthritic pain. In this study forty patients with hip, knee, spine, or hand OA were randomly assigned to receive acupuncture or non-acupoint stimulation. Each patient received a total of eight treatments. In this study no difference was found between real point and non-acupoint stimulation in subjective outcomes. Berman et al (2000) in a review article of randomized controlled trials for OA symptoms, has also shown no difference between acupuncture and "sham" acupuncture. However, none of these studies have been sufficiently powered to detect a difference between actual and sham intervention. Furthermore, in all of the studies both groups improved.[38] This may show that insertion of needles to any area of the body has analgesic effects. In 2001 Singh et al assessed seventy-four patients with OA of the knees with twice weekly treatments. Acupuncture reduced pain at four, eight, and twelve weeks, and at four weeks follow-up. Patients improved across the spectrum; however, those who were least symptomatic were most likely to return to a near-normal level of function and to report the absence of chronic pain. Comparing acupuncture to drug therapy has yielded mixed results, some showing superior outcome. One result showed no difference in outcome in cervical spine OA compared to diazepam (Junnila 1982; Berman et al 1995; Thomas et al 1991).

In general, OA in TCM is categorized by all the basic Painful Obstruction (Bi) syndrome categories. These often include acute and chronic stages.

1. Acute stages:

A. Attack by exterior pathogenic Wind, Cold, and Dampness.
   Wind wandering pain is treated with modification of Ledebourella Decoction (Fang Feng Tang).
   Cold painful Bi is treated with modifications of Aconite Decoction (Wu Tou Tang).
   Fixed Damp painful Bi is treated with modification of Coicis Decoction (Yi Yi Ren Tang).

B. Invasion of external pathogenic-Heat or transformative-Heat from prolonged accumulation and obstruction by Pathogenic Factors.
   Heat Bi is often treated with modifications of White Tiger plus Cinnamon Twig Decoction (Bai Hu Jia Gui Zhi Tang).

2. Chronic stages:

- Enduring Painful Obstruction leads to blockage of circulation of both Qi and Blood which accumulate with Phlegm in the channels and collaterals/net-work vessels: Accumulation of Pathogenic Factors in the channels and

---

37. The author has seen one patient with severe (bone on bone) OA of the knee and MS in which after six prolotherapy injections given by her physician, the joint space increased on x-ray, and greatly reduced symptoms were shown.

38. It must be noted that many of these studies have compromised the system of TCM/OM acupuncture in favor of fixed protocols used in modern research. Studies which allow for acupuncture to be tested on its own principles are needed. This would mean no fixed protocols and treatments may change from visit to visit. The dosage and frequency must be appropriate to the condition as well.

collaterals can be treated with modification of Peach Pit and Safflower Decoction (Tao Hong Yin) and Three-Painful Obstruction Decoction (San Bi Tang).

- Consumption of Righteous-Qi by prolonged disease: Treated often with modification of Tang Gui Decoction to Tonify the Blood (Dang Gui Bu Xue Tang), Strengthen Stride Pill (Jian Bu Wan) and Three-Painful Obstruction Decoction (San Bi Tang).
- Damage to the Organ system due to prolonged disease: Damage to the Organ systems is often treated with Angelica Pubescens and Loranthus Decoction (Du Duo Ji Sang Tang) and Restore the Right Decoction (You Gui Yin).[39]

Clinical studies on acupuncture for *rheumatoid* arthritis (RA) are considered less compelling than those of patients with OA (Kolasinski 2002). In general, RA is categorized in TCM similarly to OA, except that, clinically, Heat-types are seen more often. These often include:

1. Acute stages:
   - In early and mild cases, external Wind, Dampness and Cold patterns may be seen. Formulas such as modifications of Ephedra Decoction (Ma Huang Tang), and Warm Channels Remove Painful Obstruction Decoction (Wen Jing Juan Bi Tang) are used.
   - For Wind-Damp and Heat, modifications of White Tiger plus Cinnamon Twig Decoction (Bai Hu Jia Gui Zhi Tang) are often used.
   - Exterior Pathogenic Factors complicated with Blood-stasis are often treated with the addition of modified Drive Out Blood Stasis from a Painful Body (Shen Tong Zhu Yu Tang).
2. Chronic stages and enduring diseases affecting the Righteous-Qi and Organs:
   - For Transformative-Heat and Yin/Blood damage, modifications of Cinnamon Twig, Peony and Anemarrhena Decoction (Gui Zhi Shao Yao Zhi Mu Tang) are often used).
   - For Qi and Blood deficiency and accumulated Phlegm and Blood-stasis, modifications of Drive Out Blood Stasis from a Painful Body (Shen Tang Zhu Yu Tang), Astragalus and Cinnamon Twig Five Materials Decoction (Huang Qi Gui Zhi Wu Wu Tang) and Dang Gui Assuage Pain Decoction (Dang Gui Nian Tong Tang) are used.
   - For Organ involvement modifications of Restore the Right Pill (You Gui Wan) and Kidney Qi Pill (Shen Qi Wan) are often used.

---

39. In this author's experience, response to integrated therapies and TCM is quite varied and often depends on the joint treated. For example, patients with knee and shoulder OA often do better than patients with hip or ankle OA. Patients with severe OA often do poorly, but some get enough pain relief to delay joint replacement. Function, however, is often only minimally improved.

For additional information on TCM treatments see "Painful Obstruction (Bi) Syndromes" on page 659.

Arthritis: Other Natural Therapies

Many natural therapies have been evaluated in the treatment of arthritis. A review article on natural therapies by Pizzorno (1985) suggested that dietary and other natural interventions may be helpful for both inflammatory and non-inflammatory arthritis. Here are a few of the more popular therapies.

1. Professor Norman Childers at Rutgers University found that the elimination of the genus Solanaceae (*the night shade family of plants*) from the diet may be beneficial. This includes tomatoes, potatoes, eggplants, peppers, and tobacco. It is suggested that glycoalkaloids found in Solanaceae plants inhibit normal collagen repair in the joints, or promote inflammatory degeneration.
2. Niacinamide may provide major improvement in osteoarthritis symptoms.
3. Sulfur-containing compounds, including methionine (a sulfur-containing amino acid), are important in the maintenance of cartilage, especially proteoglycans and glycosaminoglycans (GAGs). Injectable glycosaminoglycans polysulfate and activated acid-pepsin-digested calf tracheal cartilage, as well as other glycosaminoglycans, have yielded positive results.
4. Vitamin E at 600 mg a day has shown benefit, possibly due to its membrane-stabilizing effect. This effect may be due to its ability to inhibit the activities of the lysosomal enzymes and stimulate increased deposition of proteoglycan.
5. Vitamin C between 1,000 and 3,000 mg a day can have positive effects on collagen synthesis and repair.
6. Manganese and boron supplementation may be beneficial in OA. Manganese supplementation in animal studies has shown that manganese plays a role in the synthesis of chondroitin sulfate. Boron appears to participate in hydroxylation reactions, which play a role in the synthesis of steroid hormones and vitamin D. In addition to its effects on calcium metabolism, vitamin D plays a role in the normal turnover of articular cartilage.
7. Yucca at 2 to 4 gm 3 times daily is recommended. In a double blind study, the saponin extract of Yucca showed a positive therapeutic benefit.
8. Cherries, hawthorn berries, and blueberries are rich sources of anthocyanidins and proanthocyanidins. These compounds are beneficial in enhancing collagen matrix integrity and structure.
9. Elimination of all refined carbohydrates and increased intake of fish and other "healthy" fatty acids is often recommended as part of the so-called anti-inflammatory diet. For a leaky gut large doses of l-glutamine,

deglycyrrhizinated licorice (DGL), muse paradisiac (plantain banana), ulmus fulve (slippery elm), althaea officinalis (marshmallow), probiotics, and possibly herbs that deal with infections are often recommended.

10. Ginger has been noted in ayurvedic and in OM to be useful in rheumatism.

11. Sea Cucumber has a reputation in the Far East for the management of arthritis.

12. Capsaicin is commonly used in the treatment of arthritis.

13. Articulin-F contains 450 mg of Withania somnifera root, 100 mg of Boswellia serrata stem, 50 mg of Curcuma longa rhizome, and 50 mg of a zinc complex (per capsule) are helpful in OA.

14. Intra-articular ("purified") hyaluronic acid injections may have a protective effect on cartilage damage in osteoarthritic joints.

15. Acetyl merystoleate is reported to help both osteoarthritis and RA.

16. S-Adenosylmethionine (SAMe), a metabolite of the essential amino acid methionine, functions as a methyl donor in many biochemical reactions. In vitro studies have provided evidence that SAMe stimulates the synthesis of proteoglycans by human articular chondrocytes.

17. There have been many studies showing the benefit of essential fatty acid supplements in RA.

18. The systemic effects of oral proteases and peptidases such as Serratia peptidase have been shown to help patients with RA.

19. Boswellia serrata have been used in the treatment of RA and OA.

20. Feverfew has been used for RA and other inflammatory diseases.

21. Sting Nettle extract has been shown to inhibit biosynthesis of acrachidonic acid metabolites.

22. Willow bark extracts contain salicin and other derivatives including, salicylic acid.

23. Folic acid supplementation may lower toxicity in patients treated with methotrexate for RA.

24. If one is taking pharmaceutical NSAIDs, the consumption of deglycyrrhizinated licorice or Robert's formula is recommended to protect the intestinal tract from the damaging effects of the NSAIDs.

25. Methanol extract of the twig of Cinnamomum cassia (Lauraceae), Lycopus europaeus (Lamiatae) and the flower of Chrysanthemum indicum (Asteraceae), and water extracts of the rhizome of Polygonum cuspidatum (Polygonaceae) have shown to inhibit the xanthine oxidase. It may therefore be used to treat gout.

26. A vegan diet has been shown to be helpful for some RA patients.

27. While not a "natural" compound, Doxycycline has been shown to protect articular cartilage (Schnitezer 2004). Celecoxib a pharmaceutical COX-2 inhibitor has been shown to protect articular cartilage as well.

Other treatments that have been shown to be helpful:

1. Pulsed electromagnetic fields may be of benefit as shown in a double-blind study.

2. Exercise therapy is very important.

3. Photopheresis may be helpful in seronegative psoriatic arthritis and RA.

4. Counseling and special stress management skills are helpful for RA patients.

5. Photonic and laser therapy may be useful.

Arthrosis/Osteoarthritis

NIACINAMIDE. According to Dr. Kaufman treatment with niacinamide usually results in an increase in joint mobility (measured objectively), as well as subjective improvements in joint discomfort, inflammation, and pain. Although its mechanism of action is not known, niacinamide does not appear to act merely as an anti-inflammatory agent or analgesic. Improvement usually occurs after three to four weeks of treatment. Kaufman observed that niacinamide was most effective when taken in frequent, divided doses—250mg taken six times per day was more effective than 500mg taken three times per day. Time release niacinamide capsules, 400mg three twice a day, is the modern version of his regime. The condition is controlled, but not cured, so it is necessary to continue with the treatment for long periods. Kaufman also suggested it is occasionally useful in rheumatoid arthritis. Niacinamide is generally well tolerated and appears to be relatively safe for long-term use. Liver damage and glucose intolerance are possible side effects of this treatment; thus periodic liver function and glucose tolerance tests are warranted. A test at three months and one year, and the absence of deterioration, are considered adequate safeguards. Hepatic dysfunctions with doses under 3gm per day are unlikely. Some patients receiving long-term niacinamide treatment maintained improved joint function (as demonstrated by an increase in joint range index) for as long as twenty years. However, patients who stopped taking the vitamin gradually reverted to their pre-treatment status. A recent double-blind study (Jonas et al 1996) supports Kaufman's observations. In that study, seventy-two patients with OA of at least five years' duration were randomly assigned to receive niacinamide (500 mg six times per day) or a placebo for twelve weeks. Outcome measures included global arthritis impact, pain, joint mobility, and erythrocyte sedimentation rate (ESR). Global arthritis impact improved by 29% in patients receiving niacinamide and worsened by 10% in patients given a placebo (p = 0.04 for difference between groups). Although pain levels were not different in the two groups, patients on niacinamide reduced their anti-inflammatory medication by 13%, compared to a slight increase in medication in the placebo group (p = 0.014 for difference between groups). ESR in the treatment group was reduced by 22% compared with placebo (p < 0.005) and increased joint mobility (as measured by the joint range index) by 8.0 degrees, compared with 3.5 degrees in the placebo group (p = 0.04).

GLYCOSAMINOGLYCAN. Glycosaminoglycan (GAGs) injections into the knee in a double-blind, placebo-controlled trial showed immediate decrease in the pain after the injections of 43% with the GAGs and 33% with the placebo. Pain relief in the GAGs versus the placebo was not different at other intervals. At six weeks the Lequesne Index decreased 20% after the GAGs and 9% after the placebo. At ten weeks the Lequesne Index decreased 24% after the GAGs and 13% after the placebo. The decrease in the Lequesne Index at thirteen weeks was 31% after the GAGs and 15% after the placebo. Other measured parameters tended to be more favorably influenced by the GAGs than placebo. Minimal side effects occurred in approximately 8% of the cases (Pavelka, Karel et al 1995).

CHONDROITIN SULFATE. Chondroitin sulfate (CS) is a term used to denote a group of structurally similar polysaccharides, typically comprised of sulfated and unsulfated residues of glucuronic acid and N-acetylglucosamine. CS is one of the components of proteoglycans, the macromolecules that contribute to the structural and functional properties of joint cartilage. There is evidence that CS stimulates the synthesis of proteoglycans by chondrocytes (Gaby *ibid*). CS has been compared to nonsteroidal anti-inflammatory drugs (NSAIDs) in a randomized, multicenter, double-blind study, using 400mg chondroitin sulfate three times per day. Patients treated with NSAIDs had rapid and plain reduction of clinical symptoms, which reappeared after the end of the treatment. In the CS group, however, the therapeutic response appeared later in time *but lasted up to three months* after the end of treatment. Chondroitin sulfate had a slow but gradual increase in clinical activity in osteoarthritis, and these benefits lasted after the end of treatment (Morreale, Manopulo, Galati, et al 1996).

GLUCOSAMINE SULFATE. Glucosamine, which is produced in the body from glucose, is a precursor molecule in the synthesis of proteoglycans. Glucosamine has been reported to stimulate proteoglycan synthesis in vitro, to inhibit its degradation, and to rebuild experimentally damaged cartilage. Glucosamine sulfate (GS) stimulates cartilage regeneration, protects against joint destruction (in vivo), and alleviates the symptoms of knee osteoarthritis. GS is not an analgesic; it takes several weeks before a symptomatic relief can be obtained. The usual dose is 500mg three times per day. GS has been shown to help knee arthritis when injected (Reichelt, Forster, Fischer et al 1994) and when taken orally (Lopes Vaz 1982). Scanning electron microscopy performed on the cartilage obtained from patients receiving GS showed a picture more similar to healthy cartilage. Patients in the placebo group showed a typical picture of established OA (Drovanti, Bignamini, Rovati 1980). A newly published study in the journal *Menopause* (2004) reported a disease-modifying effect for GS in the treatment of knee OA in postmenopausal women. After three years, women taking 1500 mg/day of crystalline GS experienced no, or minimal, joint space narrowing as compared to placebo (6.9% vs 20.6% in the placebo group had more than 0.5mm narrowing). Scores for pain and function were improved for GS over placebo, but stiffness scores were similar between the two groups. Recently, concern has been expressed about the potential for GS to induce insulin resistance, because it can do so when used in animals via intravenous infusions. The relevance of this to humans is not clear (Baron et al 1995).

GLUCOSAMINE SULFATE VS CHONDROITIN. According to Alan Gaby (*ibid*) there has been an ongoing debate concerning whether GS or CS is the preferable therapeutic agent, or whether these compounds should be used in combination. Orally administered GS has been shown to be well-absorbed. On the other hand, CS is a relatively large molecule and is presumably hydrolyzed in the intestinal tract prior to being absorbed. While some CS does appear to be absorbed intact, the proportion of an oral dose that is absorbed is said to be small. Some have argued that CS is largely broken down in the gastrointestinal tract and then reassembled after being absorbed. If that is true, administering CS is merely an expensive way to obtain precursor molecules. Since GS serves as a precursor to, and appears to promote the synthesis of, CS, administering GS may be a less expensive method of increasing the CS content of joint cartilage. On the other hand, it is conceivable that the small amount of CS that does get absorbed (or perhaps one of its byproducts of partial digestion) exerts beneficial effects that cannot be duplicated by giving GS. To date, there have been no studies comparing the efficacy of GS and CS, or comparing the combination to either compound by itself. Until such studies are done, the choice of which regimen to use remains a matter of individual preference.

It is this author's observation that GS, CS or the combination of both is mostly helpful symptomatically in the early stages of OA of the knee. Patients with more severe disease more often than not report little or no benefit, although GS may slow down the progression of the disease.

GINGER. Ginger has been noted in ayurvedic and OM to be useful in inflammation and "rheumatism." Ginger has been shown to be helpful in 261 patients with knee osteoarthritis and moderate-to-severe pain, in a randomized double-blind, placebo-controlled, multicenter, parallel group, six-week study. It showed that *ginger extract* containing 255mg and 500-1,500mg of dried galanga rhizomes given twice daily can result in a reduction in knee pain on standing. Evaluating secondary efficacy variables showed a consistently greater response in the ginger extract group compared with the control group. There was a reduction in knee pain on standing, a reduction in knee pain after walking fifty feet, and a reduction in the Western Ontario and McMaster Universities osteoarthritis composite index that was greater in the ginger group compared with the placebo group. The change in global status and reduction in intake of acetaminophen were greater in the ginger extract group. The subjects who received ginger extract had more gastrointestinal complaints than the placebo group. These GI complaints were mostly mild (Altman and Marcussen 2001).

Ginger also has been shown to be helpful in inflammation and rheumatism in a study of twenty-eight patients with rheumatoid arthritis, eighteen with osteoarthritis, and ten with muscular discomfort using *powdered ginger*. In the arthritic patients, over 75% had varying degrees of relief from pain and swelling. All of the patients with muscular discomfort had pain relief. There were no reported side effects with regard to ginger consumption from three months to two and one half years. Doses ranged from 50gms of raw fresh ginger daily, to 3 or 4 gms of powdered ginger, per day (Srivastava and Mustafa 1992).

Ginger is known to act as a dual inhibitor of both cyclooxygenase and lipoxygenase; it can inhibit leukotriene and prostaglandin synthesis and can reduce carrageenan-induced raw-paw edema in animal models of inflammation. Ginger has also been shown in *in-vitro* studies to inhibit the production of tumor necrosis factor through inhibition of gene expression in human osteoarthritic synoviocytes and chondrocytes (Hamilton 2001).

SEA CUCUMBER. Sea Cucumber has a reputation in the Far East for the management of arthritis. The scientific name is *Pseudocolochirus axiologus*. The creature contains a multitude of biologically active chemical moeities, one of which, holothurin, is effective against arthritis and some against cancer. The dose is 500mg BID with food (Dorman, personal communication).

CAPSAICIN. The following information comes from a practitioner perspective article by Deal and Chad (1994). Capsaicin is commonly used in the treatment of arthritis. Topical capsaicin (extracted from chili papers) may be beneficial in: diabetic neuropathy, post-herpetic neuralgia, post-mastectomy pain syndrome, reflex sympathetic dystrophy, and other musculoskeletal pain. Purified capsaicin has its effect on type C-fibers sensory neurons. It depletes substance P, a neurotransmitter of pain, from type C-neurons. Substance P is involved also in the exacerbation of the inflammation of arthritis. When type C-neurons are repeatedly exposed to purified capsaicin, they cease to synthesize, store, and release substance P. The pain impulses are diminished. Substance P and prostaglandin PG2 levels in synovial tissue decrease with regular joint application of topical capsaicin. Patients suitable for capsaicin therapy include those with one or two painful joints. Two strengths of topical capsaicin are available: 0.025% and 0.075%. For most patients with mild to moderate pain, 0.025% strength is a logical place to start. Patients should be instructed to apply a small amount of capsaicin to the skin covering the affected joint. For example, for a knee, a pea-size dab of cream is sufficient. Capsaicin should be applied three to four times a day. Once pain relief has been established with four times a day, it can be reduced to two times a day, depending on pain relief. Patients should be directed to wash their hands thoroughly after applying capsaicin cream, because inadvertent transference can cause temporary burning and stinging in the eyes or other sensitive mucous membranes (a roll-on is available). Relief usually occurs within a few days. Adverse effects can be burning and stinging. The burning may be as short lived as two to four days or may last. It is often worsened after bathing while exercising or perspiring. Topical anesthetics such as lidocaines before application of the cream may reduce burning. The patient should be instructed to continue applications for at least two weeks before evaluation of efficacy. No apparent systemic effects, including drug-drug-food reactions, have been reported.

A recent systematic review of topical capsaicine by Mason et al (2004) concluded that topically applied capsaicine has moderate to poor efficacy in the treatment of chronic musculoskeletal or neuropathic pain, but may be useful for some patients.

In this author's experience, capsaicin role-on (which also contains Boswellia serrata and Methyl-sulfonyl-methane, or MSM) has been somewhat useful in arthrosis, rheumatoid arthritis, tendinitis of most tendons, including epicondylitis, and bursitis. Patient compliance, however, can be problematic due to burning, especially when taking a shower or bath.

ARTICULIN-F. Forty-two patients with OA were randomly assigned to receive, in double-blind fashion, either an Ayurvedic preparation (Articulin-F) or a placebo for three months, and the alternate treatment for an additional three months. A capsule of Articulin-F contains 450mg of radix Withania somnifera, 50mg of rhizome Curcumae longa, 50mg of a zinc complex and 100mg of Boswellia serrata stem. Two capsules three times per day were given after meals. Compared with the placebo, Articulin-F significantly reduced the severity of pain and the disability score. Side effects included nausea (n = 2), dermatitis (n = 3), and abdominal pain (n = 3), none of which required discontinuation of treatment (Kulkarni et al 1991).

ANTIOXIDANTS. Antioxidant intake may be protective against the *progression* of osteoarthritis and development of pain, but not in *prevention* of osteoarthritis. A study that evaluated 640 participants found the incidence and progression of osteoarthritis in eighty-one and sixty-eight knees respectively. There was no significant association between the incidence of arthritis and any nutrient. There was a threefold reduction in the risk of osteoarthritis progression found for both the middle tertile and the highest tertile of vitamin C intake. This related mostly to a reduced risk of cartilage loss. Those with high vitamin C intake also had a reduced risk of developing *knee pain*. A reduction in the risk of osteoarthritis progression was seen for beta-carotene and vitamin E intake, but they were less consistent. A high intake of antioxidant nutrients, particularly vitamin C, may reduce the risk of cartilage loss and disease progression in people with osteoarthritis (McAlindon, Timothy et al 1996).

Vitamin E may be helpful and compares favorably to NSAIDs. Scherak, Kolarz, Schodl, Blankenhorn (1990) studied fifty-three patients with OA of the hip or knee and were treated for three weeks with vitamin E (d-alpha-tocopheryl acetate 400mg three times per day, equivalent to approximately 600IU three times per day) or diclofenac (50mg three times per day). Both treatments appeared to be equally effective in reducing the circumference of knee joints and walking time, and in increasing joint mobility. Machtey and Ouaknine (1978) studied twenty-nine patients with OA at various sites in a single blind fashion. Patients were randomly assigned to receive either 600mg of vitamin E per day or a placebo for ten days, and then the alternate treatment for an additional ten days. 52% percent of the patients reported a reduction in pain while receiving vitamin E, compared with only 4% receiving placebo (p < 0.01). Although the mechanism of action of vitamin E against OA is unknown, vitamin E has been reported to have anti-inflammatory activity and may also inhibit prostaglandin synthesis. Vitamin E may also help stabilize lysosomal membranes, thereby inhibiting the release of enzymes believed to play a role in inflammation and in the pathogenesis of osteoarthritic joint damage.

MANGANESE. Animal studies have shown that manganese plays a role in the synthesis of chondroitin sulfate, an important component of articular cartilage. Manganese deficiency has been found to cause a cartilage metabolism disorder in farm animals. This condition is said to resemble Mseleni joint disease, an OA-like disease endemic to a remote part of Zululand, where dietary intake of manganese is believed to be low. It is not known whether manganese deficiency plays a significant role in the pathogenesis of OA; however, one cannot rule out the possibility of subtle manganese deficiency in Western societies. According to Pfeiffer, modern farming techniques deplete manganese from the soil, resulting in lower concentrations of manganese in food. In addition, individuals who consume refined grains (such as white bread) obtain only half as much manganese in their diet as those who eat whole grains (Gaby *ibid*).

BORON. Boron appears to participate in hydroxylation reactions, which play a role in the synthesis of steroid hormones and vitamin D. In a double-blind study, twenty Australians with OA were randomly assigned to receive boron (6mg per day as sodium tetraborate decahydrate) or a placebo for eight weeks. Of those receiving boron, 50% improved, compared with 10% of those given the placebo. Because of the small sample size, this difference was not statistically significant. When the five subjects (25%) who dropped out of the study (mostly because of clinical deterioration) were excluded from the analysis, 71% of those in the boron group improved, compared with 12.5% of those in the placebo group (p < 0.05). No side effects were seen, and there were no significant changes in common laboratory parameters. These results suggest boron supplementation may be helpful for individuals with OA whose diets are likely to be low in boron (the soil in Australia is low in boron). Further research is needed to confirm this preliminary study and to determine whether individuals with a higher dietary intake of boron can benefit from supplementation. The average American diet provides approximately 1-2mg of boron per day, primarily from fruits, vegetables, and nuts; however, according to German research, intake can vary from 0.3 to 41mg per day. While the capacity of boron to increase estrogen levels might raise concerns about possible cancer risks with boron supplementation, there is no evidence that populations with a high intake of boron (such as the French) have an increased incidence of hormone-related cancers (Gaby *ibid*).

HYALURONIC ACID. Intra-articular ("purified") hyaluronic acid injections may have a protective effect on cartilage damage in osteoarthritic joints. This occurs by the removal of noxious substances from the joint space through the lymphatic system (Ghosh, Peter et al 1995). However, a five year follow-up study of the relationship between hyaluronic acid and osteoarthritis of the knee showed that *higher* hyaluronic acid levels were significantly related to disease duration, minimum joint space and previous surgery at *entry-baseline* of patients studied. The data suggested that hyaluronic acid levels predict disease outcome of osteoarthritis of the knee, and confirmed that a serum level of keratin sulfate was not a useful prognostic marker for osteoarthritis (Sharif, Mohammed, et al 1995). Hyaluronic acid is also available in oral form and is reported to be helpful for OA.

ACETYL MERYSTOLEATE. Acetyl merystoleate (CMO) is a product obtained from mice. In the 1970's Dr. Dehl, working at the NIH, discovered that mice do not ordinarily suffer from arthritis; they have a metabolic product CMO, which is peculiar to their species. Dr. Dehl has "cured" his own arthritis and that of friends with this product. It seems that there are at least three sources of this material with varying degree of purity. As far as Dr. Wright was able to determine in July 1996, the best comes from Dr. Dehl and his daughter. The name they use is *Myristin*. It is recommended that one capsule be taken twice daily for five days (only). This may need to be repeated once at most. Benefits from Myristin has been reported in other health problems including emphysema, chronic bronchitis and hypertension. Other animals that contain this substance are sperm whales and male beavers. (Dorman, personal communication).

S-ADENOSYLMETHIONINE (SAME). A metabolite of the

essential amino acid methionine, SAMe functions as a methyl donor in many biochemical reactions. In vitro studies have provided evidence that SAMe stimulates the synthesis of proteoglycans by human articular chondrocytes.

Extensive clinical trials, that enrolled approximately 22,000 patients suggest that SAMe is as effective as NSAIDs in the treatment of OA, but is better tolerated. In one study, 734 patients with OA were randomly assigned to receive, in double-blind fashion, a placebo, SAMe (1,200 mg per day), or naproxen (750 mg per day) for thirty days. The reduction in pain and improvement in function were similar in the SAMe and naproxen groups, and both active treatments were significantly more effective than the placebo. For most parameters measured, naproxen was significantly more effective than placebo by day fifteen, whereas with SAMe statistical significance was not seen until day thirty. SAMe was better tolerated than naproxen, both in terms of physicians' ($p < 0.025$) and patients' ($p < 0.01$) assessments, and in terms of the number of patients with side effects ($p < 0.05$). There was no difference between SAMe and placebo in the number of side effects.

In a study involving seventy-six patients, 1,200 mg per day of SAMe was significantly more effective than placebo at relieving pain. The same dose of SAMe was also as effective as indomethacin (150 mg per day) and ibuprofen (1,200 mg per day), as assessed by standard scoring systems for various clinical parameters.

Crystalline SAMe degrades rapidly upon exposure to heat or moisture, and some of the imported raw material has been said to be partially decomposed upon arrival. Therefore, it may be preferable to use the enteric-coated, pharmaceutical-grade tablets imported from Europe rather than other preparations being sold in the United States (Gaby *ibid*).

Concerns about SAMe and some cancers have been raised. SAMe may stimulate the growth of melanomas by supporting synthesis of spermidine or spermine, which are needed for mitosis (Gutman et al 1990). SAMe as a precursor of polyamines is essential for melanoma proliferation or spreading. There is a compound reported by CIBA-GEIGY, CGP 48662, which is an inhibitor of SAMe decarboxylase and is described to have "broad antiproliferative and antitumor activity." A group at Anderson Cancer Center working with the same SAMe decarboxylase inhibitor and seven different human melanoma cell lines demonstrated varying levels of cytostasis in vitro, depending on cell line. Based on this, two cell lines were introduced into nude mice then treated with CGP 48662. In the case of highly metastatic but CGP 48662 sensitive lines, these mice had significantly reduced size of cutaneous lesions and number of lung metastases was seen. Thus suppression of SAMe may be therapeutic in some cancer patients (Potts personal communication).

DMSO. DMSO has been used in the treatment of arthritis. It has the ability to be quickly absorbed when applied to the skin as well as to increase the absorption of other medication when applied together. It has been suggested that Acetyl merystoleate (CMO) applied directly over the affected part of the body with DMSO is particularly helpful. The concentration of DMSO in water needs to be balanced carefully. At present, 70% seems the optimal. If the concentration is too high, it is apt to be hydroscopic, and, if too low, it would not carry the substance through the skin into circulation. It has also been found that mineral deficiency contributes to degenerative arthritis, both osteoarthritis and rheumatoid arthritis. The best of both worlds, therefore, seems to add some minerals to the DMSO at the same time. Vanadium, chromium, selenium, boron, and others are included in what has become the Tahoma (Dr. Wright's) clinic dispensary's routine. The capsule of the Myristin oil can be opened, applied to the skin, and then rubbed in with *"DMSO with minerals."* The skin surface needed might be as much as the front of the whole thigh on both sides (Dorman, personal communication). MSM and DMV are related compounds that may be taken orally, topically or by injection. DMSO can be used to extend and increase by as much as 1000 fold the strength and penetration of injected steroids. A very small dose of steroid can then go a long way (Brown and Eke personal communication).[40]

PULSE ELECTROMAGNETIC FIELDS. A double-blind pilot study involving twenty-seven patients with osteoarthritis, predominantly of the knee, were treated with pulsed electromagnetic fields that consisted of eighteen half-hour periods of exposure to an extremely low frequency (less than 30 Hz). The varied pulsating electromagnetic fields averaged ten to twenty gauss of magnetic energy, and each coil current was up to two amps. The pulsed phase duration was sixty-seven ms, including fifteen micropulses with a pause duration of 0.1 second. These sessions occurred at a frequency of three to five per week and extended over approximately one month. Twenty-five of the twenty-seven patients completed the study. In patients with active treatment, there was an average improvement of 34% at midpoint, 36% at the end of treatment and 47% one month later. The placebo group showed an average improvement of 8% at midpoint, 10% at the end of treatment, and 14% one month later. No toxicity was noted. The authors conclude that the decreased pain and improved functional performance of these patients treated with pulse electromagnetic fields suggest that this modality has potential as an effective means of improving symptoms in osteoarthritic patients (Trock and David et al 1993).

EXERCISE. The Arthritis Foundation states that physical therapy may be the most valuable treatment for the estimated 16 million people in the United States who have osteoarthritis. Systematic reviews and subsequent RCTs have found that both exercise and education may help reduce the burden

---

40. A solution made of 50 cc 0.5% procaine or lidocaine mixed with 10 mg of triamcinolone and 1/2 to 1 cc of pharmaceutical DMSO can be used to treat neuropathic pain felt in sensitive muscles quite successfully (Klein 2004).

of pain and disability in people with hip or knee osteoarthritis, and had the strongest evidence for any of the non-invasive or chemical interventions (i.e., strongest evidence for physical medicine interventions). Practitioners should prescribe a low impact exercise program that involves keeping the joints flexible, preserving the strength of the muscles on which the joints depend for their stability, and protecting diseased joints against further damaging stresses. Those with osteoarthritis may benefit by doing exercise in the morning. Trying to achieve ten repetitions is beneficial, but if the pain persists they can go down to five repetition of each of the affected joints. If they have no pain they should work toward twenty or more repetitions (Hamilton *ibid*). These should include both stretching and strengthening movements.

DOXYCYCLINE. Although not a "natural" substance, doxycycline may reduce OA progression, as it is known to inhibit activity of matrix metalloproteinases (MMPs). This activity in not related to antibacterial activity, and a family of chemically modified tetracyclines that have no anti-infective characteristics has been developed. Doxycycline itself has been tested for its ability to prevent tissue matrix degradation in the clinical setting of periodontitis. The doses needed to prevent the progression of gingival MMPs (20 mg orally twice daily) do not provide clinically meaningful antimicrobial activity. In a human study, doxycycline was compared to placebo for inhibition in collagenous and gelatinous (MMPs) activity in the removed cartilage of patients undergoing joint replacement surgery, with one group receiving doxycycline preoperatively, taking 100 mg twice daily. Doxycycline was shown to reduce enzyme activity to a significant degree compared with the values obtained from the placebo-treated individuals. It can also inhibit C-reactive protein (CRP).

CELECOXIB. Although not a "natural" substance, the cyclooxygenase-2 (COX-2) inhibitor celecoxib as been shown to "enhance the rate of synthesis of both hyluronan and proteoglycans, and concomitantly reduce the net loss of these two glycosaminoglycans." It may therefore have protective affects on osteoarthritic cartilage (Manicourt et al 2003). If the findings of this study are replicated, this NSAID may become the preferred pharmaceutical in the treatment of arthritis.

Rheumatoid and Inflammatory Arthritis

ESSENTIAL FATTY ACIDS. Greenland Eskimos and the Japanese population have a relatively low incidences of inflammatory disease. This may be related to their consumption of cold-water marine fish. There have been many studies showing the benefit of essential fatty acid supplements in Rheumatoid arthritis (RA) patients. Positive effects of altering dietary essential fatty acids on dosage and usage of nonsteroidal anti-inflammatory (NSAIDs) drugs in rheumatoid arthritis have been shown (Belch et al 1988). The effect from NSAIDs is mediated through inhibition of cyclo-oxygenase (COX) enzymes, thereby decreasing production of the two-series prostaglandins (PGs). The lipoxygenase enzyme is not affected, however, allowing leucotriene (LT) production, e.g., LTB4 (an inflammatory mediator). Treatment with evening primrose oil (EPO), which contains gamma-linolenic acid (GLA), leads to production of the one-series PGs, e.g., PGEI, which has fewer inflammatory effects. GLA can inhibit LT production as well. Eicosapentaenoic acid (EPA, fish oil) treatment provides a substrate for PGs and LTs, which lead to less inflammation (Dorman personal communication). Patients deficient in essential fatty acids are often thirsty and have dry skin and hair.

A number of studies, including placebo-controlled studies, have shown GLA to be an effective treatment for rheumatoid arthritis in doses ranging from approximately 500 mg to 6 gm of GLA from borage oil or primrose oil.[41] Fatty acids can regulate *cell activation, immune responses,* and *inflammation*. Fatty acid supplementation appears to be well tolerated and is an effective treatment for diseases characterized by *acute* and *chronic inflammation* (Rothman, Deborah et al 1995). Omega-3 fatty acids (fish oils) produce moderate benefit in RA, but much less than Naproxen (NSAID).

An in-vitro study showed that incorporation of omega-3 fatty acids into articular cartilage chondrocyte membranes results in a dose-dependent reduction in the expression and activity of proteoglycan degrading enzymes. The expression of inflammation induces cytokines and cyclooxygenase-2 (COX-2), but not the constitutively expressed COX-1. Omega-3 fatty acid supplementation can specifically affect regulatory mechanisms involved in chondrocyte gene transcription. Omega-3 fatty acid supplementation can affect molecular mechanisms that regulate the expression of catabolic factors involved in articular cartilage degradation (Curtis, Hughes, et al 2000). GLA is also helpful in treating neuropathic pain, mostly helping in repairing the nerves.

PROTEASE AND PEPTIDASE ENZYMES. Several studies refer to the systemic effects of oral proteases and peptidases such as Serratia peptidase (SP). Some studies show repression of edema and repression of blood-vessel permeability induced by histamine or bradykinin. These enzymes also affect the kallikrein-kinin system and the complement system, thus modifying the inflammatory response. Clinically, SP has been used as an anti-inflammatory agent in the treatment of RA, traumatic injury, and post-operative inflammation, as well as in chronic sinusitis, to improve the elimination of bronchopulmonary secretions and to facilitate the therapeutic effect of antibiotics in the treatment of infections. In the urological field, SP has been used successfully for cystitis and epididymitis (Dorman personal communication). Bromelain is a proteolytic enzyme that comes from the stem of the pineapple plant. It has long been used to reduce swelling and inflammation. Bromelain is used at 80-320 mg/day.

BOSWELLIA SERRATA. Gum resin extracts of Boswellia ser-

---

41. However some studies show that only evening primrose oil, or pure GLA work.

rata have been used in the treatment of RA. The terpenoids and gum resin are potent anti-inflammatory compounds that inhibit 5-lipoxygenase. In evaluating more than 260 individuals with RA, Boswellia extract was found to be effective. Boswellia extract is a disease-modifying agent and can replace other disease-modifying therapies. Early use is beneficial. Therapy is well-tolerated and shows high levels of safety for early use and long-term therapy. The long-term effects of Boswellia extracts on the joints and the anatomy, however, are not yet clear. Dose ranges are three 400 mg tablets two or three times daily (Etzel 1996).

FEVERFEW. Tanacetum parthenium (feverfew) has been used for RA and other inflammatory diseases. Volatile oils are its chief constituents along with sesuiterpene lactones, especially with parthenolide being most active (Goenewegen and Knight 1986). Extracts rich in sesuiterpene lactones can produce dose-dependent inhibition of thromoxane B2 and leukotriene B4, and thus have anti-inflammatory effects (Summer 1992). Feverfew can be prescribed at 25-150 mg/day of dried powdered leaf, or 150-250 mg/day of standardized extracts.

STING NETTLE. Sting Nettle (Urtica Dioica) flower extract has been shown to inhibit the biosynthesis of acrachidonic acid metabolites in vitro. Extracts have shown strong concentration-dependent inhibition of cyclooxygenase-derived reaction. A phenolic acid isolate from the extract inhibits the synthesis of leukotriene B4 in a concentrated dependent manner (Obersties and Giller 1996). Extracts of the leaf have been recommended for arthritic pain. The dose is usually 750 mg/bid.

In eighteen self-selected patients with joint pain who used nettle sting, all except one were sure that the nettles had been very helpful, and several considered themselves cured. There were no side effects, except a transient urticarial rash. Nettle sting is a useful, safe, and an inexpensive therapy that may be beneficial for joint pain (Randall et al 1999).

WILLOW BARK EXTRACT. Willow (Salix) bark extracts contain salicin and other derivatives including salicylic acid. The extract is an NSAID except that fewer side-effects have been reported as compared to aspirin or other pharmaceutical drugs. In a study of low back pain, patients received oral willow bark extract at 120 mg/day (low dose), or 240 mg/day of willow bark extract (high dose) in a four-week blinded trial. The percentage of pain-free patients in the last week of treatment was 39% in the group receiving the high-dose extract, 21% in the group receiving the low-dose extract, and 6% in the placebo group. The response rate in the high-dose group was evident after one week of treatment. Significantly more patients in the placebo group required pain medication during each week of the study (Chrubasik et al 2000).

CINNAMOMUM, CHRYSANTHEMUM, LYCOPUS POLYGONUM AND GOUT. The enzyme xanthine oxidase catalyzes the oxidation of hypo-xanthine to xanthine and then to uric acid, which plays a crucial role in *gout*. Studies of 122 TCM plants, selected according to the clinical efficacy and prescription frequency for the treatment of gout and other hyperuricemia-related disorders, showed the most active to be the methanol extract of the twig of Cinnamomum cassia (Lauraceae) (IC(50), 18 microg/ml). The activity of this extract was followed by those of the flower of Chrysanthemum indicum (Asteraceae) (IC(50), 22 microg/ml) and the leaves of Lycopus europaeus (Lamiatae) (IC(50), 26 microg/ml). Among the water extracts, the strongest inhibition of the enzyme was observed with that of the rhizome of Polygonum cuspidatum (Polygonaceae) (IC(50), 38 microg/ml). The IC(50) value of *allopurinol* used as a positive control was 1.06 microg/ml. The study demonstrated that the affects of these medicinal plants used for the treatment of gout were based, at least in part, on the xanthine oxidase inhibitory action (Kong et al 2000).

FOLIC ACID. Folic acid supplementation may lower toxicity in patients treated with methotrexate for RA. Folic acid, however, does not seem to improve treatment efficacy. Low blood folate levels and increased mean corpuscular volumes are associated with substantial methotrexate toxicity. Daily dietary intakes of more than 900 nmol or 400 ug of folic acid were associated with less methotrexate toxicity (Morgan Sarah et al 1994).

SELENIUM. Plasma selenium levels were found to be significantly lower in RA patients than in healthy controls. Selenium appears to be an important factor in RA. The low selenium values in RA are probably not just a nonspecific consequence of inflammation, but also a sign of depletion of stores or redistribution of total body selenium (Kose, Kader, et al 1996).

EXERCISE. A study of dance-based exercise programs in individuals with RA showed dance-based exercise to be a safe and efficient activity to improve physical fitness and psychological well-being in individuals with RA. Positive changes in depression, anxiety, fatigue, and tension were observed after the twelve-week exercise program. These findings provide evidence in favor of aerobic exercise in individuals with rheumatoid arthritis. It is of primary interest to note that a weight-bearing activity with limited ground impact does not provoke short term adverse effects on the joints (Noreau, Luc et al 1995).

VEGAN DIET. A study evaluating sixty-six patients with RA with disease duration between two and ten years and that were on stable doses of NSAIDs, oral glucocorticoids of =7.5 mg of prednisolone, disease-modifying rheumatic drugs, and 1 mg/day of vitamin B12 and 50 mcg/day selenium, was made by (Hafstrom, Ringertz, Spangberg et al 2001). The vegan diet contained vegetables, root vegetables, nuts and fruits, and, since no gluten was permitted, buckwheat, millet, corn, rice, and sunflower seeds. Unshelled sesame seeds in the form of sesame milk were used as a source of calcium. Subjects on the non-vegan diet consumed a variety of foods from all food groups. Nine (40.5%) of the subjects in the vegan group fulfilled the American College of Rheumatology (ACR) 20-improvement criteria compared with one (4%) patient in the non-vegan group. The immunoglobulin G antibody levels against gliadin and beta-lactoglobulin decreased in the responder subgroup in the vegan diet-treated patients, but not in the other analyzed groups. No reversing of radiological destruction was noted. This study suggested that a vegan diet may have positive benefits on the signs and symptoms of rheumatoid arthritis.

The positive changes in a vegetarian diet in RA patients appears to be due to changes in the bacterial flora (Kjeldsen-Kragh, Jens 1996).

PHOTOCHEMOTHERAPY. Eight patients with *psoriasis* and seronegative arthritis received photopheresis for twelve weeks, followed by photopheresis plus psoralen-ultraviolet A irradiation (PUVA) for another twelve weeks. Four patients had marked improvement of joint symptoms that lasted more than twelve months after the therapy. These responders had a higher CD4:CD8 ratio than poor responders prior to therapy (Vahlquist, Carin, et al 1996). Photochemotherapy may be used for RA, as well (Haberman, Herbert 1995).

COUNSELING. Counseling and special stress-management skills in RA patients may result in less helplessness, less pain, and greater mobility continuing several months after completion, compared to those who had no counseling. There is evidence that the coping capacity of persons with RA are severely challenged by major life stresses associated with the disease (Tamkins 1996).

Dr. Dorman's general recommendations for RA are (personal communication):

1. Identify and avoid food allergens;
2. Zinc (picolinate or citrate), 30 mg, 2-3 times a day;
3. Copper, 2-4 mg/day;
4. Niacinamide, as for osteoarthritis, in selected cases;
5. Fish oil, 6-15 g/day;
6. Evening primrose oil, to supply 750-1,500 mg/day of gamma-linolenic acid;
7. Vitamin E, 800 IU/day;
8. Selenium, 200-300 µg/day;
9. Hydrochloric acid, 40-70 grains per meal, if hypochlorhydric;
10. Vitamin C (buffered) 1-10 g/day. Watch for exacerbation of joint pain and reduce dose if this occurs;
11. Vitamin K, 50-100 mg, 3 times a day;
12. Bromelain, 3-4 capsules, 3 times a day on empty stomach;
13. Ginger;
14. Chicken or type II cartilage.

Traumatic or Acute Arthritis

"Traumatic arthritis," capsulitis or synovitis have identical meanings and all may follow injury to any joint. However, they are more common in joints with some degree of pre-existing arthrosis. In all of these conditions, the inflammation of the entire capsule results from recent trauma. X-rays are not diagnostic in traumatic arthritis, and bony changes may take time to show (Ombregt et al *ibid*). In a joint with pre-existing damage, the trauma may be minor and the patient may not be able to recall a cause. The clue to this type of "traumatic arthritis" is pain of sudden onset in a middle-aged or elderly patient who presents with a capsular pattern (Cyriax *ibid*). Often the initial pain is very mild and may disappear to only reappear suddenly, for no apparent cause, after a week, at which point the pain can be quite severe (most often seen at the shoulder).

In children, trauma to a growing cartilage is dangerous, because it is invisible on x-ray, difficult to diagnose, and may lead to epiphysiodesis (premature union of the epiphysis with the diaphysis) and axial deviation of the limb (Barral and Croibier *ibid*).

With a single acutely-inflamed joint (monoarthritis), even if traumatic, the possibility of infection must be considered (a joint tap and fluid analysis may be necessary). An infected joint must be treated aggressively in order to avoid serious disability. If the soft tissue over a joint shows signs of infection. The practitioner never needles (acupuncture) the soft tissue through to the joint capsule; this can *infect the joint (*unless tapping the joint for analysis, in which case strict sterile technique is used).

TREATMENT OF TRAUMATIC ARTHRITIS. In treating recent trauma, it is essential to restore full range of movement as soon as possible, especially in middle-aged and elderly people, as post-traumatic adhesions are apt to form. Movements should be performed up to the point of discomfort but not to the point of causing pain. All possible movements should be attempted one by one, and a small but definite increase in range should be achieved each day. If this (together with other treatments such as herbs and acupuncture) fails, or if the patient feels pain in the absence of movement, especially at night, and if there is a wide reference of pain and an inability to lie in bed on the affected joint, intra-articular steroid injections may be needed. For a patient that refuses injections, slight painless distraction techniques with the joint in the neutral position can be tried. A variation in depth and timing in the technique is helpful. This is performed daily for the first week and every other day thereafter. *Forced movements* should not be performed in traumatic arthritis of the following peripheral joints (Ombregt et al *ibid*):

- *Elbow.* Passive mobilization of a recent post-traumatic stiffness is likely to aggravate rather than help, and com-

monly results in decreased range. Also, it may increase the chances of developing myositis ossificans.
- *Hip.* Traumatic arthritis is best treated by bed rest.
- *Interphalangeal* and *metacarpophalangeal* joints of hand and foot. These joints respond poorly to any forced movement.
- *Lower radioulnar* joint. No forced movement or active exercises should be used, as they are likely to aggravate the condition.
- Joints *not under voluntary control*. These joints do not develop adhesions. Therefore, forced movements are not needed and are often harmful. Rest and support are good alternatives.

Other treatments such as functional techniques, acupuncture, and herbs are useful for both the acute and chronic stages. Muscle energy can be used in the chronic stage. In the chronic stage (Ombregt et al *ibid*), stretching the capsule requires many repetitions of long, steady, pushes, maintained for a minute or so (as long as the patient can bear it). No increase in range can be expected for several visits, and persistence is required. Heating the joint prior to treatment is helpful.[42]

Spondylosis (Degenerative Arthritis of the Spine)

Spondylosis is an almost universal condition that occurs with aging. Many people who have x-ray findings of spondylosis are pain free and only manifest stiffness. Numerous studies have shown no relationship between low back pain and lumbar spondylosis, so that a person with only mild radiographic changes may have much more pain than one with advanced degenerative disease. However, this gradual degenerative condition of all aspects of the vertebral functional unit can predispose one to somatic dysfunction and to myofascial pain, especially if a segment is unstable. When spondylosis is severe, it may lead to narrowing of the spinal canal and intervertebral foramen. Compression of the cauda equina and nerve roots may result and surgery may be needed (Brown *ibid*).

Patients are usually over fifty years of age and may have a history of spinal trauma. Pain is usually local and may radiate to the buttocks (if the trauma was to the lumbar region) or arms (if the trauma was to the cervical region). Neuralgias or claudication may be seen in severe cases. Pain is aggravated by activity and by sitting. Posain and morning stiffness are common. Examination is often consistent with instability and a capsular pattern (limitation of all movements except flexion) may be seen (Brown *ibid*).

---

42. In traumatic and "steroid sensitive" arthritis, response to treatment with TCM methods is often slow. In the shoulder, for example, the use of steroid injections can shorten recovery with little risk of joint damage and may prevent the formation of adhesions and frozen shoulder. Systemic adverse effects however cannot be ignored and should be fully explained to the patient.

IMAGING. Ligament and fascia attenuation leading to and associated with the degeneration of the intervertebral joints, the zygoapophyseal joints, and the uncovertebral joints, with radiological manifestations, sometimes are labeled together as spondylosis. The radiological inventory of abnormalities includes:
- Disc space narrowing;
- Osteophyte formation anteriorly and posteriorly at the disc level;
- Osteophyte formation at the uncovertebral joints of Luschka (cervical spine);
- Bone spurs anteriorly at the zygoapophyseal joints.

It is suggested here that these are indirect manifestations of ligament and fascial attenuation. Severe narrowing of the spinal canal can damage the cord and cause spondylotic myelopathy. Posterior vertebral spurs usually make an important contribution to this disease. It is only through radiographic studies that this can be assessed accurately. The CT study is best for imaging bony abnormalities, but an MRI gives more accurate information about the spinal canal and neuroaxis attenuation (Dorman and Ravin *ibid*).

Because the differential diagnosis of spondylotic myelopathy includes single and multiple disc herniation, an MRI is often most helpful. When evaluating for spondylosis, it is important to remember that the degree of neurological deficit rarely coincides with the area of greatest degenerative change demonstrated on x-ray. The patient should be treated not the x-ray.

Treatment

Treatment is directed to the instability and to myofascial and vertebral (somatic) dysfunctions, and is often effective. Usually acupuncture, periosteal needling, and manual therapy are sufficient. If significant instability is found (usually in the sacroiliac joints, and the lumbosacral and cervical regions), prolotherapy can be considered. Both oral and topical herbs can be used and are helpful when integrated within total patient care.

An empirical *guiding* herbal formula for spondylosis of the cervical and thoracic spines is:

Pueraria Lobata (Ge Gen) 30g
Radix Paeonia Lactiflorae (Bai Shao) 15g
Radix Atragalus Membranaceus (Huang Qi) 15g
Radix Codonopsis Pilosulae (Dang Shen) 12g
Rhizoma Ligusticum Wallicii (Chuan Xiong) 9g
Semen Persica (Tao Ren) 9g
Flos Carthmea Tinctorius (Hong Hua) 9g
Resina Olibani (Ru Xiang) 6g
Resina Myrrhae (Mo Yao) 6g
Radix Salviae Miltorrhiza (Dan Shen) 12g
Pollen Typhoae (Pu Huang) 10g
Panax Pseudoginseng (San Qi) 6g
Spica Prunellae (Xia Ku Cao) 12g
Radix Clematidis (Wei Ling Xian) 6g
Radix Gentiana Macrophyllae (Qin Jiao) 12g
Rhizoma seu Radix Notopterygii (Qiang Huo) 6g
Cortex Phellodendri (Huang Bai) 6g
Radix Reumanniae (Sheng Di Huang) 9g
Lumbricus (Di Long) 6g
Eupolyphaga (Tu Bie Chong) 3g

For severe pain add: Radix Aconiti (Fu Zi) 12-30g[43]

Another empirical *guiding* formula for neck, arm, and head pain from cervical spondylopathy is:

    Herba Pyrolae (Lu Xian Cao) 20g
    Pueraria Lobata (Ge Gen) 30g
    Radix Angelica Sinensis (Dang Gui) 9g
    Radix Salviae (Dan Shen) 12g
    Ramulus Mori (Sang Zhi) 9g
    Fructus Hordeum Vulgare (Mai Ya) 12g
    Radix Rehmanniae (Sheng Di Huang) 9g
    Rhizoma Drynariae (Gu Sui Bu) 9g
    Herba Cistanchis (Rou Cong Rong) 9g
    Pollen Typhae (Pu Huang) 9g
    Caulis Millettiae (Ji Xue Teng) 12g
    Periostracum Cicadae (Chan Tui) 6g

An empirical *guiding* formula for acute and severe neck pain due to spondylopathy without secondary neuralgia or headache is:

    Radix Aconiti Agrestis (Cao Wu and Chuan Wu) 6g
    Eupolyphagae Seu Opisthoplatiae (Tu Bie Chong) 4g
    Lumbricus (Di Long) 6g
    Semen Sojae (Dan Dou Chi) 15g
    Moschus Moschiferi (She Xiang) 0.1g

An empirical *guiding* formula for the lower spine spondylopathy is:

    Colla Cornus Cervi (Lu Jiao Jiao) 9g
    Tortosie Plastron glue (Gui Ban Jiao) 9g
    Rhizoma Dioscoreae (Shan Yao) 12g
    Fructus Corni (Shan Zhu Yu) 12g
    Fructus Lycii (Gou Qi Zi) 9g
    Semen Cuscutae (Tu Si Zi) 12g
    Cortex Eucommiae (Du Zhong) 12g
    Angelica Sinensis (Dang Gui) 9g
    Rhizoma Corydalis (Yan Hu Suo) vinegar fried 12g
    Myrrh (Mo Yao) 6g
    Achyranthes Bidentata (Niu Xi) 12g
    Rhizoma Ligustici (Chuan Xiong) 6g
    Lumbricus (Di Long) 9g
    Eupolyphaga seu Opisthoplatia (Tu Bie Chong) 6g
    Aconitum Kusenzoffii (Cao Wu Tou) 6g
    Poriae (Fu Ling) 15g
    Semen Plantaginis (Che Qian Zi) 9g
    Radix Angelica Pubescentis (Du Huo) 12g
    Radix Gentianae (Qin Jiao) 12g
    Cortex Lycii Radicis (Di Gu Pi) 15g
    Rhizoma Alismatis (Ze Xie) 6g

For severe pain add: Radix Aconiti (Fu Zi) 12-60g

For a sensitive patient that cannot tolerate the above formula, an alternative is:

    Rhizoma Atractylodis (Bai Zhu) 12g
    Cortex Eucommiae (Du Zhong) 12g
    Radix Sileris (Fang Feng) 9g
    Angelica Sinensis (Dang Gui) 9g
    Squama Manitis (Chuan Shan Jia) 12g

An empirical *guiding* formula to treat spondylopathy with sciatica is:

    Treated Rhizoma Arisaematis (Zhi Nan Xing) 9g
    Radix Paeonia Lactiflorae (Bai Shao) 15g
    Radix Atragalus Membranaceus (Huang Qi) 15g
    Rhizoma Drynari (Gu Sui Bu) 15g
    Rhizoma Cibotii (Gou Ji) 12g
    Cortex Eucommiae (Du Zhong) 12g
    Rhizoma Ligustici (Chuan Xiong) 6g
    Flos Carthami (Hong Hua) 9g
    Rhizoma seu Radix Notopterygii (Qiang Huo) 9g
    Rhizoma Atractylodis (Cang Zhu) 9g

---

43. A large dosage of Fu Zi is often key for successful herbal intervention. If needed, Shi Gao or a large dose of Sheng Di may be added to counteract side-effects. The herb must be cooked for at least three hours especially if a large dosage is used.

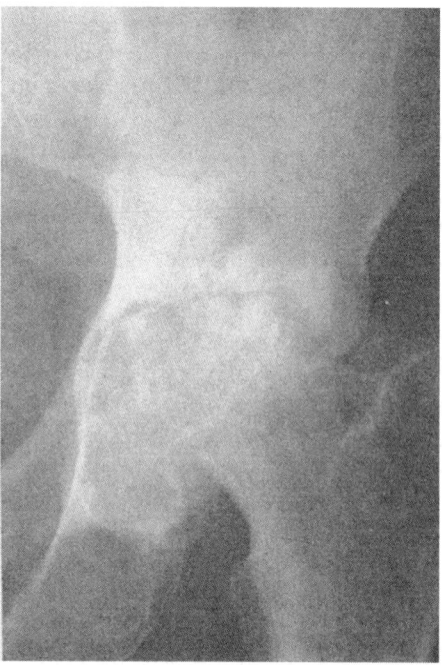

Figure 11-6: Complications from avascular necrosis. Note the collapse of the femoral head with an irregular contour and osteonecrosis.

    Radix Phelodendri (Huang Bai) 9g
    Semen Persicae (Tao Ren) 12g
    Radix Stephaniae (Fang Ji) 9g
    Rhizoma Corydalis (Yan Hu Suo) 15g
    Radix Angelica Pubescentis (Du Huo) 12g
    Radix Gentianae Scabae (Long Dan Cao) 6g
    Massa Fermentata (Shen Qu) 6g
    Ramulus Cinnamomi (Gui Zhi) 6g
    Resina Myrrhae (Mo Yao) 6g
    Resina Olibani (Ru Xiang) 6g
    Lumbricus (Di Long) 6g
    Eupolyphaga (Tu Bie Chong) 9g
    Panax Pseudoginseng (San Qi) 9g

For severe pain add: Radix Aconiti (Fu Zi) 15-60g

Avascular Necrosis

Avascular necrosis (aseptic necrosis, Figure 11-6) refers to a progressive disruption of circulation that eventually leads to a collapse of the bone structure if not treated in time. It is seen in children and young adults as the result of injuries and various genetic bone disorders. Later in life, it occurs as the result of drugs (most often from corticosteroids and alcohol) and secondary to chronic diseases (e.g., systemic lupus) that affect the vascular system, or as a result of a history of injury. The most common joint to be affected is the hip. It is seen in patients complaining of pain and restricted motion of the hip. The pain is worsened with activity and improved by rest; one or both hips can be involved; in cases other than traumatic injury, one side is affected first, and the other may develop the condition later. Prompt diagnosis is imperative because once severe, the only treatment available is joint replacement (Brown *ibid*).

TREATMENT: In the early stage, complete rest and core decompression may work and prevent the need for joint

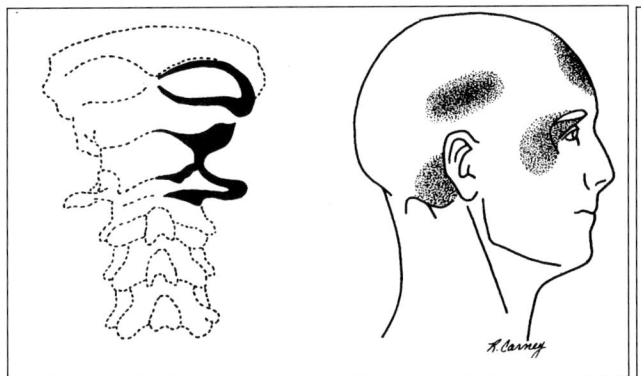

Referred patterns from upper cervical soft tissues

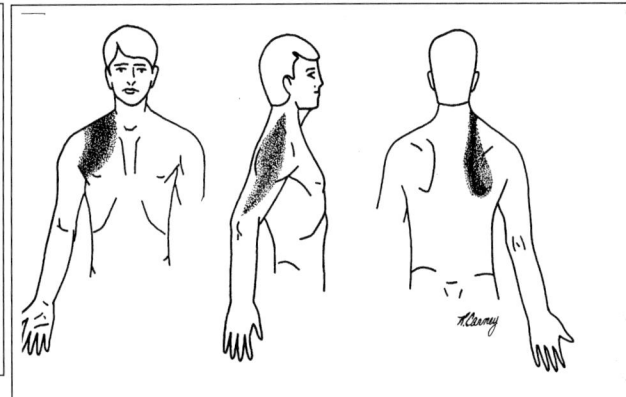

Referred patterns from the tip, front and back of C7 transverse process

Figure 11-7: Referred pain from soft tissue attachments (courtesy of Dorman and Ravin 1991).

replacement. According to Dr. Saputo (personal communication) photonic stimulation has completely relieved pain associated with aseptic necrosis in several patients. He does not know if actual bone regrowth has occurred. The following herbal formulas have been reported to be affective and may be incorporated:[44]

> Radix Salviae Miltiorrhizae (Dan Shen) 10g
> Fructus Cnidii (She Chuang Zi) 10g
> Colla Cornus Cervi (Lu Jiao Jiao) 10g
> Radix Angelicae Sinensis (Dang Gui) 10g
> Semen Sinapis Albae (Bai Jie Zi) 15g
> Achyranthes Bidentata (Niu Xi) 15g
> Rhizoma Drynariae (Gu Sui Bu) 20g
> Radix Astragali (Huang Qi) 15g
> Sanguis Draconis (Xue Jie) 15g
> Herba Epimedii (Yin Yang Huo) 30g
> Rhizoma Polygoni (Huang Jing) 30g
> Os (Gu; preferably a hip joint from sheep)
> (Cordyceps Sinensis powder caps (Dong Chong Xia Cao) 3-15g)

Or powdered:

> Cordyceps Sinensis (Dong Chong Xia Cao) 9-15g
> Radix Angelicae Sinensis (Dang Gui) 12
> Fructus Cnidii (She Chuang Zi) 10g
> Radix Dipsaci (Xu Duan) 12g
> Rhizoma Polygoni (Huang Jing) 30g
> Rhizoma Drynariae (Gu Sui Bu) 12g
> Copper Pynites (Zi Ran Tong) 6g
> Acacia seu Uncaria (Er Cha) 2g
> Eupolyphaga seu Opisthoplatia (Tu Bie Chong) 4g
> Herba cum Radix Asari (Xi Xin) 6g
> Radix Astragali (Huang Qi) 15g
> Radix Poligoni Multihlori (He Shou Wu) 15g
> Rhizoma Cibotii Barmometz (Gou Ji) 9g
> Cortex Eucommiae (Du Zhong) 12g
> Fructus Lycii (Gou Qi Zi) 12g
> Caulis Millettiae (Ji Xue Teng) 12g
> Radix Salviae Miltiorrhizae (Dan Shen) 10g
> Panax Pseudoginseng (San Qi) 15g
> Flos Carthami (Hong Hua) 9g
> Plastrum Testudinis (Gui Ban) 15g
> Carapax Trionysis (Bie Jia) 30g
> Concha Margaritifera Usta (Zhen Zhu Mu) 30g
> Buthus Martensi (Quan Xie) 6g
> Agkistrodon Acutus (Bai Hua She) 9g
> Colla Cornus Cervi (Lu Jiao Jiao) 10g

---

44. It must be noted that the window for conservative treatment of avascular necrosis is quite short, and therefore close monitoring is needed. Also, the author does not have any experience with these herbal formulas and therefore can not testify as to their usefulness.

> Achyranthes Bidentata (Niu Xi) 15g
> Flos Caryophylli (Ding Xiang) 3g

Take 15-20g per day with soup made from bone.

Ligamentous Disorders

Ligamentous injuries may be acute and traumatic in origin or chronic degenerative in character. There remains much controversy about the treatment of both acute and chronic ligamentous injuries. Even in severe ligamentous tears, studies show a good outcome with surgical and non-surgical care. In chronic pain patients (Dorman *ibid*), ligament laxity and partial tears are frequent but unrecognized sources of pain.

Normal ligaments are usually not tender when palpated. If they are injured or are stretched due to joint dysfunction, they can become sensitive and often painful. The pain of acute ligament sprains (tears) is usually felt several minutes or hours after the injury as swelling *(OM: blockage)* develops. This delay in pain is commonly seen with disc nuclear ruptures and other soft tissue injuries, especially whiplash.

Ligamentous laxity and insufficiency can result from:

- Injuries (acute overstretch);
- Poor physiologic posture or structure;
- Muscular weakness that leads to stresses on the ligaments;
- Loss of mobility at one aspect of a joint, or other joints elsewhere being stressed, resulting in other parts of the joint being overstressed;
- Degenerative joint processes that cause diminished joint volume. This results in a relative increase of ligament length. The ligament is too long to hold the joint tightly because the joint volume is decreased. This is seen commonly in degenerative disc disease.

Ligaments are especially susceptible to hysteresis (Bogduk and Twomey *ibid*) and tissue creep, particularly

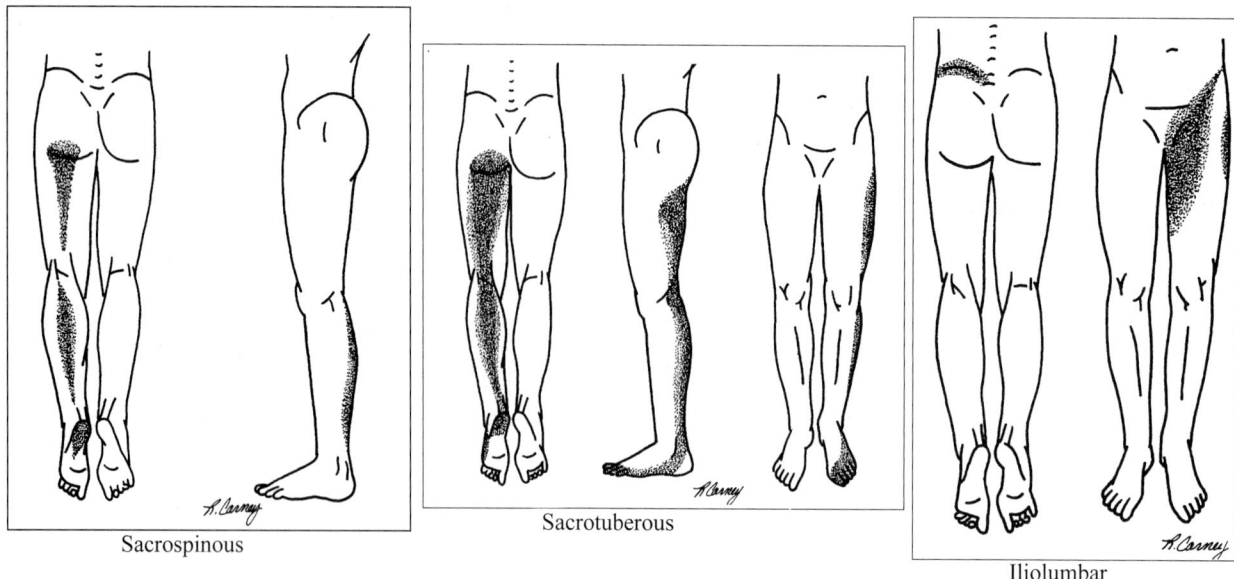

Figure 11-8: Referred pain from low back and pelvic ligaments (courtesy of Dorman and Ravin 1991).

when fatigued. Hysteresis (elastic energy loss after prolonged or repetitive loading) can become permanent and result in an increase of tissue length, called "set." Set can occur easily if a ligament is stretched 4% behind the point of which all crimp or slack is removed. Hysteresis can affect joint capsules, annulus fibrosus, and all other ligaments.

When the above structures are fatigued, they are more vulnerable to injury from inconsequential or unexpected activity. Following tissue fatigue and hysteresis, the mechanoreceptors and proprioceptors (Type I and II) compensate, and adaptation occurs in order to minimize the risk of tissue failure. Type I and II afferents habituate to stimuli and may not continue to discharge (if hysteresis or tissue fatigue is chronic). Eventually, this common occurrence may lead to partial or complete inability of tissues to accommodate. This leaves the ligament vulnerable to injury. Sensitization (the reduction of transmission threshold) and dorsal horn responses to Type I and II mechanoreceptive sensory input as though it were painful input may result (Liebenson 1996).

Symptoms

Ligamentous pain may be felt locally or distally and in various patterns. Hackett et al (1991) has mapped many of these reference patterns in his book. Figure 11-7 through Figure 11-8 show a few pain patterns related to ligaments.

Posain and Nulliness

The hallmark of ligament pain is positional pain, for which Dorman has coined the term "posain." Posain is the experience of increased pain when any position, such as sitting, or standing in one place, is held for a long period. Another important symptom of ligamentous laxity and insufficiency is the referral of a numb-like ache, which Dorman calls "nulliness." Nulliness is commonly mistaken for neurogenic symptoms, such as sciatica or carpal tunnel syndrome.

Ligamentous pain is aggravated by activity/load that strains the ligament and is alleviated by rest. Often ligamentous pain is worse in the morning due to posain *(OM: Qi/Blood, Cold congestion, poor nourishment)*. Injured ligaments are tender under pressure and/or stretching. Frequently, the pain and its referred pattern can be reproduced by needle stimulation (acupuncture) and are abolished by application of a local anesthetic. Injured and loose ligaments generally present clinically as hypermobile or unstable joints. *Further stretching of such ligaments should be avoided.*

Instability and Ligamentous Insufficiency

Clinical instability is a common cause of ongoing pain refractory to treatment. Ligamentous laxity may result from trauma, repeated injuries (including excessive therapeutic manipulation), and degenerative changes (Biering-Sonrenson 1984). Increased spinal mobility has been shown to correlate with increased low back difficulties. In patients with idiopathic low back pain, spinal flexibility was inversely correlated with functional recovery (Lankhost et al 1985). Patients with congenital hypermobility often develop muscle tightness around hypermobile joints, as the body attempts to stabilize the joint. This tightness is associated with muscle weakness. Vigorous stretching often results in increased pain and the development of trigger points (Brown *ibid*). Joints most susceptible to ligamentous insufficiency are the sternoclavicular, acromioclavicular, sacroiliac, symphysis pubis,

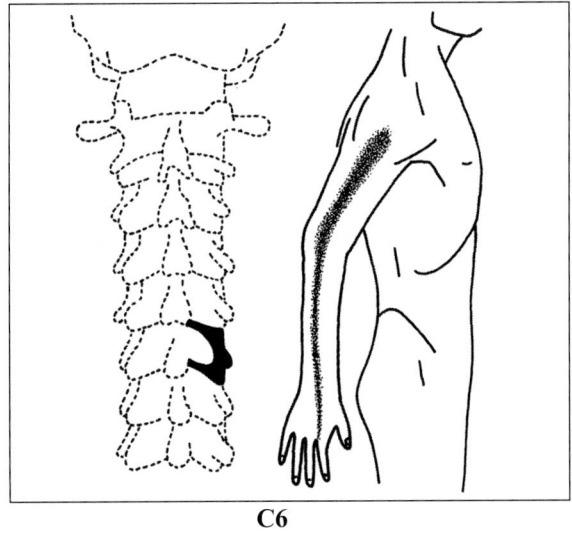 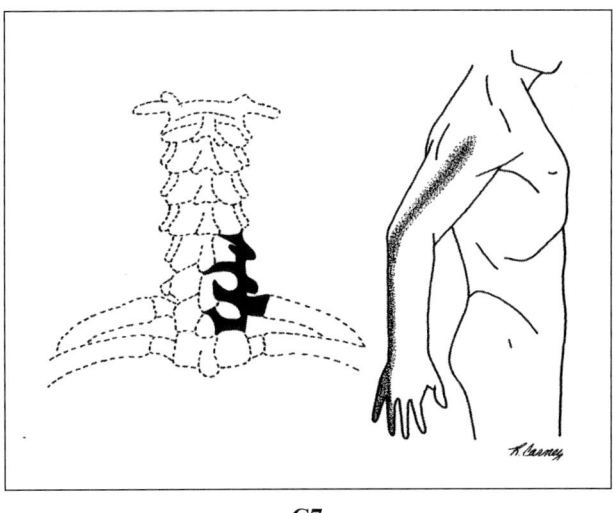

Figure 11-9: Referred pain from ligaments and soft tissue bony attachments (courtesy of Dorman and Ravin 1991).

knees, tibiofibular (superior and inferior), ankles and, sometimes, the shoulders (Cyriax *ibid*). Even simple sprains can have far reaching effects (Figure 11-1).

Clinical signs of lumbar and pelvic instability include (Dorman (*ibid*); Basmajian and Nyberg (*ibid*); Paris (*ibid*):

- Posain and morning ache that recurs later in the day, after fatigue and stress;
- Catching and "giving way";
- Shaking of the lumbar spine on forward bending, with more difficulty in returning to an upright position than in going into flexion. The patient often needs to assist himself by grasping the thighs;
  As apposed to discogenic pain which is often more severe during flexion;
- Increased occurrence of bony subluxation;.
- Involuntary muscle guarding;
- Abnormal lumbosacral rhythm (tendency to maintain lumbar lordosis during flexion);
- Increased pain when maintaining extreme range of motion;
- With spondylolisthesis (a forward slip of a part or a whole vertebra), sometimes a visible step-off can be seen in the lumbar spine when the patient is standing. It may become reduced when the patient lies down.
- With instability of the sacroiliac joint, patients report, at times, a sudden giving way or sudden falls. Dorman has named this phenomenon the "slipping clutch syndrome." (Dorman 1994).

Neurogenic Inflammation

When ligaments are lax, the joint is more likely to shift from its normal position, resulting in even more stresses on the richly innervated ligaments.

Recent research using immune-histochemical techniques suggests that, when ligaments and other connective tissues in the spine that receive a supply of small diameter fibers become irritated, an initiation of "neurogenic inflammation" occurs and commonly affects pain and sympathetic receptors. Neurogenic inflammation results from release of neuropeptides that interact with fibroblasts, mast cells, and immune cells in the surrounding connective tissues (Levine et al 1993). Neurogenic inflammation is thought to be a major factor in degenerative diseases and back pain chronicity (Garrett et al 1992; Weinstein 1992).

Treatment of Ligamentous Disorders

Ligamentous injury is best treated in a global manner designed to encourage *functional* tissue repair. Long immobilization is usually not advisable. In the more acute stage it is essential not to re-injure during the first part of the granulation stage, about ten days; however, studies have shown that ligaments heal better and stronger under functional loading than they do during rest. Loading/movement should be started on day eleven or so post injury.

In chronic stages of sprains and for patients with ligamentous laxity, the following treatments should be used: manual therapies to address joint dysfunctions and encourage tissue approximation; periosteal acupuncture or prolotherapy to induce ligamentous hypertrophy; exercise to strengthen, stretch, and educate muscles; and herbal and nutritional therapies to correct metabolic and possible constitutional deficiencies. Because ligaments are poorly vascularized, periosteal acupuncture or prolotherapy are usually needed to initiate fibroblastic locomotion and repair. Both ligaments and tendons show evidence for intrinsic cellular fibroblastic activity which induces "motion" and remodelling from within, facilitating the unity of injured tendon and ligament ends. When the ligament is significantly and chronically lax, however, an extrinsic injury by injection or dry-needling is often needed to initiate healing. Movement during the stage of collagen deposition aligns newly generated collagen fibrils in the direction of stress and prevents the formation of scars. Movement also stimulates proteoglycan synthesis, which is important in the lubrication of connective tissue and in the maintenance of the critical distance between pre-existing fibers. It may be most effective to start mobilization from the onset, before the newly generated fibrils develop crosslinks in an abnormal and irregular pattern, i.e., scar tissue. Even with severe grade III sprains, conservative treatment with partial immobilization so that unwanted movement does not take place during the recovery can be effective (Lackie 1986, Dorman *ibid*, Ombregt et al *ibid*).

Ligamentous Laxity

Periosteal acupuncture and prolotherapy are particularly helpful in treating chronic pain from ligamentous laxity. Because treatment for instability and ligamentous insufficiency can be painful, the practitioner can give the patient an analgesic before beginning. Also, the patient must understand that this process increases local inflammation and (usually) pain, and that the inflammation is required in order to rebuild tissues. Trigger points are treated at the same time.

TO TREAT THE LUMBAR SPINE AND PELVIS

Prepare the patient's skin and insert a 30-gauge needle at midline to stimulate the interspinous and supraspinous ligaments. Contact the spine and stimulate the periosteum. Be careful not to enter the cord.

1. Needle the lumbosacral ligaments.

2. Needle about 1-5 cm from midline down to the base of the lamina and try to reach the ligamentum flavum. It may be difficult to feel the ligament. However, the small amount of blood spilled probably will reach the ligament and induce inflammation. Peck the lamina as thoroughly as possible.

3. Needle the iliolumbar ligament attachments at the iliac crest with a 28-gauge needle inserted at the medial end of the iliac crest. Walk the needle by repeated insertions and withdrawal to skin level until reaching the anterior aspect of the ilia. It may be necessary to curve the needle before insertion so that it curves under and then up toward the anterior ilial wall. Leave the needles under the iliac crest and stimulate the area electrically or manually.

4. Needle the attachments of the sacrotuberous and the sacrospinous ligaments onto the medial edge of the sacrum (with the patient sidelying).

5. Next, attend to the sacroiliac (SI) ligaments, penetrating all nodules, and stimulate the periosteum covering the entire joint.

6. Needle the surfaces of the PSIS and ilia. Stimulate the periosteum.

7. Needle the deeper aspects of the ilia and interosseous sacral ligaments. This stimulates the periosteum.

8. Select several 3-inch needles and needle the deep superior aspect of the SI joint from above directing the needles downward and slightly laterally toward the SI joint. Make sure the needle penetrates the joint and is within the interosseous ligaments. Leave the needles in place (Figure 11-11).

9. Place several needles at the midline of the sacrum directing them toward the attachments of the posterior SI ligaments and leave them in place.

10. Connect the positive pole (again some patients do better with the negative pole) of a monopolar electrical stimulator to these needles and leave it on for as long as conditions allow (the longer the better, up to two hours). An electromagnetic pulse stimulator which magnetizes the needles may be placed under the patient. This may help in healing (although one study has shown this to reduce blood circulation, which may be detrimental).

11. Follow with laser stimulation which *may* increase ATP.

At the end of the treatment, the practitioner must re-evaluate the patient's lumbosacral mechanics, because muscle spasm and vertebral dysfunction may set in. The practitioner should correct these before sending the patient home.

TO TREAT THE CERVICAL SPINE:

1. Identify the affected segments.

2. Keep the patient's head flexed maximally and rotated slightly.

3. Use a lateral approach to needle the articular pillars, facets, lateral tubercles (transverse process) and spinous processes.

    Peck at the periosteum, using one needle repeatedly at all locations. (It is possible to treat both sides simultaneously by using a posterior approach. However, this tends to be more painful, and the patient's reactions can cause greater difficulty in controlling the needle and in sensing where the needle tip is located; Figure 11-12).

4. Identify the locations that best reproduce the target symptoms and leave the needles in place for one hour. (Do this only if sites are close to bone, not muscular tissue.)

Ligamentous Disorders

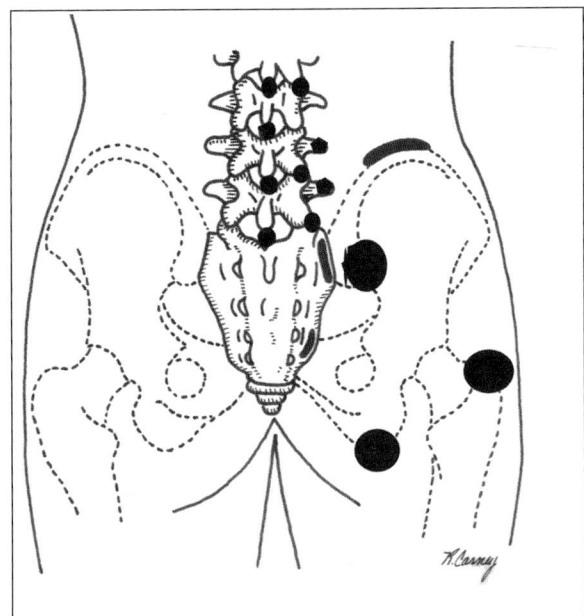

Figure 11-10: Important areas (ligaments) to treat for low back pain with instability.

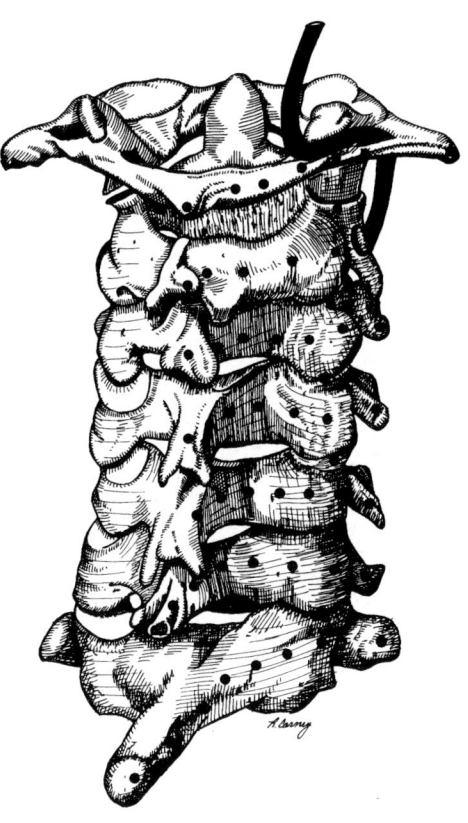

Figure 11-12: Important sites used in dry needling and prolotherapy (With permission Dorman and Ravin 1991).

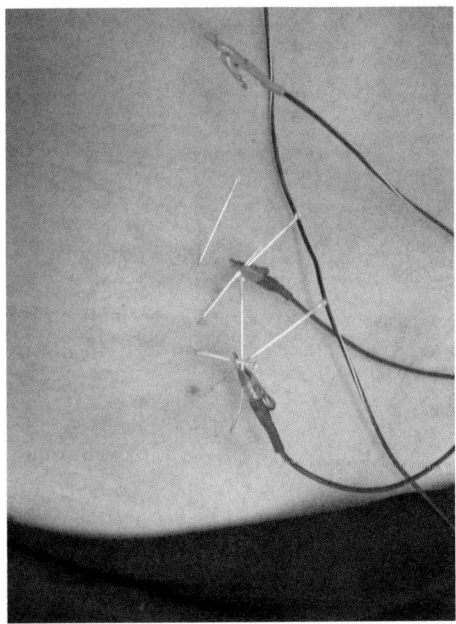

Figure 11-11: Several 3 inch 30-gauge needles inserted deeply into the interosseous sacral ligaments (at SI joint). The needles are connected to a mircoamp stimulator.

Connect a monopolar electrical stimulator with the anode (+) locally (some patients do better with the (-) pole locally). Stimulate for as long as possible. At least one hour.

It *may* be helpful to use an electromagnetic pulse devise placed under the patient. This may magnetize the needles and may help in healing.

Laser stimulation at the end of treatment *may* be helpful in healing.

5. Tell the patient to expect healing pain for a day or two following treatment.

TO TREAT THE THORACIC SPINE

1. The patient is supine, or in the lateral recumbent position, and the spine is flexed (to open the facets).

2. Needle all ligamentous periosteal junctions, including the interspinal, flava (between vertebral arches) and intertransverse ligaments.

3. First identify the edge of the vertebral bodies and leave a needle there as a marker. Do the same thing at one of the transverse processes (which may be difficult as well as dangerous) and at several rib angles. These needles are used as guides for needle depths. Finally, treat all of the above structures.

4. The needle used to treat the ligaments and facets is pointed inferiorly to minimize the danger of penetrating the cord.

5. The needle should penetrate the facets. When correctly needling a facet joint, the needle-feel is as though a tough capsule were first being penetrated, and then as though the needle were losing resistance as the joint is penetrated.

6. Needle all rib angles in symptomatic areas.

When the needle is directed superiorly and laterally, great care must be used as it may bend and, taking its own course, penetrate the cord. Only one side is needled at a time, so that, if an accidental pneumothorax occurs (puncture of the lung, letting air in to the pleural cavity), the patient will still have one fully-functional side.

Treatments for ligamentous laxity are repeated once a week or every other week. During the week between treatments, the patient must continue stabilization exercises. Lasting results often require six to fifteen treatments. If, after eight treatments, no response is evident, the practitioner should refer the patient for injection prolotherapy, although often improvement is only evident 2-3 months after treatment has ended. The patient should understand that aggravation and healing pain can be expected after the treatment.

Caution: For the needling to be effective (in the cervical, thoracic, or lumber spine), the patient must not take anti-inflammatory agents such as aspirin, ibuprofen, and naproxen for several months.

TCM Herbal Therapy

In TCM, many ligamentous disorders fall within hit medicine and Painful Obstruction (Bi) syndromes. Treatment is often directed at clearing the channels and collaterals, moving and nourishing Blood, and regulating the Liver.

An empirical, general *guiding* formula for ligamentous laxity that can be used both orally and topically is:

> Herba Lycopodium (Shen Jin Cao) 15g
> Os Draconis [calcined] (Duan Long Gu) 12g
> Cornu Bovis Carbenisatus (Niu Jiao) 15g
> Cortex Eucommiae (Du Zhong) 12g
> Fasciculus Vascularis Luffae (Si Gua Luo) 12g
> Sanguis Draconis (Xue Jie) 12g
> Radix Achyranthis Bidentatae (Niu Xi) 12g
> Radix Notoginseng (San Qi) 9g
> Cortex Acanthopanacis (Wu Jia Pi) 9g
> Rhizoma Dioscorea Bishie (Bi Xie) 12g
> Rhizoma Notopterygii (Qiang Huo) 9g
> Cortex Albizziae (He Huan Pi) 20g
> Calis Polygoni Multiflori (Ye Jiao Teng) 9g
> Rhizoma Bletillae (Bai Ji) 9g
> Rhizoma Drynariae (Gu Sui Bu) 12g
> Radix Dipsaci (Xu Duan) 12g
> Copper Pynites (Zi Ren Tong) 6g
> Acacia seu Uncaria (Er Cha) 2g
> Eupolyphaga seu Opisthoplatia (Tu Bie Chong) 4g

For post-traumatic laxity (post laxation), variations of Relaxing Sinews and Activating Blood Decoction (Shu Jin Huo Xue Tang) can be used:

> Rhizoma Notopterygii (Qiang Huo) 9g
> Radix Ledebouriellae Sesloidis (Fang Feng) 9g
> Herba seu Flos Schizonepetae Tenuifoliae (Jing Jie) 6g
> Radix Angelicae Pubescentis (Du Huo) 12g
> Radix Angelicae Sinensis (Dang Gui) 12g
> Radix Dipsaci (Xu Duan) 12g
> Pericarpium Citri Reticulatae (Qing Pi) 5g
> Radix Achyranthis Bidentatae (Niu Xi) 12g
> Cortex Acanthopanacis (Wu Jia Pi) 12g
> Cortex Eucommiae (Du Zhong) 12g
> Flos Carthami (Hong Hua) 9g
> Fructus Citri Aurantii (Zhi Qiao) 6g.

For Kidney-deficiency and ligamentous laxity, nine grams twice a day of Jin Gang Wan (Diamond Pill) can be used:

> Herba Cistanchis (Rou Cong Rong) 250g
> Cortex Eucommiae (Du Zhong) 250g
> Semen Cuscutae (Tu Si Zi) 250g
> 2 pig kidneys

If there is also bone failure/arthrosis, Niu Xi Wan (Achyranthis Bidentatae Pill) can be added:

> Radix Achyranthis Bidentatae (Huai Niu Xi)
> Cortex Eucommiae (Du Zhong)
> Radix Ledebouriellae Sesloidis (Fang Feng)
> Ramulus Cinnamomi (Gui Zhi)
> Rhizoma Dioscoreae (Bi Xie)
> Herba Cistanchis (Rou Cong Rong)
> Fructus Tribuli (Bai Ji Li)
> Pig kidney

Nutritional Support

It is advisable to make sure that patients treated for ligamentous laxity are well-nourished. A supplement of good quality proteins with extra proline, glycine, lysine, vitamin C, magnesium, and zinc are especially helpful.

Myofascial Disorders

Muscular and postural balance may be the outward and visible expression that vital communication and "energy" flow are functioning freely. Most musculoskeletal disorders are accompanied by myofascial reactions. These may not require direct treatment because "myofascial syndromes" are often *secondary* to other dysfunctions. Since muscles often react to painful stimuli with so-called "spasm" or tightness, the practitioner must assess the significance of this reaction.

Muscle responses range from contracture, spasm, and hypertonicity, to atrophy and hypotonicity. Striated muscle reactions (spasm, tension) serve to identify the lesion and amplify the experience of pain, and therefore are important diagnostically. Contractile unit disorders usually are characterized by increased muscle tone, accompanied by diminished plasticity and flexibility anywhere within the musculotendinous body. Pathology or dysfunction can either affect the entire muscle or just a few longitudinal bundles within the muscle. The muscle then becomes painful (Myalgia). Muscles act as pumps, moving fluids, blood, and lymph, dysfunctional muscles may cause decreased oxygenation of cells and tissue, and the muscle itself may become congested. If allowed to continue in this state, not only might the muscle lose its ability to relax, but fibromyositis (fibrositis) may develop. Fibromyositis is a pathological condition in which the elastic fibers in the muscle are lost and do not regenerate. It can lead to permanent contractures (Dvorák *ibid*). It has been suggested that some emotional states can lead to postural and muscular adaptations that would not be resolved until the somatic frame/structures have been addressed. At the same time, it is said that patients may suffer from emotional pain provoked by muscular and postural dysfunctions. In other words, physical patterns may be solidified from psychological attitude and vice vera. When muscular efficiency is optimal, the expenditure of energy by the body in activities such as walking or running is minimal. Good balance therefore may leave more energy available for other vital functions such as thought, digestion, circulation, tissue maintenance, repair, defense against disease, etc. (Travell and Simons *ibid*; Oschman *ibid*).

Myalgia can also be secondary to conditions such as viral infections. In these condition tissue texture changes are often lacking but they can initiate the trigger-point phenomenon that will then alter tissue texture. Long-term myalgia due to neuropathy, spasm, or guarding may lead to accumulation of waste products locally. When this develops, the muscles loose elasticity, become edematous, and often feel firm and doughy (Brown *ibid*).

Fascia

The fascial organ constitutes a single structure. The implications of deformation in that structure for producing extensive effects throughout the body are clear. One example of such effects is in the fascial divisions within the cranium. The tentorium cerebelli and falx cerebri are commonly warped during birthing difficulties. This may happen if the fetus remains in the birth canal for too long or too short a time or if there is forceps delivery. This warping is noted by craniosacral therapists to affect total body mechanics through its influence on fascia, and therefore on the musculature. (Chaitow *ibid*).

Fascia is continuous throughout the body and can provide support and communication to muscles, joints, vessels, nerves, and organs *(OM: Fascia has been associated with the Triple Warmer system)*.[45] Through the fascial planes, and microscopically through tensegrity and piezo-electricity, the fascia may enable communication between every single cell of the body.[46] Fascia functions as a tension member within the somatic frame. As muscles broaden, they stretch the fascia that surrounds them. This in-turn provides support and protection to the muscle. Consequence of the widespread continuity of fascia, its distortion or damage can have effects in a distant, seemingly unrelated area.

> Many of the layers of fascia, whether subcutaneous or investing, merge together and/or have common points of attachment. The fasciae that separate and ensheathe the external and internal abdominal oblique muscles merge posteriorly. They also merge with the thick connective tissue, thoracolumbar fascia, which continues upward, encasing and separating the erector spinae, the deep muscles of the back. Anteriorly the fascia of the abdominal muscles merge, split, and reflect to contribute to the inguinal anatomy and abdominal aponeurosis. These fascia are continuous with connective tissue sheets that flow over the crest of the pelvis and become the fascia lata of the thigh. The fascia of the thigh is continuous, in turn, with the crural fascia of the leg (Towns *ibid*.)

The stretching of fascia distributes some of the load, as fascia is continuous throughout the body and stores elastic energy. This allows the body frame to withstand forces that would otherwise be bone-crushing. Fascia is susceptible to plastic deformation (Greenman 1996) and therefore is thought to have a "memory." Hence, fascia can maintain a distorted shape for a long time, even after muscle spasm or neuromuscular tension ceases. Another aspect of fascial memory function is the imprinting of sudden physical trauma, with some of the kinetic energy of the traumatic force being stored as potential energy in the collagen (Mitchell *ibid*). Often during myofascial release the patient will recall an old injury. Collagen (Mitchell *ibid*) is a piezo-electric material; when deformed, it can generate an electric current and magnetic field that may also maintain its shape. Tension, compression, and movement may cause the crystalline lattices of the connective tissues to generate bioelectric signals. This has been described as a semiconducting communication network that can convey its signals to every part of the body (Oschman *ibid*). Ida Rolf (1962), the developer of Rolfing, puts the importance of the fascia into perspective thus (Chaitow *ibid*):

> Our ignorance of the role of fascia is profound. Therefore even in theory it is easy to overlook the possibility that far-reaching changes may be made not only in structural contour, but also in functional manifestation, through better organization of the layer of superficial fascia which enwraps the body. Experiment demonstrates that drastic changes may be made in the body, solely by stretching, separating and relaxing superficial fascia in an appropriate manner. Osteopathic manipulators have observed and recorded the extent to which all degenerative changes in the body, be they muscular, nervous, circulatory or organic, reflect in superficial fascia. Any degree of degeneration, however minor, changes the bulk of the fascia, modifies its thickness and draws it into ridges in areas overlying deeper tensions and rigidities. Conversely, as this elastic envelope is stretched, manipulative mechanical energy is added to it, and the fascial colloid becomes more "sol" and less "gel." As a result of the added energy, as well as of a directional contribution in applying it, the underlying structures, including muscles which determine the placement of the body parts in space, and also their relations to each other, come a little closer to the normal.

FASCIAL PATTERNS. According to Zink (Kuchera and Kuchera 1993) there are four crossover sites where fascial

---

45. Many oriental exercises and meditations, which often use focused abdominal breathing and gentle and subtle movement, may produce their effects by directed fascial movements.

46. It has been shown that when non-conducting materials such as plastics are formed as a tensegrity icosahedron tub, they can become conductive.

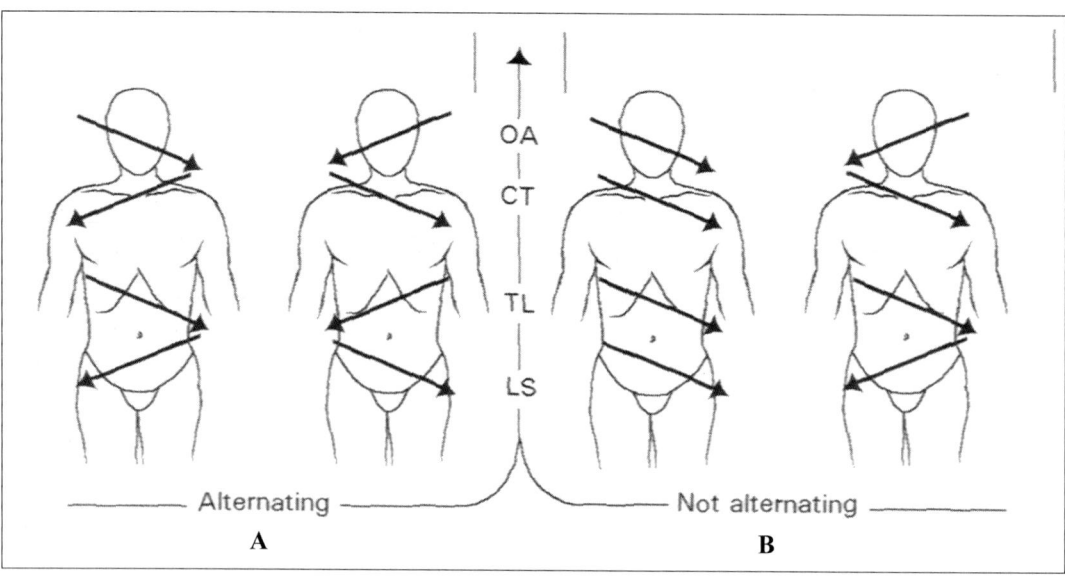

Figure 11-13: Compensated pattern (A). Uncompensated pattern (B). Patients with uncompensated patterns often need additional treatment (From Kuchera WA and Kuchera ML, Osteopathic Principles in Practice, KCOM press 1993, with permission).

tensions can be noted: occipitoatlantal (OA), cervicothoracic (CT), thoracolumbar (TL), and lumbosacral (LS). These sites are tested for their rotation and sidebending preferences in two ways. One is by placing the palm on the patient testing fascial drag. The other is to motion test the loaded area for rotational preferences. One example is flexing the neck until slight resiliency is felt at the physiological barrier of complete cervical flexion and then testing the *range* of rotation. Fascial adaptations can be divided into compensated and uncompensated patterns (Figure 11-13).

- *Compensated patterns.* These represent positive adaptive modifications that alternate in direction from one area to the next, i.e., the atlanto-occipital, cervicothoracic, thoracolumbar, and lumbosacral areas. There are two compensated patterns. The common one goes from the right upper OA towards the left CT, towards the right TL, towards the left TS. The uncommon compensated pattern would be the reverse starting at the upper left OA.

- *Uncompensated patterns.* These do not alternate. They are commonly the result of trauma and represent negative adaptive modifications.

Uncompensated patients are more likely to have poor reactions to stresses of any kind, heal more slowly than normal, and have a lower level of health. Thus (Chaitow *ibid*) uncompensated patterns suggest that there is poor adaptation, that the patient may not respond to more specific manual therapies, and that the patient may require a more general rehabilitation.

Ward (1997) described a "tight–loose" concept as one way of visualizing the body and its fascia. Evidence for inappropriately tight or loose areas, relative to each other, are sought in large or small areas in which interactive asymmetry exists. For example, commonly, a tight sacroiliac or hip is noted on one side, while the contralateral side is loose. A tight SCM and loose scalenes frequently are noted ipsilaterally. One shoulder may test as tight and the other loose (Chaitow *ibid*).

Areas of dysfunction commonly involve vertical, horizontal, and encircling (also described as crossover, spiral, or wrap-around) patterns of involvement. Ward describes a typical *wrap-around pattern*. This pattern is associated with a *tight* left low back area, which ends up involving the entire trunk and cervical area, evolving to compensate for loose, inhibited, areas or vice versa. Tightness in the posterior left hip, SI joint, lumbar erector spinae, and lower rib cage is associated with looseness on the right low back; tightness of the lateral and anterior rib cage on the right, tight left thoracic inlet posteriorly, and tight left craniocervical attachments involving jaw mechanics (Chaitow *ibid*).

Janda (*ibid*) also described myofascial patterns that he calls the *crossed pattern syndrome*.

Pattern Dysfunctions of Postural and Phasic Muscles

Myofascial shortening/tightness and weakness often develop in predictable patterns that have been described by Janda. There are upper and lower crossed syndromes. Patterns include often altered muscle firing and *substitution* of muscle use (Janda *ibid*).

The upper crossed syndrome shows the following characteristics:

- The neck extensors are short and deep flexors are weak.

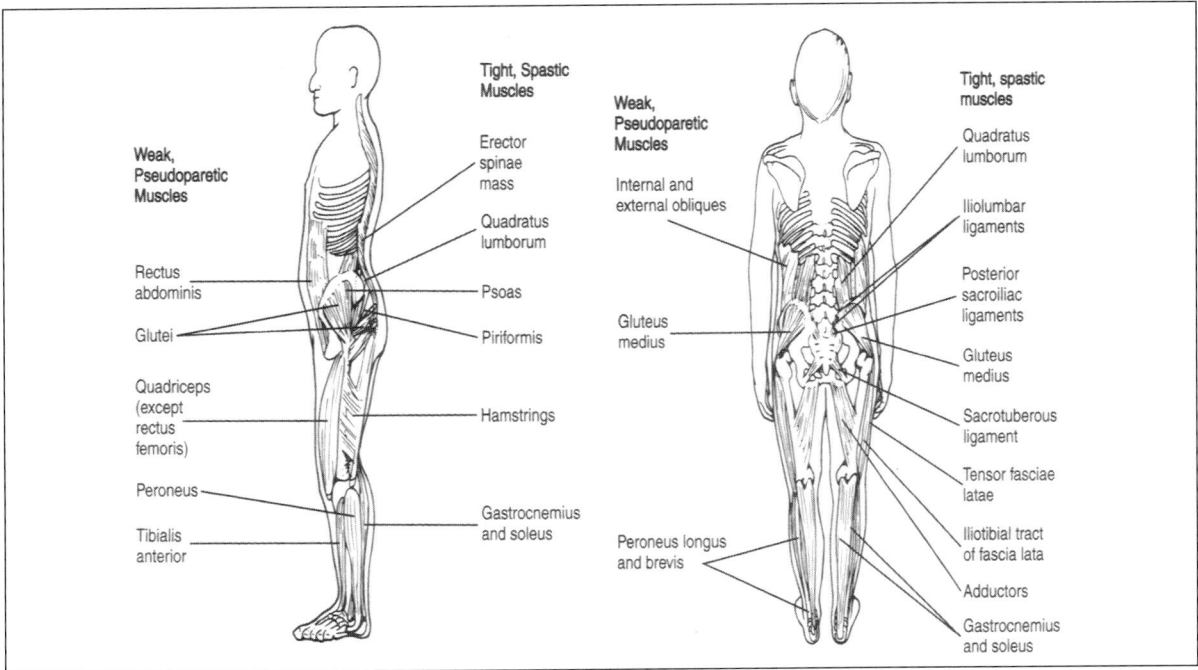

Figure 11-14: Myofascial cross patterns of weak and tight muscles (From Kuchera WA and Kuchera ML, Osteopathic Principles in Practice, KCOM press 1994, with permission).

- On one side the pectoralis major and minor, upper trapezius, levator scapulae, sternocleidomastoid, and often the scalenes are all tight and short, while the lower and middle trapezius, serratus anterior, and rhomboids are all weak and inhibited.
- This creates a posture with forward head, straightening of the cervical curve, extension of the upper cervical spine, increased kyphosis of the cervicothoracic junction, and internal rotation of the shoulder joint.

The lower crossed syndrome shows the following characteristics:

- The hip flexors, iliopsoas, rectus femoris, TFL, short adductors, quadratus lumborum, and erector spinae group of the trunk all tighten and shorten, while abdominal and gluteal muscles are weak and inhibited.
- This creates a posture with anterior pelvic tilt (usually the right side) and increased lumbar lordosis. Often "functional" hypermobility and poor control of L4-5 and L5-S1 exist in the sagittal and coronal planes.

A review of Tom Myers' fascial trains (Myers 1997, 2001) shows clear similarities with the TCM Sinew channels.

Treatment of Subcutaneous Fascia

Fascial restrictions can be treated with subcutaneous needling, guiding the needle in the restricted direction. Several insertions and withdrawals, in a fan-like distribution, may be needed to release the restrictions. Often this is all that is needed.

Using light palpation, the practitioner may encounter hard or soft nodules in fascial layers that should be needled (especially in the sacroiliac areas). Often, needling these nodules cause sharp local pain and referred pain to the areas of the patient's complaints. Cross-fiber and effleurage massage is integrated to separate the nodules from surrounding tissues and to reduce swelling. In addition, either a bleeding and cupping technique or a moving-cup technique is helpful and can be incorporated.

Myofascial release techniques can be used by stacking up tension (by finding a combination of movements that tightens up the fascia) and asking the patient to take a deep breath and hold it for several seconds. Other activating forces such as wiggling the fingers or toes are used while the patient holds his/her breath. When the patient exhales, tension is stacked up again and the process is repeated.

Indirect techniques can be used by an opposite procedure, stacking up movements that lead to increased tissue softening or compliance. Adding a compression force is helpful.

These techniques should be applied at least weekly until distorted fascial patterns are resolved or cease to change, possibly indicating an intractably fixed state.

Causes of Contractile Unit Pain/Disease

Contractile unit pain (the muscles and their attachments) and disease may be due to:

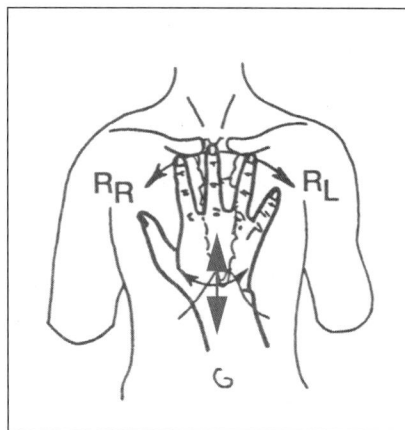

Figure 11-15: Facial assessment. The practitioner, after pressing the fascia, moves his/her hand in all possible directions noting which directions/combinations increase tension and which result in increased tissue compliance. Treatment that engages the restrictions are called direct methods while those that move away from tension are called indirect methods (From Kuchera WA and Kuchera ML, Osteopathic Principles in Practice, KCOM press 1994, with permission).

- Direct injury (burns, contusions, exertional rhabdomyolysis, seizure-related rhabdomyolysis, injection-related local myopathy and fibrosis) or infection (pyomyositis);
- Secondary infections in other associated areas (bacteria, viral, protozoal, and parasitic);
- Reflexively to somatic dysfunctions, most often ligament and joint disorders;
- Neurological dysfunctions such as chronic or acute injury to nerves as well as Gunn's "neuropathic pain" due to so-called mild denervation;
- Postures that chronically stress muscles, especially those being asked to function eccentrically for excessive periods. These muscles are being made to function as straps and may develop deformation.

Other conditions that can cause muscle pain and/or weakness are (Kagen 2000; Gunn *ibid;* Janda *ibid;* Simons, Travell and Simons *ibid*):

- Reflex sympathetic dystrophy (complex regional pain);
- Electrolyte (potassium, phosphate) abnormalities;
- Defects in carbohydrate metabolism (McArdle disease, Tarui disease, glycogen storage disorders);
- Defects in lipid metabolism (carnitine palmityl transerase deficiency, carnitine deficiency states);
- Thyroid or adrenal dysfunction;
- Malignancy;
- Inflammatory disorders (polymyalgia rheumatica, dermatomyositis, myositis, initial stage of various connective tissue diseases [scleroderma, sarcoidosis], and vasulitis syndrome);
- Osteomalacia;
- Osteoarthritis;
- Visceral disorders;
- Nutritional deficiencies;
- Sleep disorders;
- Psychological disorders;
- Parkinson's disease.
- Genetic conditions of muscular dystrophy (Duchenne, Becker phenomenon, myotonic, facioscapulohumeral, limb-girdle) and periodic paralyses from potassium disorders;
- Drug and medication-induced myopathies (alcoholic, cocaine, heroin, diuretics, corticosteroids, lipid-lowering drugs, and penicillins);
- Other rare myopathies (central core disease, nemaline myopathy, myotubular myopathy).

Muscle Functioning and Anatomical Changes in Chronic Disorders

With chronic dysfunctions and pain, muscles have been shown to have changed characteristics.

In chronic low back pain populations, EMG recordings have shown abnormalities (Wolf and Basmajian 1979). Muscle fiber physiology in patients with chronic cervical dysfunction has been shown to transform from "slow oxidative" to "fast glycolytic" (Unlig, Weber and Grob 1995). In patients with chronic low back pain, histologic evidence of type I fiber hypertrophy on the symptomatic side, and type II fiber atrophy bilaterally, were documented by Fitzmaurice et al (1992). In patients with acute low back pain, unilateral wasting has been documented in the multifidus muscle by Hide et al (1994). They further showed that atrophy was isolated to one dysfunctional segment and was not thought to be disuse-related.

Muscles are susceptible to psychogenic influences. Waersted, Eken, Westgaard (1992, 1993) have demonstrated that a small number of motor units in a muscle may display almost constant or repeated activity when influenced psychogenically. Using the trapezius muscle and surface EMG, they demonstrate low amplitude levels of activity when individuals were inactive. This small pool of low-threshold motor units may be under considerable load for prolonged periods. If tension-provoking factors are frequently present and the subject, as a result, recruits the same motor units repeatedly, an overload may follow, possibly resulting in a *metabolic crisis*.

Muscles that are being used as straps (i.e., are working excessively) may become undernourished, develop triggerpoints, show reduced functionality, become weakened, along with increased metabolic crisis, toxicity, and fibrosis (Simons, Travell and Simons *ibid*).

It is clear from these and other studies that muscle activity and form are affected in chronic pain sufferers. This does not

Myofascial Disorders

elucidate the underlying cause or whether muscles are a major primary source of chronic pain.

Muscle Spasms

Muscle spasm is defined as an involuntary sudden movement or muscular contraction that prevents lengthening of the muscles involved. Spasm is often due to pain stimuli to the lower motor neuron system and is not usually related to pain arising from the spasmed muscle. As a matter of fact, it is now known that muscle spasm has no relation to pain, and in fact muscle pain trends to inhibit, not facilitate, reflex contraction of the same muscle. Spasms may be tonic (sustained) or clonic (alternating with relaxation). There is increased electrical activity in the muscle. However, many practitioners clinically consider muscle spasm as increased tension without significant muscle shortening and electrical activity. This is more properly called tension. Travell and Simons (*ibid*) suggest that this occurrence of taut muscle bands is the result of sustained intrinsic activation of the contractile mechanisms of the muscle fibers, without motor unit action potential stimulation (electrical activity). The term "spasm" is therefore often misused.

Early and Late Spasms

Muscle spasms can be divided into early and late spasms. Early spasms occur at the beginning of the range of motion, almost as soon as movement is initiated. They are associated with inflammation. Late spasms, which occur at or near the end of the range of movement, are due to joint dysfunction, most often caused by instability of the joint.

MUSCLE TENSION. Excessive skeletal muscle tension may arise from limbic system dysfunction and may result in pain (Janda 1991). The limbic system is thought to be involved with abnormal behavior including depression, irritability, anxiety, and sleep disorders with associated muscle tension and tenderness. Chronic tension may cause pain that is felt either as sharp and well localized, or as a dull ache that is not as well localized. The pain is affected by muscle activity and is associated frequently with both deep and superficial tenderness and tightness. Longstanding tension may lead to tendinitis and fibrosis (Gunn *ibid*; Dvorák *ibid*).

Tight muscles may be stronger or weaker than normal, depending on the amount of tension. According to Janda (1993), moderately tight muscles are stronger than normal, but pronounced tightness leads to "tightness weakness." Maintaining a fixed position for a long duration often causes muscle tension, stiffness, and pain. A ligamentous or tendinous source should always be considered. Patients should be encouraged to move frequently and to vary their activity, especially if they have to use the same movements repeatedly.

Increased tension, tone, and vasoconstriction in the muscle or tendon may result in relative hypoxia, accumulation of metabolites, abnormal growth of connective tissue, and degenerative changes, all of which may lead to fatigue, stress-atrophy, and tissue weakening (Travell and Simons *ibid*). The resulting increase in motor unit recruitment leads to altered patterns of muscle contraction and increased vulnerability to injury. The injured muscles in turn remain even more vulnerable to dysfunction and pain. They are often shortened, especially after immobilization or protective behavior. Therefore, restoration of normal muscular function and length is important (Brown *ibid*).

A sedentary life style can result in overuse of postural muscles and overloading of ligaments, encouraging the development of tightness. Tense muscles should always be stretched before activity or before strengthening is attempted. Stretching tight muscles may result in improved strength of the inhibited antagonistic muscles (Janda *ibid*).

MUSCLE SPASM IN ARTHRITIC AND DYSFUNCTIONAL JOINTS. The source of pain in the arthritic joint has not been definitively established. Muscle spasm is probably a protective reaction to stretching of a painful joint capsule. The capsule, not the muscle, may be the major source of pain. This is evident in joints where no muscle spans the joint, such as the acromioclavicular, sternoclavicular and sacroiliac joints. When these joints are stretched, they are as painful as other arthritic joints that are under muscle control (Cyriax *ibid*). When arthritic joints are at rest, the muscles usually are relatively relaxed and spring into spasm when the joint capsule is stretched or under load. This is called *involuntary muscle guarding*. In contrast, *voluntary muscle guarding* is seen in chronic unstable joints where muscle hypertrophy develops. Here the muscles appear bulky and spasmed, during both weightbearing and non-weightbearing positions, often on the side opposite the instability (Paris *ibid*).

Cyriax identified the "*capsular pattern*," a limitation of movement, specific to each joint, that occurs as a reaction to arthritis and capsulitis. This pattern results from a reflexive protective spasm of muscles guarding the joint (involuntary guarding), which occurs upon initiation of passive or active movement in a particular direction. In later stages, the contracted capsule can restrict movement in the identical specific vectors that were initially inhibited by spasm.

According to Janda (*ibid*), it is not known whether dysfunction of muscles causes joint dysfunction and pain or vice versa. However, he points to the undoubted fact that they influence each other.

Steiner (1994) discussed the role of muscles in disc and facet syndromes as a strain involving body torsion, rapid stretch, and loss of balance that may produce a *myotatic stretch reflex response* and thus *spasm*. The muscles contract to protect against excessive joint movement, and spasm may result if there is an exaggerated response following a strain. This may limit the vertebrae movement and approximate a pair of vertebrae by pulling them closer to each other, and may result in compression and possibly bulging of the intervertebral discs. Strong muscle contraction may force the articular facets together. Bulging discs might then press on a nerve root, producing discogenic pain. Articular facets, when forced together, produce pressure on the intra-articular fluid, pushing it against the confining facet capsule, which may becomes stretched and irritated. The sinuvertebral capsular nerves may therefore become irritated, provoking muscular guarding, and initiating a self-perpetuating process of pain-spasm-pain (Chaitow *ibid*). Gunn (*ibid*) uses similar mechanisms to explain the development of spasms from *neuropathic hypersensitivity,* secondary to joint and vertebral degeneration.

MUSCLE SPASM IN BURSITIS. Although movement is limited in a particular direction, usually no frank muscle spasm occurs in cases of bursitis. The limitation (to avoid pain) is voluntary in that the patient limits the motion in response to pain, but is actually capable of further movement (Cyriax *ibid*). Characteristically, however, tender motor points are palpable, and treatment of them may render an effective response (Gunn *ibid*).

MUSCLE SPASM IN INTERNAL DERANGEMENT. Blockage of movement caused by internal derangement usually is due to a combination of mechanical reasons and muscle spasm (Cyriax *ibid*).

MUSCLE SPASM IN NERVE ROOT COMPRESSION. Muscle spasm associated with the spine often serves to protect the nerve roots. Irritation of the nerve root, not the muscle, is probably the direct cause of pain. In lumbar disc disease, this can be demonstrated clearly by increased leg pain during neck flexion, which pulls on the nerve root but does not affect the leg muscles. Also, epidural anesthesia, which does not affect the leg muscles, allows for increased range in the straight leg raise test (SLR) (Cyriax *ibid*).

MUSCLE SPASM AND THE DURA MATER. In conditions that affect the dura mater, muscle spasm functions to protect the dura. In meningitis, the muscle spasm holds the neck in extension, as this keeps the dura in its shortest position. In the lumbar region, protective spasms of the hamstring muscles guard the theca from getting pulled via the sciatic nerve or keep the patient deviated so that pressure is minimized at the nerve (Cyriax *ibid*).

MUSCLE SPASM IN DISLOCATION AND FRACTURE. In the case of dislocation and fracture, muscles go into constant spasm. This may prevent reduction without first administering anesthesia (Cyriax *ibid*).

MUSCLE SPASM IN MUSCLE AND TENDON RUPTURE. When a partial rupture of the muscle belly or tendon occurs, the torn fibers go into spasm, leaving the unaffected fibers in a normal state. Therefore, function is affected only partially. With complete tendon rupture, the muscle belly usually does not go into spasm; (Cyriax *ibid*) however, contractures may develop with time.

PERMANENT MUSCLE SPASM/CONTRACTURE. Schmidt has shown that nociceptive afferent stimulation via a gamma loop (vicious cycle) can affect skeletal muscles significantly, and that it can lead to permanent elevation of muscle tone. Even though muscle spasm and tension may be secondary at first, the muscle can develop intrinsic dysfunction that remains independently of the original cause. The cycle (Fassbender 1980) of nociceptive (painful) stimulation and chronic contractile unit dysfunction require treatment to avoid the long term sequelae of muscle damage and hypertrophy.

Should Muscle Spasm Be Treated?

There is much controversy regarding the significance of muscle spasms and tension. According to Cyriax, Ongly, Dorman, and others, muscle spasm and *myofascial trigger points* (other than traumatic) are mostly secondary reflex conditions that do not require direct treatment. They stress the role of discs, ligaments, and tendons in musculoskeletal disorders and pain.

Ligaments and tendons are supporting structures and are maximally affected by mechanical forces. They have a poor blood supply (although they do have one) and, therefore, are susceptible to injury and to the development of chronicity. These factors result in tissue damage and are seen as the overriding element responsible for *chronic* musculoskeletal pain. The above authors consider muscle tension, spasm, and trigger points as manifestations secondary to ligamentous relaxation, tendinitis, joint dysfunction, subluxation, and disc disease. According to Cyriax, instead of treating muscles, the primary lesion should be addressed, and then muscle "spasms" and pain will resolve by themselves. It must be remembered, however, that if normal muscle function is affected (regardless if primary or secondary), the balanced action acting across joints to provide support and to relieve load on the above-mentioned "inert" tissues is lost.[47] This loss may result in inert tissue overload and damage (to non-contractile tissues). A dysfunction in a given muscle places additional demand on the same myotatic unit (muscles sharing the same functional responsibility). Stability is then almost totally dependent on the ligaments, which fall victim to creep and hysteresis. Therefore, attention to muscle function and health is important regardless of root causes.

According to Edward Stiles DO (personal communication), during a public demonstration Dr. Simons (of Travell and Simons) localized a number of active myofascial trigger points in a patient after which Dr. Stiles diagnosed and treated somatic dysfunctions. Treatment was given to restricted spinal joints, not to the muscles, and resulted in the disappearance of all of the trigger points. In the second addition of Travell and Simons' *Myofascial Pain and Dysfunction: The Trigger Point Manual,* discussions of somatic dysfunctions have been added.

---

47. Tendons and ligament stem cells, however, contain a small amount of actin and myosin (the filaments responsible for motion in muscles) and have been described as not completely "inert."

Others believe muscles should be treated directly because, for example, the treatment may prevent the development of other lesions (such as tendinitis) that they see as secondary to muscle tension.

Gunn (1989) and Travell and Simons (1983) emphasize the role of muscles as causative factors in chronic disability and pain. Gunn states that:

> ... when pain is present, it is practically always accompanied by muscle shortening in peripheral and paraspinal muscles, spasm and/or contracture with tender painful focal areas in muscles, and autonomic and trophic manifestations of neuropathy. Muscle spasm and shortening is the key to musculoskeletal pain of neuropathic origins...

Cyriax (*ibid*), on the other hand, states:

> ... In orthopedic disorders, the muscle spasm is secondary and is the result of, not the cause of, pain; it causes no symptoms of itself...The treatment of muscle spasm is of the lesion to which it is secondary; it never of itself requires treatment in a lesion of moving parts...

Cyriax points out that muscle spasm is only rarely a source of chronic pain. His supporting example is the effect of epidural anesthesia in disc disease. Even though the anesthesia cannot reach the muscles, it reduces the pain and relaxes the muscle spasms. Cyriax also cites Conesa, who administered a muscle relaxant to treat spasmed, stiff, and painful shoulders, and, while he obtained relaxation of the muscles, it did not affect the pain or range of motion (Cyriax *ibid*).

Steiner (1994) discussed the role of muscles in disc and facet syndromes and describes a possible sequence of events as follows: A strain involving body torsion, rapid stretch, loss of balance, etc., produces a myotatic stretch reflex response in, for example, a part of the erector spinae. The muscles contract to protect excessive joint movement, and spasm may result if there is an exaggerated response and they fail to assume normal tone following the strain. This limits free movement of the attached vertebrae, approximates them and causes compression and, possibly, bulging of the intervertebral discs and/or a forcing together of the articular facets. Bulging discs might encroach on a nerve root, producing disc-syndrome symptoms. Articular facets, when forced together, produce pressure on the intra-articular fluid, pushing it against the confining facet capsule, which becomes stretched and irritated. The sinuvertebral capsular nerves may therefore become irritated, provoking muscular guarding, initiating a self-perpetuating process of pain–spasm–pain. Steiner further states: From a physiological standpoint, correction or cure of the disc or facet syndromes should be the reversal of the process that produced them, eliminating muscle spasm and restoring normal motion (Chaitow *ibid*).

Others point out that muscles that are in spasm ache due to the production of metabolic by-products and the activation of stretch-sensitive tissues. A sustained contraction of only 4% of the maximum voluntary contraction has been shown to lead to negative effects (Andersson 1990; Sato at el 1984).

Gunn (1976, 1977) suggests that mild neuropathy can lead to muscle spasm (contracture/tension), shortening, and supersensitivity that can then lead to tendinitis, bursitis, and joint restriction, treatment of which may be effective. Often these conditions are accompanied by sensory, motor, and autonomic findings that suggest functional and/or pathological alterations in the peripheral nerves. This also affects muscles (swelling, contracture, and hypersensitivity). Gunn (1989) suggests that dry needling of muscles which are affected by such nerve pathology can result in healing of the nerves and can give long term relief from pain. Certainly, the "truth" involves elements of each of these theories.

Treatment

In general, muscles heal well from injury. This may be due to the presence of satellite (stem) cells in skeletal muscles, which, when activated, provide a new cell population for muscle regeneration by transforming into myoblasts (Strohaman et al 1989), hypervascularity, and high nerve supply (Weintraub 1999) which are found in muscles. Treatment of contractile unit disorders may include: stretching, neuralmotor re-education, massage, acupuncture/electroacupuncture, electrical stimulation (faradic, micro-current, interferential, high or low volt, H-wave, etc.), countertension positional release, muscle energy techniques, and medications. Acupuncture, via the release of growth factors may be helpful in the late stages. Strained muscles are often weak and tight. It is important to rehabilitate both of these aspects as stretching or strengthening alone often results in continued pain and dysfunction. In general, muscles should be stretched before they are strengthened. According to Janda (*ibid*):

> Clinical experience, and especially therapeutic results, support the assumption that (according to Sherrington's law of reciprocal innervation) tight muscles act in an inhibitory way on their antagonists. Therefore, it does not seem reasonable to start with strengthening of the weakened muscles, as most exercise programmes do. It has been clinically proven that it is better to stretch tight muscles first. It is not exceptional that, after stretching of the tight muscles, the strength of the weakened antagonists improves spontaneously, sometimes immediately, sometimes within a few days, without any additional treatment.

Therefore, for example, to treat a patient's protruding abdomen should be done by first stretching the tight lumbar and abdominal muscle, before initiating abdominal strengthening.

According to Weintraub (*ibid*), for a chronically injured structure, treatment strategies should include:

- Increase oxygenation;
- Raise metabolic rate (energy level of the tissue);
- Ensure adequate vascular and lymphatic flow;

- Reduce inflammation (See "Perpetuating Factors" on page 669);
- Normalize the electromagnetic climate of the body region;
- Restore normal mechanics to the adjacent joints;
- Establish normal, balanced patterns of afferent input from the joint and tension/ligament;
- Restore an adequate quantity of its ground substance (ratio of ground substance to fiber);
- Reestablish the normal mobility and alignment of the individual fibers and their bundles.

Muscle Weakness

One of the major causes of musculoskeletal disorders is muscle weakness. Lack of muscle strength or balance can lead to excessive loads on the ligamentous structures supporting joints, which may degenerate and increase joint dysfunctions. Kraus showed that the majority of low back pain sufferers, in whom no "pathology" was identified, failed six basic tests for minimal muscular fitness (Bonica *ibid*). In general, muscles become weak for many reasons. According to Dr. Blaich, some of the common internal causes of muscle weakness are:

- Dysfunction of the nerve supply (nerve interference between the spine and the muscles);
- Impairment of lymphatic drainage;
- Reduced blood supply;
- Abnormal pressure in the cerebrospinal fluid affecting the nerve-to-muscle relationship;
- Blockage of an acupuncture meridian;
- Chemical imbalance;
- Organ or gland dysfunction.

Muscle weakness and degeneration of traumatic origin can result from direct trauma, or from injury to the muscle's blood or nerve supply. With immobilization there is decrease in muscle strength, most dramatically during the first week. After two weeks in a plaster cast, there is 20% loss of maximum strength (*ibid*).

Another important cause of muscle weakness or inhibition is somatic dysfunction at the associated vertebral levels. Resisted muscle testing may show a weak myotomal chain. Weakness should be differentiated as being secondary to tightness within the weak muscles or their antagonists. Treatments are often helpful that are directed to the associated vertebra (manual therapy or acupuncture), and to the muscles (manual stretches, strength exercises, and/or needling therapy to motor, trigger, or acupuncture points). According to Dr. Goodheart (the founder of Applied Kinesiology), if a specific muscle is weakened by being slightly separated from the bone, a manual procedure of firm, goading pressure on the attachment points of the weak muscles can result in an immediate response "turning on" the muscle (see "Applied Kinesiology" on page 509).

Other common causes are inhibition by other tight muscles, inactivity, poor nourishment and obesity.

Exercise programs are widely recommended to prevent the development of spinal pathology, to decrease pain, and to increase function. In some long-term follow-up studies, exercise was shown to effectively relieve 60-80% of patients who had low back pain (Kraus 1988). However, patient compliance and motivation are often problematic as many participate only in passive treatments.

Muscle Paralysis

Muscle paralysis can be due to upper or lower motor neuron lesions,[48] or may be due to intrinsic muscle diseases. Paralyzed muscles display decreased strength and altered tone in the affected muscle. They may be hypotonic (flaccid) or hypertonic (spastic), depending on the location of the lesion. Interruption of a spinal lower motor neuron,[49] or cells of the anterior horn, nerve roots or peripheral nerves interferes with the circuit to the muscle. The muscle loses normal innervation and nourishment.

FLACCID PARALYSIS. Korr found that nerves and neuromuscular synapses supply trophic substances to muscles (the delivery of proteins by exoplasmic flow, both antegrade and retrograde). When a nerve is deactivated it loses this nourishing function, which can lead to muscle atrophy. The nerve can be compromised by structural pressure at the nerve root, along the course of the axon and in the target tissue. This can have major effects on muscles, tendons and ligaments which have rich nervous supply. Denervated muscles lose the normal tone, control and tendon reflexes. This condition called flaccid paralysis, may be seen in conditions such as carpal tunnel syndrome, disc disease, poliomyelitis and other lower motor neuron paralysis (anterior horn cells of the spinal cord and the spinal and peripheral nerves) (*OM: Flaccid paralysis [Zhong] can be caused by weakness of Spleen/pancreas/Stomach, Dampness/Phlegm [numbness], Liver and Kidney weakness, Essence and Blood depletion*).

SPASTIC PARALYSIS. Interruption of upper motor neuron signals (suprasegmental in brain or spinal cord) also diminishes muscle control, but without damaging the lower motor neurons. Innervation and nourishment of the muscle remains uninterrupted. Therefore the muscle still receives input from the ventral horn motor neurons (from spinal cord). Although voluntary control over the muscle is lost, the muscle still has intrinsic tone and can become spasmed. This is called spastic paralysis. Tendon reflexes can still be elicited, as the cord is

---

48. Multiple sclerosis, strokes, brain tumors and Parkinson's are examples of upper motor neuron disorders that lead to spastic paralysis. Hyperreflexia can also be seen in pernicious anemia.

49. Poliomyelitis, amyotrophic lateral sclerosis (ALS) and nerve root palsy are examples of lower motor neuron diseases that lead to flaccid paralysis.

Table 11-2: Motor Impairments

Lower Motor Lesion	Upper Motor Lesion	Cerebellar
Muscle bulk decreased	Muscle bulk normal	Muscle bulk normal
Muscle weakness	Muscle weakness, characteristic distribution	Muscle tone decreased
Muscle tone decreased	Muscle tone increased, spasticity	Reflexes not applicable
Tendon reflex loss or diminished	Exaggerated tendon reflexes, clonus	Extensor planter response (Babinski)
Flexor planter response (normal)	Extensor planter response (Babinski)	Tremor on movement
Fasciculations (visible muscle twitching)	Loss of abdominal reflexes	Ataxic gait
Trophic changes in skin and nails	No muscle wasting	Coordination impaired
Foot drop (weakness gait)	Spastic gait	
Coordination normal	Coordination impaired	

intact, and are hyperactive (because of decreased regulation from descending brain or spinal cord, i.e. upper motor neuron fibers). The muscle resists passive stretching. Clonus may be seen (*OM: Spastic paralysis [Zhi] is mostly associated with internal-Wind, Liver Yin/Blood-deficiency with Wind, or Phlegm combined with Wind*).

Acupuncture has been shown to effectively treat patients with symptoms related to sequelae of strokes and muscle weakness (Li and Jin 1994). In a study done at Boston University, acupuncture was effective in a specific type of stroke, and resulted in significant savings in patients care (Naeser et al 1994). For characteristic motor impairments see Table 11-2.

Wasting (Wei) Syndromes—TCM

The main causes of wasting and paralysis seen in orthopedic practices are Spleen/pancreas and Stomach deficiency, a general deficiency of Qi and Blood, deficiency of Yin of the Liver and Kidneys and interruption of the channels and colleterals. Excessive causes are Dampness, Phlegm, and Blood-stasis.

While originally atrophy/wasting (Wei) syndromes were mostly associated with Heat (mostly invasion of Wind-Heat in Lungs and later Interior-Heat injuring the Spleen and Stomach), in the Tang dynasty Painful Obstruction (Bi) came to be associated with wasting and limpness. Obstruction can lead to the development of a wasting syndrome by *obstructive depletion* of Essence, Blood, Nutritive-Qi, and Yin. Wei syndromes, characterized by decreased muscular mass and strength, are seen in biomedical diseases such as multiple sclerosis and flaccid paralysis (Tan Huan), from motor-neuron disease or peripheral neuronal disorders such as radiculopathy. They are also seen in muscular atrophy from primary muscular disorders such as myasthenia gravis, viral infections such as poliomyelitis, and from strokes. Hemiplegia caused by strokes (Wind-strike) is mainly due to retention of Wind and Phlegm in the channels of the limbs on one side (often with underlying disorders of the Liver, Yin, Qi, Blood, Phlegm, and Wind).

Since Wei-atrophy conjures the image of withered and wilted tissues, it *may* correspond to some *instability syndromes*. The sinews (and therefore ligaments) are said to be lax, with impaired *motor* function and weakness. Mild "paralysis" is said to consist of weakness of the extremities and is often associated with the Spleen/Stomach. Severe paralysis is often associated also with the Liver and Kidneys (mostly deficient-Yin and Essence).

The *Classic of Internal Medicine* describes five types of wasting syndromes, one for each of the Yin Organs and its related tissue: skin, sinews, flash, vessels, and bones. Wasting syndromes were mostly attributed to Heat/Fire damaging the Lungs, body Yin-Fluids and were probably first discerned by examining disorders such as polio or infantile paralysis (which often begin with a fever).

The *Classic of Internal Medicine* also associated wasting syndromes with Yang-Ming (Stomach/Large Intestine) Dampness:

> When a person is submerged in dampness, [because] his work has to do with water, and if some [Dampness] stays [in the body], or when someone's place of living is damp, and his muscles and the flesh are soggy, obstruction [develops with] numbness. This develops into flesh limpness.

A discussion of paralysis in the same text shows a complex sense of lower extremity paralysis *(Biomedical: possibly related to innervation and circulation)*. It is also said in the *Classic of Internal Medicine* that "the ancestral sinew[50] rules the binding of the bones and the free movement of the joints."

The Yellow Emperor asked:

> Why is it maintained that only the Yang-Ming should be used to treat paralysis? Qi Po answered: The Yang-Ming is the sea of the five viscera and the six bowels; it is in charge of moistening the ancestral sinew. The ancestral sinew is in charge of the lumbar bones and the function of the lumbar joints. The Chong channel is the sea of the channels and vessels. It is in charge of irrigating the rivers and valleys [of the sinews], and it meets with the Yang-Ming in the ancestral sinew. The Yin and Yang meet in the ancestral sinew, and they travel upward along the abdomen to meet at the Qi Jie (Qi fairway), where the Yang-Ming is the master. All these channels belong to the

---

50. "Ancestral sinew" usually refers to the penis or, in this case, *perhaps* to the perineum (meeting of Yin and Yang CV-1 and GV-1), pelvic floor, and spine in general.

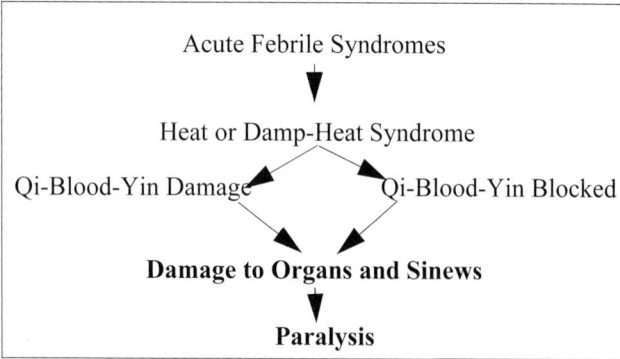

Figure 11-16: Externally contracted Wei-Syndrome

Girdle channel and are linked with the Governing channel [possibly referring to spinal system]. For this reason, when Yang-Ming is empty, the ancestral sinew will be relaxed (impotence), the Girdle channel cannot draw together, and the person will suffer paralysis of the legs with an inability to walk.[51]

As acute febrile wasting syndromes evolve, Deficiency becomes predominant. It often begins with Damp-Heat (or Dampness with pre-existing Deficiency), that leads to stasis and ecchymosis with Damp-stagnation. Qi and Blood are blocked, which leads to the shriveling of the sinews and muscles, as well as a deficiency of the Spleen/pancreas and Stomach which do not transport Qi to the limbs. Later, the Liver and Kidneys are involved, and the tonification of the Spleen/pancreas, Liver, and Kidneys is appropriate. Retained Pathogenic Factors can result in a combined Deficiency/Excess syndrome, Damp-Heat/Phlegm and Blood-stasis being the most common Excesses which result in pain and weakness. Wind can result in spasticity (Zhi or Zhi Zhong) and is often associated with biomedical upper motor lesions but can be a cause of stiffness in Painful Obstruction (Bi) syndromes associated with paralysis. When treating Wind; Essence, Fluids, Blood, and Yin are said to need nourishment often.

---

51. An interesting interpretive "translation" by Kendall (2002) is: The Yangming (stomach) vessel is the sea of the five viscera (zheng) and the six bowels (fu). It is responsible for lubricating the ancestral muscle, and the ancestral muscle is responsible for binding the bones and muscles of the lumbar region. The thoroughfare vessel (chong/aorta) is the sea of the main distribution vessels, responsible for irrigating the streams and valleys (referring to the skeletal muscles), and it joins the yangming (stomach) vessel at the ancestral muscle (meeting of external iliac and inferior epigastric arteries). The yin and yang vessels meet to empty the ancestral muscle. Their meeting is at the vital substance street (external iliac artery and vein), and the yangming (stomach) vessel is the chief of the vital substance street (Qichong, St-30). All these vessels depend upon the belt (dai) vessels (subcostal veins), which are collateral branches of the governing (du) vessel. Therefore, when the yangming (stomach) vessel is in deficiency the ancestral muscle will be relaxed. The belt (dai) vessels will not pull the other vessels together, and, therefore, the person will suffer paralysis of the legs and not be able to walk.

Spinal cord injury first leads to atrophy, wasting, and paralysis due to a severing of the channels and network-vessels, but it eventually leads to weakness of the Spleen/pancreas, Stomach, Liver, and Kidney as well.

Wasting syndromes of insidious onset such as myasthenia gravis, muscular dystrophy, and multiple sclerosis are attributed often to endogenous and independent causes such as excessive sex, overwork, irregular diet, trauma, and unbalanced emotions. These factors can also lead to sudden paralysis, as seen in Wind-strike *(Biomedical: strokes/brain attacks)*. The atrophy is often due to the malnourishment of sinew, bones, and flesh. A slowly developing condition often starts with Dampness or Phlegm, with numbness or tingling being predominant. Later, symptoms of Spleen/pancreas and Stomach deficiency increase, and a weakness of the extremities with difficulty in gait develop. As the condition progresses, the Liver and Kidneys fail to nourish the sinews and bones, and more severe pathological manifestations are seen with atrophy, wasting, and possible deformity (often associated with Damage to Essence or weak constitutional Essence). Gait becomes even more difficult or impossible. Internal-Wind and dryness of Blood, Essence, and Yin lead to spasticity. Blood-stasis and Phlegm lead to numbness and pain.

In general, Wei-atrophy syndromes are divided into Fire/Heat, Damp-Heat, Spleen/Stomach-deficiency (with Blood-deficiency and/or Qi-deficiency), Liver/Kidney exhaustion, and Phlegm-Dampness. Some patients present with combined tetanic and atrophy symptoms, or tetany evolves into Wei-atrophy syndrome. The etiology is often Fire/Heat, or Phlegm-Fire producing Wind, which may or may not be seen with an underlying Deficiency. In chronic cases there is often combined Deficiency and Excess syndrome. Atrophy secondary to trauma is often said to be due to Blood-stasis. Blood-stasis causing Wei-atrophy can also result from static-Blood "flowing" into the back region before the lochia has been eliminated.

Treatment of Wei Syndrome

Treatment is based on the type and stage of the syndrome. In *orthopedic practice*, treatment often involves modifications of Hidden Tiger Pill (Hu Qian Wan), Arouse Wasting/Wilting and Secure the True Pill (Qi Wei Gu Zhen Wan), Nourishing Yin and Moistening the Muscle and Sinews Decoction (Zi Zao Yang Rong Tang), Nourishing Yin and Marrow Decoction (Zi Yin Bu Sui Tang), and Four-Substance Decoction with Safflower and Peach Pit (Tao Hong Si Wu Tang). Acupuncture often emphasizes points on the Governing (Du), Girdle (Dai) and Yang-Ming channels.

Tendinitis, Tendinosis, and Tendon Strains

Historically, *tendinitis* has been used as a catchall term. There is, however, mounting evidence that distinguishes between the acute traumatic inflammatory type of tendinitis, and the more insidious process of chronic tendon degeneration that should be called tendinosis. The rate of collagen metabolism in the tendons is relatively slow, and normally there is a balance between breakdown and synthesis. Degenerated tendons show decreased protein synthesis, replication, storage, and contractility. There is visible discoloring of the tissue and loss of the mirror-like gloss of normal tendon surface. Other signs of attempted regeneration, such as granulation, are seen. If granulation is insufficient, necrosis and calcification may result. A shift of pH towards alkalosis together with a diminished metabolism may increase the level of calcium and phosphate ions and cause crystallization and calcification of the tendon.[52] These changes can be due to aging or repetitive use. In sports injuries, they can be due to immobilization, which leads to cell atrophy. Additionally, degeneration may be due to decreased nutrition, diminished endocrine hormonal influences, persistent inflammation, and longstanding corticosteroid therapy (Brown *ibid*). Dysfunction may result from changes either within the tendon or in the surrounding tissues of the tendon (paratendon) (Ombregt et al *ibid*).

What is often diagnosed as tendinitis should probably be called tendinopathy (or tendinosis) since often there is no clinical evidence for the diagnosis of inflammation. Light microscopy reveals collagen separation in patients with tendon pain and an absence of inflammatory cells. Anti-inflammatory medications often provide only short-term pain relief, and no evidence for longer lasting benefit exist (BMJ 2002). Increased blood circulation by the application of *topical nitric oxide* (topical nitroglycerine) improves outcomes in tennis elbow (Barclay 2003). Topical glyceryl trinitrate (nitric oxide donor; 1.25 mg glyceryl trinitrate/24 hours, Nitro-Dur patch) has also been shown to significantly improves outcomes, of tennis elbow, Achilles tendinopathy, and supraspinatus tendinopathy (Vogin 2004).

General diseases such as gout, rheumatoid arthritis, tuberculosis, syphilis, and influenza are also predisposing factors. In sports, a cold climate, bad equipment, and wrong training (e.g., lack of warming-up, stretching, too progressive an increase of load, duration of exercise, bouncing exercises, and jerky muscle contractions) may all be disastrous (Ombregt et al *ibid*). Other predisposing influences are excessive vibration or repetitive use (Brown *ibid*).

Blood supply to tendons is compromised at the sites of tendinous friction, torsion, or compression. Such areas are found particularly in the supraspinatus, achilles, and tibialis posterior tendons. Many tendons have a "critical zone" at the junction between two groups of blood vessels that lead to poor vascular and oxygen supply. The insertion of a tendon into bone involves a gradual transition from tendon to fibrocartilage to lamellar bone. Very few blood vessels cross the tenoperiosteal junction. After the age of twenty-five, the vascularization of tendinous tissues decreases and eventually is reduced by about 30% (Brown *ibid*). Overuse may disturb

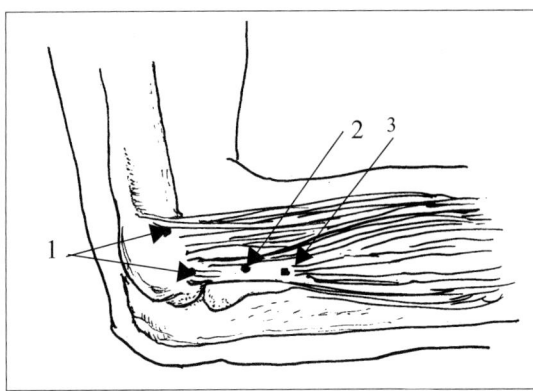

Figure 11-17: Lesion sites in tendinitis: 1) Tenoperiosteal. 2) Tendon body. 3) Tendinomuscular junction.

the arterial circulation to tendons. This in turn influences the metabolic processes, and, in the long run, result in degeneration with necrosis, and calcium deposits. From that moment on, a normal load may strain the tendon and tear some fibers. In general, tendinous lesions can be classified as follows (Ombregt et al *ibid*):

- Overuse tendon injury (tendinitis);
- Peritendinitis (tenosynovitis, tenovaginitis);
- Tendinosis;
- Tendinitis with peritendinitis;
- Local swelling of a tendon;
- Complete rupture.

Tendinitis occurs at the tendinous attachments, tendon body, or musculotendinous junction (Figure 11-17). Continued inflammation can lead excessive adhesion, fibrosis, and scarring. The lesions (and scarring) may occur anywhere, but most commonly they are found in the tenoperiosteal junction, the point of maximal mechanical tension with the poorest vascular supply (Noyes and Torvik et al 1974). Ruptures, however, seem to occur most often in the musculotendinous junction, especially in the Achilles tendon (Garrick and Ebb *ibid*). A small rupture of several fibers can lead to a self-perpetuating inflammation because healing is constantly interrupted by use and re-injury. Adhesions can develop. Partial tear of tendons can be found in several areas (Cyriax *ibid*): the deep articular aspect of the tendon, the superficial aspect, or halfway between the two, within the central portion of the tendon, or at the musculotendinous junction. Partial ruptures (tendinitis) are painful and often do not resolve spontaneously. With complete ruptures, a sharp pain is felt at the moment of injury and is immediately followed by inability to perform the movement actively. Often there is no pain after the initial injury. Ruptures occur predominately at the shoulder, wrist, and heel. In the shoulder, partial tears are quite common and are seen in asymptomatic populations as well. Ruptures of Achilles, tibialis posterior (Ombregt et al ibid), and biceps at the elbow are also quite common. In sports, traumatic tendon injuries often occur when there is a sudden

---

52. Localized anode (+) electrostimulation may be used to balance the pH.

unanticipated stretching of an already contracted muscle (Garrick and Ebb *ibid*).

Tenosynovitis and Tenovaginitis

Tenosynovitis occurs when tendons that are covered by a sheath become roughened and inflamed. It is commonly seen with occupational overuse or strain. In this condition, crepitus (a crackling sound or a grating feeling) is often elicited by movement. Tenosynovitis is commonly seen at the ankle or the wrist. Continued inflammation can lead to excessive adhesion, fibrosis, and scarring.

When a tendon sheath becomes severely inflamed without the finding of crepitus, the condition is called *primary tenovaginitis*. Tenovaginitis can occur from overuse but can also occur spontaneously. This is a lesion of the tendon sheath itself and is often associated with considerable swelling and tenderness, as is commonly found in the tendon sheath of the abductor pollicis longus and extensor pollicis brevis (de Quervain's disease). Tenovaginitis is also commonly found in the tibialis posterior tendon.

Other causes, such as infection (gonorrhoea, tuberculosis) or inflammatory disease (rheumatoid, gout), should be excluded when tenosynovitis or tenovaginitis is suspected. Coarse crepitus is a warning sign that points to rheumatoid disease or tuberculosis (Ombregt et al *ibid*).

Treatment of Tendinous Lesions

Mechanical overload seems to be the main cause of collagen degeneration in tendinosis. In athletes, training errors are a common cause, but, in some instances, a more subtle mechanism underlies tendinosis. It is important to assess all of the equipment being used (e.g., running shoes, tennis racket), examine movement biomechanics (e.g., running, throwing motion, stroke pattern), and to diagnose and treat any muscle imbalances. The importance of biomechanical correction cannot be overemphasized. Load-decreasing devices such as braces and orthotics may be needed. Patient education is very important in order to prevent the further frustration that comes from continuing activities that promote the degeneration of collagen. Appropriate strengthening may require a reasonable period of relative rest and attention to stretching. Once the tendinosis cycle is broken, the patient uses modalities that optimize collagen production and maturation. *Eccentric* muscle training should be emphasized, as it may result in tendon strengthening by stimulating mechanoreceptors in tenocytes to produce collagen (Figueroa 2002; see page 489).

Tendinitis, tendinosis, and tenosynovits can also be treated by cross-fiber massage, which can be started with light massage the day after the injury. Cryotherapy or heat and other mobilization techniques may be used in chronic degenerative tendinosis. Patients with chronic tendinosis may not respond to cross-fiber massage, and draining (effleurage/milking) type massage strokes in the direction of the heart (or away from the periosteum towards the muscle) may be helpful. The tendon is slowly "milked" with overlapping and repeated strokes until swelling is reduced. The strokes must by in the direction of the heart (i.e., direction of lymphatic vessels) when possible. The appropriate Chapmen's (neurolymphatic) reflexes are assessed and treated if needed (see "Chapman Reflexes" on page 498) to encourage lymphatic drainage. Exercises begin only when inflammation is reduced at about the third week post injury (in acute tendon strain). At times, tenovaginitis may only respond to a steroid injection. Occasionally surgical intervention is necessary. Laser or other photonic stimulation may be helpful. The lesion as well as any triggers within the muscle and appropriate segments should be treated.

In TCM, most tendinous disorders are part of Painful Obstruction syndromes. Tendinosis is often due to taxation-deficiency of Qi and Blood. Qi and Blood stasis are often seen as well. Calcific tendinosis often manifests with symptoms of Phlegm and Blood-stasis and is more difficult to treat than acute tendinitis. Important herbs in treating tendons are: Herba Lycopodii (Shen Jin Cao), Radix Asari (Xi Xin), Radix Aconiti Carmichaeli (Chuan Wu) and Radix Aconiti Kusnezoffii (Cao Wu) Fructus Chaenomelis (Mu Gua), Radix Paeoniae Alba (Bai Shao), Ramulus Cinnamomi Cassiae (Gui Zhi), Radix Dispaci Asperi (Xu Duan), Cortex Eucommiae Ulmoidis (Du Zhong), Rhizoma Gusuibu (Gu Sui Bu), Radix Astragali Membranaceus (Huang Qi), Ramulus Loranthi (Sang Ji Sheng), Succus Bambusae (Zhu Li), Fasciculus Vascularis Luffae (Si Gua Luo), Semen Vaccariae Segetalis (Wang Bu Liu Xing), Concha Arceae (Wa Leng Zi), Pollen Typhae (Pu Huang), Gummi Olibanum (Ru Xiang), Caulis Polygoni Multiflori (Ye Jiao Teng), Lumbricus (Di Long), and Vinegar (especially for calcific tendinosis).

Needle Therapy for Tendinous Lesions

When treating tendinous lesions acupuncture at the muscle belly or using distal point systems can be started immediately regardless of acuity. In the acute phase, strong local stimulation should be avoided. The most commonly used acupuncture points for tendinous lesions are: GB-34, Lu-5, LI-10, Correct tendons (a combination of two points 77.01-02 and 77.03), Liv-3, 8, UB-18, 17, 21, and regionally related points. Distal points are stimulated making sure that the needle contacts tendinous tissues ("like treats like").

If muscular dysfunction and pain are due to tendon *inflammation*, the practitioner can do the following:

1. He/she can needle the tendon periosteal junction, using a thin needle (gauge 36-38) locally around the tendon but not through it. Needling through it may lead to unnecessary inflammation and pain.

2. He/she can advance the needle slowly and take several seconds to reach the periosteum, paying constant attention to needle feel in order to prevent unnecessary

injury and muscular reactions. Once the periosteum is reached, one should gently peck the periosteum.

3. He/she can repeats this process as needed.

4. He/she can needle musculotendinous junction and trigger/motor points.

5. He/she can withdraw the needles or connect a *unipolar* microcurrent electrical stimulator with the anode (+) pole placed locally at the injured tendon and the cathode (-) held by the patient or connected to a motor point (or one can reverse the polarity if doing otherwise seems to irritate), to an ear point corresponding to the muscle, or to a distal point on the Sinew channel that passes through the muscle, or to the Accumulation point on the related Main channel. The motor or triggers at the affected or antagonist muscle(s) are addressed.

   Stimulation is maintained for one to five minutes only. A biphasic (AC) current or a positioning of the cathode (-) just distally or across to the injured site can be tried as well. Some patients do better with local tendinous tissues cathode (-) stimulation and proximal anode (+) stimulation at the appropriate vertebral segment. Follow with laser or photoic stimulation as it *may* help stimulate ATP, NO, and thus circulation and healing.

NOTE: Cross-fiber (friction) or effleurage massage can be applied before or after the treatment. Effleurage at the end of treatment can minimize post-treatment soreness.

Tendon and Muscle Insufficiency and Weakness

Chronic enthesopathy (attachment tenderness) is often due to tendon insufficiency. To treat the tendinous insertion, the tendon-periosteal junction is needled more vigorously than when treating tendon inflammation, and/or the anode (+) of a *monophasic* stimulator is connected locally, and the cathode (-) just distally (either miliamp or microamp stimulator). Some patients respond better to local cathode (-) application, and experimentation may be needed. (Studies are conflicting as to the which electrode leads to grater tissue proliferation.) The ionization and burn that can occur at the needle tip (mostly at the [-] cathode) can probably increase the inflammatory response which is needed to activate fibroblasts (only if monophasic or DC stimulation is used). The treatment lasts thirty to sixty minutes or longer. A bipolar (AC) current can be used, as well. At times, inserting a 30 gauge needle through the tendon is helpful and may resolve chronic cases.

Laser therapy by increasing ATP and by affecting NO levels may help in healing and increase blood-circulation to the tendon.[53]

Myosynovitis

Myosynovitis is a painful condition arising from a muscle due to overuse. In severe cases it is accompanied by crepitus on movement. Myosynovitis seems to occur rarely in: brachialis, quadriceps, hip adductors, and pectoralis muscles (Cyriax *ibid*).

Fibromyalgia and Myofascial Pain Syndrome

Fibromyalgia syndrome (FMS) is a controversial syndrome that was first recognized in 1987 by the American Medical Association (AMA). It is a rheumatologic diagnosis with a rather precise diagnostic criterion. FMS must be distinguished from Myofascial Pain Syndrome (MPS) even though they share several characteristics: both are affected by cold weather and may involve increased sympathetic nerve activity, resulting in conditions such as Raynaud's phenomenon. They both have tension headaches and paraesthesia as major associated symptoms (Donaldson et al 2001). Muscles (Chaitow *ibid*) that contain areas that feel like "a tight rubber band" are found in about 30% of patients with FMS, and in more than 60% of patients with MPS. Patients with FMS have reduced muscle endurance than do patients with MPS. Muscles in FMS patients tend to feel soft and doughy as compared to the tense, taut bands felt in MPS. FMS may be more of a systemic or medical disorder—possibly a component of chronic fatigue syndrome; and about 75% of patients of chronic fatigue syndrome meet the criteria of FMS; however, substance P levels are normal in MPS and chronic fatigue syndrome and not in FMS. MPS is more likely to be a musculoskeletal (orthopedic) condition. FMS occurs often as a development of chronic MPS, and 20% of MPS patients also have FMS. 72% of FMS patients have active trigger points (TPs) (Gerwin 1995).[54] Patients with FMS often are hypermobile while patients with MPS are often hypomobile, at least at the affected region. This differentiation is important, since the prognosis of each of these is very different. Both MPS and FMS may be caused by a variety of conditions which include: endocrine disorders, allergies, neoplasms, connective tissue diseases, infections, nutritional, as well as joint and ligamentous dysfunctions.

MPS is a painful condition felt by some to be due to myofascial trigger point activation, either by direct causes or as a reactive mechanism to other dysfunctions. The pain of MPS is better localized than the pain from FMS. The pain may be

---

53. Outcomes in the treatment of tendinosis varies greatly and often depend on location. Outcomes after using integrated methods for the treatment of tennis elbow (lateral epicondylitis) are often satisfactory. In the shoulder, however, in cases of impingement (i.e., with bone-spurs at the acromioclavicular joint, with acromial impingements often due to abnormally small space from the type of acromian, and with calcified tendons) surgical intervention is needed if the patient is to resume painless *sport* activities. Day pain and function can often be improved using non-surgical methods. However, often night pain and pain after vigorous activity remain. In the shoulder (and for many other tendinous lesions) good rehabilitation exercises that address both tightness and weakness are imperative and often are the key to success.

54. Although FMS patients often do not have local twitch responses at painful muscles (see below).

Table 11-3: Fibromyalgia and Myofascial Pain Syndrome

Symptoms and Signs	Fibromyalgia	Myofascial Pain Syndrome
Muscles with a tight band found in	30% of patients with FMS	60% of patients with MPS
Reduced muscle endurance	more in with FMS	less in MPS
Tension headaches	same	same
Pain affected by cold weather	same	same
Increased sympathetic nerve activity, resulting in conditions such as Raynaud's phenomenon	more in FMS	less in MPS
Substance P levels	elevated in FMS	normal in MPS
Abnormal levels of neurotransmitters and hormone responses	common	less common
Chronic fatigue	common in FMS	not common in FMS
Hypermobility	common	less common
Hypomobility	less common	more common
Internal medical problems such as: irritable bowel syndrome, dysmenorrhea, interstitial cystitis, depression, anxiety, mitral valve prolapse, and restless leg syndrome	common	less common
Myofascial trigger points	found in 72% of patients	found in 100% of patients
Wide-spread tenderness and painful skin role	found in 100% of patients	less common
Sleep disorder	very common	less common
Allodynia and hyperalgesia	common	not common
Cognitive difficulties	common	not common

confined to a large area and involve several separate sites; however, it is often unilateral with a defined pattern of distribution. MPS is associated with focal tenderness; FMS is associated with widespread tenderness. MPS is seen equally in males and females, whereas about 80% diagnosed with FMS are females (Donaldson et al *ibid*). The patient is often awakened from sleep by pain in both MPS and FMS, but chronic fatigue is not a common complaint in MPS patients. MPS does not produce morning stiffness as often as FMS does. Tension headaches are a common associated symptom in both. Prognosis for MPS is very favorable, and the condition responds well to techniques described in this text. In the MPS paradigm, emphasis is on short and tight muscles as causative factors of pain and dysfunctions. Table 11-3 compares FMS and MPS.

Myofascial Pain Syndrome (MPS) and Trigger Points

Myofascial pain syndrome (MPS) is defined as: "pain and/or autonomic phenomena referred from active trigger points with associated dysfunction." Travell and Simons (1982) describe a myofascial trigger point (TP) as a small locus in the muscle that is strikingly different from its surroundings and is sensitive to mechanical stimulation. This kind of muscle trigger point must be distinguished from "trigger points" in nonmuscular tissue such as: ligaments, fascia, scars, periosteal, bone, and skin. Kawakita, Miura, and Iwase (1991) suggested that trigger points may be more related to the fascia than the muscle. They used dry needling, pressure algometry, pulse algometry, and ultrasonic tomography to come to these conclusions. They related trigger points to inflammation in fascia. There is a close relationship between the distribution of tender spots and acupuncture points (Liu, Varela

Fibromyalgia and Myofascial Pain Syndrome

and Osutald 1957), and, according Melzack et al (*ibid*), nearly 80% of all trigger points are in the same positions as known acupuncture points. This, however, has been criticized (Birch 2003). The distribution of pain from trigger points does not relate directly to the Main acupuncture channel pathways, but many similarities are found with the Sinew channels.[55] The majority of trigger points are said to be located on or near the following acupoints (Pomeranz ibid): SI-10-13, 15; TW-13, 14; UB-12-17, 28, 29, 36-41, 48, 49, and GB-27, 30. However, myofascial triggers are often found near or on many other acupuncture points (except that trigger points are said to feel as indurated tissues and acupuncture points as holes). If "trigger points" are defined as triggers within muscle bellies, skin, scars, fascia, tendons, ligaments, capsules, and periosteum, as Travell and Simons do, most pressure sensitive acupoints (and certainly Ashi points) can be considered as "trigger points."

The prevalence of such tender areas, in both symptomatic and asymptomatic populations, results in a debate as to the significance of *myofascial pain syndromes* and myofascial trigger points. Trigger points are often classified as:

ACTIVE TRIGGER POINTS. Trigger points can be either active or latent. Active trigger points are painful and symptomatic at the time of examination. When stimulated, they reproduce the patient's symptoms easily. They can cause a pattern of referred pain at rest and/or on motion that is specific to the muscle. An active trigger point can limit full lengthening of the muscle and weaken the muscle.

LATENT TRIGGER POINTS. Latent trigger points cause dysfunction but do not produce pain at the moment of examination, i.e., they are quiescent with respect to spontaneous pain and are painful only when palpated. They have a higher threshold and require considerably more stimulation to elicit their typical reference. Sola and Kuitert (1955) found among 200 asymptomatic young adults that 54% had focal tenderness representing *latent myofascial trigger points*.

SATELLITE TRIGGER POINT. Active trigger points often result in satellite triggers in embryonic tissues of the same segmental levels and/or referred pain areas *(OM: often seen in distribution that is very similar to the sinew and main channels).* In time these will produce their own satellites.

PRIMARY TRIGGER POINTS. These are trigger points that have been activated by an acute or chronic overload of the muscle in which they are found.

SECONDARY TRIGGER POINTS. These are trigger points that have been activated as a result of dysfunction or trigger points in another muscle. They are often found in functionally related muscles, synergistic substitutes, or antagonists to the primary involved muscle. *(OM: and often manifest in Yin Yang channel relationships of sinew and main channels).*

FALSE TRIGGER POINTS. These are trigger points that are sensitive to palpation and that refer pain but that *does not correspond with known referred MPS trigger point patterns and/or the patient's symptoms*. They may produce a known referral pattern, but only when the pressure required to evoke this response is greater than indicated on the myofascial pain index (MPI).

Activating Forces

The main *direct* activating forces of TPs are: Injury to muscles, tendons, and/or joints; chronic stresses on muscles; and lengthy periods of hypothermia or exposure to environmental drafts and cold.

The main *indirect* activating forces are: Other trigger points; visceral diseases; nutritional deficiency; food and inhalant allergies with high histamine states; periodic hypoglycemia; arthritic joints; postural or anatomical stresses (e.g., short leg); emotional stress.

Latent trigger points can be activated by: Overstretching, inactivity, or momentary overtaxing of the involved muscle. Other activation causes are: Increased metabolic demands in short tight muscles, which may lead to ischemia and irritating metabolites which activate the trigger points; inhibition of antagonist muscle by over active tight agonist leading to fatigability and weakness; deconditioned muscles.[56]

MYOFASCIAL TP PAIN IS CHARACTERISTICALLY AGGRAVATED BY (Simons, Travell and Simons *ibid*):

- Strenuous use of the muscle, especially in the shortened position;
- Passively stretching the muscle;
- Pressure on the TP;
- After positioning; the muscle being in a shortened position for prolonged periods (such as after sleep);
- Sustained or repeated contraction of the muscle;
- Cold, damp weather, viral infections, and periods of marked nervous tension;
- Exposure to cold draft, especially when the muscle is fatigued.

MYOFASCIAL TP PAIN IS DECREASED BY (Simons, Travell, Simons *ibid*):

- A short period of rest;

---

55. The Sinew channels were not looked at by Melzack. Birch's analysis emphasized literature review of text-book point indications and therefore ignored the common practice of using local "points" based on palpation as "local" points (which he then classifies as Ashi points). Also, the practice of many myofascial therapists of treating referral zones and "satellite trigger points" often corresponds to distal points in acupuncture, which are used to treat similar regions. Trigger points are also associated with visceral syndromes (symptoms) and their location is often similar to the description of acupoint functions (especially in spine and abdomen).

56. Lack of muscle conditioning and protective action can lead to some muscles becoming overactive while others are inhibited, resulting in joint stress and increased muscle fatigue.

- Slow, steady *passive stretching* of involved muscles, particularly when the muscle is warmed in the shower or bath;
- Moist heat applied over the TP. The pain is not relieved if heat is applied to the reference zone;
- *Short* periods of light activity with movement (but not by isometric contraction);
- Specific myofascial therapy.

REFERRED PAIN AND VARIOUS OTHER EFFECTS OF TRIGGER POINTS. Pain referred from a myofascial TP does not follow a simple segmental pattern. Frequently, but not always, the pain occurs in the same dermatome, myotome, or sclerotome of the TP. It usually does not include the entire segment and often includes other segments (Travell and Simons *ibid*). According to Bonica (*ibid*), trigger-point pain referral patterns are related to sympathetic C-fibers distribution. The pain is *characterized* as being steady, deep, and aching, and rarely as burning. Two "skin muscles," the platysma and palmaris longus, refer a needle-like pricking sensation superficially. Throbbing pain is more likely be due to vascular disease or dysfunction than secondary to TP. Occasionally, a TP initiates sharp (lancinating) or lightning-like stabs of pain (Simons, Travell and Simons *ibid*).

Travell and Simons also report other symptoms that can be "caused" by TPs, such as: dizziness (including postural dizziness), tinnitus, diarrhea, decreased gastric motility, dysmenorrhea, spatial disorientation, localized vasoconstriction (cold limb), perspiration, change in sweat pattern, pilomotor activities (goose flesh), dermatographia, excessive lacrimation, cardiac arrhythmias, nasal secretion, disturbed weight perception, and positional pain (similar to posain caused by ligaments).

MPS (and fascial organ dysfunctions) may have far-reaching effects. For example, TPs located at the anterior and posterior axillary folds within the underlying muscles are said to result in lymphatic stasis that affects the chest/breast and upper arm structures. Scalene and SCM TPs are said to entrap many of the thoracic inlet structures, especially the subclavian vein and lymphatic trunk. TPs in pectoralis muscles may result in cardiac dysfunction with supraventricular tachyarrhythmias. Pectoralis TPs may also arise as a consequence of coronary artery insufficiency, treatment of which is considered to be an important factor in reducing reflex coronary artery spasm (Kuchera and Kuchera 1992).

Travell and Simons (*ibid*) have mapped and described each muscle trigger reference pattern in their book (Figure 11-18; Figure 11-19).

Mechanisms.

The "integrated trigger point hypothesis" has evolved to integrate information from electrophysiological and histopathological data. The *energy crises* component was developed to account for (Simons, Travell and Simons *ibid*):

- The absence of motor unit electrical activity in muscles with TPs when the muscle is at rest;
- The fact that muscles with TPs are often activated by overload;
- The sensitization of nociceptors in the TP;
- The effectiveness of almost any treatment that restores muscle length.

The concept of energy crises postulates a vicious cycle of events that appears to contribute to the development of myofascial trigger points. Either trauma or sudden marked increase in endplate release of *acetylcholine* can result in increased release of *calcium* concentration outside of the *sarcoplasmic reticulum*,[57] possibly due to a mechanical rupture of the sarcoplasmic reticulum or the muscle cell membrane. The function of the sarcoplasmic reticulum is to store and release ionized calcium, which induces the shortening activity of contractile tissues, which, in turn, causes sarcomere shortening. The excess calcium from injury or a marked increase in activity produces a maximal contraction of a *segment* of a muscle, which in turn results in an energy demand and a choking-off of local circulation. This *ischemia* and energy crisis results in a failed re-uptake of calcium into the sarcoplasmic reticulum, complicating the cycle. It is now apparent that sustained contraction is due to abnormal depolarization of the postjunctional membrane. This can continue indefinitely based on enduring the release of acetylcholine from dysfunctional nerve terminals (Simons, Travell and Simons *ibid*).

Travell and Simons (*ibid*) concluded that since *no* EMG activity is found in taut bands associated with myofascial TPs, the muscle tightness cannot correctly be called spasm/contraction and does not involve motor unit activity. They suggested the term *endogenous-contracture* for this condition. As discussed above, it is now thought more likely that an abnormal depolarization of the postjunctional membrane is responsible for the sustained contractile activity. This may continue indefinitely, based on continuing excessive acetylcholine release from a dysfunctional nerve terminal. Therefore, continued maximal contracture of the muscle fibers can persist without motor unit action potentials. When combined, the evidence from the integrated trigger point hypothesis shows that a TP is essentially a region of many dysfunctional *endplates*, and that each dysfunctional endplate is associated with a section of muscle fiber that is maximally contracted: *a contraction knot* (Simons, Travell and Simons *ibid*).

Hubbard and Berkoff (1993) on the other hand, using a dual channel monopolar needle electromyogram (EMG), showed a 1 mm foci that sustained very high spontaneous EMG activity and that was stimulated by sympathetic fibers. This rejects the extrafusal endplate theory covered above. Areas just 1 cm adjacent to these foci were EMG silent.

---

57. A net of tubules and sacs in muscle that store calcium.

Fibromyalgia and Myofascial Pain Syndrome

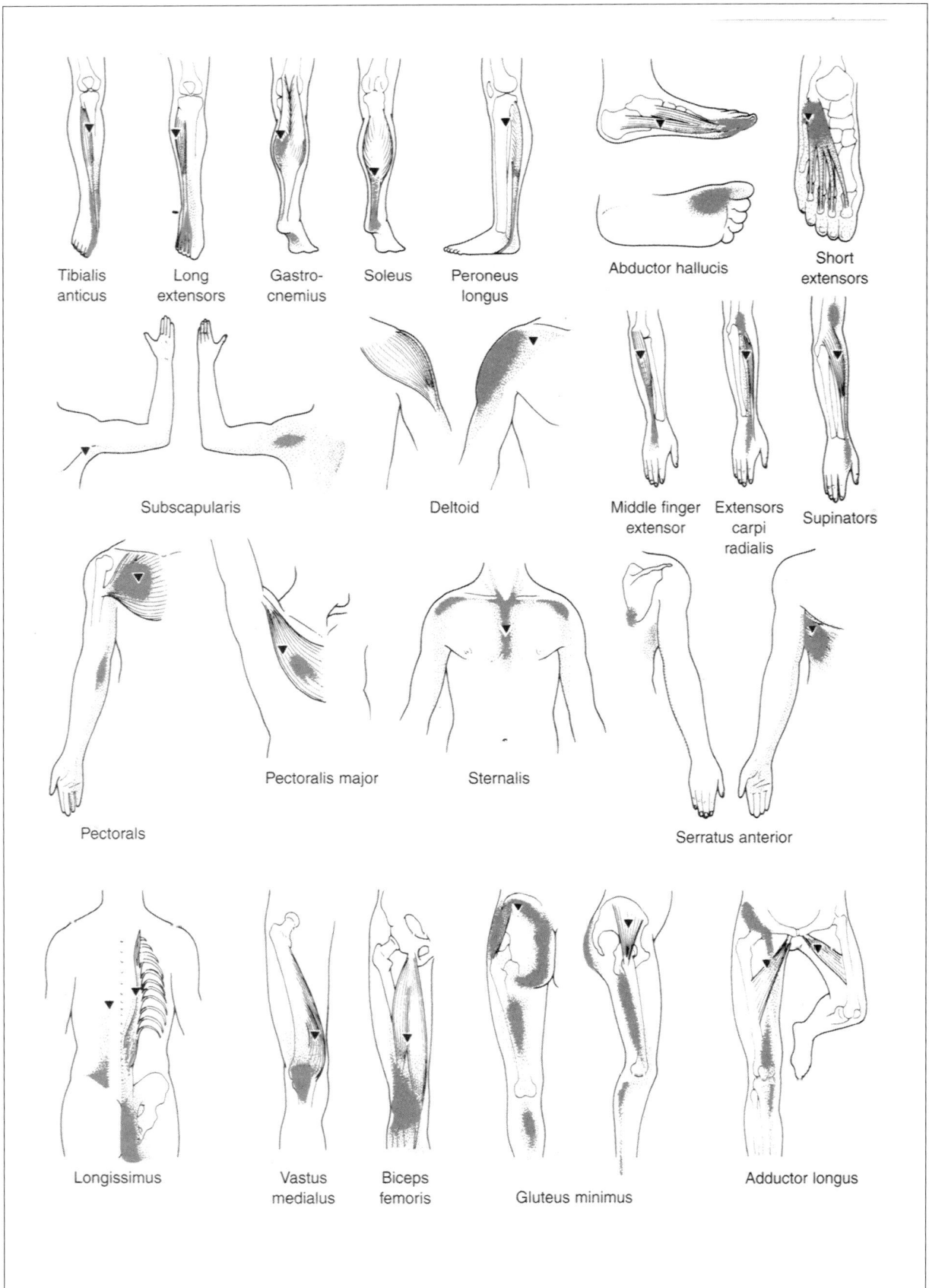

Figure 11-18: Referred pain from myofascial trigger points (with permission Chaitow 2001).

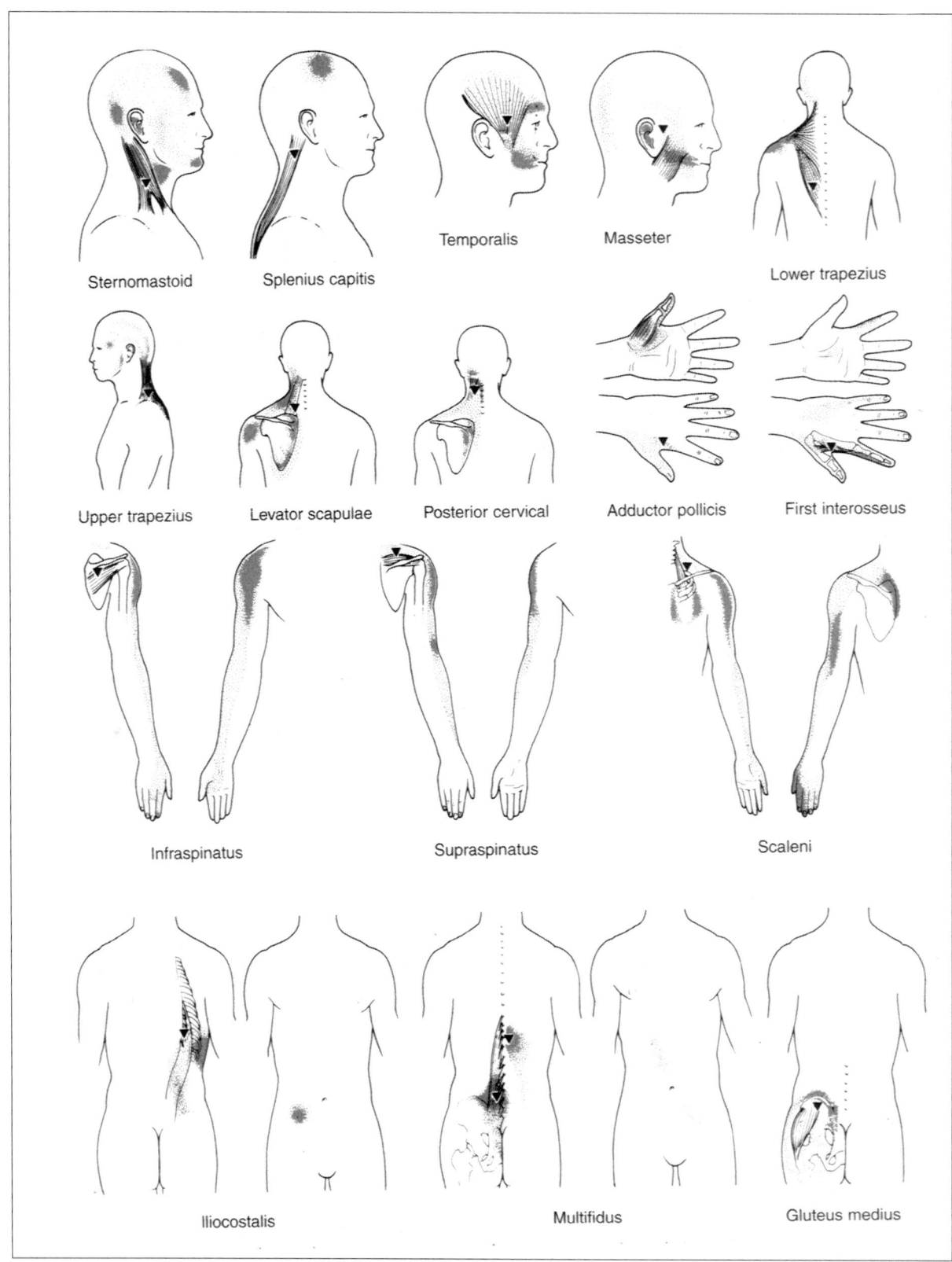

Figure 11-19: Referred pain from myofascial trigger points (with permission Chaitow 2001).

Another study by these researchers demonstrated muscle spindles in this 1 mm area. Injection of a medication that acts on sympathetic nerves was effective. However, this issue is not yet resolved, and an extensive review of the electrodiagnostic characteristics of TPs in the second edition of Simons, Travell and Simons *Myofascial Pain and Dysfunction* suggests that the critical TP abnormality appears to be a neuromuscular dysfunction at the motor endplate of an extrafusal skeletal muscle fiber. Active triggers are usually found within the endplate zones (Simons, Hong, Simons 1995).

Galletti and Procacci (1966) have reported that a stellate ganglion block (anesthesia of a sympathetic ganglion in the neck) resolved pain and tenderness associated with active TPs in the deltoid. This suggests that the sympathetic nervous system affects TP activation. Gunn (*ibid*) postulates that trigger points are supersensitive areas in the muscle secondary to intrinsic dysfunction within the neuromuscular complex—mostly due to a neuropathic origin in degenerative disc disease. This may explain why trigger points are so common, since degenerative disc disease is almost universal with aging (Miller, Schamtz and Scjultzis 1988).

It has also been suggested that an acute over stretch of a muscle, such as during an injury, can result in a sudden elongation of its intrafusal fibers (spindles and other proprioceptors) which then simulate the CNS to produce a reflex contraction and shortening. This tension may result in reciprocal inhibition of the antagonist muscle. Since the antagonist may have been in an already shortened position during the injury, its spindles may become silent, resulting in an increased loss of proper proprioception. Treatment of the muscles is often suggested (Gunn *ibid*, Travell *ibid*, Jones *ibid*).[58]

HISTOLOGICAL EVIDENCE. Studies of muscles with trigger points both in MPS and FMS have been inconclusive. Some studies reported negative findings, while others found changes (Glogowski and Wallraff 1951; Miehlke, Schulze and Eger 1950).

Hendriksson et al (1982) reported that muscle tissue biopsies from tender areas of patients with primary fibromyalgia show a "moth-eaten" appearance. He also reported that in these patients, adenosine triphosphate (ATP) and phosphocreatine were reduced, lactate values were normal, and glycogen was below normal. He concluded that TPs may be due to a primary metabolic disturbance or to an overload secondary to muscle tension.

Schroder and others reported that muscle biopsies in FMS patients revealed moderate type II fiber atrophy. This type of atrophy, however, is also associated with disuse of striated muscles. The authors concluded that muscle biopsy does not contribute to the diagnosis of FMS.

Lindman reported capillary structure irregularities in tender points in the trapezius muscle in both FMS patients and controls. These irregularities were seen more commonly in the FMS patients.

In MPS, Reitinger et al (1996) found large, rounded, darkly-staining muscle fibers and a statistically significant increase in the average diameter of muscle fibers in the myogelosis biopsies, compared to nonmyogelotic control biopsies from the same muscle. Biopsies were done on fresh cadavers with still-palpable nodules of myogelosis.[59]

Increased open space around such "giant round fiber" in patients with MPS may result in a local severe *energy crisis*. The space may contain substances that can sensitize adjacent nociceptive nerves. Additionally, biopsies show abnormally small fibers surrounding the giant fiber in the muscle knot, that may result from strong contraction elsewhere in that muscle knot (Simons, Travell and Simons *ibid*).

Trigger Point Examination

Examination for TP's reveals:

1. Painful, shortened muscles, both on passive and active stretching.

    The optimal length of a muscle for examination is at a position that is slightly longer than the position of ease. The position of the uninvolved muscle fibers are still slack, but the taut band fibers is under slight tension. The stretch may be on the verge of discomfort, but should not cause any pain. Optimal tension is usually about two-thirds of the muscle's normal stretch range of motion but may be only one-third or less with active TPs (Simons, Travell and Simons *ibid*).

2. Strong isometric contraction testing (resisted movements) may be painful when tested in the shortened position, and muscles often appear weak.

3. Cross-fiber palpation often evokes a "jump sign" and/or the local twitch response (LTR). This is best achieved at the same position as described above for examination. Travell and Simons suggest three types of palpation techniques. *Flat palpation* is performed by direct finger pressure across the muscle fibers and is suggested for muscles with underlying structures such as bone. *Pincer palpation* is done by holding the muscle between the thumb and fingers. Groups of muscle fibers are rolled

---

58. The clinical observation that local anaesthesia to acutely (and often chronic) shortened muscles or their antagonists (either at trigger points or motor point) does not result in significant and lasting clinical improvement, brings many of these theories into question. For example, with inversion sprains of the ankle, the evertor muscles are often stretched resulting in "facilitation, tenderness, shortening and sensitivity around their motor or trigger points." The invertor muscles may become inhibited. Treatment to these muscles, however, more often than not, does not resolve the clinical presentation. If the injured ligaments are injected and joint dysfunction addressed, muscle dysfunctions usually resolve immediately on their own. Patient recovery is faster than when the muscles are the main focus of treatment.

59. Myogelosis is a condition with hardened areas or nodules within muscles.

between the tips of the digits to detect taut bands and fibers, to identify tender points in the muscle, and to elicit local twitch responses. *Snapping palpation* is performed by placing a fingertip against the tense band at a right angle to the direction of the band, and suddenly pressing down while drawing the finger back so as to roll the underlying fibers under the finger.

The *psoas syndrome* illustrates well the mechanical-linkage of the musculoskeletal system and possible multiple triggering factors in MPS. For more information on perpetuating factors see page 669.

Psoas Syndrome

Psoas muscle spasm can cause more disability than a spasm in any other muscle of the back (Kuchera and Kuchera 1992). Summarizing the acute *psoas* syndrome, Kuchera and Kuchera say:

> It commonly starts during a prolonged slump sitting on a hard chair or sitting in a very soft chair, while leaning over a desk, while working stooped forward for a long time, or while doing sit-ups.

Because in all of these conditions the psoas is shortened, the intrafusal spindle fibers tighten up so they can better monitor the (*now shortened*) muscle length. Then a rapid change in muscle length occurs, usually when the patient returns to the upright posture. This leads to a protective spasm as the shortened *reset* spindles try to protect the muscle. This occurs because the newly rest spindles now monitor the muscle as being suddenly overstretched. (The receptors within the muscle have been reset as a consequence of prolonged shortening.)

At first, both *psoas* muscles are usually involved, causing the patient to forward bend in the typical lumbago posture. If sidebending is introduced during the upright recovery from sitting, a nonneutral (Type II) lumbar dysfunction at T12, L1 or L2 can occur (usually FRS, which is the key in the psoas syndrome; See "Osteopathic Medicine" on page 460),[60] with spasm in one *psoas* being more evident than in the other. A lumbar list (sidebend) is seen. A compensatory neutral group dysfunction (Type I, scoliotic curve) is seen in the rest of the lumbar spine. This dysfunction may result in a nonneutral sacral response, usually a *left on right* oblique axis. The right forward flexion test is positive and sacral asymmetry is increased in lumbar extension. A torsional dysfunction of the sacrum leads to a *piriformis* muscle irritation, which in turn may cause leg pain and "sciatica."[61]

Patients with *chronic psoas* tightness/weakness often have muscle imbalance between the anterior pelvic rotators (*psoas* and other *hip flexors*) and the posterior pelvic rotators (*erector spinae, abdominals, gluteals,* and *hamstrings*). Usu-

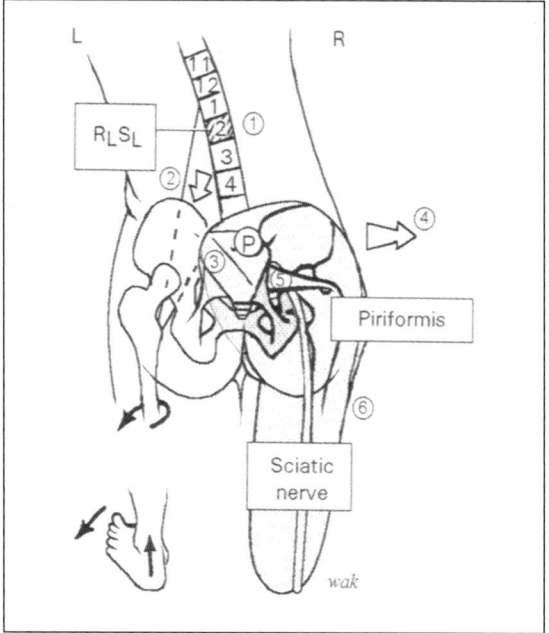

Figure 11-20: Psoas syndrome (From Kuchera WA and Kuchera ML, Osteopathic Principles in Practice, KCOM press 1993, with permission).

ally the lumbar lordosis is increased, unless *psoas* is in spasm flexing the trunk, and then the lumbar curve may decrease. The thoracolumbar paravertebral musculature and fascia are shortened, and a compensatory increase in thoracic kyphosis is seen often. The head is often held forward and the cervical curve may flatten (Janda *ibid*). Often the right leg, (or) on the side of predominate *psoas* tightness, is long and the *hamstring* (*biceps femoris*) is also tight. The knee is often held in slight flexion. The foot on that side is often pronated and externally rotated. These changes can easily result in an increase of torsional/shearing forces and may produce the failure of the annulus fibrosus fibers of the discs. In the upper and mid-lumbar levels, near the apex of the lordosis, disc extrusion may occur, with a consequent stretching or compression of the neural plexus. This may result in pain referred to the lower back, buttocks, and/or proximal lower extremities without accompanying neurological findings (Bachrach *ibid*).

Treatment of MPS

The goal of treatment is to reach a normal resting muscle length without pain or effort—any treatment that does not achieve this will only achieve temporary relief, since the muscles will *reactivate* when re-stressed. Travell and

---

60. The key to treat FRS dysfunction at T-12 is the muscle energy technique called the 500 step technique.

61. In this author's experience, this type of presentation, especially if accompanied with severe *painful twinges*, is due often to discogenic lesions. The psoas muscle has direct attachments to the lumbar discs and reacts with spasm. Often these patient's improve significantly when treated with an epidural injection which result in recovery in a much shorter period than if treated with manual and/or acupuncture therapies.

Simons (*ibid*) suggest as treatment methods spray-and-stretch or ice massage (which they suggest is the most effective noninvasive method), compression, massage, puncture (injection or dry needling), ultrasound, moist heat, electrical stimulation, and nutritional supplementation. Thus, successful treatment depends on removing the primary TP, its associated and satellite TPs, and any underlying or perpetuating factors. It must be reiterated that many times "trigger points" resolve spontaneously when joint dysfunctions and ligamentous insufficiency, or other triggering phenomena, are treated.

With *spray-and-stretch* the spray (or ice cube) sweeps are applied in one direction only, covering first the full length of the muscle and then covering the complete pain reference zone. It is important to cover both attachments of the muscle to bone as well as the TP. The bottle is held at an angle on thirty degrees from the skin at a distance of about eighteen inches. The rate of sweep is approximately four inches per second, making sure only the skin, not the muscle, is cooled. At the end of stretch-and-spray, the muscle should be warmed with moist heat and taken through its entire range of motion.

Ischemic compression is a manual compression of a trigger point which is said to deactivate it. The practitioner may apply pressure using his/her thumb, knuckle, or elbow to a relaxed muscle that has been stretched to the point of discomfort. Moderate pressure is applied at first, and, as the discomfort is beginning to subside, the pressure is gradually increased. Compression lasts for about one minute and is between 9-13 kg of pressure.

A "stripping" massage is suggested which consists of stroking massage where a digit is slowly moved along the muscle to encroach upon the area of the trigger point so that the trigger point is "milked" of its fluid content (called effleurage massage). Pressure is light and movement slow at first but increased with each successive stroke. This is thought to produce ischemia and mobilize metabolites. Once this occurs, active hyperaemia follows in the region of the trigger point. *Cross-fiber massage* can be helpful as well.

Ultrasound may be used to both diagnose and treat trigger points. Ultrasound can produce thermal and mechanical effects that may alter membrane permeability and improve local microcirculation. Ultrasound heads are usually available in two frequencies: 1 MHz is used for deep penetration (up to 3 cm), and 3 MHz for a more superficial muscle (penetration of 1cm).

Moist heat appears to be the most effective form of heat in myofascial therapy. It can be applied after needling therapy to minimize soreness and before and during stretching exersises. It can be applied by heat packs, by bathing, or by showering.

Dry needling with mild stimulation directly into the trigger point is recommended.

Electrical stimulation is only recommend if applied mildly.

Before *passive stretching* is taught to the patient, care should be taken to assess for tendinous or periosteal inflammation. This avoids placing more tension on already distressed connective tissue attachments. Tendinitis should be treated before *strong* passive stretches are applied.

For other treatment details, see "Release by Countertension-Positioning and Related Techniques" on page 487, "Muscle Energy Techniques" on page 489, "Myofascial Release Techniques" on page 496.

Integrative Therapy of Myofascial Pain

Treatment of myofascial tissues using protocols described here are often very helpful. When treating musculoskeletal disorders, treatment can begin with stimulation of the appropriate Sinew channel. Often the Sinew channel is stimulated by needling one fen proximal to the channel's Well point followed by the termination point. Then a layered acupuncture approach that directs treatment from superficial external layers to deeper somatic tissues can be used (see "The Sinew Channels" on page 300). Another approach is to needle distal points in combination with manual therapies and/or patient exercises (see "Tong/Lee-style Acupuncture" on page 350). Ear, Wrist/Ankle, or any other "holographic or imaging systems" can be used at the same time (Figure 11-18).

In *Simple Questions,* the appropriate level to be needled is illustrated in the discussion on Deep Punctures:

> When disease is in the sinews.... needle the sinews, between the muscle layers without hitting the bone. When the disease is in the skin and muscles.... needle the big and small spaces, and needle deeply several times to generate heat. Take care not to injure the sinews and bone. When the disease is in the bones.... needle deeply, taking care to neither injure the vessels nor the muscles. The needle path is through the big and small spaces. When the bones are warmed, the disease ends.

This classic reference supports many of the needle techniques proposed in this text. Treatment design, at the time of its composition, was based on tissue pathology and the insertion of needles directly into the affected area, not just into "acupuncture points." Acupuncture and local dry needling is an art that requires practice. The practitioner must apply an exacting amount of stimulation. Too much can cause undue pain and inflict injury, and too little can render the treatment ineffective. When using the following recommended techniques a thorough knowledge of anatomy is essential.

Muscle shortening and tension/spasm often respond to needling, either when treated directly or when the antagonists to the spasmed muscle, or the contralateral muscle is needled *(OM: i.e., Yin/Yang and channel therapies).* Spasmed muscles may also respond to strategic acupuncture points on the channel system (Table 5-20 on page 316). Generally, contracted, shortened, or spasmed muscles respond quickly to treatment, both qualitatively and symptomatically. Usually the problem resolves/improves in one to three treatments. Relapse rates depend on the causative factor and the amount of fibrosis/pathology/impingement/instability. Often periosteal acupuncture, manual therapy, and rehabilitation exercises are necessary to obtain long-lasting results. It should be understood that as long as a tight band (of ropy and tight muscular and tendinous tissues) is maintained by *neural facilitation*, treatment can positively alter the tone and soften the tissue. This neurological or mechanical facilitation (which is causing the tight muscles) is evident because the tight, abnormally-hard-tissue changes *immediately* after treatment. Often treatment of an abnormal or facilitated vertebra (or any restricted joint) also softens such bands, even when no direct treatment is applied to the muscle, again showing that such tightness is secondary and is probably due to neural facilitation. However, once tissues are truly fibrotic and calcified (which may also result in ectopic firing of the muscles), changes from treatment are more subtle and often qualitative only. Occasionally, the tissue does change dramatically after repeated treatments. When it does, this suggests that some reversal is still possible. (Research should continue to advance such healing techniques, which possibly activate myofascial stem cells.)

It is also important to assess for muscle weakness. The weakness of a muscle can be due to inhibition by tight muscles in the antagonist group, or to lack of stimulation within its own mechanisms. It is therefore important to assess both the myotomal group (or Sinew channel) of muscles related to the weak muscle and their antagonists (often related to Yin-Yang relationships of Sinew channels). Both tightness and weakness can result from somatic dysfunction and facilitated segments in the related vertebra that must be assessed (and often relate to back-Shu and Alarm-Mu systems/circuits in TCM). Treatment of the appropriate vertebra is important. Occasionally, a tight muscle is caused by a weakened antagonist, in which case weakness should be addressed first. (The reversal is more common, i.e., tight agonists result in weak antagonists and tightness is treated first.)

Following examination of the superficial integument and testing for muscle length (page 513) and weakness, the practitioner palpates deeper fascia and muscles to look for altered tissue texture such as: superficial or deep nodules, tight bands or "doughy" muscle, severed tissues, fibrotic changes (scars often found in chronic conditions), restricted fascial layer motions, and trigger-Ashi-Kori-indurated and motor points. The tenoperiosteal junctions and the musculotendinous junctions of involved muscles are often a site of trouble and should be palpated carefully. (They contain golgi tendon organs, stimulation of which often relaxes the muscles.) Palpation of the muscle belly should be perpendicular (cross-fiber) to the muscle fibers, stroking the fibers gently. When assessing deep-lying muscles, the practitioner should proceed palpation by going deeper, slowly and progressively, keeping overlying muscles relaxed (when possible). Stroking should begin only after the desired depth is reached. To determine tendon tenderness, the practitioner palpates the tendon along the direction of the inserting fibers and also perpendicularly, to define the tendon's borders (although cross-fiber stroking may be needed in mild cases). To determine whether tenderness lies in superficial or deep structures, the practitioner can palpate the area during the contraction and relaxation of the superficial muscle overlying the area, if possible. Pain that is more pronounced when the muscle is tense suggests that the superficial muscle is at fault.

Muscle "spasms" and/or myofascial triggers manifest as indurated tissue lying parallel to the fibers involved, spindle-shaped tissue thickening, pressure-evoked (by plucking) muscle twitches and bundles that can be moved at a right angle to the rest of the muscle fibers. Often, *active* tight fibrous bands are *very fine* and lie within a broader tense muscle bundle. A point of maximal tenderness within such fine bands is sought for treatment and is often found at mid-muscle over motor points. Direct needling of wider bands is often unhelpful and may result in unnecessary discomfort. In chronic conditions, fibrotic changes are often found, and these "scars" can become very sensitive, as abnormal facilitation occurs, and these small scars may become a major cause of enduring pain and dysfunction.

Fascial layer motions can be assessed by gentle sheer movements applied by the practitioner to the skin/fascia (Figure 11-15), or by applying pressure over symmetrical areas and then asking the patient to move the joints underlying the pressing hands. A restricted fascia will result in increased movement of the practitioner's hand on the affected side (similar to the flexion tests page 473).

Objective tissue changes are more significant than elicitation of pressure pain. The practitioner must establish the source of pain, because the location of pain may not correlate directly with the underlying lesion that is responsible (i.e., referred tenderness is a common phenomenon). Therefore, tissue texture and not pressure pain should dictate treatment (although in TCM, Ashi-points are defined as being pressure-producing pain and are often used to treat pain).

Locate Hyperactive Motor Points and Bands

Once dysfunctional muscles are identified (by a review of the patient's history, *pain drawings*, functional length/tension, weakness assessments, and palpation), the practitioner locates all hyperactive motor/trigger, Ashi-sensitive, or Kori-indurated (koketsu) points in the involved muscles. (About 80% of acupuncture points are found at the same areas as motor points.) The practitioner can:

- Palpate to identify tender areas (ashi points) and trigger points in the areas where motor points are located;

- Apply an electrical stimulator to the skin with sufficient voltage to cause a muscle contraction, but not strong enough to cause twitching in multiple locations when applied to non-motor points;

- Check skin impedance with a point locator to identify active skin over the points;

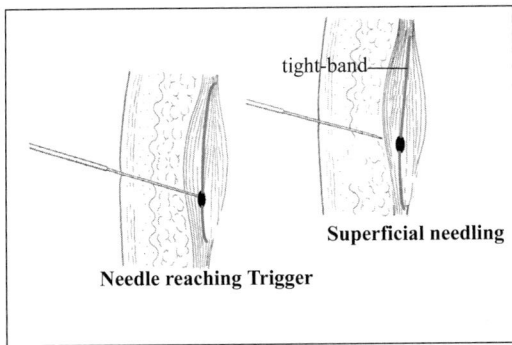

Figure 11-21: Trigger point needling.

- Use thermography to identify abnormally hot or cold areas/muscles.

Trigger point needling is an acquired art. The point must be accurately located and manually *stabilized*. This is done with the practitioner's non-needling thumb. Firm pressure is applied just to the side of the tight-band/Kori so that when the needle approaches the trigger, the muscle fibers do not roll away.

The strongest response to the needle is usually just at the outer edge of the tight band, i.e., the area most likely to produce a muscle twitch (Figure 11-21). However, tight/spasmed muscles also often respond to cross-fiber horizontal needle techniques, which may or may not contact the myofascial trigger. (This is often described as *through and through* acupuncture, which connects more than one acupuncture point/channel with one needle.) The needle may be inserted into the muscle belly or just under the skin. The SCM and scalene muscles, for example, often relax when a needle is inserted just over and across the entire muscle width. This technique may be difficult to perform when needling deep lying muscles.

Another helpful technique is to insert the needle into the tight band with the needle parallel to the muscle fibers. The needle is then rotated in various ways while the non-needling hand palpates for ease and softening of the tight band. Only needle movements that decrease tone are used (see page 487).

Needling Hyperactive Motor/Trigger/Ashi Points and Fibrotic Tissues

TREATMENT LEVEL 1

Once the hyperactive points are located, the practitioner can: do the following:

1. He/she can mark the points.
2. He/she can activate the appropriate Sinew channel;
3. He/she can treat the appropriate spinal segments (or TCM channel- Organs, Shu-Mu points, etc.) associated with neural and sympathetic supply to the involved muscles/joints. The importance of treating the appropriate segments cannot be over emphasized, as often these are the roots of the peripheral dysfunctions and/or triggers. Sympathetic (vertebral) levels can be stimulated superficially and gently. Levels associated with the primary motor and sensory innervation may both be needled deeply down to lamina, especially if motion testing shows dysfunction (i.e., vertebral fixation). There are many ways of assessing for vertebral dysfunction or fixation. With the patient prone, one can use passive motion assessment of various related vertebral segments, feeling for motion barriers. (For more detail see "Functionally Oriented Screen Tests" on page 470.) There may be a group of vertebra (two or more) resisting rotation to one side. Sidebending may be felt to be more restricted toward the rotated vertebrae or to the other side (i.e., neutral dysfunction, most commonly). Or there may be a single vertebral segment that resists rotation and sidebending to the same side (i.e., non-neutral dysfunction). A quick medially-directed pressure applied to the *spinous processes* may serve as a screen rotation for noting levels that resist such pressure. Pushing on the spinous processes from the left side medially will rotate the vertebra to the left (i.e., rotate the front of the vertebral body). Alternatively, the practitioner can push downwards on the transverse processes on the right and left. Pushing on the left transverse process will rotate the vertebra to the right and vice versa. To assess sidebending, the practitioner translates the motion segment to the left and right, placing his/her thumbs between two vertebrae (see upper Figure 11-22).

Compliance to the applied pressure is assessed. The practitioner can also use this technique by applying quick, rocking, massage-like movements that mildly mobilize the segment. At the same time he/she pays attention to feedback from each vertebral level, noting those that resist the pressure. Vertebrae that are found to be stiff and resistant to such pressure can be treated by using sustained finger pressure applied while having the patient breathe in and out deeply. This is often effective when Tuina-like rocking movements fail to restore proper segmental motion. It may be helpful to address vertebral dysfunctions manually before needling peripheral tissues and triggers, although, frequently, needling the appropriate vertebral levels is effective as well. For a more detailed assessment of vertebral functions see "Joint Dysfunctions and Manual Medicine Models" on page 461).

A quick deep insertion into the Hua Tuo Jia Ji points (i.e., in the deep intrinsic muscles) on the restricted side can be tried after (or before) the vertebra is mobilized. The opposite side is stimulated gently at a more

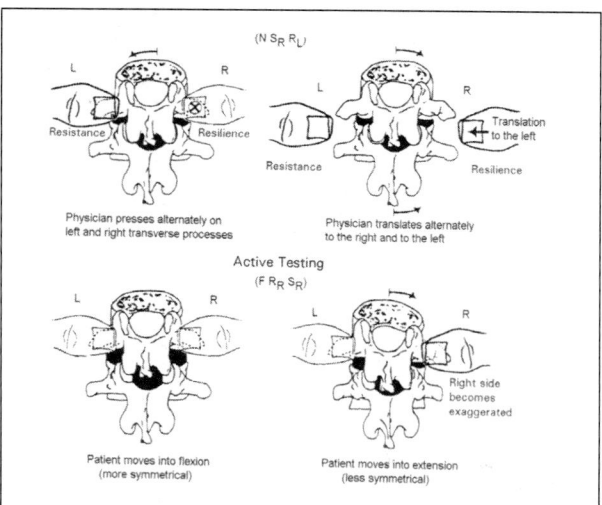

Figure 11-22: Passive and active assessments of spinal joint functions. With passive assessments, resistance or compliance to pressure applied by the practitioner is assessed to determine restrictions. To assess *rotation*, ventrally directed pressure is applied alternatively on the left and right transverse processes. Pressing down on the left transverse process will rotate the vertebra to right and vis versa (upper left). It is also possible to press medially on the spinous process from the left and right sides. Pressing medially from the left side will rotate the vertebra to the left and vis versa. To assess *sidebending*, the practitioner's thumbs are used to translate the vertebral segment from the right and left sides. Pressing from the right side medially will sidebent the segment to the right (upper right). With *active assessments* the patient performs flexion and extension of the spine and the position of the transverse processes are assessed visually. Both the left and right transverse processes should move forward in flexion and backward in extension (From Kuchera WA and Kuchera ML, Osteopathic Principles in Practice, KCOM press 1993, with permission).

superficial level. The motion is then tested, and, if no improvement is seen, the needles are reversed. This process resolves vertebral dysfunctions in about 50% of the time. A more detailed understanding of the particulars of the segment behavior, i.e., flexion or extension restriction/fixation, is needed in the other 50%. Manual therapy techniques or more detailed needling are then necessary. For specific needling techniques, see "Orthopedic Integration, Neuroanatomical Acupuncture" on page 277. For manual techniques see "Osteopathic Treatment Methods" on page 484.[62] An advantage of

---

62. At times the patient may have a stubborn segment that resist treatment or that often get refacilitated. It may be helpful to give the patient two tennis balls taped together, or other commercial wedge, which is placed under the spine and the patient lies on top. However, since often the cause is ligamentous laxity, in such patients this may increase the instability even when "feels" good to the patient. Another approach is to have the patient lie supine on the floor with a paperback book of 1" thickness under their buttock, and a tightly rolled-up towel about 3 and 1/2" diameter placed under the head and thoracic spine. The patient rest on this for 20 minutes a day. This will help address postural problems and reduce the increased sacral tilt and anterior displacement of sacral load so commonly seen in patients.

using needles to treat spinal restriction is that many levels can be treated at the same time, and the patient can be left on the treatment table freeing the practitioner to attend to other patients.

4. He/she can use 30-38 gauge needles, depending on how much stimulation is needed, and treat the peripheral triggers. Initially the practitioner can use the needle to lightly stimulate the outer subcutaneous tissues at the site *right over* the triggers (Figure 11-21). A very shallow circumduction movement of the needle at this depth is performed, making sure that no pain is felt by the patient. It is also possible to insert the needle farther in the direction that shows superficial tissue drag-resistance. The needle(s) may or may not be left in place. If the area around the needle is red, the needle may be left in place until skin color returns to normal. Because the needle(s) are inserted very superficially, the patient can mobilize the affected area at the same time, or else manual therapy may be used. Full ROM should be attempted by the patient or practitioner.

   This shallow insertion technique may elicit muscle twitches, possibly through abnormal sympathetic pathways, or by stimulating motor nerves as they pass through fascia. Shallow needling also stimulates A-δ (IIIb) and large-caliber A-β fibers, activating Wall and Melzack's "gate" and descending inhibitory pathways. Through normal feedback mechanisms, the pain threshold increases and may also result in the relaxation of the muscle, both of which make the remainder of the treatment, if needed, more comfortable for the patient.

NOTE: Often light/superficial treatment is sufficient for obtaining a clinical response and trigger deactivation. If some positive affect is achieved, this process is repeated in the next few sessions.[63]

If needed the practitioner can do the following:

5. He/she can hold the muscle band firmly and advance the needle slowly to the band's outer edge, paying attention to needle-feel. Proceed slowly to avoid the possibility of the patient feeling great pain or experience some other reaction.

6. If a muscle twitch occurs, he/she can take out the needle or poke a few more times to elicit several twitches. The needle is *not* rotated. Usually no further needle stimulation is needed at that site.

7. He/she can explore the muscle attachments and needle if needed.

TREATMENT LEVEL 2

---

63. Mark Seem advocates needling only at the superficial fascia while compressing the fatty tissue over a muscle using a thin Japanese needle. This must also be considered when using so-called superficial needles as "sham" control in acupuncture studies.

Fibromyalgia and Myofascial Pain Syndrome

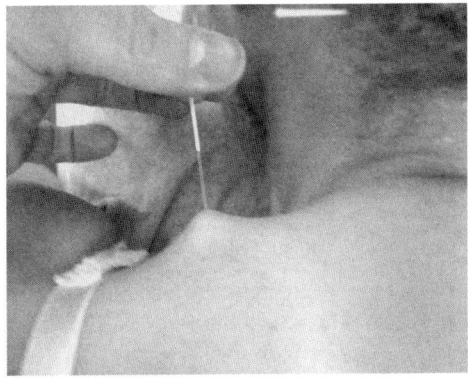

Figure 11-23: Counterclockwise rotation with a slight tug.

If the patient does not respond to mild treatments, the practitioner can do the following:

1. Treat the triggers again, stimulating the points more vigorously.
2. Needle in several directions to cover the entire area of the tight band around the trigger. Insert the needle slowly and withdraw quickly.

Or:

A. He/she can rotate the needle gently counterclockwise, until feeling a slight tug on the fibers, and then pull gently on the needle (Figure 11-23). Often this elicits a deep or referred ache and several more muscle twitches. (This is done in order to put the muscle fibers under tension, hence stimulating the Golgi apparatus to inhibit spindles.)
B. He/she can gently needle musculotendinous junctions.
C. He/she can remove needle or leaves the needle in place one to ten minutes. When the muscle relaxes, he/she can remove the needle(s) gently.
D. He/she can needle muscular attachments gently.
E. He/she can repeat segmental treatments.

TREATMENT LEVEL 3

If the patient does not improve following the above moderate stimulation, the practitioner can do the following:

1. He/she can needle the active lesions even more vigorously, to cause local bleeding. Bleeding releases growth factors, thereby treating hemodynamically-disturbed areas and possibly transforming some overactive muscle fibers into nonpainful tissues. To avoid adhesions, movement and cross-fiber massage are incorporated.
2. If hard-like tissue is found, possibly from strong, deep muscles spasms seen most often in deep vertebral muscles, he/she can needle throughout the muscle, gently rotating the needle back and forth, for no more than one eighth of a turn, until feeling a "letting go" sensation at the tip of the needle. One should not remove the needle until the muscle relaxes and the needle can penetrate the tissue and be withdrawn without force. A quick electrical stimulation can help loosen the muscle.

Or:

A. One can needle at the trigger site and at the two ends of the muscle. Connect an electrostimulator at alternating low and high frequency (2-100 Hz.) for twenty minutes to fatigue the muscle. If this is uncomfortable to the patient, then use only 2 Hz stimulation.
B. One may use a triangular (bleeding) needle, acuptomy needle, or scalpel to cause more extensive bleeding. (This technique is used by biomedical orthopedic practitioners as well as TCM doctors, and is called "acuptomy."[64, 65] Fibrotic tissue may need to be cut.
C. All fibrous areas are needled and warmed by moxa or fire needle, or, even better, with diathermy. Diathermy has deeper penetration and can actually increase tissue temperature to a much higher degree. (Diathermy is applied before the needles are inserted.)
D. One may repeat segmental treatments.
E. For patients with significant weakness, especially if associated with pathology such as knee arthritis, a home muscle stim unit can be used for one half to one hour per day to increase muscle strength, avoiding aggravation that may occur from physical exercise. When muscle strength and stability is increased, the patient should be taught appropriate rehabilitation exercises.

Weak muscles often respond better to needles placed along the muscle fibers, as apposed to muscle tension, which is often better treated cross-fiberally. A needle is placed near the motor points and at each end of the muscle. Electrostimulation at low frequency (2-20Hz) can be added using ramped intensity setting which result in a comfortable muscle contraction. Related muscle points (e.g., St-36) are needled, making sure the needles are within the muscular tissues. Again, laser stimulation *may* help in healing and can follow acupuncture.

---

64. For acuptomy Prof. Zhu Hanzhong designed special acupuncture needles with a cutting edge.
65. In general, the author has found cross-fiber needle stimulation (transversely across the entire width of the muscle) to be the most potent needling method for treating muscular tension and shortening. A 30 gauge needle works best, although a thin gauge needle can be used as well. The muscle is placed at its stretch barrier. Electrostimulation can be added. This technique may result in post-treatment soreness, but, if the patient is cooperative and stretches the muscle, good clinical outcome is often achieved.

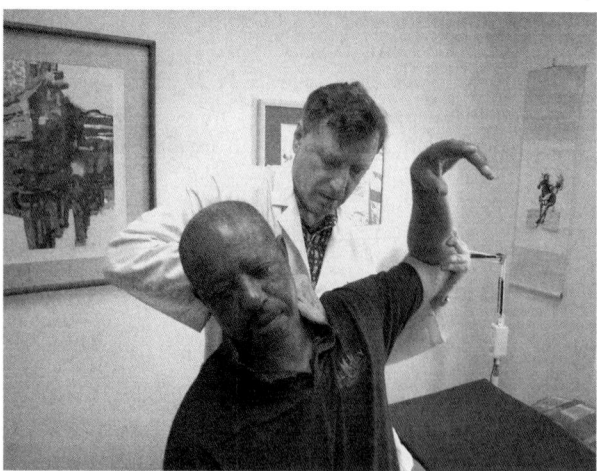

Figure 11-24: First rib mobilized following dry needling of cervical spine muscles. This is the end position after performing a functional technique for inhalation restriction.

Post Treatment Care

After acupuncture and dry needling, the muscles should be passively (i.e. by the practitioner) lengthened to their full range. Pre-stretch surface cooling using fluorimethane or ice may be integrated. Only the skin, not the muscle, should be cooled, using strokes in one direction, first on the entire muscle and then in areas of referred symptoms. Moist heat, drinking plenty of water, and effleurage massage can be helpful in preventing post-treatment soreness.

At times shortened muscles can be treated by post-isometric stretch techniques, but should follow a passive lengthening by the practitioner first. A routine often followed by the author is first to move the muscle to maximal length, then, with the affected joint(s) supported (at stretch barrier) to ask the patient to contract the muscle isometrically. After this contraction the muscle is stretched a little more (using post isometric relaxation). Then the muscle is put in the maximally shortened position, and the patient is asked to activate the antagonists which reciprocally inhibit the treated muscle(s).

Manual therapies to address joint dysfunctions, which sometimes set in as a result of strong-muscle, tendon, or ligamentous needle stimulation, may be necessary. After needling and stretching, the patient should perform at least three *active full ROM* movements of the affected joints and muscles to help normalize function and coordination. Walking backwards may be helpful to break up old patterns.

The practitioner should encourage the patient to rest and use moist-heat to reduce post-treatment soreness for twenty-four hours. Heat should be applied at the trigger sites only, not to the entire muscles. Patients with tendinitis may do better with ice or "contrast" therapy (page 541). Heavy exercise should be avoided after treatment. Appropriate rehabilitation can be started in a week or so. The patient should avoid using maximum effort or being too zealous in performing physical activities and should increase the prescribed routine slowly. As part of the treatment, the practitioner must teach good body mechanics. Both weakness and tightness should be addressed. Proper breathing is taught if needed, especially to patients with upper quarter disorders. So-called "paradoxical" breathing should be corrected by the patient's learning to synchronize the contraction of the diaphragm with the contraction of the intercostal muscles.

Fibromyalgia and Myofascial Pain Syndrome

Table 11-4: Motor Points In Commonly Affected Muscles (Geiringer 1993)[a]

Muscle	Point Location	Figure
PARASPINALS, CERVICAL (ERECTOR SPINAE)	Adjacent to the cervical spine, in vertical line with the midpoint of the nuchal ridge. Deep to trapezius.	
SPLENIUS CAPITIS	Near the region where the upper border of the upper trapezius crosses the splenius capitis, at midbelly, deep to trapezius.	
PARASPINAL, LUMBOSACRAL, AND THORACIC (ERECTOR SPINAE)	The point midway between the PSIS and the midline corresponds to the low lumbar paraspinal muscles. The points for more proximal or distal levels are through the same points and along the line parallel to the spine. The needle is directed perpendicular to the skin and somewhat medially, toward the deeper paraspinal layers.	
TRAPEZIUS UPPER	Superior border of the shoulder, immediately medial to the AC joint.	
TRAPEZIUS MIDDLE	Directly medial to the medial edge of the scapular spine.	
TRAPEZIUS LOWER	In mid-muscle about level with T7.	
RHOMBOID MAJOR	At the level of the midpoint of the medial scapular border, midway between the border of the high thoracic (T1-T4) spinous processes.	
RHOMBOID MINOR	Midpoint of the line connecting the superior medial scapular border and the cervical prominence.	
LEVATOR SCAPULA	Midpoint of the line connecting the superior medial scapular border and the nuchal line. Also just above the medial superior border of the scapula.	

Table 11-4: Motor Points In Commonly Affected Muscles (Geiringer 1993)[a]

Muscle	Point Location	Figure
Pectoralis Major (sternal portion)	Anterior axillary fold, in direct vertical line with the coracoid process.	Pec major
Supraspinatus	At the medial one-third of the scapular spine, immediately superior to the scapular spine.	Supraspinatus, Teres minor, Infraspinatus
Infraspinatus	Halfway between the scapular spine and the inferior tip of scapula, midway between the lateral and medial borders of scapula.	
Teres Minor	Immediately lateral to the middle third of the lateral scapular border.	
Deltoid Posterior	Midpoint of the line connecting the distal scapular spine and the deltoid insertion.	Deltoid post, Triceps long head, Triceps lat, Latissimus dorsi
Latissimus Dorsi	Posterior axillary fold, directly lateral to the inferior tip of the scapula.	
Triceps, Long Head	At the level of the midshaft of the humerus, just medial to the posterior midline of arm.	
Triceps, Lateral Head	Distal one-third of the arm, directly in line with the lateral epicondyle.	
Deltoid Anterior	Midpoint of the line connecting the lateral one-third of the clavicle and the deltoid insertion.	Deltoid anterior, Biceps, Brachialis, Pronator Teres
Biceps Brachii	Middle one-third of the arm, directly into and paralleling the muscle belly, approaching biceps from its lateral side.	
Brachialis	In the distal one-third of the arm, in the groove between the biceps and triceps. Needle directed down and medially toward the anterior aspect of the humeral shaft or between the two heads of biceps.	
Pronator Teres	With the index finger in the antecubital fossa pointing proximal, pronator teres is the first muscle medial to your finger, immediately distal to the antecubital vein.	

Fibromyalgia and Myofascial Pain Syndrome

Table 11-4: Motor Points In Commonly Affected Muscles (Geiringer 1993)[a]

Muscle	Point Location	Figure
Supinator	In the proximal 20% of the dorsal forearm, in the groove between the radial wrist extensors (movable), and extensor digitorum communis (not movable), deep against the radial bone.	
Flexor Carpi Radialis	With index finger in the antecubital fossa, pointing proximal. The muscle is the first medial to the finger at the level of the apex of the antecubital fossa.	
Flexor Digitorum Profundus, Ulnar Head	In the middle one-third of the forearm, immediately ventral to the ulnar shaft.	
Flexor Carpi Ulnaris	Middle third of the forearm, superficial and directly medial.	
Flexor Pollicis Longus	In the middle of the ventral forearm, just distal to the convergence of the carpi radialis and brachioradialis, virtually at midline.	
Flexor Digitorum Superficialis	At mid-forearm, halfway from the ventral midline to the medial border of the forearm.	
Pronator Quadratus	Just anterior to the distal ulnar shaft, perpendicular to it. Insert needle horizontally to meet the thick medial border of the muscle.	

Table 11-4: Motor Points In Commonly Affected Muscles (Geiringer 1993)[a]

Muscle	Point Location	Figure
ABDUCTOR DIGITI QUINTI	Directly at the medial border of the hand, at the midpoint between the distal wrist crease and the metacarpophalangeal crease.	
ABDUCTOR POLLICIS BREVIS	Parallel to the first metacarpal shaft, in line with the mid-shaft of the extended first phalanx of the thumb.	
ADDUCTOR POLLICIS	Immediately proximal to the metacarpophalangeal joint, in the groove between the metacarpal bone and the first interosseous muscle.	
GLUTEUS MEDIUS	At the midpoint and just posterior to a parallel line between the ASIS and greater trochanter. A second point is one inch distal to the midpoint of the iliac crest.	
GLUTEUS MAXIMUS	Midpoint of the line connecting the PSIS and greater trochanter.	

Table 11-4: Motor Points In Commonly Affected Muscles (Geiringer 1993)[a]

Muscle	Point Location	Figure
Piriformis	Midline between the inferior aspect of the PSIS and the greater trochanter of femur, deep.	
Quadratus Femorus	Midway between the tubercle of femur and ischial tuberosity, deep.	
Iliopsoas	Immediately distal to the inguinal ligament, halfway between the femoral artery pulse and the ASIS. Needle directed laterally, away from the neurovascular bundle.	
Rectus Femoris	At the midpoint of the line connecting the ASIS and the superior pole of the patella, slightly lateral to midline of thigh.	
Vastus Lateralis	Mid-thigh, directly lateral in the visible and palpable groove between the external hamstring and vastus lateralis.	
Vastus Medialis	The distal 20% of the medial thigh. Where the oblique fibers of the muscle are angled at nearly 45° toward the patella.	
Adductor Magnus	Upper one-third (or midway) of thigh, immediately posterior to the media border of the thigh.	
Adductor Longus	On a line connecting the medial distal epicondyle of femur and mid-inguinal ligament, just medial to sartorius muscle at upper one-quarter of thigh.	

Table 11-4: Motor Points In Commonly Affected Muscles (Geiringer 1993)[a]

Muscle	Point Location	Figure
Biceps Femoris	At mid-thigh, there is a palpable groove from the iliotibial band between the vastus lateralis and the external biceps (external hamstrings). Needle is inserted just posterior to (i.e., above in the prone position) the groove and parallel to the femur.	
Biceps Femoris Short Head	At the level of the superior crease of the popliteal fossa, immediately medial or lateral to the tendon of the biceps femoris long head.	
Semimembranosus and Semitendinsus	At mid-thigh, at or just medial to the midline and immediately subcutaneous.	
Popliteus	At midbelly about two finger breaths below the popliteal crease and slightly medially from the midline, over mid-tibial shaft.	
Gastrocnemius, Medial Head	Medial border of the leg, junction of the upper and middle thirds, and superficial.	
Gastrocnemius, Lateral Head	Midway between the fibular head and the posterior midline of the leg, and superficial.	
Soleus	At the junction of the middle and lower thirds of the leg, immediately adjacent (either medial or lateral) to the posterior midline.	
Flexor Hallucis Longus	At the lateral edge of the Achilles tendon about two finger breaths above the malleolus.	
Flexor Digitorum Longus	At the medial edge of the Achilles tendon about two finger breaths above the malleolus.	

Table 11-4: Motor Points In Commonly Affected Muscles (Geiringer 1993)[a]

Muscle	Point Location	Figure
Tibialis Anterior	At the junction of the middle and upper thirds of the leg, one-quarter of the distance from the tibial shaft to the lateral border of the leg.	
Extensor Digitorum Longus	At the junction of the upper and middle thirds of the leg, half of the distance from the tibial shaft to the lateral border of the leg.	
Extensor Hallucis Longus	At the junction of the middle and lower thirds of the leg, one-third of the distance from the tibial shaft to the lateral border of leg.	
Tibialis Posterior	At the junction of the middle and lower thirds of the leg, under the medial tibial shaft along the bone and deep, where the muscle lies against the interosseous membrane.	
First Dorsal Interosseous (Foot)	In the mid-dorsal web space between the first and second toes. Insert needle angled slightly laterally.	
Peroneus Longus	At the junction of the upper and middle thirds of the leg, directly below the fibular head.	
Abductor Digiti Quinti (Foot)	At the lateral border of the foot, locate the base of the first met bone, the prominence of which is easily felt. Insert needle immediately proximal to, and to the plantar side of the prominence, parallel to the long axis of the foot.	
Abductor Hallucis	Halfway between the prominence of the navicular and the plane of the sole. Insert needle parallel to the long axis of the foot.	

a. Many muscles have more than one motor point. Motor points are the most likely to develop reactions and tenderness from dysfunctions and are the most likely to become trigger points. Many are located in the same area as acupuncture points.

Fibromyalgia Syndrome

According to a consensus document on fibromyalgia syndrome (FMS)—the Copenhagen Declaration (Jacobsen, Samsoe, Lund, 1993)—FMS is a painful, non-articular condition predominantly involving muscles, and is the commonest cause of chronic widespread musculoskeletal pain. FMS affects an estimated 3-6 million persons in the US, most of whom are women between the ages of thirty and fifty (Goldenberg 1994), or about 2-3.3% of the North American population (Donaldson et al 2001). It was only in 1987 that FMS was recognized by the American Medical Association (AMA) as a distinct condition that is responsible for significant disability. Many, however, still do not believe FMS to be a distinct condition. They consider it a "garbage diagnosis" for many separate disorders, including "just being" a variety of a chronic affective (somatization) disorder. Some also think that FMS and related disorders such as chronic fatigue syndrome (CFS) and irritable bowel syndrome, represent the end of a continuum of pain amplification rather than a unique or discrete disorder. Most patients who meet the criteria for FMS also meet the CDC criteria for CFS (Clauw 1999). FMS, however, is a chronic disorder and is relatively unchanging, which most likely represents a distinct entity involving a disorder of the nervous system. FMS can be a source of substantial disability (Kaplan, Schmidt and Cronan, 2000). This is especially true if the patient has had it for a long time without adequate medical support. Nearly everyone with FMS exhibits reduced coordination skills and decreased endurance abilities, although some of this may be due to co-existing chronic myofascial pain (Starlanyl and Copeland 2001). In FMS the pain often is bilateral, variable, and generalized (involving all four quadrants). The pain cannot be explained by peripheral mechanisms only, and neural plasticity with *CNS sensitization* and *reduced pain threshold* probably playing a major role. FMS has been described as widespread allodynia and hyperalgesia (Russell 1998). In allodynia, nonpainful sensations are translated into pain sensations. Hyperalgesia means that pain sensations are amplified. FMS and disorders such as restless leg syndrome, primary dysmenorrhea, migraines, tension headaches, post-traumatic stress disorder (PTSD) etc., have been grouped under the name, "Central Sensitivity Syndromes," or sensitivity within the spinal cord and brain.

Patients often complain of fatigue, poor quality of sleep, morning stiffness, and increased perception of effort. Muscular pain increases during repetitive muscular activity and usually eases on cessation. FMS is frequently associated with other medical conditions such as: irritable bowel syndrome, dysmenorrhea, headaches, subjective sensation of joint swelling (Baldry *ibid*), interstitial cystitis, depression, generalized anxiety, mitral valve prolapse, restless leg syndrome, chronic fatigue syndrome, and myofascial pain syndrome (MPS). Seniors (Starlanyl and Copeland *ibid*) are more troubled by fatigue, soft-tissue swelling, and depression. In younger people, discomfort after minimal exercise, low-grade fever or below-normal temperature, and skin sensitivity are also common (*ibid*).

Common symptoms are: generalized pain that may be dull, deep, achy, or at times sharp, throbbing, shooting—especially if associated with other pathologies. There are often increased morning symptoms of stiffness, fatigue, and pain. (*OM: Often these symptoms are associated with Dampness, Cold/Yang-deficiency, and poor Blood circulation in TCM, in FMS patients.*) Other common symptoms are dizziness and/or light-headedness, "spaciness" or "brain fog" (cognitive difficulties), which can be due to orthostatic hypotension and/or hypovolemia (*OM: Often these last symptoms are associated in FMS patients with Phlegm, Central-Qi-deficiency with Clear-Yang not rising, Blood-deficiency, unstable-Yang or Wind*),[66] photophobia, ocular complaints (dry eyes, poor focus), stress intolerance, depression, sleep disturbances (including early morning awakening (*OM: Often associated in FMS patients with Liver-Blood and Liver-Qi*), digestive symptoms of bloating, gas, cramping, diarrhea and/or constipation (*OM: Often associated with Dampness or Qi-stagnation in FMS patients*), palpitations, easy sweating or night sweats (*OM: Often associated in FMS patients with Qi-Yin-Blood-deficiency or Damp-Heat*), urinary symptoms, respiratory symptoms, and allergic symptoms (*OM: Often Kidney related in FMS patients*). A reduced threshold of the nervous system can result in sensitivity to odors, sounds, lights, and vibrations that others don't even notice (*OM: often due to easy arousal of Yang, Wind or Phlegm in FMS patients*).

Dellenbach et al (2001) have suggested that many women with chronic pelvic pain are suffering from what they call *pelvic-fibromyalgia*. Pelvic pain is a frequent and difficult problem because, despite the quality and diversity of diagnostic procedures, no relevant etiology will be found in 30-40% of all cases. It has been proposed that in many cases the dominant pain is not visceral but parietal. In many of these patients, the pelvic envelope is more painful than the pelvic content. In these cases, one can evoke the diagnosis of pelvic-fibromyalgia; it is quite similar to classic FMS. This

---

66. Some patients with FMS and up to 90% of patients with chronic fatigue syndrome may suffer from a *neurally mediated hypotension* (NMH), a condition characterized by an abnormal drop in blood pressure in response to prolonged standing, exposure to warm environments, or vigorous exercise. These patients usually feel dizzy and may suffer from syncope and palpitations. Some patients may feel muscle pains, nausea, sweating, abdominal pain, blurred vision, or severe itching. Assessment may need to be done with a head-up tilt table test performed by a cardiologist in a hospital. The patient is placed on a tilt table and brought up to seventy degrees for forty-five minutes. If no significant drop in blood pressure occurs, an adrenalin-like drug is given intravenously This usually brings out the latent positives. Some patients can be diagnosed by an office orthostatic blood pressure test. First, blood pressure and pulse are taken after lying flat. Then, after standing against a wall for ten minutes without being stimulated, the blood pressure and pulse are taken again. Fainting, extreme dizziness, or a fall in blood pressure (or marked increase in pulse rate) may indicate the presence of NMH and treatment may be tried. Treatment usually includes increased salt and water intake to increase plasma volume. Licorice, drugs, that reduce adrenaline receptor sensitivity, or medications that increase blood pressure may be needed (Bouch 2001).

form of pain actually is the somatization of a past and difficult issue that will be revealed very slowly and progressively in the realm of a multidisciplinary, i.e. simultaneous physical and psychological approaches.[67] In the majority of cases these women have a history of physical, moral, or sexual trauma inflicted by family members or a third party. Taking in to account the physical dimension of body pain at the same time as psychotherapy will considerably enhance the efficiency of treatment. In the experience of the study authors, 70% of all women will be "cured" using this approach.

FMS caused by trauma or another precipitating event such as serious (often infectious) illness tends to be more severe and have a worse prognosis than idiopathic FMS (Romano 2000).[68] *Basal autonomic states* of FMS patients are characterized by increased sympathetic and decreased parasympathetic tone with associated increased resting heart rate, reduced heart rate variability (especially remaining-active-at-night frequency domains, and cortisol or heart rate variability), deranged response to orthostatic stress,[69] and a high incidence of Raynaud's syndrome (Donaldson et al 2001). Thus, FMS may be a *sympathetically mediated syndrome* with alterations in the feedback loops interconnecting the hypothalamus-pituitary-adrenal axis.

The prognosis of FMS is much less favorable than MPS, and patients often respond only temporarily to treatment. Reeves (1994), however, reported that prolotherapy was successful in resolving symptoms in more than 75% of his patients with "severe fibromyalgia." OM and other natural approaches, preferably in concert, can be very helpful. Cures, however, are few.

Mechanisms of FMS

In general, FMS is thought to be a disorder of the nervous system involving activation of larger myelinated fibers, which are recruited (by chemical amplification in the spinal cord) to rapidly transmit stimuli to the dorsal horn area of the spinal cord. Because these fibers are so large and transmit signals so rapidly, stimuli that are normally not painful are perceived as painful—allodynia (Russell 1999). Animal studies (Mense 1990) have shown that activity in central nociceptive neurons that receive input mainly from muscles are more under central inhibitory control than central nociceptive neurons receiving input from the skin. This central inhibition may explain why treatment to the CNS with antidepressants often is helpful in FMS patients. Furthermore, a review article presented by Henriksson at the Second World Congress on MPS and FMS states that there are a fairly large number of studies that indicate that FMS patients either have a disturbance of pain modulation or a disturbed function of other regulatory systems. He further cites studies that implicate serotonin metabolism and deficiency, a marked increase of substance P in CSF, lower levels of cortisol,[70] epinephrine and norepinephrine following exercise by patients than in control groups, enhanced pituitary release of ACTH, low metenkephaline levels, and lower levels of serum IGF-1. Finally, Henriksson cites a few reports of immunological disturbances in FMS, for example, a defect in the interleukin-2 pathway. Elevated levels of nerve growth factors may account for high substance P in CSF (Russel *ibid*). Patients with FMS (Bennett 1990) produced excessive lactic acid, which may add to their discomfort after exercise.

Recently, information from PET scans has shown a dysfunction in thalamic activity. Compared to healthy individuals, FMS patients have significantly lower resting-state levels of regional cerebral blood flow in the thalamus and caudate nucleus (Mountz et al 1995, Kwiatek et al 1997). About twenty-two percent of all patients with FMS have a deformity in which the cerebellum and medulla oblongata are impacted into the foramen magnum and upper spinal canal, known as Arnold-Chiari malformation (Russell *ibid*). Twenty-two percent of all patients that presented to the emergency room with whiplash injury show symptoms of FMS within three months (Buskila et al 1997). This may be due to the development of disturbances in CSF circulation and spinal canal size (and which may explain why many such patients respond to cranial osteopathy).

Because many fibromyalgia patients relate a history of acute febrile and congestive respiratory episodes prior to the onset of their illness, a viral cause has been suggested. Tyler (1997) studied ten random fibromyalgia patients with blood testing to determine if viral infections could play a part in the development of fibromyalgia. Screening volunteers for antibodies to influenza type A viral antigen yielded positive results in nine of ten patients. Only three of ten patients with FMS in a similarly aged and sex-matched group demonstrated positive responses to influenza type B. With the positive results obtained, it appears that influenza type A viral infection, which primarily strikes the respiratory and autonomic nervous systems, might be involved in the development of fibromyalgia. In the FMS cases tested, the patients related a history of upper respiratory infection along with associated neurological symptoms prior to the onset of fibromyalgia symptoms. Retroviruses where also found in muscle tissues at a higher rate in FMS patients than in controls.

Bacterial overgrowth in the small intestine was evaluated in 815 individuals using the lactulose hydrogen breath test. Of these, 152 individuals had the diagnosis of FMS, of whom twenty-nine, who had concurrent inflammatory bowel disease, were excluded. Out of the 123 subjects with FMS syndrome, 96 (78%) tested positive for small intestinal bac-

---

67. It is a common experience of acupuncturists and body-workers that such histories are revealed during treatments.

68. Information on treatment here reflects the author's experience with patients in this category.

69. Usually low blood pressure and lightheadedness or "blacking out" on standing.

70. Licorice (Gan Cao) supplementation is often useful in these patients, especially before exercise.

terial overgrowth as diagnosed by the lactulose hydrogen breath test. Of those treated with antibiotics, 57% reported global improvement in their FMS symptoms. The data suggested that bowel symptoms in FMS may be caused by small intestinal bacterial overgrowth. Associations have been made between FMS symptoms and the bacterial species, *Chlamydia* and *Borrelia burgdorferi*. In animal models, small intestinal bacterial overgrowth can result in bacterial translocation to mesenteric lymph nodes and can produce systemic effects. These systemic effects are believed to be mediated by endotoxins from Gram-negative bacteria. These endotoxin effects may explain the soft tissue hyperalgesia that is seen in FMS, since injections of the endotoxin into lab animals results in similar hyperalgesia. The authors conclude that the intestinal symptoms of FMS patients may be related to small intestinal bacterial overgrowth, and treatment of small intestinal bacterial overgrowth can result in overall improvement in intestinal symptoms (Pimentel, Chow, Hallegua, Wallace, and Lin 2001).

Patients with genetic factors that predispose them to hyper-coagulability may be especially susceptible to the effects of microbes. Abnormal coagulation can result in the accumulation of soluble fibrin monomer (SFM) that leads to the formation of a dense film that settles on the inner surface of capillary walls. These deposits form a protective coat that covers microbes living in blood vessel walls, thereby making it difficult for the immune system to attack and destroy them. SFM may also make it difficult for nutrients to pass through thickened blood vessel walls to get into cells, as well as for waste products to pass from the cells into the blood stream. This may explain why so many organ systems and regions are involved in FMS (Saputo 2004).

Some authors suggest that FMS is a somatization syndrome due to depression; however, research suggests otherwise (Stiles and Landro 1995). Their data showed that the cognitive dysfunction that reflects a presumed compromise of the right hemisphere (which is present in major depression) is not found in primary FMS. They concluded that this finding would suggest that primary FMS and depression are different conditions. Cianfrini observed SPECT brain imaging during stimulation of tender points in FMS, chronic fatigue patients, depressed patients, and a control group. He found that both FMS and chronic fatigue patients (with FMS) had significant increases in bilateral regional cerebral blood flow in the somatosensory cortex and the anterior angulate cortex following pressure stimulation at three right-sided tender points. However, healthy controls and depressed patients only showed significant regional cerebral blood flow increases in the contralateral thalamus, somatosensory cortex, and anterior angulate cortex. Croft et al. (1994) have noted that many tender points are also found with depression, chronic fatigue, anxiety disorders, and other symptoms of a somatic nature and not part of this list, including pain. Other symptoms seen in both FMS and depression include poor sleep, fatigue, morning stiffness, poor concentration and poor immediate recall (Donaldson et al *ibid*).

Other hypothetical candidates for causal factors in FMS include: central neurotransmitter imbalances, thyroid hormone resistance, stress-related physiological changes, psychopathology, psychosocial factors, and disturbance of alpha stages of sleep (Donaldson et al *ibid*).

In conclusion, any of the above causes of FMS are thought by most authors to cause a disorder of the nervous system involving CNS sensitization and the activation of larger myelinated fibers that are recruited (by chemical amplification in the spinal cord) to rapidly transmit stimuli to the dorsal horn area of the spinal cord. In CNS sensitization, the nervous systems undergoes remarkable changes, often after an initial painful stimulus at the periphery (or after an emotional stress) so that subsequent stimuli, even if normal, registers as pain and/or altered sensations.

Differential Diagnosis

Several conditions can mimic fibromyalgia. Some examples include (Jacobsen, Samsoe and Lund 1993):

- Hypothyroidism
- Widespread malignancy
- Polymyalgia rheumatica
- Osteomalacia
- Generalized osteoarthritis
- Early Parkinson's disease
- Initial stage of various connective tissue diseases.

Diagnostic Criteria

The American College of Rheumatology criteria for the classification of fibromyalgia are:

1. History of widespread pain, extending into the sides of the body, and pain above and below the waist.

2. Axial skeletal pain must be present. Low back pain is considered lower segment pain.

3. Pain must also be present in eleven of eighteen tender sites on digital palpation of an approximate force of 4kg. At (Figure 11-25):
   — The suboccipital muscle insertions
   — Anterior aspects of the intertransverse spaces of C5-C7
   — Midpoint of the upper border of the trapezius
   — Origins of supraspinous above the scapula
   — Upper lateral aspects of the second costochondral junction
   — 2 cm distal to the lateral epicondyle
   — The upper outer quadrants of the buttocks in the anterior fold of the gluteal muscle
   — The posterior aspect of the trochanteric prominence of the greater trochanter
   — Medial fat pad proximal to the joint line of the knee.

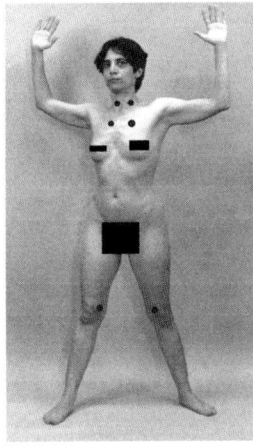
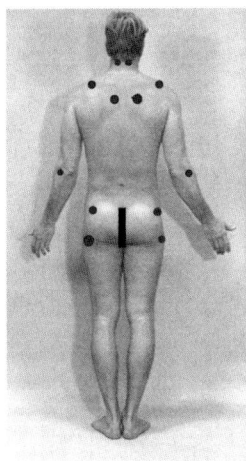

Figure 11-25: Tender points in FMS patients.

The diagnostic criteria suggested by Yunus et al. 1981 and Moldofsky et al. 1975 are:

- Widespread aching of more than three months duration
- Cutaneous and subcutaneous sensitivity as demonstrated by skin roll
- Morning fatigue stiffness with disturbed sleep
- Absence of laboratory evidence of inflammation or muscle damage
- Bilateral tender points in at least six areas.

Fibromyalgia and TCM

Because fibromyalgia presents with a variety of symptoms and fatigue is a common complaint, the disorder often falls within TCM internal medical and Painful Obstruction classifications. Stress, poor sleep quality, poor diet, insufficient rest, and unresolved emotions (such as fear, anger, frustration, depression, anxiety) or trauma can influence Organ functions, deplete True-Qi, Blood, and Fluids, all of which may result in stagnation of Qi and Blood, formation or retention of Dampness, Phlegm, Wind, and symptoms and signs of FMS. Blood loss may injure the Liver, Blood and Qi, which then may fail to nourish the sinews. The muscles may tighten and loose their strength. FMS with a primary syndrome of Blood-deficiency is more commonly seen in females, as blood is lost with the menses. Blood-stasis may be seen in chronic diseases and secondary to trauma.

Although FMS is not necessarily an externally contacted disorder, many FMS patients present with a history of infectious disease, injury, and/or severe medical conditions in which Pathogenic Factors often play a major role. FMS may be best described by six TCM clinical presentations:[71]

1. Retention of Pathogenic Factors
2. Latent Pathogenic Factors
3. Pathogenic Factors between the Interior and Exterior (Shao Yang)
4. Part of Organic or other internal disorder with or without externally contracted Pathogenic Factors. General stress depleting the Righteous and Organs, resulting in Pathogenic Factors and Organic disorders with Liver, Spleen, and Heart involvement being the most common. The Lungs and Kidneys are affected often, as well.
5. Trauma injuring Qi, Blood, and related tissues and Organs
6. Hemorrhage.

FMS often begins following an infectious or other medical disease, which can lead to retained Pathogenic Factors. It may also result from trauma, blood loss, chronic stress, or chronic disease. Stress, trauma, and retained Pathogenic Factors are said to result in obstruction, and often secondary unstable Yang (such as Yin-Fire, Empty-Heat, endogenous-Wind, and deficient-Yang rising). Unstable Yang can manifest as a facilitated sympathetic nervous system and depressed parasympathetics. This autonomic nervous dysfunction often manifests with increased pulse rate (both day and night) that tends to be variable at *rest* (frequent changes in rate strength and quality with little stimulation, which, in TCM, is often associated with weakness), wiry pulse (often with Shao Yang syndrome), decreased circulation with trophic edema, and increased red skin responses on various areas (the skin remains red when scraped or when a needle is inserted, due to poor circulation from excessive sympathetic activity, or is red due to histamines), increased fascial tissue sensitivity demonstrated by pinching or rolling the skin, tender muscles, nodulations in muscles, hypochondriac tension (felt in abdominal [Hara] evaluation), thoracic inlet/outlet tension (felt at and around the SCM muscles), and reactions

---

71. Flaws and Sionneau (2001) state, that in their view the "core" disease mechanism of FMS is Liver-Spleen disharmony. They list the following patterns:

    Liver-Spleen disharmony, that they treat with Rambling Powder -+ (Xiao Yao San);

    Damp-Heat, that they treat with Pinelliae Drain the Heart Decoction -+ (Ban Xia Xie Xin Tang);

    Qi and Yin-vacuity with Liver-depression and Fire Effulgence, that they treat with Heavenly Emperor Supplement the Heart Elixir -+ (Tian Wang Bu Xin Dan Jia Jian);

    Spleen-Kidney-Yang Vacuity with Liver-Depression, that they treat with Supplement the Center and Boost the Qi Decoction (Bu Zhong Yi Qi Tang), plus Restore the Right +- (You Gui Yin);

    Spleen-Qi and Yin and Yang vacuity with Heat and Liver-depression, that they treat with Supplement the Center and Boost the Qi Decoction (Bu Zhong Yi Qi Tang) and Two Immortals Decoction +- (Er Xian Tang);

    Blood-stasis, that they treat with Body Pain Dispel Stasis Decoction +- (Shen Tong Zhu Yu Tang);

    Phlegm Nodulation, that they treat with Disperse Scrofula pills (Xiao Luo Wan) and Two Aged Decoction +- (Er Chen Tang).

at the Kidney/Chong channels. The organs/Organs can become congested and dysfunctional. The patient is often oversensitive to stimulations such as noise, odors, light, and stress (often when Phlegm or Liver disorders are seen).

The main pathogenic factor seen clinically in FMS patients is Dampness, often with underlying Deficiency. Transformative-Heat and Yin-Fire/unstable Yang are common complicating factors. The severity of muscle aches is often related to the level of pathogenic Dampness or Phlegm. With time, Blood-stasis and more severe and fixed pain can develop. There are five distinct risk factors for Dampness, Phlegm, and related conditions are: 1) Improper treatment; 2) Fever/Heat/Fire/Cold and other Pathogenic Factors; 3) Damage to the Spleen/pancreas and Liver; 4) Damage to the Lungs; 5) Kidney Yin, Yang, Essence or True-Qi-deficiency. I will discuss each of these in turn.

1. Improper treatment.

    A common clinical iatrogenicity is due to excessive use of tonifying methods in a patient with Pathogenic Factors.[72] This is said to result in further penetration of Pathogenic Factors (often the development of Phlegm) and increased symptoms of Deficiency, stagnation, and Heat. In such cases, the proper treatment would be to eliminate pathogens. This may then result in the recovery of the patients' Righteous-Qi. In some patients a combined approach is warranted.

    Excessive or improper use of cold medicines or antibiotics is said to be capable of damaging the Spleen/Stomach and may result in Dampness and Phlegm. It may drive Exterior Wind-Cold Pathogenic Factors inside/Interiorly, which become hidden or turn into Heat. With hidden-Heat, the patient becomes ill later, when another infection sets in or life stresses increase. Latent-Heat disorder is said to be more common in a patient with a Deficient constitution or condition, especially Yin.

    Excessive or improper use of hot and spicy medicines or foods are said to thicken and consume Fluids that may transform into Phlegm and mucus, and lodge internally, or within the joints and muscles. This may result in pain and obstruction. Hot and spicy medicines are also said to be capable of injuring Yin, resulting in deficient-Yin Empty-Heat and difficulties with sleep.

    The excessive use of Qi-moving medicines is said to be capable of injuring Qi and may result in stagnation due to lack of movement from Qi-weakness. Qi-stagnation may then result in *local* transformative-Heat and inflammatory signs. Deficient-Qi may result in eventual weakness of Blood. The sinews may tighten and the patient's sleep become affected with increased dreams. Because many Qi-moving herbs are spicy, they can injure the Yin and Blood, as well.

    The excessive use of Blood-moving medicines is said to be capable of injuring both the Qi and Blood, again, resulting in obstruction due to lack of vitality.

    An inappropriate use of diuretics can injure Yin, Yang, or True-Qi or drive Pathogenic Factors inside/Interiorly. Pharmaceutical anti-histamines and some expectorants can result in thickening mucus and Phlegm-Heat.

2. Fever/Heat/Fire/Cold and other Pathogenic Factors.
    Any fever, Heat, and stagnation may damage the Fluids, which congeal and thicken and do not flow. Excessive *Coldness* from external or internal causes is said to be able to congeal the Fluids, as well.

    These common clinical presentations may result in the development of "Trigger Points" (Ashi-sensitive-Kori-tight bands) in muscles that generally feel soft, soggy, and *nodular* with low general tone. Dual Dampness and Yin-deficiency may develop. Blood-stasis is a secondary complication seen frequently. When Blood-stasis is significant, the patient may develop abdominal reactions at the left lower quadrant, visible darkened blood vessels, skin discoloration (especially lips in early stage), choppy or slippery/wiry pulse, and a hard area or point (fibrous tissue) within the muscular taught band (Kori), often at the motor points (usually at midpoint of muscle), and fixed pain that is worse at night or during inactivity. If Phlegm and Blood-stasis combine and stagnate, the patient may develop bony swellings, spurs, and inflamed and hard calcified bursae. Insertional or calcific tendinitis may develop.

    Deficient-Yin patients may show a tight radial blood vessel or a quick, thready-wiry pulse. A pounding pulse[73] may be seen in both Deficient and Excess conditions with Pathogenic Factors. A significantly weak patient may present with a pounding pulse, which may be slow or fast. The blood vessel wall tends to be tight in Excessive conditions and softer in Deficient patients (at least in Yang-deficiency and Dampness). As the patient's strength is increased, the underlying (Organ) pulse may become more evident. The tongue often shows signs of Dampness and Phlegm. Signs of Blood-stasis may or may not be seen.

3. Damage to Spleen/pancreas and Liver.
    Pathogenic Factors may damage the Spleen/pancreas disturbing the transforming and transporting functions of the Spleen. These patients may have digestive symptoms and may be sensitive to foods. They often feel bloated and have epigastric or lower abdominal discomfort and gas. The area around the umbilicus and between CV9-12 may be tight and sensitive. A pulse around the umbilical region may be visible or palpable. The degree of Dampness or Phlegm is often seen on the tongue coat, but not always.

---

72. Many of the author's patients were taking herbs such as Ginseng, either self-prescribed or given by other health-care practitioners.

73. Not a classical pulse description but seen quite frequently.

Similar presentations may be seen in patients with prior weakness of the Spleen/pancreas and a tendency to develop or retain Dampness. This condition is often secondary to poor dietary habits and/or excessive stress. Signs and symptoms are similar, but the patient has a long history of weak digestion and/or fatigue. The patient, at times, just reports fatigue or sleepiness after eating and mild bloating. The tongue coat may be normal, but the tongue body is often swollen and pale. The right middle pulse tends to be soft or weak.

Spleen/pancreas weakness is also said to result in deficiency of Blood, which then may weaken ("fail to lubricate") the Liver and may result in Liver Qi-stagnation/congestion. The Liver then may fail to nourish the sinews. The muscles and sinews may develop tension and weakness. Liver-congestion Qi-stagnation may result in variable and poorly localized pains and leave the patient susceptible to emotional stress and aggravation. Because Qi (or Phlegm/Dampness) stagnation is said to slow circulation, Blood-stasis or transformative/congested-Heat may develop. When Qi-stagnation becomes severe and rebels, swelling (usually not substantial or changing) may develop. Heat may congeal Fluids, which become Phlegm. When Phlegm and Blood join, muscles may become fibrotic and lose flexibility, possibly permanently. With Qi-stagnation, the patient's symptoms may frequently change.

Liver-congestion is a common condition. Liver/wood congestion/stagnation is an Excessive condition and may result in over-regulation of Spleen/earth (according to five-Phases theory). This disharmony is another risk factor of Spleen/pancreas failing to transform and transport, which may result in Dampness.

4. Damage to the Lungs.
Pathogenic Factors can disturb the Lung's descending function, which normally directs Fluids to the Kidneys (often after respiratory infections). This results in dryness, edema, and Qi-dysfunction: the Lungs are said to control Qi, which is the motive force behind Fluids and Blood. The failure of the Lungs to control Qi and vessels may lead to a pooling of Blood or Fluids in the lower body and may become visible as varicose veins or edema.

These patients more commonly show signs of upper edema (Phlegm) under eyes (baggy eyes), face, and sinuses, and tenderness/induration at Lu-1, GB-21, and UB-13 (upper back) *areas*. Upper arm and shoulder symptoms are common. Patients may or may not have other respiratory symptoms. The tongue coat may show signs of Dampness/Phlegm and may also show Dryness at the root.

5. Kidney Yin, Yang, Essence, or True-Qi deficiency.
The Kidneys are the source of Yin and Yang and can influence most of the bodily systems that may lead to FMS. It is Kidney-Yang that is the origin of Spleen-Yang, the catalyst within the Spleen that is in charge of transformation and transportation (digestion and metabolism). The Kidneys are the root of Qi, and healthy functional breathing requires the Kidneys to accept and root Qi. The Fire/force of the Heart and Triple Warmer come from the Kidneys. Therefore, both Blood and Fluid circulation are ultimately dependent on healthy Kidney function. The Fluids that travel with Defensive-Qi (via Triple Warmer) at the Cuo Li (the space between the skin and muscles/membranes/interstice) are rooted in Mingmen (Kidney-Yang), and therefore depend on the Kidneys for motility and warmth. The creation of Blood is also ultimately dependent on healthy marrow and Kidneys, because the Kidneys warm the Spleen/pancreas; they motivate, moisten and nourish the Liver; they root the Lungs and warm the Heart. All of these functions are needed to form Blood. The Kidneys are said to be in charge of Fluids; therefore, Dampness and other Fluid dysfunctions can result from Kidney disorders.

Patients with Kidney (Essence or True-Qi) weakness may have a long history of poor health and general physical weakness, especially poor physical and mental *endurance*. These may be due either to constitutional factors or chronic illness. The lower abdomen of such patients may be soft at the surface and tense deep inside, with excessive pulsations palpable. Kidney points at or just below the umbilicus may be tight and tender. The patient's complexion may be dull, and, especially in women, the area around the mouth and eyes may be green and dark. Tenderness and tightness/indurations may be felt especially at UB-52 (quadratus lumborum), CV4-6, K-7, and K-3. Phlegm develops due to a lack of vitality. This may be "unseen Phlegm," *affecting non-mucus membranes* and lacking many of the usual signs of Phlegm such as a greasy and slimy tongue coat, especially in Kidney-Yin-deficient patients. The pulse at the proximal positions may reflect weakness.

Latent Pathogenic Factors are said to be seen most commonly in Deficient patients who do not have a *clear* history/onset of infectious disease. An insufficiency of the patient's True-Qi, Kidney-Qi, Yin and Essence (Righteous) is said to result in Pathogenic Factors entering the Interior. This may be seen without the development of superficial symptoms (due to the absence of a struggle between the weaken antipathogenic-Qi and the pathogens) or with only mild symptoms. Later, symptoms of Heat, irritability, digestive disturbances, fatigue, and possibly muscle pain may develop.[74] Yin-deficient patients may tend to develop a complex syndrome with symptoms of Heat, Cold, and Dampness. Yang-deficient patients may tend to develop a Cold syndrome with Dampness; however, local Fire may be seen.[75] In FMS patients, if treatments that usually work in

---

74. Muscle pains are not classically among of the symptoms associated with hidden-latent Pathogenic Factors. However, Latent/hidden Pathogenic Factors are said to "reside in the bones/marrow, Cou Li *(membranes, space between the skin and muscles)*, and muscles."

"latent-Heat" prove effective, the patients may or may not show the classic syndrome of latent or retained Pathogenic Factors (such as infection, irritability, digestive symptoms and signs, etc.). Signs may be felt in the tissue texture of muscles and joint end-feels. They usually include "rheumatic" type changes and little or no systemic symptoms and signs.

Pathogenic Factors may be retained at the Shao Yang level (between the Exterior and Interior), especially in stressed patients. The patient is said to be temporarily deficient (from stress) and therefore unable to dispel the external Pathogenic Factors. The Pathogenic Factors are often weak, as well. The main manifestation is alternating or combined symptoms of Heat and Cold or cyclical symptoms (or changing symptoms and/or symptoms that are sometimes present sometimes not). FMS patients with Shao Yang syndrome may not show the classic (Shang Han Lun) syndrome. They do not have to have Exterior symptoms or a history of external Pathogenic Factors. They do, however, often present with both Interior and Exterior symptoms and have relatively strong, muscular physiques, but not always.[76] They often complain of temperature disregulation, saying that "since they have been sick" their internal temperature has not been right—sometimes they feel excessively cold or hot, or just uncomfortable when external temperature is extreme. They often feel nauseous and have a bad taste in the mouth, especially in the morning. They may feel relatively fine when rested, but when fatigued or stressed they develop symptoms. Clinical experience (of the author) suggests that this condition is slightly more common in male patients. Secondary Yin-deficiency, Liver-stagnation, and Blood-stasis may be complicating factors. The soft tissues, muscles, and joints of these patients have a tighter feel compared with the more Deficient patient. The patient usually appears to be physically strong. The subcostals and possibly the epigastric and right lateral abdomen areas may be tight, sensitive, and may show tight bands and indurations. (They often develop extensive congestions that may be anywhere within the three Warmers.) The pulse is wiry.

Treatment

FMS is notoriously unresponsive to standard biomedical treatment. Education is probably one of the most important aspects in its management. The patient must understand that being out of condition contributes to myofascial pain. Therefore, an exercise program that includes stretching, strength building, and aerobic conditioning is extremely important. However, patients should not over-exercise and should conserve their energy. A one-day rest between exercise sessions may be prudent. The patient's sleep quality must be improved, as altered sleep patterns are probably the most important clinical facet of FMS. Patients should try to sleep at least eight hours per day. Sleep hygiene is important. Having the patient observe regular bedtime hours and encouraging them to regulate their daily activities (such as rest and meals) can be helpful. Patients should avoid caffeine for eight hours, large meals for four hours, and exercise for six hours before sleep (Bennett 1999).

The standard of care (in the US) is treatment with antidepressant medication, despite a great deal of research showing that in most instances depression is a result, rather than a cause of the condition (Block 1993, Duna and Wilke 1993). The effectiveness of this treatment has much to do with improvement in sleep. Possibly this treatment results in reduced substance P formation by increasing serotonin control and by modulating pain in other ways. Lower doses are usually used than for depression. NSAIDs are of marginal value, with propionic acid derivatives (Daypro, Orudis) possibly the most effective[77] of these drugs. Analgesics, especially Tramadol, a drug that is a weak opioid and that also inhibits reuptake of norepinephrine and serotonin, have been advocated. The muscle relaxants levodopa, carbidopa, and quinine are sometimes used for restless leg syndrome or muscle cramps (Bennett *ibid*).

An alternative pharmaceutical treatment using the OTC expectorant guaifenesin (Robitussin) has been suggested to be helpful for FMS and chronic fatigue syndrome by Dr. Amand. The basic theory behind this protocol is that FMS is a manifestation of a genetic anomaly that affects the body's ability to excrete phosphates (and perhaps other minerals) effectively. Guaifenesin is said to excrete phosphates, and, to a lesser degree, oxalates and blood calcium. Progression is said to be cyclical, beginning with exacerbation of symptoms followed by good days, generally within a few months. An average reversal rate is said to be about one year for every two months of the proper dosage. Dr. Amand recommends a starting dose of 300mg BID. Within a week, the patient is said to feel significantly but tolerably worse, if the patient is not taking salicylates. Salicylates must be avoided in the form of any aspirin-related compounds including herbs. Other NSAIDs and Tylenol are okay. This dosage suffices for 20% of all patients. If there is no increase in symptoms in that time, the dose is increased to 600mg BID. This dose is maintained for three to four weeks. In 70% of the patients 1200mg/day suffices. The upper dose range is 3600mg/day.

Other treatments may include physical medicine procedures such as acupuncture, manual therapies (especially muscle energy, functional, counter-strain and cranial techniques), ultrasound, and heat. Internal interventions such as

---

75. These patients are treated mainly as Deficient Cold.

76. Minor Bupleurum Decoction (Xiao Chai Hu Tang) in some Japanese traditions is used more for "weak confirmations." This formula is then used to strengthen the patient's constitution and is taken for long periods. In the author's experience, many of the above FMS patients respond to modifications of Xiao Chai Hu Tang or Da Chai Hu Tang and therefore *may* be categorized as Shao Yang.

77. Although recently, Wallace et al. has shown increased levels of three cytokines (inflammatory mediators): IL-6, IL-8, and IL-1Ra in FMS patients.

herbal and nutritional therapies are often helpful. Psychotherapy (especially Cognitive Psychotherapy), biofeedback, and other relaxation exercise techniques, and EEG biofeedback may be helpful.

Osteopathic approaches have been shown to be helpful in treating patients diagnosed with FMS. Stotz and Kappler (1992) treated patients using a variety of Osteopathic approaches. Goldenberg (1993) measured the effects of Osteopathic manipulative therapy (OMT) on the intensity of pain reported from tender points in eighteen patients who met all of the criteria for FMS. Each patient had six treatments. Over a one year period, twelve of the patients responded well, and their tender points became less sensitive (14% reduction verses a 34% increase in the six patients who did not respond). Activities of daily living were significantly improved, and general pain symptoms decreased. Lo et al (1992) studied nineteen patients with all of the criteria of FMS. The patients were treated once a week for four weeks using OMT. At the end of treatment 84.2% of the patients had improved sleep, 94.7% reported less pain, and most patients had fewer tender points on palpation. Rubin et al. (1990), in a study involving thirty-seven patients with FMS, tested the differences resulting from using drugs only (ibuprofen, alprazolam), Osteopathic treatment (including strain-counterstrain and muscle energy) plus medication, OMT plus a placebo, and a placebo only. Drug therapy alone resulted in significantly less tenderness than did drugs and osteopathy, or the use of placebo and OMT, or placebo alone. Patients receiving placebo plus Osteopathic manipulation reported significantly less fatigue than the other groups. The group receiving medication and (mainly) osteopathic soft tissue manipulation showed the greatest improvement in their quality of life. Jiminez et al. (1993) selected three groups of FMS patients, one of which received OMT, another had OMT plus self-teaching (study of the condition and self-help measures), and a third group received only moist-heat treatment. The group with the lowest level of reported pain after six months of care was the one receiving OMT, although benefits were also noted in the self-teaching group.

Acupuncture has been shown to be helpful in FMS. Berman, Ezzo, Hadhazy, and Swyers (1999) conducted a search for the key words "acupuncture" and "fibromyalgia." They selected all randomized or quasi-randomized controlled trials, or cohort studies of patients with FMS who were treated with acupuncture. Seven studies (three randomized, controlled trials and four cohort studies) were included; only one was of high methodologic quality. The high-quality study suggests that real acupuncture is more effective than sham acupuncture for relieving pain, increasing pain thresholds, improving global ratings, and reducing morning stiffness of FMS, but the duration of benefit following the acupuncture treatment series is not known. Some patients report no benefit, and a few report an exacerbation of FMS-related pain. Lower-quality studies were consistent with these findings.

Sprott, Franke, Kluge, and Hein (1998) performed acupuncture therapy on FMS patients and established a combination of methods to objectify pain measurement before and after therapy. Acupuncture treatment of patients with FMS was associated with decreased pain levels and fewer positive tender points as measured by VAS and dolorimetry. They also showed a decreased serotonin concentration in platelets and an increase of serotonin and substance P levels in serum after treatment. These results suggest that acupuncture therapy is associated with changes in the concentrations of pain-modulating substances in serum.

Sprott, Jeschonneck, Grohmann, Hein (2000) have shown that, besides normalization of clinical parameters, acupuncture results in improvement in microcirculation above "tender points."

Zborovskii and Babaeva (1996) showed that 9.6% of 1240 patients making complaints of osteomuscular pains had clinical signs of *primary* fibromyalgia (PFM). They suggested therapies that combine the use of dimexide with NSAIDs and sessions of acupuncture to promote the normalization of dysfunctions.

Targino et al (2002), in a review of the literature on the use of acupuncture as an adjunct or chief treatment for patients with fibromyalgia, compared it with other clinical experience. He found that traditional acupuncture gives positive scores in the Visual Analogue Scale, Myalgic Index, number of tender points, and improvement in quality of life based on the SF-36 questionnaire.

Insomnia, depression, and Raynaud's are common in FMS patients. These related symptoms can be treated. For example, Montakab (1999) has shown acupuncture to be helpful for insomnia. Forty patients with primary difficulties in either falling asleep or remaining asleep were diagnosed according to TCM, assigned to specific diagnostic subgroups, and treated individually by a practitioner in his private practice. The patients were distributed at random into two groups, one receiving *true acupuncture*, the other needled at *non-acupuncture* points for three to five sessions at weekly intervals. The outcome of the therapy was assessed in several ways: first by an objective measurement of the sleep quality, and second by polysomnography in a specialized sleep laboratory, performed once before and once after termination of the series of treatments. Additional qualitative results were obtained from several questionnaires. The objective measurement showed a statistically significant effect only in the patients who received the true acupuncture.

Evaluation of the effects of a standardized acupuncture treatment in *primary Raynaud's syndrome* showed a significant decrease in the frequency of attacks from 1.4 day-1 to 0.6 day-1, $P < 0.01$ (control 1.6 to 1.2, $P = 0.08$). The overall reduction of attacks was 63% (control 27%, $P = 0.03$). The mean duration of the capillary flowstop reaction decreased from 71 to 24 s (week 1 vs week 12, $P = 0.001$) and 38 s (week 1 vs week 23, $P = 0.02$) respectively (Appiah, Hiller, Caspary, Alexander, Creutzig 1997).

Acupuncture has been used successfully to treat *depression*. For example, Allen et al (1998) treated thirty-eight women between eighteen and forty-five years of age. The patients were randomly assigned to one of three treatments: receiving specific acupuncture treatment (n=12), receiving nonspecific acupuncture treatment (n=11), or being on a waiting list (n=11). Patients who were in the nonspecific treatment group received eight weeks of nonspecific treatment first, and then eight weeks of specific treatment. Patients on the waiting-list group waited eight weeks before receiving eight weeks of specific treatment. Each eight-week treatment regimen was comprised of twelve treatment sessions: two sessions a week for the first four weeks, followed by once per week thereafter. Of the women, 64% experienced full remission. Patients receiving specific acupuncture treatments improved significantly more than those receiving the placebo-like nonspecific acupuncture treatments, and marginally more than those in the waiting-list condition. Results from this small study suggest acupuncture can provide significant symptom relief in depression at rates comparable to those of psychotherapy and pharmacotherapy.

In general, however, a review study by Sim and Adams (1999) stated that there is little *empirical* evidence for the effectiveness of physical and other non-pharmacological approaches to the management of FMS. Although a number of studies have been conducted concerning such approaches, many of these are uncontrolled. Moreover, relatively few randomized controlled trials of appropriate size and methodological rigor have been carried out. Sim and Adams reviewed evidence presented under the headings of: exercise, EMG biofeedback training, electrotherapy, acupuncture, patient education, self-management programs, multimodal treatment approaches, and other interventions. They concluded that it is hard to reach firm conclusions from the literature, owing to the variety of interventions that have been evaluated and the varying methodological quality of the studies concerned. Nonetheless, in terms of specific interventions, *exercise therapy* has received a moderate degree of support from the literature and has been subjected to more randomized studies than any other intervention.

It is this author's experience that no one style of medicine or technique is effective in the majority of FMS patients (except perhaps exercise). An integrated approach is superior to any single intervention.

Acupuncture

Acupuncture is best utilized to address the patient's physical presentation with analysis based on palpation techniques. Pulses are balanced by four-needle technique or other channel therapies; abdominal presentations such as subcostal tension are addressed with techniques utilizing the Chong, Yin Wei, Liver, and Pericardium channels. Since the pathogenesis and obstruction in MPS patients manifests mostly in the muscles (even when associated with internal Organic syndromes), muscle triggers/Kori-Ashi points are released in

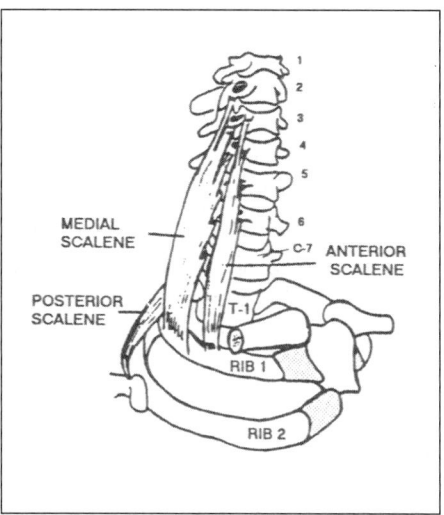

Figure 11-26: Scalene muscles and upper ribs (From Kuchera WA and Kuchera ML, Osteopathic Principles in Practice, KCOM press 1993, with permission).

affected and related areas. A gentle technique that results in *mild* muscle twitches is used first. The Sinew channels in the affected areas are sedated (trigger release), and the paired Main channel may be tonified. Moxa can be used on areas with poor muscle and skin tone when they are found within the same muscle that has indurated triggers. Moxa can also be used to vitalize Deficient channels. Blood-stasis is treated mainly via Chong and Liver channels, UB-17, LI-11, Sp-10, and 21; Dampness via the Spleen/pancreas, Lung, and Kidney channels. Microsystems such as ear and wrist/ankle can be used at the same time for further symptomatic relief. Since distortion of body image (sensation of swelling without swelling, sensation of shrinking without shrinking) and difficulty describing symptoms are common in FMS patients, Sp-4, Lu-7, UB-11, St-37, and 39 are used often. Sp-21 can be used for "total body" pain.

Acupuncture is also helpful in treating the patient's mood and sleep, which are extremely important to address. Poor sleep which is one of the most important perpetuating factor seen in these patients can be treated. H-7, P-6, Amnien, Yinteng, Du-20 and the French ear points: wrist, stress control, tranquilizer, and master cerebral and Chinese ear Shenman points may be used. A study on the effects of acupressure, manual acupuncture, and laserneedle acupuncture on the EEG bispectral index and spectral edge frequency showed that stimulation at Yinteng results in EEG similarities induced by acupressure and general anaesthesia. All of the interventions reduced scores on tests of sedation based on verbal reports (Litscher (2004).

Manual Therapy

In all FMS patients, the thoracic inlet/outlet must be carefully evaluated by assessing soft tissue tension and length, respiratory functions, and proper joint play. Treatment can

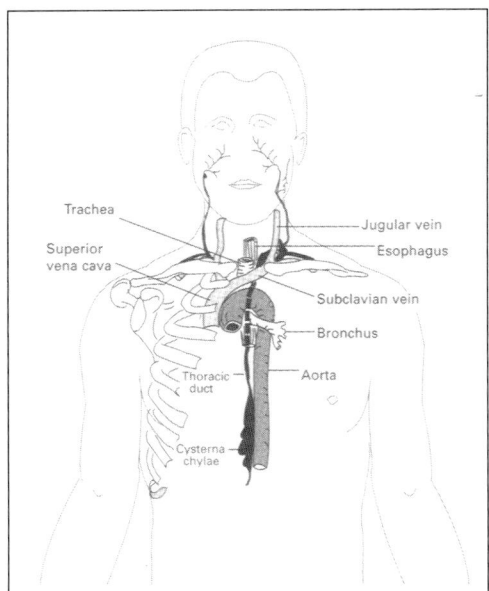

Figure 11-27: Lymphatic and circulatory organs related to thoracic structures (From Kuchera WA and Kuchera ML, Osteopathic Principles in Practice, KCOM press 1994, with permission).

begin with trigger release, but if the function of any of the above structures does not improve, other techniques such as muscle energy, indirect/functional, and cranial techniques should be incorporated. For example, it is common for the first rib to subluxate due to scalene muscle tension (due to stress), with a sudden sidebending of the neck (Figure 11-26). The rib lodges above the transverse process of the first thoracic vertebra. Subluxation results in poor rib-cage function. Release of scalene muscle tension, on its own, will not restore the rib to its proper location. One must use manual therapy to restore rib-cage function.

Also, good diaphragm and abdominal muscle tone are important in maintaining the abdominal viscera in proper position and for proper venous drainage via the diaphragmatic pump. Poor rib-cage function and/or somatic dysfunction can result in disturbances of circulation, poor muscle tone, and disturbances of organ functions. Innervation to many organs and trunk musculature is provided via the thoracic segments. It has been suggested (Chaitow *ibid*) that poor "drooped posture" can result in diaphragm and abdominal muscle relaxation, which cease to support abdominal organs. The disturbances of circulation resulting from a "low diaphragm and ptosis" may give rise to chronic passive congestion in one or all of the organs of the abdomen and pelvis. Furthermore, the drag of these "congested organs" on their nerve supply, as well as the pressure on the sympathetic ganglia and plexuses, probably cause many irregularities in their function, varying from partial paralysis to overstimulation. Proper rib-cage and spinal functions are therefore extremely important, as they control respiration, lymphatic and blood circulation, and nervous and organ functions, all of which are necessary for FMS patients to recover. Good *manual*

functional evaluation is therefore suggested, regardless of the treatment style used.

TCM Herbs

As noted above, FMS caused by trauma or another precipitating event such as serious illness tends to be more severe and have a worse prognosis than idiopathic FMS. The information below mainly reflects this author's experience and is based by and large on patients within this category. It is the author's experience that FMS patients are often sensitive and do not tolerate strong, spicy, hot, or cold formulas. They tend to develop side-effects (even with so called individually patterned appropriate formulas) and are often non-compliant, especially if prolonged herbal therapy is needed. A mild approach to herbal formula design is often preferable. The most difficult aspect is to decide between the elimination of Pathogenic Factors, tonification, and harmonization. Although, by following traditional theory, one usually eliminates Pathogenic Factors before tonifying, this is not always the best clinical approach in FMS patients. Also, as stated in the *Classic of Internal Medicine,* "When Pathogenic Factors converge, the Qi becomes Deficient in that location...Deficient Qi allows for Pathogenic Factors." Therefore, patients that seem to have infectious-like symptoms (such as cold and flu) should be carefully assessed to determine whether the syndrome is truly Internal (miscellaneous/internal diseases), External, or combined. When there are no *clear* Exterior symptoms or signs (such as stuffy or runny nose, body aches and floating pulse), an Interior cause is possible. In patients with clear, acute Exterior Pathogenic Factors (or hidden-latent ones), a mildly clearing formula can be used first. In hidden-latent Heat, a small to moderate dose of Fructus Gardenia (San Zhi Zi) and Bombyx Bartryticatus (Jiang Can) can be prescribed. For symptoms/signs of Yin-deficiency, Radix Scrophulariae (Xuan Shen), Radix Rehmanniae (Sheng Di) and Radix Pancis Quinquefolii (Xi Yang Shen) can be used. Some deficient patients, especially if they develop Exterior syndromes often, do better with a harmonizing or combined Exterior releasing formulas with mild tonification from the start. Even with these patients, however, one must carefully analyze their condition, and, most often, use only small amounts of tonic herbs. Patients who feel sick often, complaining of throat discomfort, fatigue, and aching, but do not have clear symptoms or signs of Exterior syndrome, may do better with a Qi-tonifying and Damp-transforming approach.

The following are treatment strategies based on common clinical presentations seen by the author. These formulas are based on disease diagnosis (biomedical FMS) and are modified for symptoms and TCM pattern discriminations.

To improve sleep and general physical condition and to eliminate Pathogenic Factors in FMS patients, a modification of Sour Jujube Decoction (Suan Zao Ren Tang) can often be used. The following formula gently regulates the Liver (by clearing Heat, nurturing Blood, and ensuring free flow), strengthens Spleen/pancreas without being warm or spicy, and gently regulates Qi and Blood flow, leading Pathogenic Factors to the surface and helping settle the spirit:

> Semen Ziziphi Spinosae (Suan Zao Ren) 12g
> Radix Puerariae (Ge Gen) 9g
> Poria (Fu Ling) 12g
> Rhizoma Ligustici Wallichii (Chuan Xiong) 6g
> Folium Perillae (Zi Su Ye) 3g
> Semen Coicis (Yi Yi Ren) 15g
> Rhizoma Pinelliae (Ban Xia) 6g
> Rhizoma Corydalis (Yan Hu Suo) 9g
> Rhizoma Dioscoreae Hypoglaucae (Bei Xie) 12g
> Piperis Kadsurae Caulis (Hai Feng Teng) 12g
> Bulbus Lilii (Bai He) 9g
> Radix Salvia Miltiorrhizae (Dan Shen) 9g
> Concha Margaritifera Usta (Zhen Zhu Mu) 15g
> Rhizoma Anemarrheanae (Zhi Mu) 2g
> Radix Glycyrrhizae (Gan Cao) 3g
> Fructus Ziziphi Jujubae 12 pieces

Modifications:

1. For insomnia with imbalance of Defensive and Nutritive-Qi, use Cinnamon Twig Decoction (Gui Zhi Tang) to be taken at a different time than the main formula.

2. For insomnia with agitation and retained Wind-Heat, remove the Piperis Kadsurae Caulis (Hai Feng Teng). Add Semen Sojae Praeparata (Dan Dou Chi) 9g, and Fructus Gardeniae (San Zhi Zi) 5g.

3. For insomina, agitation, early or frequent awakening, and Empty-Heat from febrile disease or other causes, remove Piperis Kadsurae Caulis (Hai Feng Teng). Add Gelatinum Asini (E Jiao) 12g and Rhizoma Coptidis (Huang Lian) 4g, Rhizoma Anemarrheanae (Zhi Mu) 6g, Bulbus Lilii (Bai He) 9g.

4. For insomina due to Defensive-Qi not entering the Organs, add Pinelliae (Ban Xia) 20g (note high dose), Coicis (Yi Ren) 20g.

5. For chronic and more severe insomnia, add Rhizoma Pinelliae (Ban Xia) 12g, Caulis Bambusae in Taeniis (Zhu Ru) 9g, Spica Prunellae Vulgaris (Xia Gu Cao) 6g, Fructus Aurantii Immaturus (Zhi Shi) 3g, Os Draconis (Long Gu) 20g.

6. For Yin and/or Kidney-deficiency, add Fructus Schisandrae (Wu Wei Zi) 6g, Semen Cuscutae (Tu Si Zi) 9g, Rhizoma Dioscoreae (Shan Yao) 15g, Radix Pseudostellariae (Tai Zi Shen) 6g.

7. For Liver Yin-deficiency, add Flos Chrysanthemi (Ju Hua) 9g, Semen Cuscutae (Tu Si Zi) 9g, Fructus Lycii (Gao Qi Zi) 9g.

8. For Liver Qi-stagnation, add Flos Chrysanthemi (Ju Hua) 9g, Herba Abri (Ji Gu Cao) 3g, Tuber Curcumae (Yu Jin) 6g, Fructus Hordei Vulgaris Geminatus (Mai Ya) 20g.

9. For Spleen and Qi-deficiency, add Rhizoma Dioscoreae (Shan Yao) 9g, Radix Ginseng (Ren Shen) 6g.

10. For unstable and deficient-Yang harassing the Heart or non-communication between Heart and Kidneys, add Cortex Cinnamomi Cassiae (Ru Gui) 6g, Rhizoma Coptidis (Huang Lian) 2g.

    If due to Yin-deficiency Empty-Heat, remove Piperis Kadsurae Caulis (Hai Feng Teng) and add Gelatinum Asini (E Jiao) 12g and Rhizoma Coptidis (Huang Lian) 4g.

11. For poor appetite, add Endothelium Corneum Gigeraiae Galli (Ji Nei Jin) 9g.

12. For digestive symptoms with Dampness and bloating, add Pericarpium Arecae Catechu (Da Fu Pi) 6g, Herba Eupatorii Fortunei (Pei Lan) 6g.

13. For Damp-Heat, add Rhizoma Coptidis (Huang Lian) 4g.

14. For Cold pain, add Rhizoma Corydalis (Yan Hu Suo) 12g, Radix Clematidis Chinensis (Wei Ling Xian) 6g, Rhizoma Zingiberis Officinalis (Gan Jiang) 5g, Ramulus Cinnamomi Cassiae (Gui Zhi) 3g.

15. For Blood-stasis or history of trauma, add Radix Cyathulae (Chuan Niu Xi) 9g, Excrementum Trogopterori Seu Pteromi (Wu Ling Zi) 6g, Radix Salvia Miltiorrhizae (Dan Shen) 12g, Radix Puerariae (Ge Gen) 9g.

16. For joint pains and stiffness from transformative-Heat, add Piperis Kadsurae Caulis (Luo Shi Teng) 12g, Ramulus Mori Albae (Sang Zhi) 9g, Ledebouriellae/Siler (Fang Feng) 6g, Flos Carthami (Hong Hua) 6g, Radix Rubrus Paeoniae Lactiflorae (Chi Shao) 6g, Ramus Lonicerae Japonicae (Ren Dong Teng) 12g.

17. For severe fatigue after exercise, add Radix Glycyrrhizae (Gan Cao) 1g (one hour prior to exercise in capsule form), Fructus Lycii (Gao Qi Zi) 12g, Semen Cuscutae (Tu Si Zi) 12g, Fructus Mori Albae (Sang Shen Zi) 15g, Salt 0.15g.

18. For weak immune system with frequent colds or respiratory allergies, add Radix Astragali (Huang Qi) 9g, Radix Ginseng (Ren Shen) 3g, Rhizoma Atractylosis Macrocephalae (Bai Zhu) 3g, Radix Ledebouriellae (Fang Feng) 6g, Fructus Schisandrae (Wu Wei Zi) 3g, Radix Glehniae Littoralis (Bei Sha Shen) 4g.

    If with Phlegm-Heat, add Radix Scutellariae Baicalensis (Huang Qin) 6g, Rhizoma Coptidis (Huang lian) 3g.

19. For excessive sweating due to Qi/Yin-deficiency, add Radix Ephedrae (Ma Huang Gen) 9g, Concha Ostreae (Mu Li) 15g.

20. For upper edema, add Cortex Mori Albae Radicis (Sang Bai Pi) 12g, Sclerotium Polypori Umbellati (Zhu Ling) 9g, Ramulus Cinnamomi Cassiae (Gui Zhi) 3g, Rhizoma Atractylosis Macrocephalae (Bai Zhu) 3.

21. For headaches, add Ramulus Uncariae Cum Uncis (Gou Teng) 9g, Rhizoma Gastrodiae Elatae (Tian Ma) 6g, Radix Ligustici Wallichii (Chuan Xiang) 9g.

22. For psychiatric symptoms, add Herba Pycnostelmae (Liao Diao Zhu) 6g, Rhizoma Acori Graminei (Shi Chang Pu) 3g.

23. For muscle cramps (especially calf or nocturnal) and restless legs, add Radix Paeoniae Alba (Bai Shao) 12g, Ramulus Cinnamomi Cassiae (Gui Zhi) 4g, Radix Glycyrrhizae (Gan Cao) 4g, Fructus Chaenomelis Longenariae (Mu Gua) 9g, Semen Persicae (Tao Ren) 6g, Os Draconis (Long Gu) 15g.

24. For fibrotic muscles and sinews, add Semen Persicae (Tao Ren) 6g, Radix Cyathulae (Chuan Niu Xi) 9g, Bulbus Fritillariae Thunbergii (Zhe Bei Mu) 12g, Concha Ostreae (Mu Li) 20g, Radix Clematidis Chinensis (Wei Ling Xian) 6g.

25. For severe tension, spasms, and pain, add Agkistrodon Deu Bungarus (Bai Hua She) 6g, Scolopendra Subspinipes (Wu Gong) 6g, Buthus Martensi (Quan Xie) 5g.

26. For discogenic symptoms add: Fructus Arctii (Niu Bang Zi) 30g, Tripterygium Wilfordii (Lei Gong Teng) 12g.

For patients with generalized muscle pain, mild articular signs, but no *significant* difficulty with sleep and energy (more likely to be extensive MPS) use:[78]

Rhizoma Dioscoreae Hypoglaucae (Bie Xie) 12g
Radix Puerariae (Ge Gen) 9g
Radix Clematidis Chinensis (Wei Ling Xian) 6g
Piperis Kadsurae Caulis (Hai Feng Teng) 12g
Cortex Erythrinae (Hai Tong Pi) 12g
Gentianae (Qin Jiao) 12g
Semen Coicis (Yi Yi Ren) 20g
Semen Cuscutae (Tu Si Zi) 12g
Radix Cyathulae (Chuan Niu Xi) 9g
Rhizoma Corydalis (Yan Hu Suo) 9g
Herba Lycopi Lucidi (Ze Lan) 6g
Aquama Manitis Pentadactylae (Chuan Shan Jia) 12g
Concha Margaritifera Usta (Zhen Zhu Mu) 15g
Fructus Hordei Vulgaris Geminatus (Mai Ya) 20g
Rhizoma Ligustici Wallichii (Chuan Xiang) 6g
Pseudoginseng (San Qi) 6g

If more Wind and Blood-deficiency, use:

Radix Gentianae (Qin Jiao) 6g
Radix Ledebouriellae (Fang Feng) 9g
Ramulus Uncariae Cum Uncis (Gou Teng) 6g
Radix Paeoniae Alba (Bai Shao) 6g
Semen Cassiae Torae (Cao Jue Ming) 12g
Semen Ziziphi Spinosae (Suan Zao Ren) 12g
Flos Chrysanthemi Morifolii (Ju Hua) 6g
Fructus Hordei Vulgaris Germinatus (Mai Ya) 12g
Semen Biotae Orientalis (Bai Zi Ren) 9g
Radix Clematidis (Wei Ling Xian) 6g
Radix Glycyrrhizae Uralensis (Gan Cao) 3g

Modifications:

1. For muscle cramps and tightness, add Radix Paeoniae Alba (Bai Shao) 12g, Ramulus Cinnamomi Cassiae (Gui Zhi) 4g, Radix Glycyrrhizae (Gan Cao) 4g, Fructus Chaenomelis Longenariae (Mu Gua) 9g.

2. For upper body symptoms, add Radix Puerariae (Ge Gen) 6g, Rhizoma Curcumae (Jiang Huang) 9g Ramulus Cinnamomi Cassiae (Gui Zhi) 6g (for Cold), Ramulus Mori Albae (Sang Zhi) 9g (for Heat).

3. For lower body symptoms, add Radix Achyranthis Bidentatae (Huai Niu Xi) 12g, Radix Stephaniae Tetrandrae (Fang Ji) 6g, Ramulus Loranthi Seu Visci (Sang Ji Sheng) 12g. For Wind-Damp add Radix Angelica Pubescentis (Due Huo).

4. For swelling in joints or superficial edema, add Herba Lycopi Lucidi (Ze Lan) 6g.

For patients with Damp-Heat depleting Kidney and Liver-Yin (i.e., primary pathology of Damp-Heat), often seen with Spleen-deficiency and Stomach-Heat (this is a very common presentation that may be due to hidden/lurking pathogens), use:[79]

Rhizoma Atractylodis (Cang Zhu) 6g
Radix Atractylodis (Bai Zhu) 9g
Rhizoma Dioscoreae Hypoglaucae (Bie Xie) 12g
Radix Astragali (Huang Qi) 9g
Herba Eupatorii Fortunei (Pei Lan) 12g
Ramus Lonicerae Japonicae (Ren Dong Teng) 12g
Tuber Curcumae (Yu Jin) 9g
Bombyx Bartryticatus (Jiang Can) 6g
Radix Scrophulariae (Xuan Shen) 6g
Radix Rehmanniae (Sheng Di) 12g
Radix Glehniae Littoralis (Bei Sha Shen) 4g
Poria (Fu Ling) 12g
Herba Lophatheri (Dan Zhu Ye) 12g
Radix Ledebouriellae (Fang Feng) 6g
Semen Coicis (Yi Yi Ren) 15g
Radix Glycyrrhizae (Gan Cao) 1g

If there is also a Qi-deficiency, use a variation of Master Li's Decoction to Clear Summer-Damp-Heat and Augment the Qi (Li Shi Qing Shu Qi Tang):

Radix Astragali Membranaceus (Huang Qi) 12g
Radix Rehmanniae (Sheng Di Huang) 9g
Radix Polygoni Multiflori (He Shou Wu) 9g
Radix Ginseng (Ren Shen) 3g
Rhizoma Atractylosis (Cang Zhu) 6g
Ramus Lonicerae Japonicae (Ren Dong Teng) 12g
Rhizoma Atractylodes Alba (Bai Zhu) 9g
Radix Ophiopogonis (Mai Dong) 12g
Cortex Phellodendri (Huang Bai) 9g
Rhizoma Anemarrhenae (Zhi Mu) 6g
Radix Angelica Sinensis (Dang Gui) 6g
Radix Puerariae (Ge Gen) 20g
Massa Fermentata (Shen Qu) 9g
Pericarpium Citri Reticulatae (Chen Pi) 6g
Pericarpium Citri Reticulatae Viride (Ching Pi) 4g
Fructus Schisandrae (Wu Wei Zi) 6g
Fructus Mume (Wu Mei) 6g
Rhizoma Cimicifugae (Sheng Ma) 5g

---

78. This formula is also good for postural phase of pain.

79. This is one of the commonest presentations seen by the author. Symptoms may include any of the typical symptoms seen in FMS patients. There are *signs* of Damp-Heat and Yin-deficiency.

Honey-fried Radix Glycyrrhizae (Zhi Gan Cao) 3g

For a patient that is Kidney and Heart deficient and is depressed, stressed, anxious, fatigued, but does not have any digestive issues and is not particularly sensitive, use:

>Radix Puerariae (Ge Gen) 20g
>Radix Rehmanniae (Sheng and Shu Di Huang) 15g each
>Radix Dioscoreae (Shan Yao) 15g
>Poria (Fu Ling) 12g
>Cortex Mountan Radicis (Mu Dan Pi) 9g
>Rhizoma Alismatis (Ze Xie) 9g
>Cortex Cinnamomi Cassiae (Rou Gui) 3g
>Ramulus Cinnamomi Cassiae (Gui Zhi) 6g
>Radix Aconiti Praeparata (Fu Zhi) 3g
>Radix Astragali Membranaceus (Hunag Qi) 12g
>Radix Glycyrrhizae (Gan Cao) 9g
>Fructus Tritici (Xiao Mai) 20g
>Cortex Albizziae (He Huan Pi) 15g
>Bulbus Lilii (Bai He) 9g

For external Wind attack or retained Wind pathogenic factor, use:[80]

>Flos Chrysanthemi (Ju Hua) 6g
>Flos Puerariae (Ge Hua) 6g
>Folium Perillae (Zi Su Ye) 3g
>Caulis Perillae (Su Gen) 4g
>Poria (Fu Ling) 12g
>Fructus Hordei Vulgaris Geminatus (Mai Ya) 15g
>Herba Artemisiae Capillaris (Yin Chen Ho) 3g
>Ramulus Uncariae Cum Uncis (Gou Teng) 6g
>Radix Glycyrrhizae (Gan Cao) 1g

Modifications:

1. For Heat, add Radix Cynanchi Atrati (Bai Wei) 2g, Fructus Forsythiae Suspensae (Lian Qiao) 9g.

2. For symptoms of infection, add Herba Traxaci Cum Radice (Pu Gong Ying), 12g, Herba Houttuyniae Cordatae (Yu Xing Cao) 12g, Herba Andrographis Paniculatae (Chuan Xin Lian) 6g.

3. For high fever, add Gypsum (Shi Gao) 20g, Rhizoma Phragmitis Communis (Lu Gen) 12g.

4. For Wind-Cold, add Radix Ledebouriellae (Fang Feng) 9g.

5. For Damp-Heat-Phlegm, add Radix Astragali (Huang Qi) 3g, Rhizoma Dioscoreae Hypoglaucae (Bi Xie) 12g, Herba Artemisiae Capillaris (Yin Chen Hao) 12g, Bulbus Fritillariae Cirrhosae (Chuan Bei Mu) 9g, Radix Scutellariae Baicalensis (Huang Qin) 6g.

6. For Damp-Cold, add Rhizoma Dioscoreae Hypoglaucae (Bi Xie) 12g, Rhizoma Atractylodis (Cang Zhu) 3g, Rhizoma Zingiberis Officinalis Recens (Sheng Jiang) 6g, Angelica Pubescentis (Due Huo) 9g.

7. For sinus symptoms, add Fructus Xanthii (Cang Er Zi) 15g, Periostracum Cicadae (Chan Tui) 9g. If also forehead headache, add Radix Angelicae (Bai Zhi) 6g.

8. For severe pain, add Angelica Pubescentis (Due Huo), Rhizoma Corydalis (Yan Hu Suo) 12g, Radix Clematidis Chinensis (Wei Ling Xian) 9g, Radix Angelicae (Bai Zhi) 3g.

9. For digestive symptoms, add Fructus Hordei Vulgaris Geminatus (Mai Ya) 15g, Pericarpium Arecae Catechu (Da Fu Pi) 6g, Herba Eupatorii Fortunei (Pei Lan) 6g. If with symptoms of Stomach Heat, add: Bambusae In Taeniis (Zhu Ru) 9g, Rhizoma Phragmitis Communis (Lu Gen) 12g.

10. For Shao Yang symptoms, add Radix Bupleuri (Chi Hu) 4g, Radix Scutellariae Baicalensis (Huang Qin) 6g, Radix Ginseng (Ren Shen) 3g.

11. For hoarseness, scratchy, or sore throat, add Radix Platycodi Grandiflori (Jie Geng) 9g, Radix Glycyrrhizae (Gan Cao) 3g, Semen Sterculiae Scaphingerae (Pang Da Hai) 12g.

12. For severe sore throat, add Fructus Lasiosphaerae (Ma Bo) 1.5g, Radix Isatidis Seu Baphicacanithi (Ban Lan Gen) 9g.

13. For ear pain, add Radix Scutellariae Baicalensis (Huang Qi) 9g, Radix Bupleuri (Chi Hu) 3g, Radix Gentianae Scabrae (Long Dan Cao) 6g.

14. For strong Interior Heat and irritability, add Fructus Gardeniae Jasminoidis (Zhi Zi) 6g.

15. For constipation, add Rhizoma Rhei (Da Huang) 4g.

16. For insomnia with agitation due to Wind-Heat, add Semen Sojae Praeparata (Dan Dou Chi) 9g, Fructus Gardeniae (San Zhi Zi) 5g.

For a patient that has Shao-Yang symptoms and signs and is depressed, stressed, fatigued, with mostly upper body pain or changing and conflicting signs and is not particularly sensitive, a modification of Miner Bupleuri Decoction (Xiao Chi Hu Tang) can be used:[81]

>Radix Bupleuri (Chi Hu) 10g
>Radix Scutellariae (Huang Qin) 10g
>Rhizoma Pinelliae (Ban Xie) 15g
>Rhizoma Zingiberis Officinalis (Sheng Jiang) 6g
>Radix Glycyrrhizae (Gan Cao) 4g
>Fructus Ziziphi Jujubae (Da Zao) 9g
>Rhizoma Ligustici Wallichii (Chuan Xiang) 6g
>Piperis Kadsurae Caulis (Hai Feng Teng) 12g
>Radix Pseudostellariae (Tai Zi Shen) 12g
>Radix Astragali (Huang Qi) 15g

---

80. This is a rather mild formula that can be used in weak and sensitive patients.

81. This and other "harmonizing" formulas are often helpful in patients who suffer from cyclical disorders including pain. Often there is a conflict between their Righteous-Qi and Pathogenic Factors, with *both* mostly being mild or weak. There are often signs of both Deficiency and Excess; the dominance of each may change frequently. While such formulas may not be appropriate during *active* stages of the disease, they can be used to prevent attacks. Harmonizing formulas tend to both strengthen the patient and address Pathogenic Factors.

Rhizoma Atractylodis Alba (Bai Zhu) 6g
Radix Ledebouriellae (Fang Feng) 9g

For a patient that, due to weakness, manifests diverse and confusing symptoms and is generally sensitive, addressing Central-Qi first may be helpful. Minor Construct the Middle Decoction (Xiao Jian Zhong Tang), a modification of Cinnamon Twig Decoction (Gui Zhi Tang), can be used, as it can gently nourish Central and Righteous-Qi (Yin and Yang). It harmonizes the Defensive and Nutritive-Qi and can outthrust pathogens.

Maltose (Yi Tang) 18g
Ramulus Cinnamomi Cassiae (Gui Zhi) 9g
Radix Paeoniae (Bai Shao) 18g
Honey-fried Radix Glycyrrhizae Uralensis (Zhi Gan Cao) 6g
Rhizoma Zingiberis Officinalis Recens (Sheng Jiang) 9g
Fructus Zizyphi Jujubae (Da Zao) 12 pieces

As the patient's strength increases, other issues become clearer and are then addressed.

Nutritional and Other Natural Therapies

A recent study by Teitelbaum et al (2001) has shown that treatment of perpetuating factors is helpful in FMS and chronic fatigue syndrome (CFS). These factors include:

- Hormonal deficiencies of thyroid, adrenal, and ovarian/testicular hormones.
- Opportunistic infections, especially parasitic and fungal.
- Sleep disorders that were treated aggressively.
- Nutritional inadequacies and subclinical abnormalities (these are important and should be treated).

A good healthy diet is important in FMS and when treating other chronic musculoskeletal disorders. The patient should avoid simple carbohydrates and sugars as these can result in insulin resistance and pain sensitization. An assessment for food allergies should be made using an elimination diet or blood tests. Assessment for hormonal levels is helpful, as some patients benefit from DHEA, testosterone, and/or growth hormone supplementation.

Some patients suffer from toxicity and should be evaluated for pesticide, formaldehyde, solvents, and heavy metal toxicity, all of which can result in pain and cognitive symptoms. The ability of the liver to detoxify can be tested. Oral DMSA at dosages of 10mg/kg-30mg/kg per day can be used to chelate lead, mercury, arsenic, copper, silver, cadmium, tin, nickel, zinc, thallium, manganese and bismuth. Because chelation is achieved via the kidneys, kidney function must be assessed by a 24 hour urine challenge and clearance test before starting treatment. Treatment is done for 3-5 days followed by an off cycle of 9-14 days. The more sensitive the patient the longer the off cycle. Phase I and Phase II liver detoxification support (mainly with n-acetyl-l-cysteine, silymarin, alpha lipoic acid and SAMe), vitamin and mineral supplementation, and other supporting therapies for the bowls are used during the off cycle period.

In patients with gasrointestinal symptoms, the use of deglycyrrhizinated licorice, bismuth salts, Oregon grape extract, l-glutamine, and probiotics are often helpful. Antibiotics may be used if needed.

Many patients with FMS seem to be deficient in magnesium and calcium. Dr. Hans Neiper popularized the use of magnesium aspartate. Another researcher, Guy Abrahams, studied magnesium maleate in a controlled trial in patients with FMS. He found that the magnesium passes well into the cells and the mitochondria. The extrapolation of the effect to other aliphatic fractions, such as aspartate, glycinate, and citrate (which is the cheapest) is by implication and has not been confirmed. Myer's cocktail (intravenous) is used with an emphasis on magnesium and calcium, as tolerated, remembering that high concentrations of magnesium tend to give a flush and may precipitate hypotension. The success rate is about 50%, which is superior to that achieved in conventional medicine. Women who receive this preparation sometimes experience a pleasant vaginal warmth. The addition of oral lithium can offer a synergistic benefit (Dorman, personal communication). A malic acid-magnesium supplement can be helpful. Since oral absorption of magnesium is not optimal, a magnesium oil can be used topically.

A good multi-vitamin and mineral supplementation can be helpful. Methyl-sulfonyl-methane (MSM), capsaicin, devil's claw, glucosamine, curcumin and baswellia have been reported to be helpful. For restless legs and nocturnal leg cramps, oral potassium, calcium, and magnesium may be helpful. Because some patients feel better when pregnant, the use of the hormone relaxin has been promoted.

For depression, 5-HTP (a precursor for serotonin), SAMe, and St. John's wort (inhibits reuptake of both serotonin and norepinephrine) are used. For sleep and anxiety disorders: kava, chamomile, valeriane, GABA, l-theonine (all of which can help increase GABA; l-theonine can decrease neurotransmitter excretion as well as increase alpha wave production in the occipital and parietal regions) and Garum armoricum (Stabilium; which has been shown to have anti-anxiety effects similar to valium without side-effects) or pharmaceutical medications can be used.

N-acetylcysteine can be useful for Raynaud's phenomenon and systemic sclerosis. In sixteen women and six men who received a two-hour loading dose of 150 mg/kg of N-acetylcysteine intravenously, followed by fifteen mg/kg/hour for five days, there was a significant reduction in the frequency and severity of Raynaud's phenomenon attacks compared with pretreatment values. Active digital ulcers were significantly less in number at follow-up visits, totaling 25.18% of baseline count on day thirty-three from the beginning of infusion (Sambo, Amico, Giacomelli, et al 2001). L-arginine can affect NO activity and result vasodilation and is therefore also useful in the treatment of Raynaud's phenomenon. Together with ornithine, l-arginine can support growth hormone levels and muscle mass. Ornitine has been shown to support healthy nitrogen balance which is important in muscle protein support (Luigi et al 1999). The use of dl-phenylalanine can be used for neurotransmitter and endorphin support. L-phenylalanine is a precursor to tyrosine, which converts to norepinephrine, epinephrine, dopamine and tyramine, which are all excitatory in their effects. D-phenylalanine may regulate endorphins by decreasing enkephalin degradation and may relax the muscles and joints and increase the pain threshold. DL-phenylalanine (which contains both l-phenylalanine and d-phenylalanine) may also increase the analgesic effects of acupuncture. Because dl-phenylalanine and SAMe are excitatory, some patients cannot tolerate them and may suffer from increased anxiety and insomnia, especially if their inhibitory neurotransmitters levels are low.[82] These patients should be first treated with amino acids that support GABA, serotonin and other inhibitory neurotransmitters. Taurine, glycine, 5HTP, N–acetylcysteine, and l-theanine are used for three weeks at which point dl-phenylalanine (or l-tyrosine), l-glutamine and SAMe are added.[83]

The author has been able to treat many patients with FMS, successfully integrating the above suggested treatments even in patients with chronic and enduring history.

Nerve Disorders

To one degree or another, nerves are always affected in painful conditions. Much investigation has focused on the pathophysiologic events occurring in the peripheral nerves and in the spinal cord. Most recently, the advent of functional neuroimaging has demonstrated alterations in brain activity associated with neuropathic pain as well.

Neuritis and Neuropathy

Neuritis or inflammation of a single nerve (mononeuritis) or multiple nerves (polyneuritis) and/or polyneurapathy/neuropathy may result from five general causes:

1. Mechanical causes:
   - Compression (the most common attended to by the orthopedic practitioner);
     Pressure palsy, which in turn may be caused by discs, tumors, stenosis, casts, crutches or any prolonged pressure such as seen when alcoholics pass out leaning on an arm ("Saturday night palsy");
   - Contusions and trauma;
   - Violent or repetitive muscular activity or forcible overexertion of a joint;
   - Hemorrhage into a nerve;
   - Exposure to cold or radiation.

2. Toxic causes:
   - Heavy metals and other toxic substances such as: lead, strychnine,[84] arsenic, mercury; alcohol; carbon tetrachloride;
   - Medications such as: hexobarbitol, sulfonamides, taxol, cisplatine, vincristine, and over dosing of vitamin B6.

3. Infections (which may be localized and/or primary or secondary to): tetanus, tuberculosis, diptheria, malaria, or various viral infections, such as Bell's palsy;

4. Metabolic causes:
   - Nutritional deficiencies (vitamin B12 deficiency);
   - Diabetes;
   - Hypothyroidism;
   - Toxemias of pregnancy.

5. Vascular or Collagen Vascular causes:
   - Rheumatoid arthritis;
   - Systemic lupus erythematosus;
   - Sarcoidosis;
   - Peripheral vascular disease.

In upto one third of patients with painful polyneuropathy, the underlying cause is never found. While patients with polyneuropathy often describe their pain in terms such as burning, sharp, raw skin, electriclike, deep aching, freezing, walking on glass and itchy. Allodynia and hyperalgesia are less common in polyneuropaphy than other neuropathic pain syndromes.

Pressure on Nerves

Pressure on nerve roots causes pain that the patient feels in all or any part of the relevant dermatome, depending on the severity of the impairment. Pressure on a large nerve trunk is usually painless and results only in distal paresthesia ("pins and needles"). Paresthesia that results from pressure on a nerve root occurs while the pressure remains and stops when the pressure is removed. Paresthesia that results from pressure on a nerve *trunk,* in contrast, occurs when the pressure is removed, such as a leg "falling asleep." Paresthesias can also occur during pressure on small peripheral nerves, as is seen in carpal tunnel syndrome, for example. Prolonged pressure on nerves can result in nerve palsy and, depending on duration, may be irreversible.

---

82. "Neuroscience urine test" can be used to evaluate neurotransmitter levels.

83. These therapies can be used to treat patients with other chronic pain syndromes as well.

84. Strychnine poisoning can occur when prescribing Semen Strychnotis (Ma Qian Zi) in large doses, or for prolonged periods. Ma Qian Zi is an herb used in TCM for pain and can be used safely and at times very effectively. For example, according to *Assemblage of Experiences on Bone-setting*, treated Ma Qiang Zi made into a pill and covered with Cinnabar (Zhu Sha), also a toxic substance (mercury), taken at 0.3g-0.6g with a decoction of Eucommiae (Du Zhong) 3g is useful in treating acute lumbar sprain. It is often used in Die Da pills (pills for traumatic injuries) as found in *Complete Records of Holy Relief.*

Nerve Disorders

Paresthesia and Numbness

Pins and needles, tingling, and numbness are important symptoms because they almost always implicate the peripheral nervous system in functional or organic disorders. In primary disorders of peripheral nerves (intrinsic disorders), the pins and needles come and go without any relationship to movement (Cyriax *ibid*). Pins and needles are also seen in trauma, pregnancy, anemia, B12 deficiency, rheumatoid arthritis, tumors, and multiple sclerosis. Paresthesia or hyperalgesia that are due to nerve injury may be provoked by stroking the affected dermatome. This is in contrast to Dorman's nulliness, i.e., the numb-like sensation felt distally due to ligament dysfunction, which is alleviated by stroking and massage.

The lesion or nerve pressure almost always occurs proximally to the area of paresthesia, numbness, or pain. Thus, if movement of the foot, for example, provokes the pins and needles in the foot, the lesion *may not be* in the ankle or foot but proximally in the limb or even the spine (Ombregt et al *ibid*). When the sensation of pins and needles is present but no movement evokes or aggravates the symptoms, a systemic or central nervous system involvement must be considered.

PARESTHESIA AND NUMBNESS IN TCM: In general, numbness is associate more with Phlegm and paresthesias more with Deficiency patterns. The most common patterns are: Phlegm obstructing the channels, Dampness in the channels, Wind-Phlegm, Liver-Blood-deficiency, internal-Wind (less commonly external-Wind), and Qi and Blood stagnation.

- Phlegm retention can block the channels and vessels, resulting in lack of nourishment and the development of numbness. The patient may report a numb-like feeling but neurological testing (testing for true altered sensation) may be negative or positive. The numbness (or numb-like sensation) is accompanied by a feeling of heaviness, often chest oppression, phlegm in chest, throat, or sinus symptoms (but is not mandatory), and other signs or symptoms of Phlegm. Swellings may or may not be seen. Because Phlegm is often associated with Qi-stagnation, symptoms of numbness may come and go.

- Dampness in the channels can also block circulation and result in numbness or tingling. There is often swelling (in soft tissues or joints), a feeling of being bound-up, or a feeling of heaviness and fatigue, and other symptoms and signs of Dampness. Occurrence often depends on whether Dampness is due more to Cold or Heat.

- Wind-Phlegm is associated mostly with unilateral numbness and/or paralysis. Dizziness, headache, or other symptoms in the head (tinnitus, pain, paralysis, or "fogginess"), nausea, phlegm in mucus membranes, and other symptoms and signs associated with Wind and Phlegm (and Cold or Heat) may, or may not, be seen.

- Liver-Blood-deficiency is associated more with paresthesias (tingling) than numbness, although it can be a cause

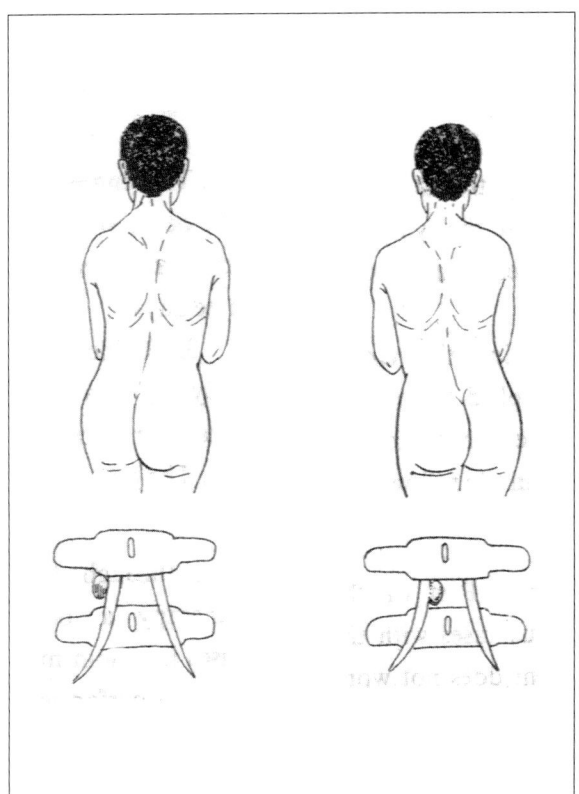

Figure 11-28: Depending on the location of the disc material, on the medial or lateral aspect of the nerve root, the patient's list may be to the right or left. A list may be also seen in patients with internal disc derangement, backward sacral torsion, or psoas syndrome with FRS dysfunction at T12.

of numbness as well. There is often tingling in the hands and feet, visual floaters ("flowery vision"), and pale or dull complexion. This pattern is more common in women than in men. Other symptoms and signs of Liver patterns and Blood patterns are seen depending on accompanying symptoms and signs. The symptoms are often worse after or during heavy exercise.

- Internal-Wind is associated frequently with unilateral numbness or paralysis. There is usually tremors or spasms and symptoms in the head region (severe dizziness, headaches, tinnitus, etc.). Other symptoms and signs depend on accompanying patterns and often involve Liver syndromes of Excess or Deficiency types.

Stagnation of Qi and Blood is associated more with tingling but can also cause numbness. The numbness/tingling is often improved by mild to moderate activity and aggravated by inactivity, fatigue, and is thus worse at night or early in the morning. Other symptoms depend on associated patterns and predominance of Qi or Blood stagnation. (With a predominance of Blood-stasis there is more pain, especially night pain).

Nerve Root Compression

A nerve root with impaired mobility, such as from external pressure due to disc herniation, may be painful, and the affected area may suffer limited range when stretched. For example, a straight leg raise (SLR) stretches the L4-S2 nerve roots via the sciatic nerve and can cause pain when these roots are entrapped. A list may be present (Figure 11-28).

Compression of nerve roots (called radicular pain) is said to be accompanied classically by:

- Pain in the region supplied by the nerve;
- Radicular loss of sensitivity, according to the dermatome;
- Motor loss in muscles innervated by the corresponding roots;
- Deep tendon reflex changes.

NOTE: Tenderness is often present in the muscles of the entire myotome supplied by both the anterior and posterior rami, as the nerve root is often affected before it branches (Gunn *ibid*).

Neuropathic Pain

Neuropathic pain, which is less common than nociceptive pain, can be caused by trauma or disease-evoked damage affecting the peripheral nerves, posterior roots, spinal cord, or certain regions of the brain. Neuropathic pain usually results from prolonged damage to peripheral nerve tissue. Tasker (1991) proposed that the term "deafferenation pain" be used for all conditions that are commonly called "neuropathic pain."

The effects of, and interaction with, sympathetic nerves can occur with repetitive strain and ligamentous laxity, and can result in neuropathic pain and inflammation. Viscerosomatic convergence may also be involved in reflex sympathetic dystrophy (now known as complex regional pain) as occurs for example, in the upper limb following an episode of cardiac pain (Bonica *ibid*). Sprouting of peripheral nerves after injury, although not always involving deafferenation, can result in convergence of low threshold mechanoreceptors and nociceptors, leading to abnormal nociceptive output from mechanoreceptors (Willis 1993, Willard *ibid*). Woolf et al (1992) have shown that sciatic nerve section or crush produces a long-lasting rearrangement in the organization of primary afferent central terminals, with A-fibers sprouting into lamina II, a region that normally receives only C-fiber input. The mechanism of this A-fiber sprouting has been thought to involve injury-induced C-fiber transganglionic degeneration combined with myelinated A-fibers being conditioned into a regenerative growth state. Mannion et al (1996) studied whether C-fiber degeneration and A-fiber conditioning are both necessary for the sprouting of A-fibers into lamina II. Local application of the C-fiber-specific neurotoxin capsaicin to the sciatic nerve has previously been shown to result in C-fiber damage and degenerative atrophy in lamina II. Mannion et al have shown that 2 weeks after topical capsaicin treatment to the sciatic nerve, the pattern of B-HRP staining in the dorsal horn is indistinguishable from that seen after axotomy, with lamina II displaying novel staining in the identical region containing capsaicin-treated C-fiber central terminals. These results suggest that after C-fiber injury, uninjured A-fiber central terminals can collaterally sprout into lamina II of the dorsal horn. This phenomenon may help to explain the pain associated with C-fiber neuropathy.

Neuroplasticity, changes that occur in the nervous system and may develop within seconds and become permanent, has been demonstrated for many different aspects of the nervous system. These include: gene expression, neurotransmitter and neuropeptide transmission, receptor type, receptor affinity, synaptic activity, and CNS neuronal receptive field (Galer and Dwokin *ibid*).

Patients with large-fiber neuropathy may complain of poor balance and nighttime falls because they are unable to sense the position of their feet when walking. Because small-fiber peripheral fibers relay sensation of thermal and sharp pain (painful heat and cold), patients with small-fiber neuropathy may burn themselves or step on a sharp object without sensing it.

Neuropathic pain is felt often as a continuous and burning-like pain, which is *independent* of *posture* or *movement*. The patient is extremely pressure- and touch-sensitive.

Neuropathic pain is commonly seen with (Wall *ibid*; Bonica *ibid*):

- Complex regional pain syndrome (CRPS-I);
- Causalgia (now called CRPS-II);
- Post-herpetic neuralgia;
- Stroke;
- Multiple sclerosis (MS);
- Spinal cord injury;
- Amputations.

Neuropathic pain from "mild" denervation is frequently associated with autonomic dysfunction such as (Gunn and Milbrandt 1978):

- Pilomotor reflex (seen as goose flesh when the skin is exposed to cool air) in the dermatome, with associated spondylosis;
- Vasomotor disturbances, (seen as vasoconstrictor action with pallor and cynotic skin);
- Sudomotor reflex (seen as increased tendency to perspire);
- Trophic disturbances (seen as trophic edema).

Gunn (1992) suggests that neuropathic pain is common and can be due to spondylosis and "prespondylosis," with denervation supersensitivity due to nerve deafferenation.

Complex Regional Pain Syndrome

In 1994, the IASP Task Force on Taxonomy renamed reflex sympathetic dystrophy (RSD) as "complex regional pain syndrome, type-I (CRPS-I)" and causalgia as "complex regional pain syndrome, type-II (CRPS-II)." These were renamed because the term RSD was inaccurate in several respects:

- A reflex responsible for the condition has never been identified.
- Most patients with this condition do not have sympathetically maintained pain (SMP).
- Dystrophic changes do not develop in most patients who have this condition.

The only difference between CRPS type-I and CRPS type-II is the etiology: Type-I is associated with a soft-tissue injury or immobilization; type-II follows a well-defined large peripheral nerve injury. Thus CRPS-I can be thought of as evolving from the old term RSD and CRPS-II from the term causalgia. CPRS-I usually starts with neuropathology of the A-δ and C-fibers caused by acute or repetitive trauma. Damage to efferent nerves causes visible physical changes that are well described in CPRS/RSD literature. In addition, one may see patients with similar or identical symptoms without detectable nerve damage, such as is seen in post-sprain reflex sympathetic dystrophy (Bennett 1994; Woessner *ibid*). CPRS/RSD is a poorly understood condition and the role in it of the autonomic nervous system is not clearly understood (Bonica *ibid*; Wall *ibid*). Nerve damage can occur via an infinite number of mechanisms and result in several outcomes, i.e., hyperesthesia and/or hyperalgesia, paresthesias and/or allodynia, or hypoesthesia; the ultimate hypoesthesia is the complete inability to experience any pain at all (Woessner *ibid*). Currently, neuropathic pain is subdivided into three categories summarized in Table 11-5.

THE ROLE OF SYMPATHETIC NERVOUS SYSTEM. Even though the observation is debatable, considerable evidence indicates that the sympathetic nervous system (SNS) is commonly, and/or partly involved in chronic pain and in so-called sympathetically maintained pain. When used diagnostically in conjunction with CRPS/RSD, sympathetically maintained pain should be implicated only if the patient responds to sympathetic blocks or other treatment such as phentolamine infusion. This involvement is apparently due to post-injury nociceptor activity that is modulated by catecholamines, particularly norepinephrine (Wall *ibid*). Inflammatory mediators such as bradykinin, interleukin-8, prostaglandins, and norepinephrine also have been shown to require the post-ganglionic sympathetic neuron for expression of hyperalgesia. Behavioral studies in rats point to a contribution of the sympathetic post-ganglionic terminals in the hyperalgesia of cutaneous inflammation and in the severity of arthritis (Levine and Taiwo 1994). Some researchers have postulated that norepinephrine and inflammatory mediators have an indirect effect through the release of prostaglandins (Wall *ibid*). Recent understanding, however, has de-emphasized the sympathetic nervous system and hence the name for reflex sympathetic dystrophy has been changed to complex regional pain syndrome (CRPS).

Table 11-5: Common Types of Neuropathic Pain
(Galer and Dworkin *ibid*)

TYPE	FOUND IN
PERIPHERAL	• Carpal tunnel syndrome • Complex regional pain syndrome • HIV sensory neuropathy • Meralgia paresthetica • Painful diabetic neuropathy • Phantom limb pain • Postherpetic neuralgia • Postthoracotomy pain • Trigeminal neuralgia • Radiculopathy
CENTRAL	• Central poststroke pain • HIV myelopathy • Multiple sclerosis pain • Parkinson's disease pain • Spinal cord injury pain • Syringomyelia
CANCER ASSOCIATED	• Chemotherapy-induced polyneuropathy • Neuropathy secondary to tumor infiltration of nerve compression • Phantom breast pain • Postmastectomy pain • Postradiation plexopathy and myelopathy

As early as 1947, Korr described the contributions the sympathetic nervous system makes to chronic pain (including contributions other than causalgia and reflex sympathetic dystrophy). However, Korr's opinion remains disputed. Schott (1994) suggests that the clinical phenomena that imply sympathetic nerve involvement in pain might be attributed more satisfactorily to effects of neuropeptides that afferent C-fibers have released. Neither neurophysiological studies of nociceptors in rats nor psychophysical studies in humans have provided conclusive confirmation of the role of sympathetic efferents in inflammatory pain and hyperalgesia (Raja 1995). However, as previously stated, sympathetic innervation has been observed in most soft tissues and bones, including the vertebral bodies, discs, dura mater, and spinal ligaments (Ahmed et al *ibid*). This finding supports the possibility of sympathetic contribution to pain. Recent information has also shown NMDA receptor cells in peripheral joints (Brown personal communication).

Chronic hyperactivity of the sympathetic pathway may result in clinical manifestations such as: hyperhydrosis (excessive perspiration), cold and wet skin, vasospasm, cyanosis, and edema. In the early stage of CRPS/RSD (or acute injury), the skin may be hot and dry but not edematous, despite the fact that sympathetic hyperacitvity results in constriction of blood vessels and stimulation of the sweat glands. This is probably due to over-powering by local chemical injury-related factors (inflammation). Later on, the sweat gland activity may decrease (possibly due to decreased nutrition); the chemical effects may have been neutralized and the cells and torn vessels healed. At this point the skin is often cool, pale, and either dry or wet. Depending on the severity of the disorder, further trophic shifts may be seen, such as changes in skin thickness and texture, loss of hair, shortening of tendons, atrophy of muscles, osteoporosis, and other degenerative changes in bone. Abnormalities can be shown on bone and thermo scans.

Long-term sympathetic hyperactivity may be deleterious to certain sensitive tissues. At the very least, the result is vaso-constriction (in some tissues), and therefore reduced blood supply and nutrition. Edema may also be caused by *microvasodilation* and passive congestion of blood and fluid (Mitchell *ibid*). Some studies in animal models of neuropathic pain and clinical observations have confirmed these observations and point to a role the sympathetic nervous system plays in certain chronic pain states (Raja *ibid*). It has been suggested that emotional disturbances, because they influence the autonomic nervous system, may cause vaso-constriction in muscles and the development of myofascial trigger points (Travell and Simons *ibid*, Janda *ibid*).

Another important consequence of sympathetic hyperactivity is a reduced threshold of several types of receptors and sense organs that are influenced by sympathetic impulses. Many such afferent fibers may then exaggerate their discharge, causing them to report a greater intensity of stimulation than actually occurred. This can cause the patient to be hypersensitive (Willard *ibid*).

REFLEX SYMPATHETIC DYSTROPHY (RSD). RSD has been used to describe a collection of polymorphic pathologic signs in conjunction with vasomotor and pseudomotor disturbances, triggered by trauma and a variety of stresses. As previously stated, RSD is now called *complex regional pain syndrome type-I* (CRPS-I). Although not clear, predisposing factors may be disturbances of the autonomic nervous system, metabolic disturbances (hypertriglyceidemia, diabetes), and psychological disturbances (depression, anxiety). Pain is of the inflammatory or mechanical type. Diagnosis may be difficult especially in atypical or monosymptomatic cases and if bony changes are not seen on x-ray. Bony changes may take months to develop. RSD/CERPS-I is fairly common, but many atypical cases escape detection. In about 50% of cases there is no obvious etiology. The other 50% of cases are associated with trauma, surgical procedures, immobility from a cast, or various nontraumatic causes such as from nervous system disorders, cardiovascular disorders, pleuropulmonary disorders, endocrine disorders, tumors, pregnancy, and from medications (Barral and Croibier *ibid*).

Several recent studies have failed to show abnormal sympathetic activity in CRPS patients. In addition, most CRPS patients do not respond to treatments that reduce sympathetic

Table 11-6: CRPS-I and CRPS-II

SYMPTOMS	SIGNS
Unilateral pain most often in one foot or one hand (although can be present in any body part covered by skin). The pain does not follow peripheral nerve or dermatomal distribution. Typically the entire hand or foot is involved. • Deep aching • Burning • Shooting • Skin sensitivity In area of pain (at least 2 of the following symptoms): • Sense of edema • Sense of temperature changes (hot and/or cold) • Sense of Increased or decreased sweating • Sense of weakness • Feeling limb is disconnected from body • Motor neglect	Signs do not follow peripheral nerve or dermatomal distribution. Abnormal painful perceptions in area of pain: • Allodynia • Hyperalgesia May have sensory deficits within the area of pain. In area of pain (at least 2 of the following signs): • Edema • Skin color changes • Temperature changes (hot and/or cold) • Increased or decreased sweating • Dystrophic changes • Weakness • Tremors • Dystonia • Lack of spontaneous movement of involved limb

tone in the involved region. The explanation currently favored by most authors is that the entire nervous system may be involved in the development and maintenance of CRPS, including the PNS, the CNS, and their sensory, motor, and autonomic system (Galer and Dworkin *ibid*).

Patients with suspected CRPS-I (RSD) should be asked several questions regarding symptom localized to the painful area:

• Edema or sense of swelling;
• Skin color changes;
• Temperature changes (abnormal cold or hot);
• Sudomotor activity (abnormal sweating or dryness);
• Motor abnormalities (weakness, tremor);
• Motor neglect (the need to focus all mental and visual attention to move a limb voluntarily);
• Cognitive neglect (the sense of the body part not being connected or part of the body).

Symptoms and signs associated with CRPS-I and CERPS-II are summarized in Table 11-6.

TREATMENT OF NEUROPATHIC PAIN

True neuropathic pain, including CRPS, can be difficult to treat especially once established (after one year or so). It is therefore very important to address acute pain as early as possible, and to make sure effective analgesia has been provided. Studies have shown that early analgesia, or preemptive analgesia, can reduce the incidence of chronic pain and neuropathic pain syndromes. While "alternative/natural" approaches may be tried, effective analgesia must be achieved because within hours the CNS may be permanently affected. The use of opioid based medication may be used. Local anaesthetic injection have been shown to prevent sensitization and phantom limb syndrome in patients undergoing lower-extremity amputation under epidural anesthesia as compared to only general anesthesia. A single dose of 40-60 mg/kg of rectal acetaminophen has a clear morphine-sparing effects in day-case surgery in children, if administered at the induction of anesthesia. NSAIDs by blocking prostaglandins may also prevent sensitization and therefore should be considered (Gudin ibid). For other suggested therapies see "THE MANAGEMENT OF SPRAINS, STRAINS AND TRAUMA" on page 537.

Most CRPS patients require a multidisciplinary model of care, in which a strong rehabilitative component is emphasized. According to Klein (2004) many patients suffering from allodynia have high levels of C-reactive protein that should be treated. A highly-sensitive serum C-reactive protein test is suggested. All underlying conditions, biomechanical and "energetic," must be addressed. Proper nutrition may play a role, as proteins, carbohydrates, fats, vitamins, and minerals are all building blocks for tissues and cells. Nutritional precursors are needed to allow the body to metabolize appropriate bi-products for cure and normalization of function and structure. High dose nutritional supplementation may also have pharmacological effects beyond proper nutrition. Intravenous Magnesium has been reported to be effective.[85] Omega fish oils (6 to 3 ratio of 4 to 1),[86] glucosamine and Gingko are important as well. Glucosamine may play a role, because collagen has been shown to form the sheaths around nerves. DL-phenylalanine has been shown to facilitate the production of endorphins and enhance acupuncture. B6 and B12 are commonly used to treat neuropathic pain both orally and by injection. Homeopathic Traumeel[R] can be helpful when used topically, orally, and by injection (Dorman personal communication). Low dose tetracycline (25mg BID), vitamin C and E, DHEA, DHA, ACE inhibitors, Nattokinase (support fibrinolytic activity) and statin medications can be used to reduce C-reactive protein levels and general inflammation.

Pharmacological (oral) and injection therapy may provide benefit, especially in the *acute* stage, and it is essential to let the affected region *rest* as well (Bonica ibid, Wall ibid, Brown ibid). Ketamin injected into peripheral joints is now being experimented with to address possible peripheral windup (Brown personal communication). Pharmaceutical drugs such as membrane stabilizers (anticonvulsants), antidepressants and antiarrhythimics can be helpful and are frequently needed. If needed opioids may be used. Topical 5% lidocaine patches have been shown to help in chronic cases (use upto 4 patches per 18-24 hours).

Medium frequency stimulation via alternating current of 20,000 Hz may be helpful by regulating cyclic AMP, and by masking pain via electric neuron blockade (Woessner ibid). Alternating between low, medium, and high frequencies using electromagnetic stimulators may be helpful. When used in conjunction with acupuncture, the needles may be magnetized and may increase clinical effects.[87]

Other treatments including: transcranial (Alphastim[R,] or LISS[R]) and body electrostimulation; auricular therapy; acupuncture; yoga and other body movement therapies; imagery; and a whole range of psychological techniques may be particularly helpful in "central" pain (Woesner ibid). Acupuncture may be of value in diabetic neuropathy (Abuaisha et al 1998). Acupuncture has long been used to relieve pain and is known to do so, in part, by controlling the activities of the autonomic nervous system. Ko et al (2002) studied the cDNA microarray analysis of the differential gene expression in neuropathic pain in an animal model. and after electroacupuncture. Dot-blotting results showed that the opioid receptor sigma was among effected genes. Interestingly, electroacupuncture restored these to normal expression level. They concluded that this indicates that opioid-signaling events are involved in neuropathic pain and the analgesic effects of electroacupuncture.

When treating neuropathic pain, all manual therapies should be performed as gently as possible and at a distance from the inflammatory nerves. Osteopathic approaches may include (Kuchera and Kuchera ibid):

- Treating all somatic dysfunctions using techniques that restore normal motions to joints or reduce stress on somatic tissues. This decreases somatic afferent input to the cord. Treatment of somatic dysfunctions is especially important in the thoracolumbar region (the sympathetic outflow region).

- Treating Chapman's points by finding positive anterior points and then treating the posterior points with circular soft tissue manipulation between the transverse processes, in areas that correspond to the anterior Chapman reflex points for the organ being treated.

- Inhibiting collateral ganglion by carefully applied midline abdominal pressure until a fascial release is palpable. The pressure is applied over the collateral sympathetic ganglion that is related to the organ with hypersympathetic activity. These ganglia are located between the xiphoid process and the umbilicus and lie just anterior to the aorta (see page 335).

---

85. Intravenous and topical Magnesium are often helpful in many painful conditions, especially FMS and MPS.

86. High dose GLA (500mg of GLA) from evening primrose oil (not borage or black currant unless especially processed) has been reported to be effective in the treatment of diabetic neuropathy, both improving pain and nerve function. Initially, however, pain may increase for some time as nerve function begins to improve. Borage and black currant oils are said to contain substances that for some reason block the positive effects of GLA.

87. This however often results in bleeding at the needle sites.

- Manipulating the ventral abdomen to relieve congestion around the nerves, plexi, and receptors in the affected tissues or organs. This reduces visceral afferent input to the spinal cord.

Herbal therapy, both topical and oral, is of value and should be focused on reducing vascular stasis and increasing circulation. Radix Shefflera (Qi Ye Lian) is said to be especially effective for neuropathic pain; (however, it is only of limited value in the author's experience). Radix Coculi (Mu Fang Ji) is also said to be used for all forms of neuralgia. Radix Polygonii Multiflori (He Shou Wu) is said to be capable of regenerating healthy nerves. Caulis Milletiae Seu Spatholobi (Ji Xue Teng) and other Blood moving herbs are used commonly as well.

The Treatment of Modern Western Diseases with Chinese Medicine (2001) lists five main patterns for peripheral neuropathy:

1. Damp-Heat invasion and excessiveness pattern for which they suggest Four Wanders Powder with Added Flavors (Si Miao San Jia Wei) and acupuncture at Sp-10, 9, 6, St-36 and regional points.

2. Lung-Stomach Fluid damage pattern is treated with Clear Dryness and Rescue the Lung Decoction (Qing Zao Jiu Fei Tang) and with Boost the Stomach Decoction (Yi Wei Tang). Acupuncture to St-44, St-36, TB-6, K-6, GV-14 and regional points.

3. Spleen-Stomach deficiency/vacuity weakness pattern is treated with Ginseng, Poria, and Atractylodes Powder with Additions and Subtractions (Shen Ling Bai Zhu San Jia Jian). Acupuncture at Sp-6, 10, St-36, UB-20, 21 and regional points.

4. Liver-Kidney insufficiency pattern is treated with Hidden Tiger Pills with Additions and Subtractions (Hu Qian Wan Jia Jian). Acupuncture at Sp-6, 10, K-3, 7, St-36 and regional points.

5. Spleen-Kidney insufficiency with Cold-Dampness pouring down pattern is treated with Ephedra, Aconite, and Asarum Decoction (Ma Huang Ju Zi Xin Tang) with Ginseng and Atractylodes Decoction (Shen Zhu Tang). Acupuncture at Sp-6, K-3, UB-20, 21, 23, GV-4 and regional points.[88]

In addition Flaws and Sionneau suggest that Liver-depression (congestion), Qi-stagnation, Spleen-deficiency, Qi/Yin-deficiency, Damp-Heat, and Qi and Blood stasis are common with the above patterns. For Blood-stasis in the network-vessels, they suggest adding worm and insect ingredients. Additionally, deep acupuncture (1-1.5 cun) is suggested at Ba Feng (M-LE-8) or Ba Xie (M-UE-22).

Topical herbal hot soaks are suggested to treat Damp-Heat and Blood-stasis using: Herba Siegesbeckiae (Xi Xian Cao) 100g, Caulis Milletiae Seu Spatholobi (Ji Xue Teng), Caulis Loncerae Japonicae (Ren Dong Teng), Folium Artemisiae Argyii (Ai Ye) 60g each, Cortex Radicis Acanthopanacis Gracilistylis (Wu Jia Pi), Herba Impatientis Balsaminae (Tou Gu Cao) 30g each,[89] Flos Carthami Tinctorii (Hong Hua), Radix Sophorae Falvescentis (Ku Shen) and Resina Myrrhae (Mo Yao) 20g each.

Disc Disorders

Pain in the low back usually starts after age twenty-five, when early changes within the discs begin to develop. Similar changes in other structures of the vertebral column usually occur much later in life (Ramani 1985), although preceding muscular weakness and ligament laxity is probable. Patients with herniated discs in the lumbar spine manifest a premature degeneration in the interspinous ligament (Yahia, Garzon, Strykowski and Rivard 1990). Studies in mice genetically predisposed to disc degeneration also suggest that the extracellular matrix components are often normal, and that degeneration is due to abnormal extrinsic factors such as paraspinal muscle weakness (Hopwood and Robinson 1973). Disc injuries may affect either the annulus alone, or the annulus, nucleus, dura and/or nerve roots (Figure 11-29).

Disc pathology is probably the most common cause of nerve root impingement seen in the practitioner's office. In the past, many low back symptoms were attributed to nerve compression by the disc. This has led to a large number of disc surgeries and was called the "disc dynasty" by McNab (Brown *ibid*). Chemical pain from minor tears in the annulus fibrosus (due to torsional and compression injuries) may explain some of the elusive pain syndromes seen without

---

88. Although Flows, Sionneau, and some Chinese authors report that locally applied acupuncture is helpful for neuropathy, it is this author's experience that patients with severe symptoms often do better with other acupuncture approaches. For example, bleeding and cupping Tong-style points DT.05 (UB first line points from T2 downward every one inch and UB-43), cranial points, Hand Five Gold (33.08), Hand Thousand Gold (33.09), and Five Tigers (11.27, mainly #2, 3) often is tolerated better. GV-16 can be used for feet insensitivity. When local sensitivity is reduced, local points are added. Some diabetic patients have only mild neuropathic symptoms and can tolerate local needles quite well. Sp-9 is needled to connect to GB-34 (2-3 inch needle). Electrostimulation is then connected between points at the feet and Sp-9. Cranial stimulation using acupoints or the LISS stimulator is helpful. Laser therapy, (infrared or red diode) starting proximally at the spine and working down the extremity, including stimulation of femoral nerve at the groin area, Liv-3, K-1 and St-36 is reported to work well. Thermography guided photonic or laser stimulation is reported to work particularly well (Saputo personal communication). Hamaza et al (2000) reported on the successful use of percutaneous electrical nerve stimulation (PENS) for the treatment of diabetic neuropathy. PENS is essentially the same as electroacupuncture. Their protocol included the placement of 32 gage needles to a depth of 1-3 cm, into areas which are essentially St-36 connected to UB-60 (stimulating L4-5, S1-2 segments), Sp-6 connected to Sp-9 (stimulating L3-S2 segments and cutaneous branch of sciatic tibial nerve) and Liv3 connected to Liv-3 (deep perioneal nerve). They used a biphasic square wave at 15 and 30 Hz every 3 seconds, stimulation of upto 25mA to patient tolerance with a pulse width of 0.5 ms and in a continuos duty cycle.

89. AKA, Speranskiae seu Impatients.

Disc Disorders

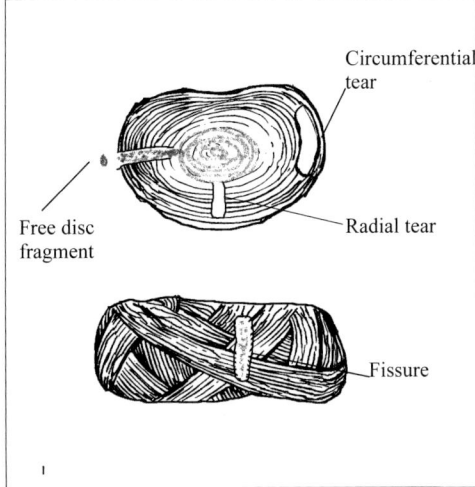

Figure 11-29: Disc tears.

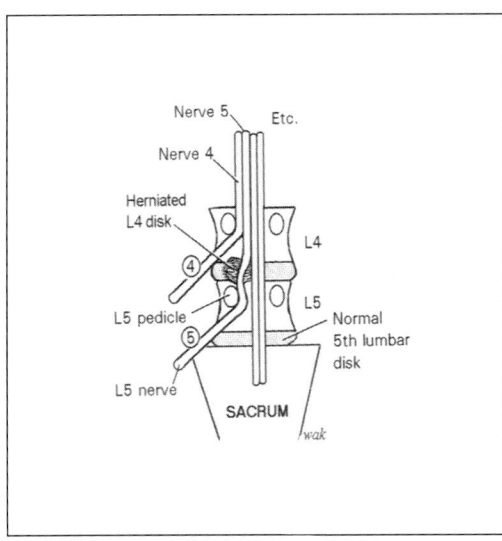

Figure 11-30: Herniated disc. Depending on the location in the lumbar spine towards which the disc herniates, it may impinge differently and result in different clinical patterns (From Kuchera WA and Kuchera ML, Osteopathic Principles in Practice, KCOM press 1994, with permission).

mechanical pressure on the dura or nerve roots (Bogduk 1990), and may yet bring about a new disc dynasty. Several new techniques, including provocation CT discography, are being explored to elucidate these theories.

Many physicians now think that the majority of chronic low back pain patients, refractory or only partially responsive to treatment protocols including prolotherapy, other injection therapies, and manual therapies are suffering from these types of disc lesions (Klein, Eek, Derby and Brown personal communication).

Disc Biochemistry

The role of biochemistry in patients with back pain due to disc disorders is receiving increasing attention and importance. This may result in improved treatments as more knowledge accumulates.

Glucosaminoglycans

Herniated discs show a fall of total GAGs (*glucosaminoglycans*) and an increase in lower molecular weight sugar fractions of glycoproteins of the nucleus and annulus. There is also a premature appearance of proteins and non-collagenous protein in the nucleus. Age-related disc degeneration results in a fall of total GAGs as well (Brown *ibid*).

Phospholipase A2 (PLA2)

Franson et al (1992) demonstrated an increase in PLA2 in prolapsed disc fragments. PLA2 is an enzyme that controls the liberation of arachidonic acid (important in the inflammatory cascade) from membranes. PLA2 in circulation is inflammatory itself, as it can cause inflammation when liberated. Expression of inflammatory mediators is achieved by PLA2 releasing fatty acids from lipid membranes. These can be converted to prostaglandins and leukotrienes, which are potent inflammatory mediators (Willburger and Wittenberg 1994). PLA2 can be secreted by disc tears (which may be visualized only by special dye studies) making the disc and the immediate environment irritable, causing discitis. Willburger and Wittenberg suggest that, since the prostaglandin release from a sequestrated disc is rather low, the inflammatory effect might actually be due to immunologic reactions, since nuclear material is a foreign substance in the circulatory system.

Intradiscal pH

The intradiscal pH in symptomatic patients with disc pathology is often more acidic than in patients with similar radiological disc findings who are nonetheless asymptomatic (Mooney 1989). This change in pH can cause pain and may explain why some people with similar pathologies (as seen by MRI) have pain while others do not. Smoking lowers the intradiscal pH (Hambly and Moony 1992). Localized acidosis may explain segmental and non-segmental pain.

The Degenerative Cascade and Discs

In the early *postural* stage, the patient is usually around thirty years old (may be younger) with discs that show decreased water content and:

- Decreased height;
- Decreased turgor;
- Ligamentous strain;
- Change in axis of rotation in anterior (discs) and posterior (facets) columns;
- Pain that usually does not refer below the upper buttock;
- Usually no dural signs.

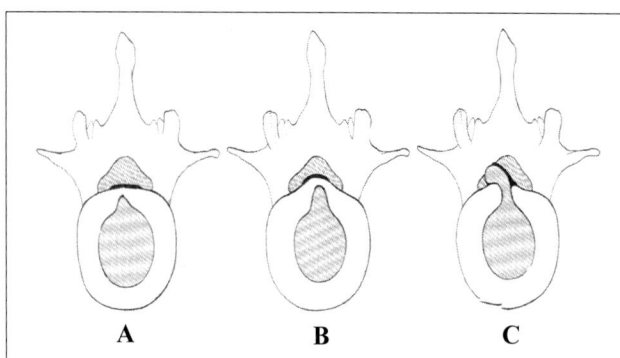

Figure 11-31: Disc pathologies. (A) shows internal disc derangement; (B) shows bulging disc without perforating the annulus; (C) shows herniation of disc material through the annulus into the spinal canal (disc prolapse).

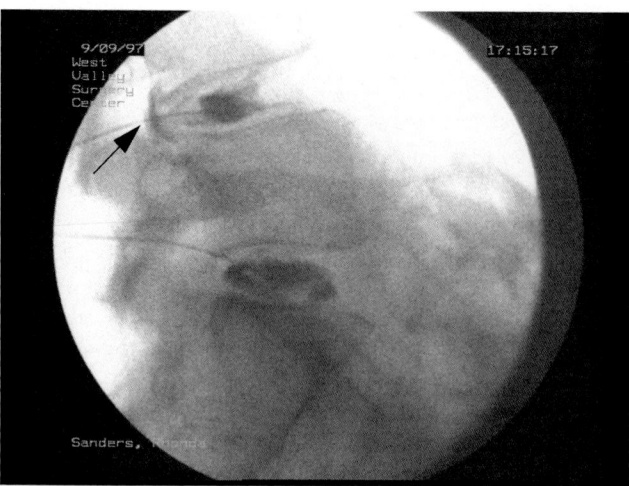

Figure 11-32: Two level discogram. Note the dye remains at the center of the disc at L5. At L4, note crescent shape dye print at the posterior annulus (arrow), indicating a fissure.

Later, in the *instability* stage, discs develop fibrotic degeneration. This is seen in patients around thirty to fifty years of age. Instability manifests with:

- Concentric tears;
- Radial tears;
- Traction spurs;
- Cysts;
- Posterior displacement; bulging, protrusion, prolapse;
- Hypermobility and joint subluxations of anterior and posterior columns;
- If symptoms are from the posterior column (facets) only, pain usually is unilateral without dural tension signs. If both the anterior and posterior column are involved, one may see midline pain and dural tension signs.

In the *stabilization* stage, the patient is usually fifty to sixty years old and there is often reduced symptoms and:

- Marked reduced disc height and disc dryness;
- Disc resorption;
- Fissures and cavities (which may cause continued pain);
- Circular and anterior protrusions;
- Gross osteophytosis (which may cause impingement and continued pain);
- Spondyloarthrosis developing in the anterior and posterior columns which may lead to stenotic pain.

Stages of Disc Injury

Disc injuries can be divided into four stages based on the condition of the annulus and nucleus (MacNab 1977):

1. The first stage refers to a *protrusion* of the disc without rupture of the annulus. This is also called "disc bulge" or "internal derangement." This is a partial radial annular tear; nuclear material has been extruded into it. The posterior longitudinal ligament (PLL) is intact.

2. The second stage is called *extrusion*. Here, the nuclear material reaches the epidural space. The PLL, however, is still intact.

3. The third stage, *disc prolapse/herniation,* involves ruptures in the annulus fibers, with expulsion of nuclear material that breaks through the PLL into the vertebral canal. There is still connection of nuclear material with the disc (Figure 11-31).

4. The last stage, *sequestration,* involves the separation of a disc fragment from the disc proper, which, at this point is free in the spinal canal.

Disc bulges, ruptures, and extrusions are seen in 28-50% of *asymptomatic* populations, and correlate poorly with clinical findings (Jensel et al 1994; Rothman et al 1984). This is probably due to differences in biochemical reactions and inflammatory responses among patients.

Disc Derangement

The first and second stages of disc disease (disc protrusion and disc bulge) are also called "internal disc derangement" or "disruption" (IDD). Disc derangements can be further divided into four stages by CT discography (Figure 11-32) (Aprill and Bogduk 1992).

- *Grade 0.* In grade 0 the contrast medium is strictly confined to the nucleus with a normal perimeter.
- *Grade 1.* A disrupted nucleus extends into the inner third of the annulus.
- *Grade 2.* The nucleus enters the middle third of the annulus. Grade 2 may or may not be painful, because the

affected middle third of the annulus has irregular nerve supply.

- *Grade 3.* The nuclear material has full access to the nerve endings in the outer third of the annulus and therefore produces pain.
- *Grade 4.* There is further annular disruption with vertical annular rupture — sometimes called fissures. Grade 4 annular disruptions show as high-intensity zones (HIZ) in the annulus with T2-weighted magnetic resonance images. These high intensity zones have been shown to have a high correlation (86%) with symptoms reproduced by provocation discography.

DIAGNOSIS OF DISC DERANGEMENT. While low tech techniques such as the use of vibration may be a simple and possibly useful tool in the diagnosis of internal disc derangements, more often a discogram is needed. Yrjama and Vanharanta (1994) report good correlation between sensitivity to vibration applied to the lumbar spinous processes by a standard electric toothbrush shaft (Braun) (with a blunt head instead of the brush) and provocation discography.

The intervertebral disc can be injected with contrast, local anesthetic, or other substances. Although observing the effect of a local anesthetic injection on pain and function (analgesic discography) can potentially provide useful information, the clinical utility of this has not been well defined. The effect of an applied mechanical and/or chemical stimulus on pain (provocative discography) does have demonstrated clinical utility. In addition to provoking pain that can be compared to the patient's clinical symptoms, injecting contrast into the disc may demonstrate pathology that is not otherwise revealed on conventional imaging studies (Figure 11-32). The purpose of discography is to determine whether the intervertebral disc is a source of clinical symptoms. While interpretation of the radiologic images obtained at the time of discography is important, in contemporary practice, discography is primarily a provocative clinical test, rather than a radiologic imaging procedure (Derby *ibid*).

Acute Disc Injury

Disc injuries generally occur when the patient performs an awkward or unguarded movement. Commonly, a sudden sensation that something "popped" in the back occurs. Sometimes a noise is heard.

Degenerative Disc Disease

Degenerative disc disease is almost universal with aging (Miller, Schamtz and Scjultz 1988) and is not necessarily symptomatic. Disc degeneration is demonstrated with equal incidence in subjects with or without pain (Nachemson 1992). Differentiating between patients that have stable or unstable segments is helpful. Nachemson, however, questions the reliability of segmental instability and isolated disc resorption as causative factors in low back pain.

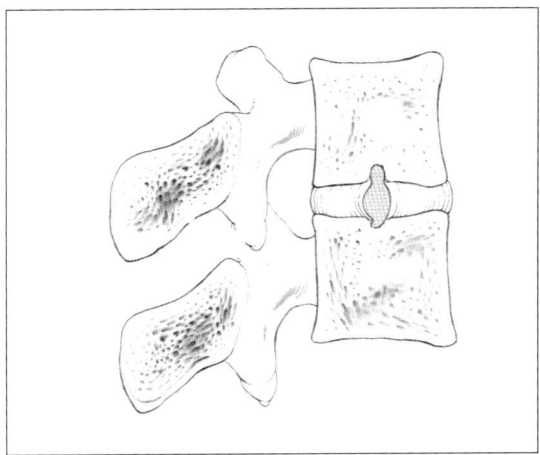

Figure 11-33: Disc herniation into the vertebral body, called a Schmorl's node. It is often not painful and may actually increase stability at the motion segment.

Smoking has been shown to increase the rate of disc degeneration (Battié et al *ibid*; Helms and Nachemson *ibid*). Individuals with at least one Trp3 allele in the COL9A3 (collagen IX) gene, are about three times more likely to develop lumbar disc disease (Leena Ala-Kokko et al 2001).

The risk factors for lumbar disc degeneration was studied in a five-year follow-up study of forty-one asymptomatic individuals who were evaluated by longitudinal magnetic resonance imaging (Elfering, Semmer et al 2002). Forty-one percent of the subjects showed a deterioration of disc status in that time period. In ten individuals, the progression of disc degeneration was one grade or more. There was only a *weak correlation between progressive disc degeneration and low back pain development* during this five-year follow-up period. Multiple logistic regression analysis showed that the extent of the disc herniation, the lack of sports activities, and night shift work were significant predictors for disc degeneration during follow-up, when control was used for the number of degenerated discs at baseline, gender, age, and body mass index.

Gunn (*ibid*) postulates that spondylosis/prespondylosis and degenerative disc disease are contributing factors to the unavoidable degenerative cascades that affect the nervous system. He claims spondylosis/prespondylosis may lead to mild segmental denervation and neuropathic pain. Others suggest that the internal chemistry of the disc, which is largely based on the relationship between mucopolysaccharides production and the water content in the disc, may at times lead to pain. The water content is reduced with aging and with degenerative disc disease and may be responsive to dysfunction and lack of normal motion. Dysfunction may lead to disruption of the disc chemistry and pH (Mooney *ibid*).

When discs degenerate, both function and regenerative qualities within the surrounding joint are affected: normal motion is necessary for joint, soft tissue, and disc nourishment. Disc degeneration has been shown to increase loads on

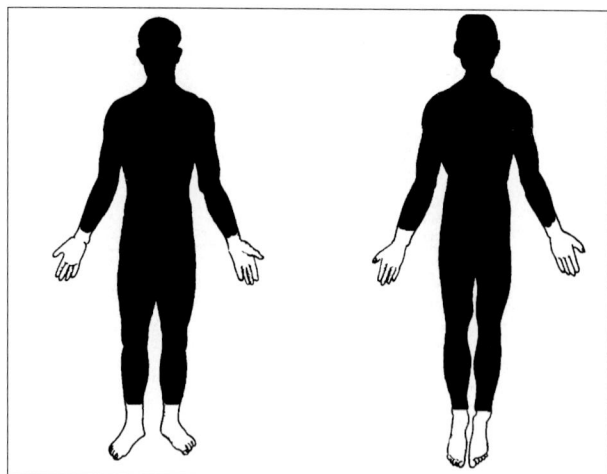

Figure 11-34: Cyriax's extrasegmental disc or dural pain distribution.

the facets, and is associated with muscle weakness (Brown *ibid*).

The Dural Concept

Cyriax's *dural concept* states that pain can arise due to *subluxation* of a disc fragment that impinges on dura, dural sleeves, or nerve roots. Newer information shows this pain to be mechanical or chemical. Dural pain is often extrasegmental and thus does not follow dermatomal distribution. Research has demonstrated that dural pain may spread over *eight segments* (dermatomes) with great overlap between adjacent and contralateral dura mater (Goen, Baljet and Drukker 1988). Usually there are both articular and dural signs. Articular signs of joint dysfunction are:

- Movement to one or more directions increases symptoms and signs.
- Movement in one or more directions is pain free or with minimal symptoms.

Dural signs are:

- Straight leg raise (SLR) positive with increased symptoms on ankle dorsiflexion (lumbar spine);
- Slump test often positive (lumbar or thoracic);
- Neck flexion test may be positive (thoracic);
- Painful coughing, sneezing, and/or defecation (lumbar);
- Strong twinges of pain and loss of power with movement and loading.

ANNULAR LUMBAGO. Annular lumbago is characterized by pain following a trivial activity, which results in a *sudden* "snap" in the back and often *immediate* pain. This occurs when a few annular fibers rupture with or without dural irritation. The pain may arise from the outer annular fibers which are innervated. Often the key for diagnosis is immediate pain. This pain usually follows bending, sitting for a long time, picking up an object, etc. The pain is usually central (midline) first. Later, pain may radiate to abdomen, groin and/or legs but not to the foot. Often the patient presents with a list, usually forward and sideways bent.[90] The pain is vague in distribution, (as opposed to radicular pain, which presents with a clear edge and distribution). The pain (Brown *ibid*):

- has characteristic twinges that may be severe and "breath-taking." When twinges are severe, they may be even felt when the patient is turning over in bed, which the patient may take some time to accomplish;
- is aggravated by sitting and forward-bending or forward-postures;
- often decreases or centralizes with extension;
- increases when getting up from sitting or bed;
- possibly increases with coughing and sneezing;
- often responds to manual therapy fairly quickly. Usually the patient is better within days or weeks.

According to Cyriax (*ibid*), extrasegmental pain reference:

- of cervical disc origin may be perceived all the way from the head to the mid-thorax;
- from mid and low-thoracic disc lesions, may radiate to the base of the neck;
- from the low lumbar disc levels may reach the lower thorax (posteriorly), the lower abdomen, the upper buttocks, the sacrum, and the coccyx. It does not extend to the upper limbs or hands. However, it often reaches down to the lower limbs and ankles, but not to the feet (Figure 11-34).

NUCLEAR LUMBAGO. The onset of a nuclear lumbago is *slower*, which is the key to diagnosis. The nucleus is a thick viscus substance that moves slowly. The annular fibers rupture and movement of the nucleus towards the dura or nerve roots may take some time. Usually, the patient reports slight immediate back pain following injury or movement that becomes severe in hours, the next morning, or within days. The patient reports *severe*, painful twinges (often "breath taking"), increased pain with coughing, and increased and *peripheralization* of pain with *extension*. Flexion is often painful, as well. Dural signs are common. Pain may or may not improve in days, weeks, or months. It is often segmental (dermatomal) in distribution (Brown *ibid*).

ANTERIOR DISC PROTRUSIONS. Traditionally, anterior disc protrusion is not thought to result in symptoms. However,

---

90. A similar presentation is seen with acute FRS dysfunction at T12, and a backward sacroiliac torsion. There is usually psoas muscle spasm. Here however, usually, there is no *severe painful twinges* with a sense of a loss of power. Clinically, severe twinges are most commonly seen with discogenic pain, and, if it takes the patient great effort to move, manual therapies should be performed with great care, as aggravation of symptoms is likely.

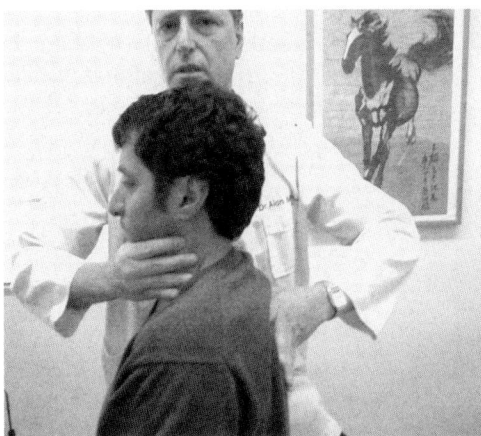 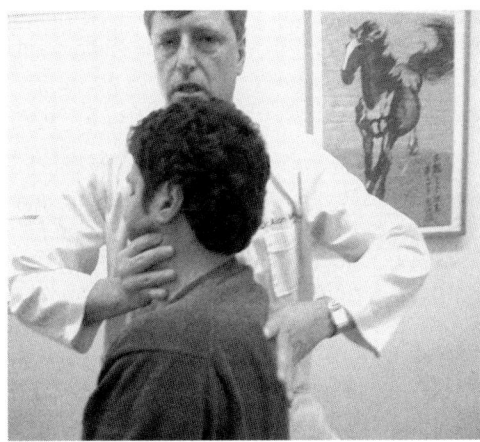

Figure 11-35: Patient treated for disc derangement with McKenzie forced retraction, and retraction rotation techniques.

the afferent fibers to the sympathetic ganglia are present in all anterior vertebral structures, including the anterior longitudinal ligament (ALL), the peripheral fibers of the annulus fibrosus, the vertebral body, and its periosteum. Also, a major autonomic branch extends posteriorly from the sympathetic ganglion or gray ramus communicate to join the recurrent meningeal nerve, that together form the paravertebral autonomic neural plexus. Therefore, symptoms arising from anterior protrusions are likely (Bachrach 1997).

SELF-REDUCING DISC LESION. This term is used in patients that only feel pain after sitting for some time. Often the patient wakes up in the morning pain free but feels pain later in the day following a period of sitting. The longer the patient sits the longer it take for him/her to recuperate upon lying down. It is thought to be caused by the gradual dehydration of the disc that follows prolonged sitting, as well as posterior migration of the whole intra-articular content of the disc as a result of prolonged kyphosis (Ombregt et al *ibid*). This condition may also represent ligamentous laxity and postural loading. With ligamentous pain the patient may also complain of posain (pain when not moving and morning ache). Treatment with stabilization exercises, frequent extension exercises, avoidance of prolonged sitting, periosteal acupuncture, or prolotherapy are often helpful.

Diagnosis and Treatment of Disc Disease

There are two types of lumbar spinal pain: radicular pain and axial pain (Bogduk 1997). Radicular pain results from mechanical compression and/or chemical irritation of a nerve root. Establishing an anatomic diagnosis for patients with radicular pain is important, as there are treatments, such as selective nerve root blocks and surgery, that are directed towards specific pathology and have excellent outcomes in *well selected* patients. The source of radicular pain, typically either a herniated nucleus pulposus or lateral spinal stenosis, can be definitively diagnosed at surgery; therefore, there is a gold standard that can be used to assess the validity of diagnostic studies. Consequently, the ability of both clinical findings and imaging studies to diagnose the site of pathology is well-defined. A precision diagnostic injection may be indicated when imaging studies suggest that more than one nerve root may be responsible for a patient's symptoms. In that circumstance, a selective epidural injection may be useful. In contrast to radicular pain, the relationship between spinal pathology and lumbar axial pain is uncertain. There are a number of anatomic structures which are potential sources of pain, including myofascial tissues, synovial joints, and the intervertebral discs. While discogenic pain is felt by many to be an indication for surgical fusion, outcome studies have demonstrated variable results (Derby 2004), and conservative therapies work for many patients.

Nerve compression from disc protrusions can lead to radiculopathy. However, to diagnose leg or buttock pain as being due to mechanical nerve root compression by a disc (apart from internal disc derangements), there must be:

- A true positive SLR with dural tension signs (L4-S2), positive knee flexion in L3 lesions;
- Weakness of the appropriate muscles (depending on degree of compression);
- Loss of sensation (depending on degree of compression);
- Sluggish reflexes (depending on degree of compression).

An MRI finding without these signs can be misleading, as both buttock and leg pains can originate from other myofascial and ligamentous structures. A discogram may be needed to diagnose internal disc disease.

Stenotic back and leg pain can be due to direct pressure from intrinsic or extrinsic factors. There is usually decreased spinal canal or foraminal space with pressure on nerve roots in (Brown *ibid*):

- within the spinal canal (cauada equina);

- lateral recess, formed by the superior articular process, lamina, posterior aspect of vertebra, or disc and posterior longitudinal ligament;
- foramina.

In the case of internal disc derangement and *chemical discitis*, one may or may not see the above signs and symptoms of compression. Symptoms and signs depend on the amount of swelling and chemical reaction.

Various treatments have been tried for chemical disc pain. It has been postulated that treatment with tetracycline may be effective, as it can inhibit the enzymes responsible for abnormal disc pH; however, this does not seem to be born out clinically (Klein 1995). Heating the discs with intradiscal electrothermal annuloplasty (IDET or IDEA) has been tried with some success. Longer periods of thermocoagulation directly at the annulus and nucleus is being evaluated and may be helpful in about 50% of patients; however, it can be quite painful (Derby 1997). Currently intradiscal nucleoplasty using a radiofrequency device that can break up the bonds in the nucleus with low temperature, followed by an intradiscal injection of glucose, glucosamine, and chondroitin sulfate are the preferred method. This technique seems to cause less of a flair-up while being more effective than IDET (Derby, Brown and Eek personal communication). The overall satisfaction of nucleoplasty is 89% (Sharp 2002, Chen 2002, Singh 2002).

When the nuclear material is truly extruded and there is nerve root compromise, the patient may need surgery, but in most cases conservative treatment can be as effective as surgery. Surgical intervention for low back pain has been estimated to be helpful in only 1% of patients (Waddell 1987). Conservative treatment is effective even in patients who have radiculopathy (Saal and Saal 1989). In a two years follow-up of properly-selected patients who had disc herniation, no difference in outcome was shown between patients who had been treated surgically and patients who had been treated conservatively (Weber 1983). In a study reported at the American Back Society meeting in 1997, patients with disc herniations were examined to see if MRI studies would predict treatment outcomes. It seems that psychosocial factors such as worker compensation can effect outcomes negatively both for conservative and surgical care. In conservative care patients the MRI studies did not have any predictive value regarding outcome. Short duration of symptoms, low standing chronic symptoms of back pain, and no litigation are favorably associated with conservative care outcomes. On the other hand, predictions of surgical care are greatly dependent on the size of the disc herniations. Most patients with *big* disc herniation (over 6mm at AP plane) did well with surgical interventions. The size of the disc was almost ten times more predictive of outcome than worker compensation or litigation. Outcomes in patients with smaller discs is a toss-up. Just as many patients did well as did poorly. Patients with positive dural tension signs did bet-

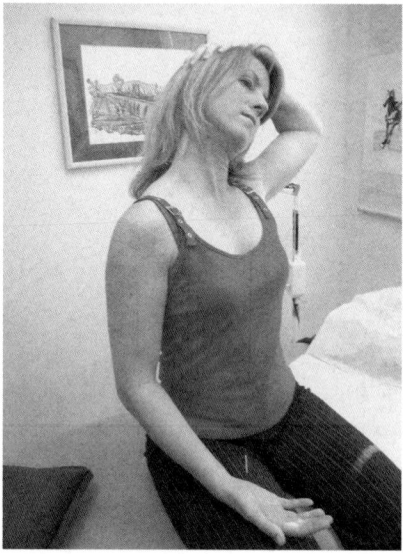

Figure 11-36: Patient treated using Tong-style acupuncture (Double Child and Double Immortal 22.01-22.02) with self sidebending-extension McKenzie exercises for discogenic periscapular pain.

ter with surgical interventions than patients that did not have dural tension signs.

Nuclear pain does not respond as well as annular lumbago to high velocity manipulations (Cyriax *ibid*). Acupuncture and other less forceful therapies such as muscle energy and functional techniques may be tried. However, often the patient cannot tolerate any movement in the acute stage. Traction can be helpful for some patients. The use of newer traction devices such as the distraction, reduction, stabilization (DRS) device that can selectively apply distraction traction forces has been reported to be very efficacious, and MRI studies have shown both reduction and rehydration of discs (Shealy and Leroy 1998).

Epidural injection, selective nerve root blocks, or oral steroid dose pack can be very helpful for both *acute* annular and nuclear disc pain. Injections combined with McKenzie exercises seem to shorten the course of recovery and give rapid relief of pain. Both should be used *early*, within hours to days of onset, as the outcome is much better than if used later (as is so commonly done).

Acupuncture using gentle techniques may be useful, but strong stimulation at local points should be avoided when the patient suffers from severe painful twinges and moves slowly.[91] To maximize acupuncture's usefulness, it should be performed daily. In this author's experience, local spinal points should be stimulated on the contralateral side of the pain, and extremity points may be stimulated ipsilaterally. High frequency (5,000-10,000 Hz) alternating with low frequency (2-4 Hz) stimulation can be added and connected from one side to the other (spinal points on the nonpainful side with extremity points on the other).[92] Short needle retention may be best in severe cases (in and out). At times bleeding and cupping techniques provide relief but should not be used if there is skin hyperalgesia. Acupuncture and herbs are used also to address underlying constitutional or systemic patterns. All spinal dysfunctions should be addressed, when possible. In more chronic cases local needling of intrinsic muscles is helpful and may (Gunn *ibid*) decrease pressure on nerves and discs from spasmed muscles.

In general "sciatica" (discogenic or not) has been divided in TCM into:

1. *Wind-Damp-Cold,* which is treated with variations of Licorice, Ginger, Poria, and Atractylodis Decoction (Gan Jiang Ling Zhu Tang) and acupuncture points such as LI-4, TW-5, GB-30, 31 St-36, Sp-6, ear-sciatica and regional points;

2. *Qi-stagnation Blood-stasis,* which is treated with variations of Drive Out Blood Stasis from a Painful Body Decoction (Shen Tong Zhu Yu Tang) or Smooth the Flow of Qi and Invigorate the Blood Decoction (Shun Qi Huo Xue Tang). Acupuncture to UB-40 (bleed), 17 (bleed), LI-10, Liv-3, LI-4, Sp-10 and regional points are used;

3. *Qi and Blood deficiency,* which is treated with variations of Eight-Treasure Decoction (Ba Zhen Tang) and acupuncture points such as S-36, Sp-6, LI-11, LI4, Liv-3, K-3, GB-39, 34, 30, and regional points are used;

4. *Liver-Qi-stagnation and Yin/Blood-deficiency,* which are treated with Rumbling Powder (Xiao Yao San) with Restoring the Right Decoction (You Gui Yin). Points such as Liv-3, LI-4, UB, 17, 18, 40 (bleed) and regional points are used;

5. *Kidney-Essence-deficiency with Blood-stasis,* which is treated with Supplement the Kidneys and Invigorate the Blood Decoction (Bu Shen Huo Xue Tang) or Restoring the Right Decoction (You Gui Yin) with Smooth the Flow of Qi and Invigorate the Blood Decoction (Shun Qi Huo Xua Tang). Points such as K-3, 7, Lu-8, GB-39, 30, SP-10, UB-17, 23 and regional points are used;

6. *Accumulation of Phlegm and stasis of Blood,* which is treated with Two-Cured Decoction (Er Chen Tang) with Smooth the Flow of Qi and Invigorate the Blood Decoction (Shun Qi Huo Xue Tang). Points such as St-40, 36, TW-6, LI-4, Sp-3, 6, 9, UB-17, GB-30 and regional points are used. For more information, see Table 5-31 on page 330.

Empirical *guiding* formulas for discogenic pain are:

Fructus Arctii Lappae (Niu Bang Zi) 30g
Radix Angelicae Pubescentis (Du Huo) 12g
Rhizoma Cibotii Barmometz (Gou Ji) 9g
Semen Persicae (Tao Ren) 9g
Rhizoma Drynari (Gu Sui Bu) 9g
Bombyx Batryticatus (Bai Jiang Can) 12g
Rhizoma et Radix Notopterygii (Qiang Huo) 12g
Cortex Eucommiae Ulmoidis (Du Zhong) 15g
Radix Dipsaci Asperi (Xu Duan) 9g
Flos Carthami (Hong Hua) 9g
Lumbricus (Di Long) 12g
Radix Rehmanniae Glutinosae (Shu Di) 12g
Radix Angelica Sinensis (Dang Gui) 9g

For severe pain, add: Radix Aconiti (Fu Zi) 15-60g;

For severe leg pain (sciatica) add: Radix Paeoniae (Bai Shao) 30g;

For Phlegm and Stasis use:

Fructus Arctii Lappae (Niu Bang Zi) 30g
Semen Sinapis Albae (Bai Jie Zi) 9g
Lumbricus (Di Long) 9g
Lycopi (Ze Lan) 9g
Radix Achyranthis Bidentatae (Niu Xi) 12g
Radix Clematidis (Wei Ling Xian) 9-15g
Rhizoma Artsiaematis (Dan Nan Xing) 9g
Radix Glycyrrhizae (Gan Cao) 9g
Radix Salvia (Dan Shen) 9g
Radix Angelica Sinensis (Dang Gui) 9g

For severe pain add: Radix Aconiti (Fu Zi) 15-30g;

For Blood-stasis from Cold use:

Lumbricus (Di Long) 9g
Honey-fried Herba Ephedrae (Zhi Ma Huang) 3-6g
Cortex Cinnamomi Cassiae (Rou Gui) 3g
Herba cum Radix Asari (Xi Xin) 3g
Radix Angelicae Sinesis (Dang Gui) 9g
Flos Carthami (Hong Hua) 6g
Cortex Phellodendri (Huang Bai) 6g
Radix Morindae (Ba Ji Tian) 12g
Lignum Sappan (Su Mu) 9g
Radix Glycyrrhizae (Gan Cao) 3g
Gelatinum Cornu Cervu (Lu Jiao) 6g
Semen Persicae (Tao Ren) 6g

For both Cold and Heat, add Rhizoma Anemarrheanae (Zhi Mu) 20g;

For Kidney-Yin-deficiency back pain add Polygoni (Shou Wu) 15g.

For severe pain and inflammation (mostly in acute stage) add Tripterygium Wilfordii (Lei Gong Teng) 15g, Radix Aconiti (Fu Zi) 15g.

PATIENT EDUCATION AND PROPHYLACTICS. Disc derangements and extrusions are often preceded by one or more low back pain attacks, probably representing some degree of ligamentous laxity, segmental instability, or other somatic dysfunctions and restrictions. Therefore, patients with simple back pain should be educated about the possibility of developing acute disc disorders and what to do when they occur.

---

91. Even though studies show that vertebral disc lesions or entrapment syndromes are responsive to acupuncture (Thomas and Lundeberg 1994, for example), in this author's experience, results of treatment using TCM or modern acupuncture techniques are often disappointing in patients with *severe nuclear* disc pain. They are often disappointing in patients with chronic pain due to internal disc *fissures* as well. Progress is slow and may not clearly shorten the course of recovery. Pain reduction is often minimal, although some patients do quite well with integrated therapies (manual, herbs, and acupuncture). Frequent treatments are necessary. Patients with disc fissures often do not "heal," and only palliative effects can be expected. However, a course of treatment is appropriate as some patients do quite well. Intra-disc procedures can be considered, but, again, they cannot guaranty long-term relief (only in about 50% of patients), though in some patients, relief can be quite dramatic.

92. High frequency stimulation results in a nerve block of short duration (mostly during therapy) but may also prevent sensitization. Some authors have stated that crossing the spine with electroacupuncture is "dangerous," however, this author has never seen problems with this technique.

They should be taught the principles of the McKenzie exercise system (page 526; Figure 11-35). Early application may reduce the extent of herniation. Because in TCM the "root" of back pain and spinal strength is said to be dependent on Kidney function and a free flow of Qi and Blood. Patients may benefit from prophylactic treatments that strengthen the Kidneys (and spine) and insure a free flow of Qi and Blood. Manual therapies that result in improved spinal function and exercises to strengthen and stabilize the spine are important, as well.

Facet Disorders

The role of facets in pain is controversial. Mooney and Roberston (1976) have shown that an injection of the facets with hypertonic saline under specific radiographic control can lead to pain. The facet capsule can be sprained, in which case it will probably elicit pain. Trauma from excessive stress to the joint and ligaments may cause the ligaments to pull tightly on the joint, leading to joint locking (Mennell 1952). With small ligamentous tearing, even greater restrictions may be seen (Turek 1984).

Facet Meniscus

The facet joint contains a meniscus, or can develop one by damage to cartilage that remains attached to the external capsule. The process of meniscus formation is called "intra-articular inclusion." A meniscus, in the knee, for example, can get trapped and cause pain and facet meniscal entrapment may provoke similar mechanisms (Bogduk *ibid*).

PLA2 and Prostaglandins

PLA2 and prostaglandins, both of which are pro-inflammatory, can be released by the facet joint (Willburger and Wittenberg 1994). Prostaglandins can sensitize nociceptors, making the joint more sensitive to pain from normal motions.

Facet Degenerative Disease

The facets may develop marked osteoarthrosis, with possible ligamentous or capsule insufficiency. This may lead to pain and referred nulliness. Eventually, this leads to decreased efficiency of intervertebral joint and disc functions, increasing the possibility disc injury. Roaf (1977) suggested that degeneration of the facet joint results in reduced stability of the intervertebral disc and a decrease in the forces that can cause tears in the disc fibers.

The degenerative processes within the facet joint, like other synovial joints, can yield a synovial cyst that can emerge and create an extradural compression. This may cause a mechanical or chemical irritation of the nerve endings. Degenerative changes may also lead to foraminal stenosis (Brown *ibid*).

The Facet Syndrome

Sprain of the facet (facet syndrome) can lead to hemarthrosis and capsulitis of the facet. Symptoms usually consist of localized sharp pain with little or no radiation initially, involuntary muscle guarding, spasms, and motion restriction. The pain is aggravated by all movements except flexion. Extension with side bending toward the painful side is especially painful (Kraft and Levinthal 1951).

When more than one segment is involved, a flattening of the normal spinal curve may be seen, more commonly in the thoracic and lumbar areas. Painful and tender muscle guarding with neutral vertebral dysfunctions[93] often are evident above and below the restricted site (Helbig and Lees 1988).

The criteria of facet syndrome diagnosis consist of (Bonica *ibid*):

- back, buttock and groin pain (or higher if in thoracic or cervical areas);
- well-localized paraspinal tenderness;
- pain reproduction with extension and rotation toward the painful side;
- significant x-ray evidence of facet arthrosis;
- strong correlation of pain relief by a facet block.

Clinically, pain from the facet joints can often be indistinguishable from disc pain and can mislead the practitioner.

Types of Facet Dysfunction

Paris (*ibid*) describes facet dysfunctions as occurring in painful and non-painful blocks.

PAINFUL BLOCK. A painful block is an acute condition that is initially felt as a sharp local pain, accompanied by simultaneous postural deviation. The onset of acute painful facet block and postural deviation is immediate, in contrast to disc nuclear lesions, which take some time to lead to postural deviation.[94]

A NONPAINFUL BLOCK. A nonpainful block is also an acute condition in which the back is effectively stuck in a laterally deviated (list) position away from the blocked facet.[95]

With internal derangement of the facets or discs, most frequently the joints lock in flexion. As stated before, this typical antalgic posture also can be due to spasm of the psoas, spasm of the deep aspect of the quadratus lumborum, extension spinal joint restrictions, and backward torsions of SI joint (see "Joint Dysfunctions and Manual Medicine Models" on page 461).

---

93. A group of vertebrae which are sidebent to one side and rotated to the opposite sides.
94. Clinically, this presentation is more likely to be due to internal disc derangement, backward sacral torsion, or psoas syndrome with FRS dysfunction at T12.
95. Facet dysfunctions often accompany sacroiliac dysfunctions.

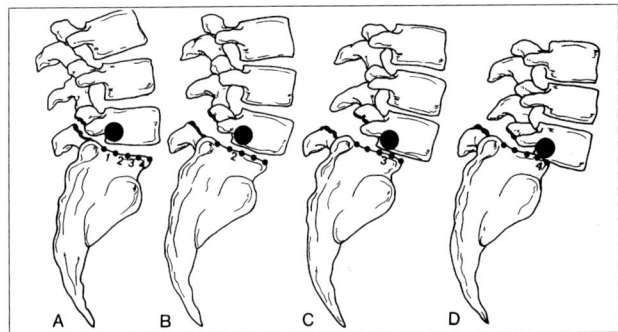

Figure 11-37: Spondylolisthesis, first through grade four (With permission Dorman and Ravin 1991).

TREATMENT. Whether painful or not, facet disorders are treated with manual therapy and/or acupuncture. Thrust manipulation may result in a residual facet inflammation that should be treated accordingly. In the non-acute period, the facet joint capsule and the surrounding ligaments can be needled to stabilize the joint. This may be difficult to perform accurately in the low back without fluoroscopic control. Steroid, Sarapin, or proliferant injections may be needed. In TCM, facet disorders are treated as back and leg pain.

Spondylolysis-Spondylolisthesis

Spondylolysis is a stress fracture and separation of one part of the vertebra, the *pars interarticularis.* Listhesis of the vertebrae always indicates ligament attenuation and instability. The pedicle of the vertebral body and the superior articular pillar can slide anteriorly, while the spinous process, the laminae, and the inferior articular pillar are held posteriorly. This, or a slip of the entire vertebra (due to facet or ligament pathology), can be seen at any age. It may be congenital, traumatic, or degenerative. However, recent studies have shown that the lytic defect develops principally during childhood and adolescence (Figure 11-37 through Figure 11-40), (Brown *ibid*).

Spondylolisthesis can be separated into several types, the most common of which is fatigue separation of the pars interarticularis. A congenital arrangement in which the facets are somewhat horizontal (in a sagittal plane) may result in a slippage forward of one side of the vertebra. Degeneration of the facets and of other ligaments may account for the remaining types. Spondylolisthesis is found in about 5% of asymptomatic populations and mostly affects the low back, but can also be found in the cervical spine. Degenerative spondylolisthesis in the lumbar spine occurs predominantly in females and often at the L4-L5 junction (Brown *ibid*).

Spondylolisthesis may or may not cause pain, and, when it does, it is often intermittent. When felt in the lumbar spine, the pain comes on after prolonged standing, is aggravated by activity, and usually is felt in the low back. However, it can radiate to the buttock, outer thighs, and legs as well. Usually, the pain is bilateral and often is relieved by lying or sitting. Squatting often is restful (Dorman *ibid*). (Squatting is thought by some to be the reason back pain is less common in countries in which toilet seats are not used).

Hamstring tightness, limited flexion, and marked lordosis is common (before age 50). The resulting excess lordosis may shift gravitational loads more to the posterior element, less on vertebral bodies and discs and more on the facet joints, wearing them out. The nerve roots may rub over a bony ledge (Brown *ibid*).

Inspection often reveals a step-like abnormality that may be seen on standing or during motion, and that may disappear in the prone position. If the step remains the same between standing and lying, it may be considered stable and it is less likely to cause symptoms or to progress (Brown *ibid*).

In symptomatic patients, the interspinous ligaments over the segments are tender. Bilateral leg pain is common and is aggravated by standing and is alleviated by flexion. Spinal claudication syndrome should be considered (Paris *ibid*).

CERVICAL SPINE. Unstable degenerative spondylolisthesis of the cervical spine is rare (Deburge et al 1995). Usually the slips occur at the C3-on-C4 or C4-on-C5 levels, immediately above a stiff lower-cervical spine. The two clinical patterns are neck pain alone or neck pain with neurological involvement that causes cervicobrachial pain or myelopathy. Symptoms and signs of instability are:

- paresthesia and neurological signs of the upper limbs;
- bilateral symptoms, simultaneous or alternating in both limbs;
- symptoms crossing the midline;
- chronic and persistent pain;
- symptoms relieved by immobilization.

IMAGING. This lesion is of the pars interarticularis and can be identified on the AP and lateral x-ray. These views are relatively high in radiation and should be used sparingly and with forethought. The oblique image demonstrates the lesion and is identified as the "collar of the scotty dog" (Figure 11-40). In degenerative spondylolisthesis the degree of anterior displacement usually is not more than about a fourth of the lower vertebral body width (first or second degree). In the cervical spine stress x-rays may be needed. Listhesis of the vertebrae always indicates ligament attenuation and usually is noted in flexion or extension. In forward spondylolisthesis of a vertebra on the one below, the major attenuation is to the posterior restraining structures, and vice versa. It is likely that the zygoapophyseal capsular ligaments also are injured, and that all restraining structures are affected to some extent (Dorman and Ravin *ibid*).

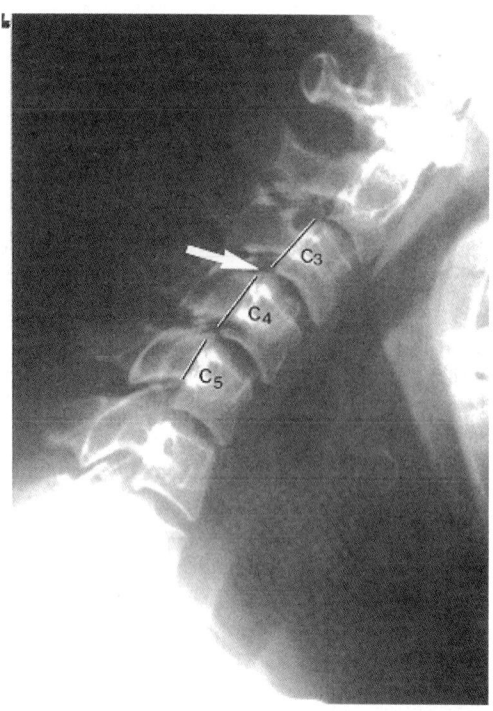

Figure 11-38: Lateral view of cervical spine with anterior listhesis in flexion of C3 on C4. The arrow points to the site of the anterior displacement.

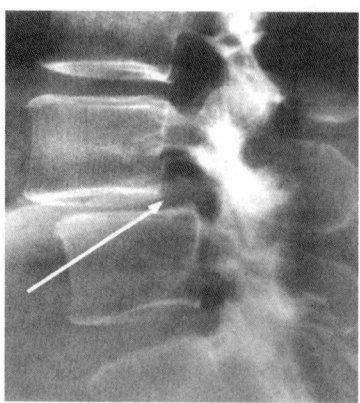

Figure 11-39: Degenerative spondylolisthesis at L4. Note that the arrow points to the area of anterior displacement of L4 on L5.

Treatment of Spondylolisthesis

Treatment in the lumbar spine is directed to decreasing lordosis, correcting vertebral dysfunctions, stabilizing the segment and correcting abnormal muscular patterning. Periosteal acupuncture, prolotherapy, electric stimulation and herbal application to the interspinous ligaments can be helpful. Selective nerve root blocks can be used for leg pain. All lumbopelvic, thoracic, leg and hip muscles should be assessed and treated. Often the hamstrings and quadratus lumborum are involved and should be treated. Post-isometric stretches and countertension release may be helpful.

Orthotics with negative heels or heel lifts may be helpful, both to address an un-level sacral base and to decrease lordosis (Paris *ibid*). Bracing and corsets may be necessary during acute phases but should be removed as soon as possible as they weaken the supporting muscles of the back (Magora 1976). The use of a Levator™ has been advocated (Jungmann 1992) to aid in decreasing postural decompensation as measured by the pelvic index, reducing the lumbosacral angle and transferring postural stress off the posterior tissues (Kuchera and Kuchera *ibid*).

In patients who have a recent soft tissue injury to the cervical spine and minimal or no neurologic deficits, a temporary improvement in symptoms following manual treatment may indicate instability. In such cases, *further manual treatment is contraindicated* until serious instability is ruled out.

In TCM, spondylolysis and spondylolisthesis are treated as spinal and extremity pain.

Stenosis

Spinal and lateral foraminal stenosis can be seen in older patients who often are heavy framed, obese, and out of shape. Symptoms and signs are variable but often include transient neurological and neurovascular symptoms brought on by activity. Often symptoms are relieved by assuming a forward (flexed) posture (Brown *ibid*).

Neurogenic Claudication

Neurogenic claudication is due to hypoxia (lack of oxygen) of the nerve roots from compression. Symptoms of burning, weakness, and "pins and needles" (tingling) are often felt first when the patient is walking downhill (because of increased lordosis which results in a reduced foramen space) and are less related to the distance walked. Symptoms are relieved by sitting and leaning forward (Paris *ibid*).

Vascular Claudication

Vascular claudication, not an orthopedic disorder, is a cramplike pain caused by poor blood circulation. The onset of vascular claudication is gradual, with a fairly predictable symptomatic pattern. The onset of a cramping ache occurs during walking a predictable distance and ceases rapidly while resting (Paris *ibid*).

Treatment of Neurogenic Claudication

The objective of treatment of neurogenic claudication is to open the narrowing of the canal and/or foramen. In mild disorders of lumbar spine this can be achieved by reducing the patient's lordosis; using lower or negative heels in their shoes. The obese patient should be encouraged to lose weight and to strengthen the abdominal muscles (Paris *ibid*).

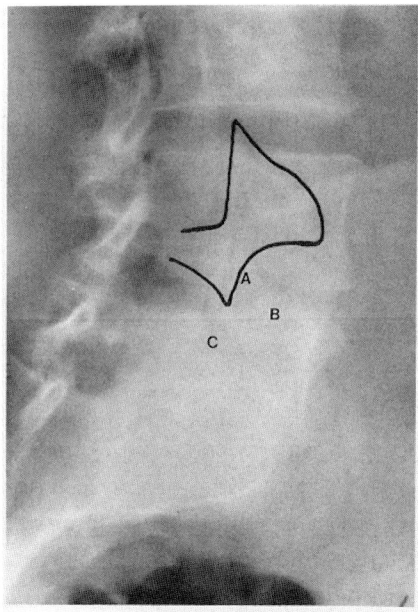

Figure 11-40: Oblique views of the lumbar spine with "collar on the dog," which is the area of no bone in the pars interarticularis (C). The normal dog is outlined on the vertebra above.

Lumbosacral stabilization and ligamentous strengthening may be helpful in some patients. All forward sacral and ERS dysfunctions should be addressed.

In patients with unilateral symptoms, placing a heel lift under the opposite leg sometimes is effective, as it produces sidebending to that side, opening the involved neural foramen (Paris *ibid*). In more severe cases, surgery is often necessary. Acupuncture often has only a temporary analgesic effect but which some patients find very helpful. Selective nerve blocks and epidural blocks may be beneficial, but, often, only temporarily, although in some patients the response can last for a long time.

Vascular claudication (not an orthopedic condition) can be treated with blood thinners or angioplasty. Herbal and nutritional therapy can be of great help.

In TCM, neurogenic claudication from stenosis is often manifested with patterns of excess type pain. In the elderly there is usually a combination of Deficiency and Excess. Treatment is the same as for spondylosis and outcomes vary greatly.[96]

Thoracic Outlet Syndrome

Thoracic outlet syndrome (TOS) is a poorly defined group of symptoms that may be due to compression of the brachial plexus and subclavian artery, resulting in neuropathy. The brachial plexus is spatially related to other important structures in the arm, axilla, and roots of the neck. The ventral rami of the spinal nerves that form the brachial plexus pass through and among the scalene muscles of the neck; the cords of the brachial plexus surround the brachial artery; and the nerves derived from the cord pass around and among the muscles of the arm, all of which must be understood. Diagnosis using current clinical and electrophysiological criteria is difficult. This syndrome can lead to vascular compromise and may be associated with an anomalous cervical rib (McCarthy, Yao, and Schafer et al 1989; Towns 2003). A variety of anatomical anomalies, most commonly a cervical rib, have been used to justify surgery, which is only successful in about 50% of cases, even though symptoms of TOS appear first in early adulthood (Simons, Travell, Simons *ibid*). Often cervical spine and/or first rib dysfunctions and postural disorders are present. Many anatomical "anomalies" such as cervical ribs, anomalous first ribs, or fibrous bands are seen among asymptomatic individuals, as well (Lindogren 2001).

Traumatic history was found in 86% of 668 patients undergoing surgery for TOS (Sanders and Pearce 1989). The mechanisms are probably due to the development of swelling and adhesions in the fascia or fibrous bands of the anterior and/or middle scalenes (Cailliet 1988).

Symptoms

Thoracic outlet syndrome can cause a variety of symptoms, often presenting with nocturnal symptoms of paresthesia in the arms or hands, possibly bilaterally. This sensation, which may awaken the patient at night, is a phenomenon of release of pressure on the brachial plexus nerve trunk. Normal daytime activity causes compression of the brachial nerve from the weight of the arms or contracted myofascial structures and leads to mechanical pressure on the brachial plexus. During sleep, the tension is relaxed, and this causes the onset of paresthesia (Cyriax *ibid*). Neural symptoms (Simons, Travell, Simons *ibid*) most commonly are felt in ulnar or ulnar/median distribution. The patient may show hyperesthesia to light touch, pinprick, and temperature change in the little finger.

In patients with thoracic outlet syndrome that did not respond to conservative therapy for over seven to twelve months, Liu, Tahmoush, Roos, and Schwartzman (1995) found a compressive brachial plexopathy from abnormally-attached or enlarged scalene muscles that affected the upper trunk of the brachial plexus. In some patients, at least one fibrous band compressed the lower trunk of the brachial plexus, as well. The patients had pain and sensory changes in a brachial plexus distribution, aggravation of pain with use of the affected extremity, pain on palpation over the brachial plexus, no intrinsic hand muscle atrophy, and normal nerve conduction in studies. Electromyography (EMG) showed mild chronic neuropathic changes in some patients.

Liu et al concluded that neurogenic thoracic outlet syndrome can occur from cervical band and scalene muscle

---

96. Surprisingly, some patients with severe stenosis respond satisfactorily to TCM methods with enough pain reduction so that surgery may be delayed. However, full recovery to normal activity cannot be expected.

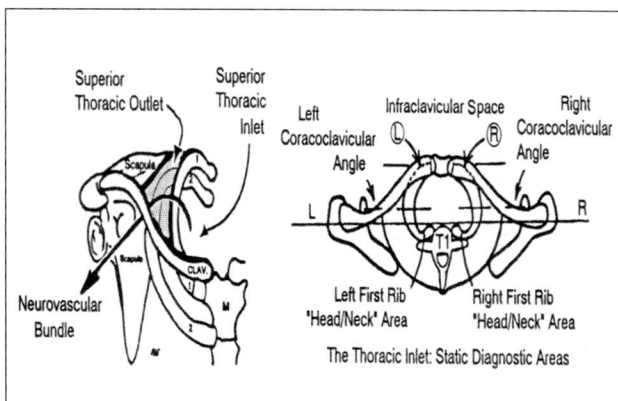

Figure 11-41: Thoracic inlet and outlet (From Kuchera WA and Kuchera ML, Osteopathic Principles in Practice, KCOM press 1993, with permission).

anomalies without intrinsic hand muscle atrophy from abnormalities such as the presence of cervical ribs or enlarged C7 transverse processes and can occur with or without abnormalities of EMG readings.

MYOFASCIAL PSEUDO TOS. According to Simons, Travell, and Simons (*ibid*) trigger points in scalenes, pectoralis major, latissimus dorsi, teres major, subscapularis, and, possibly, trapezius, levator scapulae, and pectoralis minor muscles are capable of giving symptoms that mimic TOS. Articular and ligamentous disorders often perpetuate myofascial symptoms.

Examination and Diagnosis

No good examination for thoracic outlet syndrome exists. Tests designed to obliterate radial pulses are not specific for TOS, as they can be positive in normals and in patients with other diagnoses. Arteriography has limited value except in patients with signs of pronounced compression. Neurophysiological examination should primarily be used to exclude nerve compression at sites more distal than the thoracic outlet; for example, ulnar nerve entrapment at the elbow (Lindogren *ibid*). The practitioner can:

1. Ask the seated patient to abduct his arms to 90°; Externally rotate his hands so that they face the ceiling, keeping the shoulders retracted, then open and close his hands rapidly for three minutes. The exam is positive if symptoms and fatigue are produced on the symptomatic side while the asymptomatic side remains unchanged.

2. Ask the patient to carry a 5-lb. weight in each hand for three minutes. The examination is positive if symptoms are reproduced on the symptomatic side.

3. Ask the patient to rest the patient's arm on the patient's head for several minutes. If paresthesia occurs after several minutes, the patient is likely to be suffering from thoracic outlet syndrome.

4. With the patients cervical spine in neutral position, rotate the spine maximally away from the side being examined. In this position, gently flex the spine as far as possible, moving the ear towards the chest. A bony restriction totally blocking this movement is said to indicate a positive test (the cervical rotation lateral flexion-test [CRLF-test]).

5. Order an x-ray, which is needed to diagnose a cervical rib.

Treatment

Treatment is directed to the underlying condition and may present a clinical challenge. Therapy should restore the function of the upper thoracic aperture. Exercises should start with shoulder girdle stabilization. They should include appropriate stretches to restore movement of the whole shoulder girdle and provide more space for the neurovascular structures. Attention to the cervical spine is important, as movements of the upper and lower cervical spine are often restricted in these patients. Exercises that aim to activate the anterior, middle, and posterior scalene muscles are the most important, because they may help correct dysfunction of the first rib. Other stretches and strengthening exercises are administered according to physical findings. This protocol will yield good long-term results in over 80% of the patients (Lindogren *ibid*). McKenzie assessment and treatment can be helpful. Other treatments may consist of manual therapies, acupuncture, dry needling, and herbs. In some cases (Cyriax *ibid*), simple, frequent shoulder shrugging is all that is required to alleviate symptoms. Local heparin injection may be tried in patients that do not respond (Ellis personal communication). If symptoms are severe and are unresponsive to less invasive treatment, surgical intervention might be necessary, but only if a cervical rib is present which is rare.

Whiplash

The term *whiplash injury* was used first by Crowe in 1928 to describe neck injuries that are due to automobile rear-end collisions. Whiplash is a nonspecific term that neither conveys the character of the injury nor indicates a diagnosis. It refers to cervical hyperextension-flexion injury, also called acceleration-deceleration syndrome. It must be understood, however, that whiplash injuries (automobile or other) can effect other regions of the spine and extremities, as well. Another current term used for injuries due to low-speed, rear-end collision is LoSRC.

Automobile accident injuries are common, and their clinical importance tends to be *underestimated*. Even mild and moderate whiplash can cause tears of muscles, tendons, ligaments, and joint capsules. The threshold (for male subjects) seems to be at 5mph for mild cervical strain injury, which is caused by a rapid compression-tension cycle directed through the musculoskeletal neck (McConnell et al 1993). At the same time, according to Sarno (2004) pain following automobile accidents is rare in under developed countries and therefore may be a social rather than a medical phenomenon.

In a review of thirty-two studies from 1980 to 1994, Nordhoff (1996) found that about 40% of automobile accident victims have long-term and persistent symptoms. The upper neck, the weakest part of the spine, is most vulnerable to this form of trauma (Tsuchisashi et al. 1981). Whiplash can occur due to other traumas such as sports injuries as well.

Whiplash may cause injury to many structures because the direction of collision is variable and the seat belt provides a pivot line that tends to lead to torsional strains. While the use of seat belts prevents serious injuries and saves lives, their use does increase the risk of sprain/strains in the neck and low back (Orsay et al 1990). Because the cervical system is linked mechanically to the rest of the spine, concomitant brain, spinal cord, facet, and peripheral nerve injuries are probable and common (Ward *ibid*). The most commonly involved tissues are probably the cervical ligaments and muscles. In severe trauma, the anterior longitudinal ligament can rupture, which causes the upper facets to move downward on the lower facets, markedly relaxing the ligamentum flavum. This sliding of the vertebrae can damage the spinal cord and can even cause death (Cyriax *ibid*). Traumatic syrinx, a pathological, tube-shaped cavity in the brain or spinal cord, also has been noted on MRIs secondary to traumatic cord injury (Brown 1995).

Mechanisms of Injury

For diagnosis and treatment of whiplash injury, determining the direction and mode of an injury may be important.

Rear-End Collision

During a rear-end collision (Figure 11-42), the trunk accelerates forward, leaving the head relatively behind, resulting in hyper-extension injury. Even low-velocity rear end collisions can cause significant injuries to muscles, ligaments, discs, and even vertebral body fractures (Dunn and Blazar 1987). Low speed rear-end collisions can cause more symptoms than higher speed front-end collisions (Hyde 1992):

- The eight to fifteen pounds of the head whips backward into hyperextension. The excessive extension is probably due, in part, to the unopposed movement of the neck that occurs because ventral muscles that usually protect against hyperextension do not have time to react. Hyperextension leads to stretch injury of the anterior structures such as the anterior longitudinal ligament, anterior disc herniation, joint infringement into the intervetebral foramen, fracture of the cervical vertebrae, and compression injury of the facet structures posteriorly.
- Usually flexion follows, limited by the seat belt and by the chin hitting the chest. As the head hits the head rest and the soft tissues are stretched, the head is whipped forward. Release of elastic energy from the head rest, recoil of the car seat and soft tissues, and the stretch reflex (reflex contraction) of the ventral (flexors) muscles are contributing factors. The head will *whip* forward, because of the preset cervical flexors tension, and because of their reactive forceful contraction (reactive to forceful stretch). Also, the timing of flexor muscle recoil appears to have an additive affect with the recoil affects of the seats, so that the head thrusts forward violently. Hyperflexion results in posterior soft tissues injury (Dorman 1997).

Forward Collision

Forward collision (often called deceleration injury) (Figure 11-42) causes cervical hyperflexion, which can be followed by hyperextension. The hyperflexion leads to trauma of the posterior cervical ligaments, most often at C5-C6 (Jackson 1958), subluxation and sprain of the facets, capsular tears, and posterior disc herniation.

Pathology

Little "direct" information is available on the pathological processes of *non-fatal* whiplash injuries. MacNab reports damage to the longus colli muscles and widespread soft tissue contusion in the neck, including anterior longitudinal ligament tears, sympathetic nerve involvement, and bruising of the esophagus (MacNab 1964, 1973).

Long-Term Degenerative Changes

Long-term x-ray follow-up shows an increased rate of degenerative changes in patients who originally had normal x-ray findings. Typically, these changes are confined to one or two segments at the C5-6-7 level, as compared to the non-traumatic, diffuse degeneration pattern seen in the elderly. Pre-existing degenerative disease *does not* seem to contribute significantly to prolonged symptoms in cases of whiplash injuries (Meenen, Katzer, Dihlmann, Held, Fyfe and Jungbluth 1994). However, other studies find a high correlation between pre-existing cervical spondylosis and persistence of pain after whiplash injury (Miles et al 1988).

DISC LESIONS. Whiplash injuries often result in an S-shaped configuration (flexed at upper spine and extended at lower spine) in one-tenth of a second, resulting in significant sheer forces at the discs, with disruption and tearing on the annular fibers (Ono et al 1997; Croft 2000). Postmortems also show common isolated avulsions of the annular fibers from the rim of the cervical vertebral body, with annular ruptures extending into the central disc, usually at C5-C7 (Jónsson 1991; Eliyahu 1989). Fatal disc lesions have been reported as well. Hinz (1968) demonstrated that, in forty-one cases of fatal whiplash, the most common lesion was a disc rupture, usually at the C3-C4 level.

FACET LESIONS. In a diagnostic block study of patients who

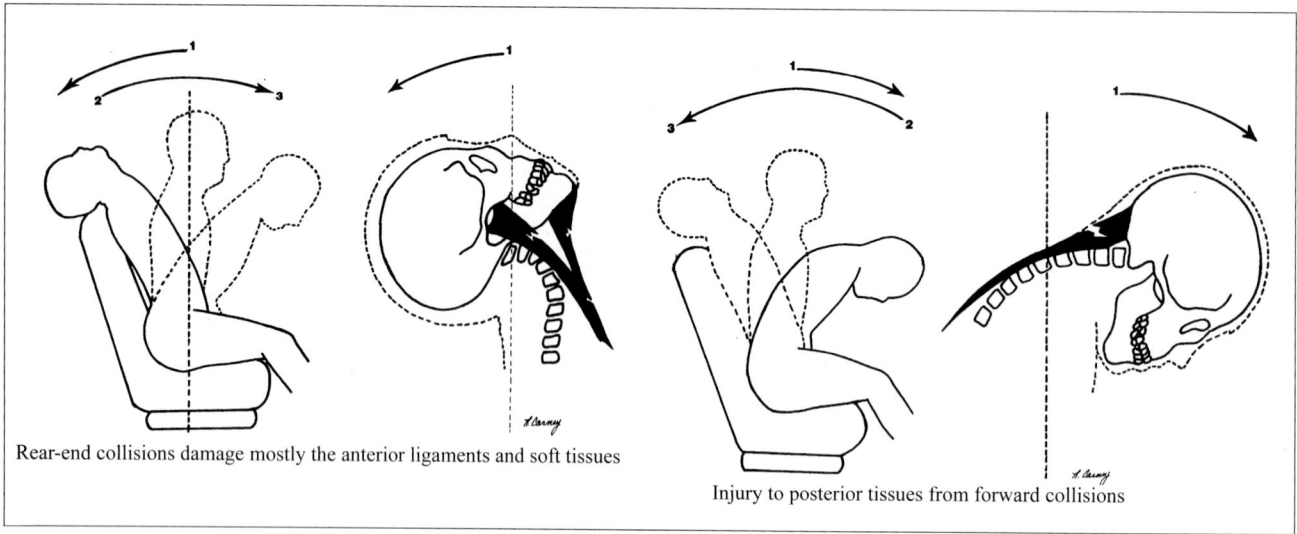

Figure 11-42: Whiplash injuries (courtesy of Dorman and Ravin *ibid*).

had chronic neck pain following whiplash injury, Barnsley et al (1995) reported that the prevalence of cervical facet joint pain occurred in 54% of patients. Barnsley concluded that cervical facet joint pain was the most common source of chronic neck pain following whiplash. The sudden S-shaped forces at the cervical spine can result in instantaneous change of the axis of C5 on C6 resulting in facet jamming and structural changes (Ono et al *ibid*; Croft *ibid*).

TYPE OF IMPACT. In rear-end collisions, replica studies of *hyperextension* injury show that the greatest deformation (about 57%) occurs in the longus colli. The scalenus anterior muscle was deformed in 21% and was more common than deformations in the sternocleidomastoid, longus capitis, and scalene posterior muscles (Deng and Goldsmith 1987).

MacNab (1971) has implicated (in hyperextension injuries) the sympathetic plexus, anterior longitudinal ligaments, with separation of cervical discs, trapezius, splenius capitis, semispinalis capitis, scaleni, longissimus capitis, rectus capitis, rhomboid, inferior and superior oblique capitis, and longus capitis.

Hyperflexion neck injuries produce primarily ligamentous-disc injuries (Yoganandan et al 1989). A replica study showed that the splenius cervicis and splenius capitis muscles bear the greatest deformation, about 50%, (Deng and Goldsmith 1987). If the neck is flexed at the time of impact, the T-1 to T-4 areas will bear the greatest stress (Pintar et al 1989).

Rotational spinal soft tissue injuries affect primarily the ligaments and zygoapophyseal (facet) joints complex (Yoganandan et al *ibid*).

Side collisions result in sidebending injury. Side collisions tend to affect the middle-to-upper neck regions more than other crashes. A replica side collision study showed the longus capitis bearing the majority (57%) of deforming forces. (Sidebending in the cervical spine is always coupled with rotation).

Diagnostic Limitations

When whiplash occurs, diagnosis is complicated by the fact that currently available imaging techniques are deficient in visualizing the soft tissues. Ultrasound, which is being explored as a diagnostic tool, may be valuable for documenting swelling in soft tissues. Woltring et al (1994) suggest that helical axis may provide objective assessment of joint pathology and dysfunction. This would help significantly in assessing whiplash injuries and settling litigation issues. Currently, in many cases the patient's complaints are dismissed because "objective" evidence is lacking and ulterior motives such as litigation are suspected. The evidence that litigating prolongs recovery from automobile accidents is unconvincing (Mendelson 1982, 1984). At the same time, claims of persistent pain following car accidents are less common in undeveloped countries (Sorno *ibid*).

POOR CORRELATION WITH MRI FINDINGS. In studies in which patients were examined clinically and by MRI, Pettersson et al (1994) reported that twenty-six of thirty-nine cases of whiplash neck injury showed changes on the MRI. Twenty-five of those cases showed disc lesions, of which ten were identified as disc herniations and one was identified as a muscle lesion. The correlation between the MRI findings and the clinical symptoms and signs was poor.

Initial Findings After Injury

In studies of the relationship between accident mechanisms and initial findings after whiplash injury, Sturzenegger et al

(1994) found that the passenger's position in the car, use of a seat belt, and the presence of a head restraint showed no significant correlation with findings. Rotated or inclined head position at the moment of impact was associated with a higher frequency of multiple symptoms, with more severe symptoms, and signs of musculoligamental-cervical strain and neural involvement, particularly radicular damage. Unprepared occupants had a higher frequency of multiple symptoms and more severe headache. Rear-end collision was associated with a higher frequency of multiple symptoms, especially of cranial nerve or brainstem dysfunction. Sturzenegger et al concluded that three features of accident mechanisms were associated with more severe symptoms:

- An unprepared occupant;
- Rear-end collision, with or without subsequent frontal impact;
- Rotated or inclined head position at the moment of impact.

Because whiplash can cause a variety of symptoms that can manifest at different times, the practitioner must stay alert for possible long-term complications.

DELAY IN SYMPTOMS. Pain due to whiplash usually begins several hours, days, or even weeks (typical of ligamentous pain) after the accident (Hirsch, Hirsch and Hiramoto 1988). Unless the practitioner obtains a thorough history for trauma, this delayed onset of symptoms can cause the practitioner to miss the precipitating mechanism of injury (which may be important to understand for medilegal reasons as well as clinically). In a study of 5,000 patients, 25% showed significantly-prolonged onset of symptoms that were secondary to whiplash injury. In more severe injuries, the pain usually was immediate. In the delayed group, the most frequently reported symptom was headache (Balla and Karnaghan 1987). Upper-extremity radiating symptoms may not appear until several months after injury (Bogduk *ibid*).

HEADACHE FOLLOWING WHIPLASH. Headache following whiplash injury has been reported to occur in 48-80% of patients (Norris and Watts 1983). In a study of the prevalence of third occipital nerve headache among whiplash patients, Lord et al found that a third occipital nerve block was effective in patients whom the diagnosis was positive. These patients were significantly more likely to be tender over the C2-3 facet joint (Lord, Barnsley, Wallis, Bogduk and 1994). Anderson (2001) finds that successful disc surgery to joints from C4 to C7 can help as well. Surgical intervention however should be considered very rarely.

PROGRESSION OF SYMPTOMS. Following whiplash injury the victim typically complains of a wide variety of symptoms. Immediately after the injury, the only complaints usually are of shock and anxiety without pain, probably due to stress analgesia. Later, general aching, mild neck pain, occipital pain, headache, limitation of cervical movement, and perhaps blurred vision, tinnitus, and dysphagia are seen.

Often these symptoms intensify with time. Unless treated properly, they can last for years. Most patients who require medical attention and then recover, do so within the first two years (Gargan and Bannister 1990).

Injuries of the upper cervical spine develop earlier. Often they are accompanied by sympathetic/cranial/central involvements such as headache, tinnitus, diaphoresis, dizziness, altered sensorium and blurred vision. This may be due to the sympathetic afferents from the cranial vessels, which pass their sensory information through the upper cervical roots (Lambert and Bogduk et al 1991), or from brain or spinal cord injury. These symptoms were described first in 1926 as the *Barré-Lieou syndrome*,[97] in which a series of symptoms including headache, vertigo, tinnitus, and ocular problems were associated with post-traumatic disc prolapse at the C 3-4 level.

Other symptoms reported at various stages of whiplash include: anxiety, fatigue, irritability, insomnia, and flashbacks (Dalal and Harrison 1993). Dysphagia or discomfort on swallowing may be seen in up to 30% of patients (Norris and Watt 1983). Usually this is due to injury of ventral soft tissues. Low back pain may be seen in 57-71% of patients (Foreman and Croft 1988).

IMPAIRMENT OF ATTENTION. In their evaluation of attention and memory function of patients two years following a whiplash injury, Stefano and Radavov (1995) found no memory impairment in symptomatic patients. However, symptomatic and matched asymptomatic individuals had differing levels of attention. In tasks that required divided attention, symptomatic patients had difficulties that could not be explained as having occurred due to use of medicines that might affect ability to perform divided-attention tasks.

POST-CONCUSSION SYNDROME. Head injuries from mild traumas (and whiplash) can lead to chronic symptoms or "post concussion syndrome" in as many as 50% of patients (Alves et al 1986). Symptoms often include cognitive, behavioral and pain complaints (Alves and Jenttner 1986).

DELAYED RECOVERY. In their study of the predictive relationship between psychosocial factors and the course of recovery in patients who have whiplash injury, Radanov et al (1994) found that patients who remained symptomatic at one year had:

- significantly higher ratings of initial neck pain and headache;
- a greater variety of subjective complaints;
- higher scores on the "nervousness" scale from the personality inventory;
- worse well-being scores;
- poorer performance with regard to focussed attention.

---

97. Bensky (2003) has recommend Frigid Extremities Powder (Si Ni San) plus Salviae (Dan Shen) for post whiplash pain and disorientation.

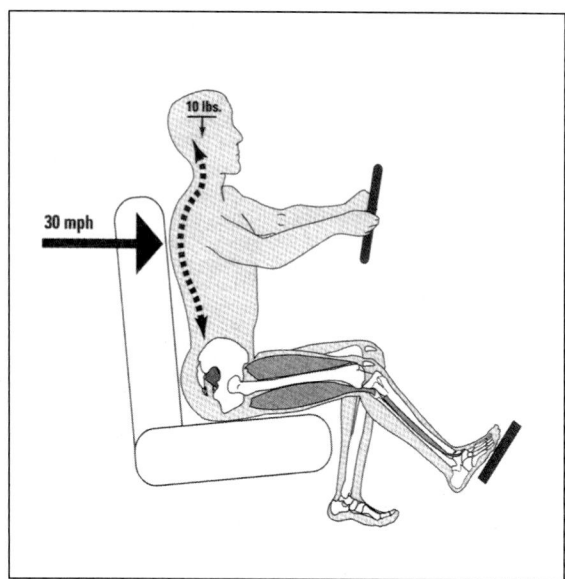

Figure 11-43: Mechanism of sacral injury in whiplash. The recoil from the car seat transfers pressure onto the sacrum, often resulting in flexed left sacrum. Rotation of the ilia via leg pressure can also result in SI injury (courtesy of Mitchell 1999).

The study's regression analysis revealed that the initial variables that correlated significantly with poor recovery at one year were: higher age, complaint of sleep disturbances, and higher intensity of initial neck pain, and headache.

Treatment of Whiplash Injury

Treatment for acute whiplash can consist of compression, icing and bracing of the neck as soon as possible.[98] Microscopic capillary bleeding in deep neck muscles has been shown to persist up to two to five days after motor vehicle collision injuries (Aldman 1987); therefore, the use of Panax Pseudoginseng (San Qi) and Pollen Typhoae (Pu Huang) should be considered. Bracing for a prolonged period has been shown to cause muscle atrophy, joint contracture, and prolonged rehabilitation (Ruskin 1984). Treatment can include indirect techniques to relax muscles, acupuncture, :laser, electromagnetic therapy, and herbs for pain control, preventing swelling, bleeding, and blood stasis. Bracing and cervical collars can be used:

- for severe neck pain (in patients who have severe spasm, suspected fracture, and ligamentous instability);
- temporarily during activities that aggravate pain;
- during sleep.

Thrust manipulation is only rarely used to restore function and free entrapped tissues. When mild signs of disc involvement (such as partial articular pattern and joint dysfunction) are present without radicular signs, direct and/or indirect cervical manipulation can be helpful. However, the practitioner must be sure of the diagnosis and the technique, because serious instability may exist. Acupuncture can be used early for its analgesic effect and resulting improved mobility. Exercise should be started as soon as possible but must not be too vigorous. Range of motion exercises, within the pain-free range, should be done for the first two weeks, allowing muscles and ligamentous tissues to go through the initial inflammatory phase.

Warning: Thrust manipulation in a patient with instability can have catastrophic consequences.

NOTE: The appropriateness of nonsteroidal anti-inflammatory agents (NSAIDs) use is debatable, because they inhibit inflammation and therefore interfere with the healing of wounded tissues. Some NSAIDs can also prolong bleeding. If NSAIDs are used, they should be combined with TCM hemostatic herbs. Use of these herbs will help keep to a minimum the microbleeding that occurs due to the antiplatelet action of NSAIDs. This will prevent inflammation in areas that will not benefit from inflammation. NSAID use should probably be limited to the first several days.

TREATMENT OF FACET JOINT INJURY. Injury to the cervical facet joints is thought to be a common problem following whiplash injury. Barnsley et al (1994) report that following whiplash injury, injection of betamethasone into the facets is *not* effective. This study indicates that, if the facets are involved, the pain probably is due to mechanical dysfunctions and ligamentous laxity and not just inflammation.

Thermal ablation of the nerve that supplies a symptomatic facet can result in complete relief of symptoms, both physical and psychological, in *chronic* post whiplash patients (Bogduk 1997).

TREATMENT OF CHRONIC-STAGE WHIPLASH. To treat chronic-stage whiplash, the practitioner should address all mechanical and myofascial/ligamentous components globally. Integrated neuromusculaoskeletal release and myofascial release techniques that incorporate cranial nerve activities are particularly important in patients suffering from cognitive symptoms (Ward *ibid*). Rehabilitation should involve (Fitz-Ritson 1995) exercises that address coordination of eye-head-neck-arm movements, coordination of the entire vertebral column, and returning the "phasic" component of the musculature to functional levels.

Exercise must be started at a very low level and gradually increased at patient tolerance. Too vigorous or fast progression often results in pain and poor patient compliance.

Acupuncture can have a 71% to 91% positive clinical response (Su and Su 1988). Acupuncture has been used successfully in combination with manual medicine techniques (Pearson 1990). Any OM Organic and Pathogenic Factors are addressed.

---

98. Some researchers say that the neck should not be kept immobile. The author prefers only early bracing, but finds that immobilizing the neck during sleep periods is helpful at later stages.

Biofeedback can be helpful especially for headaches. The patient learns to relax the suboccipital muscles, the temporomadibular joint, and the rectus capitis posterior minor (Hack et al 1995).

Electromagnetic therapy is useful (Thuile and Walzl 2002).

Prolotherapy is effective in many patients that have failed to respond to the above therapies. For patients with continued upper neck and head pain, altologous blood can be injected under fluoroscopy to the upper cervical and occipital ligaments (Brown, Eke and Derby personal communication).

Mushroom Phenomenon

This condition (described by Cyriax) is found in elderly patients who complain of almost immediate severe pain upon standing up and walking. The pain quickly resolves when the patient is lying down. Radiographic studies show significant disc-space narrowing. Cyriax believed that the pain is due to laxity of the posterior longitudinal ligament protruding posteriorly while the patient is weight-bearing. When the patient lies down the ligament is pulled forward or tightened, pressure on the dura is relieved, and the pain subsides (Cyriax and Cyriax *ibid*).

Treatment

According to Hackett et al (1991) some of these patients benefit from prolotherapy. Treatments similar to that of spinal or foraminal stenosis may be tried.

Iliocostal Friction Syndrome

Hirschberg et al (1992) suggest that patients with iliocostal friction syndrome may have their lower ribs rub against the iliac crest, which may cause severe pain at the lower chest margin, or in the low back, hip, and groin with radiation into the chest and thigh. Symptoms are aggravated by mobility, such as changing the position of the body from lying to sitting or standing, and are more severe when the patient bends or twists the spine. The syndrome may be detected clinically by palpation of the iliac crests, which are extremely tender and are in contact with the lower ribs.

Pathological conditions that may lead to reduction of the distance between the ribs and the ilia are severe dorsal kyphosis, scoliosis, and compression fracture. The structures irritated by iliocostal friction are the tendons of the muscles inserting at the iliac crest and the lower rib cage, the abdominal and quadratus lumborum muscles.

Treatment

Compression of the lower four ribs, pushing them to the inside and away from the iliac crest can be achieved by a strong three-inch elastic belt. The belt is positioned immediately above the iliac crest and adjusted tightly enough to move the ribs away from the iliac crest. Periosteal acupuncture or proliferant injections at the iliac crest may help.

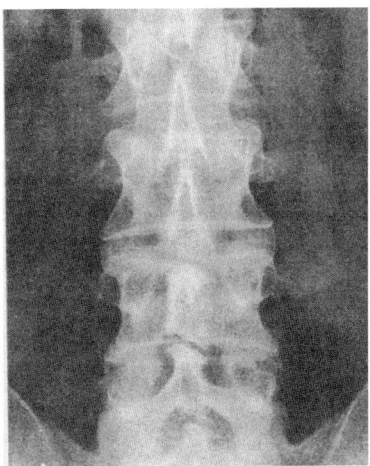

Figure 11-44: Kissing spine. Note the closely opposed spinous processes and the articular cortex at their tips.

Kissing Spine (Basstrap's Disease)

In 1924 Basstrap described the "kissing spine" condition in which the spinous processes of the lumbar spine encroach on each other. This may give rise to arthritis and sclerotic changes, which may be painful, but usually are not. Normal aging and degeneration of the discs can lead to approximation of the spinous processes (which may impinge on one another, especially when the spine is extended) and produce pain that is relieved by forward bending. It is most common in people with large spinous processes, small disc spaces, and excessive lordosis. Other factors may include facet arthrosis, neuromuscular disorders, thoracic kyphosis, thoracolumbar gibbus, obesity, and congenital hip dysplasia (Sartorius, Resnick, and Tyson et al 1985). Although this syndrome is controversial, surgical intervention has been suggested. Others have also suggested desensitization through proliferant injections (Dorman personal communication).

Treatment

Within the context of this book, treatment includes the correction of any sacral and vertebral dysfunction, especially those that increase lordosis (flexed sacrum and restriction of lumbar flexion, i.e., ERS dysfunctions). Tight myofascial layers (especially dorsal) are stretched, and this is followed by strengthening of abdominal and psoas muscles in order to reduce lumbar lordosis. Dry needling using the same principles is appropriate. Often the interspinous ligaments are sensitive and may be needled. Topical herb packs are especially helpful. Negative heels in the shoes can be used to reduce lordosis.

Periosteal Lesions

Periosteal lesions are common and can refer pain in a non-segmental distribution and to a sizable area (Kellgren 1949; Inman and Saunders 1944). Tears often appear secondary to trauma or strains in the periosteum, where soft tissues are attached to bone. Vagler and Krauss describe periosteal changes in organic disease and treat them by massage.

Periostitis, or inflammation of the periosteum, is a condition caused by chronic or acute infection or trauma, and is characterized by a tenderness and swelling of the affected bone, pain, fever, and chills. In severe cases, blood or an albuminous serous exudate forms under the membrane. In syphilitic infections periostitis may occur as an early symptom (Brown *ibid*).

Treatment

Periosteal lesions can be treated by massage, periosteal acupuncture, electric stimulation, and, if needed, by injection or surgery. Infections are treated medically.

Scar Tissue and Interference Fields

It is advisable to check scars for triggers, as they can act as low level antagonists and activate other pain mechanisms. Prolonged immobilization of muscles or joints, injuries, infections, and surgeries can all result in the formation of scar tissue. When joints are immobilized, collagen fibers will be laid down at random and form scars. Scars can interfere with fascial load distribution, often adhering tissues that should move independently. Scar tissue tends to be weaker than normal tissue; the amount of ground substance and proteoglycan content is reduced so that water content is affected. The ratio of normal ground substance to collagen fibers is reduced, which results in reduced metabolism and denser and less pliant tissues. There may also be abnormal infiltration of nervous tissues. Neural therapists consider scars as capable of neural irritation, constituting an "interference field" that may lead to numerous symptoms including pain. (Sites of active [possibly occult] infection found especially in teeth, tonsils, appendix, and gallbladder can also be a site of an interference field.)[99] Scar tissue formation (Wall and Gutnick 1974) may provoke pain mechanisms without involvement of the nociceptive system. Referred pain or numbness has been reported in skin and scar triggers, and the sensations are felt nearby or remotely. Travell and Simons (*ibid*) report burning, prickling, and "lightning-like" jabs of pain from cutaneous scars.

Stacher found scars to have higher skin resistance than adjacent, undamaged tissue. Scar tissue has a resistance of 120-500 kilo-ohms above that of the surrounding skin. Skin resistance in a non-active scar (not producing symptoms) is mostly uniform over the scar, whereas an active scar there may have as much as 600-1500 kilo-ohms of variation. Active scars (sites) are often painful when pinched. It is important to remember that many scars are deep and not visually accessible. Palpation for scar tissue is therefore important.

Treatment

Scars are treated by massage, myofascial release techniques, functional techniques, acupuncture, herbs, and, if needed, by injection with 1% buffered procaine with no preservative. The active scar is surrounded by needles that are inserted at the edge of the scar about 1 cm apart (when visible). If the scar crosses an acupuncture channel, a point above and below the scar is added on the channel. An electrical stimulator or ion cord may be connected to "push" Qi through the scar. It is sometimes helpful to thread a needle just below the surface along the scar's edges. The scar is then mobilized. Deeper scars should be explored with the needle, followed by manual therapy. At times fibrotic muscle-bands need to be cut for pain to disappear. This is best done with a thin scalpel (cataract blade) under local anesthesia. Triangular and cutting acupuncture needles can be used as well. The muscle must be mobilized hourly by having the patient voluntarily contract the muscle placed in its shortened position. This is done to prevent the rescaring and adhering of tissues. Functional techniques can be very helpful when treating scar tissue; the scar is mobilized in the directions of ease in all planes (see "Dynamic Functional Techniques," page 484). Because scars are still pliable, a quality that increases when scar tissue is heated, it is advisable to heat the area prior to acupuncture or manual therapy. A ginger hot pack has been recommend. Laser or electromagnetic therapy to the scar may be helpful. Propolis (a product from bees) used topically has anesthetic effects. Herbs can be used topically as well. An empirical topical paste for scar tissue can be used as a hot pack. Its contents are:

> Galla Chinensis (Wu Bei Zi) 90g
> Fructus Evodiae Rutaecarpae (Wu Zhu Yu) 15g
> Radix Caulis/Folium Schefflera (Qi Ye Lian) 30g
> Herba Speranskiae seu Impatients (Tou Gu Cao) 100g
> Rhizoma Homalomenae Occultae (Qian Nian Jian) 30g
> Radix Angelica Sinensis (Dang Gui) 30g
> Radix Rubrus Paeoniae Lactiflorae (Chi Shao) 30g
> Gummi Olibanum (Ru Xiang) 15g
> Resina Myrrhae (Mo Yao) 15g
> Flos Carthami (Hong Hua) 15g
> Vinegar, enough to cover herbs
> Honey, enough to make a past
> The powdered ingredients are first cooked in water until becoming a thick paste. Vinegar is than added and the formula cooked again until pasty. Finally, honey is mixed in to form a final paste. The paste is applied directly on the scar.

---

99. Neural therapy is a German system that uses anaesthetic injections to regulate the autonomic nervous system and treat many medical conditions.

For a highly symptomatic scar, a topical application of Secretio Bufonis (Chan Su) can be used as an anesthetic. Hua Tuo's Powder Containing Venenum Bufonis (Qiong Su San) may be used topically. (A tincture of this formula is most effective as an anesthetic.) Its contents are:

    Venenum Bufonis (Chan Su) 3g
    Rhizoma Pinelliae (Ban Xia) 2g
    Radix Aconitii (Chuan Wu) 6g
    Radix Rhododendri Mollis (Yang Zhi Zhu) 2g
    Fructus Piperis Nigri (Hu Jiao) 6g
    Fructus Piperis Longi (Bi Ba) 6g
    Pericarpium Zanthoxyli (Chuan Jiao) 6g

If symptoms persist, injection therapy with procaine may be necessary.

Bursitis

The bursal sac serves as a cushion between bony prominences, tendons, and fibrous tissues. It also protects articular and periarticular structures from extrinsic trauma. Bursitis occurs when the synovial fluid within the bursa becomes inflamed, leading to painful stimulation of nerve endings.

Bursitis occurs most often in the shoulder but can be seen in several locations, including the knee, olecranon, retrocalcaneal, iliopsoas, trochanteric, ichial, and bursa of the first metatarsal head (bunion) (Cyriax *ibid*). The olecranon and prepatellar bursae are also susceptible to exogenous infection because of their superficial locations. Bursitis may be one of the most common musculoskeletal syndromes seen in daily practice. The etiology of bursitis is unknown but can result from trauma, infections, crystalline deposit diseases, and other inflammatory arthritis. The affected area is often red, swollen, and warm. This may not be evident or palpable if the bursa is deep (Arromdee and Matteson 2001).

The most common causes of bursitis are repetitive microtrauma or macrotrauma, extension of inflammation from the surrounding structures, including, adjacent tendons, muscle, fascia, skin, and joint synovium. Infection from straphylococcus aureus accounts for approximately 80% of all cases of septic bursitis and should be suspected when there is a history of skin abrasion or other skin lesion, such as cellulitis. Suspect a hematogenous source when blood cultures are positive or when noncutaneous pathogens are cultured from the bursal fluid (Arromdee and Matteson *ibid*).

Clinical diagnosis of bursitis (especially chronic) may be difficult to make, and technical evaluation such as ultrasonography, MRI, radiographs, and anesthetic injections may be needed to confirm a diagnosis (Ombregt et al 1995). There is usually a qualitative difference between chronic and acute bursitis, especially in the shoulder. Chronic bursitis is *not* a continuation of the acute process. Acute subdeltoid bursitis is not related in any way to chronic subdeltoid bursitis. Acute subdeltoid bursitis comes on suddenly and is one of the most painful disorders seen in orthopedic medicine patients. The pain is most severe in the first seven to ten days. It usually completely resolves on its own within six weeks. There may be a tendency for recurrence within five years at one or both shoulders. Chronic bursitis is chronic at the onset (Cyriax *ibid*). There are many bursae in the body that can be affected:

SHOULDER AREA. Shoulder pain that originates from other sources is often wrongly attributed to bursitis. Between the acromion and the rotator cuff lies the *subdeltoid* bursa, which helps cushion the tendon from the bone. This fluid-filled space can become inflamed, leading to pain and limitation of motion in a noncapsular pattern.

A second bursa, the *subcoracoid* bursa, is located between the coracoid process and the pectoralis major muscle. An acromioclavicular (AC) joint lesion sometimes is difficult to differentiate from chronic subdeltoid bursitis. Subdeltoid bursitis can be acute or chronic. Passive and active elevation are the most painful movements. Resisted movement may or may not be painful. All passive movements are painful often at end range. When the subcoracoid bursa is inflamed, the pain is usually felt locally in the outer infraclavicular area and does not radiate. Passive external rotation is often painful. The pain disappears when the test is repeated with the arm abducted to the horizontal (Cyriax *ibid*).

ELBOW AREA. At the lateral elbow, *epicondylar* and *radiohumeral* bursitis can cause a vague ache that can be mistaken for tennis elbow.

Olecranon bursitis can occur with repetitive pressure, a fall on a bent elbow, and various other conditions such as gout, rheumatic disease, and tuberculosis. Often conservative treatment is not effective (Ombregt et al *ibid*).

HIP AREA. Bursitis can result in noncapsular limitation. Several bursae around the hip joint can be affected clinically.

Gluteal bursae are involved most frequently. Pain is felt at the gluteal or trochanteric area, spreading to outer or posterior thigh. The pain is not related to sitting but increases with walking and stair-climbing. Typically, painful passive internal rotation and passive abduction are seen. Resisted external rotation or resisted abduction may be painful, as well.

Trochanteric bursa often can become inflamed. Pain is felt at the trochanteric area, spreading to the lateral aspect of the knee, especially while running or stair-climbing. External rotation with hip and the knee flexed is very painful and sometimes limited.

Psoas bursitis pain is felt in the groin area. Passive adduction with the hip in flexion is most painful. External rotation and flexion are painful at end range.

Ischial bursitis pain is felt at the ischial area as soon as the patient is seated (Ombregt et al *ibid*).

KNEE AREA. Many bursae are found around the knee; all can become inflamed.

The *prepatellar* bursa is the most frequently affected. Prepatellar bursitis is seen most often in patients who kneel repeatedly, as brick layers do. The front of the knee is swollen between the skin and the patella. Severe swelling can limit flexion due to pain that results from stretching the bursa.

Another common location of bursitis is under the *medial collateral ligament*. The pain, which is over the medial joint line, becomes worse with activity and eases with rest. Flexion can be limited with a soft end-feel. Valgus strain and lateral rotation are painful. A solid swelling, which can be mistaken for bone, can be palpated under the ligament.

Pes anserinus bursitis can be found over the medial collateral ligament. It also can occur in the space between the tendons of the sartorius, gracilis, and semitendinosus muscles.

A bursa between the *iliotibial tract* and the *lateral condyle* can form in long-distance runners, skiers, and cyclists. When inflamed, pain is felt over the lateral aspect of the knee while walking or running. A painful arc can be seen at 30° of flexion. Swelling can be felt between the condyle and the iliotibial tract (Ombregt et al *ibid*).

ANKLE FOOT AREA. *Achilles* bursitis can cause limitation in the noncapsular pattern. Pain is elicited when the bursa is squeezed between the posterior side of the tibia and the upper surface of the calcaneus at the extreme of passive plantiflexion. The condition should be differentiated from a posterior tibiotalar impingement of the trigonum (a large posterior tubercle of the posterior talus or an accessory bone) and from Achilles tendinitis (Ombregt et al *ibid*).

Treatment

Bursitis is treated by first addressing any accompanying joint dysfunction and myofascial pain or tension, or any other underlying conditions such as gout, or biomechanical imbalances, such as short leg. Herbal, NSAIDs, electromagnetic, laser, and acupuncture therapy can be helpful. If needed, the bursa can be drained or injected. Surgical consultation may be needed in refractory cases and in septic cases. Early diagnosis of septic bursitis and appropriate antibiotic or antifungal therapy are essential.

In TCM, bursitis is categorized as a Painful Obstruction (Bi) syndrome. The local area can be treated with a seven-star needle followed by cupping to draw-out blood. Both oral and topical herbs are used. Often treatment is directed at transforming Phlegm and breaking-up Blood-stasis. Fragrant and drying herbs such as Moschus Moschiferi (She Xiang), Rhizoma Atractylodes (Cang Zhu) and insects are often used. Acute bursitis (often of the shoulder) is usually attributed to severe Wind-Cold and Blood-stasis patterns and treated with modification of Remove Painful Obstruction Decoction (Juan Bi Tong). In chronic cases both attacking and tonification may be used simultaneously.[100,101]

An empirical *guiding* topical and oral formula for upper body bursitis is:

   Rhizoma seu Radix Notopterygium (Qiang Hou) 9g
   Rhizoma Curcumae Longae (Jiang Huang) 20g
   Radix Salviae Miltiorrhizae (Dan Shen) 15g
   Rhizoma Ligusticum (Chuan Xiong) 9g
   Radix Glycyrrhizae (Gan Cao) 6g
   Radix Ledebouriellae Sesloidis (Fang Feng) 9g
   Rhizoma Atractylodes (Cang Zhu) 9g
   Rhizoma Atractylodes Macrocephalae (Bai Zhu) 6g

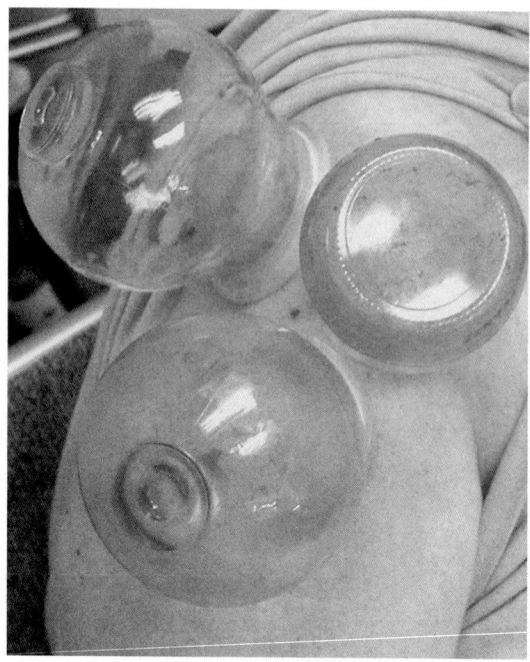

Figure 11-45: Cupping used to treat subdeltoid bursitis.

   Poria Cocus (Fu Ling) 15g
   Rhizoma Alismatis (Ze Xie) 9g
   Semen Coicis (Yi Yi Ren) 25g
   Lumbricus (Di Long) 9g
   Scolopendra Subspinipes (Wu Gong) 6g
   Herba cum Radix Asari (Xi Xin) 5g
   Moschus Moschiferi (She Xiang) 0.1

An empirical *guiding* topical or oral formula for lower body bursitis is:

   Radix Stephaniae (Fang Ji) 15g
   Semen Coix (Yi Yi Ren) 25g
   Semen Plantaginis (Che Qian Zi) 15g
   Herba Plantaginis (Che Qian Cao) 20g
   Semen Sinapis Albae (Bai Jie Zi) 12g
   Aconitum Carmichaeli (Chuan Wu Tou) 6g
   Aconitum Kusnezoffii (Cao Wu Tou) 6g
   Herba cum Radix Asari (Xi Xin) 5g
   Lumbricus (Di Long) 9g
   Scolopendra Subspinipes (Wu Gong) 6g
   Radix Angelicae Pubescentis (Du Huo) 12g
   Achyranthes Bidentata (Niu Xi) 12g
   Fructus Lycii (Gou Qi Zi) 9g
   Flos Carthami (Hong Hua) 9g
   Moschus Moschiferi (She Xiang) 0.1

---

100. It is this author's experience that the *acute variety* of shoulder bursitis does not respond quickly enough to TCM methods, and a local injection of steroids is suggested. This can resolve the *severe* pain quickly, which otherwise may last for a week or two. Also, palpable heat is often seen in acute cases and cooling herbs and Tripterygium Wilfordii (Lei Gong Teng) can be used with some benefit. When bursitis is seen with inflammatory arthritis (acute or chronic) cooling herbs and Tripterygium Wilfordii (Lei Gong Teng) can be used and is beneficial in many cases.

101. In the elderly there is usually degenerative malnourishment of sinews and accumulation of Pathogenic Factors. Combined attacking and tonifying methods may be needed.

Painful Obstruction (Bi) Syndromes

In Chinese Medicine the word "Bi" has many meanings, and it may indicate the presence of Pathogenic Factors blocking the limbs, channels, collaterals/network-vessels and/or Organs. The phrase "Bi or Painful Obstructive Syndromes (which has also been translated as: "Obstructive syndromes," "Impediment patterns," or "Rheumatic patterns") describes painful disorders including muscular and bony disorders. Painful Obstruction (Bi) syndrome describes biomedical disorders such as: rheumatic diseases, painful local and systemic inflammatory conditions (rheumatoid arthritis, lupus etc.), painful soft tissue disorders, painful metabolic disorders, painful neural disorders, and some traumatic injuries. In general, *inflammatory disorders* fit most closely the syndromes characterized in TCM as Wind-Damp-Cold (or Heat), while degenerative conditions (osteoarthritis/arthrosis/DJD) more closely fit syndromes of Liver/Kidney-deficiency and Blood-Phlegm-stasis causing degenerative weakness, stiffness, and pain.[102] However, clinically, Painful Obstruction Syndromes are complex and *multiple* patterns are often the rule. Pathogenic Factors may include: Wind, Cold, Heat, Dampness, Phlegm and Blood-stasis. Other bodily functions such as Qi, Blood, Yin, Yang, Kidney, Liver and Spleen/pancreas are often affected, and Deficiency-Excess mixed patterns are common as well. There is often general weakness, disharmony of Organs with Pathogenic Factors, and/or generation of Bi-disease from abnormalities of the Defensive and Nutritive-Qi.[103] Therefore, many of the formulas that have been developed to treat Painful Obstruction (Bi) syndromes are composed of herbs with opposite natures: hot and cold, supporting and attacking, surface resolving and deep penetrating, etc. Careful assessment of symptoms and signs is needed to ascertain which pathogens are primary and which are secondary or tertiary and their relationships.

The *Classic of Internal Medicine/Simple Questions* devoted an entire chapter to Bi syndromes (Painful Obstruction) and Bi is related in this classic to external Pathogenic Factors, mostly Wind, Cold, and Dampness, with Dampness being at the center of the complex.[104] Both external and internal Heat and Deficiency syndromes are described. Clinically, endogenous and exogenous factors are often seen at the same time. Painful Obstructive disorders have been further elaborated throughout the history of TCM and were given names such as: *moving/Wind-Bi, painful/Cold-Bi, burning/Hot-Bi, fixed/Damp-Bi, inflexible/Liver-Bi, bone/Kidney-Bi, sinew/Liver-Bi, muscle/flesh-Spleen-Bi, blood/vessel/Heart-Bi, skin/Lung-Bi, multiple-Bi*, and several Deficient type Bi syndromes. According to Li Gong Zuo, Sinew-Bi is similar to Wind-Bi; Vessel-Bi is equivalent to Heat-Bi; Muscle-Bi is intimately related to Damp-Bi; Skin-Bi may be classified into moving/Wind-Bi and Heat-Bi (Cheung 1998).

These categories of Bi syndromes describe not only the affected tissues but also a pattern of symptoms. For example, *The Systematic Classic of Acupuncture & Moxibustion* states:

> The Yellow Emperor asked: Circulatory Bi travels around the body upwards and downward, following the [affected] channel up and down. [It attacks] the left and right sides at the corresponding places with no intermission. I would like to learn where this pain lies, in the blood vessels or in the partings of the flesh, and how it comes about in this way. It moves [so swiftly] that there is no time for one to insert the needle, and the time it takes for the pain to build up is [so brief] that it has come to an [abrupt] stop before a treatment is decided upon. What causes it to behave in such a way?

> Qi Bo answered: This is multiple Bi rather than circulatory Bi. [The pains] are fixed in location, alternately erupting and then ceasing in succession, with the left responding to the right and the right to the left. However, [the Bi] is incapable of moving, only starting and stopping [in a fixed location]. To needle this, treat the painful place even once then pain there will cease in order to prevent it from recurring...

> ...Circulatory Bi lies within the blood vessels, following the vessels up and following the vessels down, but it does not travel from left to the right or vice versa, nor does it have a fixed location. For pain travelling from above to below, one must first needle points below to thwart it and then needle points above to eliminate it. As for the pain travelling from below to the above, one must first needle points above to thwart it and then needle points below to eliminate it...

> ...Bi that lies within the bone causes heaviness. If it lies in the vessels, it causes congestion and failure of Blood flow. If it lies in the sinews, it results in the ability to contract but inability to stretch. If it lies in the flesh, it causes insensitivity. If it lies in the skin, it causes Cold. In the case of any of these five patterns, there is no pain. Any type of Bi may give rise to hypertonicity when coming in contact with Cold, and to slackness when coming in contact with Heat.

In the *Classic of Internal Medicine* (*Simple Questions*), Bi syndromes affecting the sinews and bones are also described as difficult to cure, suggesting that Bi syndromes presented a clinical challenge at the time. Characteristically, at the onset, Painful Obstruction (Bi) syndromes are mani-

---

102. Some sources state that in order to qualify as a Bi-syndrome, there must be combined Wind-Damp-Cold pathogens. There may be a predominance of one, but all three must be involved.

103. To treat the Nutritive-Qi, in Bi-syndromes, bleeding techniques are often used, while to treat the Defense-Qi, regular needling is used often. Bi-disease in the Nutritive-Qi is characterized by Cold and Heat, diminished Qi, and disharmonious flow of Blood up and down. Bi-disease generated in the Defense-Qi is characterized by Qi pain that intermittently comes and goes, oppression and fullness, and strong borborygmus due to Wind-Cold encroaching upon the Stomach and Intestines (*The Systematic Classic of Acupuncture & Moxibustion*).

104. Interestingly the biomedical word "rheumatism" is derived from the term "rheum" which means phlegm and watery secretion.

fested as pain, soreness, numbness, and impaired movement. Numb-like sensation is often said to be due to Qi/Blood-deficiency or Cold-Bi, while true numbness (lack of sensation) *may* be more due to chronicity and deep penetration with Damp-Phlegm and Blood-damage, or stasis, causing malnutrition of the skin, which may also lead to painless numbness. In general, numbness is caused by:

- Congested Pathogenic Factors (especially Phlegm and Blood) which block the network-vessels;
- Righteous-Qi blocked and "hidden" by pathogens;
- Spleen/pancreas-Qi that is Hot and Stomach is Dry damaging Yin-Fluids;
- Defensive and Nutritive aspects that are depleted and cannot flow.

Painful Obstruction and Pathogenic Factors affect Qi and Blood circulation (and Nutritive and Defensive-Qi functions), and with time result in disruption of nourishment to the sinews—numbness and weakness may ensue, and *Atrophy/Wilting* syndromes may develop. Patients with "rough and coarse" skin and weak muscles are said to have a tendency to contract Bi-diseases. At the onset, Painful Obstruction (Bi) syndromes affect mainly the channels. However, if not treated effectively, Painful Obstruction can affect the Organs and even become fatal. For example, unresolved *vessel* Bi is said to be capable of affecting the Heart (Heart or chest Bi), and to cause symptoms of irritability with epigastric throbbing ("below the Heart," CV-14 or Heart Alarm point), rebellious-Qi (rising of Qi, panting, and pressure in the chest) and fear, as commonly seen with heart disease.[105]

The *Classic of Internal Medicine* says:

> The five Yin Organs are related to the five tissues where a chronic disease can settle in. In bone Bi syndrome the pathogenic factor reaches the Kidneys; in sinew Bi syndrome it reaches the Liver; in Blood vessel Bi syndrome it reaches the Heart; in muscle Bi syndrome it reaches the Spleen; and in skin Bi syndrome it reaches the Lungs.

Therefore, any prolonged Bi of an associated tissue will eventually affect the Organ associated with it. Many Organ Bi and polyarthralgia syndromes may correspond to systemic biomedical disorders such as: chronic or acute rheumatic fever, rheumatoid arthritis, psoriatic arthritis, lupus, gout, and lyme disease, among others.[106]

Theoretically, Exterior Painful Obstruction (Bi) disorder is mainly caused by exposure to adverse environmental conditions such as dampness, cold or wind. The Pathogenic Factors (Die-Qi, Wind-Cold-Damp) are said to jointly enter the body mostly via the pores, entering the Yang channels and then penetrating the deeper channel and vessel systems.

Characteristically, the acute type has a quick and progressive on-set which begins with symptoms associated usually with external Wind, Cold, and Damp (superficial/Exterior syndromes)—or viral and infectious-like disease. Clinically, however, unless the symptoms are clearly inflammatory, patients with arthritic or other pain syndromes (even in acute onset) only occasionally convey such a history. This may be due to lack of awareness (or slower onset) and may be explained by an *expansion* of the theory of latent pathogenic factor: pathogens enter deeply due to weak antipathogenic-Qi without causing a superficial syndrome. When there is exogenous-Wind attack, if the patient's anti-Pathogenic Factors are strong, a simple Exterior syndrome should develop and the condition should resolve without development of a Bi syndrome. If, however, there are other complicating factors, pathogens may lurk and Obstruction can develop.[107]

In general, Painful Obstructive (Bi) syndromes are said to develop in patients with constitutional weakness or when Defensive-Qi is weak or the surface is open while sweating. Parasitic or Warm-diseases can infect patients regardless of constitution or state of anti-pathogenic forces. Even in Hot-type arthralgias, the majority of traditional discussion was in terms Wind-Damp-Cold disease, which transforms into Heat (Huo-Hua) or into Damp-Heat.[108] Cold, Wind, and Dampness can cause stagnation or slowing of circulation within the channels and network-vessels and may then transform into Heat or Damp-Heat. Or a pre-existing internal-Heat may combine with external or internal Wind-Damp-Cold pathogens to become a mixed Cold and Hot syndrome. Patients with Yang-deficiency constitution are susceptible to the effects of windy, cold, and damp environments and tend to develop Cold-Damp Bi-syndromes. Patients with Yang-fullness or deficient-Yin constitution are susceptible to the effects of windy, damp, dry, and warm environments and tend to develop Damp-Heat Bi-syndromes. Patient with Kidney-Yin-deficiency are especially susceptible to latent/hidden Pathogenic Factors.[109] Retained or lurking Pathogenic Factors are often a result of stressful lifestyles that suppress immunity/anti-pathogenic forces.[110]

The magnitude and resolution of pain often reflects the relative strength and struggle between Pathogenic Factors

---

105. Recently, an infectious and/or inflammatory origin to cardiovascular disease has been suggested by modern biomedicine as well.

106. Polyarthralgia is a variety of conditions that can result in multiple joint pains, swelling, and possibly joint deformity.

107. Recently, infectious agents other than acute bacterial infections have been associated with rheumatoid arthritis (RA), lyme disease, and possibly osteoarthritis. For example, epidemiologic findings support the idea that HTLV-I infection is a risk factor for RA. These findings suggest that approximately 13% of the cases of RA in females living in Nagasaki are associated with HTLV-I infection [Eguchi, Origuchi, Takashima, Iwata, Katamine and Nagataki 1996.] Minocycline—an antibiotic—can be effective in about 50% of patients with RA if started early in the course of the Disease [O'Dell 1998]. Mycoplasma has been associated with both inflammatory and non-inflammatory arthritis. Of course, lyme, several enterically associated arthritic disorders, viral arthritic disorders (from hepatitis, mononucleosis and rubella) and gonococcal arthritis are infectious.

108. Possibly influenced by the eighteen hundred year-old classic *On Cold Damage.*

109. Symptomless until pathogens surface due to stress or new Exterior syndrome.

110. With retained Pathogenic Factors the patient feels ill for an unusual duration; the Pathogenic Factors as well as the patient are often weak.

and Righteous-Qi (anti-Pathogenic Factors). In healthy people whose anti-pathogenic-Qi is strong, a "battle" takes place in the Exterior layers between the Pathogenic Factors and the Defensive and Righteous Qis. The pathogens often reach only the outer Tai-Yang, or possibly only the Shao-Yang (intermediate) channels and tend to not affect deeper tissues. The pain will be relatively acute and moderately strong.

In cases where the anti-Pathogenic Factors are weak and/or the patient is feeble or old, the pathogens may enter deeply into the network-vessels, tissues, and Organs. First the muscles and joints will be affected, but with time *skin-obstruction* will affect the Lungs, *vessel-obstruction* the Heart, *sinew-obstruction* the Liver, *muscle/flesh-obstruction* the Spleen, and *bone-obstruction the Kidneys*. Often the pain will be milder and Deficient in character, but chronic. A more complex *mix* syndrome is then the rule.

Thus, in general, Excess/Full pain in Bi syndromes is associated mostly with Pathogenic Factors and impairment of free-flow of Qi and Blood in the channels and vessels, while Deficient/Empty pain is associated mostly with the malnourishment of sinews, muscles, and bones from insufficiency of Qi and Blood, and is often associated with Kidney and Liver Organ weakness.

Constitutional patterns seen in TCM (usually related to Organ diagnosis) can be developed into a differential diagnosis based on Painful Obstruction (Bi) etiology and further analysis of key pathologic factors: Wind, Damp, Cold, Heat, and Stasis/Congestion.

- *Wind* often refers to the sudden onset, mobility, and variability of symptoms. Wind-dominant arthralgia affects first the upper body and corresponds mostly to the *early stages* of arthritis. Internal-Wind can result in severe pain, tightness, spasms, and headaches, and is not often related to early-stage arthritis. Internal-Wind can be caused by Deficiency (mostly of Yin and Blood) or stirred by extreme-Heat. To treat combined internal and external Wind, herbs that address both may be needed, and, especially in chronic cases, so-called herbs that "track" Wind are used. Stiffness and rigidity caused by Liver-Wind is seen especially in the elderly.

- *Dampness* refers to the worsening of the symptoms in damp weather, the *initiation* of the disease, or the worsening of symptoms after exposure to damp environments, and the accumulation of Fluid. Dampness-dominated arthralgia affects most often the lower parts of the body and is said to be characterized by *heaviness*, swelling; stiffness, and the *feeling of being bound up* in the joints, limbs, chest, or head. Numbness is said to result from Dampness obstructing Qi and Blood, especially when congealed into Phlegm. Dampness-dominated syndromes are said to correspond often to a *middle stage* of arthritis; however, external-Dampness can be an etiological factor in early stages as well. Dampness and Phlegm can also refer to the contraction and limitation of the movements of the joint due to an obstructing of the sinews and muscles. It refers to swelling as well.[111] While Cold-Dampness is usually thought of as being the most common cause of Painful Obstruction syndromes, Dan-xi said, "Of the six Qi (Pathogenic Factors), disease caused by Damp-Heat amounts to eight or nine out of ten cases."[112]

- *Cold* often refers to the *degree* of pain and stiffness, and to the initiation and worsening of symptoms with exposure to cold; improvement by the application of heat; and impaired circulation with feeling cold, or with cold extremities. Cold is associated also with interior-Cold (mostly Kidney-Yang-deficiency) and aging. Cold-dominated arthritis affects the extremities (hands and feet) where circulation is poorest. Interior-Cold is associated often with the lower back and knees (Kidneys), and then is commonly seen in *arthrosis* (DJD) and back pain.

- *Hot*-type-arthralgia may be initiated by exposure to a hot environment (especially summer-Heat) and then manifest as pain with redness and Heat of the joints. It can also result from Cold and Dampness transforming into Heat or Damp-Heat. Heat-dominated arthritis may be seen in both *early* and *late* stages of arthritis (and can be traumatic as well).[113] Internal-Heat is often due to Empty-Heat from Yin/Blood-deficiency, or from congested/transformative-Heat (depressive-Heat) secondary to stagnation and stasis from Deficiency or Excess. *Rapid-onset* of Heat dominated arthralgias, usually without Exterior symptoms and signs, may result from lurking pathogens, especially Spring-Wind. It is also important to realize that for example: Blood-stasis, Yin/Blood-deficiency, or severe Yang-deficiency can all result in Heat and feverish symptoms.

- *Blood* is said to become static when the disease is chronic and enduring. Eventually the initiating factors (e.g., Wind or Dampness) become less dominant, and *mixed* Deficiency and Excess (and mixed Blood-stasis and Phlegm) are more dominant. When treating chronic and advanced diseases there may be more emphasis on dispersing static-Blood than when treating an earlier and more *variable* phase of the disease. Wind-Dampness tends to vary while Blood-stasis is fixed and enduring.

In summary, Painful Obstruction (Bi) syndromes are generally divided into three major stages:

1. *Exterior/Superficial stage*. Pathogenic Factors affect the channels, and symptoms and signs are moderately acute/new. If the patient is strong, the syndrome will resolve, often on its own.

2. *Intermediate stage*. There is more involvement of bodily tissues, with symptoms and signs becoming more severe and chronic, or recurrent. The patient's Righteous-Qi

---

111. Joint effusion is often responsible for limited movements in arthritic joints.
112. This statement pertains to Dampness in general, not to Painful Obstruction Syndromes.

(anti-Pathogenic Factors) is weak, or Pathogenic Factors are strong.

3. *Deep stage*. Organ and Righteous-Qi in general have been strongly affected; there is gross tissue deformation, and symptoms and signs are chronic, often milder (but may be severe with *exacerbations*) and usually difficult to resolve. The patient is generally Deficient (although the Deficiency may be difficult to demonstrate and therefore should not be assumed); the Pathogenic Factors stagnate and result in proliferation of tissues and complex syndromes. Atrophy may be setting in.

Treatment of Bi Syndrome

Treatment of Painful Obstruction (Bi) syndromes (musculoskeletal disorders) in TCM generally includes both internal (herbal) and external (acupuncture, heat, and manual) therapies. Treatment is generally aimed at expelling Pathogenic Factors and mobilizing *obstructed or stagnant* Qi and Blood. Since Deficiency may be at the root, herbal treatments that nourish the Blood, harmonize the Defensive and Nutritive-Qi, warm the Yang, and treat underlying Organic disorders are often integrated.

Manual therapies are important, and, in the text *On the Origin and Further Course of Medicine,* Hsu writes:

> If evil [influences] have entered the sinews, the bones, the muscles or the flesh, then the illness [resulting from this intrusion] is a morphological one, and the [thermo] influences and flavor [influences] of drugs will show no effect.[114] Hence [in such cases] one must apply [therapeutic] methods such as needling and cauterization...As long as they [the illness] flow through the [main] conduits and the network [vessels], as well as through the viscera and bowels, there is no other way to eliminate them except through the intake of drugs.

As we can see, according to Hsu, when disease affects *form* and *structure*, herbal medicine may not be sufficient. In the *Classic of Internal Medicine,* acupuncture is mentioned much more frequently than herbal medicine as treatment of choice for difficult Painful Obstruction.[115] Acupuncture using the Divergent channels and other manual therapies are then important. Hsu also recommends using external ointments, spooning (scraping; Gua Sha), and soaking to treat accumulations, Blood-stasis, and when the illness "assumes" a physical shape. Herbal therapy often involves:

- Expelling Pathogenic Factors: Wind, Cold, Damp, Phlegm, Blood-stasis, Heat, or cooling Hot-Blood.
- Regulating local tissues: relaxing sinews, vitalizing or regulating network-vessels and Blood, softening masses, dispersing entanglements, and moving Qi and Blood to arrest pain.
- Supporting Righteous-Qi and bodily functions: fortifying Spleen/pancreas, moistening Yin and nourishing Blood, warming the Kidneys and assisting Yang, tonifying the Liver and Kidneys and invigorating the sinews and bones.

Treatment of Painful Obstruction According to TCM Pattern Diagnosis

The following discussion covers commonly seen clinical presentations which often consist of mixed clinical patterns. Integration of these TCM treatments is often helpful in the management of musculoskeletal disorders. The herbal formulas on their own may be insufficient clinically. Painful Obstruction (Bi) Syndromes (musculoskeletal) are due in general to *external* pathogenic Wind, Cold, Damp, and/or Heat which obstruct the channels and collaterals/network-vessels, causing blockage of Qi and Blood circulation. Bi syndromes manifest as pain, soreness, aching, numbness or heaviness of muscles, sinews, and joints, and/or swelling and burning pain.

While theoretical simple classifications are found in text books (e.g., Cold-Bi, Wind-Bi, Damp-Bi, Hot-Bi), in reality distinct diagnostic classifications are difficult to make and are seldom seen in the clinic. Identifying the inter-relationships of the various possible patterns is most important. Flexibility in treatment and timing is essential. Herbal and acupuncture medicine can be helpful in the treatment of articular and soft-tissue rheumatological disorders. The *Classic of Internal Medicine* states:

---

113. Many of the author's patients with Bi syndromes have some type of Heat complicating their patterns. These include Wind-Heat, Damp-Heat, stagnation/depressive-Heat, Blood-stasis- Qi-stagnation-transformative-Heat (or lurking pathogens), and Blood-Heat. Because these can be seen with underlying Cold and Deficiency, care must be taken when designing herbal formulas. If stasis and/or Heat is secondary to a root condition of Deficiency (often Kidney-Yang, Yin and Yang, or Qi) it may be necessary to place emphasis on tonification or neutral formulation. Zhu Liang-chun recommends, in complex syndromes when there is obstinate Painful Obstruction, the use of Herba Epimedii (Yin Yang Huo), 15g, Rhizoma Curculiginis Orchioidis (Xian Mao), 10g, Fructus Lycii Chinensis (Gou Qi Zi), 10g, Placenta Hominis (Zi He Che), 6g, and Radix Glycyrrhizae (Gan Cao), 5g to strengthen the Kidneys (and treat the root disorder) so that Evil and Righteous can be separated (Bi). He states that because the patient is often already Yang-Qi-deficient and debilitated, the disease evils (pathogens) lodge in the channels and network-vessels blocking Qi and Blood. The pathogens/evils may sink and enter the bone marrow (i.e., deep aspects or Kidney sphere as they are already weak), becoming fixed and unremovable. Phlegm and stasis join and obstruct, congeal, and stagnate influencing Qi and Blood (and stagnation can easily transform into Heat). Evil and Righteous become like mixed oil and flour, and swelling and pain become chronic. Therefore, there is an aspect of Righteous-deficiency as well as of evil (pathogenic) excess to this condition, even when there are *Exterior* signs and joint swelling (Wan 2000).

114. This shows that the idea of pathology versus functional dysfunction may have been understood, and explains why TCM is usually more effective in functional disorders.

115. Throughout most of recorded Chinese medical history, herbal medicine has been considered the mainstay therapy in Chinese medicine. During the Han period, when "natural laws" were integrated into medicine (as described in the *Classic of Internal Medicine*), acupuncture discussion dominated the Confucian literature.

When needling Painful Obstruction (Bi) syndromes, first one has to palpate the six channels below and observe Emptiness and Fullness, [to see] whether Blood-stasis is in the big (Main) network-vessels and if [the vessel] is obstructed in its flow, [or whether there is] Emptiness with the pulse being entrapped and empty. Harmonizing is done by restoring the connection (freeing the flow) using [the] hot pack [method].[116]

For all of these reasons, close examination of the patient's condition is always important before initiating a treatment protocol. The treatment of pain in TCM is predicated most often on the saying, "If there is free flow there is no pain." Therefore, formulas and treatments that restore flow are used.

All herbal formulas in the following section are used regularly by the author. They are derived from the formulary of Guangzhou Municipal Hospital, physicians in that hospital, general literature, and the author's experience. Commentary regarding physical findings reflects the author's experience. Finally, it is the author's experience that patients with a history of a sudden onset of *nontraumatic* articular pain (which may have occurred just before an examination or some time previously) often suffer from syndromes in which Cinnamon Twig, Peony and Anemarrhena Decoction (Gui Zhi Shao Yao Zhi Mu Tang) can be used as a guiding formula, and which can be modified for predominance of Wind, Cold, Heat, Dampness, or stasis.[117] If the onset of articular pain is more insidious, a close analysis of the patient with a view to the predominance of Deficiency or Pathogenic Factors is important.

Wind-Dampness

Articular and soft tissue syndromes are often said to be variations of Wind-Damp Obstruction. In its pure personation, this pattern is usually seen in the beginning stages of the disease. Patients may suffer from joint pains that increase with changing weather, and during rainy days. When there is a predominance of Wind, there would be migrating joint pains. Under this condition, it is common to add Blood herbs to Painful Obstruction Wind formulas, because it is said that "to treat Wind," one should "first treat Blood." Depending on the patient's constitution, Organ health, other Pathogenic Factors, and anatomical variations, symptoms and signs can vary. Depending on severity and acuteness, soft tissue and joint end-feels may range from normal to slightly tight and limited. Since this pattern is more common in the beginning stages of Painful Obstruction (especially with Wind predominance), it is not uncommon to see fairly normal joints and muscles. A patient with Wind-Damp pathogens may show a thick, white tongue coat. Other patients may have a swollen tongue with a thin white coat. The pulse may be slow, slippery, wiry, or soft. A representative formula is Remove Painful Obstruction (Juan Bi Tong) which can be used with the appropriate variations given below.

> Radix et Rhizoma Notopterygii (Qiang Huo) 9g
> Radix Angelicae Pubescentis (Du Huo) 9g
> Radix Gentianae (Qin Jiao) 12g
> Ramulus Mori (Sang Zhi) 12g
> Caulis Piperis (Hai Feng Teng) 12g
> Radix Angelica Sinensis (Dang Gui) 9g
> Radix Ligustici (Chuan Xiong) 6g
> Radix Paeoniae Alba (Bai Shao) 15g
> Radix Paeoniae Rubra (Chi Shao) 9g
> Gummi Olibanum (Mo Yao) 3g
> Ramulus Cinnamomi (Gui Zhi) 9g
> Herba cum Radix Asari (Xi Xin) 3g

For severe pain add Zanthoxylum Netidom (Ye Di Jin Niu) 30g.

For predominance of Dampness with increased swollen joints and muscles, fatigue, strong aggravation from weather changes or during cold rainy days use:

> Semen Coicis (Yi Ren) 15g
> Rhizoma Atractylodis (Cang Zhu) 9g
> Radix Stephaniae Tetrandrae (Fang Ji) 12g
> Ramulus Cinnamomi (Gui Zhi) 9g
> Radix Angelicae Pubescentis (Du Huo) 12g
> Caulis Piperis (Hai Feng Teng) 12g
> Radix Angelicae Sinensis (Dang Gui) 12g
> Caulis Akebiae (Mu Tong) 6g
> Radix Astragali (Huang Qi) 15g
> Poriae Cocos (Fu Ling) 15g
> Caulis Spatholobi (Ji Xue Teng) 15g

For severely swollen joints with joint effusion and a capsular pattern of restriction remove: Radix Angelicae Pubescentis (Du Huo), Rhizoma Atractylodis (Cang Zhu), Radix Stephaniae Tetrandrae (Fang Ji). Add: Exocarpium Citri Rubrum (Ju Hong) 9g, Herba Laminariae (Kun Bu) 20g, Semen Sinapis Albae (Bai Jie Zi) 12g, Prepared Rhizoma Arisaematis (Dan Nan Xing) 12g and Spina Gleditsiae (Zao Jiao Ci) 12g.

Acupuncture

Commonly used points and methods are: Sedation techniques at LI-11, 8, 4, TW-5, 10, UB-12, 13, GV-14, 16, GB-20, 31, Lu-7 and Ashi points. Tonification technique at St-36. For predominance of Dampness, use sedation technique at Sp-9, CV-9, Lu-7, GB-34, St-40 with tonification technique at UB-20.

Wind-Damp-Cold

This pattern is most often seen as a progression of the first pattern or in patients with pre-existing Yang-deficiency, but again is rarely seen in its pure presentation. When there is a predominance of Cold, the pain will be more severe than Wind-Damp and may affect the low back and lower extremities (although any joint can be affected). The pain improves with warmth and movement. The tissues feel *tight* and the joints are *stiff* because of the tightening affect of Cold. There

---

116. Hot packs were usually made from cloth bags containing medicinals that have been warmed and applied to the painful area.

117. Ingredients are: Cinnamomi (Gui Zhi) 12g, Ephedrae (Ma Huang) 6g, Aconiti (Fu Zhi) 6-30g, Anemarrhenae (Zhi Mu) 4-20g, Paeoniae (Bai Shao) 12g, Atractylodes (Bai Zhu) 12g, Ledebouriellae (Fang Feng) 12g, Zingiberis (Sheng Jiang) 6g, Glycyrrhizae (Gan Cao) 3g.

is usually little or no swelling, but, if Dampness predominates, there can be swelling and joint effusion. Wind-Damp-Cold is often seen with *arthrosis,* especially in the early stages. Joint end-feel may be normal or hard depending on acuteness and underlying pathology. Since endogenous Cold-Dampness is often accompanied by Spleen or Kidney-Yang-deficiency, the muscles (flesh) and/or bones, or both, may be involved. With Spleen involvement, the patient may have digestive symptoms and pain, mostly in the muscle. When the Kidneys are involved, the bones are affected. Pain is often felt throughout the limbs and deep in the joints and low back. The condition is then usually seen in later stages. The urine may be scanty but clear or profuse and clear. Representative formulas are Prepared Aconite Decoction (Fu Zi Tang), Minor Invigorate the Collaterals Special Pill (Xiao Huo Luo Dan) and Aconite Decoction (Wu Tou Tang) which can be used with the appropriate variations.

> Radix Aconiti Carmichaeli Praeparata (Zhi Chuan Wu) 9-30g[118]
> Radix Aconiti Kusnezoffii Praeparata (Zhi Cao Wu) 9-30g
> Honey-fried Herba Ephedrae (Zhi Ma Huang) 9g
> Ramulus Cinnamomi (Gui Zhi) 12g
> Rhizoma Zingiberis (Gan Jiang) 9g
> Radix Astragali (Huang Qi) 15g
> Poriae Cocos (Fu Ling) 15g
> Rhizoma Dioscoreae Hypoglaucae (Bei Xie) 15g
> Myrrha (Mo Yao) 3g
> Honey-fried Radix Glycyrrhizae (Zhi Gan Cao) 6g

For severe pain add Zanthoxylum Netidom (Ye Di Jin Niu) 30g.

For joint swelling add Rhizoma Artisaematis (Tian Nan Xing) 6g, Semen Coicis (Yi Yi Ren) 30g, and Spina Gleditsiae (Zao Jiao Ci) 12g.

For psoriatic arthritis:

> Radix Astragali (Huang Qi) 20g
> Ramulus Cinnamomi (Gui Zhi) 12g
> Radix et Rhizoma Notopterygii (Qiang Huo) 15g
> Radix Angelica Sinesis (Dang Gui) 15g
> Flos Carthami (Hong Hua) 10g
> Semen Persicae (Tao Ren) 10g
> Radix Gentianae (Qin Jiao) 15g
> Olibanum (Ru Xiang) 9g
> Honey-fried Radix Glycyrrhizae (Zhi Gan Cao) 6g
> Kochiae (Di Fu Zi) 12g
> Zaocys (Wu Shao She) 15g

For Rheumatoid arthritis with a predominance of Cold use:[119]

> Herba Ephedrae (Ma Huang) 4g
> Radix Stephaniae Tetrandrae (Fang Ji) 12g
> Cortex Cinnamomi (Rou Gui) 4g
> Fried Squama Manitis (Chuan Shan Jia) 6g
> Cornu Cervi Degelatinatum (Lu Jiao Shuang) 6g

> Radix Rehmanniae (Shu Di Huang) 30g
> Rhizoma Zingiberis (Gan Jiang) 4g
> Fried Semen Sinapis Albae (Bai Jie Zi) 15g
> Radix Aconiti Lateralis Praeparata (Fu Zi) 15-30g

For painful Swelling, Blood-stasis and ecchymosis add: Rhizoma Curcumae Longae (Jiang Huang) 12g, Rhizoma Zedoriae (E Zhu) 9g, Herba Lycopi (Ze Lan) 15g.

For dry mouth or to prevent side-effects from Aconiti (Fu Zi) add: Cortex Phellodendri (Huang Bai) 12g, Rhizoma Anemarrhenae (Zhi Mu) 15g,[120] Rhizoma Rhei (Da Huang) 6g.

Acupuncture

Acupuncture with moxa can be used. Commonly used points and methods are: Sedation technique at LI-4, TW-5, UB-12, 13, GB-30, 31, 35, St-34 and Ashi points. Moxa at St-36, GV-4, CV-4, 6, UB-20 and GV-14.

Wind-Damp-Cold—Interior Heat

This pattern is commonly seen in the clinic and may present in patients with joint and soft tissue pains and symptoms of Wind-Cold-Damp, but with *signs* such as tongue, lips, eyes, or pulse showing Interior-Heat. These are patients with Exterior Bi-syndromes and excess-Heat internally. Often, Heat is lodged in the Large Intestines and Stomach due to dietary habits or from Liver and Gall Bladder stagnant-Qi with transformative-Heat. This pattern can also be seen in patients with Yin-deficient constitutions. The joints and soft tissues are *not* red, hot, or particularly swollen. The patient's bowels and urine may show signs of Heat. There may be red eyes, mouth sores, red chapped lips, and thirst. There may be hidden pathogens with Exterior Wind-Damp-Cold, especially in patients with weak immune systems (Yin/Yang-deficiency, weak Defensive/antipathogenic-Qi). Depending on acuteness, the soft tissues and joint end-feel may be tight, shortened, normal, or sometimes overly loose and weak. The tongue body may be red, dry, and possibly with a yellow or off-white coat. The pulse may be rapid, overflowing, slippery, or tidal, or may be deep and forceful. This pattern is also said to develop from warm and dry formulas, and/or pharmaceutical drugs, particularly steroid medications. A representative formula is Major Notopterygium Decoction (Da Qiang Huo Tang) which can be used with the appropriate modifications:

> Gypsum (Shi Gao) 25g
> Radix et Rhizome Notopterygii (Qiang Huo) 9g
> Radix Gentianae (Qin Jiao) 12g
> Radix Angelica Pubescentis (Due Huo) 9g
> Radix Clematidis (Wei Ling Xian) 9g
> Radix Ledebouriellae (Fang Feng) 9g
> Radix Rehmanniae Glutinosae (Sheng Di Huang) 15g
> Semen Gardenia (San Zhi Zi) 6g
> Radix Scutellariae (Huang Qin) 9g
> Radix Angelicae Sinesis (Dang Gui) 12g

---

118. Aconiti (Chuan Wu, Cao Wu, and Fu Zi) are often used in very high doses to achieve the desired effect in pain syndromes. They should be cooked for over two hour to reduce their toxicity, especially if used in large doses. To balance their drying effects, high doses of Rehmanniae (Sheng or Shu Di) and Anemarrhenae (Zhi Mu) can be added. If symptoms of Stomach Heat or thirst develop, Shi Gao may be added. At high doses they should be used short-term only.

119. As can be seen the fact that RA is an inflammatory type arthritis does not mean that it is treated with cooling formulas in TCM.

120. Anemarrhenae (Zhi Mu) is an important herb for treating pain as it can clear connecting/network-vessels Heat, nourish Yin, clear Dampness, arrest pain, and calm the patient.

Radix Paeoniae Rubrae (Chi Shao) 9g
Radix Salvia (Dan Shen) 15g
Cortex Moutan Radicis (Mu Dan Pi) 6g
Herba cum Radix Asari (Xi Xin) 3g

For constipation add: Radix et Rhizoma Rhei (Da Huang) 9g

For severe pain add: Radix Paeonia Alba (Bai Shao) 30g, Radix Glycyrrhizae (Gan Cao) 9g

For muscle spasms add: Zaocys Dhumnades (Wu Shao She) 3g, Buthus Martensi (Quan Xie) 3g, Scolopendra Subspinipes (Wu Gong) 3g (note lower doses).

Caulis Spatholobi (Ji Xua Teng) 15g
Flos Lonicerae Japonicae (Jin Yin Hua) 15g
Radix Rehmanniae (Shu Di) 30g
Cortex Dictamni Radicis (Bai Xian Pi) 30g
Fried Semen Sinapis Albae (Bai Jie Pi) 12g
Radix Aconiti Lateralis Praeparata (Fu Zhi) 12g

For strong Heat with elevated ESR add: Rhizoma Smilacis Glabrae (Tu Fu Ling) 15g, Gypsum (Shi Gao) 20g.

For significant Cold with normal ESR add: Herba Ephedrae (Ma Huang) 6g, Herba Asari (Xi Xin) 4g, Herba Cistanches (Rou Cang Rong) 12g, Rhizoma Zingiberis (Gan Jiang) 9g.

Acupuncture

Commonly used points and methods are: Sedation technique at GV-14, LI-11, 4, St-25, UB-12, TW-5, GB-34, SP-9, 10 and Ashi points, followed by tonification at St-36, Sp-6, UB-20.

Acupuncture

Commonly used points and methods are: Sedation technique at LI-11, 4, St-25, TW-5, GB-34, SP-9, 10 and Ashi points, followed by tonification at St-36, Sp-6, UB-20, 23.

Cold or Deficiency Transforming Into Heat

This pattern is also commonly seen and may present in patients that are generally Deficient or whose Interior is Cold. Both Deficients and Interior Coldness can result in poor vitality of body milieu leading to accumulations-transformation-Heat. It may be difficult to ascertain if Deficiency of transformation-Heat is predominant. Often Heat signs may obscure the underlying Deficiency. The patient is often restless, slightly thirsty, or just complains of dryness, weakness, evening fevers (a feeling of warmth) and may have night sweats. The pain is often mild to moderate and becomes worse after activity, possibly accompanied by heat symptoms and signs, but may improve with heat application as well. The tongue and lips are dry and possibly red. The pulse tends to be thready and rapid. A modification of Angelicae Sinesis Pluck Pain Decoction (Dang Gui Nian Tong Tang) may be used:

Radix Angelicae Sinesis (Dang Gui) 9g
Rhizoma seu Radix Notopterygii (Qiang Huo) 9g
Wine prepared Radix Sophorae (Ku Shen) 9g
Radix Puerariae (Ge Gen) 9g
Rhizoma Atractylodis (Cang Zhu) 9g
Radix Atractylodis Alba (Bai Zhu) 9g
Radix Ledebouriellae (Fang Feng) 9g
Rhizoma Anemarrhenae (Zhi Mu) 9g
Cortex Phelodendri (Huang Bai) 6g
Rhizoma Alismatis (Ze Xie) 9g
Rhizoma Cimicifugae (Sheng Ma) 3g
Radix Ginseng (Ren Shen) 3g
Herba Artemisiae Capillaris 15g
Radix Achyranthis Bidentatae (Huai Niu Xi) 9g

For Rheumatoid arthritis with mixed Heat and Cold, from Cold transforming into Heat (or exterior Cold interior Heat), and internal confinement of Damp-Toxins, seen in either the acute or chronic stages with severe pain, rigidity and/or joint deformity use:

Wine prepared Rhizoma Rhei (Da Huang) 6g
Squama Manitis (Chuan Shan Jia) 6g
Spina Gleditsiae (Zao Jiao Ci) 15g
Radix Stemonae (Bai Bu) 24g
Cortex Cinnamomi (Rou Gui) 4g

Wind-Damp-Cold—Chronic Disease—Blood-stasis, Qi-stagnation

This pattern is one of the most commonly seen in clinical practice and presents in patients with chronic painful arthralgias. The pain patterns are mixed, showing characteristics of Wind-Damp-Cold and Blood-stasis-Qi-stagnation. Often the patient shows signs of Deficiency as well. Since chronic disease often results in Blood-stasis, and since it is said: "to treat Wind first, treat Blood...when Blood moves, Wind resolves," Blood moving herbs are added, especially with a history of trauma or in chronic disease—with or without clear signs of Blood-stasis (i.e., pulse tongue signs). Because Qi moves the Blood and Qi and Blood are mutually dependent, herbs that regulate Qi are added as well. It is important to remember that this pattern may be seen in patients with or without *clear signs* of Blood-stasis (tongue and pulse) and/or with or without fixed pain. Soft tissues are often hardened (fibrous) and less flexible. There are signs of long-term hypoxia. Muscular and tendinous triggers have a more defined edge that can be palpated and often feel hard. Joint end-feels are often hard and may or not be painful. This pattern is sometimes seen in patients with instability as well. Joint end-feels are then often hard and ROM may be abnormally increased or decreased. There are often painful twinges and sudden, transient loss of strength. The following type of formula can be used in patients with Painful Obstruction (Bi) syndrome that has not responded to Wind-Damp obstruction formulas and/or chronic Cold type formulas. The representative formula is Drive Out Blood Stasis from a Painful Body Decoction (Shen Tong Zhu Yu Tong), which can be used with the appropriate modification. If used topically vinegar can be added:

Radix Gentianae (Qin Jiao) 12g
Rhizoma Ligustici Wallichii (Chuan Xiang) 9g
Semen Persicae (Tao Ren) 9g
Exrementum Trogopteri seu Pteromi (Wu Ling Zhi) 12g
Rhizoma Corydalis (Yan Hu Suo) 12g
Rhizoma et Radix Notopterygii (Qiang Hou) 6g
Radix Angelica Dahuricae (Bai Zhi) 9g
Radix Clematidis (Wei Ling Xian) 9g

Radix Angelica Sinensis (Dang Gui) 9g
Radix Paeoniae Rubrae (Chi Shao) 9g
Radix Salvia (Dan Shen) 15g
Cortex Moutan Radicis (Mu Dan Pi) 6g
Herba cum Radix Asari (Xi Xin) 3g
Myrrha (Mo Yao) 3g
Lumbricus (Di Long) 9g
Rhizoma Cyperi (Xiang Fu) 9g
Radix Astragali (Huang Qi) 15g
Radix Cyathulae Officinalis (Chuan Niu Xi) 9g

For symptoms of muscle spasms or cramps, add: Agkistrodon (Bai Hua She) 6g, Scolopendra (Wu Gong) 3g, Buthus Martensi (Quan Xie) 5g, Radix Paeoniae (Bai Shao) 20g.

Acupuncture

Commonly used points and methods are: Sedation technique at UB-17, 18, 57, Sp-10, 8, LI-11, 4, 15, TW-11, GB-41 and Ashi points. After sedation, the same points are moxaed with direct-skin moxa or by warming the needles. For deficiency add: Sp-6, UB-23, 20, GV-4, CV-17.

Another common combination is GV-14, 12, 11 and two extra points 4-finger breadths lateral to GV-12, and two extra points 4-finger breadths lateral to GV-11. Bleeding and cupping UB-43 is helpful as well.

Wind-Phlegm-Obstruction—Chronic Disease/ Numbness

While Phlegm is said to be quite common, this pattern is seen mostly when neural involvement results in numbness. The pattern is seen when puffy swelling, numbness, tremors, and possibly itchiness are predominant. Phlegm usually results from constitutional weakness of the Spleen/pancreas, or from dietary irregularities that damage the digestive functions of the Spleen and Stomach. Phlegm can also arise from Heat or Cold congealing Fluids and from Qi-stagnation that fails to move Fluids. Phlegm obstruction can block Nutritive-Qi and Blood with resulting numbness and swelling. Other symptoms such as light headedness, dizziness, vertigo, chest discomfort, or nausea may or may not be seen. Soft tissues and joint capsules are often nodular, soft with very sensitive subcutaneous tissues as demonstrated by skin-rolling (page 217). Nodules are moveable but may feel hard. The muscles in general lack tone. Joint end-feels may be hard or soggy, depending on the amount of effusion and may or may not be painful. The tongue may be dark and swollen, and its coat may be greasy. The pulse may be wiry, slippery, or soft. A representative formula is Pinellia, Atractylodis Macrocephalae, and Gastrodia Decoction (Ban Xia Bai Zhu Tian Ma Tang) and can be used with the following variations:

Rhizoma Pinellia (Ban Xia) 9g
Rhizoma Gastrodiae (Tian Ma) 9g
Rhizoma Artsiaematis (Tian Nan Xing) 9g
Rhizoma Atractylodis Alba (Bai Zhu) 9g
Poriae Cocos (Fu Ling) 15g
Rhizoma Zingiberis (Sheng Jiang) 6g
Pericarpium Citri Erythrocarpae (Ju Hong) 6g
Fructus Zizyphi Jujubae (Da Zao) 4g
Radix Ledebouriellae (Fang Feng) 6g
Rhizoma Acrori Graminei (Shi Chang Pu) 6g
Radix Clematidis (Wei Ling Xian) 9g
Herba Artemisiae (Yin Chen Hao) 12g

For symptoms consisting of muscle spasms, add: Agkistrodon (Bai Hua She) 5g, Buthus Martensi (Quan Xie) 4g, Scolopendra Subspinipes (Wu Gong) 3g.

For severe pain, add: Zanthoxylum Netidom (Ye Di Jin Niu) 30g.

For joint swelling or nodules, add: Semen Coicis (Yi Yi Ren) 30g, Bulbus Fritillariae Thunbergii (Zhe Bei Mu) 15g, Concha Ostreae (Mu Li) 20g.

For pronounced numbness, add: Radix Paeoniae Rubrae (Chi Shao) 9g, Radix Ligustici (Chuan Xiang) 9g, Radix Angelica Sinensis (Dang Gui) 9g, and Folium Clerodendri Trichotomi (Chou Wu Tong) 9g.

Acupuncture

Commonly used points and methods are: Sedation technique followed by moxa at St-40, 36, UB-13, 43, 20, 59, CV-12, GV-3 and Ashi points. Sedation technique at GB-20, 31, 33, 38, Lu-7, LI-4, 11, TW-5. Tonification technique at St-36, UB-20.

Qi-Stagnation-Cold

This pattern is quite common and presents mainly in patients with morning pain or with *posain*. Soon after the patient gets up from bed and moves, as warmth and nourishment return to tissues, the pain *disappears or is greatly reduced* at the affected joint *until the next morning,* or until a posture is again maintained for a prolonged period. Often the patient can perform most daily activities pain free (or with mild pain), as is commonly seen in self-reducing disc with morning low back pain. The patient may or may not show other symptoms of Qi-stagnation and Cold. Joint and soft tissues are often cold and contracted *only* during symptomatic periods. During symptomatic periods, joint end-feel may be hard (or just tight) and may or may not be painful. Some patients with morning pain who also suffer from pain that is worse after heavy exertion (especially fixed back pain) may have "Kidney-taxation pain." A representative formula is Modified Minor Invigorate the Collaterals Special Pill (Jia Wei Xiao Huo Luo Dan) and can be used with the following variations:

Radix Aconiti Carmichaeli Praeparata (Zhi Chuan Wu) 9g
Radix Aconiti Kusnezoffii Praeparata (Zhi Cao Wu) 9g
Ramulus Cinnamomi (Gui Zhi) 12g
Fructus Alpiniae Oxyphylae (Yi Zhi Ren) 9g
Rhizoma Cypri (Xiang Fu) 9g
Radix Lindrae (Wu Yao) 12g
Rhizoma Zedoriae (E Zhu) 9g
Rhizoma Sparganii (San Leng) 9g
Radix Paeoniae Alba (Bai Shao) 30g
Fasciculus Vascularis Luffae (Si Gua Luo) 15g
Flos Caryophylli (Ding Xiang) 3g
Lumbricus (Di Long) 12g
Cortex Phellodendri (Huang Bai) 4g
Radix Gentianae (Long Dan Cao) 4g

For a sensitive patient or with minor pain and disability, take out: Radix Aconiti Carmichaeli Praeparata (Zhi Chuan Wu) and Radix Aconiti Kusnezoffii Praeparata (Zhi Cao Wu).

For fatigued patients with a sense that great effort is needed to accomplish physical activity and when pain increases by activity (Kidney-taxation encumbrance pain) Young Maid Pill (Qing E Wan) can be used by itself or added to the above formula. This formula contains Psoralea (Bu Gu Zhi), Cortex Eucommia (Du Zhong), Walnut (Hu Tao Rou) and Garlic (Da Suan).[121]

Acupuncture

Commonly used points and methods are: Sedation techniques followed by moxa at Liv-3, 2, LI-4, UB-18, GB-34, 30, 35, 41, 43 and Ashi points. Tonification and moxa at CV-4, GV-4, 14, UB-23, 52, St-36.

Wind-Damp-Heat

This pattern is mainly seen in the acute or early stages of Bi-syndromes and usually presents in patients with *active* inflammation. The joints are warm, swollen, and have a hard end-feel that is painful. There is usually a capsular pattern. Patients often complain of pain that is severe. The muscles are often *lax* when *not* under load, but spring into spasm when the affected joint *is* under load. In severe cases, muscle weakness and wasting/atrophy may be seen. The pulse may be rapid and soft, or rapid and slippery, or wiry. The tongue may be red and have an off-white or yellow greasy coat. A representative formula for the early stage is Disband Painful Obstruction Decoction (Xuan Bi Tang) and the following variations can be used:

Gypsum (Shi Gao) 25g
Semen Coicis (Yi Yi Ren) 20g
Excrementum Bombycis Mori (Can Sha) 9g
Rhizoma Pinelliae (Ban Xia) 9g
Fructus Forsythiae (Lian Qiao) 9g
Fructus Gardeniae (Zhi Zi) 9g
Radix Gentianae (Qin Jiao) 12g
Radix Ledebouriellae (Fang Feng) 9g
Ramulus Cinnamomi (Gui Zhi) 9g
Herba Ephedra (Honey fried is preferable) (Ma Huang) 6g

When Damp-Heat is chronic or severe, a modification of Four-Marvel Pill (Si Miao Wan) and Relax the Channels and Invigorate the Blood Decoction (Shu Jing Ho Xue Tang) can be used. This formula can be used for lumbar or lower extremity disorders. The author often uses variations of the formula below for patients with radiculopathy from disc disease. Some patients do well when Minor Invigorate the Collaterals Special Pill (Xiao Huo Luo Dan) is given at the same time:

Cortex Phellodendri (Huang Bai) 12g
Rhizoma Arisaematis (Tian Nan Xing) 6g
Semen Coicis (Yi Yi Ren) 20g
Rhizoma Atractylodis (Cang Zhu) 12g
Radix Achyranthis Bidentatae (Niu Xi) 12g
Lumbricus (Di Long) 12g
Bombyx Batryticatus (Jiang Can) 9g
Radix Paeoniae Alba (Bai Shao) 20g
Radix Angelicae Sinensis (Dang Gui) 9g
Rhizoma Anemarrhenae (Zhi Mu) 9g
Rhizoma Dioscoreae Hypoglaucae (Bei Xie) 15g
Rhizoma Dioscoreae Nippnicae (Chuan Shan Long) 20g
Radix Gentianae (Long Dan Cao) 6g
Radix Paeoniae Rubrae (Chi Shao) 9g
Poriae Cocos (Fu Ling) 12g
Radix Glycyrrhizae (Gan Cao) 6g
Herba cum Radix Asari (Xi Xin) 3g

For symptoms of muscle spasms and numbness, add: Fructus Chaenomeles (Mu Gua) 9g, Radix Ligustici (Chuan Xiong), Cortex Lycii Radicis (Di Gu Pi) 20g, Agkistrodon (Bai Hua She) 9g, Scolopendra (Wu Gong) 3g, Buthus Martensi (Quan Xie) 4g.

For Damp-Heat psoriatic or rheumatoid arthritis:

Rhizoma Atractylodis (Cang Zhu) 10g
Cortex Phellodendri (Huang Bai) 12g
Radix Gentianae (Qin Jiao) 15g
Dictamni (Bai Xian Pi) 20g
Semen Coicis (Yi Ren) 20g
Smilax (Tu Fu Ling) 30g
Rhizoma et Radix Notopterygii (Qiang Huo) 15g
Flos Carthami (Hong Hua) 10g
Semen Persicae (Tao Ren) 10g
Olibanum (Ru Xiang) 10g
Polyporus (Zhu Ling) 15g
Radix Cyathulae (Chuan Niu Xi) 20g
Sophorae (Ku Shen) 12g

For Heat-toxin psoriatic arthritis:

Flos Lonicerae Japonicae (Jin Yin Hua) 30g
Herba Traxaci Mongolici cum Radice (Pu Gong Ying) 20g
Fructus Forsythia Suspensae (Lin Qiao) 20g
Radix Isatis seu Baphicanthi (Ban Lan Gen) 20g
Radix Rehmanniae Glutinosae (Sheng Di) 20g
Rhizoma Anemarrhenae (Zhi Mu) 15g
Dendrobii (Shi Hu) 15g
Gypsum (Shi Gao) 60g
Radix Paeoniae Rubrae (Chi Shao) 20g
Miltiorrhizae Salviae (Dan Shen) 20g
Cortex Moutan Radicis (Dan Pi) 20g
Bubali (Shui Niu Jiao) 30g

For Wind-Heat psoriatic or rheumatoid arthritis:

Flos Lonicerae (Jin Yin Hua) 20g
Tripterygium Wilfordii (Lei Gong Teng) 20g
Radix Rehmanniae Glutinosae (Sheng Di) 30g
Rhizoma Anemarrhenae (Zhi Mu) 15g
Serpentis (She Tui) 10g
Radix Dendrobii (Shi Hu) 15g
Gypsum (Shi Gao) 30g
Radix Paeoniae Rubrae (Chi Shao) 20g
Miltiorrhizae Salviae (Dan Shen) 20g
Cortex Moutan Radicis (Dan Pi) 20g
Kochiae (Di Fu Zi) 20g

Acupuncture

Commonly used points and methods are: Sedation techniques/bleeding at GV-14, 10, UB-18, Sp-10, 9, LI-11, 4, St-44, Well (distal/ nail) and Ashi points.

---

121. These patients often suffer from ligamentous pain. The pain is worse in the morning, better with movement or slight exercise, worse with strain, and is usually felt in a fixed location. There may be a numb-like sensation, as well. Young Maid Pill (Qing E Wan) is often cooked or baked with Pork kidneys.

Wind-Damp-Heat—Chronic Disease, Blood-stasis

This pattern is seen most often in the middle to late stages of rheumatoid or other chronic *inflammatory* type arthritis. The joints are swollen, red, painful, and possibly *deformed*. Joints often show a combination of hard and soggy end-feels. Soft tissues and muscles are often weak and lack tone, or they can be shortened, painful, congested, and hard. The pulse and tongue may or may not show signs of Heat and Dampness. Modification of Two-Marvel Powder (Er Miao San), or Free the Channels and Stop Pain Decoction (Tong Jing Zhi Tong Tang) can be used.

> Cortex Phellodendri (Huang Bai) 15g
> Rhizoma Atractylodis (Cang Zhu) 12g
> Lumbricus (Di Long) 12g
> Caulis Lonicerae (Ren Dong Teng) 15g
> Radix Clematidis (Wei Ling Xian) 9g
> Cortex Cinnamomi (Gui Pi) 6g
> Rhizoma Arisaematis (Tian Nan Xing) 9g
> Radix Gentianae (Long Dan Cao) 12g
> Poriae Cocos (Fu Ling) 15g
> Radix Gentianae (Qin Jiao) 12g
> Semen Persicae (Tao Ren) 12g
> Flos Carthami (Hong Hua) 6
> Rhizoma Ligustici Wallichii (Chuan Xiang) 6g
> Radix Angelicae Dahuricae (Bai Zhi) 9g
> Herba cum Radix Asari (Xi Xin) 3g

For acute flare, take out: Radix Ligustici (Chuan Xiang) 6g, Radix Angelicae Dahuricae (Bai Zhi) 9g, Cortex Cinnamomi (Gui Pi) 6g. Add: Gypsum (Shi Gao) 25g, Flos Loncerae (Jin Yin Hua) 12g, Caulis Lonicerae (Ren Dong Teng) 15g, Fructus Forsythiae (Lian Qiao) 9g, and Ramulus Cinnamomi (Gui Zhi) 9g

For Joint deformities and spasms, take out: Cortex Cinnamomi (Gui Pi), Radix Gentianae (Long Dan Cao), Flos Carthami (Hong Hua), Radix Angelicae Dahuricae (Bai Zhi), and Herba cum Radix Asari (Xi Xin). Add: Radix Paeoniae Rubrae (Chi Shao) 9g, Radix Paeoniae Alba (Bai Shao) 20g, Angelica Sinesis (Dang Gui) 15g, Agkistrodon (Bai Hua She) 6g, Scolopendra (Wu Gong) 3g, Buthus Martensi (Quan Xie) 4g, Eupolyphaga seu Opisthoplatia (Tu Bie Chong) 4g, Herba Epimedii (Yin Yang Hou) 9g, Rhizoma Frynari (Gu Sui Bu) 12g, and Radix Polygonum Multiflorum (He Shao Wu) 12g.

An alternative for rheumatoid arthritis is:

> Herba Oldenlandiae Diffusae (Bai Hua She She Cao) 20g
> Radix Rehmanniae Glutinosae (Sheng Di Huang) 15g
> Herba Oldenlandiae Diffusae (Tu Fu Ling) 12g
> Radix Paeoniae Alba (Bai Shao) 12g
> Radix Paeoniae Rubrae (Chi Shao) 9g
> Semen Coicis (Yi Yi Ren) 20g
> Caulis Lonicerae (Ren Dong Teng) 15g
> Caulis Sinomenii (Qing Feng Teng) 9g
> Radix Clematidis (Wei Ling Xian) 9g
> Herba Pyrolae (Lu Xian Cao) 20g
> Lumbricus (Di Long) 6g
> Ramulus Cinnamomi Cassiae (Gui Zhi) 6g
> Radix Glycyrrhizae (Gan Cao) 3g

For severe cases, add Tripterygium Wilfordii (Lei Gong Teng) 12g.

For *gout* add Herba Oldenlandiae Diffusae (Tu Fu Ling) 20g, Rhizoma Dioscoreae Hypoglaucae (Bei Xie) 15g, Cortex Fraxini (Qin Pi) 9g.[122]

For rheumatoid or psoriatic arthritis, or fibromyalgia with Wind-Heat (Dampness) and Blood-deficiency, a guiding *mild* approach is:

> Radix Gentianae (Qin Jiao) 6g
> Radix Ledebouriellae (Fang Feng) 9g
> Ramulus Uncariae Cum Uncis (Gou Teng) 6g
> Radix Paeoniae Alba (Bai Shao) 6g
> Semen Cassiae Torae (Cao Jue Ming/Jue Ming Zi) 12g
> Semen Ziziphi Spinosae (Suan Zao Ren) 12g
> Flos Chrysanthemi Morifolii (Ju Hua) 6g
> Fructus Hordei Vulgaris Germinatus (Mai Ya) 12g
> Semen Biotae Orientalis (Bai Zi Ren) 9g
> Radix Clematidis (Wei Ling Xian) 6g
> Radix Glycyrrhizae Uralensis (Gan Cao) 3g

Or:

> Semen Ziziphi Spinosae (Suan Zao Ren) 12g
> Poriae (Fu Ling) 9g
> Herba Artemisiae Capillaris (Mian Yin Chen) 8g
> Radix Trichosanthis (Tian Hua Fen) 9g
> Radix Glycyrrhizae Uralensis (Zhi Gan Cao) 4g
> Fructus Hordei Vulgaris Germinatus (Mai Ya) 10g
> Ramulus Uncariae Cum Uncis (Gou Teng) 6g
> Rhizoma Anemarrhenae (Zhi Mu) 5g
> Semen Beninacasae (Dong Gua Ren) 12g
> Semen Cassiae Torae (Cao Jue Ming/Jue Ming Zi) 12g
> Radix Aurantii (Zhi Ke) 6g
> Ramulus Taxilli (Ji Sheng) 6g
> Rhizoma Corydalis (Yan Hu Suo) 9g

Acupuncture

Commonly used points and methods are: Sedation techniques/bleeding at GV-14, 10, UB-17, Sp-10, 9, LI-11, 4, Well (distal-nail) and Ashi points. Use cupping/bleeding at UB-43 and over swollen areas. Tonify St-36, Sp-6, CV-4, UB-20.

Wind-Damp-Cold—Weakness of Liver, Kidneys, Qi, and Blood

While this pattern is said to occur in the majority of elderly patients, clinical utility of herbs to treat such patients has been limited in this author's experience and observation of other practitioners. The Invasion of the Sinews and bones by Pathogenic Factors implies, to some extent, a weakness of the Liver and Kidneys, which control these tissues. Formulas that address the Liver, Kidneys, Qi, and Blood are frequently used. This pattern is seen most often in elderly patients or in patients with chronic arthrosis. The main symptoms are Cold-pain in the back and knees, and generalized stiff joints. Some patients may complain of a sense of numbness/ache and a feeling fatigue or heaviness. The pain improves with heat and may worsen in changing weather or rainy days. The joints and soft tissues are cold and not particularly swollen, except in more severe stages and then are very difficult to adequately treat (severe DJD). Joints usually show a hard end-feel. Depending on chronicity, soft tissues may be tight or lack normal tone. Bony outgrowths (spurs) are common. The pulse may be weak (deep, fine, soft, thready) or hidden (not obvious, very deep). The tongue may be pale. A representative formula is Angelica Pubescens and Sangjisheng

---

122. Qin Pi can be used for RA, rheumatic myositis, and gout. It can increase the excretion of uric acid via the urine.

Decoction (Du Huo Ji Shen Tong) and the following modifications can be used:

> Angelicae Pubescentis (Due Huo) 12g
> Ramus Loranthi (Sang Ji Sheng) 12g
> Radix Gentianae (Qin Jiao) 12
> Radix Ledebouriellae (Fang Feng) 9g
> Radix Ligustici (Chuan Xiong) 9g
> Radix Rehmanniae (Shu Di Huang) 12g
> Ginseng (Ren Shen) 6g
> Radix Achyranthis Bidentatae (Niu Xi) 12g
> Ramulus Cinnamomi (Gui Zhi) 9g
> Radix Paeoniae Alba (Bai Shao) 15g
> Fructus Lycii (Gou Qi Zi) 9g
> Radix Dispsacus (Xu Duan) 9 g
> Radix Polygonum Multiflorum (He Shao Wu) 12g
> Stamen Nelumbinis (Lian Xu) 3g

For severe pain, add: Zanthoxylum Netidom (Ye Di Jin Niu) 30g.

For Swelling, add: Semen Coicis (Yi Yi Ren) 20g and Rhizoma Dioscoreae Hypoglaucae (Bi Xie) 12g.

For psoriatic arthritis with Liver and Kidney deficiency, Blood-stasis and Wind-Dampness:

> Radix Rehmanniae Glutinosae (Sheng Di) 20g and (Shu Di) 20g
> Radix Angelicae Sinensis (Dang Gui) 15g
> Cortex Eucommiae Ulmoidis (Du Zhong) 12g
> Fructus Corni Officinalis (Shan Zhu Yu) 12g
> Fructus Lycii (Gou Qi Zi) 15g
> Radix Gentianae (Qin Jiao) 15g
> Rhizoma seu Radix Notopterygii (Qiang Huo) 12g
> Flos Carthami (Hong Hua) 10g
> Semen Persicae (Tao Ren) 10g
> Olibanum (Ru Xiang) 10g
> Rhizoma Ligustici Wallichii (Chuan Xiong) 12g

Acupuncture

Commonly used points and methods are: Sedation technique at LI-4, TW-5, UB-12, 13 and Ashi points. Tonification and Moxa at St-36, Sp-6, K-3, 7, GV-4, CV-4, 6, UB-20, 18, 23, GV-14.

Damage of Yin and Essence with Cold-Damp

This pattern is commonly seen in the clinic and is not easily addressed. The patient complains of arthritic pains with local signs of Dampness and Cold (or aggravation in cold weather), but the pulse and tongue and possibly other symptoms and signs show Damage to Yin. There usually is joint deformity. Modification of Yang-Heartening Decoction (Yang He Tang) can be used:

> Radix Aconite Lateralis (Fu Zi) 15-30g
> Radix Scrophulariae (Xuan Shen) 30g
> Radix Rehmanniae (Shu Di) 30g
> Colla Cornu Cervi (Lu Jiao Jiao) 12g
> Cortex Cinnamomi Cassiae (Rou Gui) 5g
> Fried Rhizoma Zingiberis (Pao Jiang) 2g
> Semen Sinapis Albae (Bai Jia Zi) 6g
> Herba Ephedra (Ma Huang) 3g
> Radix Glycyrrhizae (Gan Cao) 3g

Acupuncture

Commonly used points and methods are: Sedation techniques at K-3, Sp-9, GB-34, Sp-10, UB-43. Tonification at St-36, UB-23, 18, Sp-6.

Perpetuating Factors

Perpetuating factors for MPS and other musculoskeletal disorders are numerous; an understanding of them is mandatory for successful clinical management. Simons, Travell and Simons (*ibid*) list at least six major categories of perpetuating factors for MPS:

1. Mechanical stresses, divided mainly into structural and postural;
2. Nutritional inadequacies;
3. Metabolic and endocrine inadequacies;
4. Psychological factors;
5. Chronic infections;
6. Other.

Short Leg Syndrome

Many structural and postural factors can affect the musculoskeletal systems. Differences in leg length are common and are often overlooked, with some 23% (McCarthy and MacEwen 2001) of the general population having a discrepancy of 1cm or more. A short leg results in an unleveled sacral base and postural compensations (usually spinal curvature or pelvic rotations) which may have significant consequences. One must differentiate between primary anatomic leg length differences and secondary/functional variations (not true leg length). According to Greenman 50% of failed low back patients suffer from a short leg. Primary (anatomic) leg length discrepancy has been shown to correlate with the frequency of back pain (Friberg 1985). Leg length discrepancies, however, are seen in asymptomatic populations, as well. If the difference is larger than 5mm and symptomatic, it should be treated; although, to attain "peak physical performance" in athletes patient with smaller differences may be treated. Some patients with as little as 1.5 mm (1/16 inch) leg length differences may suffer clinical symptoms (Kuchera 2003). Clinical measurement of leg length has been shown to be inaccurate compared with x-ray measurements (Morscher and Finger 1977). Still, a tape measurement can be helpful (Beattie et al 1990).

Apparent leg length (secondary to pelvic dysfunction) can be demonstrated after movement of the pelvic ring. This can be accomplished by checking for changes in leg lengths between the sitting and the supine positions. The gluteus medius is usually weak on the short leg side.

Adaptations to Short Leg

Leg length differences generally cause the pelvis to tilt to the side of the short leg, with lumbar sidebending to the opposite side or to the long-leg side. Rotation occurs toward the convexity of the curve. However, atypical adaptations also can be seen and may be more symptomatic. Although each per-

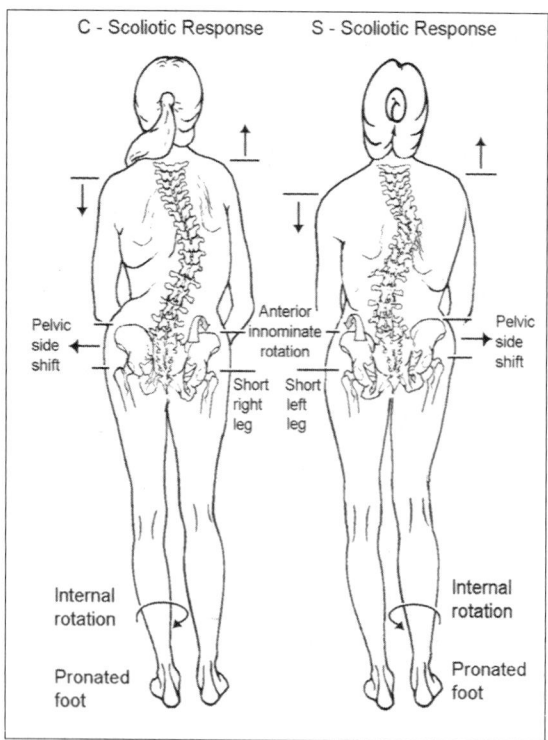

Figure 11-46: Adaptation to short leg, C-scoliotic and S-scoliotic responses (From Kuchera WA and Kuchera ML, Osteopathic Principles in Practice, KCOM press 1993, with permission).

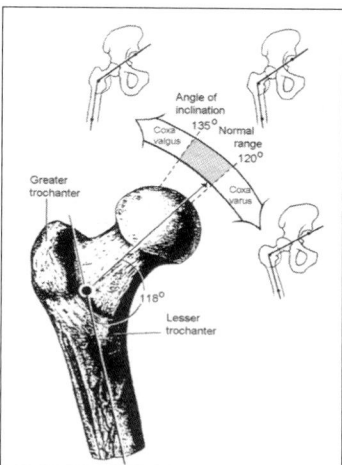

Figure 11-47: Coxa valgum and valgus (From Kuchera WA and Kuchera ML, Osteopathic Principles in Practice, KCOM press 1993, with permission).

A short leg is responsible often for recurrent joint dysfunctions anywhere in the spine and even the cranium. It should be suspected if the standing trochanteric plane is unlevel and there is no clinical evidence of shear. If, after somatic dysfunctions have been treated, the standing flexion test is still positive and sitting flexion is negative, a short leg should be suspected (Kuchera and Kuchera *ibid*).

Assessment of Short Leg

Short leg syndrome is best assessed by a standing x-ray. In one study of standing patients with known radiographic leg length inequality, the wrong extremity was identified as being short in 13% of the clinical observations; more than half of the 196 clinical estimates of leg length were incorrect by more than 3/16 of an inch (Kuchera *ibid*). Figure 11-48 show the proper landmarks needed to assess leg length by x-ray.

The office assessment begins with the patient standing with feet slightly apart. (If the feet are together, the leg that the patient favors may appear longer). The practitioner compares the levelness of both iliac crests, PSISs or ASISs, greater trochanter of both femurs, and gluteal folds carefully. He repeats these observations several times to assure that the findings are reproducible, as it is easy to make mistakes. Palpation has been shown to have poor inter-rater reliability in several studies (Potter and Rothstein 1985; Mann, Glassjenn-Wray and Nyberg 1984). Greater trochanter height in the standing patient is probably the most reliable sign of the above-mentioned landmarks; however, errors are still possible with unilateral coxa varus or coxa valgus. Frequently one side of the patient is smaller than the other, including the feet. The patient may report having to use two different size shoes.

The practitioner can also compare the levelness of the PSISs when the patient is standing, forward-bent, and seated. When the PSISs (or iliac crests) are unlevel when standing

son will adapt differently, in general, the lumbosacral angle is increased by 2-3°. The innominate rotates anteriorly on the side of the short leg and posteriorly on the other side in order to equalize the leg length (Basmajian and Nyberg 1993). The foot is often pronated on the long side. Often this compensation masks the apparent length differences (Kuchera and Kuchera 1993). Scoliotic curves develop to keep the eyes level (Figure 11-46).

The pelvic obliqueness that results from a short leg stresses the ligaments and muscles of the back, pelvis, hip, and possibly the neck. With time, muscle adaptation, shortening, and dysfunction develop and lead to tendon inflammation and ligament insufficiency.

Tissues on the concavity shorten and demonstrate increased electromyographic activity. Tissues on the convex side lengthen. Patients with coronal plane postural imbalance develop tight abductors on one side and tight thigh adductors on the contralateral side. Associated horizontal plane imbalance often results in tight hamstrings on one side and tight rectus femoris on the other thigh. The iliolumbar ligament on the convex side is the first to react and show symptoms, since it is affected by both sacral and innominate rotations. The sacroiliac ligaments of the side of the convexity may also become stressed and tender to palpation and may refer pain down the lateral side of the leg. Often the patient has sciatic-like pain and hip pain on the long leg side. (Kuchera *ibid*).

Perpetuating Factors

but become level when the patient is seated, the probability of leg length difference is high. If they remain uneven, pelvic dysfunction or structural asymmetry is likely. Then, with the patient supine, one measures the length between the patient's ASISs and lateral malleoli to assess for structural differences, and from the umbilicus to the medial malleoli for functional differences. Figure 11-49 shows tape measurement from the ASIS to the malleolus for anatomical leg length.

Having the standing patient swing one leg and then the other is sometimes helpful. It may be more difficult when the patient is standing on the short-leg side, and when the trunk sidebending is greater. According to Greenman the short leg is found most often on the left side.

When an anatomic difference is suspected, elevate the patient's heel using a shim, and re-evaluate all of the findings. If spinal scoliosis remains after the hips are level, the problem may be due to sacral (pelvic) asymlocation or primary scoliosis. With primary scoliosis, when the patient is flexed forward, one usually sees increased prominence at the rib cage area.

Treatment of Short Leg Syndrome and Postural Compensations

If compensatory mechanisms are overwhelmed, treatment of postural decompensation should include some combination of sound education, functional orthotics, specific exercises, manual therapies, and acupuncture or prolotherapy. Clinically, one should first treat all somatic (mechanical) dysfunctions, including myofascial shortening and spasm, before making a final conclusion and prescribing a heel lift. Leg length discrepancies in children between one-and-a-half and fifteen years of age can be corrected (cured) by using heel-lifts for three to seven months (Redler 1952). Accord-

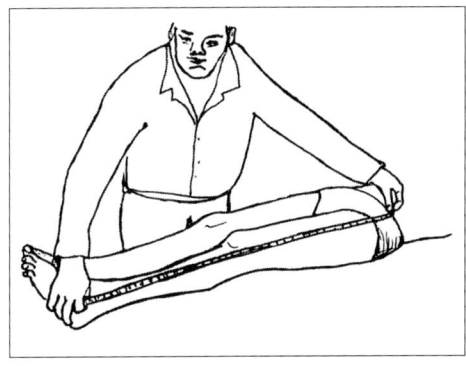

Figure 11-49: Tape measurement of leg length.

ing to Greenman (personal communication), bone growth can be stimulated in children by having them jump on the short leg.

Education should include proper use of footwear, including the reduction of high heels, promotion of functional arches and heel support, and correction of pronation (i.e. good footwear). Other useful education includes proper lifting techniques, specific exercises designed first to rest and then to functionally enhance ineffective soft tissue structures, and dietary counseling when necessary for appropriate weight distribution (Kuchera 2003).

LIFT THERAPY. Typically, treatment of short leg syndrome involves lifts inserted in the patient's shoe or incorporated into a functional orthotic. Some studies show that an 80% reduction in subjective pain and other posture-related symptoms can be expected as a result of properly balancing the sacral base with lift therapy to within 1 mm of levelness. It is therefore best to use lifts based on x-ray findings of an

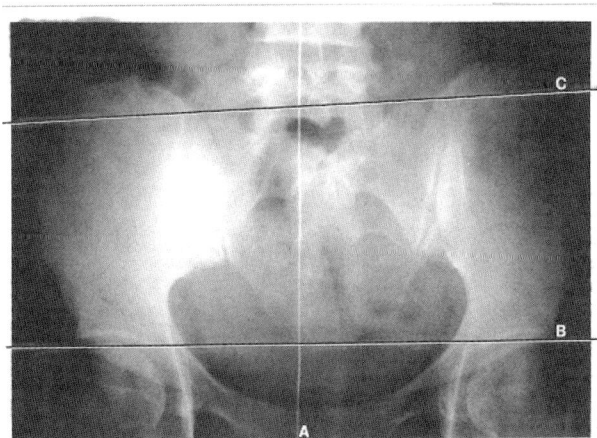

Line A is a true vertical line (a plum line). Line B shows that the legs are of equal length. Line C, which is a sacral line, shows an unlevel sacral base which is not due to short-leg syndrome.

Figure 11-48: Standing x-ray of pelvis with visual aids.

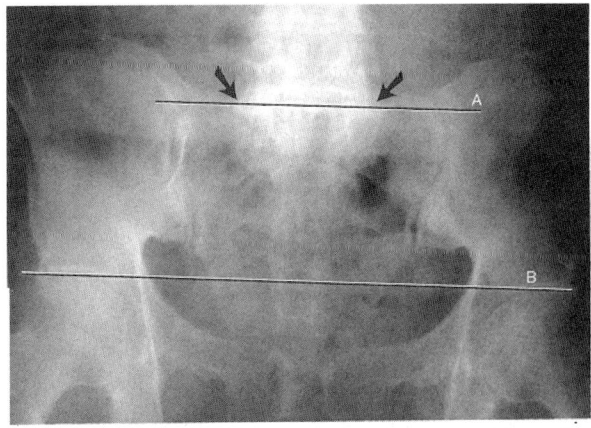

A tilt to the left due to short leg. Line A is a sacral base line and is parallel with the line across the femoral heads, which is the B line. The black arrows point to the sacral notches, which are a good location to establish the sacral base. Note line B is at different heights over the left and right femoral heads

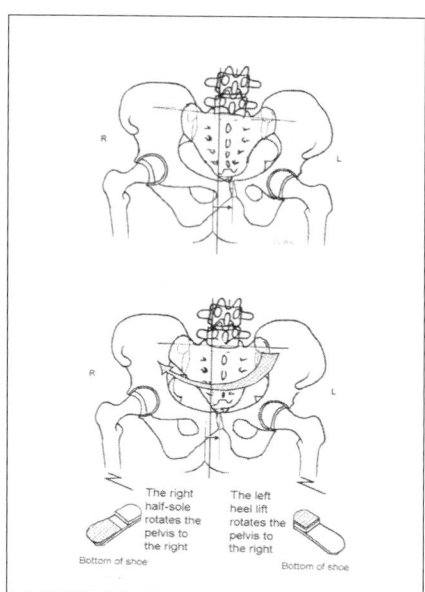

Figure 11-50: Anterior and posterior lift (From Kuchera WA and Kuchera ML, Osteopathic Principles in Practice, KCOM press 1993, with permission).

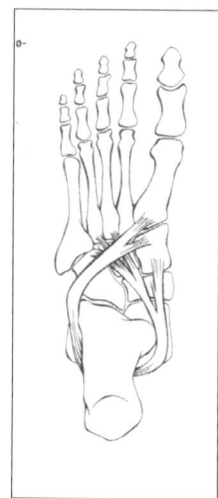

Figure 11-51: Tendinous arrangement that supports the foot (courtesy of Mitchell 1995).

unlevel sacral base. The lift is designed to restore the sacrum to the horizontal and is inserted under the leg on the depressed sacral base side. This is especially true if there is a compensatory *curvature* that side bends to the *opposite side of the short leg*. In the less common situation where the curve has its concavity towards the side of the short leg, it may be necessary to lift the side of the long leg. This first effects a change in the lumbar scoliosis and also relieves some of the pelvis and lumbar strain (Kuchera *ibid*).

The heels should be rased slowly with no more than an one eighth of an inch at a time (every two weeks). A fragile patient (arthritic, osteoporotic, elderly, or in severe pain, etc.) should begin with a one sixteenth of an inch lift and raised no faster than one sixteenth of an inch every two weeks.

Anterior (forefoot) lift therapy rotates the pelvis toward the same side; heel lifts may rotate the pelvis away from the lift side. Treatment of both planes may be warranted, as side bending and rotation are biomechanically linked. A heel lift pushes that side of the pelvis anteriorly in the horizontal plane because the lift is behind the axis of motion (i.e., rotates the pelvis away from the side of the heel lift). Anterior sole (forefoot) lifts are in front of the axis and so they rotate that side of the pelvis posteriorly in a horizontal plane (i.e., rotate the pelvis toward the side of the sole lift). The use of anterior sole lift is fairly new and should be used with caution (Kuchera *ibid*).

Small Hemipelvis

A small hemipelvis is associated with back pain (Lowman 1941). In this condition the pelvis is vertically smaller on one side than on the other, both when the patient is seated and when standing. The patient sits crookedly and leans toward the small side, and often sits cross-legged to cantilever the low side. A see-saw affect tilts the spine in both standing and sitting positions (Travell and Simons 1983).

Assessment

Assessment is done with the patient seated on a hard, flat surface. The feet are supported high enough so the patient can slip his fingers between his thighs and the front edge of the table. The practitioner observes and checks the same landmarks as when examining for a short leg. Since somatic dysfunction of the pelvis can result in similar findings, the patient is asked to rock and stress his pelvis. If findings do not change, a small hemipelvis should be considered (Travell and Simons *ibid*).

TREATMENT. If a small hemipelvis is found, the patient should use a sit-pad to compensate while seated.

Short Upper Arms

According to Simons, Travell and Simons (*ibid*), short upper arms in relation to the torso height is not an uncommon source of muscle strain and perpetuation of trigger points, especially in the shoulder region.

Assessment

The standing patient's elbows should reach the iliac crests.

TREATMENT. Compensate for short limbs with use of furnature.

Foot Abnormalities

Poor foot function is probably one of the most common perpetuating factor in musculoskeletal pain syndromes, and foot *orthotic therapy* often should be used. The feet are an important contributor to the body's general mechanics and often are a *primary* source of myofascial and skeletal pain. The foot has had to achieve a highly specialized mechanical apparatus in order to counterbalance the gravitational pull, thus keeping the body erect and being able to use energy economically to propel the body forward. Three aspects of foot function must be present for this to occur (Horwitz 1995):

1. Stability must be maintained as the feet carry the total body weight, which is spent on a single foot 17% of gait.
2. Feet must be able to function as shock absorbing mechanisms that decelerate the body as it falls forward during gait.
3. Feet must function as a sprinkled lever to propel us forward in a way that conserves energy.

The foot structures are acted upon by hard, unyielding surfaces and by the rotations and translations of the trunk and leg that are needed to advance the body forward. Therefore, as the interface between the body and the ground, the feet are subjected to tremendous stresses and loads that, in turn, can amplify any gait or postural-effects from dysfunctional feet.

Pes Planus

Abnormal pronation is probably the most common of all biomechanical foot problems. This so-called "flat-foot" (see next section) can occur congenitally or can result from functional or traumatic etiologies (Valmassy 1996).

CONGENITAL ETIOLOGIES:

1. Gastrocnemius equines (shortening) or gastrocnemius solius equines.
2. Tipples (foot and ankle) calcaneovalgus (flexible).
3. Congenital convex pes (foot) valgus, vertical talus (rigid).
4. Peroneal spastic secondary to tarsal coalition (rigid).
5. Ankle valgus secondary to oblique ankle joint mortise.
6. Ligamentous laxity.

FUNCTIONAL ETIOLOGIES:

1. Compensated forefoot varus.
2. Compensation for transverse plane deformities.
3. Malinsertion of posterior tibial tendon with or without accessory navicular.
4. Limb length discrepancy.

TRAUMATIC ETIOLOGY:

1. Posterior tibial dysfunction. Complete or partial rupture of the posterior tibial tendon leads to progressive

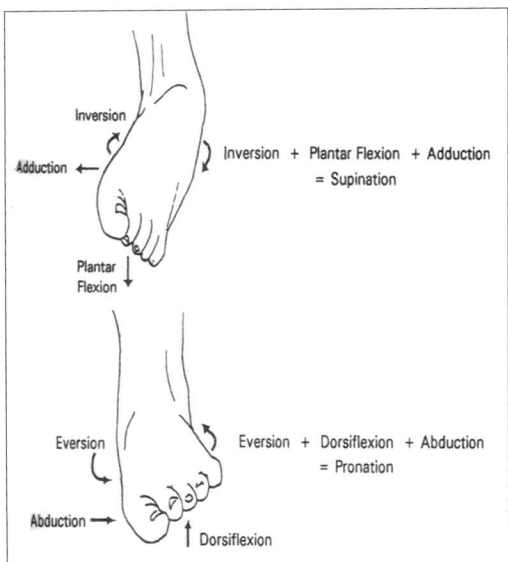

Figure 11-52: Foot motion terminology (From Kuchera WA and Kuchera ML, Osteopathic Principles in Practice, KCOM press 1993, with permission).

flattening of the arch along with associated abduction of the forefoot relative to the rearfoot.

THE LOIS FOOT: Pes Valgo Planus was named "Lois" by Dr. Horwitz. Lois is a low arch foot which is often referred to as a "falling arch" foot. Although a Lois foot looks like a low arch foot, it should never be considered a flat-foot. The Lois center of gravity is higher on the back than "Heidi's" (Cavus high-arched foot). In modern times, the Lois foot presents with reduced skin proprioception and ligamentous resiliency. With loss of proprioception and the reciprocal ground reaction force, the muscles fatigue more quickly and become irritated easily. As the ligaments loose strength, the Lois foot weakens. The muscles that hold up the arch also weaken, and the arch collapses. The internal collapse of the long-limb arch allows the pelvic girdle to internally sublux and rotate on the sacrum. In response to the sacral torque, the back, neck, and head become unstable.

For a Lois patient to pull his/her legs from the ground while walking, he/she must hyper-rotate and sideband the middle lumbar spines. This movement weakens the lumbar ligaments and causes the *costa-lumbar fascia* and associative muscles (*quadratus lumborum and erector spinalis*) to become spastic and shortened on the long-limb side, as a means of lifting the other leg from the ground. A predictable domino effect in the upper torso causes a sidebend and misalignment to the osteoarticular and ligamentous structure of the lumbar and lower thoracic spines, shoulder, and neck.

The implosion of the medial or spring-arch causes protective muscular splinting, plantar fasciitis, and other muscle imbalances. These are often associated with Janda's *Untercross pattern*. As the foot structure slides forward and downward, the navicular can no longer act as the keystone to the foot. This causes the following in the foot's domelike structure:

- The cuboid-calcaneal joint rotates, subluxes, and collapses on itself.
- The peroneus brevis, tertius, and longus muscles no longer have the necessary fulcrum in the foot to help stabilize the leg and low back. This results in gluteus maximus weakness, and lateral band, or tensor fascia pain.

Myofascial and structural disorganization are almost always associated with this foot lesion. X-ray examination of a Lois foot reveals a calcaneal inclination angle of 12 to 18°, measured on a weight bearing x-ray with the beam aimed at the talo-navicular joint.

The patient who has a Pes Valgo Planus or Lois foot has the following physical manifestations and complaints:

- Stands straight.
- Has hypokyphotic thoracic spine.
- One shoulder rotated anteriorly and sometimes painful.
- Unilaterally tight iliopsoas and piriformis muscles.
- Torqued pelvis.
- Temporal headaches.
- A one-sided stiff neck that at times is painful when bent.
- Hip and mid-back pain, lumbar 2-5 pain that radiates down the outside of the leg.
- Medial knee pain.
- Chronic shin splints.
- Chronically sprained ankles.
- Arch pain or plantar fasciitis.
- Heel pain.

Orthotics therapy for a Lois foot should stabilize the mid-tarsal joints of the foot and realign the body's coronal plane. This helps in weight transference and muscle balance. Ideally, the feel of the foot ground is imitated, helping restore the lost proprioception. The orthotics should end at the toes or sulcus and should be made from a combination of Pelite and Crepe, cork, or thin elastic plastic. Many podiatric physicians use a more rigid orthotic, (e.g. rigid plastics; the more flexible the foot the more rigid the orthotic and vice versa). This is useful if the practitioner does not use prolotherapy. However, the use of rigid orthotics can result in three unwanted effects:[123]

1. Disuse atrophy of the intrinsic muscles of the foot from the immobilization.
2. Loss of the skin's proprioception from the unyielding concrete-like composite of the orthotic.

---

123. A wide flexible devise with deep heel cups, 4/4 post, 2-4 mm Curbi skive, 2 degree inversion, and EVA bottom fill is a good compromise which addresses the need for stability as well as proprioception. A K-wedge or reverse Morton's extension (a 5-2 extension) is needed often to address functional hallux limitus

3. Loss of shock absorption causing unrecognized symptoms in areas such as the knee, hip, and back.

Pes Cavus

A *highly* arched-foot can cause even more significant pathologic changes than the low-arched foot. The Cavus foot type leads to a marked abnormal distribution of stresses through the foot, abnormal weightbearing and ground contact, and decreased foot mobility and shock absorption. A host of secondary compensatory mechanisms may occur. The Cavus foot tends to be rigid with decreased ankle dorsiflexion (osseous block) and limited pronation. It can lead to increased tendency to lateral ankle instability, with associated ankle sprains and digital contractions (Valmassy *ibid*).

Patients with this type of feet need to be neurologically evaluated for Charcot-Marie-Tooth disease, Friedreich's ataxia, poliomyelitis, Roussey-Levy syndrome, spina bifida, myelodysplasias, spastic monoplegia or paraplegia, polyneuritis, muscle dysplasia, trauma, angioma of the medulla or other spinal cord tumors, arthrogryposis, congenital lymphedema, and congenital syphilis, because they can all result in cavus type deformity (Valmassy *ibid*).

The cavus foot may be classified as two types: the anterior pes cavus and the posterior pes cavus. The *anterior pes cavus* is characterized by sagittal plane plantarflexion of the forefoot relative to the rearfoot. The *posterior pes cavus* is characterized by rearfoot compensation which occurs as a result of a forefoot equinus, usually resulting in a high calcaneal inclination angle, and is often referred to as pseudoequinus. There is an apparent clinical lack of ankle joint dorsiflexion (often with failure to achieve 10° of dorsiflexion while loaded). Other associated conditions that should be considered are (Valmassy *ibid*):

CONGENITAL:

1. Congenital plantarflexed first-ray deformity.
2. Spasm of peroneus longus.
3. Spasm of posterior tibialis.
4. Weakness of peroneus brevis.
5. Weakness of peroneus longus.
6. Clubfoot deformity.
7. Metatarsus adductus.

FUNCTIONAL:

1. Uncompensated rearfoot varus.
2. Partially compensated rearfoot varus.
3. Compensated rigid forefoot valgus.
4. Limb length inequality (on short leg).

THE HEIDI FOOT: Dr. Horwitz has named the Talapi Equino Varus (cavus) foot "Heidi." A patient who has a Heidi foot tends to be muscularly stiff, probably a good runner, comfortable in high heel shoes, and unlikely to stand for any period of time. X-rays show a calcaneal inclination angle of greater than 18°. This angle is measured weight-bearing, with the beam aimed at the talo-navicular joint. According to Dr. Horwitz, a patient who has a Heidi foot can present with some of the following physical characteristics and complaints:

- Stiff neck with limited and painful forward bending.
- Extended neck that sits forward on the thoracic spine.
- Slouched stance with a hyperkyphotic thoracic spine.
- Reduced and painful shoulder movement on extension.
- Internally rotated shoulders.
- Bilateral tight iliopsoas and piriformis muscles.
- Hyperlordotic lumbar spine.
- Balanced stance over the balls of feet (standing on the toes and having difficulty bringing heels to the ground).
- Shortened plantar fascia.
- Occipital or frontal headaches.
- Coccyx pain that mimics a sciatic lesion by radiating down the back of the legs.
- Posterior knee pain.
- Chronic Achilles tendinitis.
- Burning in the balls of the feet.

Orthotic therapy for a Heidi foot should help bring the ground to the body and to treat the lack of shock absorption in Heidi foot. This can be accomplished by using an orthotic that raises the heel cephalically with materials that absorb the shock generated by the foot striking the ground. A *Pelit* and *Crepe* combination orthotic, or a semi-rigid plastic orthotic, ending behind the metatarsal heads, generally accomplishes both goals.

Functional Hallux Limitus/Sagittal Plane Blockade

Functional hallux limitus (FHL) is a momentary locking of the great toe joint just at a time when the body moves past the planted foot. This results in limited extension of the toe during the propulsion phase of gait, as well as limitation of hip extension with *sagittal plane gait dysfunction*. The limitation of the big toe dorsiflexion is seen during weight-bearing only; usually, secondary to a dorsiflexed first ray which results in deformity of the first metatarsophalangeal joint (MTPJ) in which the base of the proximal phalanx of the hallux is subluxed plantarly upon the first met-head. With loss of first MTPJ extension, the pivot needed for propulsion is lost. Further trauma to the joint can result in proliferative changes which ultimately can lead to ankylosis of the first MTP, called hallux rigidus (Brown *ibid*). Hallux limitus is associated with (Valmassy *ibid*):

1. Partially compensated forefoot varus.

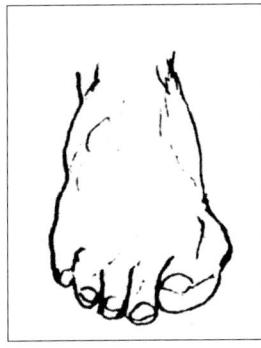

Figure 11-53: Hallux valgus.

2. Compensated forefoot varus.
3. Forefoot supination.
4. Flexible forefoot valgus.
5. Compensated congenital gastrocnemius equinus.
6. Compensated transverse plane deformity.

Scherer (2001) summarizes the pathomechanics of *hallux valgus* (Figure 11-53) and hallux limitus (which are often seen together) as starting with an everted calcaneus or a flexible forefoot valgus which drives the medial column of the forefoot into the ground. This creates an increased dorsiflexory moment on the first ray. As the first ray dorsiflexes the big toe joint becomes limited in its range of motion, and, as the heel comes off the ground in gait, the rigid hallux is driven into the sole of the shoe causing the irritation to the skin and the dislocation of the joint.

According to Prior (1999):

> First MTPJ dorsiflexion is accompanied by ankle plantarflexion. A failure of this to occur results in early knee joint flexion (prior to heel strike of the swing limb) and thus reduced hip joint extension. Insufficient hip joint extension prevents the hip flexors gaining mechanical advantage and thus removes their ability to initiate motion via a swing of the limb. As a result, the gluteals and quadratus lumborum on the contralateral side become active in order to help pull the weightbearing leg into swing. This will destabilize the contralateral lower back and sacroiliac joint and may predispose to piriformis overactivity. Furthermore the position of the hip at the time of hip flexor activity means that the leg effectively acts as a dead weight. As the hip flexors are unable to accelerate the leg forwards, they effectively pull the leg downwards, exacerbating the effect of the dead weight. This results in lateral rotation on the spine and trauma to the intervertebral discs. Whilst this abnormal function is of low magnitude, it is its repetitive nature that causes the problem over a sustained period of time. The average person takes 5000 steps per day, or 2500 per foot,

thus subtle imbalances are repeated thousands of times per day.

A hallux limitus therefore results in secondary alterations and adaptations that have profound abnormal biomechanical effects up the lower kinetic chain causing problems at the feet, knee, hip, pelvis, lumbar, thoracic, and cervical spines (Brown *ibid*). The most notable feature of FHL is *limited hip extension* during gait, which normally extends approximately 15° by the end of single support phase. This allows the torso to remain erect, and it positions the limb so it can be lifted easily for the next swing phase. With mechanically inefficient motions (which may be due to FHL), myogenic overuse, degenerative disease, and neurogenic hypersensitivity often develop. For example, hip and lower limb extension are needed for the sacrum to properly nutate, so that self-bracing at the sacroiliac joint can take place (Vleeming *ibid*). For this to occur, the *biceps femoris* muscle must relax during the midstance portion of gait, so that the sacrotuberous also relaxes, thus allowing the sacrum to nutate forward.[124] According to Dananberg (*ibid*) FHL blocks this action. The *psoas* and *piriformis* then may bear a significantly higher load. Because lumbar discs have little tolerance to twisting motions and FHL can result in excessive torquing movements at the lumbar spine, the discs may be injured.

THE POSSIBLE CAUSES OF HALLUX LIMITUS ARE (Valmassy *ibid*):

1. Hypermobility of the first ray, in conjunction with eversion of the foot caused by abnormal subtalar joint pronation (cavus foot).
2. Immobilization of the first ray, which may occur secondary to longstanding abnormal subtalar joint pronation.
3. Excessively long first metatarsal.
4. Dorsiflexed first ray (metatarsus primus elevatus).
5. Degenerative joint disease.
6. Trauma.

In summary, the most common cause of FHL is a forefoot that is everted relative to the ground by abnormal subtalar joint pronation. The first ray is hypermobile, and ground reaction maintains it in a dorsiflexed position during propulsion (Brown *ibid*).

Orthotic therapy with a Kinetic Wedge™ (a type of reverse Morton's extension with a first MTPJ clip), which is designed to restore normal timing and sagittal plane function on the first MTPJ is said to be effective. A reverse Morton's extension can be used, as well (Figure 11-54). The purpose of the orthotic therapy is to hold the calcaneus perpendicular

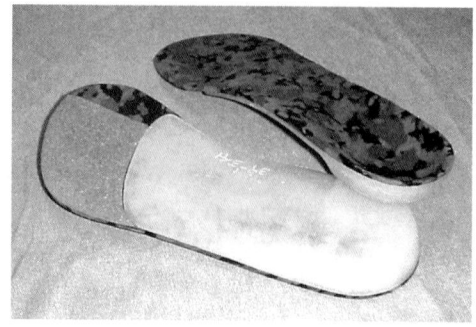

Figure 11-54: Reverse Morton's extension.

and allow the first ray to drop below the second, third, and fourth metatarsals. If the first MTPJ becomes stiff, mobilization may be required.

Morton's Foot

Dr. Morton has characterized a short first and long second metatarsal (toe) as being dysfunctional; however, it may be a normal variant seen in asymptomatic populations as well. According to Dr. Morton, when this dysfunction occurs more weight is shifted to the second metatarsal. This makes the foot rock excessively, and often it produces a callus.[125] To compensate, some patients modify their gait so the affected foot is slightly toed-out at heel strike and during the stance phase of the gait. The ankle and subtalar joints pronate excessively during the stance phase. Excessive pronation leads to the knee swinging toward the other knee as the leg undergoes excessive internal rotation (with possible increasing knee valgus). Excessive wear on the lateral heel and medial side of the sole of the shoe may be seen (Morton 1955, 1935). The resulting gait may activate trigger points in the *gluteus medius* and *posterior gluteus minimus*, which laterally rotates the thigh at the hip. Pain refers to the low back and posterior thigh and calf, and may look like radiculopathy. Excessive foot rocking may strain the peroneus longus muscle with trigger point activation and ankle pain, possibly resulting in an entrapment of the peroneal nerve against the fibula. This produces numbness and tingling across the dorsum of the foot and sometimes motor weakness with foot drop (Travell 1975, 1952).

This type of foot dysfunction is said to be capable of perpetuating myofascial pain syndromes in the low back, thigh, knee, leg, and dorsum of the foot. The patient often reports a history of ankle sprains and weakness (Simons, Travell, Simons *ibid*). Morton's foot should not be confused with a Morton's neuroma, a growth on the nerve at the foot (Figure 11-56).

---

124. The biceps connect directly to the sacrotuberous ligament and can change its tension.

125. A callus under the middle metatarsal correlates to abnormal weight bearing patterns at the foot but not necessarily to a Morton's foot. It is a common finding with functional hallux limitus as well.

Perpetuating Factors

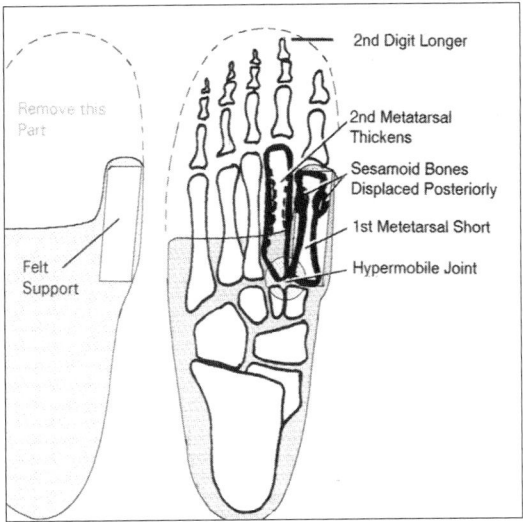

Figure 11-55: Morton's foot (R). Morton's extension (L) (From Kuchera WA and Kuchera ML, Osteopathic Principles in Practice, KCOM press 1994, with permission).

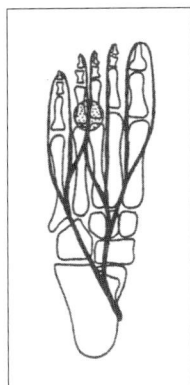

Figure 11-56: Morton's neuroma (From Kuchera WA and Kuchera ML, Osteopathic Principles in Practice, KCOM press 1994, with permission).

Orthotic therapy for Morton's foot usually involves an extension incorporated in a custom orthotic distal to the device itself. A Morton's extension can also be incorporated into the shoe directly, or as an adjunct to a longitudinal arch pad. Care must be paid however, as patients with "Morton's foot" often develop functional hallux limitus, and a Morton's extension can limit hallux dorsiflexion even more. Thus, even with a short first and long second metatarsal, one may need to use a Kinetic Wedge™ or a reverse Morton's extension. Patients with dosiflexed first phalange may do well with a Morton's extension if it does not result in functional hallux limitus.

Additional Foot Disorders

The following are descriptions of some commonly seen foot disorders. While not necessarily perpetuating chronic musculoskeletal pain syndromes, any foot dysfunction and/or pain has wide ranging affects on gait and therefore on whole body mechanics. This section is based on a course given by ProLab Orthotics (Sherer 2001), and the California Collage of Podiatric Medicine. For additional information on pathology-specific orthotic therapy see page 530.

POSTERIOR TIBIAL DYSFUNCTION. Posterior tibial dysfunction (PTD) is fairly rare but seems to appear with a consistent clinical presentation. PTD is sometimes referred to as "acquired unilateral flat-foot" or "advanced tibialis posterior tendinitis." Surgical procedures designed to repair or reinforce the PT tendon are rarely successful. Rearfoot fusion seems to relieve the symptoms but presents a broad spectrum of complications. The majority of symptoms are secondary to midtarsal joint subluxation and to overuse syndrome of the remaining flexors and intrinsic muscles. Steroid use, rheumatoid arthritis, chronic synovitis, and obesity seem to be most of the primary etiologies creating the rupture or attenuation of the tibialis posterior tendon. The pathomechanics pathway, following dysfunction of the tendon, is midtarsal joint instability, supination of the long axis, medial arch collapse, eversion of the heel from the subtalar joint pronation, and, finally, forefoot abduction at the T-N joint. A secondary or false equinus also develops, and the subtalar joint (STJ) axis becomes more horizontal and more medial.

A specially designed orthotic gives considerable symptomatic relief and functional support and should be tried (Figure 11-57).

PLANTAR FASCIITIS. Heel pain, plantar fasciitis, and heel spur syndrome are probably the most common complaints seen in any foot specialist's office. The pathology behind the symptoms is always a stretching of the plantar fascia caused by a supination of the midtarsal joint, remembering that as the rearfoot everts the forefoot must invert on the rearfoot, stretching the plantar fascia like a bowstring. The pull on the plantar fascia can cause chronic pain. The plantar fascia's pull on the calcaneal periosteum can cause acute pain. It is essential to rule out the other diagnoses that cause heel pain. Some possibilities are: calcaneal stress fracture, infracalcaneal neuropathy, Reiters syndrome, ankylosing spondylitis, gout, tarsal tunnel syndrome, and rheumatoid arthritis (Figure 11-58). While most patient's with heel pain or plantar fasciitis over pronate, in some patients the rearfoot is stable and not everted on stance. The heel pain is then likely to be caused by dorsiflexion of the first ray due to a flexible forefoot valgus or plantarflexed first ray, both of which increase the force under the forefoot.

Literature accounts of successful treatment with orthotics ranges in the high 80% of positive outcomes.

TARSAL COALITION: Most of the pain from tarsal coalition is thought to be secondary to peroneal brevis spasm and jamming of the lateral subtalar joint in the body's unconscious effort to immobilize the subtalar and midtarsal joints. Making a diagnosis of a middle facet or calcaneal navicular bar is difficult, and managing this pathology conservatively or post fusion is extremely difficult.

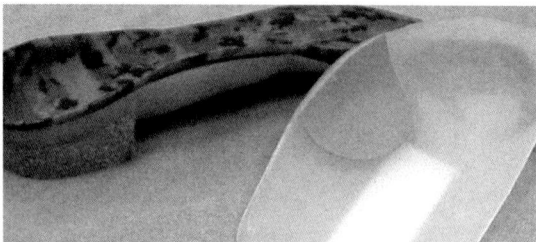

Figure 11-57: Orthotic for posterior tibialis dysfunction.

TARSAL TUNNEL SYNDROME: Tarsal tunnel syndrome is similar to carpal tunnel syndrome and both disorders symptoms are due to nerve compression. The pathology produces arch discomfort of an unusual quality that includes sharp pain, paresthesia, tingling of the plantar foot, and a knife point sensation in the heel upon palpation of the nerve under the medial retinaculum. The pathomechanic pathway includes a subtalar pronation, an unusually flexible foot, a lengthening of the foot, and a stretching of the flexor and adductor hallucis brevis. The stretching of the intrinsic muscles narrows both the porta pedis and the tarsal canal.

Orthotic therapy can be useful.

ACHILLES TENDINITIS: The relationship between Achilles tendinitis and flexible flat-foot, especially when related to equinus, is understood. The universally accepted concept is that the more flexible the foot, the harder the gastroc-soleus muscles must work to create heel off. Achilles tendinitis is, therefore, an overuse syndrome in the flexible flat-foot. The primary complaint is persistent and recurrent posterior ankle pain, especially in the morning. The point of maximum tenderness is often at the upper portion of the tendon, the myotendious junction. Pain at the insertion is often associated with arthropathies or systemic disease rather than the overuse syndrome of tendinitis. A lack of dorsiflexion with this pathology is common. If the tendon never gets stretched out, it will shorten. If the forefoot can dorsiflex on the rearfoot at the midtarsal joint, why would the Achilles tendon ever need to be stretched to its full length? Stability of the midtarsal joint is therefore crucial for successful management.

Orthotic therapy can be helpful.

CHONDROMALCIA PATELLA, PATELLAR FEMORAL PAIN SYNDROME. While not a foot disorder, chondromalcia patella as well as many other patello-femoral pain syndromes (and other knee problems) are commonly believed to relate to poor foot biomechanics. This syndrome is a clinical condition of complex symptoms, characterized by peripatellar pain and crepitation of the knee with activity. The symptoms of anterior or posterior knee pain are usually exacerbated by stairs and frequently occur upon standing after prolonged sitting. Interestingly, the age span of patello-femoral pain syndromes ranges from active prepubescent to geriatric. Although the exact etiology of the problem has not

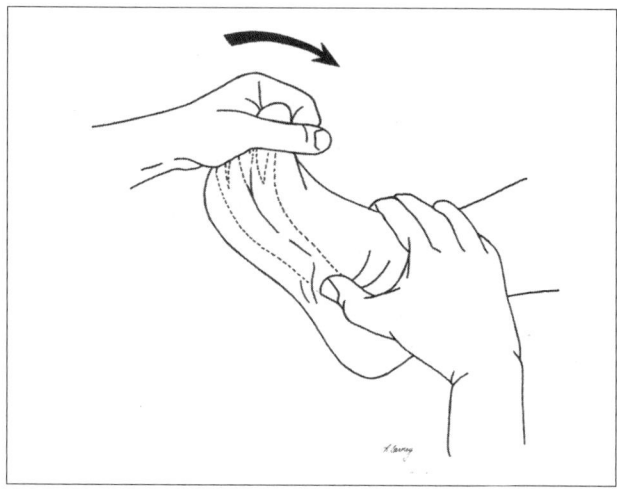

Figure 11-58: Palpation of plantar fascia (courtesy of Dorman and Ravin *ibid*).

been established, most literature suggests that excessive subtalar and midtarsal motion is associated with the symptoms. The pathology suggested by several studies is an "abnormal coupling" between the axial rotation of the leg and the pronation of the foot. A simple way of looking at the pathomechanics is that the more the subtalar joint pronates and the more the midtarsal joint coalesces, the more the leg internally rotates behind the patella. The patella's position and articulation with the femur is designed for sagittal plane motion of extension and flexion. The abnormal transverse motion of the femur behind the patella is what causes the softening, fibrillation, fissuring, and ultimate erosion that exposes the subchondral bone. Symptoms can sometimes be reproduced by non-weight-bearing lateral distraction of the patella.

Orthotic therapy is helpful and should be used early in the development of these conditions.

Postural Stresses

Many postural and gravitational stresses can perpetuate myofascial pain syndromes and other musculoskeletal disorders. Misfitting furniture, poor postures, abuse of muscles, sustained muscular contractions, immobility, and repetitive movements are listed by Simons, Travell, and Simons (*ibid*). Activities that can increase stress on the musculoskeletal system include prolonged sitting or sleeping in poorly designed or poorly manufactured furniture, ineffective ergonomics, unphysiologic positioning at a computer station or when reading, overly kyphotic (slouched) or "stiff-back" postures, poor footwear and foot positioning, poor body mechanics when lifting, bending, dressing, and many ordinary daily activities.

Gravitational forces often stress the sagittal plane. Compensations and the righting reflex[126] often stress the coronal plane. Often gravity encourages the sacral base to rotate

Perpetuating Factors

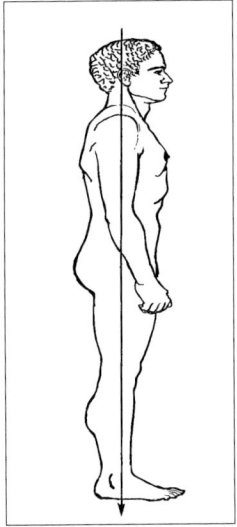

Figure 11-59: Optimal posture.

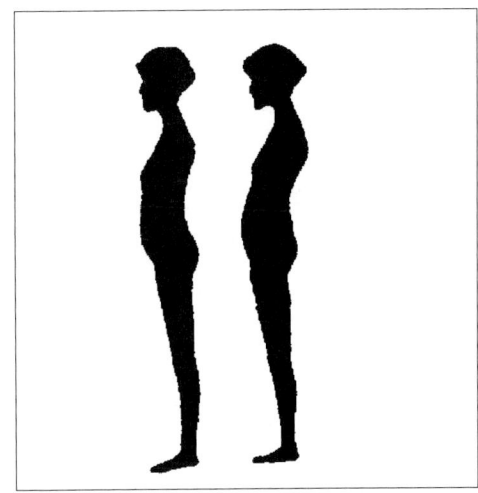

Figure 11-60: Adaptation to forward head posture or foot dysfunctions.

anteriorly and the innominates to rotate posteriorly. If compensatory mechanisms are overwhelmed and fail, the patient develops symptoms and pain, that stresses the ligamentous-fascial organ, often affecting the illiolumbar ligament first. Somatic dysfunction may result in a facilitated cord segment and visceral symptoms (Figure 11-61). Sagittal plane decompensation (increased or decreased spinal curves)[127] is often seen with *extension mechanic prevalence in the craniosacral mechanism*. The extension phase is often accompanied by loss of energy and psychological depression. In general, a person with a decompensated posture requires a period of rest before exercise is effective (Kuchera and Kuchera *ibid*).

When the ligamentous-fascial organ is healthy, one should be able to withstand many of the above stresses painlessly. However, once injured (or to prevent reinjury) the patient must reduce stress on injured tissues.

Forward Head Posture

Although often not symptomatic, non-optimal postures may result in abnormal stresses and accommodation in the musculoskeletal system. Many sagittal and coronal postural compensations result in forward head posture and vice versa. When head posture is "optimal" (Figure 11-59), the apex of the lordotic cervical curve is usually at C4-5, and the head's center of gravity is at a point just anterior to the cervical spine and just superior to the temporomandibular joint. This changes when the head is held forward. The lower cervical segments flex and, for the head to remain looking forward, the apex of the cervical lordosis shifts upward. This may result in increased compression forces on the lower cervical segments, which can lead to pathology of the lower segments (Figure 11-60).

According to Shaw (1992), forward movement of the head results from any joint dysfunction that affects the parallel plane of the eyes and ears, and from occlusion of the mandible in its horizontal plane. These new planes are maintained at the expense of normal function almost anywhere in the musculoskeletal system. Forward head posture can result in significant effects on the entire musculoskeletal system. Such posture also can be secondary to any dysfunction as far down as the feet.

Forward head posture is commonly associated with either a general increase in thoracic kyphosis or with "dowager's hump," i.e., an increased, localized kyphosis at the cervicothoracic area. However, especially if the patient is standing, in order to maintain the body's center of gravity the upper thoracic spine might extend (losing its usual kyphosis) and may appear to flatten.

DEVELOPMENT OF FORWARD HEAD POSTURE. Although forward head posture is most obvious in mature patients, usually the condition begins early in life when posture becomes habitual. Gravity tends to exert a force on the head and neck (and sacrum) making them shift forward. Because the head can weigh as much as fifteen pounds, poor posture during many daily activities such as working at computers and/or reading, and even postural laziness and emotional disturbances such as poor self-esteem and depression, can perpetuate this tendency. Poor (Simons, Travell, Simons *ibid*) foot function and standing posture with weight on the heels tends to shift the head forward as a counterweight, with the

---

126. A reflex that makes sure the plane of vision remains strait.

127. Patients often develop spondylolisthesis at about age six, which causes no problems until age thirty-five or so. Of the estimated 5% of the population with spondylolisthesis, approximately half are asymptomatic. One of the most consistent physical findings in patients under the age of thirty is tight hamstrings. In contrast, patients over age fifty with degenerative spondylolisthesis can easily touch their toes without bending their knees or obliterating their lumbar lordosis (Kuchera and Kuchera *ibid*).

resulting loss of normal cervical and lumbar lordotic curves.

EFFECTS OF FORWARD HEAD POSTURE. Forward head posture can result in many joints being maintained at their extreme range. This can result in reduced motion and, therefore, reduce regenerative activities at the joint. This probably leads to degenerative changes in the joint complex. Abnormal resting joint positions may also lead to some ligaments being stretched continuously, resulting in hypersensitivity and loss of tensile strength. Unbalanced posture alters weight-bearing, causing (Janda *ibid*) muscle compensations with shortening in some groups, and causing the muscle's antagonistic group to be inhibited and stretched.

One adaptation seen clinically is that the *suboccipital* muscles, *levator scapulae*, and the upper fibers of *trapezius* and *sternocleidomastoid* fatigue and shorten as they work harder to maintain the head upright. The upper *flexors* then can become inhibited, stretched, and weak.

Another clinical presentation is the *hyperactivity* of the upper *flexor* muscles and of the *sternocleidomastoid* and *scalene* muscles, which accentuates forward head posture. This hyperactivity can stretch and facilitate the *suboccipital* neck *extensors* and the *levator scapulae*, which often develop trigger points at their attachments to the scapula (Ayub, Glasheen-Wray, Kraus 1984).

PROTRACTION OF THE SHOULDER GIRDLE. According to Shaw (*ibid*), the shoulder girdle (scapula) is the positional foundation of the head and neck. The shoulder girdle can protract, elevate, and internally rotate, causing a round-shouldered appearance. This dysfunction shortens the upper fibers of the *trapezius* and *levator scapulae*, elevating the scapula and leading to increased thoracic convexity and abduction. The result is a shortening of such muscles as the *teres major* and, reciprocally, an inhibition of the *lower fibers* of the *trapezius* and *rhomboids*. The extension by the head on the atlas (for maintaining the visual plane) causes the *suprahyoid* and *infrahyoid* muscles to stretch and pull the mandible. This can give rise to temporomandibular joint disorders. Other types of compensation are possible as well. Therefore, attention to shoulder girdle positioning and muscle balance is important in chronic neck pain patients.

SYMPTOMS. Because forward head posture can affect such a variety of structures, symptoms can vary greatly. Headaches and myofascial pain are common, and temporomandibular joint disorders are seen (Ayub, Glasheen-Wray, Kraus *ibid*). Because the thoracic spine can compensate by either decreasing or increasing its kyphosis (depending on how the lumbar spine and lower extremities compensate for the load), many patients develop low back pain, as well.

According to Janda (*ibid*), temporomandibular joint (TMJ) problems and facial pain can be analyzed in relation to the patient's whole posture. He suggests that the muscular pattern associated with TMJ problems result from hyperactivity and tension in the *temporal* and *masseter* muscles, resulting in the reciprocal inhibition of the *suprahyoid*,

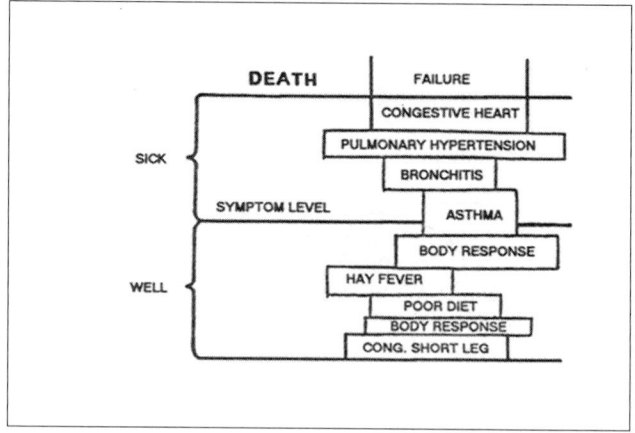

Figure 11-61: Posture and function interdependency (From Kuchera WA and Kuchera ML, Osteopathic Principles in Practice, KCOM press 1993, with permission).

digastric, and *mylohyoid* muscles. The external *pterygoid* in particular often develops spasm. This imbalance between jaw *adductors* and jaw *openers* modifies the position of the TMJ condyle and leads to a consequent redistribution of stress on the joint, leading to degenerative changes. The postural pattern in a TMJ syndrome [and forward head posture] might involve (Chaitow *ibid*):

- hyperextension of knee joints;
- increased anterior tilt of pelvis;
- pronounced flexion of hip joints;
- hyperlordosis of lumbar spine;
- Rounded shoulders and winged (rotated and abducted) scapulae;
- cervical hyperlordosis;
- forward thrust of head;
- compensatory over-activity of upper trapezius and levator scapulae;
- forward thrust of head resulting in opening of mouth and retraction of mandible.

TREATMENT. The best treatment approach is global, addressing joint dysfunctions, pelvic obliquities, foot mechanics, and myofascial adaptations. Postural training often is helpful; however, changes in tissue and general habits can take a long time. Postural training may not work in patients who have significant physiological tissue alterations. TMJ problems can be treated effectively with acupuncture (Rosted 2001). St-6, St-7, SI-18, GV-20, GB-20, UB-10, LI-4 and auricular points are often recommended. After needles are inserted, they should be manipulated manually to achieve the De-Qi sensation and left in situ for thirty minutes. Abnormal Sinew and Extra channel functions are often treated. Muscle energy and cranial osteopathic techniques are particularly useful for TMJ pain.

Postural awareness and alteration can often be achieved by teaching the patient to pay attention to the *position of his/her chin and shoulder girdle*. One method for affecting this condition is frequent tucking-in of the chin, while elongating the spine through visualization.

For patients who have *shortening* of the *suboccipital* muscles and inhibition of the *flexor* muscles, exercises to stretch the *suboccipitals* and strengthen the *flexors* tend to be helpful. Because this type of patient often has increased thoracic kyphosis, it may be necessary to stretch the *pectoral* muscles and strengthen the *rhomboids*. The patient may need to keep the scapula retracted. If the *flexor* muscles are shortened clinically, and if the *suboccipital* and *levator* scapula develop trigger points, the practitioner should needle them and stretch the *flexors* (Shaw *ibid*, Janda *ibid*).

Nutritional Inadequacies

According to Simons, Travell, and Simons (*ibid*) vitamin and mineral deficiencies, especially in patients with poor dietary habits, who drink alcohol or have chronic co-morbid diseases, can result in myofascial pain. This is found in nearly half of their patients. Vitamin B1, B6, B12, folic acid, vitamin C, calcium, magnesium, iron, and potassium are of particular interest. Insulin resistance, protein deficiency and a high glycemic diets may result in increased pain sensitivity.

Metabolic and Endocrine Inadequacies

According to Simons, Travell, and Simons (*ibid*), any compromise of the energy metabolism of a muscle appears to aggravate and perpetuate MPS. Anemia, hypometabolism, hypothyroidism and other thyroid disease, hypoglycemia, and gouty diathesis are of particular concern.

Excess estrogen can sensitize nociceptors and thus reduce the pain threshold.[128]

Psychological Factors

According to Simons, Travell, and Simons (*ibid*), a number of psychological factors can contribute and perpetuate MPS. Especially important are depression, tension, caused by anxiety, the "good sport" syndrome, sleep, secondary gain, and learned illness behavior. For more information see page 144.

Chronic Infection

According to Simon, Travell, and Simon (*ibid*), infection due to viral or bacterial disease as well as some parasitic infestations can prevent recovery from myofascial pain syndromes. Viral illnesses including influenza, and especially herpes simplex, can perpetuate myofascial pain syndrome. Absorption of bacterial or viral toxic products may result in the development of trigger points when a minor mechanical stress is added. Common locations are abscessed tooth, sinuses, and the intestinal and urinary tracts. The erythrocyte sedimentation rate may be increased. Fish tapeworm, giardiasis, and amebiasis can perpetuate myofascial pain syndromes, as well.

Other Factors

According to Simon, Travell, and Simon (*ibid*), factors such as allergies, radiculopathy, and chronic visceral disease can prolong treatment. Allergic rhinitis seems to perpetuate myofascial pain syndrome, and patients seem to respond to treatments only temporarily. They recommend avoidance of exposure to the allergens. They also recommends the use of antihistamine therapy.

Medical Conditions

Many diseases can manifest with pain and need to be considered. A partial list to consider in patients with pain is (Ombregt et al *ibid*; Brown *ibid;* Merck *ibid,* Opipari et al 2003):

1. Urinary infection and stones are common in patients with back pain. Renal disease may result in pain at the flanks and upper lumbar regions, which may be sensitive to percussion and may radiate to the thigh. Calculi (stones) or other obstructive diseases often radiate pain to the groin, testes, and thigh. Prostatitis commonly refers pain to the back and sacrum.

2. Retroperitoneal masses such as lymphomas, GYN disorders, and aneurysms may refer pain to the back. Excessive perspiration is often an early sign of lymphomas. A bruit (a friction-like sound) may be heard over an aneurysm, and, often, a pulsating mass can be felt on palpation. Gynecological diseases often refer pain to the lumbosacral region.

3. Rectosigmoid diseases can refer an ache to the low back. The character of such pain may or may not change with defecation.

4. Infectious conditions may lead to back pain. Gonococcal, staphylococcal, syphilitic, tubercular, and viral infections should be kept in mind. Osteomyelitis (often seen in younger patients), brucellosis (in farm workers), tuberculosis (in immune deficient patients) should be kept in mind.

5. Inflammatory conditions such as rheumatoid arthritis (RA), Reiter's syndrome, psoriatic arthritis, and ankylosing spondylitis can give rise to back and other joint pains. RA usually gives rise to bilateral migratory pains in joints and muscles, with signs of inflammation such as red, hot, swollen, tender, and enlarged joints. RA, ankylosing spondylitis,[129] psoriasis[130] and Reiter's

---

128. DIM and I3C can be used to treat estrogen dominance.

disease[131] are unlikely to present with primary spinal involvement. In RA, lupus, systemic sclerosis, and dermatomyositis the small joints (e.g. metacarpophalangeal joints) are usually affected. Reactive type arthritis (e.g. peripheral joint involvement in ankylosing spondylitis, ulcerative colitis, Reiter's syndrome, sarcoidosis and psoriatic arthritis) usually affect a few large joints (shoulder, hip, or knee) symmetrically. Some inflammatory conditions (especially RA) can affect the transverse ligament in the cervical spine permitting the odontoid process of the axis to sublux. Reiter's syndrome affects mostly lower spine.

6. Connective tissue and collagen vascular diseases such as Ehlers-Danlos syndrome, Marfan's syndrome, and some of which are inflammatory such as lupus, progressive systemic sclerosis, dermatomyositis, and polymyalgia Rheumatica are kept in mind.

    Patients with Ehlers-Danlos are often very flexible (both their skins and joints) and are susceptible to joint sprains/strains, early arthritis and joint dislocations. They heal poorly and often develop "paper thin" scars.[132]

    Patients with Marfans tend to be tall with arm span exceeding height. They are also often hyperflexible and have backward curvature of the legs at the knee (genu recuvatum), flat-feet and kyphoscoliosis. The most serious danger they face is due to cardiovascular changes with weakness of the aortic media in areas subject to greatest hemodynamic stress, which may lead to rupture. Systemic lupus erythematosus is an inflammatory connective tissue disorder of unknown etiology occurring predominately in young women. Articular symptoms ranging from intermittent arthralgias to acute polyarthritis, some for months or years, may be seen before other manifestation of the disease. Progressive systemic sclerosis is a chronic disease of unknown etiology, characterized by diffuse fibrosis, degenerative changes, and vascular abnormalities in the skin (scleoderma), articular structures, and internal organs. There is often overlap with syndromes such as sclerodermatomyositis (muscle weakness indistinguishable from polymyositis) and mixed connective tissue disease. Polymyalgia Rheumatica is a disease of unknown etiology seen with pain and stiffness in proximal muscle groups without permanent weakness or atrophy. It is a fairly common disease occurring in a female-to-male ratio of 4:1. The onset may be sudden or gradual; pain and stiffness may appear symmetrically in the neck, back, or shoulder or pelvic girdle muscles.

7. The bony skeleton is the second most common metastatic site of malignancy in terms of frequency. Over 80% of the metastatic tumors originate within breast, prostate, lung, kidney, and thyroid gland. Colon cancer can also result in metastasis. Microscopically, at autopsy, a much higher rate of metastasis to bone is present than noted clinically, with in excess of 80% in breast and prostate, 50% in thyroid, and 40% in lung and kidney cancers. Other malignancies such as esophageal cancers frequently refer pain to the neck and upper extremities. The spine is involved most often with a reducing order of frequency extending from lumbar to dorsal to cervical areas of the spine. Back pain is often the first indication of metastatic disease. Malignant diseases are seen usually in patients over fifty years of age. Primary spinal tumors, most commonly osteosarcomas, affect younger patients. Multiple myelomas, the most common primary malignant bone tumor, and chondrosarcomas are seen in older patients as well. Early metastatic disease can be difficult to detect because the physical signs can be subtle and radiographs can be negative. Bone scan abnormalities require radiographic, CT, or MRI confirmation of metastases. Deposits in the upper cervical spine and the upper thoracic vertebrae are difficult to detect because often nerve sequelae are absent.

    The peripheral joints may be involved with malignancy by either a primary tumor or metastatic process to the bone or synovium. This presents as a picture of asymmetric arthritis, or diffuse articular changes caused by an indirect, humoral-related process as in hypertrophic osteoarthropathy. Leukemia in children can be present as localized or diffuse bone pain associated with joint swelling and pain. Both primary and metastatic disease has been reported in a variety of soft tissues including muscles.

    Warning signs are:

    - Pain that awakens the patient at night and that is unrelieved by rest;
    - Expanding or rapidly-increasing pain;
    - Any new or increasing pain in an elderly patient;
    - Constitutional symptoms such as weight loss, fever, excessive sweating and/or fatigue;
    - True muscular spasm that increases with sidebending away from the painful side;
    - History of cancer or smoking. A family history of cancer;
    - Major neurological signs without significant root pain;
    - Involvement of several roots;
    - Severe bone tenderness when percussed.

8. Primary benign tumors in the spine occur more often in children than adults. The most common are giant cell tumors, aneurysmal bone cyst, osteoblastoma

---

129. A progressive disease in which the joint and/or its surrounding tissue becomes fixed; usually seen in young adults; four times more common in the white population than in the black population.
130. A dermatological and arthritic disorder.
131. A triad of arthritis with fever, conjunctivitis, and urethritis.
132. Patients with Ehler-Danlos syndrome respond well to prolotherapy, but treatment needs to be repeated often.

haemangioma, osteochondroma, osteoid osteoma and eosinophilic granuloma.

9. Neurofibromatosis (von Recklinghausen's disease) is a condition that results in tumors of nervous tissue that may appear on the skin or in the optic and acoustic nerves. Other manifestations include multiple soft tissue pendunculated fleshy tumors and café-au-lait-pigmented macules (café-colored plaque or patches) associated with pain confined to radicular pattern. Symptoms often start in the periphery and progress proximally.

10. Metabolic destructive processes such as osteoporosis and osteomalacia should be suspected in elderly kyphotic patients, or in patients in whom minor injuries cause severe localized pain. Paget's disease (osteitis deformans) is seen in three percent of adults over forty years. Ninety percent of patients are asymptomatic. Ochronosis is a rare condition marked by dark pigmentation of cartilage, ligaments, fibrous tissue, skin, and urine. Twice as common in males as in females, this condition is seen in mid-life and in patients with hyperparathyroidism.

11. Paresthesia (numbness and tingling) requires consideration of conditions such as diabetes, peripheral neuritis, nerve entrapment, transitory ischemic attack (TIA), strokes, and pernicious anemia.

12. Scapular and shoulder pain can be felt in pleurisy and in conditions that irritate the diaphragm such as ectopic pregnancy, gallbladder disease, and in inferior myocardial infarction.

13. Neuralgic amyotropy is an uncommon disorder seen more frequently in the cervical spine than at other spinal levels. The onset can be sudden, with central or bilateral severe neck pain that later radiates to both upper limbs. After a while the pain remains in one arm only. Movement is possible and paresthesias uncommon. The pain may be aggravated by coughing or deep breathing.

14. Herpetic neuralgia can present as pain before cutaneous lesions are visible.

15. Trigeminal neuralgia presents as severe paroxysmal (sudden bouts of second-long lacerating) facial pain in the distribution of the trigeminal nerve. This can be aggravated by cold air, shaving, chewing, and other movements, but it is unaffected by cervical movements. Other symptoms of trigeminal neuralgia include muscle spasms, flushing of the face, lacrimation, and increased salivation.

16. Mononeuritis should be considered especially in patients with a history of trauma or viral infections.
    Long thoracic nerve. Discomfort mostly over the scapular and upper arm area with limitation of active arm elevation and a positive scapula-winging test.
    Spinal accessory nerve. Ache and weakness similar to long thoracic nerve neuritis except that resisted approximation of scapula is weak due to trapezius muscle weakness. There is no scapular winging.
    Suprascapular nerve. Constant pain in the scapular area and upper arm, movements of neck and scapula are normal, there is weakness of supraspinatus and infraspinatus.

17. Organ diseases of the gall bladder, pancreas, spleen, or apex of the heart; any irritation of the diaphragm, and/or ectopic pregnancy frequently refer pain to the scapular and shoulder regions. However, scapular/shoulder pain is unlikely to be the only presenting symptom. Renal, urinary, pelvic, and digestive disorders often refer pain to the back.

18. Depression and anxiety disorders are common contributing factors in patients with pain. Patients who have been diagnosed with fibromyalgia syndromes score much higher on anxiety and depression scales. Pain tends to be variable and is associated with fatigue, sleep disorders, head, and other aches, and the inability to cope with stress.

19. Vascular disorders are an important element in the diagnosis of pain, especially in the cervical spine. Potential of vascular compromise is inherent in certain mechanical therapies and other treatments of the neck. The differential diagnoses of vascular conditions include:

PREDISPOSING FACTORS	OTHER FACTORS
• hypertension	• diabetes
• fibromuscular dysplasia	• neoplasm
• oral contraceptive use	• arteritis
• arteriopathy	• multiple sclerosis
• cervical spondylosis	• aneurysm
• arteriosclerosis	• bony congenital abnormalities
• congenital asymmetry of the posterior circulation	• neurofibromatosis
• history of previous neck trauma	• steroid treatment
• cardiovascular disease	
• osteoarthrosis	
• segmental hypermobility	
• smoking	

Sudden arterial occlusions (as in coronary artery disease with angina), thoracic outlet syndrome, arteritis. intermittent claudication by ischemia secondary to arteriosclerotic plaque progression, which can cause the patient to complain of pain in the extremities on exertion (uncommon in the upper extremities), Raynaud's disease/phenomenon that may result in extremity pain that is secondary to vasospasm. Basilar syndrome is a condition that affects the posterior cerebral and vertebral arteries. The risk factors that may result in vascular disease are summarizes below.

20. Headache, a common symptom of cervical dysfunction, can be due to mechanical, muscular, ligamentous and/or none-orthopedic/musculoskeletal causes. An acute new headache can be serious. The practitioner should consider

conditions such as an impending CVA (cerebral vascular accident), subarachnoid hemorrhage, infections, malignant hypertension, arteritis, poisoning, intracranial tumor and trauma. Migraine headaches are believed to have a vascular origin[133]: in the prodromal phase (before headache begins), intracranial blood vessels constrict, and characteristic visual and/or sensory disturbances occur. In the second phase, the blood vessels dilate, which results in acute unilateral headache. Migraine headaches can be precipitated by cervical spine mechanical dysfunctions.

---

133. These theories are now changing, and migraine is thought to be also serotonin and other mediators related.

References

Works Cited

A

Abad-Alegria F, Pomaron C, Aznar C, Munoz C, Adelantado S. Objective assessment of the sympatholytic action of the Nei-Kuan acupoint *Am J Chin Med* 29:201, 2001.

Adams MA, Dolan P, Hutton WC The lumbar spine in backward bending. *spine.* 13:1019, 1988.

Adems MA, Dolan P. Posture and spinal mechanisms during lifting. *2ed interdisciplinary world congress on low back pain.* The integrated function of the lumbar spine SI joins 1995.

Aigner N et al. Laseracupuncture for Patellar Tendinitis in Performance Athletes. *Akupuncktur Theorie und Praxis* 24:11, 1996.

Akai M, Oda H, Shiraski Y, Tateishi T. Electrical stimulation of ligament healing: An experimental study of the patellar ligament of rabbits. *Clin Orthop.* 235:296, 1988.

Akermark C, et al. Glycosaminoglycan Polysulfate Injections in Lateral Humeral Epicondylagia: A Placebo-Controlled Double-Blind Trial. *International Journal of Sports Medicine* 16:196, 1995.

Akeson WH, Amiel D, Woo SL-Y. Immobility effects on synovial joints, the pathomechanics of joint contracture. *Biorheology.* 17:95, 1980.

Aldman B. Injury Biomechanics. Government/Industry Meeting and Eposition. Washington, DC: *Society of Automotive Engineers*, 1987; SP-731.

Alfano AP et al. Static magnetic fields for treatment of fibromyalgia: a randomized controlled trial. *J Altern Complement Med.* 7(1):53, 2001.

Allen JJB, et al. The Efficacy of Acupuncture in the Treatment of Major Depression in Women. *Psychological Science* 9:397, 1998.

Altman RD, Marcussen KC. Effects of a Ginger Extract on Knee Pain in Patients With Osteoarthritis. *Arthritis Rheum* 44:2531, 2001.

Alvarez OM, Gilbereath RL. Thiamine influence on collagen during the granulation of skin wounds. *J Surg Res* 32:24,1982.

Alvarez OM, Gilbereath RL. Thiamine influence on collagen during the granulation of skin wounds. *J Surg Res* 32:24,1982.

Alvarez OM, Gilbereath RL. Thiamine influence on collagen during the granulation of skin wounds. *J Surg Res* 32:24,1982Alves WM et al.: Understanding posttraumatic symptoms after minor head injury. *J Head Trouma Rehabil.* 1:1, 1986.

Alves WM. Motor vehicle head injuries: damage and outcome. *In: Crash Injury Impairment and Disability*: Long Term Effects. International Congress and Exposition; paper 860423. Detroit, Mich: Society of Automotive Engineers; SP-661:167-176, 1986.

American Medical Association. *Standard Nomenclature of Athletic Injuries*. AMA Chicago, 1976.

Amiel D, Woo S et al. The effects of immobilization on collagen turnover in connective tissue. *Trans Orthop Res Soc* 6:85, 1981.

Ammon HPT, Mack T, et al. Inhibition of Leukotriene B4 Formation in rat Peritoneal Neutrophils by Ethanolic extract of the Gum Resin Exudate of Boswellia Serrata. *Planta Medica* 57:203, 1991.

Andermann G and Dietz M. The influence of an endogenous macromolecule: Chondroitin Sulfate (CSA), *Eur.J.Drug Metabol. Pharmacol.*, 7,11,1982.

Anderson AV. Cervicogenic Processes: Results of Injury to the Cervical Spine. The Pain Practitioner 11:9, 2001.

Andersson S. Physiological mechanisms in acupuncture. In: Hopwood V, Lovesey M, Mokone S (edi) *Acupuncture & Related Techniques in Physical Therapy*. Churchill Livingstone 1997.

Andersson S. The functional background in acupuncture effects. *Scandinavian J of Rehab Med* (suppl) 29:31, 1993.

Angelica sinensis research unit, Second Teaching Hospital of Hubei Medical College. *Health J of Jubei* 5:64, 1977.

Annand JC. Pantothenic acid and osteoarthritis. Letter. Lancet 2:1168,1963;

Annand JC. Osteoarthrosis and pantothenic acid. Letter. *J coll Gen Pract* 5:136,1962.

Appiah R, Hiller S, Caspary L, Alexander K, Creutzig A. Treatment of primary Raynaud's syndrome with traditional Chinese acupuncture. *J Intern Med* 241:119, 1997.

Aprahamian M et al. *Am J Clin Nutr* 578:89,1985.

April C, Bogduk N.:High-intensity zone: a diagnostic sign of painful lumbar disc on magnetic resonance imaging. *Br J Radiol.* 65:361, 1992.

Aprill C. et al: Discografic outcomes predicted by centralization of pain and directional preference. A prospective study. *Presented at the Eighth Annual International Intradical therapy Society Meeting*, San Diego, Calif, 1995.

Arpaia MR et al. Effects of Centella asiatica extract on mucopolysaccharide metabolism in subjects with varicose veins. *Int J Clin Pharmacol Res* 10:229-,1990.

Arromdee E, Mattesom EL. Bursitis: Common condition, uncommon challenge. *J Musculoskel Med* 18:213, 2001.

Asmundson GJ, Taylor S. Role of anxiety sensitivity in pain-related fear and avoidance. *J Behav Med* 19:577, 1996.

Auaisha BB et al. Acupuncture for the treatment of Chronic Painful Peripheral Diabetic Neuropathy: A long-Term Study. *Diabetic Research and Clinical Practice* 39:115, 1998.

B

Bachrach RM: Psoas dysfunction/insufficiency, sacroiliac dysfunction and low back pain. In: Vleeming, Mooney, Dorman, Snijders, Soeckart *Movement Stability and Low Back Pain* Churchill Livingstone 1997.

Baker BA: The muscle trigger: evidence of overload injury. *J Neurol Orthop Med Surg* 10:129, 1989.

Baker d, Daito M.: *Proc. R Soc. Lond. B.* 212,1981.

Baker DM. Penniculitis. *Lancet. 2: 75,* 1951.

Backer M., Hammes M.G., Valet M., Deppe M., Conrad B., Tolle T.R., Dobos G. Different modes of manual acupuncture stimulation differentially modulate cerebral blood flow velocity, arterial blood pressure and heart rate in human subjects. *Neurosci Lett* 333(3):203, 2002.

Balagot RC et al. Analgesia in mice and humans by D-phenylalanine: Relation to inhibition of enkephalin degradation and enkephalin levels. *Adv Pain Res Ther* 5:289,1983.

Baldry PE. Acupuncture, *Trigger Points and Musculoskeletal Pain* (2ed ed) Churchill Livingstone 1993.

Balgent, Michael, Leigh, Richard. *The Dead Sea Scrolls Deception.* Simon and Schuster, New York, 1991.

Balla, J., Karnaghan, J. Whiplash Headache. *Clin Exp Neurol* 23:179, 1987.

Banks AR. A rationale for prolotherapy. *J Orthop Med* 13:54, 1991.

Bann RT, Woods PH: An attempt to estimate the size of the problem. *Rheumatol Rehabil* 14:121,1975.

Bannister G et al. The management of acute acromioclavicular dislocations. *J Bone Joint Surg* 71:848, 1989.

Barclay L. 29th annual meeting of the American Orthopaedic Society for Sports Medicine held in San Diego July 29, 2003.

Barnsley L, Lord SM, Wallis BJ, Bogduk N. The prevalence of chronic cervical zygapophyseal joint pain after whiplash. *Spine* 20:20, 1995.

Barnett C, Richardson AT. The postural function of the popliteus muscle. *Ann Phys Med* 17:179, 1953.

Barnsley L, Lord SM, Wallis BJ, Bogduk N Lack of effect of intraarticular corticosteroids for chronic pain in the cervical zygapophyseal joints. *N Engl J Med* 330:1047, 1994.

Baron AD, Zhu JS, Zhu JH, et al. Glucosamine induces insulin resistance in vivo by affecting GLUT 4 translocation in skeletal muscle. Implications for glucose toxicity. *J Clin Invest* 96:2792, 1995.

Baron JB et al. Interaction Between Labyrinthine Electrical Mechanical Stimulations and Musculo-Oculo-Nucal Magnetic Stimulation on Tonic Postural Activity. Seventh International Symposium of the International Society of Postugogaphy, Houston, Texas 1983.

Barral JP, Croibier A. *Trauma, an Osteopathic Approach*. Eastland Press, 1999.

Barson PK, Solomon JD. Blood Serotonin in Chronic Pain Syndromes. Am J Pain Mang 8:49, 1998.

Basford JR. Low-energy laser therapy: Controversies and new research findings. *Lasers Surg Med* 9:1,1989.

Basic Research Group. Xian Medical Collage *Shaanxi Med J* 1:28,1972.

Basmajian JV. *Muscles Alive*. 4th Ed. Williams and Willkins, Baltimore, 1978.

Basmajian JV and Nyberg R. *Rational Manual Therapies* edi Williams and Wilkins 1993.

Bassett CAL, Michell SM, Norton I et al. Repair of non-unions by pulsing electromagnetic fields. Acta Orhopedica Belgica 44:706, 1978.

Bates CJ, Levene CI. The effect of ascorbic acid deficiency on the glycosaminoglycans and glycoproteins in connective tissue. Biol Nutr Dieta 13:131, 1969.

Battié MC et al. Smoking and lumbar intervertebral disc degeneration: as MRI study of identical twins, *spine.* 16:1015, 1991.

Battié MC, Videman T, Gibbons LE, et al. Occupational Driving and Lumbar Disc Degeneration: A Case-Control Study *Lancet,* November 2,360, 2002.

Bauman J et al. *Prostaglandins* 20:627,1980.

Beaton E, Anson BJ: The sciatic nerve and the piriformis muscle: their interrelationship a possible cause of coccygodynia. *J Bone Joint Surg* [Br] 20:686, 1938.

Beattie P et al. Validity of derived measurements of leg length differences obtained by use of a tape measure. *Phys Ther* 70 150, 1990.

Becker RO, Selden G. *The Body Electric: Electromagnetism and the Foundation of Life.* New York: William Morrow and Company, 1985.

Becker RO and Marino AA. *Electromagnetism and life*, State University of NY Press, 1982.

Beecher HK. The powerful placebo. *JAMA* Dec. 24 1955.

Beforre GH J et al. Heterozygosity for homocystinuria in premature peripheral and cerebral occlusive arterial disease. *N Eng J Med* 313:709,1985.

Beighton, P., R. Grahame, and H Brode. *Hypermobility of Joints*. Berlin, Pringer-Verlag, 1983.

Bekkering R, van Bussel R. Segmental acupuncture (in *Medical Acupuncture*) Churchill Livingstone 1998.

Belch JJ, Anseli D, Madhok R, O'Dowd, A, Sturrock RD. Effects of altering dietary essential fatty acids on requirements for non steroidal anti-inflammatory drugs in patients with rheumatoid arthritis: a double blind placebo controlled study. *Ann-Rheum-Dis* 47: 96, 1988.

Beneliyahu DJ. Chiropractic management and manipulative therapy for MRI documented cervical disk herniation. *J Manipulative*

References

Physiol Ther 17:177, 1994.

Bennett GF. Neuropathic pain In: *Textbook of pain* Wall and Melzack (ed). Churchill Livingstone (3ed ed), 1994.

Bennett R. Presentation on muscle microtrauma. First National Seminar for Patients, Columbus, Ohio, April 1990. Report in Fibromyalgia Network, May 1993.

Bennett GJ. Update on the Neurophysiology of Pain Transmission and Modulation: Focus on the NMDA-Receptor. *J Pain Symptom Mange* 19:2, 2000.

Bennet R. Treatment strategies for fibromyalgia syndrome. *The J of Musculoskeletal Med* 16:20, 1999.

Bensoussan A. *The Vital Meridian, A modern Exploration of Acupuncture*. Churchill Livingstone UK 1991.

Bateman J, Chapman RD, Simpson D. Possible toxicity of herbal-remedies *Scott Med J.* 43:7, 1998.

Bettany JA, Fish DR, Mendel FC. Influence of high voltage pulsed galvanic stimulation on edema formation following impact injury. *Pys Ther.* 69:301, 1988.

Bergmark A. Stability of the lumbar spine: a study in mechanical engineering. *Acta Orthopaedica Scandinavica* 230(suppl): 20, 1989.

Berman BM et al. Efficacy of traditional Chinese acupuncture in the treatment of symptomatic knee osteoarthritis: a pilot study. *Osteoarthritis Cartilage* 3:139, 1995.

Berman BM, Ezzo J, Hadhazy V, Swyers JP. Is acupuncture effective in the treatment of fibromyalgia? *J Fam Pract* 48:213, 1999.

Bernstein IH, Jaremko ME, Hinkley BS. On the utility of the West-Haven-Yale-Multidimensional pain inventory. *Spine* 20:956, 1995).

Bernstein Al. Vitamin B6 in neurology. *Ann N Y Acad Sci* 585:250,1990.

Bhathena S et al. Decreased plasma enkephalins in copper deficiency in man. *Am J Clin Nutr* 43:42,1986.

Bhattacharya SK and Mira SK. Anxiolytic activity of Panax ginseng roots: an experimental study. *J Ethnopharmacol* 34:87,1991.

Biella G, Sotgiu ML, Pellegata G, Paulesu E, Castiglioni I, Fazio F. Acupuncture produces central activations in pain regions. Neuroimage 14:60, 2001.

Biering-Sorenson F. Physical measurements as risk factors for low back trouble over a one year period. *Spine* 9:106, 1984.

Billow RG, Laskowski ER, Harmsen WS. Effect of magnetic vs sham-magnetic insoles on plantar heel pain: a randomized controlled trial. *JAMA* 17;290(11):1474-, 2003.

Binder HJ et al. Cimentadine in the treatment of duodenal ulcer. Gastroenterology 74: 380, 1978.

Binder et al. Pulsed Electromagnetic Field Therapy of Persistent Rotator Cuff Tendinitis. *Lancet* March 31:695, 1984.

Bing Z, Chen G, Xu R, et al. Electrical Characteristics and Specificities of Auricular Points. *Chinese Acupuncture & Moxibustion* 21:12, 2001.

Binkley and Peat.: The effects of immobilization on the ultrastructure and mechanical properties of the rat medial collateral ligament. *Clin Orthop* 203:30, 1986.

Biochem Pharm 38:3527-34;1989.

Birch S. Trigger point--acupuncture point correlations revisited. *J Altern Complement Med* 9(1):91, 2003.

Biskind MS, Marin WC. The use of citrus flavonoids in infection. II. *Am J Digest Dis* 22:4145, 1955.

Bjodal et al. Low level Laser Therapy For Tendinopathy. Evidence of a Dose-Response Pattern. *Physical Therapy Review* 6:91, 2001.

Bjodal et al. A Systematic Review of Low Level Laser Therapy With Location-specific Doses For Pain From Joint Disorders. Australian J of Physiotherapy 49:49, 2003.

Black HN. An improved technique for the evaluation of ligamentous infer in severe ankle sprains. *Am J Sports Med*:276, 1978.

Blair HT, Sharp PE. Anticipatory Head Direction Signals in Anterior Thalamus: Evidence for a Thalamocortical Circuit That Integrates Angular Head Motion to Compute Head Direction. *The Journal of Neuro Science* 15:9, 1995.

Bland JH. The cervical spine: from anatomy to clinical care. *Med Times.* 9:15, 1989.

Blankenhorn G. Vitamin E: Clinical research from Europe. *Nutr Dietary Consult.* June 1988.

Bland JH, Cooper SM. Osteoarthritis: A review of the cell biology involved and evidence for irreversibility. Management rationally related to Known genesis and pathophysiology. *Semin Arthritis Rheum* 14:106,1984.

Blau JN, MacGregor EA. Migraine and the neck. *Headache* 2:88, 1994.

Blechman AM, Oz MC, Nair V, Ting W. Discrepancy between claimed field flux density of some commercially available magnets and actual gauss meter measurements. *Altern Ther Health Med.* 8(1):22, 2002.

Blood S. Treatment of the sprained ankle. *Journal of the American Osteopathic Association* 79: 689, 1980.

Blum LW et al. Peripheral neuropathy and cadmium toxicity. *Pa Med* 92:54,1989Baker D. Banks R. The muscle spindle. In: Engel A, Benker B. eds. *Myology*. NY: McGraw-Hill, 1986.

BMJ 2002; 7338(324):626-7.

Bogduk, N., Aprill, C. On the Nature of Neck Pain, Discography and Cervical Zygapophyseal Joint Blocks. *Pain* 54:213, 1993.

Bogduk N, Tynan W, Wilson AS. The nerve supply to the human lumbar intervertebral discs. *J Anat* 132:39,1981.

Bogduk N. A reappraisal of the anatomy of the human erector spinae. *J Anat* 131:525, 1980.

Bogduk N, Macintosh JE, Pearcy MJ.: A universal model of the lumbar back muscles in the upright position. *Spine* 17:897, 1992.

Bogduk N, Windsor M, Inglis A. The innervation of the cervical intervertebral discs. *Spine.* 13:3, 1988.

Bogduk N, Twomey LT.: *Clinical Anatomy of the Lumbar Spine*. 2nd Ed. Churchill Livingstone, Melbourne, 1991.

Bogduk N.:Pathology of lumbar disc pain. *J Manu Medi.* 5:72,1990.

Bogduk, N. The anatomical Basis for Cervicogenic Headache. *J Manipulative Physiol Ther*. 1:67, 1992.

Bogduk N. A reappraisal of the anatomy of the human erector spinae. *J Anat* 131:525, 1980.

Bogduk N. *The zygapophyseal joints—the most common source of neck pain*. American Back Society 1997.

Boline PD, Kassak K, Bronfort G, Nelson C, Anderson AV. Spinal manipulation vs. amitriptyline for the treatment of chronic tension-type headaches: a randomized clinical trial. *J Manipulative Physiol Ther* 3:148, 1995.

Bombelli R. *Structure and function in normal and abnormal hips*. 3ed ed. Springer-Verlag NY 1993.

Bonica J.J., *The Management of Pain*. lea and febinger 1990.

Borsook H et al. The relief of symptoms of major trigeminal neuralgia (tic doloureux) following the use of vitamin B1 and concentrated liver extract. *JAMA* April 13, 1940.

Bouch B. Chronic Fatigue Syndrome and Neurally Mediated Hypotension. *The American Academy of Medical Acupuncture 13th anniversary* 2001.

Bourdillon JF, Day EA, Brookhout MR. *Spinal Manipulation Butterworth Heinemann 5th edi. 1992*.

Bourguignon GJ, Bourguignon LYW. Electric stimulation of protein and DNA synthesis in human fibroblasts. *FASEB J*. 1:198, 1987.

Bower BL. Rigid subtalar Joint—a radiographic spectrum. *Skeletal Radiol* 17:583, 1989.

Bowsher D. The physiology of stimulation-producted analgesia. *J of the British Med Acupuncture Society* 2:58, 1991.

Brand P. Pain--it's all in your head: a philosophical essay. *J Hand Ther* 10:59, 1997.

Brandmuller J. Fivefold symmetry in mathematics, physics, chemistry, biology and beyond. In *Fivefold Symmetry*, Hargittai I, editor. World Scientific Singapure 1992.

Brattberg G. Acupuncture therapy for tennis elbow. *Pain* 16:283, 1983.

Brevetti G et al. Increases in walking distance in patients with peripheral vascular disease treated with L-carnitine: A double-blind, cross-over study. *Circulation* 77:767,1988.

Bridgman C, Eldred E., *Science* 143,481,1964.

Brighton CT, Pollack SR. Treatment of recalcitrant nonunion with a capacitively coupled electrical field. *J Bone Joint Surg*. 67-A:577, 1986.

Brodsky AE, Khalil MA. Update of experience with electrical stimulation for enhancement of lumbar spine fusion. *Tras Biol Repair Growth Soc*. 8:25, 1988.

Broffman M, McCullock M. Instrument-Assisted Pulse Evaluation in the Acupuncture Practice. *American J of Acup* 14(3):255, 1986.

Bronfort G, Assendelft WJJ, Evans R, et al. Efficacy of Spinal Manipulation for Chronic Headache: A Systematic Review, *J Manipulative Physiol Ther*, 24:466, 2001.

Brooks PM, Potter SR, Buchanan WW. NSAID and osteoarthritis help or hindrance. J Rheumatol 9:3, 1985.

Brouillette DL, Gurske DT. Chiropractic treatment of cervical radiculopathy caused by a herniated cervical disc. *J Manipulative Physiol Ther* 17:119, 1994.

Brown M. American Academy of Oriental Orthopedics. *Lectures* 1995; 1996.

Brown CW, Orme TJ, Richardson HD. The rate of pseudoarthrosis (surgical nonunion) in patients who are smokers and patients who are nonsmokers: a comparison study. *Spine*. 11:943, 1986.

Brown RA. Weiss JB. Neovascularisation and its role in the osteoarthritic process. *Ann Ruem Dis* 47:881,1988.

Brown CS, Ling FW, Wan JY, Pilla AA. Efficacy of static magnetic field therapy in chronic pelvic pain: a double-blind pilot study. *Am J Obstet Gynecol*.187(6):1581, 2002.

Brudnak MA, Dundero D, Van Hecke FM. Are the 'Hard' Martial Arts, Such as the Korean Martial Art, Tae Kwon-Do, of Benefit to Senior Citizens? *Med Hypotheses*, 59(4):485, 2002.

Bucci LR. Chondroprotective Agents Glucosamine Salts and Chondroitin Sulfates. *Townsend Letter for Doctors*, Jan 1994 Cohen A, Goldman J. Bromelains therapy in rheumatoid arthritis. *Pennsyl Med J* 67:27,1964.

Burke. *J of Amer Podiatrtic Med*, Nov. 2001.

Burns et al. Linking symptom-specific physiological reactivity to pain severity in chronic low back pain patients: a test of mediation and moderation models. *Health Psychol* 16:319, 1997.

Buskila et al. Increased rates of fibromyalgia following cervical spine injury: a controlled study of 161 cases of traumatic injury. *Arthritis Rheum* 40:446, 1997.

Byers CM et al. Pyridoxine metabolism in carpal tunnel syndrome with and without peripheral neuropathy. *Am J Med* 75:887,1983.

C

Cailliet R. *Neck and Arm Pain*. 3ed ed. Philadelphia: FA Davis Co; 1991.

Cailliet R. Neck and Arm Pain 12th (ed). FA Davis Company, Philadelphia, 1977.

Cailleit, R. *Low Back Pain Syndromes*. 3st Ed. Philadelphia, F.A. Davis, 1981.

Calabro, J.J., et al.: Classification of anterior chest wall syndrome. JAMA, 243:1420,1980.

Campbell SM. Clinical characteristics of fibrositis. *Arthritis and Rheumatism*. 26:817,1983.

Carey PF A report on the occurrence of cerebral vascular accidents in chiropractic practice; *J of the Canadian Chiro Ass*; 37:104, 1993.

Cats-Baril WL, Frymoyer JW. Identifying patients at risk of becoming disabled because of low-back pain. *Spine* 16:605, 1991.

Cervero F. Afferent activity evoked by neural stimulation of the biliary system of the efferents. *Pain*. 13:137, 1982.

Cervero F, Laird JMA, Pozo MA.: Selective changes of receptive field properties of spinal nociceptive neurons induced by noxious visceral stimulation in the cat. *Pain* 51:335-342, 1992.

References

Cervero F. Neurobiology of pain. *Rev Neurol* 30(6):551, 2000.

Chan SHH. What is being stimulated in Acupuncture: Evaluation of the existence of a specific substrate. *Neurosci Biobehav Rev* 8:25, 1984.

Chan TYK. The prevalence, use and harmful potential of some Chinese herbal medicines in babies and children. *Vet Hum Toxicol* 36:238, 1994

Chan TYK, Chan AYW, Critchley JAJH. Hospital admissions due to adverse reactions to Chinese herbal medicines. *J Trop Med Hyg* 95:296, 1992.

Chen YY; Hsue YT; Chang HH; Gee MJ. The association between postmenopausal osteoporosis and kidney-vacuity syndrome in traditional Chinese medicine *Am J Chin Med* 27:25, 1999.

Chen YC. Nucleoplasty for Chronic Discogenic Back Pain. Poster presentation at NASS Meating of the Americas. April 2002.

Chen GS. The effect of acupuncture treatment on carpal tunnel syndrome. *Amer J of Acup* 18:5, 1990.

Chen P et al. Relationship between cerebral cortex and acupuncture inhibition of visceral pain. In: Zhang X (ed) *Research on Acupuncture, Moxibustion, and Acupuncture Anesthesia.* Sciences Press. Beijing and Sringer-Verlag, Berlin 1998.

Chen XG, et. al. Effects of the extract of Polygonum multiflorum on some biochemical indicators related to aging in old mice. *Chinese Traditional and Herbal Drugs* 22:357, 1991.

Chen JM et al. Calcium pantothenate in arthritis conditions *Practitioner* 224:208,1980.

Cheng TO. Warfarin Danshen interaction [letter]. *Ann Thorac Surg* 67:894, 1999.

Cheung CS. *Comprehensive Management of Phlegm Fluid.* HSCC San Francisco 1996.

Cheung CS. *Deficiency Damage.* HSCC San Francisco 2001.

Chiang CY, Liu JY, Chu TH, Pai YH, Chang SC. Studies on spinal ascending pathway for effect of acupuncture analgesia in rabbits *Sci China* 18:651, 1975.

Chiang CY, Chiang CT and Chu HL. Peripheral afferent pathways for acupuncture analgesia *Sci China* 16:210, 1973.

Chaitow L. *Muscle Energy Techniques.* Churchill Livingstone, 2001.

Chaitow L. Integrated neuromuscular inhibition technique (INIT) in treatment of pain and trigger points. *British Journal of Osteopathy* 13: 17, 1993.

Christensen BV et al. Acupuncture treatment of severe knee osteoarthritis: a long-term study. *Acta Anaes Scand* 36:5, 1992.

Christie SBM et al. Observations on the performance of a standard exercise test by claudicants taking gamma-linolenic acid. *J Atheroscler Res.* 8:83,1986.

Cho et al. New Findings of the Correlation Between Acupoints and Corresponding Brain Cortices Using Functional MIR. *Proceedings of the National Academy of Science* 95(5):2,670, 1998.

Cho et al. Further Evidence for the Correlation Between Acupuncture Stimulation and Cortical Activation. *Proceedings of the International Workshop, Society for Acupuncture Research,* University of California at Irvine, May 22, 1999.

Chrubasik S, Eisenberg E, Balan E, et al. Treatment of Low Back Pain Exacerbations With Willow Bark Extract: A Randomized Double-Blind Study. *Am J Med* 109:9, 2000.

Chu J. The local mechanism of acupuncture. *Zhonghua Yi Xue Za Zhi* (Taipei) 65(7):299, 2002.

Chung JM, Lee KH, Hori Y, Endo K, Willis WD. Factors influencing peripheral nerve stimulation produced inhibition of primate spinothalamic tract cells. *Pain* 19:277, 1984.

Chusid JG. *Correlative Neuroanatomy and Functional Neurology.* 18th edition Lang Medical Publications Los Altos 1982.

Cichoke AJ, Marty L. The use of proteolytic enzymes with soft tissue athletic injuries. *Am Chiropractor*, Oct 1981.

Clark K. et al, Aged-related hearing loss and bone mass in population of rural women aged 60-85 years. Annals of Epidemiology, 5:8-4, 1995.

Clark CR. Atlanto-axial rotatory fixation with compensatory counter occipito-atlantal subluxation. *Spine* 12:488, 1987.

Clinical evidence. The United Health Foundation. Issue 5, 2001.

Clauw DJ. Questions and challenges in the diagnosis of fibromyalgia syndrome. *The J of Musculoskeletal Med* 16:7, 1999.

C T.: Experimental models of osteoarthritis: the role of immobilization. *Clin Biomech* 2:223, 1987.

Cobb JR. Outline for the study of scoliosis. *Am Acad Orthop Surg* 5:261, 1958.

Cohnheim JF. Lectures on general pathology (English translation) London 1889.

Colantuoni S et al. Effects of Vaccinium myritillus anthocyanosides on arterial vasomotion. *Arzneim Forsch* 41:905,1991.

Colachis SC, Worden RE, Bechtol CO et al. Movement of the sacro-iliac joint in the adult male: A preliminary report *Archiv Phys Med Rehabil* 44, 1963.

Cook SP, Vulchanova L, Hargreaves KM, Elde R, McCleskey EW. Distinct ATP receptors on pain-sensing and stretch-sensing neurons. *Nature* 387:505,1997.

Cordell GA, Araujo OE. Capsaicin: Identification, Nomenclature, and pharmacotherapy. *Ann Pharmacother* 27: 330,1993.

Cosyns JP, Jadoul M, Squifflet JP, De Plaen JF, Ferluga D, van Ypersele de Strihou C. Chinese herbs nephropathy: a clue to Balkan endemic nephropathy? *Kidney Int* 45:1680, 1994.

Coursin DB, Wood KE. Corticosteroid Supplementation for Adrenal Insufficiency. *JAMA* 287:236, 2002.

Cragin RB.: The use of Bioflavonoids in the Prevention and Treatment of Athletic Injuries. *Medical Times* Vol 90,No 5 May 1962.

Creagan ET et al. Failure of high-dose vitamin C therapy to benefit patients with advanced cancer. *N Engl J Med* 301:687,1979.

Creamer P; Singh BB; Hochberg MC; Berman BM. Are psychosocial factors related to response to acupuncture among patients with knee osteoarthritis? *Altern Ther Health Med* 5:72, 1999.

Crocq L et al. Treatment of astheno-depressive conditions by Manprine, Multi-center study of 248 cases assessed by Fatigue. *Psy-*

chologie Medicale 12:643, 1980.

Croft A. Whiplash. *J of American Chiro Ass*. 2000.

Curtis CL, Hughes CE, et al. n-3 Fatty Acids Specifically Modulate Catabolic Factors Involved in Articular Cartilage Degradation. *J Biol Chem* 275:721, 2000.

Cyriax JH, Cyriax PJ. *Cyriax's illustrated manual of orthopaedic medicine*, Oxford Butterworth Heinemann 1993.

Cyriax, J. *Textbook of Orthopaedic Medicine, Vol I* 8th ed. Baillère Tindall 1982.

D

Daffner RH. Stress fractures: current concepts. *Skeletal Radiol*.

Dai YR and Yin Y. Inhibition of MAO B activity by Chinese medicinal materials. *Chinese Journal of Geriatrics* 6:27, 1987.

Dai YR and Yin Y. Inhibition of MAO B activity by Chinese medicinal materials. *Chinese Journal of Geriatrics* 6:27, 1987.

Dain TR and Tin Y. Inhibition of MAO B activity by Chinese medicinal materials. *Chinese Journal of Geriatrics* 6:27, 1987.

Dan TC. Routine skin preparation before injection. *Lancet* 12:96, 1967.

DeFeudis FV. Ginkgo biloba extract (EGb 761). *Pharmacological Activities and Clinical Applications*. Paris, Elsevier, 1991.

Daffner RH. Magnetic resonance imaging in acute tendon ruptures. *Skeletal Radiol* 15:619, 1986.

Deal, Chad L. The Use of Topical Capsaicin in Managing Arthritis Pain: A Clinician's Prospective. *Seminars in Arthritis and Rheumatism* 23:48, 1994.

Dettori Ag, Ponari O. Effetto antalgico della aobamimide in corso di neuropatie periferche di diversa etopatogenesi. *Minerva Med* 64:1077,1973Dalal, B., Harrison, G. Psychiatric Consequences of Road Traffic Accidents, *BMJ* 307:1282, 1993.

Dalton S, Snyder S. Glenohumeral instability. Balliere's Clin Rheumatol 3:511, 1989.

Dau TR and Yin Y. Inhibition of MAO B activity by Chinese medicinal materials. *Chinese Journal of Geriatrics* 6:271978.

de Duve C. *A guided tour of the living cell*. Scientific American Books, New York 1984.

De Fabio A. Treatment and prevention of osteoarthritis. *Townsend Letter for Doctors*. February-March, 143, 1990.

De Vernejoul P, Albaréde P, Darras JC. Etude des Méridiens D'acupuncture Par Les Traceurs Radioactifs. *Bull Acad Nat Méd* 169:1071, 1985.

Deans et al. Neck sprain: a major cause of disability following car accidents. *Injury* 18:10, 1987.

Deburge A, Mazda K, Guigui P. Unstable degenerative spondylolisthesis of the cervical spine. *J Bone Joint Surg Br* Jan 77:122, 1995.

Deng Y-C, Goldsmith W. Response of a human head/neck/upper-torso replica to dynamic loading. I: physical model. *J Biomechanics* 5:741,1987.

Denslow, JS., Korr IM.,Krems AD. Quantitative studies of chronic facilitation in human motoneuron pools, *Amer. J. Phsiol*. 105: 229, 1947.

Depierreux M, Van Damme B, Vanden Houte K, Vanherweghem JL. Pathologic aspects of a newly described nephropathy related to the prolonged use of Chinese herbs. *Am J Kidney Dis* 24:172, 1994.

Derby R. Interadiscal Radio-Frequency Thermocoagulation - A Prospective Pilot Study. *Proceedings of the American Back Society* SF 1997.

Derby R. Precision Injection Techniques for Diagnosis and Treatment of Lumbar Disc Disease, 2004.

Dettori AG, Ponari O. Effetto antalgico della cobamamide in corso di neuropatie periferiche di diversa etiopatogenesi. *Minerva Med* 64:1077,1973.

Deyo RA, Diehl AK, Rosenthal M. How many days of bed rest for acute low back pain?. *N Engl J Med*. 315:1064, 1986.

D'Ambrogio K, Roth G *Positional Release Therapy*. Mosby, St. Louis 1997.

D'Ambrosio E et al. Glucosamine sulphate: A controlled clinical investigation in arthrosis. *Pharmatherapeutica* 2:504,1981.

Di Renzi L et al. [On the use of injectable crataegus extracts in therapy of the lower extremities]. *Voll Soc Ital Cardiol* 14:577,1969.

Dieck GS et al. An epidemiologic study of the relationship between postural asymmetry in the teen years and subsequent back neck pain. *Spine* 10:872, 1985.

Dihlmann Wolfgang. *Diagnostic Radiology of the Sacroiliac Joint*. Yearbook Medical Publishers Inc.: Chicago and london 1980.

Dodge CR, Jimenez SA. Glucosamine sulfate modulates the levels of aggrecan and matrix metalloproteinase-3 synthesized by cultured human osteoarthritis articular chondrocytes. *Osteoarthritis Cartilage* 11(6):424, 2003.

Donaldson S et al. The Neural Plasticity Model of Fibromyalgia. Theory, Assessment, and Treatment. *Practical Pain Management* May June:12, 2001.

Donelson R, Silva G, Murphy K. Centralization phenomenon: Its usefulness in evaluating and treating referred pain. *Spine* 15:211,1990.

Dong JC, Li J, Zuo CT. Influence of needling at yin-yang meridian points on cerebral glucose metabolism. *Zhongguo Zhong Xi Yi Jie He Za Zhi* 22:107, 2002.

Don Tigny R L. Sacroiliac dysfunction: Recognition and treatment. First Interdisciplinary *World Congress on Low Back Pain and its Relation to the Sacroiliac Joint* San Diego. November 5-6, 1992.

Dorman TA, Ravin TH. *Diagnosis and Injection Techniques in Orthopedic Medicine*. Williams and Wilkens, 1991.

Dorman TA. Failure of self-bracing at the sacroiliac joints: The slipping clutch syndrome. *J of Othrop Med*. 16:49, 1994.

Dorman T A, Buchmiller JC, Cohen RE, Lively AJ, Peffall SM Stein JB Brown R. Energy Efficiency During Human Walking. *J Orthop Med*. 1993.

Dorman TA. *A new understanding of whiplash*. American Back Society 1997.

Dorman, T.A., Cohen R E., Dasig D., Jeng S., Fischer N., Dejong, A. Energy Efficiency During Human Walking; Before and After Prolotherapy. *J Orthop Med* 17:1, 1995 (accepted).

Dorman T, et al. The effective of Garum Amoricum (Stabilium) on Reducing Anxiety in College Students. *J of Advan in Med* 8:193, 1995.

Dorman HL, Gage TW. Effects of electroacupuncture on the threshold for eliciting the jaw depressor reflex in cats. *Arch Oral Biol* 23:505, 1982.

Dowling RJ et al. Use of fat emulsions, in M Deitel, Ed. *Nutrition in Clinical Surgery*. Baltimore, Williams and Wilkins, 1985.

Dragomirescu C, et al. L'action de l'acupuncture sur les composants sanguins et les principales fonctions de défense organique. *Revue Internationale d'Acupuncture*, 2:16, 1961.

Dreyfuss P, Michaelsen M, Fletcher D. Atlanto-occipital and lateral atlanto-axial joint pain patterns. *Spine* 19:1125, 1994.

Drovanti A, Bignamini AA, Rovati AL. Therapeutic activity of oral glucosamine sulfate in osteoarthrosis: a placebo-controlled double-blind investigation. *Clin Ther* 3:260, 1980.

Duchenne GB. *Physiology of motion*, translated by E.B. Kaplan. J.B. Lippincott, Philadelphia, 1949.

Dulabon RPB et al. Infrared thermography: a rapid, portable, and accurate technique to detect experimental pneumothorax. *J Surg Res* 120(2):163, 2004.

Dung HC: Anatomical features contributing to the formation of acupuncture points. *Amer J Acup* 12:139, 1984.

Dvorák, J., Schmeider, E., Rahn, B. Biomechanics of the Craniocervical Region: the Alar and Transverse Ligaments. *J. Orthop. Res.* 6:452, 1988.

Dvorák j. CT-Functional diagnostics of the rotatory instability of upper cervical spine. *Spine* 12:197, 1987.

Dvorák, J.M., Panjabi, M., Grber, M., Wichmann, W. CT-Functional Diagnostics of the Rotary Instability of Upper Cervical Spine. I: An Experimental Study on Cadavers. *Spine* 12:195, 1987.

Dvorák, J., Dvorák, V. *Manual Medicine Diagnostics*, 2nd ed. Thieme Medical Publishers, Inc. 1990.

Dvorák J, Baumgartner J, Antinnes JA: Frequency of complications of manipulations of the spine. *Eur Spine*. 2;136, 1993.

Dyson-Hudson TA, Shiflett SC, Kirshblum SC, et al. Acupuncture and Trager Psychophysical Integration in the Treatment of Wheelchair User's Shoulder Pain in Individuals With Spinal Cord Injury. *Arch Phys Med Rehabil* 82:1038, 2001.

E

Eguchi K, Origuchi T, Takashima H, Iwata K, Katamine S, Nagataki S. *Arthritis Rheum* 39:463, 1996.

Egund, N. et al.: Movements in the sacroiliac joints demonstrated with Roentgen stereophotogrammetry. *Acta Radiol. Diagn* 19:5, 1978.

Egund N, Olsson TH, Schmid H et al. Movement in the sacro-iliac joints demonstrated with Roentgen stereophotogrammetry. *Acta Radiologica Diagnosis* 19:83345, 1978.

Ehrenpreis S. Potentiation of acupuncture analgesia by inhibition of endorphin degradation. *Acupunct Electrother Res Int J.* 8:310, 1993.

Elfering A, Semmer N, et al. Risk Factors for Lumbar Disc Degeneration: A 5-Year Prospective MRI Study in Asymptomatic Individuals. *Spine*. 27:125, 2002.

Eliyahu DJB. Disc herniations of the cervical spine. *Am j Chiro Med*. 3:93, 1989.

Epstein NE. Technical note: "Dynamic" MRI scanning of the cervical spine. *Spine* 13:937, 1988.

Ernst M, Lee MHM. Sympathetic vasomotor changes induced by manual and electrical acupuncture of Hoku Point visualized by thermography. *Pain*, 21:25, 1985.

Etzel, R. Special Extract of Boswellia serrata (H 15) in the Treatment of Rheumatoid Arthritis,. *Phytomedicine* 3:91, 1996.

F

Fam A G et al.: Stress fractures in rheumatoid arthritis. J. Rheumatol., 10:722, 1983.

Fan YJ et al. Information on Medical Sciences and Technology, *Guangxi Institute of Medical and Pharmaceutical Bulletin* 11:56, 1965.

Fan SG, Qu ZC, Zhe QZ, Han JS. GABA: antagonistic effect on electroacupuncture analgesia and morphine analgesia in rat. *Life Sci* 31:1225, 1982.

Farfan H F. *Mechanical Disorders of the low back*. Philadelphia, LeaandFeber, 1973.

Fassbender HG. Der rheumatische Schmerz, *Med.Welt* 36:1263, 1980.

Feng GH. *Jiangxi Yirao* (Jiangxi Medical J) 6:26, 1961.

Fields RD. The Other Half of the Brain. *Scientific American* Apr, 55, 2004.

Fiexner, Abraharn. *Medical Education in the United States and Canada* A report to the Carnegie Foundation for the Advancement of Teaching, 1910.

Figueroa JS. *Epicondylitis Lecture*. AOA convention Oct 2002.

Fitz-Ritson D. Phasic exercises for cervical rehabilitation after "whiplash" trauma. *J Manipulative Physiol Ther* 18:21, 1995.

Fitzmaurice R, Cooper RG, Freemont AJ: A histo-morphometric comparison of muscle biopsies from normal subjects and patients with ankylosing spondylitis and severe mechanical low back pain. *J Pathol* 163:182, 1992.

Flohe L. Superoxide dismutase for therapeutic use: clinical experience, dead ends and hopes. *Mol Cell Biochem* 84: 123,1988.

Flohe L et al. Effectiveness of superoxide dismutase in osteoarthritis of the knee joint. Results of a double blind multi-center clinical trial, in WH Bannister, JV Bannester, Eds. *Biological and Clinical Aspects of Superoxide and Superoxde Dismutase*. New York, Elsevier/North Holland,1980.

Foley-Nolan et al. Pulsed High Freuency (27 MHz) Electromagnetic Therapy for Persistent Neck Pain: A Double-Blind, Placebo-Controlled Study of 20 Patients. Orthopedics 13(4):445, 1990.

Foreman RD, Ohata CA. Effect of coronary artery occlusion on thoracic spinal neurons receiving viscerosomatic inputs. *Am. J. Physiol*. 238:H666, 1980.

Foreman SM. *Whiplash Injuries*. Williams and Wilkins, 1988.

Foreman SM, Croft AC. Whiplash Injuries, *The Cervical Acceleration/Deceleration Syndrome*. Williams and Wilkins 1988.

Forese RV et al. Licorice-induced hypermineralocorticoidism. *N Engl J Med* 325:1223,1991.

Franson RC, Saal JS, Saal JA. Human disc phospholipase A2 is inflammatory. *Spine*. 17:S129, 1992.

Friberg O. Clinical symptoms and Biomechanics of lumbar spine and hip joint in leg length inequality. *Spine* 8: 643, 1985.

Fredman H, Becker RO, Bachman C. Geomagnetic parmameters and psychiatric hospital admissions. *Nature* 200:626, 1965.

Frost FA, Jessen B, Siggaard-Andersen J. A controlled, double-blind comparison of mepivacaine injection versus saline injection for myofascial pain. *Lancet* 1:499, 1980.

Fukui S, Ohseto K, Shiotani M, Ohno K, Karasawa H, Naganuma Y, Yuda Y. Referred pain distribution of the cervical zygapophyseal joints and cervical dorsal rami. Pain 68:79, 1996.

Fuller RB. *Synergetics*. New York 1975.

Fulgham DD. Ascorbic acid revisited. *Arch Dermatol*, 113:91,1977Fairbank et al.: The Oswestry Low Back Pain Index, *Physiotherapy* 66:271, 1980.

Furlan AD, Brosseau L, Imamura M, Irvin E. Massage for Low-back Pain: A Systematic Review within the Framework of the Cochrane Collaboration Back Review Group. *Spine* 1;27(17):1896, 2002.

Furtado D, Chicorro V. *Rev Clin Espan Madrid* 5:516,1942.

G

Galer BS, Dworkin RH. *A Clinical Guide to Neuropathic Pain*. The McGrow-Hill Companies, 2000.

Garfinkel MS et al. Yoga-Based Intervention for Carpal Tunnel Syndrome: A Randomized Trial. *JAMA* 280:1601, 1998.

Gargan MF, Mannister GC. Long term prognosis of soft tissue injury of the neck. *JBJS* 72-B:901, 1990.

Garrick JG, Ebb DR. *Sports Injuries: Diagnosis and Management*. Saunders Comp 1990.

Gatchel RJ et al. Million Behavioral Health Inventory: its ability in predicting physical function in patients with low back pain. *Arch Phy Med Rehab* 67:878, 1986).

Gattett NE et al. Role of substance P in inflammatory arthritis. *Ann Reum Dis* 51:1014, 1992.

Gaw A et al. Efficacy of acupuncture on osteoarthritic pain: A controlled, double-blind study N Engl J Med 293:375, 1975.

Gedhey EH. Hypermobile joint *Osteopathic Profession* 4:30, 1937.

Greenman DM et al. Serum copper and zinc in rheumatoid arthritis and osteoarthritis. *N Z Med J* 91:47,1980.

Gelberman et al. The effects of mobilization on the vascularization of healing flexor tendons in dogs. *Clin Orthop* 153:283, 1989.

Gerlach. H.L. Über die Bewegung in den Atlasgelenke unde deren Beziehungen du der Butsrömmung an den vertebral Arterien. *Beitr. Morpbol*, 1:104, 1984.

Gerwin RD. A study of 96 subjects examined both for fibromyalgia and myoascial pain. *Musculoske Pain* 3:121, 1995.

Ghosh, Peter, et al. Hyaluronic Acid (Hyaluronan) in Experimental Osteoarthritis. *Journal of Rheumatology* 43:22 1995.

Gilmer W, Anderson L. Reaction of the somatic tissue which progress to bone formation. *South Med J*. 52:1432, 1959.

Giles L.G., Muller R. Chronic Spinal Pain: A Randomized Clinical Trial Comparing Medication, Acupuncture, and Spinal Manipulation. *Spine* 15;28(14):1490, 2003.

Gleick J. *Chaos*. Penguin Books New York 1988.

Glogowski G, Wallraff J. Ein beitrag zur Klinik und Histologie der Muskelharten (Myogelosen). *Z Orthop* 80:237, 1951.

Gogia PP, Sabbahi MA. Electromyographic analysis of neck muscle fatigue in patients with osteoarthritis of the cervical spine. *Spine* 19:502, 1994.

Goldenberg DL. Fibromyalgia. In: Kippel JH, Dieppe PA, eds. *Rheumatology*, Mosby, St Louis 1994.

Goldenberg DL. Fibromyalgia syndrome a decade later. What have we learned? *Archives of Internal Med*. 159:777, 1999.

Golding DN. Is There an Allergic Synovitis? *Journal of The Royal Society of Medicine* 83:312, 1990.

Gollub RL; Hui KK; Stefano GB. Acupuncture: pain management coupled to immune stimulation. *Zhongguo Yao Li Xue Bao* 20:769, 1999.

Goodheart G *Applied Kinesiology Workshop Procedure Manual*, 21st edn. Privately published, Detroit 1984.

Gordon JE. *The science of structures and materials*. Scientific American Library. New York, 1988.

Gordon JE. *Structures: or Why things don't fall down*. De Capa Press, New York 1978.

Grace DL. Lateral ankle ligament injuries. *Clin Orthop* 183:153, 1984.

Gracovetsky S. *The Spinal Engine*. Springer-Verlag, New York 1988.

Grant, R. Dizziness Testing and Manipulation of the Cervical Spine, in *Physical Therapy of the Cervical and Thoracic Spine*. ed.: R. Grant 1988.

Greenman PE. *Principles of Manual Medicine*. Williams and Wilkins 1989.

Greenman PE. *Principles of Manual Medicine* (2ed edi). Williams and Wilkins 1996.

Greenman P.E. Sacroiliac Dysfunction In The Failed Low Back Pain Syndrome, *First Interdisciplinary World Congress on Low Back Pain and its Relation to the SI Joint* 1992.

Greenman P E. Clinical aspects of sacroiliac function in walking. *J Manual Med*. 5:25,1990.

Grinberg-Zylerbaum J, Ramos J. Interpersonal communication: an

References

experimental approach. *Int J Neurosci.* 36:41, 1989.

Groen GJ, Baljet B, Drukker J. The innervation of the spinal dura mater: anatomy and clinical implications. *Acta Neurochir* 99:39, 1988.

Groencewegen WA, Knight DW, Heptinstall S. *J Pharmacol* 38:709, 1986.

Guan, Yu, Wng and Liu. The role of cholinergic nerves in electroacupuncture analgesia - influence of acetylcholine, eserine, neostigmine, and hemichonum on electroacupuncture analgesia. In: Zhang XT (ed) *Research on acupuncture, moxibustion, and acupuncture anesthesia.* Science Press, Beijing 1986.

Gudin JA. Expanding Our Understanding of Central Pain. *Medscape Neurology & Nerosurgery* 6(1), 2004.

Guizhou Institute for Drug Control. Proceedings of the first symposium of the *Chinese Parmaceutical Association.* 324,1962.Galletti R, Procacci P. The role of the sympathetic system in the control of pain and of some associated phenomena. *Aceta Neurovegetativa* 28:495,1966.

Gunn CC. Tennis elbow and the cervical spine. CMA J. 114:803, 1976.

Gunn CC. "Bursitis" Around the Hip. *Am. J. Acup.* 5:53, 1977.

Gunn CC. Shoulder Pain, Cervical Spondylosis and Acupuncture. *Am J Acup.* 5:121, 1977.

Gunn CC. Tennis Elbow and the Cervical Spine. *Can Med Assoc J.* 114:803, 1977.

Gunn CC. *Treating Myofascial Pain Intramuscular Stimulation for Myofascial Pain Syndromes of Neuropathic Origin.* University of Washington 1989.

Gunn CC. Neuropathic Pain: A New Theory for Chronic Pain of Intrinsic Origin. *Annals RCPSC.* 22. 327, 1989.

Gur MD. *Lasers Med Sci* (17), 1:57, 2002.

H

Haberman, Herbert. Photochemotherapy of Rheumatoid Arthritis-Will This Be a New Therapy?", *The Journal of Rheumatology* 22:1, 1995.

Hack et al. Anatomic relation between the rectus capitis posterior minor muscle and the dura mater. *Spine* 20:2484, 1995.

Hachett G S, Hemwall, GA, Montgomery GA.: *Ligament and Tedon Relaxation treated by Prolotherapy.* Gustav A Hemwall, Publisher 1991.

Hackett GS. Ligament and tendon relaxation. Treated by prolotherapy. 3rd ed. Springfield: Charles C. Thomas Publisher, 1958.

Hachisu M et al. Analgesic effect of novel organogermanium compound. Ge-132. *J Pharmacobiodyn* 6:814,1983.

Haeckel E. *Report on the scientific results of the voyage of the H.M.S. Challenger*, Radiolaria Edinburg 18:XL, 1887.

Haker E, Lundeberg T. Acupuncture treatment in epicondlylagia: a comparative study of two acupuncture techniques. *The Clinical J of Pain* 6:221,1990.

Haldeman S, Carey P, Townsend M, Papadopoulos C. Arterial Dissections Following Cervical Manipulation: The Chiropractic Experience. CMAJ, 165:905, 2001.

Hamba XT, Toda K. Rat hypothalamic arcuate neuron response in electroacupuncture-induced analgesia. Brain Res 21:31, 1988.

Hambly MF, Mooney V. Effect of smoking and pulsed electromagnetic fields on intradiscal pH in rabbits. *Spine.* 17:S83, 1992.

Hamilton W. *Traumatic Disorders Of The Ankle.* Springer Verlag, NY, 1984.

Hamilton K. *Clincal Pearls Disc*, 2001.

Hammond DL. Control Systems for Nociceptive Afferent Processing: The Descending Inhibitory Pathways. In: *Spinal Afferent Processing.* Tony L. Yaksh Ed. NY, Plentum Press, 1986.

Hamza MA et al. Percutaneous Electrical Nerve Stimulation: A novel analgesic therapy for diabetic neuropathic pain. *Diabetes Care* 23(3) 365, 2000.

Han JS, Tang J, Zhou Z. Augmentation of acupuncture analgesia by peptidase inhibitor D-phenylalanine in rabbits. *Acta Zoologica Sinica.* 2:133, 1991.

Han JS. *The Neurochemical Basis of Pain Relief by Acupuncture*: A collection of papers 1973-1987. Beijing Medical University. 1987.

Han JS. Neurochemical Basis of Acupuncture Analgesia. *Ann. Rev. Pharmocol Toxicol* 22:193, 1982.

Han JS, Zhou ZF, Xuan YT. Acupuncture has analgesic effect in rabbits. *Pain* 15:83, 1983.

Han JS. Physiology and neurochemical basis of acupuncture analgesia, in Cheng TO (ed). *The International Textbook of Cardiology.* Pergamon Press, NY 1986.

Han JS. Recent Advances in the Mechanisms of Acupuncture Analgesia. *The World United J for TCM and Acup* 1:2, 1998.

Han JS (eds). The rationale of acupuncture analgesia. Shanghai Scientific & Technological Education Press House, 2000.

Hanck A, Weiser H. Analgesic and anti-inflammatory properties of vitamins. *Int J Vitam Nutr Res* (supp) 27:189,1985.

Hanck A, Wiser H. Analgesic and anti-inflammatory properties of vitamins. *Int J Vitam Nutr Res* (supp) 37:189,1985.

Hansen PE, Hansen JH. Acupuncture treatment of chronic tension headache: a controlled cross-over trial. *Cephalalgia* 5:137, 1985.

Hardin JG, Halla JT. Cervical spine and radicular pain syndromes, *Curr Opin Rheumatol* 2:136, 1995.

Harper P, Nuki G. Genetic factors in osteoarthrosis. In: The aetiopathogenesis of osteoarthrosis. Pitman Press 1980.

Hardy GL, Napier JK. Inter and intra therapist reliability of passive accessory movement and technique. *J Physiother* Dec:22, 1991.

Hascall VC, Hascall GK. Proteoglycans. In Cell *Biology of Extracellular Matrix*, edited by Hay ED. Penum, New York, 1981.

Hayes MA. Roentgenographic evaluation of lumbar spine flexion-extension in asymptomatic individuals. *Spine* 14:327, 1989.

Hegyi MD. *J of Medicine* 3:87, 1999.

Heine H. Anatomische Struktur der Akupunkturpunkte. *Dtsch Ztschr Akup* 31:26, 1988.

Helbig T, Lee CK. The lumbar facet syndrome. *Spine* 13:61, 1988.

Helms JM. *Acupuncture Energetics. A Clinical Approach for Physicians.* Medical Acupuncture Publishers, 1995.

Heinz, G.J., and Zavala, D.C.: Slipping rib syndrome. Diagnosis using the "hooking maneuver" *JAMA*, 237:794,1977.

Hendriksson, K.D., et al.: Muscle biopsy findings of possible diagnostic importance in primary fibromyalgia (fibrositis, myofascial syndrome). *Lancet* 2:1395, 1982.

Henriet JP. [Veno-lymphatic insufficiency. 4,729 pts. undergoing hormonal and procymidol oligomer therapy]. *Phlebolojie* 46:313,1993.

Hide JA, Stokes MJ, Saide M, et al.: Evidence of lumbar multifidus muscles wasting ipsilateral to symptoms in patients with acute/subacute low back pain 1994.

Hieber H. Die Behandlung vertebragener schmerezen und sensibilitatsstorungen mit hochdosiertem hydroxocobalamin. *Med Monatsschr* 28:545,1974.

Hilsrome C et al. Effect of ginseng on the performance of nurses on night duty. *Comp Med East West* 6:277,1982.

Hinman MR, Ford J, Heyl H. Effects of static magnets on chronic knee pain and physical function: a double-blind study. *Altern Ther Health Med.* 8(4):50, 2002.

Hinz, P. Sektionsbefunde nach Schleudertraunmen der Halswirbelsäule. *Dt. Z Med* 64:204, 1968.

Hippocrates. *The genuine works of Hippocrates.* Francis Adams, trans. Baltimore: Williams and Wilkins 212, 1946.

Hirschberg GG, Lynn P, Ramsey T. The Incidence and distribution of skinfold tenderness in subjects with cervical sprain. *The J Orthop Med* 16:52, 1994.

Hirschberg G.G., Williams K.A., Byrd J.G.: Diagnosis and Treatment of Iliocostal Friction Syndromes, *J Ortho Med* 14:35, 1992.

Hirsch, S.A., Hirsch, P.J., Hiramoto, H. et al. Whiplash Syndromes: Fact or Fiction? *Orthop Clin North Am* 3:19, 1988.

Ho M-W, Knight DP. The acupuncture system and liquid crystalline collagen fibers of the connective tissues. *American J of Chinese Med* 26(3-4):1, 1998.

Hohl M. Soft tissue injuries of the neck. *Clin Orthop.* 109:42, 1975.

Holbrook, T.L., et al.: *The Frequency of Occurrence, Impact and Cost of Selected Musculoskeletal Conditions in the US.* Chicago, American Academy of Orthopedic Surgeons,1984.

Hollinshead WH. *Functional Anatomy of the Limbs and Back.* 4th Ed. W.B. Saunders, Philadelphia, 1976.

Holm S, Nachemson A. Nutrition of the intervertebral disc: acute effects of cigarette smoking: an experimental animal study. *Uppsala J Med Sci.* 93:91, 1988.

Holm S et al. Nutrition of the intervertibral disc: Solute transport and metabolism. *Connect Tissue Tes.* 8:101, 1981.

Hopwood JJ, Robinson HC. The molecular-weight distribution of glycosaminoglycans. *Biochem J* 135:631, 1973.

Houghton PJ. The biological activity of Valerian and related plants. *J Ethnopharmacol* 22:121,1988.

Howard JMH. Magnesium deficiency in peripheral vascular disease. *J Nutr Med* 1:39,1990.

Hsieh JC et al. Activation of the hypothalamus characterizes the acupuncture stimulation at the analgesic point in human: a positron emission tomography study. *Neurosci Lett* 307:105, 2001.

Hu CJ. *Acta Academiae Medicinae Wuhan* 1:125, 1957.

Hubbard D,R. and Berkoff G,M.: Myofascial Trigger Points Show Spontaneous Needle EMG Activity. *Spine*.18:1993, 1988.

Huberti HH, Hayes WC. Patelofemoral contact pressures. *J Bone Joint Surg* 66A:715, 1984.

Hunt TK et al. Effect of vitamin A on reversing the inhibitory effect of cortisone on healing in animals and man. *Ann Surg* 170:203,1969.

Hunt V. *Infinite Mind: The Science of Human Vibrations* Malibu, Malibu 1995.

Huppin L, Scherer P. *Orthotic Therapy Communique.* Num 97, 99, 2004.

Hyde AS. Crash Injuries: How and Why They Happen. Key Biscayne, Fla: Hyde Assoc;1992.

I

Ikezono E., Ikezono T., Ackerman J. Establishing the existence of the active stomach point in the auricle utilizing radial artery tonometry. *Am J Chin Med* 31(2):285, 2003.

Imai K, Kitakoji H. Comparison of transient heart rate reduction associated with acupuncture stimulation in supine and sitting subjects. *Acupunct Med* 21(4):133, 2003.

Inman VT, Saunders JB, deCM. Referred pain from skeletal structures. *J Nerv Ment Dis* 99:660,1944.

Illingworth C. Pulled elbow. BMJ 1:672, 1975.

Ioenscu-Tirgoviste. Measurement of acupuncture injury potential by acuputometry. *Am J Acup.* 15, 1987.

Ioenscu-Tirgoviste, Pruna. The acu-point potential, electroreception and bio-electrical homeostasis of the human body. *Am J Acup.* 9, 1990.

Isaacson J. Living anatomy – an anatomic basis for osteopathic theory. *Journal of the American Osteopathic Association* 79: 752, 1980.

J

Jackson R. *The cervical syndrome.* Springfield, Charles Thomas, 1977.

Jackson R. *The cervical syndrome.* 4th ed, Charles C Thomas; Springfield, 1958.

Jacobsen S., Samsoe D.S., Lund B.; Consensus document on fibromyalgia: The Copenhagen Declaration. *J of Musculoskeletal Pain* 1:295, 1993.

Jaffe L et al. The glabrous epidermis of cavies contains a powerful battery. Am J Physiol 242:R358, 1982.

Jameson S et al. Pain relief and selenium balance in patients with connective tissue disease and osteoarthritis: A double blind selenium tocopherol supplementation study. *Nutr Res Supp* 1:391, 1985.

Janda, V.: Evaluation of Muscular Imbalance. In *Rehabilitation of the Spine* (eds) Liebenson C. Williams and Willkins 1996.

Janda V: *Muscle Function Testing*. Butterworths, london, 1983.

Janda V. Muscle spasm-a proposed procedure for differential diagnosis. *J Manual Med* 6:136, 1991.

Janda V. *Muscle strength in relation to muscle length*. NY Churchill Livingstone, 1993.

Jelnes R et al. Improvement of subcutaneous nutritional blood flow in the forefoot by hydroxyethylrutosides in patients arterial insufficiency: Case studies. *Angiology* 37:198,1986.

Jensel MC et al. Magnetic resonance imaging of the lumbar spine in people without back pain. *N Engl J Med* 2:331, 1994.

Jensen LB, et al. Effect of acupuncture on headache measured by reduction in number of attacks and use of drugs. *Scand J of Dent Res*. 87:373, 1985.

Jenzel JH. U. of Missouri School of Med.-reported in *Med Trib* 10/26/70.

Ji Y. 776 cases of pain treated with auriculoacupuncture therapy. *J Trad Chin Med* 12:275, 1992.

Ji XJ et al. *Acta Physiologica Sinica* 23:151, 1959.

Jiang MX et al. *Acta Physiologica Sinica* 22:294, 1958.

Jin Gz et al. *Acta Pharmaceutica Sinica* 5:39, 1957.

Johansson JA, Rubenowitz S. Risk indicators in the psychosocial and physical work environment for work-related neck, shoulder and low back symptoms: a study among blue- and white-collar workers in eight companies. *Scand J Rehabil Med* 3:131, 1994.

Johnstone PA, Peng YP, May BC, Inouye WS, Niemtzow RC. Acupuncture for pilocarpine-resistant xerostomia following radiotherapy for head and neck malignancies. *Int J Radiat Oncol Biol Phys* 50:353, 2001.

Jonas WB, Rapoza CP, Blair WF. The effect of niacinamide on osteoarthritis: a pilot study. *Inflamm Res* 45:330, 1996.

Jónsson H Jr., et al. Hidden cervical spine injuries in traffic accident victims with skull fractures. *J Spinal Discord*. 3: 251, 1991.

Jose A. Orcasita, assistant clinical Pharmacology, U. of Miami School of Medicine-reported in Walker M. Therapeutic effects of shark cartilage. *Townsend Letter for Doctors*, June, 1989Jackson, R. *The Cervical Syndrome*. 4th ed. Springfield. Charles C. Thomas, 1958.

Journal of the American Board of Family Practice 16(2):131, 2003.

Juhan D. *Job's Body* Station Hill Press NY 1987.

Jull G, Bogduk N. Accuracy of manual diagnosis for cervical zygapophysial joints. *Medical J Australia* 148: 233, 1988

Jungmann, M. *The Jungmann Concept and Technique of Antigravity Leverage*. 2ed ed. Rangeley, Institute for Gravitational Strain Pathology, Inc., 1992.

Junnila SY. Acupuncture therapy of prolonged pain. *Duodecim* 98:871, 1982.

K

Kaada B. Vasodilatation induced by transcutaneous nerve stimulation in peripheral ischemia (Raynaud's phenomenon and diabetic polyneuropathy). *European Heart J* 3:303, 1982.

Kagen LJ. How to evaluate the patient who has muscle disease. *J of Musculoskeletal Med* 17:407, 2000.

Kartinen JAE. Diagnostic value of stress radiography in lesions of the lateral ligaments of the ankle. *Acta Radio* 18:711; 1988.

Kamada T et al. Dietary sardine oil increases erythrocyte membrane fluidity in diabetic patients. *Diabetes* 35:604,1986.

Kamiyama T, Nouchi T, Kojiman S, Murata N, Ikeda T, Sato C. Autoimmune hepatitis triggered by administration of an herbal medicine *Am J Gastroenterol* 92:703, 1997.

Kane JA, Kane SP, Jain S. Hepatitis induced by traditional Chinese herbs: possible toxic components. *Gut* 36:146, 1995.

Kannus P. Immobilization or Early Mobilization After an Acute Soft-Tissue Injury? *The Physician and Sports Medicine* 28:55, 2000.

Kapandji I.A. *The Physiology of the Joints Vol 3 The trunk and the Vertebral Column*. Churchill Livingstone Edinburgh London and New York, 1974.

Kapandji I.A. *The Physiology of the Joints Vol 2 Lower Limb*. Churchill Livingstone Edinburgh London and New York, 1987.

Kapandji I.A. *The Physiology of the Joints Vol 1 Upper Limb*. Churchill Livingstone Edinburgh London and New York, 1974.

Karasek M, Bogduk N. Twelve-Month Follow-Up of a Controlled Trial of Intradiscal Thermal Anuloplasty for Back Pain Due to Internal Disc Disruption. *Spine*, 25:2601, 2000.

Karst M, Reinhard M, Thum P, et al. Needle Acupuncture in Tension-Type Headache: A Randomized, Placebo-Controlled Study. *Cephalalgia* 21:637, 2001.

Katayama Y, Nishi S. Peptidergic Transmission. In: *Autonomic and Enteric Ganglia: Transmission and Its Pharmacology*. Alexander G, Karczmar, Koketsu K, Nishi, eds. NY: Plenum Press 1986.

Katoh Y, Chao EY, Morrey BF. Objective technique for evaluating painful heel syndrome and its treatment. Foot Ankle. 16:60, 1984.

Kaufman W. The use of vitamin therapy to reverse certain concomitants of aging. *J Am Geriatr Soc* 3:927,1955.

Kawakita K, Miura T, Iwase Y. Deep pain measurement at tender points by pulse alagometry with insulated needle electrodes. *Pain* 44:235, 1991.

Kellgren JH.:Observation of referred pain arising from muscles. *Clin. Sci*.3:175, 1938.

Kellner G. Bau und Funktion der Haut. *Dtsch Ztschr Akup* 3:1, 1966.

Kelmes IS. Vitamin B12 in acute subdeltoid bursitis. *Indust Med Surg* 26:20,1957.

Kennedy R, Berry D. *The Sports Therapy Taping Guide*. Sprts-Medics, 1991.

Kenyon JJ, Cheng N, Blott B, Hopwood V. Studies with acupuncture using a SQUID biomagnetometer: preliminary report. *Complementary Medical Research* 6(3):142, 1992.

Kim H, Shin MS, Kim SS, Kim CJ. Acupuncture increases nitric oxide synthase expression in hippocampus of streptozotocin induced diabetic rats. *Am J Chin Med.* 31(2):305, 2003.

Kime CE. Bell's palsy: A new syndrome associated with treatment by nicotinic acid. *Arch Otolaryngol* 68:28,1958.

Kho HG, Arnold BJ. As chronische benigne Schmerzsyndrom: Moglichkeiten und Rolle der Akupunktur. *Deut Zeits Aku* 40:51, 1997.

Kho HG, Robertson EN. The Mechanisms of Acupuncture Analgesia: Review and Update. *Amer J of Acup* 25:261, 1997.

Mimura M et al. Electron Microscopical and Immunohistochemical Studies on the Induction of "Qi" Employing Needling Manipulation. *American J of Chinese Medicine* 20(1):25, 1992.

King E, Cobbin D, Walsh S, Ryan D. The Reliable Measurement of Radial Pulse Characteristics. *Acupuncture in Medicine* 20(4): 150, 2002.

Kinzler E, Kromer J and Lehamann E. Effect of a special Kava extract in patients with anxiety, tension and excitation states of non-psychotic genesis. Double blind study with placebos over 4 weeks. *Arzneim Forsch* 41:584,1991.

Kirk Hamilton. Clinical Pearls Disc 2001.

Kirkalldy-Willis WH, Burton CV. *Managing Low Back Pain* (3ed)edi Churchill Livingstone NY 1992.

Kitade T et al. Studies on the enhanced effect of acupuncture analgesia and acupuncture anesthesia, by D-phenylalanine (first report): effects on threshold and inhibition by naloxone. *Acupunct Electrother Res* 13:87,1988.

Kjeldsen-Kragh, Jens. Dietary Treatment of Rheumatoid Arthritis. *Scandinavian Journal of Rheumatology* 63, 1996.

Kleijnen J, Knipschild P. Ginkgo biloba. Lancet 340:1136,1992Knight K, Aquino J, Urban C. A re-examination of lewis's cold-induced vasodilation in the finger and ankle. *Athl Train* 15: 248, 1980.

Klein RG, Eek BJ, DeLong B, Mooney V. A Randomized Double-Blind Trial of Dextrose-Glycerine-Phenol Injections for Chronic Low Back Pain. *Journal of Spinal Disorders* 6:1 22, 1993.

Kleinhenz J, Streitberger K, Windeler J, Gussbacher A, Mavridis G, Martin E. Randomized clinical trial comparing the effects of acupuncture and a newly designed placebo needle in rotator cuff tendinitis. *Pain* 83:235, 1999.

Knight KL. Cryotherapy in sports medicine. In: Schriber K, Burke Ej, eds. *Relevant Topics in Athletic Training.* Ithaca, NY: Monument Publications; 1978.

Kober A et al. Prehospital Analgesia with Acupressure in Victims of Minor Trauma: A Prospective, Randomized, Double-Blinded Trial. *Anesth Analg* 95(3):723, 2002.

Kolasinski SL. Acupuncture for arthritis. *Alternative Medicine Alert* 5:37, 2002.

Ko JS, Na DS, Lee YH, Shin SY, Kim JH, Hwang BG., Min BI, Park DS. cDNA microarray analysis of the differential gene expression in the neuropathic pain and electroacupuncture treatment models. *J Biochem Mol Biol* 35(4):420, 2002.

Koltringer P et al. Ginkgo biloba extract and folic acid in the therapy of changes caused by autonomic neuropathy. *Aceta Med Austriaca* 16:35,1989.

Kong LD, Cai Y, Huang WW, Cheng CH, Tan RX. Inhibition of xanthine oxidase by some Chinese medicinal plants used to treat gout. *J Ethnopharmacol* 73:199, 2000.

Konovalov MN et al (trans. by Lin Y). *Chine Med J.* 49:402,1963Kamimura M. Anti-inflammatory effects of vitamin E. *J Vitaminol* 18:204, 1972.

Kopell HP, Thompson WAL. Peripheral entrapment neuropathies of the lower extremity. *New Eng J Med* 262:56, 1960.

Kopell HP, Thompson WA. *Peripheral Entrapment Neuropathies.* Krieger Publishing Co Malabar, Fl, 1976.

Korista VA, Felig P. Is skin preparation necessary before insulin injections? *Lancet* 20:1072, 1992.

Korsakova SS. Central nervous system mechanisms of pathological pain. *Zh Nevrol Psikhiatr Im* 99(12):4,1999.

Korr IM et al. Cutaneous patterns of sympathetic activity in clinical abnormalities of the musculoskeletal system. *Acta Neuroveget Bd* XXXV, Heft 4:589, 1962.

Korr IM, Wright HM, Thomas PE. Effects of experimental myofascial insult on cutaneous patterns of sympathetic activity in man, *J. Neural Transm.* 23:330, 1962.

Korr IR, Edi, The Neurobiologic Mechanisms in Manipulative Therapy; *Sustained sympathicotonia as a factor of disease.* Plenum Publishing Corp, NY, 1987.

Korr IM. The neural basis of the osteopathic lesion. *J Amer Osteo Ass.* 47:191, 1947.

Korr I.M.,Edi.: Sustained sympathicotonia as a factor in disease in. *The Neurobiologic Mechanisms in Manipulative Therapy.* Plenum Publishing Corp, New York,1978.

Korr IM et al. Cutaneous patterns of sympathetic activity in clinical abnormalities of the musculoskeletal system. *Acta Neuroveget Bd. XXXV*, Heft 4:589, 1962.

Korr I. Somatic dysfunction, osteopathic manipulative treatment, and the nervous system. *J of the American Osteopathic Ass.* 86: 109, 1986.

Kose, Kader, et al. Plasma Selenium Levels in Rheumatoid Arthritis. *Biological Trace Element Research*, 53:51, 1996.

Kotani N, Hashimoto H, Sato Y, Sessler DI, Yoshioka H, Kitayama M, Yasuda T, Matsuki A. Preoperative intradermal acupuncture reduces postoperative pain, nausea and vomiting, analgesic requirement, and sympathoadrenal responses. *Anesthesiology* 95:349, 2001.

Koslow SH et al. *The Neuroscience of Mental health II.* NIH publication 1995.

Kraus, H. Diagnosis and treatment of low back pain. *Gen. Pract.* 5:55, 1988.

Kraft, G.L.and Levinthal, O.H.,. Facet synovial impingement. *Sug Gynol Obstet* 19:439, 1951.

Kraus, H.: *Diagnosis and Treatment of Muscle Pain.* Quintessence Publishing, Chicago, 1988.

Krismer M, Haid C, Rabl W. The Contribution of Annulus Fibres

Torque Resistance. Spin 21:2551, 1996.

Kroening R, Oleson T. Rapid narcotic detoxification in chronic pain patients treated with auricular electroacupuncture and naloxon. *International J of Addiction.* 20:1347, 1985.

Kroto H. Space, stars, C60, and soot. *Science* 242:1145, 1988.

Kuchera W.A., Kuchera M.L. *Osteopathic Principles in Practice* 2ed edi KCOM Press Kirksville, Miss 1993.

Kuhn, Thomas S. *The Structure of Scientific Revolution.* The University of Chicago Press, 1962.

Kulkarni RR, Patki PS, Kog VP, et al. Treatment of osteoarthritis with a herbomineral formulation: a double-blind, placebo-controlled, cross-over study. *J Ethnopharmacol* 33:91, 1991.

Kumar A, Tandon OP, Bhattacharya A, Gupta RK, Dhar D. Somatosensory evoked potential changes following electro-acupuncture therapy in chronic pain patients. *Anaesthesia* 50:411, 1995.

Kunnasmaa KTT, Thiel HW. Vertebral Artery Syndrome: A review of the literature. *J. Ortho Med* 16:17, 1994.

Kunnasmaa KTT. Literature review of the prevalence of normal imaging modalities of the vertebrobasilar system in reported cases of cerebrovascular accidents following manipulation of the cervical spine. BSc Project *Anglo-European College of Chiropractic,* Bournemouth, England 1993.

Kuz'menko and Katz. Magnetic Field in the Treatment of Pain Syndromes of the Stumps of the Extremities. *Ortopedia Travmatologia I Protezir Ovanie* 6:8, 1982.

Kwiatek R et al. Pontine tegmental regional cerebral blood flow {rCBF} is reduced in fibromyalgia. *Arthritis and Rheumatology.* 40:S43, 1997.

L

LeBars D, Dickenson AH, Besson JM. Diffuse noxious inhibitory controls (DNIC). I. Effects on dorsal horn convergent neurons in the rat. II. Lach of effect on non convergent neurons, supraspinal involvement and theoretical implications. *Pain* 6:283, 1979.

LeBars D, Dickinson AH, Besson JM. Opiate analgesia and descending controle systems, In Bonica JJ, Lindblom U, Iggo A (eds) *Advances in pain research and therapy.* Ravin Press, NY 1983.

Lackie JM. ed. *Cell Movement and Cell Behavior.* Allen and Unwin, London 1986.

LaCourse M, Moore K, Davis K, Func M, Dorman T. A report on the asymmetry of iliac inclination: A study comparing normal, laterality and change in a patient population with painful sacro-iliac dysfunction treated with prolotherapy. *J Orthop Med.* 12:3, 1990.

Laitenen J. Treatment of cervical syndrome by acupuncture. *Scandinavian J of Rehab Med.* 7:114, 1975.

Lambert, G.A., Bogduk, N. et al, Cervical Cord Neurons Receiving Sensory Input from the Cranial Vasculature. *Cephalgia.* 11:75, 1991.

Lan C, Lai J-S, Chen S-Y, Wong M-K. Tai Chi Chuan to Improve Muscular Strength and Endurance in Elderly Individuals: A Pilot Study. *Arch Phys Med Rehabil* 81:604, 2000.

Langevin HM, Churchill DL, Fox JR, et al. Mechanical signaling through connective tissue: a mechanism for the therapeutic effect of acupuncture. *FASEV J* 15:2275, 2001.

Langevin HM, Churchill DL, Wu J, et al. Evidence of connective tissue involvement in acupuncture. *FASEV J* 16:872, 2002.

Langevin HM., Yandow JA. Relationship of acupuncture points and meridians to connective tissue planes. *Anat Rec* 15;269(6):257, 2002.

Langohr HD et al. Vitamin B-1, B-2. and B-6 deficiency in neurological disorders. *J Neurol* 225:95,1981

Lankhorst GJ, Van de Stadt RJ, Van der Korst JK. The natural history of idiopathic low back pain. *Scand J Rehabil Med* 17:1, 1985.

Lappin MS, Lawrie FW, Richards TL, Kramer ED. Effects of a pulsed electromagnetic therapy on multiple sclerosis fatigue and quality of life: a double-blind, placebo controlled trial. *Altern Ther Health Med.* 9(4):38, 2003.

Latman NS, Walls R. Personality and Stress. An Exploratory Comparison of Rheumatoid Arthritis and Osteoarthritis. *Archives of Physical Medicine and Rehabilitation* 77:796, 1996.

Larsen B et al. Stellate ganglion block with transcutaneous electric nerve stimulation (TENS): a double-blind study with healthy probands. Anasthesiol Intensivmed *Notfallmed Schmerzther* 30(3):155, 1995.

Laude D, Girard A, Consoli S, Mounier-Vehier C, Elghozi JL. Anger expression and cardiovascular reactivity to metal stress: a spectral analysis approach. *Clin Exp Hypertens* 19:901, 1997)

Lavignolle B, et al. An approach to the functional anatomy of the sacroiliac joints in vivo. *Anat Clin* 5:169, 1983.

Lavignolle B, Vital JM, Senegas J, Destandan J, Toson B, Bouyx P, Morlier P, Delorme G, Calabet A. A new understanding of the human pelvis. An approach to the functional anatomy of the sacroiliac joints in vivo. *Mat Clin* 5:169, 1983.

Lawson GE, Walden T. Nutrition and the traumatized patient. *J Council Nutrition.* 12:1 1989.

Lawrence RM. The periosteum: Neurophysiology and its role in treatment. *Annu of Sport Med.* 3:85, 1987.

Lawrence, Dana J. *Chiropractic Diagnosis and Management* Williams and Wilkins, 1991.

Laxorthes Y, Esquerré, Simon J, Guiraud G, Guiraud R. Acupuncture meridians and radiotracers. *Pain* 40:109, 1990.

Lechnyr R, Holmes HH. Taxonomy of pain patient behavior. *Practical Pain Management* 2:5, 2002.

Leduc et al. The effect of physical factors on the vasomotricity of blood and lymph vessels. In Leduc, Lievens (eds) *Lympho-kinetics.* Birkhauser Verlag, Basel, 1979.

Lee T. The genetic and embryological basis of traditional Chinese medicine including acupuncture. *Med Hypotheses* 59(5):504, 2002.

Lee MHM, Ernst M. The sympatholytic effect of acupuncture as evidenced by thermography: A preliminary report. *Ortho Rev* 12:67, 1983.

Lee CS, Tsai TL. The relation of the sciatic nerve to the piriformis muscle. *J Formosan Med Ass* 73:75, 1974.

Lee MHM, Ernst M. Clinical and research observation on acupuncture analgesia and thermography. Presented at Duesseldorfer Akupunktur Symposium. 1987.

Lee Th et al. Effect of dietary enrichment with eicosapentaenoic acid and docosahexaenoic acids on in vitro neutrophil and monocyte leukotriene generation and neutrophil function. *N Engl J Med* 312:1217,1985.

Lenot G. Note sur l'aneurine, anesthesique general. *Ann Anesthesiol Franc* 7:173, 1966.

Levine JD, Fields HL, Basbaum AL: Peptides and the primary afferent nociceptor. *J. Neurosci* 13: 2273, 1993.

Levine J, Taiwo Y. Inflammatory pain. In: *Textbook of Pain* (3ed)(edi) Wall and Melzack. Churchill Livingstone 1994.

Levin SM. *The icosahedron as the three-dimensional finite element in biomechanical support*. Proceedings of the Society of General System Research Symposium on Mental Images, Values and Reality Philadelphia 1986.

Lewis T. *Pain*. MacMillan, NY 1942.

Lewit K. *Manipulative therapy in rehabilitation of the motor system*. 2ed Ed. London, Butterworths, 1991.

Lewit K. Chain reactions in disturbed function of the motor system. *Manuelle Med* 3:27, 1987.

Lewit K. *Manipulative therapy in rehabilitation of the locomotor system, 3rd ed*. Butterworths, London, 1999.

Li Y, Chen S. A study on the reflex arc outside the central nervous system with sympathetic ganglia as the centre. *Zhen Ci Yan Jiu* 21:25, 1996.

Li Y, Jin R. Clinical study on the sequelae of cerebral vascular accident treated with temporal-point acupuncture. *Chen Tzu Yen Chiu* 19:4, 1994.

Li C, Peoples RW, Weight FF. Acid pH augments excitatory action of ATP on a dissociated mammalian sensory neuron. *Neuroreport* 7:2151, 1996.

Liao SJ, Liao MK. Acupuncture and tele-electronic infrared thermography. *Acupunct Electrother Res Int J* 10:41, 1985.

Liberman HR et al. Mood, performance and pain sensitivity: Changes induced by food constituents. *J Psychiatr Res* 17:135,1983.

Liebenson C. *Rehabilitation of the Spine*. Williams and Wilkins 1996.

Lietti A et al. Studies on vaccinium myrtillus anthocyanosides. I. Vasoprotective and anti-inflammatory activity. *Arzneim Forsch* 26:829,1976.

Lin Zj. *Chinese Medical J* 2:114,1954.

Lindenberg D, Pitule-Scodel H. Dl-kavain in comparison with oxazepam in anxiety disorders. A double-blind study of clinical effectiveness. *Fortschr Med* 108:49,1990.

Linetsky FS et al. Position Paper: Regenerative Injection Therapy, Effectiveness and Appropriate Usage. *The Academy of Pain Medicine Annual Conference* June 2001.

Lindgren KA. Is there a Thoracic Outlet Syndrome. *13th Triennial International Congress of Integrative Manual Medicine* (Congress Workbook) 2001.

Lindh, M.: Biomechanics Of The Lumbar Spine. In *Basic Biomechanics of the Skeletal System*. Lea and Febiger, Philadelphia 1980.

Lindstrand A. Diagnosis. *Acta Radiol* 18:529, 1977.

Lings S, Leboeuf-Yde C. Whole-Body Vibration and Low Back Pain: A Systematic, Critical Review of the Epidemiological Literature 1992-1999. *Int Arch Occup Environ Health* 73:290, 2000.

Linzer M, Van Atta A. Effects of acupuncture stimulation activity of single thalamic neurons in the cat. *Adv Neurol* 4:799, 1975.

Litscher G. Effects of acupressure, manual acupuncture and laser needle acupuncture on EEG bispectral index and spectral edge frequency in healthy volunteers. *Eur J Anaesthesiol* 21(1)13, 2004.

Lischer G et al. Acupuncture using laser needles modulates brain function: first evidence from functional transcranial Doppler sonography and functional magnetic resonance imaging. *Laser Med Sci* 19(1):6, 2004.

Liu Z. Meridian pharmacology research. *Meridian Forum* [in Chinese] S:1-4, 1998.

Liu JE, Tahmoush AJ, Roos DB, Schwartzman RJ. Shoulder-arm pain from cervical bands and scalene muscle anomalies.*J Neurol Sci* 128:175, 1995.

Lo K et al. Osteopathic manipulative treatment in fibromyalgia syndrome. *J American Osteopathic Association* 92: 1177, 1992.

Loh L. et al. Acupuncture versus medical treatment for migraine and muscle tension headaches. *J of Neuro, Neurosurg, and Psychiatry* 47:333, 1984.

Long T el al. *Acta Pharmaceutica Sinica*. 14:429,1979.

Lord, SM, Barnsley L, Wallis BJ, Bogduk N. Third Occipital Nerve Headache: a Prevalence Study. *J Neurol Neurosurg Psychiatry*. 57:1187, 1994.

Lopes Vaz A. Double-Blind Clinical Evaluation of the Relative Efficacy of Ibuprofen and Glucosamine Sulphate in the Management of Osteoarthrosis of the Knee in Out-Patients. *Curr Med Res Opin* 8:145, 1982.

Loser J. Pain and Suffering. *The Clinical J of Pain*. June:2000.

Lugar TA, Bhardwaj RS, Grabbe S, Schwarz T. Regulation of the Immune Response by Epidermal Cytokines and Neurohormones. *J of Dermatological Science* 13(1):5, 1996.

Lunderberg T, Laurell G, Thomas M. Effect of acupuncture on sinus pain and experimentally induced pain. *Ear Nose and Throat J* 67:565 1988.

Lunsford LD et al. Anterior Surgery For Cervical Disc Disease: Treatment Of Lateral Cervical Disc Herniation In 253 Cases. *J Neurosurg*. 53:1, 1980.

Lowman CL. The sitting position in relation to pelvic stress. *Physiother Rev* 21:3033, 1941.

Loy TT. Treatment of cervical spondylosis: electoacupuncture versus physiotherapy. *The Medi J of Australia* 2:32, 1983.

Lu FH et al. *Acta Physiologica Sinica* 5:113, 1957.

References

M

Ma SX. Enhanced nitric oxide concentrations and expression of nitric oxide synthase in acupuncture points/meridians. *J Altern Complement Med* 9(2):207, 2003.

Ma W et al. Perivascular space: possible anatomical substrate for the meridian. *J Altern Complement Med* (6):851-9, 2003.

Maciocia G. *The Foundations of Chinese Medicine*. New York: Churchill Livingstone, 1989.

Machtey I, Ouaknine L. Tocopherol in osteoarthritis: a controlled pilot study. *J Am Geriatr Soc* 26:328, 1978.

Mackenzie J. *Symptoms and their interpretation*. Shaw, London 1989.

Mackenzie MA et al. The influence of glycyrrhetinec acid on plasma cortisol and cortisone in healthy young volunteers. *J Clin Endocrinol Metb* 70:1637,1990.

Macintosh JE, Pearcy MJ, Bogduk. The axial torque of the lumbar back muscles: torsion strength of the back. *Aust N Z J Surg* 63:205, 1993.

Macintosh JE, Bogduk N, Pearcy MJ. The effects of flexion on the geometry and actions of the lumbar erector spinae. *Spine* 18:884, 1993.

MacNab I. *Backache*, Williams and Wilkins, 1977.

MacNab, I. Acceleration Injuries of the Cervical Spine. *J of Bone and Joint Surgery.* 46a:1655, 1964.

MacNab, I. Whiplash Syndrome, *J. Clinical Neurosurgery.* 20:232, 1973.

MacNab I. The "whiplash syndrome." *Orthop Clin North Am.* 2, 2:389, 1971.

Madan BR, Khanna NK. Anti-inflammatory activity of L-Tryptophan and DL-tryptophan. *Indian J Med Res* 68:708,1978.

Magora, A: Conservative treatment in spondylolisthesis. *Clin. Ortho.* 117:74, 1976.

Magidoff A. Treatment of Low Back Pain with Kiiko Matsumoto Style Acupuncture. *CJOM* 10(3), 16, 1999.

Main CJ, Spanswick CC. Personality assessment and Minnesota multiphasic inventory. 50 years on: do we still need our security blanket? *Pain Forum* 4:60, 1995.

Malarky WB et al. Influence of academic stress and season on 24-hour mean concentrations of ACTH, cortisol and beta-endorphin. *Psychneuroendocrinology* 20:499; 1995.

Mann M Glasjeen-Wray M, Nyberg R: Therapist Agreement for Palpation and Observation of Iliac Crest Heights. *Phys Ther* 64:223, 1984.

Mannoin et al. Collateral sprouting of uninjured primary afferent A-fibers into the superficial dorsal horn of the adult rat spinal cord after topical capsaicin treatment to the sciatic nerve. *J-Neurosci* 16(16): 5189, 1996.

Mao et al. High versus low intensity acupuncture analgesia for treatment of chronic pain: effects on platelet serotonin. Pain 8:331, 1980.

Maquart FX et al. Simulation of collagen synthesis in fibroblast culture by a triterpene extracted from Centella asiatica. *Connect Tissue Res.* 24:107,1990.

Marcus A. *Acute Abdominal Syndromes. Their Diagnosis and Treatment According to Combined Chinese-Western Medicine.* Boulder: Blue Poppy Press, 1991.

Marcus A, Gracer R.: A Modern Approach to Shoulder Pain Using the Combined Methods of Acupuncture and Cyriax-Based "Orthopaedic Medicine". *American J of Acupuncture* 22:5, 1994.

Mark et al. Daily Repetitive Transcranial Magnetic Stimulation Improves Mood in Depression. *NeuroReprt* 6(14):1853, 1995.

Markelova VF et al. Changes in blood serotonin levels in patients with migraine headaches before and after a course of reflexotherapy. *Zh Nervopatol Psikhiatr* 84:1313, 1984.

Martel GF, Andrews SC, Roseboom CG. Comparison of static and placebo magnets on resting forearm blood flow in young, healthy men. *J Orthop Sports Phys Ther.* 32(10):518, 2002.

Martin R M. *The gravity guiding system*. Essential Publishing Co. 2823 Cumberland Rd. San Marino, CA. 1975.

Martin R. Laser-Accelerated Inflammation/Pain Reduction and Healing. *Practical Pain Management* 3:6, 2003.

Matin P. Basic principles of nuclear medicine techniques for detection and evaluation of trauma and sports medicine. *Smin Nucl Med*:18:90, 1988.

Matin PJ. The appearance of bone scans following fracture, including immediate and long term studies. *J Nuc Med* 20:1227, 1979.

Matthews PM, et al. Enhancement of natural cytotoxicity by beta-endorphin. *J of Immunology* 132: 3046, 1984.

Matsuo K et al. Influence of alcohol intake, cigarette smoking and occupational status on isiopathic osteonecrosis of the femoral head. *Clin Orthop* 234:115, 1988.

Matsumoto K, Birch S. *Hara: Reflections on the Sea.* Brookline: Paradigm Press 1988.

Matyas T, Bach T. The reliability of selected techniques in clinical arthrometics. *Aust J Physiother* 31:175, 1985.

Maver DJ, Price DD, Rafii A. Antagonism of acupuncture hyperalgesia in man by the narcotic antagonist naloxone. *Brain Res.* 121:368, 1977.

Mazzara JT. The effect of C1-C2 rotation on canal size. *Clin Ortho Relat Res* 237:15, 1989.

McAlindon, Timothy, E., et al. Do Antioxidant Micronutrients Protect Against the Development and Progression of Knee Osteoarthritis? *Arthritis and Rheumatism* 39:648, 1996.

McCaig CD. Spinal neurite regeneration and regrowth in vitro depend on the polarity of an applied electric field. *Development* 100:31 1987.

McCarthy JJ, MacEwen GD. Management of Leg Length Inequality. *J South Orthop Assoc* 10:73, 2001.

McConnell WE et al. Analysis of Human Test Subject Kinematic Responses to Low Velocity Rear End Impacts. paper 930094. Society of Automotive Engineers, 1993.

McCann P, Wootten M, Kadaba M Bigliani L. A kinematic and electromyographic study of shoulder rehabilitation exercises. Cil Orthop Rel Res. 288:179, 1993.

McCarthy, W.J., Yao, S.J., Schafer, M.F. et al. Upper Extremity Arterial Injury in Athletes. *J Vasc Surg* 9:317, 1989.

McGeer, T. Passive Dynamic Walking. *Int J Robotics Res* 9,2.1990.

McKenzie and Jacobes In: Liebenson C. *Rehabilitation of the Spine*. Williams and Wilkins 1996.

Mcleod Dw, Revell P, Robinson BV. Investigations of Hapagophytum procumbens (Devil's claw) in the treatment of experimental inflammation and arthritis in the rat. *Br J Pharmacol* 66:140,1979.

McLennan H Von, Gilfillan K, Heap Y. Some pharmacological observations on the analgesia induced by acupuncture in rabbits. *Pain* 15:83, 1977.

McMorland G, Suter E. Chiropractic Management of Mechanical Neck and Low-Back Pain: A Retrospective, Outcome-Based Analysis. *J Manipulative Physiol Ther* 23:307, 2000.

McNair JFS. Acute locking of the cervical spine. In: Gieve GP (eds). *Modern Manual Therapy of the Vertebral Column*. Churchill Livingstone, London 1986.

McNeil Alexander, R. *Elastic Mechanism in Animal Movement*. Cambridge University Press, New York, 1988.

Medelson, G. Not "cured by verdict." Effects of Legal Settlement on Compensation Claimants. *Medical Journal of Australia*. 1:132, 1982.

Medscape. Return to The Brain-Body Connection and the Relationship Between Depression and Pain. 2003.

Meenen NM, Katzer A, Dihlmann SW, Held S, Fyfe I, Jungbluth KH. Whiplash injury of the cervical spine--on the role of pre-existing degenerative diseases. *Unfallchirurgie* 3:138, 1994.

Mehta AK, et al. Pharmacological effects of Withania somnifera rot extract on GABA receptor complex. *Ind J Med Res* 94(b):312,1991.

Mellin G. Chronic low back pain in men 54-63 years of age, correlations of physical measurements with the degree of trouble and progress after treatment. *Spine* 11:421, 1986.

Melzack R, Wall P. Pain mechanisms. A new theory. *Science* 150:971, 1965.

Melzack R. From the gate to neuromatrix. *Pain Supplement* 6:121, 1999.

Mendelson G. Follow-up studies of personal injury litigants. *Int J Law Psychiatry* 7:179, 1984.

Mense S: Physiology of Nociception in Muscles. *J Advances in Pain Research and Therapy* 17:67-85,1990.

Mennell, J. *The Science and Art of Joint Manipulation*. New York, Blakinston, 1952.

Mennell J. *Back Pain*. Little Brown. Boston 1960.

Mennell JM. *Joint Pain*. Little, Brown, Boston. 1964.

Mercer S, Bogduk N. Intra-articular inclusions of the cervical synovial joints. *Br J Rheumatol* 32:705, 1993.

Metchnikoff Eli (1848-1916). *Lectures on the comparative pathology of inflammation*. Dover publications, NY 1968. original 1893.

Michalsen A et al. Leach Therapy for Symptomatic Treatment of Knee Osteoarthritis: Results and Implication of a Pilot Study. *Alter Ther Health Med* 8(5):84, 2002.

Middleeditch A The cervical spine-safe in our hands? *World confederation for physical therapy 11th international congress book III* The Barbican center, London UK,1991.

Miehlke K, Schulze G, Eger W: Klinische und experimentelle Untersuchungen Zum Fibrositis-syndrom. *Z Rheumaforsch* 19:310, 1950.

Miles KA et al. The incidence and prognostic significance of abnormal radiology in soft tissue injury of cervical spine. *Skeletal Radiology* 17:493, 1988.

Miller BD, Wood BL. Influences of specific emotional states on autonomic reactivity and pulmonary function in asthmatic children. *J AM Acad Child Adolesc Psychiatry* 36: 669, 1997.

Miller JAA, Schamtz BS, Scjultz AB. Lumbar disc degeneration: correlation with age, sex and spine level in 600 autopsy specimens. *Spine* 13:173, 1988.

Miller J AA, Schultz A B, Andersson G B 3. Load displacement behavior of sacroiliac joints. *J Orthop Research* 5:92,1987.

Miller EJ. Chemistry, structure and function of collagen, in L manaker, Ed. *Biologic Basis of wound Healing*. NY, Harper and Row 1975.

Miller L. Neurosensitization: A pathophysiological model for traumatic disability syndrome. *J of Cognitive Rehabilitation*. 151:12, 1997.

Millinger GS. Neutral amino acid therapy for the management of chronic pain. *Cranio* 4:156,1986.

Mitchell FL Jr. In *Rational Manual Therapies* edi Basmajian JV and Nyberg R. Williams and Wilkins 1993.

Mitchell F.L. The balanced pelvis and its relationship to reflexes. *Yearbook, Academy Applied Osteopathy* 48:146, 1948.

Mitra M, Nandi AK. Cyanocobalmin in chronic Bell's Palsy. *J Indian Med Assoc* 33:129,195

Moldofsky, H., et al.:Musculoskeletal symptoms and non-Rem sleep disturbances in patients with "fibrositic" syndromes and healthy subjects. *Psychosom. Med.* 37:341,1975.

Molsberger A, Jille E. The analgesic effect of acupuncture in chronic tennis elbow pain. *British J of Rheumatology* 33:1162, 1994.

Montakab H. Acupuncture and Insomnia. *Forsch Komplementarmed* 1:29, 1999.

Montazeri K, Farahnakian M, Saghaei M. The effect of acupuncture on the acute withdrawal symptoms from rapid opiate detoxification. *Acta Anaesthesiol Sin* 40(4): 173, 2002.

Mooney V. Where is the Lumbar Pain Coming from?. *Ann Med.* 21:373, 1989.

Mooney V, and Robertson J. The facet syndrome. *Clin. Orthop.* 115:149, 1976.

Mooney V. American Association of Orthopaedic Medicine Annual Meeting 2004.

Morgan, Sarah L, et al. Supplementation with Folic Acid during Methotrexate Therapy for Rheumatoid Arthritis: A Double-Blind, Placebo-Controlled Trial. *Annals of Internal Medicine* 121:833, 1994.

Morre HHE, et al. Treatment of Chronic Tennis Elbow With Botulinum Toxin. *The Lancet* 349:1746, 1997.

Morreale P, Manopulo R, Galati M, et al. Comparison of the Anti-inflammatory Efficacy of Chondroitin Sulfate and Diclofenac Sodium in Patients With Knee Osteoarthritis. *J Rheumatol* 23:1385, 1996.

Morscher E, Finger G. Measurement of leg length. *Prog Orthop Surg* 1:21, 1977.

Morton DJ. *The Human Foot*. Columbia University Press. NY 1935.

Morton DJ. Foot disorders in women. *J Am Med Wom Assoc* 10:41, 1955.

Moses Ma, Subhalter J, Langer R. Identification of and inhibitor of neovascularisation from cartilage. *Science* 248:1408, 1990.

Mountz J et al. Fibromyalgia in women: Abnormalities of regional cerebral blood flow in the thalamus and caudate nucleus are associated with low pain threshold levels. Arthritis and Rheumatism. 38:926, 1995.

Moussard C et al. A drug used in traditional medicine, harpagophytum procumbens: No evidence for NSAID-like effect on whole blood eicosanoid production in humans. *Prostaglan Leukotri Essent Fatty Acids* 46:283, 1992.

Murad S et al. Regulation of collagen synthesis by ascorbic acid. *Proc Natl Acad Sci USA*, 78:2879, 1981.

Musaev AV, Guseinova SG, Imamverdieva SS. The use of pulsed electromagnetic fields with complex modulation in the treatment of patients with diabetic polyneuropathy. *Neurosci Behav Physiol.* 33(8):745, 2003.

Myers T. The Anatomy Trains. *Journal of Bodywork and Movement Therapies* 1: 91, (99, 134) 1997.

Myers T. *Anatomy trains: myofascial meridians for manual and movement therapists.* Churchill Livingstone, Edinburgh, 2001.

N

Nachemson AL. Newest knowledge of low back pain, *Clin Orthop* 279:8, 1992.

Nachemson, A., Elfstrom, G.: *Intravertibral Dynamic Pressure Measurement in the Lumbar Spine in Lumbar Disks: A Study of Common Movements, Maneuvers and Exercises.* Stockholm, Alwuist and Wikstell, 1970

Naeser MA, Alexander MP, Stiassny-Eder D, Galler V, Hobbs J, Bachman D. Acupuncture in the treatment of paralysis in chronic and acute stroke patients--improvement correlated with specific CT scan lesion sites. Boston University School of Medicine, MA, USA. *Acupunct Electrother Res* 19:227, 1994.

Naeser MA, Hahn KK, Lieberman B. Real vs. Sham Laser Acupuncture and Microamps TENS to Treat Carpal Tunnel Syndrome and Worksite Wrist Pain: Pilot Study. *Lasers Surg and Med* suppl. 8:7, 1996.

Naeser MA, Hahn CK and Lieberman BE. Home Naeser Laser Treatment Program for the Hand, AAOM Publication, 1996.

Naliboff BD et al. Comprehensive assessment of chronic low back pain patients and controls: Physical abilities, level of activities, psychological adjustment and pain perception. *Pain* 23:121, 1985.

Nash CL, Moe JH. A study of vertebral rotation. *J Bone Joint Surg* 51A:223, 1969.

National Medical Journal of China 7:444, 1978.

Neuberger A et al. Metabolism of collagen. *Biochemistry Journal* 53: 47, 1953

Neuhuber WL, Bankoul S. Specifics of innervation of the craniocervical transition Orthopade 23:256, 1994.

Newman NM, Ling RSM. Acetabular bone destruction related to non-steroidal anti-inflammatory drugs. Lancet:11, 1985.

Nielsen S. Radiologic findings in lesions of the ligamentum bifurcation of the midfoot. *Skeletal Radiol* 16:114, 1987.

Niccole R, Sivak-Sears *Am J Epidemiol* 159:1131, 2004).

Nicolakis P et al. Pulsed magnetic field therapy for osteoarthritis of the knee-double-blind sham-controlled trial. *Wien Klin Wochenschr.* 30;114(15-16):678, 2002.

Nordenström BEW. *Biologically Closed Electric Circuits (BCEC) Clinical, Experimental And Theoretical Evidence For An Additional Circulatory System*, 1982.

Nordenström BEW. An electrophysiological view of acupuncture. Role of capacitative and closed circuit currents and their clinical effects in the treatment of cancer and chronic pain. *Am J Acupuncture 17*:105, 1989.

Nordenström BEW: Electrochemical treatment of cancer. 1. Variable response to anodic and cathodic fields. *Am J Clin Oncol* (CCT) 12:530, 1989.

Nordhoff LS. *Motor Vehicle Collision Injuries:Mechanisms, Diagnosis and Management.* Maryland, An Aspen Publication, 1996.

Noreau, Luc et al. Effects of a Modified Dance-Based Exercise on Cardiorespiratory Fitness, Psychological State and Health Status of Persons With Rheumatoid Arthritis. *American Journal of Physical Rehabilitation* 74:19, 1995.

Norris SH, Watt I. The prognosis of neck injuries resulting from rear-end vehicle collisions. *J Bone Joint Surg* [Br] 65: 608, 1983.

Norris C. Functional load abdominal training (part 1). *Journal of Bodywork and Movement Therapies* 3: 150, 1999

Noyes F, Torvik PM, et al. Biomechanics of ligament failure: an analysis of immobilization, exercise and reconditioning effects on primates. *J Bone Joint Surg.* 56A:1406, 1974.

Nuccitelli R. The involvement of transcellular ion currents and electric fields in pattern formation. In: Malacinski GM (ed) *Pattern Formation*. Macmilan NY 1984.

O

Obertreis B, Giller K, et al. Anti-inflammatory effect of Uria dioca folia extract in comparison to caffeic malic acid. *Arzneimittelforschung* 46:52, 1996.

Obodencheva GV. Farmakologiia I Tokisikologiia 29:496, 1966.

Ochoa J, Mair EGP The normal sural nerve in man. *J. Neuropathological Berlin* 13:197, 1969.

O'Connor J, Bensky D (eds). *Acupuncture, A Comprehensive Text.* Chicago, Eastland Press, 1981.

O'Dell B et al. Zinc status and peripheral nerve function in guinea pigs. *FASEBJ* 4:2919,1990.

Oleson TD, et al. An experimental evaluation of auricular diagnosis: the somatotropic mapping of musculoskeletal pain at ear acupuncture points. *Pain* 8:217, 1980.

Ohuchi K et al. Glycyrrhizine inhibits prostaglandin E2 formation by activated peritoneal macrophages from rats. *Prostagland Metab* 70:143,1981.

O'Hara J. A double-blind-controlled study of Hexopal in the treatment of intermittent claudication. *J Int Med Res.* 13:322-27,1985.

O'Keefe RJ. *J Clin Invest.* 109:1405, 2002.

Okimasa E et al. Inhibition of Phosphatase A2 by Glycyrrhizine, an anti-inflammatory drug. *Acta Med Okayma* 37:385,1983.

Ombregt L, Bisschop P, ter Veer HJ, Van de Velde T. *A System of Orthoaedic Medicine.* Saunders, London UK 1995.

Omura Y. Pathophysiology of acupuncture effects, ACTH and morphine-like substances, pain, phantom sensation, brain mirocirculation and memory. *Acupunct Electrother Res Int J.* 2:1, 1976.

Ongley MJ, Klein RG, Dorman TA et al. A new approach to the treatment of chronic back pain. *Lancet* 143, 1987.

Orange, Lisa M. Body Mass Linked to Knee Osteoarthritis Risk in Women. *Family Practice News* 16, 1993.

Orloff S, Krieg T and Muller P: (+) Cyanidanol-3 changes functional properties of collagen. *Biochem Pharmacol* 31:3581,1982.

Ornstein R, Thompson RF. The Amazing Brain. Houghton Mifflin Company. Boston1984.

Orsay Em at al. Prospective study of the effect of safety belts in motor vehicle crashes. *Ann Emeg Med.* 19:258, 1990.

Orthopade 4:287, 1994.

Oschman JL. *Energy Medicine.* Churchill Livingstone, Edinburgh London, NY, Philadelphia, St Louis, Sydney, Toranto, 2000.

Oschman JL. A biophysical basis for acupuncture. *Proceedings of the First Symposium of the Society for Acupuncture Research,* Rockvill, MD 1994.

Otto KC. Acupuncture and substance abuse: a synopsis with indications for further research. *Am J Addict* 12(1):43, 2003.

Ouigley, Carroll. Tragedy and Hope, *A History of the World in Our time.* Collier MacMillan, London, 1966.

Owens J, Malone T. Treatment parameters of high frequency electrical stimulation as established on the electro-stim 180. *J Orthopaed Sports Phys Ther.* 4:162, 1983.

Owens EF et al. Paraspinal skin temperature patterns: an interexaminer and intraexaminer reliability study. *J Manipulative Physiol Ther* 27(3):155, 2004.

Owoeye I, Spielholx NI, Fetto J, et al. Low intensity pulsed galvanic current and healing of tentomized rat achilles tendons: Preliminary report using load-to-breaking measurements. *Arch Phys Med Rehabil.* 68:415, 1987.

P

Padova C. S-adenosylmethionine in the treatment of osteoarthritis. Review of clinical studies. *Am J Med* 83:60,1987.

Paladin F, Russo Perez G. The haematic thiamine level in the course of alcoholic neuropathy. *Eur Neurol* 26:129,1987.

Palmoski MJ, Brandt KD. Effects of some nonsteroidal antiinflammatory drugs on proteoglycan metabolism and organization in canine articular cartilage. Arthit Reum 23:1010, 1980.

Panzer DM. The reliability of lumbar motion palpation. *J Manipulative Physi Ther* 15:518, 1992.

Paris SV. Differential Diagnosis of SI joint from lumbar spine dysfunction, *First interdisciplinary world congress on low back pain and its relation to the SI joint*; 1992.

Parker GB, Tupling H and Pryor DS. A controlled trial of cervical manipulation for migraine. *Aust NZ J Med* 8:589, 1978.

Parry GJ. Sensory neuropathy with low-dose pyridoxine. *Neurology* 35:1466,1985.

Passatore M., Filippi M., Grassi C. In: *The Muscle Spindle*, Boyd I. and Gaden M.,(eds.) Macmillan, London 1985.

Patacchini R, Maggi CA and Meli A. Capsaicin-like activity of some natural pungent substances on peripheral ending of visceral primary afferents. *Arch Pharmaco* 342:72,1990.

Patterson M. *Hooked? NET: the new approach to drug cure.* Faber and Gaber London 1986.

Pavelka, Karel, Jr., et al. Glycosaminoglycan Polysulfuric Acid (GAGPS) in Osteoarthritis of the Knee. *Osteoarthritis and Cartilage* 3:15, 1995.

Pearce P. Structures in Nature as a Strategy for Design. MIT Press Cambridge 1978.

Pearson EJ. Combined manual medicine and acupuncture in neck injury. *Manual Med.* 5:19, 1990.

Pecina M. Contribution to the etiological explanation of the piriformis syndrome. *Aceta Anat* 105:181, 1979.

Pellegrino M. *Understanding Post-Traumatic Fibromyalgia.* OH: Anadem Publishing Columbus 1996.

Pennarola R et al. The therapeutic action of the anthocyanosides in microcirculatory changes due to adhesive-induced polyneuritis. *Gazz Med Ital* 139:485,1980.

Peterson B. *The collected papers of Irvin M. Korr.* Amer Acad. Osteo Indianapolis, IN 1979.

Petrou P. Double-blind trail to evaluate the effects of acupuncture treatment on knee osteoarthritis pain: a placebo controlled study. American J of Chin Med 19:95 1991.

Petrie JP, Langley GB. Acupuncture in the treatment of chronic cervical pain: A pilot study. *Clinical and Experimental Rheumatology.* 1:333, 1983.

Pettersson K, Hildingsson C, Toolanen G, Fagerlund M, Bjornebrink J MRI and neurology in acute whiplash trauma. No correlation in prospective examination of 39 cases. *Acta Orthop Scand* 5:525, 1994.

Penimak T et al. Progressive strengthening and stretching exercises and ultrasound for chronic lateral epicondylitis. *Physiotherapy*

82:522, 1996.

Penning L. Normal movements of the cervical spine. *Amer J Radiol* 130:317, 1978.

Penning L, Wilmick JT. Rotation of the cervical spine—A CT study in normal subjects. *Spine* 12:732, 1987.

Penning L, Wilmick JT. Rotation of the cervical spine—A CT study in normal subjects. *Spine* 12:732, 1987.

Perharic L, Shaw D, De Smet PAGM, Murray SG. Possible association of liver damage with the use of Chinese herbal medicine for skin disease. *Vet Hum Toxicol* 37:562, 1995

Perri FS, Reichmanis M, Marino A, Becker RO. Environmental power frequency magnetic fields and suicide. *Health Physics* 41:267, 1981.

Piesse JW. Vitamin E and peripheral vascular disease. *Int Clin Nutr Res*, 4:178,1984.

Pietri-Taleb F, Riihimaki H, Viikari-Juntura E, Lindstrom K. Longitudinal study on the role of personality characteristics and psychological distress in neck trouble among working men. *Pain* 2:261, 1994.

Pimentel M, Chow EJ, Hallegua D, Wallace D, Lin HC. Small Intestinal Bacterial Overgrowth: A Possible Association With Fibromyalgia. *J Musculoskeletal Pain* 9:107, 2001.

Pintar FA, et al. Kinematic and anatomical analysis of the human cervical spinal column under axial loading. In: Proceedings of 33rd Strapp Car Crash Conference, P-227, 892436. Washington, DC: Society of Automotive Engineers: 191, 1989.

Pipitone N, Scott DL. Magnetic pulse treatment for knee osteoarthritis: a randomized, double-blind, placebo-controlled study. *Curr Med Res Opin.* 17(3):190, 2001.

Pizzorno Joseph E., Jr. Natural Medicine Approach to Treating Osteoarthritis. *Alternative and Complementary Therapies* 93:95, 1995.

Pomeranz B, Cheng R, Law P. Acupuncture reduces electrophysiological and behavioral responses to noxious stimuli: Pituitary is implicated. *Exp Neurol.* 54:172, 1977.

Pomeranz B, Paley D. Electroacupuncture hypalgesia is mediated by afferent nerve impulses: An electrophysiological study in mice. *Exp Neuro* 66:398, 1979.

Pomeranz B, Nguyen P. Inrathecal diazepam suppresses nociceptive reflexes and potentiates electroacupuncture effects in pentobarbitol rats. *Neurosci Lett* 77:316, 1987.

Potter N, Rothstein J: Inter-tester Reliability for Selected Tests of the Sacro Iliac Joint. *Phys Ther* 65:1671,1985.

Pray R, Pray JJ. Topical Devices and Products for Pain. *US Pharmacist* 28(1), 2003.

Prestman AS. *Electromagnetic Fields and Life*. NY, NY, Plenum Press, 1970.

Preyde M. Effectiveness of Massage Therapy for Subacute Low-Back Pain: A Randomized Controlled Trial. *CMAJ*, 162:1815, 2000.

Prince JP. The Use of Low Strength Magnets on EAV points. *American J of Acup* 3(2):125, 1983.

Prino G. Pharmacological profile of Ateroid, *Mod. Probl. Pharmacopsychiatry*, 23, 68,1989.

Prior T. Biomechanical foot function: a podiatric perspective (part 2). *Journal of Bodywork and Movement Therapies* 3: 169, 1999

Prodigal genius: The Life of Nicola Tesla. John J O'Neill. Angriff Press. P.O.Box 2726, Hollywood CA 90078.

Prudden, Jf and Balassa LL, The biological activity of bovine cartilage preparations, *Sem Arth Ruem.*, 17:35, 1987.

Prudden JF, Allen J. The clinical accelerating of healing with a cartilage preparation; a controlled study. *JAMA* 192:352,1965.

Q

Qian L, et al. Effects of Electroacupuncture on Gastric Migrating Myoelectrical Complex in Dogs. *Dig Dis Sci* 44:56, 1999.

Qin L, Au S, Choy W, et al. Regular Tai Chi Chuan Exercise May Retard Bone Loss in Postmenopausal Women: A Case-Control Study. *Arch Phys Med Rehabil* 83:1355, 2002.

Quirin H. Pain and vitamin B1 therapy. *Bibl Nutr Dieta* 38:708, 1986.

R

Radanov P, Sturzenegger M, Di Stefano G. Prediction of recovery from dislocation of the cervical vertebrae (whiplash injury of the cervical vertebrae) with initial assessment of psychosocial variables. *Orthopade* 23:282, 1994.

Raja SN. Role of the sympathetic nervous system in acute pain and inflammation. *Ann Med* 2:241, 1995.

Ramani, P.S., et al.: "Role of Ligamentum Flavum in the Symptomatology of Prolapse Lumbar Intervertebral Discs," *J. Neurol. Neurosurg.* 38:550,1975.

Randall C, et al. Nettle Sting of Urtica dioica for Joint Pain - an Exploratory Study of This Complementary Therapy. *Complementary Therapies in Medicine* 7:126, 1999.

Reeves KD. Treatment of consecutive severe fibromyalgia patients with prolotherapy. *The J of Orthop Med.* 16:84,1994

Reddy CK, Chandrakasan G, Dhar SC. Studies on the metabolism of glycosaminoglycans under the influence of new herbal anti-inflammatory agents. *Biovhemical Pharmacol* 20:3527,1989.

Reichelt A, Forster KK, Fischer M, et al. Efficacy and Safety of Intramuscular Glucosamine Sulfate in Osteoarthritis of the Knee. A Randomized, Placebo-Controlled, Double-Blind Study. *Arzneimittelforschung* 44:75, 1994.

Reider B, Marshall J, Warren R. Clinical characteristics of patellar disorders in young athletes. *Am J Sports Med* 9:4, 1981.

Rejhole V. Long term studies of anti-osteoarthritic drugs: An assessment. Semin Arth Rheum 17:35,1987.

Redler I. Clinical significance of minor inequalities in leg length. *New Orleans Med Surg J.* 104:308, 1952.

Ren MF, Tu ZP, Han JS. The effect of hemicholine, choline, atropine and eserine on electroacupuncture analgesia in rats, in Han JS (ed) *The Neurochemical Basis of Pain Relief by Acupuncture; A*

Collection Papers. Med Sci Press Beijing 1987.

Reshentinkova AD. *Sovetskaia Meditisina* 2:23, 1954.

Richardson C et al. *Therapeutic exercise for spinal segmental stabilization in low back pain.* Churchill Livingstone, Edinburgh, 1999.

Richez, Chamay and Bieler. Bone Changes Due to Pulses of Direct Electric Microcurrent. *Virchows Arch. Abt. (A Path Anat.)* 357:11, 1972.

Richmond, FJ, Abrahams,VC: What are the proprioceptors of the neck? Progr. *Brain Res.* 50:245, 1979.

Rivett HM. Cervical Manipulation: Confronting the Spectre of the Vertebral Artery Syndrome. *J. Ortho Med* 16:12, 1994.

Rheumatoid Arthritis Coordinating Research Group, First Teaching Hospital. *Acta Academae Medicinae Wuhan* 6:51, 1977.

Roaf R. *Spinal Deformities*. Philadelphia: JB Lippincott Co; 1977.

Rogers F, Bossy J. Activation of the defence system of the body of animals and men by acupuncture and moxibustion. *Acupuncture Research Quarterly* 5:47, 1981.

Roland M, Morris R. A study of the natural history of low back pain. Part I. Development of a Reliable and sensitive measure of disability in low back pain. *Spine* 8: 141, 1983.

Rolf I. Structural dynamics. *British Academy of Osteopathy Yearbook* 1962, Maidstone, 1962.

Rollnik JD et al. Repetitive transcranial magnetic stimulation for the treatment of chronic pain - a pilot study. *Eur Neurol.* 48(1):6, 2002.

Romano T: Fibromyalgia update. *The pain practitioner*. 10:2, 2000.

Rong M. Comparing observations of treatments of periarthritis of the shoulder by acupuncture and massage. *Chin Acupun and Moxib* 6:3, 1986.

Ronningen, Langeland N. Indomethacin treatment in osteoarthritis of the hip joint. *Acta Orthop Scand* 50:169, 1979.

Rosenberg ZS. Ankle tendons: Evaluation with CT. *Radiology* 166:221, 1988.

Rosted P. Literature Survey of Reported Adverse Effects Associated with Acupuncture Treatment. *Amer J Acupu* 24:1, 1996.

Rosted P. Practical recommendations for the use of acupuncture in the treatment of temporomandibular disorders based on the outcome of published controlled studies. *Oral Dis* 7:109, 2001.

Rotariu O et al. Stimulating the Embolization of Blood vessels using Magnetic Microparticles and Acupuncture Needle in a Magnetic Field. *Biotechnol Prog* 20(1):229, 2004.

Rothman, Deborah, et al. Botanical Lipids: Effects on Inflammation, Immune Responses, and Rheumatoid Arthritis. *Seminars in Arthritis and Rheumatism*, October, 25:87, 1995.

Rothman Rh et al.: A study of computer-assisted tomograpy. *Spine* 9:548,1984.

Royal FF. Understanding homeopathy, acupuncture and electrodiagnosis: clinical applications of quantum mechanics. *Am J Acupunctue.* 18: 1990.

Rubin B et al. Treatment options in fibromyalgia syndrome. *J American Osteopathic Association* 90: 844, 1990.

Bubnic et al. Alternative Medicine: Expanding Medical Horizons. Presentation paper 1992.

Ruch T.C., Patton H.D (eds). *Pathophysiology of pain,* Physiology and biophysics. Sanders, Philadelphia, 1965.

Rupani HD. Three phase radio nuclide bone imaging in sports medicine. *Radiology* 156:187, 1985.

Rush, Polatin and Gatchel 2000. Depression and Chronic Low Back Pain: Establishing Priorities in Treatment. *Spine* 25:2566, 2000.

Ruskin AP. *Current Therapy in Physiatry*: Physical Medicine and Rehabilitation. Philadelphia: WB Saunders Co; 1984.

Russell IJ. Fibromyalgia (Introduction). *The J of Muscuskel Med* 16:5, 1999.

Ryan GB, Majno G. *Inflammation a Scope Publication*. Upjohn Kalamzoo, 1983.

S

Saal JA, Saal JS.: Nonoperative treatment of herniated lumbar intervertebral disc with radiculopathy. *Spine* 14:431, 1989.

Sabolovic D, Michon C. Effect of acupuncture on human peripheral T and B lymphocytes. *Acupunct Electrother Res Int J.* 3: 97, 1978.

Sakai F, Ebihara S, Akiyama M, Horikawa M Pericranial muscle hardness in tension-type headache. A non-invasive measurement method and its clinical application. *Brain* 118:52, 1995.

Saldinger, P., Dvorák, B., Rahn, S., Perren, M. The Histology of Alar and Transverse Ligaments. *Spine* 15:257,1990.

Sambo P, Amico D, Giacomelli R. Intravenous N–Acetylcysteine for Treatment of Raynaud's Phenomenon Secondary to Systemic Sclerosis: A Pilot Study *J Rheumatol* 28:2257, 2001.

Sandberg M., Lundeberg T., Lindberg L.G., Gerdle B. Effects of acupuncture on skin and muscle blood flow in healthy subjects. *Eur J Appl Physiol* Jun 24, 2003.

Sanders RJ, Pearce WH. The treatment of thoracic outlet syndrome: a comparison of different operations. *J Vasc Surg* 10: 626, 1989.

Sandkuhler J. The organization and function of endogenous antinociceptive systems. *Prog Neurobiol* 50:49, 1996.

Sandler S. Physiology of soft tissue massage. *British Osteopathic Journal* 15: 1, 1983.

Sandyk et al. Magnetic Fileds in the Treatment of Parkinson's Disease. *International J of Neuroscience* 63:141, 1992.

Santini M, Ibata Y.: *Brain Res*. 33: 289, 1971.

Sawynok J, Reid A. Peripheral adenosine 5'-triphosphate enhances nociception in the formalin test via activation of a purinergic p2X receptor. *Eur J Pharmacol* 330:115, 1997.

Scherak O, Kolarz G, Schodl C, Blankenhorn G. High dosage vitamin E therapy in patients with activated arthrosis. *Z Rheumatol* 49:369, 1990. [Article in German]

Schiowitz S. Facilitated positional release. *J American Osteopathic Association* 90: 145, 1990.

Schinter TJ. Advances in Osteoarthritis Research: Investigating Subchondral Bone as Etiologic Agent and Therapeutic Target. *Medscape CME* Jan 20, 2004.

References

Schultz AB. *Biomechanics of the spine. In Low Back Pain and industrial and social disablement.* American Back Association, London 1983.

Schultz DG, Fox NH. Kenneth Snelson Buffalo, Albright-Knox Art Gallery. 1981.

Schwarzer AC, Aprill CN, Bogduk N.:The sacroiliac joint in chronic low back pain. *Spine* 20:31, 1995.

Schwarzer AC, Aprill CN, Derby R, Fortin J, Kine G, Bogduk N. The relative contributions of the disc and zygapophyseal joint in chronic low back pain. *Spine* 19:801, 1994.

Schwarzer AC, Aprill CN, Derby R, Fortin J, Kine G, Bogduk N. Clinical features of patients with pain stemming from the lumbar zygapophyseal joints. Is the lumbar facet syndrome a clinical entity?. *Spine* 19:1132, 1994.

Shapira MY, Chelouche M, et al. Tai Chi Chuan Practice as a Tool for Rehabilitation of Severe Head Trauma: 3 Case Reports. *Arch Phys Med Rehabil* 82:1283, 2001.

Shealy CN and Leroy PL. New Concepts in Back Pain Management, Decompression, Reduction, Stabilization. *Pain Management: A Practical Guide for Clinicians.* Vol 1. St. Lucie Press FL 1988.

Sheild MJ. Anti-inflammatory drugs and their effects on cartilage synthesis and renal function. *European J Rhemalol Inflam* 13:7, 1993.

Seifter E et al. Supplemental arginine: Endocrine, autocrine, and paracrine effects on wound healing. *J Am Coll Nutr* 8:437,1989.

Seitfer E et al. Influence of vitamin A on wound healing in rats with femoral fracture. *Ann Surg* 181:836,1975.

Selzer M, Spencer W A. Convergence of visceral and cutaneous afferent pathways in the lumbar spinal cord. *Brain Res.* 14:331, 1969.

Shang C. Electrophysiology of growth control and acupuncture. *Life Sci* 68:1333, 2001.

Shapiro D, Goldstein IB, Jamner LD. Effects of cynical hostility, anger out, anxiety, and defensiveness on ambulatory blood pressure in black and white collage students. *Psychosom Med* 58:354, 1996.

Sharif, Mohammed, et al. Serum Hyaluronic Acid Level as a Predictor of Disease Progression in Osteoarthritis of the Knee. *Arthritis and Rheumatism* 38:760, 1995.

Sharp L. Percutaneous Disc Decompression using Nucleoplasty. Poster presentation a 6th International Congress of Spinal Surgery. Ankara, Turky. September 2002.

Shaw, T.E.In.: Mennell J. *The Musculoskeletal System.* Anaspen Publication, Gaithersburg, Maryland 1992.

Shekelle, PG, Adams, AH, Chassin, MR, Hurwitz, EL, Brook, RH. Spinal Manipulation for Low-Back Pain. *Annals of Internal Medicine* 17:590, 1992.

Shen E, Tsai TT, Lan C. Supraspinal participation in the inhibitory effect of acupuncture on viscero-somatic reflex discharges. *Chin Med J* 1:431, 1975.

Shi GD et al. *J of Guiyang College of TCM* 1:59, 1980.

Shigata M. *J of the Pharm Socie of Jap* (Tokyo) 97:911, 1977.

Shibata M. Metabolism and Disease *Wakan Yaku* Supplement 10:687, 1973.

Shriber WJ. *A Manual of Electrotherapy*, 4th ed. Philadelphia, Lea and Febiger, 1974.

Shudo D. *Introduction to Meridian Therapy.* Seattle: Eastland Press, 1990.

Siegman AW, Snow SC. The outward expression of anger, the inward experience of anger and CVR: the role of vocal expression. *J Behav Med.* 20:29, 1997.

Sim J, Adams N. Physical and other non-pharmacological interventions for fibromyalgia. *Clin Rheumatol* 13:507, 1999.

Simon L. The importance of cyclo-oxygenase selectivity in the efficacy of NSAID therapy. *Proceedings of American Back Society,* 1997.

Simons DG, Hong CZ, Simons LS. Nature of myofaxial trigger points, active loci. J Musculoskeletal Pain 3 (Supplement 1) 1:62, 1005.

Simons DG, Travell JG, Simons LS. *Myofascial Pain and Dysfunction. The Trigger Point Manual Vol 1* (Second Edi), Williams and Willkins 1999.

Sims, J. The Mechanism of Acupuncture Analgesia: A Review, *Complementary Therapies in Medicine* 5:102, 1997.

Sin YM. Acupuncture and inflammation. *Int J Chin Med.* 1:15, 1984.

Sincair DC, Weddell G, Feindel WH, Referred pain and associated phenomena. *Brain* 71:184, 1948.

Singer R, Roy S. Osteochondrosis of the humeral capitulum. *Am J Sports Med.* 12:351, 1984.

Singh K. PDD using Nucleoplasty in the treatment of chronic discogenic pain. *Pain Physician* 5(3):250, 2002.

Singh GB, Atal CK. Pharmacology of an extract of salai guggalex Boswellia serrata, a new non-steroidal anti-inflammatory agent. *Agents Action* 18:4,1986.

Singh YN. Effects of kava on neuromuscular transmission and muscle contractility. *J Ethnopharmacol* 7:267; 1983.

Sinken BF, Wlker J. Therapeutic aspects of electromagnetic fields for soft-tissue healing. In: *Blank M (ed) Electromagnetic fields: biological intercations and mechanisms.* Advances in Chemistry Series 250. American Chemical Society, Washington DC 1995.

Smidt N, et al. Short or Long Term Advantage Seen with Steroids, Physiotherapy for Lateral Epicondylitis. *Lancet.* 359:657, 2002.

Smillie IS. The current pattern of internal derangements of the knee joint relative to the menisci. *Clin Orthop.* 51:117, 1967.

Smith MT, Pelis ML, Haythrornthwaite JA. Suicidal Ideation in Outpatients with Chronic Musculoskeletal Pain: An Exploratory Study of the Role of Sleep Onset Insomnia and Pain Intensity. Clin J Pain 20(2):111, 2004.

Smock T, Fields HL. ACTH (1-24) blocks opiate induced analgesia in the rat. *Brain Research.* 212:202, 1980.

Snelson KD. Continuous tension, discontinuous compression structures. U.S. Patent 3,169, 611, Washington Patent Office 1965.

Snijders C J, Vleeming A, Stoeckart R. Transfer of lumbosacral load to iliac bones and legs. Part I Biomechanics of self-bracing of the sacroiliac joints and its significance for treatment and exercise. *In Low back pain and its relation to the sacroiliac joint. First interdisciplinary world congress*. San Diego, Nov 1992.

Snook, S.H.: The Costs of Back Pain in Industry. *State of the Art Review. Spine*, 2:1 1987.

Sola AE, Kuitert JH, Myofascial trigger point pain in the neck and shoulder girdle. *Northwest Med* 54:980, 1955.

Solonen KA. The sacroiliac joint in the light of anatomical, roentgenological and clinical studies. *Acta Orthp Scand Suppi* 27, 1957.

Song ZY et al. *Acta Pharmaceutica Sinica* 10:708, 1963

Song ZY et al. *Acta Physiologica sinica* 22: 201, 1958.

Sorenson JRJ. Copper complexes offer a physiological approach to treatment of chronic diseases. *Progress in Medical Chemistry* Vol. 26, 1989.

Sorenson J. Copper aspirinate: a more potent anti-inflammatory and ulcer agent. *J Int Acad Prev Med* 1980.

Sopranzi N et al [Biological and electroencephalographic parameters in rats in relation to Passiflora incarnata L.] *Clin Ter* 13:329, 1990.

Srivastava KC and Mustafa T. Ginger (Zingiber officinale) in rheumatism and musculoskeletal disorders. *Med Hypothesis* 39:342, 1992.

Srivastava R Srimal RC. Modification of certain inflammation-induced biochemical changes of by curcumin. *Indian J Med Res* 81:447, 1973.

Spector TD. Bisphosphonates: potential therapeutic agents for disease modification in osteoarthritis. *Aging Clin Exp Res* 15(5)413, 2003.

Spengler, Oswald. *The Decline of the West*. Alfred A. Knopf, New York, 1932.

Sprott H, Franke S, Kluge H, Hein G. Pain treatment of fibromyalgia by acupuncture. *Rheumatol Int* 18:35, 1998.

Sprott H; Jeschonneck M; Grohmann G; Hein G. Microcirculatory changes over the tender points in fibromyalgia patients after acupuncture therapy (measured with laser-Doppler flowmetry). *Wien Klin Wochenschr* 112:580, 2000.

Stammers T et al. Fish oil in osteoarthritis. Letter. *Lancet* 2:503, 1989.

Stanish WD, Valiant GA, Bonen A, et al. The effects of immobilization and electrical stimulation on muscle glycogen and myofibrillar ATPase. *Can J Appl Sport Sci*. 7:267, 1982.

Starlanyl DJ, and Copeland ME. *Fibromyalgia and Chronic Myofascial Pain: A Survival Manual* edition 2, 2001.

Stefano G, Radanov BP. Course of attention and memory after common whiplash: a two-years prospective study with age, education and gender pair-matched patients. *Acta Neurol Scand* 91:346, 1995.

Stevens, A. Side bending in Axial Rotation of the Sacrum Inside the Pelvic Girdle. *First Interdisciplinary World Congress on Low Back Pain and its Relation to the Sacroiliac Joint*. San Diego 1992.

Stiles TC, Landro NI. Information processing in primary fibromyalgia, major depression and healthy controls. *J Rheumatol*. 22:137, 1995.

Stone S. Pyridoxine and thiamine therapy in disorders of the nervous system. *Dis Nerv Sys* 11:131, 1950.

Strohman R et al. Fibroblast Growth Factor Plays a Role in Regulating Muscle Hypertrophy. Medicine and Science in Sport and Exercise *Am Coll of Sports Medicine* 5:173, 1989.

Sturzenegger M. Headache and neck pain: the warning symptoms of vertebral artery dissection. *Headache* 34:187, 1994.

Su HC, Su RK. Treatment of whiplash injuries with acupuncture. *Clin J Pain*. 4:233, 1988.

Su XR et al. Scientific Research Compilation (*Shenyang Medical College*) 3:6, 1959.

Subotnick SI. *Sports Medicine Of The Lower Extremity*. Churchill Livingstone, NY., 1975.

Suessmann Muntner. *Moshe ben Maimon Medical Works*. Mossad Harav Kook, Jerusalem, 1957.

Suga T. Metabolism and Disease (may supp); *The References of Traditional Chinese Medicine* 4:39, 1976.

Sullivan MX, Hess WC. Cystine content of finger nails in arthritis. *J None Joint Surg* 16:1985, 1935.

Sun AY, Boney F, Lee DZ. Electroacupuncture alters cathecolamines in brain regions of rats. *Neurochem Res* 10:251, 1984.

Sun XY, Yu J, Yao T. Pressor effect produced by stimulation of somatic nerve on hemorrhagic hypertension in conscious rats. *Acta Physiologica Sinica* 35:264, 1983.

Surtees SJ, Hughes RR. Treatment of trigeminal neuralgia: Conservative management with massive vitamin B12 therapy. *N Carolina Med J* 14:206, 1953.

T

Tait RC, Chibnall JT, Margolis RB.: Pain extent: Relations with psychological state, pain severity, pain history and disability. *Pain* 41:295, 1990.

Taillard, Meyer and Garcia. *Int Orthop* 5:117, 1981.

Takeshige C, Sato M. Comparison of Pain Relief Mechanisms Between Nedling to the Muscle, Static Magnetic Field, External Qigong and Needling to the Acupuncture Point. *Acupuncture and Electro-Therapeutics Reseach* 21(2)119, 1996.

Tamkins T. Reducing Stress Eases Arthritis Pain, Depression. *Medical Tribune* 5, 1996.

Tanaka TH. Professor Nishijo's Research-Acupuncture and the Autonomic Nervous System. *North Amer J of Orien Med*. 3:8, 1996.

Taren DL et al. Increasing the breaking strength of wounds exposed to pre-operative irradiation using vitamin E supplementing. *Int J Vitam Nut Res*, 57:133, 1987.

Targino RA et al. Pain treatment with acupuncture for patients with fibromyalgia. *Curr Pain Headache Rep* 6:(5):379, 2002.

Tasker RR.: *Deafferentation pain syndromes*: pathophysiology and treatment. Raven Press, NY 1991.

Tatlow Brown BSt, Issingtone Tatlow WF. Radiographic studies of

References

the vertebral arteries in cadavers. *Radiology* 81:80, 1963.

Taube JS, Goodridge JP, Golob EJ, Dudchenko PA, Stackman RW. Processing the Head Direction Cell Signal: A Review and Commentary. *Brain Research Bulletin*, Vol. 40, Nos.5/6, 1996.

Taussig S, Batkin S. Bromelain, the enzyme complex of pineapple (ananas comosus) and its clinical application. An update. *J Ethnopharmacol.* 22:191,1988.

Taylor JR, Twomey LT. Structure and Function of Lumbar Zygapophyseal (Facet) Joints: Review. *J Ortho Med* 14-3: 71, 1992.

Thiel H, Wallace K, Donat J, Yong-Hing K. The effect of various head and neck positions on vertebral artery blood flow-a study using Doppoler ultrasound. *Clinical Biomechanics* [in press].

Thomas M et al. A comparative study of diazepam and acupuncture in patients with osteoarthritis pain: A placebo controlled study. *Am J Chin Med* 19:95, 1991.

Thomas M, Lundeberg T. Importance of modes of acupuncture in the treatment of chronic nociceptive low back pain. *Acta Anaesthesiol Scandinavica* 38:63, 1994.

Thomas M et al. Pain and discomfort in primary dysmenorrea is reduce by preemptive acupuncture or low frequency TENS. *European Journal of Physical Medicine and Rehabilitation* 5(3):71, 1995.

Thompson D. On growth and form. Cambridge University Press, Cambridge 1961.

Thuile Ch, Walzl M. Evaluation of electromagnetic fields in the treatment of pain in patients with lumbar radiculopathy or the whiplash syndrome. *Neuro Rehabilitation* 17(1):63, 2002.

Timofeev MF. Effects of acupuncture and an agonist of opiate receptors on heroin dependent patients. *Am J Chin Med* 27(2):143, 1999.

Tixier IM, et al. Evidence by in vivo and in vitro studies that binding of pycnogenols to elastin affects its rate of degradation by elastase. *Biochem Pharmacol* 33:3933,1984.

Trabrer MG et al. Lock of tocopherol in peripheral nerves of vitamin E deficient patients with peripheral neuropathy. *N Engl J Med* 317:262,1987.

Travell JG, Simons DG. Myofascial Pain and Dysfunction. *The Trigger Point Manual.* Williams and Willkins Baltimore, 1983.

Travell JG, Simons DG., *Myofascial Pain and Dysfunction The Trigger Point Manua*l. vol.II. Williams and Wilkins 1992.

Travell J, Rinzler SH. The myofascial genesis of pain. *Postgrad Med* 11: 425, 1952.

Travell J. Low back pain and the Dudley J. Morton foot (long second toe). *Arch Phys Med Rehabil* 56:566, 1975.

Travers RL, et al Boron and arthritis: the results of a double-blind pilot study. *J Nutri Med* 1:127,1990.

Tripterygium Wilfordii Coordinating Research Group of Hubei, Institute of Combined Western and Chinese Medicine et al. *Health J of Hubei* 1:72, 1979.

Trock, David H., et al. A Double-Blind Trial of the Clinical Effects of Pulsed Electromagnetic Fields in Osteoarthritis. *The Journal of Rheumatology* 20:456, 1993.

Troup JD et al. The perception of back pain and the role of psychophysical tests of lifting capacity. *Spine* 12:645, 1987.

Tsibuliak VN; Alisov AP; Shatrova VP. Acupuncture analgesia and analgesic transcutaneous electroneuro-stimulation in the early postoperative period. *Anesteziol Reanimatol* 2:93, 1995.

Tsuchisashi M. et al. Road traffic accidents and the abbreviated injury scale (AIS) in Japan. Accid Anal Prev. 13:37,1981.

Tume S. *Remedial Magnetic Therapy*. SA Collage of Natural and Traditional Medicine, Course Notes. Australia 2004.

Turek SL. *Orthopaedics*: Principles and Their Application. 4th ed. Philadelphia, J.B. Lippincott, 1984.

Tyler AN. Influenza A Virus: A Possible Precipitating Factor in Fibromyalgia? *Alt Med Rev* 2:82-86, 1997.

U

Yang YR et al. *Acta Physiologica Sinica* 8:101, 1966.

Uhlig Y, Weber BR, Grob D, Muntener M. Fiber composition and fiber transformations in neck muscles of patients with dysfunction of the cervical spine. *Orthop Res* 13:240, 1995.

Unruh AM. Gender variations in clinical pain experience. *Pain* 65:123, 1996.

Upadhaya L et al. Role of an indigenous drug Geriforte on blood levels of biogenic amines and its significance in the treatment of anxiety neurosis. *Acta Nerv Super* 32:1,1990.

Ursa Foundation. *Usng Scan Examinations in Clinical Practice* 1996.

Usichenko TI, Ivashkivsky OI, Gizhko VV. Treatment of rheumatoid arthritis with electromagnetic millimeter waves applied to acupuncture points--a randomized double blind clinical study. *Acupunct Electrother Res.* 28(1-2):11, 2003.

Y

Yamada K et al. Subchondral bone of the human knee joint in aging and osteoarthritis. *Osteoarthritis Cartilage* 10(5):360, 2002.

Yang TD. The Herbs of the Eight Extraordinary. *Acupuncture.com*.

Yelland MJ et al. Prolotherapy Injections, Saline Injections, and Exercises for Chronic Low Back Pain: A Randomized Trial. *Spine* 29(1):9, 2004.

Yi Xue Za Zhi. *Zhonghua* (Taipei) 65(7):299, 2002.

Yu YX, Bao H, Zhou ZF, Han JS. C-fibers afferents are necessary for diffuse noxious inhibitory control (DNIC) but not for electroacupuncture analgesia, in Han JS: *The Neurochemical Basis of Pain Relief by Acupuncture; A Collection of Papers.* Med Sci Press Beijing 1978.

Yu PL et al. *Hunan Yiyao Zazhi* (Hunan Medical J) 5:52, 1979.

Yu QX et al. *Chinese Pharmaceutical Bulletin* 7:567, 1959.

V

Vahlquist, Carin, et al. Treatment of Psoriatic Arthritis With Extracorporeal Photochemotherapy and Conventional Psoralen-Ultraviolet A Irradiation. *Arthritis and Rheumatism* 39:1519, 1996.

Vallo MD, Ransohoff J. Thoracic disc disease in: *The Spine*, 2ed ed. WB Saunders Philadelphia 1982.

Van Buskirk. FIMM meeting Chicago 2001.

Van Tulder M, Malmivaara A, et al. Exercise Therapy for Low Back Pain. *Spine* 25:2784, 2000.

Vanherweghem JL, Depierreux M, Tielemans C, et al. Rapidly progressive interstitial renal fibrosis in young women: association with slimming regime including Chinese herbs. *Lancet* 341:38, 1993.

Veldhuizen AG. Kinematics of the scoliotic spine as related to the normal spine. *Spine* 12:852, 1987.

Vernon HT, Mior S.: The neck disability index: A study of reliability and validity. *J Manip Phsiol Ther* 14:409, 1991.

Verrier RL, Mittleman MA. Life-threatening cardiovascular consequences of anger in patients with coronary heart disease. *Cardiol Clin* 14:289, 1996.

Vickers AJ. Statistical reanalysis of four recent randomized trials of acupuncture for pain using analysis of covariance. *Clin J Pain* 20(5):319, 2004.

Vidal Y Plana RR et al. Articular cartilage pharmacology: In vitro studies on glucosamine and non-steroidal anti-inflammatory drugs. *Pharmacol Res Commun* 10:557,1978.

Videman at al.: Changes in 35S-sulphate uptake in different tissues in the knee and hip regions of rabbits during immobilization, remobilization and the development of osteoarthritis, *Acta Orthop Scand* 47: 290, 1979.

Vicenzino B, Collins D, Wright A. The initial effects of a cervical spine manipulative physiotherapy treatment on the pain and dysfunction of lateral epicondlylagia. *Pain* 68:69, 1996.

Viidik A, Gottrup F. Mechanics of Healing Soft Tissue Wounds. in: Woo et al eds. *Frontiers in Biomechanics* Springer-Verlag NY 1986.

Vincent CA. A Controlled trial in the treatment of migraine by acupuncture. *The Clin J of Pain* 5:305, 1990.

Vitamin A supplementation may be beneficial in peripheral vascular disease (PVD) *Acta Vitaminol Enzymol* 4:15,1982.

Vleeming A. et al. Mobility in the SI-Joints in old people: A kinematic and radiologic study. *Clin Biomech* 7:170, 1992.

Vleeming A et al. Load application to the sacrotuberous ligament: Influences on sacro-iliac joint mechanics. *Clin Biomech* 4:204, 1989.

Vleeming A. *AAOM annual meeting* 1994.

Vleeming A, Stoeckart R, Volkers AC, Snijders CJ. Relation between form and function in the sacroililac joint Part I: Clinical anatomical aspects. *Spine* 15:130, 1990.

Vleeming, Volkers AC, Snijders CJ, Stoeckart R. Relation between form and function in the sacroiliac joint Part II: Biomechanical aspects. *Spine* 15:133, 1990.

Vreden SG et al. Aseptic bone necrosis in patients on glucocorticoid replacement therapy. *Netherlands J Med*. 39:153, 1991.

Vyklicky L, Knotkova-Urbancova H. Can sensory neurons in culture serve as a model of nociception?. *Physiol Res* 45:1, 1996.

W

Waersted M, Eken T, Westgaard R. Single motor unit activity in psychogenic trapezius muscle tension. *Arbete och Halsa* 17: 319, 1992.

Waersted M, Eken T, Westgaard R. Psychogenic motor unit activity – a possible muscle injury mechanism studied in a healthy subject. *J Musculoskeletal Pain* 1: 185, 1993.

Waddell G.: A new clinical model for the treatment of low back pain. *Spine* 12:634,1987.

Wan WR. Zhu Liang-chun's Thoughts on The Treatment of Knotty, Difficult Diseases. *J of Chinese Medicine*, 1:14, 2000.

Wang N, Butler JP, Ingber DE. Microtransduction across the cell surface and through the cyroskeleton. *Science* 260:1124, 1993.

Wang S-M, Peloquin C, Kain ZN. The Use of Auricular Acupuncture to Reduce Preoperative Anxiety. *Anesth Analg* 93:1178, 2001.

Wang J.D., Kuo T.B., Yang C.C. An alternative method to enhance vagal activities and suppress sympathetic activities in humans. *Auton Neurosci* 30;100(1-2):90, 2002.

Wang JS, Lan C, Wong MK. Tai Chi Chuan Training to Enhance Microcirculatory Function in Healthy Elderly Men. *Arch Phys Med Rehabil* 82:1176, 2001.

Wang K, Yao S, Xian Y, Hou Z. A study on the receptive field of acupoints and the relationship between characteristics of the needle sensation and groups of afferent fibers. *Sci China* 28:963, 1985.

Wall PD, Gutnick M. Ongoing activity in peripheral nerves: the physiology and pharmacology of impulses originating from a neuroma. *Exp Neurol* 43:580, 1074.

Ward R. *Foundations of Osteopathic Medicine*. Williams and Wilkins, Baltimore, 1997

Waxman SG, deGroot J. *Correlative Neuroanatomy* 22ed (edi) Appleton and Lange Northwalk, Connecticut 1995.

Weber H.: Lumbar disc herniation: A controlled prospective study with ten years of observation. *Spine* 8:131, 1983.

Weintraub W. *Tendon and Ligament Healing A new Approach through Manual Therapy*. North Atlantic Books, Berkeley 1999.

Weisl H. The movement of the sacro-iliac joint *Acta Mat* 23, 1955.

Webster BS, Snook SH. The cost of 1989 workers' compensation low back pain claims. *Spine* 19:1111,1994.

Wei Hui Publishing. *Chinese Medicine Secret Recipe*. Shanghai, 1990.

Weiner DS, Macnab I. Superior migration of the humeral head. *J Bone Surg* 52B:524, 1970.

Weingart, J.R., Bischoff, H.P. Doppler-Sonographische untersuchungen der a. vertebralis unter berucksichtigung Chirotherapeutisch relevanter. *Kopfpositionen Manuelle Medizin* 30:62, 1992.

Weintraub MI, Khoury A. Critical neck position as an independent risk factor for posterior circulation stroke. A magnetic resonance angiographic analysis. *J Neuroimaging* 5:16, 1995.

Weiss DS, Kirsner R, Eaglastein WH. Electrical stimulation and wound healing. *Arch Dermato*. 126:222, 1990.

Weinstein JN: The role of neurogenic and non-neurogenic mediators as they relate to pain and the development of osteoarthritis. *Spine* 105: 356, 1992.

Wenneberg et al. Anger expression correlates with platelet aggregation. *Behav Med* 22:174 1997.

Werback MR. *Nutritional Influences on Illness* (second edition) Third Line Press, Trazana, CA).

Werback MR. *Botanical Influences on Illness*, Tarzana, CA, Third Line Press 1994.

Wever R. ELF-effects on human circadian rhythms. In: *Persinger MA (ed) ELF and VLF electromagnetic field effects.* Plenum Press, NY 1974.

White AR, Ernst E. Risks Associated With Acupuncture. *Perfusion*, 15:153, 2002.

White AA, Panjabi. M.M.The basic kinematics of the spine. *Spine* 3:13, 1978.

White AA, Panjabi MM. *Clinical biomechanics of the spine.* Lippincott, Philadelphia 1978.

White AR, Resch KL, Chan JC, Norris CD, Modi SK, Patel JN, Ernst E. Acupuncture for episodic tension-type headache: a multicentre randomized controlled trial. *Cephalalgia* 20:632, 2000.

White G. Vitamin E inhibition of platelet prostaglandin biosynthesis. *Fed Proc* 36:350, 1977.

Whittingham W, Ellis WB, Molyneux TP. The effect of manipulation, toggle recoil technique for headaches with upper cervical joint dysfunction: a pilot study. *J Manipulative Physiol Ther* 6:369, 1994.

Wildy P, Home RW. Structures of animal virus particles. *Progressive Medical Virology* 5:1, 1963.

Williams KW et al. The effect of topically applied zinc on healing of wounds in animals and man. *Ann Surg* 170:203,1969.

Willburger RE, Wittenberg RH. Prostaglandin release from lumbar disc and facet joint tissue. *Spine* 19:2068, 1994.

Willis GC et al. Serial artheriography in atherosclerosis. *Can Med Assoc J.* Dec, Willis GC et al. Serial artheriography in atherosclerosis. *Can Med Assoc J.* 562:68,1954.

Willis WD.: Mechanical allodynia: A role from nocireceptive tract cells with convergent input from mechanoreceptors and nociceptors? *APS Journal* 2:23, 1993.

Woelk H. Multicentric practice-study analyzing the functional capacity in depressive patients. *4th International Congress on Phytotherapy.* Munich, Germany, Sep 10-13, 1992, abstract SL54.

Woldanska-Okonska M, Czernicki J. Influence of pulsating magnetic field used in magnet therapy and magnet stimulation on cortisol secretion in human. *Med Pr.* 54(1):29, 2003.

Woldenberg SC. The treatment of arthritis with colloidal sulphur. *J South Med Assoc* 28:875,1935.

Wolf SL, Basmajian JV.: Assessment of paraspinal electromyographic activity in normal subjects and in chronic low back pain patients using biofeedback device. In: Asmussen E, Jorgensoen K, eds. *Biomechanics* VI-B, Baltimore: University Park Press,1979.

Wolff, HD. Comments on the Evolution of the Sacroiliac Joint in Progress and Vertebral Column Research, *First International Symposium on the Sacroiliac Joint, Its Role in Posture and Locomotion.* EcL Vleeming, A. European Conference Orgairrers, Rotterdam, 1991.

Woltring HJ, Long K, Osterbauer PJ, Fuhr AW. Instantaneous helical axis estimation from 3-D video data in neck kinematics for whiplash diagnostics. *J Biomech* 27:1415, 1994.

Wong J. *Neuro-Anatomical Acupuncture.* AAMA Symposium, 1999.

Wong J et al. The therapeutic effect of 154 cases of scapulohumeral peri-arthritis treated with electroacupuncture. *Chin Acup and Moxib* 8:20, 1988.

Wybran J, et al., Suggestive Evidence for Receptors for Morphine and Methionine-enkephalins on Hormonal Human T Lymphocytes. *Journal of Immunology* 130:168, 1979.

Wyke B. The neurology of joints. A review of general principles. Clinics in Rheumatic Diseases 7:233, 1981.

Wyke BD. Neurology of the cervical spinal joints. *Physiotherapy* 65:72, 1979.

Wyke BD. Clinical significance of articular receptor system in the limbs and spine. *Proc. of the 5th Int. Congress of Manual Medicine* Copenhagen 1977.

Wynne-Davis, R.: Hypermobility. Proc. Roy. *Soc. Med* 64:689, 1971.

Wynne-Davis, R.: Hypermobility. Manipulation of the spine: In: Basmajian JV (ed). *Manipulation, traction and massage.* Paris RML., 1986.

X

Xie CW, Tang J, Han JS. Central norepinephrine in acupuncture analgesia: Differential effects in brain and spinal cord, in Takagi H, Simon EJ, (eds). *Advances in Endogenous and Exogenous Opioids: Proceedings of the Int Narcotic Res Conference / INRC*, Kodansha Sci Books, Tokyo, 1981.

Xiao M. Analysis of the historical evolution to the Tong Luo method. *The European J of Integrated Eastern and Western Medicine* 2(1):37, 2003.

Xu J, Huang X, Wu B, Hu X. *Influence of Mechanical Pressure Applied on the Stomach Meridian upon the Effectiveness of Acupuncture of Zusanli.* Acupuncture Research 19(2):137, 1993.

Y

Yahia LH, Garzon S, Strykowski H, Rivard CH. Ultrastructure of the human interspinous ligament and ligamentum flavum: a preliminary study. *spine* 15:262, 1990.

Yaksh TL, Hammond DL. Peripheral and central substrates involved in the rostrad transmission of nociceptive information. *Pain* 13:1, 1982.

Yi ZZ. *Acta Pharmceutica Sinica* 15:321, 1980.

Yin QZ, Duanmu ZX, Guo SY, Yu XM. Role of hypothalamic arcuate nucleus in acupuncture analgesia: A review of behavior and electrophysiological studies. *J Trad Chin Med* 4:103, 1984.

Ying Y, et al. Effects of acupuncture on adrenocortical hormone production. *Amer J Chin Med.* 22:160, 1976.

Yrjama M Vanharanta H. Bony vibration stimulation: a new, non-invasive method for examining intradiscal pain. *Eur Spine J.* 3:233, 1994.

Yoganandan N et al. Epidemiology and injury biomechanics of motor vehicle related trauma to the human spine. In: Proceedings of the 33rd Stapp Car Crash Conference, P-227, 892438, Washington, DC, 1989, SAE.

Yu P, Bai H, Zhang W, Wu G. Effects of acupuncture on humoral immunologic function and trace elements in 20 cases of Behcet's disease. *J Tradit Chin Med* 21:100, 2001.

Yufang Xue. Eight Treatment Methods for Complicated Patterns of Qi and Blood. *J of Chinese Medicine.*

Yunus, M et al.: Primary fibromyalgia (fibrositis): Clinical study of 50 patients with matched normal controls. Semin. *Arthr. Rheum.* 11:151,1981.

Z

Zaslawski C.J., Cobbin D., Lidums E., Petocz P. The impact of site specificity and needle manipulation on changes to pain pressure threshold following manual acupuncture: a controlled study. *Complement Ther Med* Mar 11:11, 2003.

Zang QZ et al. Abstracts of the symposium of the Chinese society of Physiology *Pharmacology* 1964. p.106

Zborovskii AB, Babaeva AR. New trends in the study of the primary fibromyalgic syndrome. *Vestn Ross Akad Med Nauk* 11:52, 1996.

Zhang Y, Seshadri S, Ellison RC, et al. Bone Mineral Density and Verbal Memory Impairment: Third National Health and Nutrition Examination Survey, *Am J Epidemiol* 154:795, 2001.

Zhang DF et al. *Jiangsu Zhongyi* (Jiangsu J of TCM) 3:23, 1965.

Zhang YZ, Tong J, Han JS. Potentiation of electroacupuncture analgesia by D-phenylalanine or bacitracine in mice. *Kexue Tongbao.* 24:1523, 1981.

Zhang Xinshu. Wrist and Ankle Acupuncture Therapy. *J Chin Med* 37:5, 1991.

Zang XT. Interaction in thalamus of afferent impulses from acupuncture point and site of pain. *Chin Med J* 93:1, 1980.

Zao FY, Meng JZ, Yu SD, Ma AH, Dong XY, Han JS. Acupuncture analgesia in impacted last molar extraction: effect of clomipramine and pargyline, in Han JS (ed) *The Neurochemical Basis of Pain Relief by Acupuncture; A Collection of Papers.* Med Sci Press, Beijing 1981.

Zhejiang Medical College. Proceedings of the national symposium on Chinese traditional anesthesia 1970.

Zhongguo Zhong. Clinical study on relation between Spleen Qi deficiency syndrome and the pancreatic exocrine function. *Xi Yi Jie He Za Zhi* 16:414, 1996.

Zhu Zong-Xiang. Research advances in the electrical specificity of channels and acupuncture points. *Amer. J. Acup.* 9:203, 1981.

Zhu Y. *Pharmacology and applications of Chinese medicinal materials.* People's Medical Publishing House. 1958.

Ziboh Va, Fletcher MP. Dose-Response effects of dietary γ-linolenic acid-enriched oils on human polymorphonuclear-neutrophil biosynthesis of leukotriene B4. *Am J Clin Nutr* 55:39,1992.

Zukauskas G et al. Quantitative analysis of bioelectrical potentials for the diagnosis of internal organ pathology and theoretical speculations concerning electrical circulation in the organism. *Acup and Electro-ther. Res Int. J.* 13:119, 1988.

Works Consulted

A

Anon. *A Barefoot Doctor's Manual.* Washington, DC: U.S. Department of Health, Education and Welfare: Public Health Service, 1974.

Anon. *The Canon of Acupuncture*: *Huangti Nei Ching Ling Shu.* Sunu K, translator. Los Angeles: Yuin University Press, 1985.

B

Becker RO, Selden G. *The Body Electric: Electromagnetism and the Foundation of Life.* New York: William Morrow and Company, 1985.

Becker S. *Blue Poppy Online Journal.*

Beijing College of Traditional Chinese Medicine, Shanghai College of Traditional Chinese Medicine, et al. *Essentials of Chinese Acupuncture.* Beijing: Foreign Languages Press, 1980.

Bensky D, Barolet R. *Chinese Herbal Medicine Formulas and Strategies.* Seattle WA: Eastland Press, 1990.

Bensky D, Gamble A. *Chinese Herbal Medicine Materia Medica.* Seattle WA.: Eastland Press, 1986.

C

Chace C. The Administration of Chinese Medicinals in the Treatment of 32 Cases of Fractured Ribs. *Traumatology and Orthopedic Research Reports*, Blue Poppy Press 2000.

Chang CG. *The Fundamentals of Moxibustion, Cupping and Bloodletting.* China Medical College 1985.

Chen Y, Deng L. *Essentials of Contemporary Chinese Acupuncturists' Clinical Experiences.* Beijing, China: Foreign Languages Press, 1989.

Chen Z-L, Chen M-F. *The Essence and Scientific Background of Tongue Diagnosis.* Long Beach: OHAI, 1989.

Cheung CS. *Deficiency Damage.* HSCC San Francisco 2001.

Cheung CS. *Comprehensive Management of Phlegm Fluid (Tan Yin).* HSCC San Francisco 1996.

Chinese-English Chinese *Traditional Medical World-Ocean Dictionary*, CIBTC China 1994.

Clavey S. *Fluid Physiology and Pathology in Traditional Chinese Medicine.* Churchill Livingstone London, 1995.

Croizier RC. *Traditional Medicine in Modern China.* Cambridge: Harvard University Press, 1980.

References

D

Dharmananda S. Treatment of Avascular Necrosis of the Femoral Head with Chinese Herbs *Institute for Traditional Medicine*, Portland, Oregon.

Dosch M. *Illustrated Atlas of the Techniques of Neural Therapy with Local Anesthetics*. HAUG, 1985.

Dosch P. *Manual of Neural Therapy According to Huneke*. Haug Publishers 1984.

E

Eckmann P. *The Book of Changes in Traditional Oriental Medicine*. Columbia, MD: Traditional Acupuncture Institute, 1987.

Ellis A, Wiseman N, Boss K. *Grasping the Wind*. Brookline, MA: Paradigm Publications, 1989.

F

Faber W, Walker M. *Pain Pain Go Away*. ISHI Press International, 1990.

Flaws B. *Sticking to the Point*. Boulder CO: Blue Poppy Press, 1989.

Flaws B, Sionneau P. *The Treatment of Modern Western Medical Diseases with Chinese Medicine*. Blue Poppy Press, 2001.

Flaws B, Zhang Ting-liang, Chace C, Helme M, Wolfe HL, and The Dechen Yonten Dzo. *Blue Poppy Essays: Translations and Ruminations on Chinese Medicine*. Boulder, CO: Blue Poppy Press, 1988.

Flaws B. Ye Tian-shi's Medicinals Entering the Extraordinary Vessels. *Blue Poppy Articles*.

G

Griffin JE, Karselis TC. *Physical Agents for Physical Therapists* (2nd ed). Springfield: Charles C Thomas, 1982.

Guillaume G, Chieu M. *Rheumatology in Chinese Medicine*. Eastland Press 1996.

Gunn CC. *Treating Myofascial Pain: Intramuscular Simulation (IMS) for Myofasical Pain Syndromes of Neuropathic Origin*. Seattle WA: University of Washington press, 1989.

H

Hammer LI. *Chinese Pulse Diagnosis. A Contemporary Approach*. Eastland Press, 2001.

Helms JM. *Acupuncture Energetics. A Clinical Approach for Physicians*. Bekeley: Medical Acupuncture Publishers, 1995.

Hoc KH, Seifert GM. *Pulse Diagnosis Li Shi Zhen*. Brookline, Mass: Paradigm Publications 1985.

Hsü TC. *Forgotten Traditions of Ancient Chinese Medicine: A Chinese View from the Eighteenth Century*. Translated and annotated by Unschuld PU. Brookline, Mass: Paradigm Publications, 1990.

Huang BS. *Treatment of Pain by Traditional Chinese Medicine*. Harbin, China: Heilongjiang Education Press, 1993.

Hui JL, Xiang JZ. *Pointing Therapy*. Shandong China: Shandong Science and Technology Press, 1990.

J

Jenkner FL. *Electric Pain-Controle*. Vienna Austria.

Jiao Shu-De. *Ten Lectures on the Use of Medicinals from the Personal Experience of Jiao Shu-De*. Translated by Creg Mitchell, Nigel Wiseman, Marnae Ergil, and Shelly Ochs: Paradigm Publications 2003.

Jirui, C. and Wang, N., editors. *Acupuncture Case Histories from China*. Seattle: Eastland Press, 1988.

K

Kaptchuk TJ. *The Web That Has No Weaver: Understanding Chinese Medicine*. New York: Congdon and Weed, 1983.

Kikutani T. *Combined Use of Western Therapies and Chinese Medicine*. Hsu H-Y, translator. Long Beach: HOAI, 1987.

L

Lade A. *Acupuncture Points: Images and Functions*. Seattle: Eastland Press, 1989.

Lee J, Cheung CS. *Current Acupuncture Therapy*. Hong Kong: Medical Book Publications, 1978.

Lee M. *Master Tong's Acupuncture*. Boulder: Blue Poppy Press, 1992.

Lee HM, Whincup G. *Chinese Massage Therapy*. Boulder: Shambhala Press, 1983.

Legge D. *Close To The Bone*. Australia: Sydney College Press, 1990.

Lennard TA. *Physiatric Procedures in Clinical Practice*. Philadelphia: Hanley and Belfus Inc. 1995.

Leonhardt H. *Fundamentals of Electroacupuncture According to Voll*. Uelzen: MLV, 1990.

Leslie C, editor. *Asian Medical Systems*. Berkeley: University of California, 1977.

Liu Yanchi. *The Essential Book of Traditional Chinese Medicine*, Volume 2: Clinical Practice. New York: Columbia University Press, 1988.

Low R. *The Secondary Vessels of Acupuncture*. New York: Thorsons Publishers, Inc., 1983.

M

Maciocia G. *The Foundations of Chinese Medicine*. New York: Churchill Livingstone, 1989.

Maciocia G. *Tongue Diagnosis in Chinese Medicine*. Seattle: Eastland Press, 1995.

Maciocia G. *The Practice of Chinese Medicine: The Treatment of Diseases with Acupuncture and Chinese Herbs*. Edinburgh:

Churchill Livingstone, 1994.

Manaka Y, Birch S. *Chasing the Dragon's Tail*. Brookline: Paradigm Publications, 1995.

Man D, Man B, Plosker H. The influence of permanent magnetic field therapy on wound healing in suction lipectomy patients: a double-blind study. *Plast Reconstr Surg*. 104(7):2261, 1999.

Mann F. *The Treatment of Disease by Acupuncture*, 2nd ed. London: William Heinemann Medical Books Ltd, 1967.

Matsumoto K, Birch S. *Extraordinary Vessels*. Brookline: Paradigm Publications, 1986.

Matsumoto K, Birch S. *Hara: Reflections on the Sea*. Brookline: Paradigm Press 1988.

Matsumoto K, Birch S. *Five Elements and Ten Stems*. Higganum: Paradigm Publications, 1985.

Mori H. *Modern Acupuncture and Moxibustion III - Locomotor*. Tokyo: Ido No Nippon Sha, 1982.

N

Naeser MA. *Outline Guide to Chinese Herbal Patent Medicines in Pill Form*. Boston: Boston Medical, 1990.

Nakatani Y. *A Guide for Application of Ryodoraku Autonomous Nerve Regulatory Therapy*. Tokyo: Japan Ryodoraku Autonomic Nervous System Society, 1972.

Nogier PMF. *From Auriculotherapy to Auriculomedicine*. Paris: Maisonneuve, 1983.

Nogier PMF. *Handbook to Auriculotherapy*. Paris: Maisonneuve, 1981.

O

O'Connor J, Bensky D, translators. Shanghai College of Traditional Medicine (Shanghai). *Acupuncture: A Comprehensive Text*. Chicago: Eastland Press, 1981.

Oleson TD. *Auriculotherapy Manual. Chinese and Western Systems of Ear Acupuncture*. Los Angeles CA: Health Care Alternatives, 1990.

Ombrengt L, Bisschop P, ter Veer HJ and Van de Velde T. *A System of Orthopaedic Medicine*. Saunders 1995.

Omura Y. *Acupuncture Medicine: Its Historical and Clinical Background*. Tokyo: Japan Publications, Inc., 1982.

P

Peigen K, Yuanping W. *Acupuncture Treatment of Neurological Disorders*. Beijing China: Traditional Chinese Medical Publishers of China, 1991.

Peilin S. *The Treatment of Pain with Chinese Herbs and Acupuncture*. Churchill Livingstone 2002.

Pomeranz B, Stux G. *Scientific Basis of Acupuncture*. Berlin: Springer-Verlag, 1989.

Porkert M. *The Theoretical Foundations of Chinese Medicine*. M.I.T. East Asian Science Series, Vol.3. Cambridge: M.I.T. Press, 1994.

Q

Quan SX. Yuan JY, Mao GY, Lin Y, translators;. *Applied Chinese Acupuncture for Clinical Practitioners*. Shangdong China: Shangdong Science and Technology Press, 1985.

R

Ross J. *Zang Fu: The Organ Systems of Traditional Chinese Medicine*, 2nd ed. Edinburgh: Churchill Livingstone, 1985.

S

Seem M. *A New American Acupuncture: Acupuncture Osteopathy*. Boulder: Blue Poppy Press, 1993.

Serizawa, K. *Clinical Acupuncture: A Practical Japanese Approach*. New York: Japan Publications, 1988.

Shima M, Chace C. *The Channel Divergences Deeper Pathways of the Web*. Boulder: Blue Poppy Press 2001.

Shou-Zhong Y. Dan-Xi, translator. *The Heart and Essence of Nan-Xi's Method of Treatment*. Boulder: Blue Poppy Press, 1993.

Shudo, D. *Japanese Classical Acupuncture: Introduction to Meridian Therapy*. Stephen Brown, translator. Seattle: Eastland Press, 1990.

Sionneau P, Gang L. *The Treatment of Disease In TCM* (Vol 1-7). Blue Poppy Press, Boulder 1996.

So J Tin Yau. *The Book of Acupuncture Points*. Brookline: Paradigm Publications, 1985.

So J Tin Yau. *Treatment of Disease with Acupuncture*. Brookline: Paradigm Publications,1987.

Stux G, Pomeranz B. *Basics of Acupuncture*. Berlin: Springer-Verlag, 1991.

T

Tan R, Rush S. *Twelve and Twelve in Acupuncture*. San Diego CA, 1991.

Tan R, Rush S. *Twenty-Four More in Acupuncture*. San Diego CA, 1994.

Tanner J. *Beating Back Pain. A practical self-help guide to prevention and treatment*. Doris Kindersley 1987.

U

US Directory Service. *Acupuncture Anesthesia* (A translation of a Chinese Publication of the same title) U.S. Directory Service, 1975.

Unschuld PU. *Nan-Ching The Classic of Difficult Issues*. Berkeley: University of California Press. 1986.

V

Veith Ilza. *The Yellow Emperor's Classic of Internal Medicine*.

Berkeley: University of California Press 1972.

W

Wallach, J: Interpretation of *Diagnostic Tests, A Handbook Synopsis of Laboratory Medicine*. Little, Brown and Cope Boston USA 1978.

Wexu M. *A Modern Guide to Ear Acupuncture*. New York: ASI Publishers, Inc. 1975.

Wiseman N, Ellis A, Zmiewaski P. *Fundamentals of Chinese Medicine*. Brookline: Paradigm Publications, 1985.

Worsley JR. *Acupuncturists' Therapeutic Pocket Book*. Columbia, Maryland: The Centre for Traditional Acupuncture, 1975.

Wu Jing-Huan. *Ling Shu or The Spiritual Pivot*. University of Hawaii Press 1993.

X

Xianmin S, et al. *Practical Traditional Chinese Medicine* and *Pharmacology: Clinical Experiences*. Beijing China: New World Press, 1990.

Xing Z. *The English-Chinese Encyclopedia of Practical Traditional Chinese Medicine: Simple and Proved Recipes*. Beijing China: Higher Education Press, 1990.

Xu X, You K, Bao X. *The English-Chinese Encyclopedia of Practical Traditional Chinese Medicine: Orthopedics and Traumatology*. Beijing, China: Higher Education Press, 1990.

Y

Yang Shou-zhong *The Heat and Essence of Dan-Xi's Method of Treatment*. Blue Poppy Press 1993.

Yang Shou-zhong, Duan Wu-Jin. *Extra Treatises Based on Investigation and Inquiry*. Blue Poppy Press 1994.

Yau PS, editor. Scalp-Needling Therapy. Revised Ed. Hong Kong: Medicine and Health Publishing Company, 1984.

Yeung H-C. *Handbook of Chinese Herbs and Formulas Vol. 1 und Vol. 2*. Los Angeles: 1983.

Yoo TW. *Lecture on KoRyo SooJi Chim: About* the *Korean Hand Acupuncture*. Korea: Eum Yang Maek Jin Publishing, 1983.

You HJ, Yuan B, Tang JS. Influence of inhibiting SI cortical neurons to electroacupuncture and manual acupuncture in the rat. Chin J Neurosci 15:301, 1999.

Yu Hui-chan, Han Fu-ru. *Golden Needle Wang Le-Ting A 20th Century Master's Approach to Acupuncture*. Blue Poppy Press 1997.

Z

Zhang YH and Ken R. *Who Can Ride the Dragon?* Paradigm Publications 1995.

Zhang R-F, Wu X-F, and Wang N. *Illustrated Dictionary of Chinese Acupuncture*. Hong Kong: Sheep's Publications, 1986.

Zang XT, editor. *Research on Acupuncture, Moxibustion, and Acupuncture Anesthesia*. Beijing: Science Press; Berlin: Springer-Verlag, 1986.

Index

17-hydroxycorticosterone 271
5-HTP 139
5-lipoxygenase 575

A

abdomen 55, 95, 220
Abdominal
    Assessment, main topic 333
    examination Japanese system 338
        confirmation and herbs 339
    oblique 191
    pain 211
abdominal (oblique and rectus) 186
    fascia 183
    muscles 183
    pain 65, 91, 389
    wall 70
abnormal
    curvature of spine 72
    flora 245
    gait patterns, table 241
abscess 224, 229
accelerant nerve 279
accelerated neural degeneration 150
ACE inhibitors and nerve disorders 637
acetaminophen 571
acetyl merystoleate (CMO) 569, 572
acetylcholine 139, 142, 271, 600
Achilles
    bursitis 658
    tendinitis and foot dysfunction 675, 678
    tendon 595
acid phosphatase 244
acidic lipids 143
acquired Essence 17
acrachidonic acid 569, 575
acromegaly 244
acromian 280
acromioclavicular 228, 229, 589, 597
    and bursitis 657
ACTH 150, 271
actin 22, 173
action potential 138, 173
activating a wave through channel system 350

active range of movement 223
acupuncture 57, 137, 138, 140, 262, 264, 265, 269, 271, 289, 291, 293, 347, 564, 577, 593, 606, 638, 656
    analgesia 272
    auricular 289
    disc disorders 644
    fibromyalgia 625
    Four Needle Technique Sedation, table 315
    Four Needle Technique to treat Cold symptoms, table 316
    Four Needle Technique to treat Hot symptoms, table 316
    Four Needle Technique Tonification, table 315
    magic Square 306
    microsystems 289
    mid-day mid-night 288, 306
    nerve disorders 637
    precaution with treatment 298
    skin preparation 298
    tendons 596
Acupuncture And Dry Needling **264, 267**
    Mechanisms
        agglutinin 275
        anti-stress effects 276
        apoptosis 275
        arcuate nucleus 272
        atrophy 275
        autonomic system 274
        B lymphocytes 275
        beta-globulin 275
        bioelectrical fields 275
        brain 272
        cerebellum 272, 273
        conductance 275
        convergence visceral and somatic 273
        descending and ascending tracts 273
        DNIC 273
        electrical effects 275

        functional magnetic resonance imaging (fMRI) 273
        gamma globulin 275
        gap junctions 275
        gray matter 273
        hyperplasia 275
        hypertrophy 275
        hypothalamus 273
        immune effects 275
        irritation zones 273
        lysozyme and immune effects 275
        met-enkephalin 275
        neurochemical 271
        neurophysiologic and other mechanisms 272
        neurophysiological 273
        non-opioid 271
        opioid system 271
        periaqueductal gray 273
        PET scans 273
        physiological 275
        raphe magnus nucleus 272
        receptive field 273
        reticular formation 274
        somatovisceral 273
        T lymphocyte 275
        temperature 274
        thalamus 272
        The Brain 272
        thermography 274
        viscerosomatic 273
        X-signal 276
acute
    flashes of pain in lumbar spine, points 332
    pain main topic 143
    inflammation 29
acutely stiff back, points 329
adaptations to short leg 669
Additional Foot Disorders 677
adenosine triphosphate (ATP) 139, 174, 175, 603
adhesion 223, 224, 228, 231

ADP 4, 86
adrenal 81, 89
    cortex 150
    exhaustion 27
    function testing 85
    functions 245
    glands 84
    insufficiency 81, 82
adrenaline 84, 150, 618
adrenocortical hormones 84
adrenocorticotropic hormone 84, 150
Adverse Events Reported on TCM Herbs 293
afferent 125, 175
afferent nerves 134
Aging 90, 562
agitation 36
agonist 22, 174, 185, 599
air 51
Akabane testing 56, 301
alanine 86
alcohol 37, 298, 578, 588, 632
algogens 139
alkaline phosphatase 244
allergic 84, 245, 597, 681
    reactions 293
    synovitis 566
Allodynia and Hyperalgesis, main topic 142
allopurinol 575
alpha motor neuron 132
alpha-endorphin 138
alprazolam and fibromyalgia 625
ALS 125
altered consciousness 389
Alzheimer's disease 125
amines, inflammation 265
amino acids 86
AMP 86
ampere 426
amphiarthrosis 187
amygdala 134
amyotrophic lateral sclerosis 125, 592
An Mo massage 544
anaerobic 174
analgesia 262, 269, 288
    acupuncture 271
anatomical barrier 222
Ancestral-Qi 14, 78, 306
    sinew 593
Ancillary Techniques 368
anemia 243
anesthesia 52, 273
    injection bursitis 657
aneurysm 222, 683
aneurysmal bone cyst 682
anger 33, 36, 76, 145
    fibromyalgia 621
angina 93, 683

angioma of the medulla
    foot dysfunction 674
ankle
    joint, central line of gravity 213
Ankle Sprain 411
ankylosing spondylitis 244, 681
annular
    fissures 253
    lumbago 642
    ruptures whiplash 651
annulospiral endings 127
annulus fibrosus 184, 580
    disc disorders 638
anorexia 6, 84
antagonist 22, 174, 185, 280, 599
antalgic postures 476
anterior
    cingulate cortex 134
    disc protrusions 642
    longitudinal ligament 181, 195
    pes cavus foot dysfunction 674
anterolateral spinothalamic tract 151
anthocyanidins 568
antibiotics 31
anti-histamines 681
    fibromyalgia 622
Anti-Inflammatory Drugs 271, 282
    side effects 555
    clooxygenase-2 (COX-2) 555
    hypertension 555
    osteoarthritic cartilage 555
antinuclear antibodies 243, 244
antiopioid substances 138
antioxidants 571
anuria 82
anxiety 34, 36, 38, 78, 145, 211, 575, 589, 598
    fibromyalgia 621
aorta 219, 222
aortic dissection 222
aortic regurgitation 222
apex of the heart 683
aponeuroses 179
aponeurosis 186, 191
appetite 40, 91
Applied Kinesiology Muscle 85, **509**, 511
apprehension tests 226
aptosis 272
arachidonic acid
    disc disorders 639
    cascade 552
arched back 55
arsenic 632
arterial occlusion 219
arterioles 63
arteriopathy 683
arteriosclerosis 39, 683
arteriosclerotic plaque 683

arteritis 222, 683, 684
Arthritis and natural therapiesic **568**
arthritis 145, 230, 424, **564**
    active/Hot 407
    capsular pattern 230
    end feel 224
    kissing spine 655
    lumbar spondylosis 577
    resisted movements 229
arthrogryposis and foot dysfunction 674
arthrosis 30, 218, 571, 664
    end feel 223
    pain 565
    degenerative joint disease 408
articular 219
    cartilage 275, 568
    crepitus 219
    infection 544
articulatory techniques
    integration to TCM practice 498
Articulin-F 569, 571
aseptic necrosis 578
Ashi 56, 220, 277, 285, 303, 489, 606, 607, 667
Aspects of Pain **143**
aspirin 552, 575
    fibromyalgia 624
Assessing Patient's Pain **155**
asthenia 86
asthma 73, 145
asymptomatic between attacks 40
atherosclerosis 344
atherosclerotic carotid arteries 222
atlantoaxoid 195
atonia 57, 65
ATP 4, 86, 140
atrophic gastritis 85
atrophy 6, 24, 30, 57, 87, 166, 213, 381, 584, 595, 603, 660, 682
Atrophy syndromes treatment 594
atypical segments 195
atypical vertebrae 194
Auricular therapy 343
    brainstem 344
    cerebrospinal 344
    cranial nerve 344
    ectodermal 344
    embryological 344
    endodermal 344
    master points 345
    mesodermal 344
    reticular formation 344
    somatotopic 344
    spinothalamic 344
Auscultation 222
Auto Immune 409
    arthritis 30
    disease 211, 244
autonomic nervous system 13, 86, 134,

276
auxiliary column cells 133
Avascular Necrosis 578
    treatment 578
axis 195
ayurvedic 570
B
Babinski sign 210, 232, 593
bacitracin 271
bacteria 244
bacteria flora 86, 576
basal ganglia striatum 140, 272
basal spinal nucleus 131
basilar syndrome 683
Basstrap's Disease 655
Beckwith's syndrome 344
Bell's palsy 632
Bence Jones protein 245
benign 211, 538, 682
    tremor 6
beta-carotene 572
beta-endorphin 138, 271
beta-lactoglobulin 576
beta-lipotropin 138
Bi Syndrome 168, 659
    Connecting channels 299
    Organs 660
bile 97
biliary disease 244
bio
    electric battery 429, 553
    electromagnetic 447
    energetic 423
    biofeedback and fibromyalgia 625, 626
    mechanical 284
    mechanics of the pelvis 505
        spinal joints 185
    medical diagnosis 205
    medical injection therapy 297
bizarre symptoms 40
black stools 389
Bladder 49
    and Divergent channels 69
bladder disease 211
bleeding 87, 293, 539
    biomedical and OM 87
bleeding and bruising 293
bloating 33
Blood **14**, 31, 39, 58, 63, 65, 69, 74, 95, 165, 168, 207, 224, 277, 284, 292, 369, 543, 544, 556, 593, 594, 660, 662
    Bi 659
    deficiency 33, 106
    depression/congestion 26
    disorders 14, 16
        table 15
    division 26
    Essence 17

    fibromyalgia 621
    Heat 43
    letting therapy 371
    musculoskeletal effects 16
    Organs 17
    Penetrating channel 70
    stagnation 42, 209
    stasis 31, 37, 38, **41**, 103, 106, 160, 167, 220, 262, 286, 299, 334, 375, 537, 594
        fibromyalgia 622, 626
blood 244
    circulation 167
    letting 541
    pressure 212, 279, 618
    vessels 39
    urine 245
blueberries 568
blurred vision 65, 385
bodily milieu 106
body aches 44
body inch 285
bone/Bone 220, 286, 311
    Bi 659
    clinging flat-access 168
    marrow 19, 134, 166
        emptiness 168
        suppression 389
    metastasis 244
    OM **166**
    scan **250**, 682
    setting 453
    spurs 39
    tumor 682
Bone and Periosteum **180**
bony congenital abnormalities 683
boron 568, 572
boswellia serrata 569, 571, 569, 574
brachial plexus 649
bradykinin 138, 139, 142, 143, 169, 574
brain 72, 89
    stem 128, 140, 151, 272
        clinical deficit 129
        nuclei 134
    tumor 592
branch 102, 262, 276, 277
brass 296
breast 55
breath 92
breathing 76, 193
broad needling 294
broken needle tips 293
bromelain 574
bronchitis 73, 572
bruit 222, 681
bulging disc 640
bunion 657
burning balls of the feet
    foot dysfunction 675

    neurogenic claudication 648
bursae 57, 225, 229
bursal 219
    crepitus 220
    sac 657
bursitis 41, 224, 230, 232, 571, 590, **657** 658
    and TCM 658
    ankle foot area 658
    knee area 657
    treatment 658
buttocks 55, 65
C
café-au-lait-pigmented macules 683
calcific tendinitis
    fibromyalgia 622
calcified bursae
    fibromyalgia 622
calcium 139, 271, 568, 575, 600, 681
    fibromyalgia 624
callus and foot dysfunction 676
caloric energy production 81
cAMP 81
Cancer
    warning signs 682
cancer 168, 209, 211, 217, 224, 243, 244, 262, 571
Cannon and Rosenblueth's law of super-sensitivity 140
capacitance 268
capillary refill time 219
capsaicin 569, 571
capsular
    pattern 224, 228, 230, 576, 589
    rupture 561
    thickenin 218
capsule 225, 230
capsulitis 230, 646
cardiac
    arrhythmias 600
    dysfunction 600
    plexus 279
    tamponade 293
cardiovascular disease 683
carotid artery 222
carpal tunnel syndrome
    posain and nulliness 580
    pressure on nerves 632
cartilage 165, 171, 186, 568, 574, 646
    type summary table 171
cauada equina and disc disorders 643
CBC 243
CD4 86
CD4/CD8 ratio 576
CD8 86
Celecoxib 569, 574
cell-to-cell communication 53
cellular
    elements 180

immunity 551
nutrition 428
polarity 275
central 144
    convergence 132
    core disease 588
    cyclic nucleotides 271
    line of gravity 213
    sensitization 132
    summation 132
    vision 213
Central-Qi 44, 46, 106
centromedian nucleus 272
cerebellum 128
    clinical deficit 129
cerebral
    cortex 272
    vertebral arteries 683
    palsy 424
    vascular accident 684
cerebrum 129, 130
    clinical deficit 130
CERPS-I and CERPS-II, table 636
cervical 94
    spondylosis 683
    spondylopathy herbs 578
Cervical Spine 194
    extension 196
    flexion 196
    sidebending 196
C-fibers 571
cGMP 81
chain joint reactions 561
channel palpation 285
Channels 6, 51
    acupuncture 51
    Conception (Ren), summery table 73
    Connecting /Vessels and Collateral Branches 63
    disorders of six energetic zones 60
    distributed 53
    Divergent
        main topic 68
    Divergent and Extra channel use 69
    Extra 69
    Extra channel use 69
    Girdle (Dai), summery table 75
    in musculoskeletal medicine 54
    less Qi and more Blood 291
    Main 65
    pattern discriminations 53
    physiologic activity summary table 50
    Qi/Blood balance, table 291
    Shao-Yang level 58
    Sinews 54
        summery table 55
    Tai-Yang level 58

Yang Linking (Wei), summery table 79
Yang Motility (Qiao), summery table 76
Yang-Ming level 58
Yin Levels 60
Yin Linking (Wei), summery table 78
Yin Motility (Qiao), summery table 77
channels 220
Channels, Meridians, Vessels **51**
Chapman's reflexes 85, 281, 335, 336, 498, 499
    nerve disorders 637
Charcot-Marie-Tooth disease
    foot dysfunction 674
charge 426
Chemical Pain Theories and Implications 138
    disc pain 644
chemical-mediated communication 126
chemotherapy 424
cherries 568
chest 55, 220
Chest and Rib Cage 414
chili papers 571
chills 65, 389
chin 65
Chinese Herbal Therapy **375**
chiropractic 500
cholecystokinin 138, 271
choleithiasis 333
cholinergic 272
chondritis 566
chondrocytes 565, 569, 570, 573, 574
chondroitin sulfate 169, 570, 572
    disc disorders 644
Chondromalcia Patella, Patellar Femoral Pain Syndrome
    foot dysfunction 678
chondrosarcomas 682
Chong 70, 336
chronic 18
    bursitis 657
    disc lesions, points 332
    fatigue syndrome 18, 31, 150
    infection 681
    pain 143, 424
    visceral disease 681
chrysanthemum indicum 569, 575
cimetidine 265
cinnamomum cassia 569, 575
circadian time 305
circles around eyes 40
circulation 299
circulatory problems 78
cirrhosis 430
clavicle 55

Clear-Yang 39, 45
clomipramine 139
clonus 593
clotting factors 87
cloy herbs 41
clubbing 87
cocaine 588
coccydynia 330
coccyx and foot dysfunction 675
Cognitive Psychotherapy and fibromyalgia 625
cognitive symptom 70
Cold 25, 26, 106
cold hands and feet 220
Cold or Deficiency Transforming Into Heat
    Bi 665
Cold Therapy 371
Cold/deficiency-stagnation-transformative/congested-Heat 105
Cold-Phlegm 39
collagen 169, 179, 180, 184, 265, 555, 568, 595, 596, 656
    vascular diseases 682
collagenous 574
collaterals 51
combination needling 294
Common Types of Neuropathic Pain, table 635
compensatory changes and asymmetry 217
complete blood count 243
Complex regional pain syndrome 588, 634
    motor tests 238
    CPRS-I 635
complexion 40
compression
    and sprain strain 539
    forces on lumbar spine 191
    trigger points 605
congealed Dampness (interarticular free body) 545
congenital
    abnormalities and asymmetry 217
    asymmetry of the posterior circulation 683
    lymphedema and foot dysfunction 674
congestion 285
Connecting channels 63, 103, 209, 290, 304
    external pathogens 299
    painful obstruction syndrome 299
    symptoms 63
    treatment 304
    treatment outside channels 299
connective tissues 74, **169**, 170, 538, 552, 561, 581, 589, 597

diseases and fibromyalgia 620
    planes 269
constitution 17
constitutional symptoms 211
Construction-Qi 16
Consumption/Taxation 36, 38
Contractile structures 538
    muscle
        contraction 173
        fibers 172
        functions 173
        postural & phasic muscles 174
        skeletal muscles 172
Contractile Unit Disorders
    acute sprains/strains 539
    causes of 587
    contracture 30
    locate hyperactive motor points and bands 606
    needle motor, trigger, ashi points 607
    patient positioning 283
    post-treatment care 610
    sprains and strains treatment 537
    tendon insufficiency treatment 597
    testing 228
        summary table 230
contrast therapy 610
control cycle 49, 51
convergence of nociceptor 153
convergence-facilitation 153
convergence-projection 153
convulsions 24, 389
copper 139, 296, 555
coronary artery spasm 600
corpus callosum 130
corpuscular 575
Corrective Exercises **517**
Correspondences of Channels, Muscles and Organs/Glands
    summery table 509
cortex 151
corticosteroids 84, 578, 588
corticotropin-releasing hormone 84, 150
cortisol 84
    acupuncture 271
    dysregulation 150
cosmic rays 423
costotransverse ligament 194
costovertebral stability 194
Cou Li 13, 25, 31, 63, 161, 220
cough 65, 73, 90
Coulomb 426
counseling 576
counter-irritation therapies 137
counternutation 199, 465
countertension positional release 487
coupling of vertebra movement, Fryette Laws 462

    summery table 462
coxa valgum 670
CPK 86
C-polymodal nociceptors 127
cranial nerves 133
    X 135
CranialSacral Osteopathic Techniques 135, 295, **499**
    fibromyalgia 627
cranial-sacral rhythms 285
C-reactive protein 574
    nerve disorders 637
creaking 219
creep 170
cri du chat syndrome 344
    cross fiber palpation 606
cross needling 288
cross-fiber massage 596
cruciform ligament 196
cryotherapy 539
crystalline
    bursitis 657
    diseases 243
    structures 425
    like protein structures 425
C-scoliotic and S-scoliotic responses 670
cubit 342
cun 285
cuneate nuclei 137
cupping 368
curcuma longa 569, 571
current of injury 125
Cushing's disease 84
Cutaneous regions 54
cyanosis 93
cyclic adenosine monophosphate 21
cyclic guanosine monophosphate 21
cyclooxygenase 571, 575
    COX enzymes 574
cyst 218, 232
cystitis 95, 574
cytokines 574
    fibromyalgia 624
cytoplasm 140
cytoplasmic
    components 140
    membrane 553

D
Dai 70, 106, 214, 290, 594
Damage of Yin and Essence with Cold-Damp 37
    Bi 669
    cupping technique 368
    depression/congestion 26
    Heat 26, 28, 29, 103, 105, 220, 221
    Heat/Phlegm 594
    Heat/toxic-abscess 168
    Phlegm 39

    tetany 26
    Warmth 29
Dampness 26, 27, 39, 105, 286, 291
    fibromyalgia 622
    trapped by Yin tonics 105
Daoist 57
Daypro and fibromyalgia 624
DC currents 275
deafferentation 34, 634
    pain 142, 634
decarboxylase 573
deceleration muscle function 173
deep
    myotonic reflex 233
    puncture 605
    reflexes 233
    skin 220
defecation 135
    and muscles 173
Defensive 102, 103, 220
Defensive-Qi 11, 19, 28, 29, 57, 63, 168, 303, 660, 662
    biomedical analogies 13
    fascia 13
Deficiency 27, 102, 103, 167, 283, 307
    accumulation-transformative-Heat 104
    Bi 659
    Phlegm 102
deficient-Blood 70
Definition of Pain Terms, table 142
deformation 171
Degenerative
    arthritis 243
    changes and asymmetry 217
    disc disease **603**, 641,
    Cascade and Discs 639
        TCM treatment 558
    foot dysfunction 676
    Joint Disease and Arthritis/Arthrosis 564
deglycyrrhizinated licorice 569
deltoid 603
demethyladrenaline 84
dendrites 125
denervation supersensitivity 143
dens 195
depolarization of muscles 173
depressed 289
Depression 26
depression 33, 36, 38, 40, 55, 78, 86, 145, 211, 269, 285, 371, 389, 575, 589, 598, 621
    fibromyalgia 625
De-Qi 269, 272, 295, 343, 441
de-Quervain's disease 52
derangements 106
dermatographia 600
dermatomal 280

dermatome 152, 207, 278, 288, 600, 633
dermatomyositis 588, 682
detoxification **246**
deviation 55
dexamethasone 271
dextrose 297
DHA and nerve disorders 637
DHEA 85
    nerve disorders 637
diabetes 145, 245, 344, 632, 683
diabetic 265
diabetic neuropathy 571
Diagnosis
    OM Pulses, summery table 109
Diagnosis (Zhen) 8
    inquiry summary table 113
    tongue 108
    visual summary table 107
    Treatment OM priorities 101
Diagnostic Process Orthopedic 207
diaphragm 56, 193, 279, 288, 337, 683
    fibromyalgia 627
diarrhea 90, 385, 389, 600
diarthrodial 186
diarthrosis 187
diathermy 302, 424
diencephalic 130
diencephalon 129
diet 36, 37
    fibromyalgia 621
difficulty standing 97
diffuse noxious inhibitory control system 288
diffusion 428
Digeorge syndrome 344
digestion 96
digestive enzymes 103
digestive symptoms
    caused by Yin herbs 105
DIM 681
dimexide and fibromyalgia 625
diphosphonates 539
diptheria 632
direct
    current 125
    needling 294
    techniques 222
direction of bind 222
direction of ease 222
Disc derangement patient education and prophylactics 645
Disc Disorders **638**
    acute injury 641
    biochemistry 639
    bulge 640
    degenerative disc disease 641
    derangement 640
    diagnosis of disc derangement 641
    disctis 644

interspinous ligament 638
intradiscal pH 639
nerve root impingement 638
paraspinal muscle weakness 638
phospholipase A2 639
stages of disc injury 640
sympathetic system 635
symptoms and treatment 643
discitis 644
discography 147
Disease Etiologies 22
    Pathogenic factors 22
disinfect skin and acupuncture 298
dislocation 453
Disorders of Six Energetic Zones 60
distinct peptide families 138
distortion 55
disturbed weight perception 600
diuretics 588
diurnal 305
Divergent Channels 32, 47, 56, 65, 68, 277, 285, 288, 290, 300
    access, reurn points 301
    directing (focusing) point 300
    other uses 300
    pathological tissues 300
    prevention of chronicity 300
    treatment 300
    use 69
    Yang 68
    Yin 68
diverticulosis 333
dizziness 6, 24, 84, 90, 91, 291, 385, 389, 600
DL-phenylalanine and nerve disorders 637
DMSO 573
dolorimetry 156
    fibromyalgia 625
Dontigny Model **505**
dopamine 86, 139, 271
dopamine beta-hydroxylase 139
doppler ultrasonic 295
dorsal horn 132, 133
dorsal roots 132
dorsiflexion 65
dowager's hump
    forward head posture 679
doxycycline 569, 574
D-phenylalanine 271, 292
drowsiness 292
dry mouth 389
Dry Needling 264, 277, 605, 610
    Strengthen Tendons and Ligaments 265
drying 37
Dryness 26, 28
Dry-Phlegm 39
Du 70, 106, 214, 594

Duchenne, Becker phenomenon 588
duodenal ulcers 265
duodenum 84
Dupuytren's contracture 87
dura mater 225, 590, 635
Dural Concept
    disc disorders 642
    signs 642
dynamic allodynia 236
dysentery 333
dysesthesia 210
dysmenorrhea 598
dysphagia 6
dyspnea 65, 78
E
ears 65
Earth 48
earth 166
Earth-type people 336
ease 223
eccentric 22
    contraction 191
ECG 52
ectopic pregnancy 211, 683
Eddison's disease 84
edema 19, 27, 28, 30, 57, 90, 93, 96, 218, 277, 571, 574
    fibromyalgia 621, 623
    pitting 28, 221
Edwards' syndrome 344
Effects of Smoking 38
efferent 125
    nerves 134
Effexor 145
effleurage 596, 610
eggplants 568
Ehlers-Danlos syndrome 555, 682
eicosapentaenoic acid (EPA) 574
Eight Extra Channels (Curious Channels Extra Vessels) 69
    herbal therapy 303
Eight Principles
    clinical use 44
    main topic 43
    muscle strain 43
elastic
    barrier 222, 224
    energy 171, 180, 185, 580
    fibers 180, 265
elastin 169, 179
Elbow 65, 95, 412
    extensors 65
electrical
    charges 424
    conduction 425
    potentials 428
    stimulation 605
Electroacupuncture 277, 289, 423, **438**
    anode 442

catecholamines 441
cathode 442
C-fibers 439
channel treatments 442
DC electricity 442
dense disperse 441
Electrical Frequencies in Electro-stimulation, table 439
fMRI 439
Han-stimulation 441
Hz 440
monoamine 441
monopolar 440
neuralgias 441
opioids 441
polarity
    of the body 442
TENS 443
Vaga 438
electroencephalgrapy (EEG) 295
electromagnetic 275, 423
    diagnostics 430
    energy 428

Electromagnetic therapy 425
    Curaton PC 436
    Diapulse 436
    equipment 436
    gauss 436
    stimulators nerve disorders 637
    whiplash 654
electromagnetism 53
electromyogram 600
Electromyography (EMG) 56, 246, 266
electron microscopy 570
electrons 424
Electrotherapy
    acupuncture-like-TENS 434, 435
    Alpha-Stim 435
    alternating current (AC) 426
    amplitude 426
    analgesia 432, 436
    anode 433
    bioelectromagnetic 435
    biphasic 433
    bone
        regeneration 432
    capacitance 427
    catecholamine 432, 436
    cathode 432
    collagen 433
    complex vibration 428
    conventional TENS 434
    direct current (DC) 426
    duty cycle 427
    electrode effects 432
    electrode effects, table 432
    electrophoresis 432
    fibroblasts 432

frequency 426, 433
fundamental frequency 428
galvanic stimulation 434
harmonic 428
healing effects of specific frequencies, table 436
high frequency stimulation 436
high-volt cathode stimulation 433
H-wave 438
Hz 436
inductance 427
interferential 434
iontophoresis 432
LISS cranial stimulator 433
local effects 432
mechanoreceptors
    electrical stimulation 432
microamp TENS 435
microcurrent 432, 438
MIRCO-Plus 438
modulation 427
monophasic 432
neurotransmitters 435
nociceptors 432
noise 427
nonsegmental 436
ohm 426
open circuit 427
osteogenesis 433
Period 426
pH 432
polypeptides 432
pulse rise time 427
pulses 427
quadripole stimulation 433
pate of current 428
resonance 428
short circuit 427
signal 427
sympathetic 436
systemic and segmental effects 432
transcutaneous stimulation-TENS 434, 438
    434
volt 426
waveforms 427
wavelength 427
EM field hazards 429
embryo 53
embryological 52, 81, 181
    developmental scheme 53
    segmental derivations, table 152
EMG 266
emphysema 73, 572
Empty-Fire 41
Empty-Heat 27, 38, 46, 103, 220
End Feel 223
    abrupt, hard stop 224
    boggy, spongy 223

empty, soft 224
hard 223
rubbery leathery 223
springy rebound 224
end-feel
    Bi 664
endocarditis 293
endocrine 86, 509, 595, 597
endocytosis 428
Endogenous Factors 32
    depression 36
    Heart 33
    pain 36
    seven affects 32
    summary table 35
endogenous-damage 32
endogenous-Dampness 28
endorphins 138
    acupuncture 271
    chemical theories pain 138
    nerve disorders 637
endotendon 179
endplate zones 176
enkephalins 138
    chemical theories pain 138
enteropathic arthritis 244
environment 37
enzymes 574
eosinophilic granuloma 683
epicondylitis 373, 571
Epidemic (Yi) 26
epididymitis 574
epidural injection and disc disorders 644
epilepsy 32, 55, 72, 76
epinephrine 139
epineurium 133
epiphysiodesis 576
epithalamus 129
epithelia 268
equilibrium 429
erection 135
ergotropic function 135
erosion 168
erythrocyte sedimentation rate 243, 570
esophagitis 424
esophagus 211
ESR
    Bi 665
Essence 17, 34, 74, 89, 103, 165, 166, 168, 224, 556, 593, 594
    acquired 17
    deficiet
        herbs 18
    inherited 17
    spirit 18, 65
    weakness 18
essential fatty acids 574
Essentials of Oriental Medicine 1
esterase 245

estrogen dominance 681
esuiterpene lactones 575
European 51, 81
evening primrose oil 574
Evidence For Spinal Physical Examination 206
evil 295
evil-Qi 60
Examination
    OM inquiry summary table 113
exercise 262, 573, 575, 592
    fibromyalgia 626
    intolerance 84
exhalation 194
Exogenous Pathogenic Factors 22
    summary table 30
exoplasmic nerve flow 18
expectorants and fibromyalgia 622
extension
    lumbopelvic 191
    spine 185
Exterior 13, 23, 24, 31, 37, 42, 53, 63, 81, 102, 165, 168, 220, 221, 262, 263, 299, 556
    fibromyalgia 621, 627
Extra Channels 69
    channel activation 303
    Conception (Ren) 73
    Governing (Du), summery table 72
    left right imbalance 290
    locomotion 300
    musculoskeletal use 303
    Penetrating (Chong) 74
    points summary table 303
    treatment 303
        design 277
    use 69
extra-articular lesion 228, 231, 232
extracellular matrix 169, 179
extrafusal fibers132
extrasegmental 276
    reference of pain 154
eye dominance 213

F

facet joints **185**, 195, 281, 561
Facet Disorders **646**
    arthropathy 217
    degenerative disease 646
    dysfunctions 646
    meniscus 646
    pain 185
    PLA2 and prostaglandins 646
    psoas 646
    quadratus
        lumborum 646
    spasm 646
    steroid 647
    syndrome 646
    treatment 647

facial edema 389
facilitated diffusion 428
Facilitated Segment 141, 217, 279, **562**
facioscapulohumeral 588
fainting 293
false-Heat 103
Fascia **180**, 585
    adaptations patterns Zink 585
        compensated patterns 586
        crossed pattern syndrome 586
        uncompensated patterns 586
        wrap-around pattern 586
    fascicle axial torque 192
    piezo-electricity 585
fascia 13, 165, 185, 191, 202, 218, 225, 598
fascicles 179
fasciculi 133
fat 220
fatal whiplash 651
fatigability 84
fatigue 27, 42, 65, 79, 91, 106, 292, 389, 575, 621
Fatty acids 174, **552**, 568
    arachidonic acid (AA) 552
    cartilage 552
    cycloxygenase enzyme (COX) 552
    delta 6 desaturase 552
    eicosapentaenoic acid (EPA) 552
    gamma linolenic acid (DGLA) 552
fear 34, 38, 78, 660
    fibromyalgia 621
Feet 411
femoral artery 222
fetus 73
fever 65, 106, 389
feverfew 569, 575
feverish 24
fibrin 265
fibroblasts 133, 169, 265, 553, 581
fibrocartilage 595
fibromascular
    hyperplasia 222
    dysplasia 683
Fibromyalgia 14, 18, 31, 38, 145, 150, 243, 261, 597, 603, **618**, 683
    ACTH 619
    allodynia 618, 619
    antidepressant 619
    anxiety 618
    Arnold-Chiari malformation 619
    caudate nucleus 619
    central neurotransmitter imbalance 620
    central sensitivity syndromes 618
    cerebellum 619
    chronic fatigue syndrome 618
    CNS sensitization 620
    cortisol 619

    cranial osteopathy 619
    depression 618, 620
    dysmenorrhea 618
    epinephrine 619
    exercise 619
    fatigue 618
    foramen magnum 619
    headache 618
    hyperalgesia 618
    hypothalamus-pituitary-adrenal axis 619
    IGF-1 619
    influenza type A 619
    influenza type B 619
    interleukin-2 619
    interstitial cystitis 618
    irritable bowel syndrome 618
    lactic acid 619
    medulla oblongata 619
    metenkephaline 619
    migraine 618
    mitral valve prolapse 618
    morning stiffness 618
    myofascial pain syndrome 618
    nerve growth factors 619
    neurally mediated hypotension 618
    norepinephrine 619
    parasympathetic 619
    PET scan 619
    physiological 620
    pituitary 619
    post-traumatic stress disorder (PTSD) 618
    prolotherapy 619
    psychopathology 620
    psychosocial 620
    restless leg syndrome 618
    retroviruses 619
    serotonin 619
    sexual trauma 619
    soluble fibrin monomer 620
    sounds 618
    stress 618
    substance P 619
    sympathetic 619
    sympathetically mediated syndrome 619
    TCM 621
    thalamic activity 619
    thalamus 619
    thyroid hormone resistance 620
    whiplash 619
Fibromyalgia & Myofascial Pain Syndrome 618
    diagnostic criteria 620
    differential diagnosis 620
    fibromyalgia mechanisims 619
    myofascial pain syndrome 598
    OM 621

fibromyositis 584
fibrositic nodules 54
fibrous elements 169
fibular 278
fight or flight 143
fingers 65
Fire 24, 33, 48
    depression/congestion 26
    rising 51
    type people 336
fire cup 368
fire needle 302, 371
fish 568
fistulous infection 41
Five Phases **48**, 50, 87, 339
    counter-regulation 51
    disorders 50
    mother affecting son 51
    over-regulation 51
    points
        influences summary table 310
        tonification sedation 297
    son affecting mother 51
    summery table 49
    treatment 309
five Qi 49
five-center-Heat 27
Fixed/Damp 659
fixed-Bi 27
Flaccid Paralysis 592
flaccidity of lateral lower extremity and spasm of medial aspect, points 331
flat-feet 682
    flexible
        foot dysfunction 678
flesh 220

flexion 190, 191
    spine 185
floaters 90
flora 103
flowery vision 90
fluctuating mass 218
Fluids 18, 37, 166, 594
    fibromyalgia 621
    Ye and biomedicine 18
fluorimethane 610
fogginess 40
Food Diseases 37
    depression/stagnation 26, 38
food-Qi 14
Foot
    Abnormalities **672**
    Biomechanics, table 200
Foot dysfunctions
    arch collapsed 70
    arch pain 674
    chronic sprained ankles 674
    drop, points 332
    falling arch foot 673
    headache Lois foot 674
    hypokyphotic 674
    Lois foot 673
    medial knee pain 674
    one-sided stiff neck 674
    pes valgo planus 673
    plantar fasciitis 674
    shin splints 674
    torqued pelvis 674
foraminal
    disc disorders 644
    stenosis 655
force closure 186
form 96
fornix 130
forward
    collision 651
    head posture 476, **679**
Foundations of Electricity and Biomagnetic Therapy **424**
Four-Divisions 58
fractal 52
fracture 210, 224, 277, 453, 538, 543, 555, 647
fragile x syndrome 344
Framingham study 36
French 56, 290
frequent urination 389
Friedreich's ataxia, foot dysfunction 674
fright 34
frontal lobe 130
frustration 33
    fibromyalgia 621
Fryette laws 462
fT3 86
full passive range 225
Functional Assessment
    aberration of weight transfer 479
    antalgic posture 476
    anterior sacral dysfunctions 476
    calf 473
    callous 480
    clavicular jump test 474
    decreased lumbar lordosis 478
    Divergent channels 479
    Faber Patrick's test 474
    femur 479
    foot varus 480
    footwear 480
    forefoot
        OM 479
        varus 480
    functional hallux limitus 478
    functional short leg 478
    hallux valgus 479
    iliopsoas 478
    instability scoliosis 479
    knee tracking 473, 478
    levator scapulae 476
    ligamentous laxity 474
    lordosis 476
    lumbar lordosis 476
    midtarsal joint 479
    Morton's foot 480
    patellar position 479
    pectoralis major 476
    pelvic
        crossed syndrome 476
        shifting 479
        tilt (oblique position) 478
    piriformis 478
    plantar myotatic reflexe 479
    pronated forefoot 479
    psoas 476
    pupillary line 476
    push-off 479
    quadratus lumborum and pelvic twist 478
    rearfoot varus 479
    rib cage respiratory motions 478
    righting reflex 476
    rotated leg 479
    scapular winging 476
    scoliosis 476, 479
    screening
        test findings 474
    Shao Yang
        channel 479
        Sinew channel 479
    short leg
        gait 478
    slew-foot 479
    spondylolisthesis 476
    squat test 473
    standing and sitting flexion tests 473
    sternocleidomastoid
        protruded head 476
    sway back 476
    Tai Yang
        Sinew channel 479
    thigh adductors 478
    tibial torsion 479
    tilted shoulders, head, upper body 476
    toe-off 480
    toe-out 479
    trapezius
        protruded head 476
    universal pattern 481
    valgus 480
    weightbearing 480
    Yang Ming Sinews channels 479
    Motility (Qiao) channel foot varus and valgus 480
    Yin Motility (Qiao) channel foot

varus and valgus 480
Functional Hallux Limitus/Sagittal Plane Blockade **675**
Functional Overlay Syndrome 146

G
GABA 139, 271
Gait 196, 199, 594
    analysis 239
    ballistic stance 197
    basic aspects, table 197
    biceps femoris 199
    bipedal support 197
    contralateral swing 197
    contralateral toe-off 197
    examination 239
    foot dysfunction 676
    gluteus medius 198
    hamstrings 199
    heel strik 197
    iliotibial tract 199
    medial hamstrings 199
    mid-stance 198
    mid-stride 197
    and Oriental Medicine 199
    peroneus longus 199
    propellant stance 197
    quadriceps 199
    rectus femoris 199
    thoracolumbar fascia 199
    tibialis anterior 199
    tibialis posterior 199
    toe-off 197, 199
    vastus lateralis 199
Gall Bladder 33, 34, 48, 52, 56, 75, 81, 87, 167, 288
gallbladder 336, 683
    disease 211
    disease and shoulder pain 683
gamma
    alpha motor (efferent) nerves 177
    aminobutyric acid 139
    globulin 275
    loop 180
    rays 423
    linolenic acid (GLA) 574
    motor neuron 132
ganglia 134, 279, 333
ganglion 141, 218
    cysts 27
gap junctions 53, 268
gastric motility 600
gastrocnemius 56, 197
gastrointestinal 74, 86
Gate Control Pain Theory 136
Gate of Fire 38, **81**
gelatinous 574
generalized aches 389
generation 89
    cycle 49

genital pain 78
genitals 65, 75
genitourinary 76
genu recuvatum 682
genus Solanaceae 568
Ghost points 322
giant cell tumors 682
Gillet's Stork test 190, 463
ginger 569, 570
gingko and nerve disorders 637
ginseng 293
Girdle (Dai) channel 70, 106, 214, 290, 594
    musculoskeletal use 303
GLA 574
glenohumeral joint 229
glial cell 126
glucocorticoids 84, 575
glucosamine 169, 565, 570
    disc disorders 644
    nerve disorders 637
glucosaminoglycans
    disc disorders 639
glucose 174, 175, 245, 570
    disc disorders 644
    intolerance 569
glucuronic acid 570
glutamate 139
gluteal
    bursitis 657
    foot dysfunction 675
glycemic index 85
glycine 86
glycoalkaloids 568
glycogen 86, 603
glycolysis 174
glycoproteins
    disc disorders 639
glycosaminoglycans 169, 568, 570, 574
goiter 40
gold 296
gold standard 205
Goldenhar's syndrome 344
golgi
    receptor 265
    tendon organs 127, 177, 266
gonadal axes 81
gonococcal 681
    arthritis 168
    infection 660
gout 30, 243, 244, 407, 569, 575, 595, 660
Governing (Du) channel 70, 106, 214, 383, 594
    Hua Tuo Jia Ji 308
    left right imbalance 290
gracilis
    bursitis 658
granulation tissue 552, 553

granulocytes 265
gravitational force 186
gravitational forces
    postural stress 678
great needling 288
greater tuberosity 280
grief 34
grinding 219
groin 77
    stones 681
ground substance 169
growth factors 265
growth hormone 17
growth retardation 244
guaifenesin and fibromyalgia 624
guarding 289
guest host acupuncture 304
gynecological diseases 681

H
hair loss 389
hallux limitus
    foot dysfunction 676
hallux rigidus
    foot dysfunction 675
haloperidol 271
hamstrings 176
hand and fingers 412
Hara
    fibromyalgia 621
harmonic oscillations 273
harmonizing 106
hawthorn 568
Head and Neck
    atlantoaxoid joint 195
    atypical segments 195
    benign tumors 682
    occipitoatloid joint 195
    paresthesia 683
    points
        for neck shoulder pain 315
        to treat movement 315
    typical segments 194
    uncovertebral joints 195
    whiplash injury 650
headache 6, 24, 65, 79, 94, 97, 265, 389
    fibromyalgia 618
    Heidi foot
        foot dysfunction 675
    myofascial pain syndrome 598
healing powers 286
Heart 33, 38, 46, 49, 56, 68, 81, 96
    Yang-deficiency 220
heart disease 211
heel pain
    foot dysfunction 674
Heidi foot
    foot dysfunction 674
helicobacter 86
hemarthrosis 217, 646

hematocrit 243
hematoma 369
hemicholine 139
hemiplegia 40, 41
hemoglobin 243
hemorrhage
    fibromyalgia 621
hemorrhoids 72, 297
heparin 169
hepatic damage 293
hepatitis 244, 293, 660
hepatitis B 293
Herbs
    and abscesses 385
    and accumulations 381
    and achy 388
    and acute flare-ups 381
    and acute injury 388
    and analgesic 383, 387, 388, 389
    and anti-inflammatory 382, 383, 385, 389
    and anxiety 380
    and aristolochic acid 386
    and aromatically transforming Dampness 389
    and aromaticaly transforming Dampness 381
    and arthralgias 386, 389
    and arthritic disorders 384
    and arthritis 381, 390
    and arthrosis 390, 668
    and atrophy 381
    and autoimmune diseases 381, 388
    and belching 382
    and beriberi 390
    and bleeding 379, 381, 384, 389
    and bloating-pain 380
    and Blood moving 381
    and Blood-stasis 378
    and bone loss 383
    and bony injuries 391
    and bowl control 391
    and burning pain 381
    and bursitis 658
    and calves 387
    and cardio-toxic 389
    and chest 381
    and clear Heat 381
    and clearing Heat transforming stasis 381
    and Clear-Yang 383, 390
    and clenched jaws 390
    and cloy 104, 389, 391
        herbs for 379
    and combinations for commonly seen musculoskeletal disorders, summery table 406
    and commonly-used in painful obstruction syndromes 381
    and conduct formulas to a particular channel, summery table 402
    and constitutional weakness 391
    and contraindications for commonly used herbs in musculoskeletal disorders, summery table 419
    and contusions 381
    and convulsions 384, 385, 390
    and COX-2 385
    and cramping 385, 387, 388, 389
    and crampy 391
    and cyanosis 384
    and cynicism 380
    and cysts 390
    and daidzein 383
    and Damp resolving 381
    and Dampness 385
    and Dampness bland draining-precipitating 386
    and death 385
    and deep venous thrombosis 381
    and degenerative joint disease 391
    and deviation of mouth 390
    and diabetes 381
    and diaphragm 380, 381
    and DIC 379
    and difficulty breathing 385
    and digestive enzymes 388
    and dig-in 384
    and discogenic pain 645
    and disorientation 385
    and dispel Dampness via the surface 386
    and dispelling stasis and generating the new 378
    and disseminated intravasclar coagulation 379
    and dissipate nodules 389
    and dissipating nodules and transforming stasis 381
    and dissolve Phlegm 385
    and distension 380
    and diuretic 387
    and dizziness 384
    and dry Dampness 381
    and dry mouth 385, 389
    and DVT 381
    and dyspnea 384
    and edema 380, 390
    and eliminating Blood-stasis 378
    and Empty-Heat 385
    and enlarged lymph nodes 381
    and Essence 391
    and estrogen 383
    and excess salivation 384
    and Exterior releasing 381
    and Exterior-Cold 385
    and facial disorders 390
    and facial neuritis 390
    and fear 380
    and fever 384
    and fibromyalgia 380, 668
    and fibromyositis 381
    and FMS 627
    and fracture 391
    and free body 381
    and generalized muscle aches 386
    and generalized pain 385
    and genistein 383
    and gout 668
    and greasy 104
    and harmonizing 43, 47, 383
    and headache 383, 384, 388
    and heart rhythm disorder 384, 385
    and heaviness 387
    and hiccups 382
    and hidden pathogenic Heat 386
    and hidden-Heat 385
    and hidden-muscle-Heat 385
    and highly toxic 389
    and hypertension 384
    and hypertonicity 388
    and hypertrophic spondylitis 387
    and hypertrophy 378
    and hypotension 384, 385
    and hypothermia 384, 385
    and immune system, suppress 388
    and incontinence 385
    and inflammation 381, 388
    and inflammatory arthritis 388
    and inflammatory diseases 381
    and inflammatory disorders 388
    and insomnia 381
    and instability phase 378
    and Interior-Wind
        spasms and/or paralysis 384
    and intoxications 383
    and intramuscular injection 384
    and involuntary salivation 385
    and isoflavonoids 383
    and Ji 381
    and Jia 381
    and joint mouse 381
    and knees 389, 391
    and leg pain 388
    and ligament laxity 386
    and Liver-congestion 383
    and low back pain 391
    and lumbar pain 391
    and lupus 388
    and malnourishment-Deficiency type pain 382
    and masses 381
    and mending soft tissues 391
    and migraine 383, 384, 388, 390

and mild 104
and mild anti-inflammatory 302
and most commonly used herbs, summery table 392
and musculoskeletal use from Warm-diseases doctrine 32
and moodiness 380
and moving pains 387
and muscle aches 388
and muscle cramping 387
and muscle pain from Spring-Warm 385
and muscle pains 387
and muscle weakness 381
and nausea 384, 385
and nephrotoxic 383
and neuralgias 386
and neuritic pains 384
and neuritis 386, 388
and neuropathic pain 381, 637
and neuropathies 382, 388
and night pain 381
and night sweats 381
and nodules 381, 390
and non-substantial swelling 380
and not to be excessively cloying 104
and nourish the Heart and calm the Spirit, but also open the collaterals/network-vessels and treat musculoskeletal pain 148
and nourishing Yin/Blood, clearing Heat, and vitalizing and transforming Blood-stasis 381
and numbness 384, 385, 387, 388, 389
and numbness of the body and extremities 385
and opening the channels and collaterals/network-vessels 385
and overdosage 385, 390
and overdose 384
and overuse pain 167
and Painful Obstruction (Bi) syndromes 383, 384, 386, 390
and papaya 388
and paralysis 380, 381, 388, 390
and paranoia 380
and Parsonage-Turner syndrome 381
and penetrate 384
and perspiration 384, 389
and phlebitis 381
and Phlegm transforming 381, 389

and photophobia 384
and poisonous 389
and poliomyelitis 389
and postural phase 378
and promote Yang-movement 382
and pulmonary edema 384
and pungent Exterior releasing 382
and purging, cracking and dispersing stasis 381
and obstinate and complex Painful Obstruction 662
and Qi moving 382
and Qi regulating 381, 391
and Qi-stagnation 391
and osteoporosis 85
and pain 302
and radix reumanniae (Sheng Di Huang and rhizoma alismatis (Ze Xie), Empty/transormative-Heat 105
and redness 384
and regulating Qi 380
and relax striated muscles 389
and respiratory depression 384
and rheumatic myositis 668
and rheumatoid arthritis 388, 664, 667, 668
and runny nose 384
and scar tissue 656
and sciatica 386
and scorpion 384
and secondary-stagnant-Heat 105
and seizures 384
and septic arthritis 381
and sequelae of stroke 381
and sequlae to acute neuritis 381
and shortened muscles 391
and shortness of breath 381
and slowed pulse 385
and snake 387, 389
and soft tissue nodules 389
and soften 389
and soles of feet 381
and somatoform disorders 149
and spasm 384, 385, 387, 390
and spicy 381
and Spleen weakness 382
and Spleen-Qi rasing 383
and sprains 381
and spurs 381, 382, 389, 390
and stabilization phase 378
and stenosis 381
and stiff tongue 384
and stiffness 384, 385, 387
and stiffness of joints 387, 388
and stop bleeding 385
and stopping bleeding transform-

ing Blood-stasis 381
and strains 381
and strengthening Yang 382
and strengthening Yang to transform Dampness 390
and subcostal 391
and substantial stagnant-Blood 378
and Summer-Heat 385
and suprascapular neuritis 381
and swelling 380, 381, 382, 385, 388, 389, 391
and swollen joints 384
and tacycardia 381
and tearing 384
and tendinitis 388
and tendinosis 388
and tendons 596
and tension 388
and thirst 389
and tight lumpy muscles 391
and tingling 384, 387
and TMJ 383
and tonic-clonic convulsions 384
and tonifying Kidney-Yang 390
and tonifying Qi and Blood transforming Blood-stasis 381
and toxic 386, 388, 389, 390
and toxicity 390
and toxins 384
and transformation/congested-Heat 388
and transforming stasis 380
and trapping pathogenic Cold 385
and traumatic injuries 385, 387, 388
and traumatic swelling 389
and treat toxicity 385
and tremors 390
and Triple Warmer 391
and trunk 391
and twitching limbs 385
and unconsciousness 384
and up-bearing and down-bearing 33
lurking pathogens 32
and uric acid 668
and vertebral hypertrophy 381
and vinegar 388
and vomiting 382, 384
and warm the channels, joints and sinews 384
and Warming 381
and warming Yang and vitalizing Blood 381
and warmth of palms 381
and weak digestion 385
and weak low back 391
and weakness 384, 388

and whiplash 654
and Wind extinguishing 381
and Wind-Damp dispelling 381, 386
and Yang lifting 390
and Yin-abscesses 385
and Yin-Fluids 381
anemarrhena (Zhi Mu) 58
Agkistrodon seu Bungarus (Bai Hua She) 387
antler glue, (Lu Jiao) 18
Astragalus (Huang Qi), and adrenal function 85
   chronic disease 102
bamboo 293
Bombys Batryticatus (Jiang Can) 32, 384
Bulbus Fritillariae Thunbergii (Zhe Bei Mu) 389
Buthus Martensi (Quan Xie) 384
Caulis Hyptis Captitatae (Mo Gu Xiao) 386
Caulis Sinomenii (Qing Feng Teng) 389
Caulis Trachelospermi (Luo Shi Teng) 388
centipede 384
Coicis Lachrma-jobi (Yi Yi Ren) 386
Cornu Cervu Parvum (Lu Rong) 391
Cortex Acanthopanacis (Wu Jia Pi) 387
Cortex Erythrinae (Hai Tong Pi) 388
Cortex Eucommiae Ulmoidis (Du Zhong) 18, 390
Cortex Mountan Radicis (Mu Dan Pi) 379
Cortex Phellodendri (Huang Bai) 385
Cyperi Rotundi (Xiang Fu) 391
Excrementum Bombycis Mori (Can Sha) 387
Faeces Trogopterorum (Wu Ling Zhi) 380
Fasciculus Vascularis Luffae (Si Gua Lao) 377
Flos Carthami Tinctorii (Hong Hua) 376
Flos Rosae Rugosae (Mei Gui Hua) 382
Folium Clerodendri Trichotomi (Chou Wu Tong) 388
Fructus Arctii (Niu Bang Zi) 383
Fructus Chaenomelis (Mu Gua) 388
fructus corni (Shan Zhu Yu) 18
fructus gardenia (Zhi Zi) 32
Fructus Liquidambaris (Lu Lu Tong) 377
fructus lycii (Gou Qi Zi) 18
Fructus Viticis (Man Jing Zi) 383
Fructus Psoraleae (Bu Gu Zhi) 391
Ginger 293
ginseng 293
   and adrenals function 85
Gummi Olibanum (Ru Xiang) 377
Gypsum (Shi Gao) 32, 58
Herba Artemisiae Anomalae (Liu Ji Nu) 379
Herba Cistanshes (Rou Cang Rong) 18, 391
Herba cum Radix Asari (Xi Xin) 383
Herba Eupatorii Fortunei (Pei Lan) 389
herba lophatheri (Dan Zhu Ye) 32
Herba Lycopi Lucidi (Ze Lan) 379
Herba Lycopodii Claviati cum Radice (Shen Jin Cao) 387
Herba Lycopodii Serrati (Jin Bu Huan) 380
Herba Pyrolae (Lu Xian Cao) 389
herba schizonepetae (Jing Jie) 32
Herba Siegesbeckiae (Xi Xian Cao) 388
Herba Solidaginis (Liu Zhi Huang) 388
Herba Speranskiae seu Impatients (Tou Gu Cao) 387
Hirudo seu Whitmania (Shui Zhi) 378
human placenta (Zi He Che) 18
Lignum Aquilariae (Chen Xiang) 382
Lignum Pini Nodi (Song Jie) 388
Lignum Sappan (Su Mu) 377, 380
Lumbricus (Di Long) 384
masses 378
Medula Tetrapanadis (Tong Cao) 386
Myrrha (Mo Yao) 377
Natrii Sulfas (Ming Fen) 384
Nidus Vespae (Lu Feng Fang) 384
Oposthoplatia (Tu Bie Chong) 378
Pericarpium Citri Reticulatae (Chen Pi) 391
Pericarpium Citri Reticulatae Viride (Qing Pi) 391
Pollen Typhae (Pu Huang) 380
Polypori Umbellati (Zhu Ling) 386
Poriae Cocos (Fu Ling) 339, 386
pseudoginseng (Tian Qi) 293
Radix Achyranthis Bidentatae (Niu Xi) 378
Radix Aconiti Carmichaeli (Chuan Wu) 385
Radix Aconiti Kusnezoffii (Cao Wu) 385
Radix Aconiti Lateralis (Fu Zi) 384
Radix Angelica Sinensis (Dang Gui) 378
Radix Angelicae Dahuricae (Bai Zhi) 383
Radix Angelicae Pubescenis (Du Huo) 387
Radix Astragali (Huang Qi) 380
Radix Bupleuri (Chai Hu) 339, 383
Radix Clematidis (Wei Ling Xian) 387
Radix Coculi (Mu Fang Ji) 386
Radix Cythulae Officinalis (Chuan Niu Xi) 378
Radix Dipsaci Asperi (Xu Duan) 391
Radix Gentianae (Qin Jiao) 388
Radix Ginseng (Ren Shen) 380
radix ledebouriellae (Fang Feng) 32
Radix Linderae Strychnifoliae (Wu Yao) 382
Radix Millettiae Reticulatae (Ji Xue Teng) 377
Radix Morindae (Ba Ji Tian) 18, 390
Radix Pseudoginseng (San Qi) 379
Radix Puerariae (Ge Gen) 383
radix rehmanniae (Shu Di Huang) 18
Radix Rehmanniae raw (Sheng Di Huang) 379, 339
Radix Rubrus Paeoniae Lactiflorae (Chi Shao) 377
Radix Sacutellariae Baicalensis (Huang Qin) 385
Radix Salviae Miltiorrhizae (Dan Shen) 376
Radix Schefflerae (Qi Ye Lian) 388
Radix Stephaniae Tetrandrae (Han Fang Ji) 386
Radix Trichosanthis Kirilowii (Tian Hua Fen) 32, 41, 389
Radix Tripteryggi Wilfordii (Lei Gong Teng) 388
Ramulus Cinnamomi Cassiae (Gui Zhi) 382
Ramulus Loranthus (Sang Ji Sheng) 389
Ramulus Mori Albae (Sang Zhi) 388
Ramus Lonicerae Japonicae (Ren Dong Teng) 388
Ramus Piperis Wallichii (Hai Feng Teng) 388

Ramus Tinosporae Sinensis (Kuan Jin Teng) 388
Rhizoma Alismatis Orientalitis (Ze Xie) 386
Rhizoma Arisaematis (Tian Nan Xing) 390
rhizoma atractylodes (Bai Zhu) 339
Rhizoma Atractylodis (Cang Zhu) 389
Rhizoma Cibotii Barmometz (Gou Ji) 18, 391
Rhizoma Cimicifugae (Sheng Ma) 390
Rhizoma Corydalis (Yan Hu Suo) 376
Rhizoma Curculiginis Orchioidis (Xian Mao) 390
Rhizoma Curcumae (E Zhu) 378
rhizoma curcumae (Huang Jiang) 32
Rhizoma Dioscoreae Hypoglaucae (Bie Xie or Bi Xie) 386
Rhizoma Dioscoreae Nipponicae (Chuan Shan Long) 388
rhizoma drynari (Gu Sui Bu) 18
Rhizoma et Radix Notopterygii (Qiang Huo) 382
Rhizoma Gastrodiae Elatae (Tian Ma) 383
Rhizoma Gusuibu (Gu Sui Bu) 391
Rhizoma Ligustici (Gao Ben) 383
Rhizoma Ligustici Wallichii (Chuan Xiong) 376
Rhizoma Pinelliae Ternatae (Ban Xia) 390
Rhizoma Rhei (Da Huang) 32, 380
Rhizoma Sparganii Stoloniferi 378
Rhizoma Typhonii Gigaantei (Bai Fu Zi) 390
Rhizoma Zingiberis (Gan Jiang) 385
Sanguis Draconis (Xue Jie) 377
Scolopendra (Wu Gong) 384
scorpio (Quan Xie) 32
Semen Arechae Catechu (Bing Lang) 391
Semen Cuscutae (Tu Si Zi) 18, 391
semen persicae (Tao Ren) 339
Semen Plantaginis (Che Qian Zi) 386
Semen Pruni Persicae (Tao Ren) 378
Spina Gleditsiae (Zao Jiao Ci) 390
spurs 378
Squama Mantitis Pentadactylae (Chuan Shan Jia) 377
Succus Bambusae (Zhu Li) 389
Thallus Algae (Kun Bu) 390
Toad venom (Can Su) 540
tortosie plastron (Gui Ban) 18
tortosie plastron glue (Gui Ban Jiao) 18
Tuber Curcumae (Yu Jin) 376
uncariae ramulus cum unicis (Gou Teng) 32
Zaocys Dhumnades (Wu Shao She) 389

Herbal Formulas
Aconite Decoction (Wu Tou Tang) 567, 664
Against Bony Hyperplasia Tablet (Kang Gu Zeng Sheng Pian) 381
Agastache, Magnolia Bark, Pinellia, and Poria (Huo Po Xia Ling Tang) 31
Angelica Pubescens and Loranthus Decoction (Du Hou Ji Sang Tang) 568
Angelica Pubescens and Sangjisheng Decoction (Du Huo Ji Shen Tong 668
Argument Great Tonify Yin Pill (Da Bu Yin Wan Jia Jie) 381
Arouse Wasting/Wilting and Secure the True Pill (Qi Wei Gu Zhen Wan) 594
Artemisia Yinchenhao Decoction (Yin Chen Hao Tang) 32
Astragalus and Cinnamon Twig Five Materials Decoction (Huang Qi Gui Zhi Wu Wu Tang) 381, 568
Augmented Four-Substance Decoction with Safflower and Peach Pit (Jia Wei Tao Hong Si Wu Tang) 381
Augmented Pinellia Atractylodis Macrocephalae and Gastrodia Decoction (Jia Wei Ban Xia Bai Zhu Tian Ma Tang) 380
Augmented Reduce Scrofula Pill (Xiao Luo Wan Jia Wei) 381
Augmented Ten-Ingredient Decoction to Warm the Gallbladder (Jia Wei Shi Wei Wen Dang Tang) 380
Boost the Stomach Decoction (Yi Wei Tang) 638
Bupleurum Powder to Spread the Liver (Chi Hu Shu Gan San) 262
Cinnamon Combination (Gui Zhi Tang) 309
Cinnamon Twig Decoction (Gui Zhi Tang) 102, 628, 631
Cinnamon Twig Decoction (Gui Zhi Tang) 106
Cinnamon Twig, Peony and Anemarrhena Decoction (Gui Zhi Shao Yao Zhi Mu Tang) 552, 568, 663
Clear the Nutritive Decoction (Qing Yin Tang) 32
Clear the Palace Decoction (Qing Gong Tang) 32
Common Cold Tea 104
Cool the Nutritive and Clear the Qi Decoction (Liang Ying Qing Qi Tang) 32
Coptis and Magnolia Bark Decoction (Lian Po Tang) 31, 32
Dang Gui Assuage Pain Decoction (Dang Gui Nian Tong Tang) 568
Disband Painful Obstruction Decoction (Xuan Bi Tang) 667
Drain Static Blood Decoction (Xie Yu Xue Tang) 381
Drive Out Blood Stasis from a Painful Body (Shen Tang Zhu Yu Tang) 568
Drive Out Blood Stasis from a Painful Body Decoction (Shen Tong Zhu Yu Tong) 665
Drive Out Blood-stasis Below Diaphragm Decoction (Ge Xia Zhu Yu Tang) 380
Drive Out Blood-stasis in the Mansion of Blood Decoction (Xue Fu Zhu Yu Tang) 380
Dryness and Rescue the Lung Decoction (Qing Zao Jiu Fei Tang) 638
Ephedra Decoction (Ma Huang Tang) 568
Ephedra, Aconite, and Asarum Decoction (Ma Huang Ju Zi Xin Tang) 638
Fantastically Effective Pill to Invigorate the Collaterals (Hou Luo Xiao Ling Dan) 380
Fixed Bi Empirical Formula (Zhuo Bi Yan Fang) 544
Fixed Damp painful Bi is treated with modification of Coicis Decoction (Yi Yi

Ren Tang) 567
Food stagnation Spleen-deficiency Tea 104
Four Wanders Powder with Added Flavors (Si Miao San Jia Wei) 638
Four-Marvel Pill (Si Miao Wan) 667
Four-Substance Decoction with Safflower and Peach Pit (Tao Hong Si Wu Tang) 594
Four-Valiant Decoction for Well Being (Si Miao Yang An Tang) 381
Free the Channels and Stop Pain Decoction (Tong Jing Zhi Tong Tang) 668
Frigid Extremities Decoction (Si Ni Tang) 381
Ginseng and Atractylodes Decoction (Shen Zhu Tang) 638
Ginseng and Carapax Amydae Pill (Ren Shen Bie Jia Qian Wan) 381
Ginseng, Poria, and Atractylodes Powder with Additions and Subtractions (Shen Ling Bai Zhu San Jia Jian) 638
Harmonize Center Tea 104
Hidden Tiger Pill (Hu Qian Wan) 381, 594
Hidden Tiger Pills with Additions and Subtractions (Hu Qian Wan Jia Jian) 638
Ten Spirit Decoction (Shi Shen Tang) 105
Honeysuckle and Forsythia Powder (Yin Qiao San) 32
Immature Bitter Orange Decoction to Guide Out Stagnation (Zhi Shi Dao Zhi Tang) 32
Jade Windscreen Powder (Yu Ping Feng San+-) 309
Jade Woman Decoction (Yu Nu Jiang Tang) 32
Kidney Qi Pill (Shen Qi Wan) 568
Ledebourella Decoction (Fang Feng Tang) 567
Left-Restoring Pill (Zuo Gui Wan) 18
Liu Wei Di Huang (Six Ingredient Radix Rehmanniae Pill) 17
Major Invigorate the Collaterals Special Pill (Da Huo Luo Dan) 380
Major Notopterygium Decoction (Da Qiang Huo Tang) 664
Master Li's Decoction to Clear Summer-Damp-Heat and Augment the Qi (Li Shi Qing Shu Qi Tang) 629
Miner Bupleuri Decoction (Xiao Chi Hu Tang) 309, 630, 624
Minor Construct the Middle Decoction (Xiao Jian Zhong Tang) 631
Minor Invigorate the Collaterals Special Pill (Xiao Huo Luo Dan) 380, 664, 667
Modified Minor Invigorate the Collaterals Special Pill (Jia Wei Xiao Huo Luo Dan) 666
Newly Augmented Yellow Dragon Decoction (Xin Jia Huang Long Tang) 32
Nourish Joint Clear Heat (inflammation) Tea 104
Nourish Liver Tea 104
Nourish Spleen Tea 104
Nourishing Yin and Marrow Decoction (Zi Yin Bu Sui Tang) 594
Nourishing Yin and Moistening the Muscle and Sinews Decoction (Zi Zao Yang Rong Tang) 594
Peach Pit and Safflower Decoction (Tao Hong Yin) 568
Pinellia, Atractylodis Macrocephalae, and Gastrodia Decoction (Ban Xia Bai Zhu Tian Ma Tang) 666
Po Sum On 549
Prepared Aconite Decoction (Fu Zi Tang) 664
Prepared Soybean and Scrophularia (Huang Qin Tang Jia Dan Dou Chi He Xuan Shen) 32
Pueraria Decoction (Ge Gen Tang) 544
Restore the Right Pill (You Gui Wan) 568
Relax the Channels and Invigorate the Blood Decoction (Shu Jing Ho Xue Tang) 381, 667
Remove Painful Obstruction (Juan Bi Tong) 663
Remove Painful Obstruction Decoction (Juan Bi Tong) 658
Restore the Right Decoction (You Gui Yin) 568
Revive Health by Invigorating Blood Decoction (Fu Yuan Huo Xue Tang) 262, 380, 544
Rhinoceros Horn and Rhemannia Decoction (Xi Jiao Di Huang Tang)32, 381
Rhubarb and Eupolyphaga Pill (Da Huang Zhe Chong Wan) 381
Right-Restoring Pill (You Gui Wan) 18
Safflower and Peach Pit (Tao Hong Si Wu Tang) 263, 381
Scallion and Platycody Decoction (Cang Chi Jie Geng Tang) 32
Scutellaria Decoction plus Prepared Soybean and Scrophularia (Huang Qin Tang Jia Dan Dou Chi He Xuan Shen) 32
Seven-Thousandths of a Pearl Powder (Qi Li San) 543, 380
Seven-Treasure Special Pill for Beautiful Whiskers (Qi Bao Mei Ran Dan) 559
Six Depressions Decoction (Liu Yu Tang) 26
Sour Jujube Decoction (Suan Zao Ren Tang) 627
Stomach-Heat food stagnation Tea 104
Strengthen Stride Pill (Jian Bu Wan) 568
Sudden Smile Powder (Shi Xiao San) 381
Sweet Dew Special Pill to Eliminate Toxin (Gan Lu Xiao Du Dan) 32
Tangkuei Decoction for Frigid Extremities (Dang Gui Si Ni San) 381
Tangkuei Decoction to Tonify the Blood (Dang Gui Bu Xue Tang) 24, 568
Ten Partially-Charred Substances Powder (Shi Hui San) 381
Ten Spirits Decoction (Shi Shen Tang) 32, 385
Three-Nut Decoction (San Ren Tang) 31, 32

Three-Painful Obstruction Decoction (San Bi Tang) 568
Tonify Blood Tea 104
Tonify Qi and Blood Tea 104
Trauma Pill (Die Da Wan) 380, 543
Two-Cured Decoction (Er Chen Tang) 31
Two-Marvel Powder (Er Miao San) 552, 668
Universal Benefit Decoction to Eliminate Toxin (Pu Ji Xiao Du Yin) 32
Wang's Decoction to Clear Summerheat and Augment the Qi (Wang Shi Qing Shu Yi Qi Tang) 32
Warm Channels Remove Painful Obstruction Decoction (Wen Jing Juan Bi Tang) 568
Warm the Gall Bladder Decoction (Wen Dan Tang) 32
White Tiger Decoction (Bai Hu Tang) 32
White Tiger plus Cinnamon Twig Decoction (Bai Hu Jia Gui Zhi Tang) 552, 567, 568
Yang-Heartening Decoction 379
Yang-Heartening Decoction (Yang He Tang) 381
Young Maiden Pill (Qing E Wan) 559, 667
Yunan White Medicine (Yunan Bai Yao) 381
Zheng Gu Shui 549
hernias 70, 43
herniation of disc 640
heroin 262, 588
herotopic bone formation 538
herpetic neuralgia 683
hertz (Hz) 426
hidden 23
    lurking Pathogenic Factors 31
    muscle-heat 32
high velocity 453
Highlights Of The Most Commonly Used Herbs In Musculoskeletal Disorders, table 392
Highly Sensitive C-reactive Protein 243
hip 75, 574, 578
Hip and Buttock
    bursitis 657
hippocampus 130, 140
histamine 139, 142, 143, 169, 369, 574
    fibromyalgia 621
histological 603
histone 86

HLA-B12 86
HLA-B15 86
HLA-B27 antigen 244
holistic 2, 261
Hollow 81, 263, 311
holothurin 571
homeostatic resonance 424
hormone imbalance 145
Hot Bi 659
Hot, Cold, Deficiency and Excess table 42
Hot-Phlegm 39
HTLV-I
    infection and Bi 660
Hua 106
humerous 280
hyaline cartilage 134, 565
hyaluronate 19
hyaluronic acid 170, 569, 572
hydroxylation 568
hyluronan 574
hyperalgesia 142, 154, 210, 238, 598, 633, 635
hyperesthesia 285
hyperextension rear-end collision 652
hyperflexion rear-end collision 652
hyperkypotic
    foot dysfunction 675
hyperlordotic lumbar spine
    foot dysfunction 675
hypermobile 224, 580
    joint 561
hypermobility 75
    possible causes of 225
hyperparathyroidism 244, 683
hypersomnia 76
hypersympathetic activity 333
hypertension 6, 424, 572, 683
hyperthermia 424
hypertonicity 65
hypertrophic osteoarthropathy 682
hypertrophy 69, 589
hypochondriac
    fibromyalgia 621
hypochondriasis 145
hypoesthesia 57
hypogastric 95
hypoglycemia 84, 145
hypomobile 217
    joints 561
hypoparathyroidism 244
hypotension 78, 84, 389
hypothalamic arcuate nucleus 271
hypothalamic-pituitary-adrenal 81, 150
hypothalamus 84, 128, 129, 130, 134, 138
hypothermia 219, 389
hypothyroidism 78, 244, 282, 588, 632
    fibromyalgia 620

hypovolemic shock 219
hypoxia 18, 389, 589
hysteresis 169, 170, 579, 590
hysteria 32, 145, 147
Hz 291
I
I Ching 306
I3C 681
iatrogenicity 37
ibuprofen 573
ice 610
ichial
    bursitis 657
icosahedron 202, 585
Ideal Conditions for Treatment 293
IDET
    disc disorders 644
idiopathic FMS 619
idiosyncratic reaction 293
ILA 187
Iliocostal Friction Syndrome 655
iliopsoas syndrome 278
iliosacral 461
iliotibial tract
    bursitis 658
ilium 187
Imaging & Radiology 247
    ankle 257
    changes on MRI & CT 255
    congenital abnormalities 252
    degenerative disc & joint disease 253
    degenerative disease 253
    dynamic studies 249
    joint dysfunctions 253
    knee 259
    limitations 249
    magnetic resonance imaging & computer-reconstructed radiographic tomography 249
    medical radiographic imaging 247
    nuclear medicine 250
    principles 248
    radiography of vertebral rotation 254
    safety 248
    shoulder and elbow 259
    spine 252
    ultrasound 250
    visceral 251
    wrist 257
immobile joint 225
immobilization 595, 656
immune cells 581
immune system 56
immunity 72
immunoglobulin G 576
Impediment patterns 659

impingement syndrome 597
impotence 65, 87, 594
impulsiveness 97
impure 95
inch 342
indecisiveness 97
Independent Factors 37
indirect techniques 222, 587
indomethacin 573
indurated 289
induration 285
inert tissues 225
infantile paralysis 593
infection 211, 333, 576
    acupuncture complications 293
    CBC 243
    ESR 243
    fibromyalgia 597
    headache acute 684
    myalgia 585
    neuritis 632
    single acute joint 576
    travel 211
infectious conditions 681
Inflammation 29
    acidity 551
    acupuncture 554
    alkalinity 551
    arachidonic acid 552, 554
    autoimmune disease 553
    bacteria 553
    bradykinin 551
    bursitis 657
    chronic 144, 552
    collagen 554
    connective tissue 553
    connective tissues 551
    Defensive Qi 29
    degeneration 595
    eicosanoids 552
    eosinophils 552
    factors influencing healing 555
    fibroblasts 552, 554
    fungi 553
    granulation tissue 552
    granulocytes 554
    growth factors 554
    heparin 551
    histamine 551
    humoral elements 551
    humoral response 551
    hypersensitivity 561
    immune cells 553
    inflammatory
        cells 552
            mediators 143, 639
    insulin-like growth factor (IGF-1) 554
    lymphocytes 552
lysosomal
    enzyme 552
macrophages 554
    chronic 552
mast cells 552, 333
manipulation 502
monocytes 554
mononuclear predominance 552
movement and healing 554
nerve disorders 636, 637
neuropeptides 553
neutrophils 552
night pain 210
NSAIDs 552
parasite 553
phagocytes 552
plasma cells 552
platelet 554
    factor 4 554
    growth factors (PDGF) 554
polypeptides 554
proteolytic enzymes 554
remodeling maturation phase 554
self-perpetuating 553
serotonin 551
spirochete 553
steroid hormones 552
synovium 565
toxins 551
transforming growth factor 554
treatment 289
vasodilation 552
virus 553
wound healing 554
Yang Ming 58
inflammation 25, 30, 31, 58, 265, 286, 302, 430, 552, 553, 571, 574, 575, 581, 592, 632
inflammatory
    arthritis 168, 668
    bursitis 657
    conditions 681
    response 63
inflexible Bi 659
influenza 595
infraspinatus 683
inhalation 193
inherited Essence 17
initiation of muscle contraction 173
injection 296
innominate 197, 187
    innominates
insomnia 6, 36, 38, 40, 42, 76, 78
    fibromyalgia 625
instability 70
    ligaments 580
    osteoarthritis 566
    twinges and giving-way 210
insulin resistance 570

integrated neuromuscular inhibition technique 489
integrated trigger point hypothesis 600
intention 264, 295
interdiscal pH 38
interference field 656
Interior 13, 24, 27, 31, 37, 42, 53, 63, 102, 165, 220, 221, 262, 263, 290, 544, 556
    fibromyalgia 621, 627
interior mammary arteries 279
intermediolateral cell columns 134
intermittent claudication 217, 683
intermuscular 269
internal
    derangement 224, 228, 231
    disc derangement 643
internal-Wind 33, 70
    paresthesia and numbness 633
interosseous 183, 186
interspinous ligament 191, 195
    disc disorders 638
interspinous ligaments 182
interstitial
    connective tissue 269
    cystitis 598
    fluids 18
intertransversarii 183, 192
intertransverse ligament 195
Intervertebral Disc 184
    anatomy 184
    nourishment 184
intestinal diseases 211
intestinal parasites 333
intestines 389
intracellular matrix 170
intracranial blood vessels 684
intracranial tumor 684
intradermal acupuncture 262
intrafusal 132
intramuscular 269
Invisible Phlegm 39
involuntary guarding 589
ion cord 368
    treatment of low back 325, 327, 328, 332
ionic bonding 425
ionic conduction 425
ionizing 430
iontophoresis, clinical use 434
iron 681
irregular heart rhythms 389
irregular menstuation 389
irritability 44, 589
irritable bowel syndrome 145, 598
irritable focus 153
ischemia 600
ischemic compression 605
ischial

bursitis 657
tuberosity 189
ischium 187, 189
isoleucine 86
isometric 174, 228
isotonic 174, 228
itching 6, 24, 40
J
Japanese 51, 56, 81, 284, 293, 295, 338, 339, 438
    acupuncture systems obtaining Qi 295
jaundice 87
jaw 65, 96
Joint **169**
    barriers **222**
    capsules
        Sinews 165
        vascular supply 561
    cartilage 171
        summary table 171
    categories 172
    connective tissue 169
    Disorders **560**
        dysfunction 556, 561
        effusion 223
        hypermobile 561
        instability 556
        intrinsic 560
        monoarthritis 566
        pathology 564
        phases of degeneration 561
        play **475**
        polyarthritis 566
        restriction 561
        somatic dysfunction 562
        stabilization phase 556
        swelling fibromyalgia 618
        vertebral dysfunctions 462
    neurophysiology 172
    OM 165
    play 560
    receptors 172, 560
        summery table 173
    synovium 172
joint destruction 31
Joint diseases
    adhesion 561
    Chain Joint Muscle Reaction, table 561
    compression
        immobilization 561
    degenerative joint disease 564
    demineralization 561
    doxycycline 565
    food sensitivities 566
    glycosaminoglycans 561
    hepatitis 566
    hyaluronic acid 567
    hypomobile 561
    immobilization prolonged 561
    lymphatic 562
    matrix metalloproteinases (MMPs) 565
    mononucleosis 566
    MRI 565
    muscle atrophy 561
    nociceptors 561
        oversensitive 566
    posain 564
    prolotherapy 567
    replacement 578
    rubella 566
    spinal 561
    traumatic arthritis 576
Joint Dysfunctions and Manual Medicine Models **461**
judgment 97
jumping 55

K
kallikrein-kinin 574
Kappa score 205
keratin sulfate 572
Ketamin and nerve disorders 637
keystone 188
Kidney 49, 60, 220, 305, 383
    atrophy 166
    Divergent channels 69
    Essence 166, 214
    Fire 26
    Heat 166
    Qi 37, 334
    Liver disorders 214
    taxation pain, Bi 666
    Yang 38, 81, 166
        deficiency 106, 168, 220, 221, 277
    Yin 81
kidney
    cancers 682
    disease 211, 244
    failure 293
    stone 245, 333
Kidneys 33, 39, 45, 81, 96, 106, 286, 556, 558, 594
kinesiology 276
Kinesiology of the Gait Cycle **197**
Kinetic wedge
    foot dysfunction 676, 677
Kissing Spine (Basstrap's Disease) 655
knee 55, 65, 89, 413, 570, 572, 573
    imaging 258
knots 56
Koketsu 606
Kori-indurated 56, 220, 285, 606
    fibromyalgia 622
Kreb cycle 4
kyphoscoliosis 682

kyphosis 192
kyphotic 214
L
L2 and L3 disc lesions, points 332
L4 and L5 disc lesions, points 332
Laboratory and Technical Testing 243
    acid phosphatase 244
    alkaline phosphatase 244
    Bence Jones protein 245
    blood tests 243
    complete blood count 243
    compressive stool analysis 245
    erythrocyte sedimentation rate 243
    detoxification profile 246
    HLA-B27 antigen 244
    neurotransmitter levels 245
    phosphorus 244
    prostate specific antigen 244
    osteomark-NTX 245
    rheumatoid factor 244
    saliva testing 245
    sensitive c-reactive protein 245
    sensitive thyroid stimulating hormone 244
    serum calcium 244
        glutamic-oxaloacetic transaminase 244
    uric acid 244
    urine tests 245
lacrimation 135, 600
lactic acid 175
lactobacilli 86
lamellar bone 595
lamina 133, 151
laminae 185
landmarks anterior/posterior 216
Large Intestine 18,49, 305
L-arginine 272
Laser Therapy, 280, 424, **447**
    acetylcholine 449
    acupuncture 449
    angiogenesis 449
    argon 448
    ATP 448
    axonal sprouting 449
    bata-endorphins 449
    biophoton 447
    bradykinin 449
    carpal tunnel syndrome 449
    C-fiber 449
    collagen 448
    COX-1 449
    COX-2 449
    C-reactive protein 449
    cytochrome c oxidase 449
    diode lasers 448
    effects of 448
    fatigue 449
    fibroblast 449

fractures 451
gas 448
general effect 448
granulation 448
helium 448
inflammation 449
infrared 448
ion 449
joint pain 448
keratinocyte 449
laser light penetration 448
lateral epicondylagia 449
leukocyte 449
ligaments and tendons 451
light energy 448
liquid 448
low back pain 448
muscle pain 448
muscle problems 450
nausea 449
neck 448
neon 448
neurotransmitters 448
nitric oxide 449
osteoarthritic 449
PGG2 449
photon 448
proinflammatory 449
prostaglandins 448, 449
protein 448
rheumatoid arthritis 449
Ruby laser 448
rypton 448
semiconductor 448
serotonin 449
spasm 449
vasodilation 449
wounds 451
Latent Heat 31, 224
latent pathogenic factors 29
    Bi 660
    fibromyalgia 621
lateral
    epicondylitis 597
    foraminal stenosis 648
    recess
        disc disorders 644
LDII 86
leaky gut 245
leaky vessels 42
learning difficulties 84
leg length discrepancies 213, 669
Lequesne Index 570
lesion 261, 284
leucotriene 574
leu-enkephalin 138
leukemia 682
leukocyte 169, 243, 245
leukocytic 265

leukocytosis 243
leukotriene 571
leukotriene B4 575
    disc disorders 639
li 74
libido 36, 90
licorice 618, 619
lidocaine 571, 573
lifestyle and OM 37
ligament insufficiency 265
ligamenta
    flava 182, 195
    nuchae 195
Ligamentous Disorders **579**
    instability 580
    insufficiency 580
    laxity 30, 282, 579
    neurogenic inflammation 553, 581
    nulliness 580
    posain 580
    sprains 537
    symptoms 580
    treatment 581
ligaments 57, **180**, 561
    elastic energy 185
    mechanoreceptors 180
    OM 165
    tension element 202
ligamentum capitus costae radiatum 194
ligand-gated 140
lightheadedness 293
likelihood ratio 205
Limb(s) Numbness 410
limbic forebrain 134
limbic system 130, 151, 589
lipid-lowering drugs 588
lipoxygenase enzyme 571, 574
Liver 33, 39, 48, 56, 60, 87, 90, 286, 288, 305, 556, 558, 594
    fibromyalgia 621, 622, 626, 627
    disorders and biomedicine 87
    Blood 166
        deficiency 166
            paresthesia and numbness 633
    congestion 86, 168
    congestion-Qi-stagnation 26, 33
    Depression 28
    Fire 46, 160
    hand 63
    Qi 28, 34
        stagnation 28, 39, 160, 214
    Wind 165
liver 336, 389
    disease 211, 244
load 170
locomotion 70
long term potentiation (LTP) 129, 292
long first metatarsal foot dysfunction 676
long thoracic nerve 683
loose bodies 39, 211
    end feel 224
loose-packed position 222
lordosis 181, 190
lordotic 214
Low Back
    acute sprain/strain 412
    extension 191
    flexion 190
    iliolumbar ligaments 188
    innominates 187
    knees pain 412
    loads on discs, table 190
    lumbopelvic ligaments, figure 189
    lumbosacral ligaments 189
    movement of spine 190
    mushroom phenomenon 655
    pelvic
        girdle 186
        motions 189
    pain 412
    points based on location of pain 330
    sacroiliac
        joint 188
        ligaments 188
    sacrospinous ligament 189
    sacrotuberous ligament 189
    sciatica, herbs 578
    sensitive patient, herbs 578
    sidebending and rotation 191
    symphysis pubis 187
low level laser therapy (LLLT) 447
lower motor neuron 592
low-level microwaves 424
lumbar 94
    list 604
    pain radiating to abdomen 75
    region 76
    spine 190
lumbodorsal fasciae 187, 188
lumbopelvic rhythm 191
lumbosacral rhythm 581
lumps, 77, 220
lung disease 430
    shoulder pain 211
Lungs 18, 39, 40, 49, 56, 160, 81, 214, 286, 305
    fibromyalgia 621
lungs 389
lupus 144, 578, 682
lurking pathogens 288
lurking/hidden 103
lycopus europaeus 569
lyme disease 660
lymph 584
    nodes 134

vessels 133
Lymphatic Drainage
    achilles tendon 475
    axillary fold 475
    epigastric 475
    gland 229
    inguinal 475
    popliteal 475
    rib cage 475
    supraclavicular 475
lymphatics 475
    stasis 600
    system 96
    trunk 600
    and Divergent channels 69
lymphocyte products
lymphocytes 143, 169
lymphomas 211, 681
lysine 86
lysosomal
    components, acute pain 143
    enzymes 29, 568
    membranes, inflammation 552

M

macrophages 169, 265
    connective tissue 169
    dry needling 265
macrotrauma
    bursitis 657
Magnafield 436
magnesium 139, 271, 681
    nerve disorders 637
Magnetic Field Deficiency Syndrome 424
Magnetic Resonance Angiography 249
Magnetic Resonance Imaging (MRI) 249
Magnetic Resonance Neurography 249
Magnetic Therapy 443
magnetism 430
magnetoencephalography 131
Main channels 209, 277, 300
    summary table 63
    treatment 299
main vessels 63
malabsorption 244
malaria 632
malignancy 588, 682
    fibromyalgia 620
malignant
    conditions 211
    hypertension 684
mammography 252
mandibular 65
manganese 568, 572
mania 40, 65
manipulation 262
Manipulation With Impulse **499**
    contraindication 502

manual diagnosis 214
Manual Therapy 288, 662
    acromioclavicular 470
    additional commonly used techniques 504
    adherent dura 502
    adhesions 453
    angiographic analysis 500
    ankylosing spondylitis 502
    antagonist 489, 500
    anterior innominate 469
    anterior torsions 468
    applied kinesiology 509
    articulatory techniques 497
    atlantoaxial
        blood flow 501
    atlantooccipital 501
    balance and hold 484
        integration with TCM practice 484
    basilar ischemia 502
    bilateral oblique subluxation 508
    bilateral symmetrical lesion 508
    blister 455
    bursitis 455
    catalepsy 502
    chafing method 458
    Chapman's points 498
        adaptation to TCM practice 499
    concentric 493
    contraindications to manipulation 502
    cord signs 502
    countertension techniques
        adaptation of TCM practice 489
    cranial technique 499
    cross-fiber massage 455
        contraindications 455
    deep transverse friction 453, 455
    dermatomal 470
    Dontigny model 505
    drop attacks 502
    dynamic functional techniques 484
    eccentric 493
    effleurage 455
    ERS 462, 467
    facilitated positional release 489
    fibromyalgia 624, 626
    fracture 502
    FRS 462, 467
    functional techniques
        adaptation in TCM practice 485
    golgi tendon organ 509
    grasping method 459
    group dysfunction 462
    haematomas 455

    head and neck
        considerations for thrust manipulation 503
    high velocity 500
    hypermobility 502
    iliac inflare 469
    iliac outflare 469
    infection 455, 502
    instability 502
        rheumatoid 503
    integrated neuromusculaoskeletal release 496
    isokinetic 493
    isolytic 493
    isometric 493
    isotonic 489, 493
    joint crack from manipulation 503
    joint dysfunctions
        common clusters 466
    kneading method 458
    left on right 468
    left-on-left 468
    lever techniques 499
    ligamentous laxity 502
    long lever techniques 500
    low back
        counternutation 465
        nutation 463
    lumbar 462
    muscle energy technique 489
    muscle energy techniques
        adaptation to TCM practice 494
    muscle fibrosis and adhesions
        muscle energy treatments 494
    muscle testing 511
    muscle weakness
        muscle energy techniques 493
    myofascial release 496
        integration to TCM practice 497
    myotomal 470
    neoplastic disease 502
    nonsteroidal anti-inflationary medications
        complications 502
    NSAIDs, complications 502
    nutational dysfunctions 466
    oblique pelvis with secondary caudad slip 508
    one finger meditation method 459
    osteopathic techniques 460
    osteoporosis 494, 502
    pelvic dysfunction 466
    perfusion abnormlities with neck movements 501
    pertrissage 453
    piezoelectric 453
    pinching method 459

piriformis 466
posterior
    backward torsions 466
posterior innominate 469
postisometric stretching 492
pressing method 459
progressive resisted exercise 494
psoriasis 455
psoriatic arthritis 502
pubic shears 468
pushing method 459
quadratus lumborum 466, 486
radicular pain 502
reciprocal inhibition 492, 500, 511
Reiter's syndrome 502
release by countertension-positioning and related techniques 487
rheumatoid 455, 502
right on left 468
right-on-right 468
rolling method 458
rotation method 459
rubbing method 459
sacral
    torsions 466
scleratomal 470
sedating 458
segmental relations 470
shaking method 460
shears 466
skin-rolling 454
spasm 453
spinal cord compression 502
spindle cells 509
Stretching 504
stretching method 460
swelling 453
sympathetic 470
tapotement 454
tendinitis 455
tennis elbow 455
thoracic 462
tonifying 458
traction and distraction 504
treatment of SIJD using Dontigny techniques 508
ulcer 455
unilateral extended sacrum 469
unilateral flexed sacrum 469
unilateral oblique pelvis 508
upper motor neuron lesion 502
upslipped innominate 469
vertebral
    artery 501
visceratomal 470
manual therapy 453, 500
Marfan's syndrome 555, 682
Marrow

meeting point 307
marrow 43, 72, 81, 286
massage 261
Massage/Manipulation **453**
masses 40
mast cell 169, 581
mastoid process 213
matrix metalloproteinases 574
McGill pain questionnaire 156
McKenzie System **526**
    anterior deviations 527
    derangement syndrome 526
    disc disorders 644
    dysfunction syndrome 526
    lateral deviations 527
    posterior deviations 526
    postural syndrome 526
    validity 527
mechanical allodynia 236
mechanoreceptors 142, 596
    acupuncture mechanisms 272
    joints 172
    ligaments 180
    pain 566
    transmitted via 151
medial
    lemniscus 137
    lower extremity flaccid, and lateral spasmed, points 331
medial collateral ligament
    bursitis 658
Medical Conditions **681**
medical lesion 208
Medical Ultrasound 250
medicinal cupping 369
medulla 134, 137
    oblongata's gracile 137
    oblongata 128
melanoma 573
membranes 31, 70, 89, 103, 161
memory 40
menstruation 73
mercury 632
Meridian Therapy **339**, 341
Meridians 51
mesenchyme 169
mesonephric tubules 81
mesonephros 81
metabolic
    destructive lesions 211
metabolic and endocrine inadequacies 681
metabolic destructive processes 683
Metal 48
metallic conduction 425
Metal-type people 335
metanephros 81
metastatic disease of cervical spine 682
metatarsophalangeal

foot dysfunction 675
metathalamus 129
met-enkephalin 138, 271
methionine 568, 573
methotrexate 569, 575
methyl 573
methylsulfonylmethane (MSM) 169
Mg 86
microacupuncture systems 52
microamp 126
microsystems 52
    fibromyalgia 626
microtrabeculae 170
microtrauma
    bursitis 657
microvaso-dilation
    nerve disorders 636
microvolt 126, 429
microwaves 423
midbrain 128
midline neutral 223
midrange 223
midstance
    foot dysfunction 676
migraine headaches 76, 77, 95, 684
Millon behavioral health inventory 159
Mingmen 26, 45, 46, **81**
Ministerial-Fire 45, 81
Minnesota multiphasic personality inventory 158
minute vessels 63
Miscellaneous diseases 37
Mitchell model 197
mitochondria 174
mitosis 573
mitral valv 222
    prolapse 598
Mixed and Complex TCM Presentations 44
mobilization 288, 289
moist heat 605
moistening-Yin 104
monoamines 271
monoarthritis 566, 576
mononeuritis 632, 683
mononucleosis 660
moon face 84
moons under the finger nails 105
morning pain 30
Morton's
    neuroma 211
Morton's foot
    foot dysfunction 676
motor 175
Motor Impairments
    table 593
motor
    nerves 134
    neuron 134, 233

neurons 175
unit 57
motor points 266, 278, 606
    fibromyalgia 622
        and Bands hyperactive, locating 606
    commonly affected muscles, table and figures 611
Motor Tests 232
    neuropathic pain 238
movement 216
    characteristics of spine, table 185
    testing 212
moxa 104, 289, 290, 293, 301, 303, 304, 305, 334, 369
    fibromyalgia 626
    mechanisms 370
MRI 205, 243, 682
    bursitis 657
    disc disorders 643, 644
    whiplash 652
mucopolysaccharides 169
mucous membrane lining 39
Muehrcke lines 87
multiconvergent cells 141, 142
multi-level analgesia 276
multiple myeloma 245, 682
multiple sclerosis 70, 592, 683
Multiple-Bi 209
murmurs 222
muscle 220
    atrophy 588
    belly palpation 218
    Bi 659
    biomedical **172**
    contracture 590
    dysfunction 590
    dysplasia
        foot dysfunction 674
    emaciation 86
    faradic 591
    fast glycolytic 588
    fibers 172
    fibrosis 588
    functions 173
    hypertrophy 588
    immobilization 589
    interferential 591
    innervation 175
    gamma loop 590
        types, table 175
    metabolism 86
    metabolic crisis 588
    micro-current 591
    sinews 165
    slow oxidative 588
    spasm 141, **589**
    spindles 132
    strains, hypomobile joints 561
    causes of 538
    tension 589
    tension members 202
    trigger-points 588
    viscous cycle 590
    weakness 592
Muscle Energy Technique 197, **489**
    fibromyalgia 625, 627
Muscle Tension/Length Testing, main topic 513
Muscles 415
    biceps femoris 183, 197
        foot dysfunction 676
    biceps 176, 189
    brachialis 597
    erector spinae 182, 186, 191
    gluteus maximus 183, 186, 187, 197, 198
        pelvic girdle 186
        scarotuberous ligament 189
    gluteus medius 197, 198
        foot dysfunction 676
    gluteus posterior minimus
        foot dysfunction 676
    hamstring 590
        medial 197
    iliocostalis
        lumborum 192
        thoracis 191
    iliopsoas 186, 515
        bursitis 657
    interspinales 191
    latissimus dorsi 183, 186, 191, 281
    levator scapulae 516
    longissimus
    capiti 182
        whiplash 652
    cervicis 195
    thoracis 182, 191
        torque 192
    longus
        capitis 183,195
        cervicis 183
        colli 183
        levator scapulae
        forward head posture 680
        longissimus capitis
        longus capitis
        whiplash 652
    multifidi 183, 191
        changes in chronic disorders 588
    pectoralis 597
    piriformis 186, 187, 197, 282
    psoas syndrome **604**
        abdominals 604
        biceps femoris 604
        erector spinae 604
        gluteals 604
        hamstrings 604
        left on righ 604
        piriformis 604
        sciatica 604
    quadratus lumborum 186, 193, 198, 210
        iliocostal friction 655
        foot dysfunction 675
        spasm points 329
        test 516
    quadriceps 56, 86, 597
        femoris 191
        squat test 473
        test 515
    rectus
        abdominus 191
        femoris 197
        testing 516
    rhomboids
        whiplash 652
    splenius cervicis
        hyperflexion 652
    sternocleidomastoid
        forward head posture 680
    scalenes 183, 195
        fibromyalgia 627
        rear-end collisions 652
    semispinalis capitis
        whiplash 652
    semispinalis 182
        thoracis 191
    semitendinosus
        pes anserinus bursitis 658
        spinalis 182
        thoracis 191
    splenius cervicis 195
        whiplash 652
    sternocleidomastoid (SCM) 56, 183
        rear-end collision 652
        test 516
    subscapularis 280, 281
    supraspinatus
        blood supply 595
        nerve 683
    tensor fascia lata
        testing 515
    teres major 281
    tibialis anterior 176, 197, 220
    tibialis posterior 595
    tonic muscles 174
    tonic stabilizing 197
    transverospinalis 183
    trapezius
        hyperextension 652
        fatigue shortening forward head posture 680
    vastus medialis 197
    white muscles 174

muscular
    crepitus 220
    dystrophy 244
    weakness 86
Musculoskeletal Medicine 165
    OM differential diagnosis 168
    OM pathology & etiology 167
    painful obstruction syndromes 659
musculotendinous junction 220, 595
mushroom phenomenon 655
myalgia 30, 584
myalgic index
    fibromyalgia 625
myasthenia gravis 60, 593
mycoplasma 660
myelinated 134, 143, 172
myelodysplasias
    foot dysfunction 674
Myers Five Major Fascial Chains 60
myocardial infarction 244, 683
myofascial pain syndrome
    Defensive Qi 14
    general 598
    thyroid function 244
    trigger points 598
Myofascial Disorders **584**
    contractile unit pain 587
    contusion 538
    early & late spasms 589
    fibromyalgia 597
    functioning and anatomical changes 588
    myofascial pain syndrome **597**
        treatment 604
    paralysis 592
    should spasm be treated 590
    spasm 589
    strain 538
        grading 538
    tendinitis 594
    tenosynovitis 596
    tension 589
    tightness weakness 589
    treatment 591
    weakness 592
myofascial pain index 599
myofascial release techniques 587
myofascial tests
    neuropathic pain 238
myofibril 173
myofilaments 173
myoglobin 174
myopathy 150, 588
myosin 22, 173
myositis 293, 588
    ossificans 538
myosynovitis 597
myotatic stretch reflex 589
myotome 280

origin of symptoms 207
    referred pain 152
    trigger points 600
myotonic 588
myotubular myopathy 588
Myristin 572

N

N-acetylglucosamine 570
naloxone 271
Naproxen 573, 574
nasal secretion 600
Naturopathic 424
nausea 40, 84, 87, 262, 293
navel 55
neck 65, 95
    and Head 414
    neck disability index 159
    pain 72
Needle Hyperactive Points 607
needle pain 292
negative ion 425
nemaline myopathy 588
neoplasm 597, 683
nerve
    membranes and opioids 138
    roots and passive testing 225
    sprouting 141
Nerve Conduction Velocity (NCV) 246
Nerve Disorders **632**
    amputations 634
    bradykinin 635
    catecholamines 635
    causalgia 634, 635
    cyanosis 635
    deafferenation 634
    denervation supersensitivity 634
    dermatome 634
    edema 634, 635
    hyperalgesia 635
    hyperhidrosis 635
    inflammation
        cutaneous 635
    interleukin-8 635
    mechanoreceptors
        neuropathic pain 634
    multiple sclerosis 634
    neuralgia 30
    neuralgic amyotropy 683
    neurally mediated hypotension 618
    neurapathies 238, 272
    neuritis 30, 70, 632
    neurofibromatosis 209, 211, 683
    neuropathic pain 141, 588, 603, **634**
        hypersensitivity 590
    neuropeptides 635
    nociceptors 634, 635
    norepinephrine 635
    pilomotor reflex 634

    post-herpetic neuralgia 634
    prespondylosis 634
    pressure on nerves 632
    prostaglandins 635
    reflex sympathetic dystrophy 635
    spinal cord injury 634
    spondylosis 634
    stroke 634
    sudomotor reflex 634
    sympathetically maintained pain 634
    threshold 634
    treatment 636
    trophic disturbances 634
    vasomotor disturbances 634
    vasospasm 635
    vertebral bodies 635
nerve fibers 127
    A-alpha 127, 132
    A-beta 127, 132, 137, 143
    A-delta 127, 132, 137, 143, 151
    A-fibers 127
    B-fibers 127
    C-fibers 127, 137, 140, 143, 151
    C-unmyelinated 132
    divided by 127
    myelinated 127
    unmyelinated 127
nerve root compression
Nerve Root Compression 175, 634
Nervous System 72, 125, 268
    afferent nerves 134
    brain 128
    brain stem 128
    cerebrum 129
    dorsal horn 132
    efferent nerves 134
    limbic system 130
    motor neurons 134
    nerve fibers 127
    neurons 125, 134
    parasympathetic 134
    peripheral nervous system 133
    reticular system 129
    spinal cord 131
        innervation 132
    sympathetic 134
    synapses 126
    ventral horn 132
network-vessels 63, 103, 106, 288
Neural Mechanisms of Pain **125**
Neurogenic claudication 648
    angioplasty 649
    cramping 648
    hypoxia 648
    oxygen 648
    treatment 648
    walking downhill 648
neurogenic hypersensitivity

foot dysfunction 676
neurogenic inflammation 553, 581
neurokinin 1 271
neurological 280
neurological disorders 72, 424
Neurological Testing **232**
    of patients with neuropathic pain syndromes 236
neuromatrix pain theory 137
    cognitive functions 137
    evaluative-cognitive dimensions 138
    sensory inputs 138
    sensory-discriminative 138
    stress system 137
neuromuscular synapse and trophic substances 592
neuropathy 265
    CBC 243
    myofascial disorders 585
    thoracic outlet 649
neuropeptides 137, 141, 581
neurophysiologic studies 246
neurosignature 138
neurotensin 139
neurotransmitter levels 245
neurotransmitters 126, 137, 142
    pain 139
neurovascular bundle 268
neutral
    joint dysfunctions 461
    spinal movments 462
neutrophils 29, 553
Newtonian 267
night pain 11, 381
night shade plants 568
nightmares 78
NIH 261
nitogen 143
nitric oxide 126, 140, 272, 595
nitrites 245
nitroglycerine 595
NMDA receptors N-methyl-D-Aspartate (NMDA) 131, 132 ,140, 141, 142
nociception 136
nociceptive 144
    pain 634
    receptors 172
nociceptors 127, 143, 144, 266, 646
    types, table 127
nocturia 82, 90
nodes 41
nodules 40, 95, 220
non-adrenergeic 272
noncapsular pattern 228
nonfatal whiplash injuries 651
nonfibrous ground substance 169
nonionizing radiation 424

nonneutral
    spinal movments 462
    vertebral dysfunctions 462
nonorganic pain, differentiating 148
nonspecific musculoskeletal complaints 145
nontraumatic articular pain 663
Noonan's syndrome 344
noradrenaline 84
norepinephrine 84, 138, 139, 141, 142, 145, 150, 271
    fibromyalgia 624
Normal Gait, main topic 196
Nourishing Qi 300
Nourishing-Qi 13, 63
noxious inhibitory controls (DNIC) 279
noxious stimuli 264
NSAID 569
NSAIDs 31, 139, 302
    fibromyalgia 624, 625
nuchal ligament 196
nuclear disc herniations 103
nuclear disc pain 280
Nuclear Lumbago 642
nuclear medicine 250
nucleoplasty
    disc disorders 644
nucleoproteins 244
nucleotides 271
nucleus 425
nucleus gracilis 140
nucleus pulposus 185
nulliness 580, 633
numbness 6, 34, 40, 41, 57, 76
nutation 187, 463
Nutrient-Qi 104
nutritional deficiencies and pain 588
Nutritional Inadequacies 681
Nutritive 106
Nutritive-division 31
Nutritive-Qi 14, 15, 16, 19, 20, 26, 27, 37, 38, 63, 91, 102, 113, 165
    in Bi-syndromes 659

O

Observation 212
obstructive disease 222
Obstructive syndromes 659
obtaining Qi 287
occipitoatlantoid 195
occipitoatloid 195
ochronosis 683
odontoid 195
odors 618
Ohm's Law 426
olecranon bursitis 657
oligoarthritis 566
omega fish oils
    nerve disorders 637
omnidirectional truss 201, 202

one-series PGs, 574
opiates 262
opioid
    fibromyalgia 624
    peptide 137
    systems 271
oral contraceptive use 683
orchitis 74
Organs TCM **81**
    Bi 660
organ degeneration 430
organ disorders 683
organic disease, history 211
Organs 63, 81
    biomedical adrenal 81
    biomedical and OM 85
    biomedical and OM Kidney systems 82
    Extraordinary 87
    Gall Bladder, summery table 97
    gate of Fire 81
    Heart/Pericardium 93
    Kidney, summery table 89
    Large Intestine, summery table 96
    Liver, summery table 87
    Lung, summery table 92
    Small Intestine, summery table 95
    Spleen/pancreas, summery table 91
    Stomach, summery table 97
    Triple Warmer, summery table 96
Original Qi, 300
Origina/Sourcel-Qi 38, 69, 81
O-ring test 276
Orthopaedic Medicine 168, 207, 261, 277, 453, 494, 500, 551
Orthopedic Assessment 205
    active movement 224
    age, occupation,sex, risk factors 208
    age/occupation 208
    antinuclear antibodies 244
    auscultation 222
    capsular pattern 230
    chronology and progression 209
    contractile unit testing 228
    coughing 210
    cutaneous trophic changes 213
    deep reflexes 233
    end feel 223
    evaluation 207
    examination 211
    extra-articular lesion 232
    gait analysis 239
    history, travel, diet, swelling, pain and perspiration 211
    internal derangement 231
    joint 222
        barriers 222
        play 223

testing 222
medical conditions 211
neurological testing 232
noncapsular pattern 231
observation 212
origin of symptoms 207
pain inquiry 209
painful arc 232
palpation 214, 215
passive motion 225, 226
patterns of passive and resisted movements 230
percussion 221
pins, needles and burning 210
posture, activity, rest, and exertion 210
resisted movement testing 228
screening
    examination 238
selective tension 224
squat test 473
superficial reflexes 233
timing of symptoms 209
twinges and giving-way 210
visceral reflexes 233
vital signs 212
orthopedics 453
Orthoses
    Achilles Tendinitis 532
    Chondromalcia Pattela or Patellow Femoral Pain Syndrome 534
    Hallux Limitus or Rigidus 532
    Heal Pain, Plantar Fasciitis 534
    Lateral Ankle Istability and/or Peroneal Tendinitis 533
    Metatarsalgia 533
    Neuroma 533
    Pediatric Flatfoot 533
    Posterior Tibialis Dysfunction 534
    Sesmoditis 534
    Tarsal Coalition 534
    Tarsal Tunnel Syndrome 534
orthostatic hypotension 84, 91
orthotic therapy
    foot dysfunction 674, 677, 678
Orthotics and Restraints **530**
Orudis and fibromyalgia 624
osmosis 428
osseous crepitus 220
osteitis deformans 683
osteoarthritic cartilage 574
osteoarthritis 564, 571, 576, 660
    contractile unit pain 588
    fibromyalgia 620
    hypermobile joints 561
osteoarthrosis 683
osteoblastoma haemangioma 682
osteochondritis dissecans 209

osteochondroma 683
osteoid osteoma 683
osteomalacia 209, 244, 588
    fibromyalgia 620
osteomyelitis 293, 681
Osteopathic 261, 277, 500, 543
    fibromyalgia 625
    lesion 562
    iliosacral disorders summery table 469
    medicine 460
    philosophy 460
    sacroiliac dysfunctions summery table 468
    treatment methods 484
    vertebral dysfunctions summery table 467
    functional assessment analysis of findings 476
osteoporosis 209
osteosarcomas 245, 682
Oswestry low back index 158, 262
ovulatory cycle 430
oxalates
    fibromyalgia 624
oxygen 139, 148, 174, 185, 266

P
p values 292
P2X-3 140
PAG 273
Paget's disease 209, 244, 683
Pain 123, 414
    visual analog scale 156
    acute 143
    all over 291
    ancillary mechanisms 140
    and emotions 36
    aspects 143
    assessment 155
    at extreme range 225
    ATP 140
    brain 130
    chemical theories 138
    chronic 143
    chronic muscular 44
    complex regional pain syndrome 634
    cramping 55
    craniocervical 279
    daytime in OM 161
    deafferenation 634
    dermatomal 153
    diffuse bone 682
    dolorimeter 156
    drawing 606
        drawing (figure) 157
    endorphins 138
    enkephalins 138
    extrasegmental 154

facilitated cord segment 141
fixed 40
from acute muscle strain 43
herbs 161
gate control theory **136**
gender variations 149
headache
headaches 70
    points 327
heel 70
    foot dysfunction 677
immediate 143
in TCM **159**
inflammatory mediators 139
intermittent in OM 161
location and treatment 162
lower extremities 279
lumbar aggravated by rotation, points 331
lumbar points based on movement summary 331
McGill pain questionnaire 156
mechanisms **136**
midline 70
migraine headache 684
Minnesota multiphasic personality inventory 158
mixed pain in OM 160
myotomal 153
neck spondylopathy, herbs 578
nerve sprouting 141
neurotransmitters 139
night 11, 40
nonorganic 148
OM pathogenesis, summary table 164
opiod peptides 138
Oswestry low back questionnaire 158
patent medicines summary table 404
patient drawing 156
perception & localization 150
perception & localization, main topic 150
peripheral
    central mechanisms 140
    mechanisms 140
phantom 131, 141
possible causes of 123
postoperative 262
presentation, summary table 153
psychological diagnosis 146
psychological influences (biomedical) **144**
psychological sequelae 144
psychophysical concepts 137
psychosomatic 70
referred **151**, 152

       in OM 160
       reflex sympathetic dystrophy 635
       regional in OM 160
       sclerotomal 153
       sensitivity 34
       sensitization 142
       sharp 40
       shifting 151
       shooting 40
       shoulder 70
       stabbing 40
       sympathetic nervous system 141
       TCM types, summary table 162
       the neuromatrix theory 137
       upper extremities 279
       upper extremity 70
       verbal scale 156
       West Haven-Yale multidimensional pain inventory 156
       Wiltse's evaluation method 156
       winddown 292
       windup 292
painful
       arc 223, 231
       obstruction 54
Painful Obstruction (Bi) syndrome 106, 167, 287, **659**, 368, 567
       fibromyalgia 621
       stages 661
       treatment 662
paired needling 294
palpating for movement 216
Palpation 214
       asymmetries 217
       contractile
           tissues 218
           tissues summary table 218
       crepitus, snaps, popping, and cracks 219
       excessive
           cold 217
           warmth 217
       findings 216
       peripheral pulses 218
       progression 216
       restrictions of tissues or movements 218
       skin and subcutaneous mobility 216
           overlying active lesions 217
       swelling 216, 218
       OM 98
       TCM 220
palpitations 6, 78, 84, 90, 93, 371, 389
palsy 70
pancreas 683
       disease 211
paradoxical breathing 518
paralysis 30, 65, 70, 592

paranoia 40
paraplegia
       foot dysfunction 674
parasitic infection 36
parasympathetic 86, 100, 295
       fibromyalgia 621
       ganglia 134
       nervous system 134
parathyroid plexuses 279
paravertebral muscles 183
paresthesia 632, 649
Paresthesia and Numbness in TCM 633
pargyline 139
Parkinson's disease 125, 588, 592
       fibromyalgia 620
pars interarticularis 647
partial articular pattern 228, 231
particles 423
passive 281
       range of movement 223
passive stretching 605
Patau's syndrome 344
patello-femoral pain syndromes 678
Pathogenic Factors 22, 32, 39, 102, 461
       Cold 25
       Dampness 27
       Dryness 28
       fibromyalgia 621, 622, 627
       Heat 26
       latent lurking 29
       Summer-Heat 28
       Wind 24
pathogenic-Qi 287
pathological barriers 222
Pathology-Specific Foot Orthotics **531**
pathomechanisms 47
Patrick's Faber test 472
pattern discriminations 5, 8
patterns of correspondences 6
pelvic
       diaphragm 186
       disease 211
       motion 189
Pelvic Dysfunctions **463**
       fibromyalgia 618
       obliqueness short leg 670
       torsion 282
pelvis 75
       anatomy 186
       compression test 478
       gravitational force 186
Penetrating 70, 336
penicillins 588
peppers 568
peptic ulcer 333
peptidases 569, 574
Percussion 221
periaqueductal gray (PAG) 134, 137
pericadial 96

Pericardium 33, 46, 56, 60
       and Divergent channels 69
       fibromyalgia 626
perineum 186
perineural glial cells 425
perineural tissues 126
periodontitis 574
periosteal 282
       acupuncture 266, 655, 656
Periosteal Lesions 656
       needling 278
periosteum 266, 538
peripheral
       joint pains 165
       nerve comprise 133, 134
       nervous system 133
           and pain 140
       neuritis 683
       vasculature 135
           disease 632
       vessels and discs 184
       vision and examination 213
peritoneal 96
peritonitis 293
perivascular space 52
pernicious anemia 683
peroneus 197
perspiration 42, 211, 274, 600, 681
Pes anserinus
       bursitis 658
Pes Cavus
       foot dysfunction 674
pestilential factors (Li Qi) 29
PGEI 574
pH 142
phagocytosis 553
phantom limb pain 141
phasic actions 197
phasic muscles 22, 174
phenolic acid 575
Phlegm 31, 37, 38, **39**, 103, 106, 224, 544
       end feel 224
       fibromyalgia 622
       Fire 594
       Heat 38, 40, 220
       masses 375
       musculoskeletal disorders 41
       nodes 167
phosphate 588
       fibromyalgia 624
phosphocreatine 603
phospholipase A2
       disc disorders 639
phosphorus 244
photochemotherapy 576
photon 423
photopheresis 569, 576
photophobia 618

phrenic nerve 279
Physical Examination **211**
physiologic barrier 222, 224
physiological medicine 2
piezo-electricity 170, 180, 425
pigment cell 169
pilomotor
    and trigger points 600
pins and needles 209
pituitary 84, 150
    acupuncture analgesia 271
    gland 130
placebo 264, 269, 292, 295, 570, 571, 572, 575
    fibromyalgia 625, 626
plain film imaging 251
planes of body 212
plantar
    response 210
    fasciitis
        foot dysfunction 677
plasma
    cells and connective tissue 169
    dry needling 265
plasticity 142
platelet 389
    derived-growth factor 266
    growth factors and dry needling 265
pleospino-reticulothalamic tract 151
pleural 96
pleurisy 683
plexi 333
plum seed Qi 40
pneumothorax 293, 298
Points Ear
    Master, Cerebral/Psychosomatic 345
    Master, Endocrine/Internal Se 345
    Master, Oscillation/Cerebral Hemispheres 345
    Master, Sensorial/Eye 345
    Master, Shen Men/Spirit Gate 345
    Master, Stress Control/Adrenal 345
    Master, Sympathetic 345
    Master, Thalamus/Pain Control 345
    Master, Tranquilizer/Valium/Hypertension 345
    Master, Zero/Solar Plexus 345
Points, acupuncture
    Accumulating (Xi) 303, 307
        summary table 307
    Alarm (Mu) 277, 288, 308
    back Shu
        and Alarm summary table 314
    back-Shu (Transport) 289, 308, 499
    based on location of back pain, table 330
    cervical stiffness, table 325
    commonly used and axillary 314
    commonly used points
        mental conditions 322
    Connecting (Luo) 299, 303, 304
        summary table 304
    embryological 308
    endocrine dysfunctions 323
        table 323
    entry and exit 304
    Five Phases
        treatment 309
        Yang channels 315
    for Extension/Flexion, table 325
    group Connecting 314
    Hua Tuo Jia Ji 298, 308
    Influential
        summary table 308
    Influential/Meeting 307
    local contralateral connections table 351
    locating 284
    low back, acute and chronic disc, table 332
    low back, based on movement, table 331
    low back, other conditions, table 330
    low back, sprain strain, table 329
    Master (meeting) 303
    master oscillation 290
    moisten sinews 288
    musculoskeletal summary table 316
    neck and shoulder, table 326
    nervous regulation, table 324
    Phlegm 288
    qualities of deep skin acupoints 269
    qualities of superficial Acupoints 268
    selecting 286
    Shu-stream 288
    Source 304
        Entry and Exit, table 305
        treatment 304
    Spring-Ying 288
    subcutaneous 285
    thoracic shoulder, table 328
    Tong-style points used in musculoskeletal disorders, table 357
    Treating Cervical movement restrictions and rotation, table 325
    Well 56, 300
    windows of the sky 322
Point Gateways and General Treatment Methods 304
Point Location and Reactivity 285
poisoning 684
poisons 36
polarity 428
poliomyelitis 592, 593
    foot dysfunction 674
polyamines 573
polyarthralgia 660
polyarthritis 566
polycythemia 243
polygonum cuspidatum 569, 575
polymorphs 265
polymyalgia rheumatica 243, 588, 682
    fibromyalgia 620
polyneuritis 632
    foot dysfunction 674
polypeptides 138, 169
polysaccharides 169, 570
polysulfate 568
polyuria 82, 90
pons 128
posain 189, 579, 581
    positional pain 564, 600
positive ion 425
post concussion syndrome 653
posterior longitudinal ligament 181, 196
posterior nutation 465
posterior arch 190
posterior knee pain
    foot dysfunction 675
posterior pes cavus
    foot dysfunction 674
posterior tibial dysfunction
    foot dysfunction 677
posterior tibiotalar impingement bursitis 658
post-ganglionic 140
    sympathetic neuron 635
post-herpetic neuralgia 211, 571
post-immobilization arthritis 218
postisometric stretch 610
post-mastectomy pain syndrome 571
post-operative inflammation 574
post-synaptic inhibition 136
postural 517
    and phasic muscles 174
        table 178
    muscles and sedentary life-style 589
    stresses 678
    syndrome 208, 209
    Yin and Yang muscles 22
Posture 213
    and TCM 214
    EMG and erector spinae 191
potassium 84, 138, 142, 143, 588, 681
potatoes 568

potential difference 426
potential space and elastic barrier 222
Potter's syndrome 344
precautions and contra-indications during application of cupping 369
pre-existing Heat 44
preganglionic
    autonomic fibers 132
    sympathetic neurons 140
pregnancy 188
prenatal-Qi 14
prepatellar bursa 657
prespondylosis 641
    disc disorders 641
pressure on nerves 632
presynaptic inhibition 127
primary respiratory system 285
prime mover muscles 185
Priorities in Treatment, OM 104
proanthocyanidins 568
procaine 573
progressive systemic sclerosis 682
proliferated Bi syndromes (osseous arthritis) 545
prolonged acute nociception 143
Prolotherapy **297,** 577, 655
    fibroblasts 297
    disc disorders 639
pronephros 81
propagated needling sensation 287
propagated sensation 52
Proper Shoes 534
propionic acid
    fibromyalgia 624
proprioceptors 186
prostaglandin 571, 572
prostaglandin PG2 571
prostaglandins 139, 574, 646
    acute pain 143
    arachidonic acid 552
    chemical pain 138
    NSAIDs 552
    phospholipase A2
        disc disorders 639
    sensitization 142
    sympathetically maintained pain 635
prostate 244
    cancer 244, 682
    low back pain 211
    specific antigen 243, 244
prostatitis 74, 681
proteases 569, 574
proteins
    deficiency 555
    urine 245
proteoglycans 568, 570, 573, 574
    degrading enzymes 574
    disc 185

nonfibrous ground substance 169
proteolysis 553
protons 424
protoplasm 53
protrusion disc stages 640
Provocative Discography 253
pruritus 57
pseudocolochirus axiologus 571
pseudomotor 274
psoas 70, 183, 210
    bursitis 657
    major test 515
Psoas Syndrome **604**
psoriasis 57, 681
    spondylitis 244
psoriatic
    arthritis 408, 569, 681
psychiatric disorders 39
psychiatric symptoms 40
psychological 264, 269
    diagnosis 146
    disorders 588
    factors in MPS 681
    influences on pain 144
psychosomatic 224
pubic
    dysfunction and pain, points 330
    symphysis 186
pubis and innominates 187
pulsed electromagnetic therapy 569, 573
pulses
    organ association table 341
    vital signs 212
punctured viscera 293
pyomyositis 588

Q

Qi 39, 51, 69, 165, 207, 283, 286, 292, 306, 309, 369, 543, 660, 662
    Ancestral 12, 14
    channel 12
    Defense 12
    Defensive 11, 19
    Defensive and biomedical analogies 13
    deficiency 10, 11
    deficiency 42
        pain 11
    division 29, 31
    fibromyalgia 621
    dynamic 289
    dysfunctions 375
    Gong 148, 295, 513
    main topic 9
    Nourishing 12
    Organ 12
    Original 12
    pain 11
    Righteous 14
    stagnation 10, 11, 26, 28, 33, 103, 220, 334
    Cold Bi 666
    transformative-Heat 662
    pain 11
    transformation 10
    transportation 10
    True 12
    types of Qi summary table 12
    wild pulse 100
Quantitative Sensory Testing (QST) 247
quantum mechanics 267
quantum theory 4, 267

R

radiant-heat 220
radiation 248
radiculopathy 643, 681
radiofriquency
    disc disorders 644
radiohumeral bursitis 657
radiotherapy 262
rapid opiate detoxification 262
raping Heat 220, 221
Raynaud's disease 683
    fibromyalgia 625
reactive arthritis 682
rear-end collision 651
rebellious-Qi 74, 660
receptive fields 273
rectal disease 211
rectosigmoid diseases 681
recurrent nerve 279
red blood cells 81
red muscles 174
red skin response 369
    fibromyalgia 621
referred pain 208
    influences 155
    main topic 151
    trigger point 600
referred tenderness 154, 208
reflex sympathetic dystrophy 571, 588, 635, 636
reflexes 233
Regional TCM Pulses, table 219
Rehabilitation
    centralization 526
    derangement syndrome 526
    dysfunction
        syndrome, McKenzie 526
    exhalation 518
    gluteus 513
    inhalation 518
    isotonic 514
    McKenzie system 526
    paradoxical breathing 518
    postural syndrome 526
    postural exercise 517
    proprioception 513
    Qi Gong 518

spinal stretch 518
stabilization postural exercises 519
Tai-Chi 513, 518
Rehabilitation and Exercise **513**
Reiter's disease 681
Reiter's syndrome 244, 681
relaxin 188
reliability scores 205
Relora 85
renal failure 6, 82
renal insufficiency 244
repetitive motion injury 209
reproduction 73, 89
residual pathogens 29
resistance 426
resisted movements 223
testing 228
respiration 173, 212
respiration at a cellular level 135
restless leg syndrome 598
restricted lumbar
extension pain, points 331
flexion, points 331
movement, points 331
rotation, points 331
restrictive
barrier 222
spinal movements 462
retained pathogenic factors 594
retaliation needling 294
retention of pathogenic factors
fibromyalgia 621
reticular formation 344
reticular system 129
reticulin 169
reticuloendothelial system diseases 245
retrocalcaneal bursitis 657
retroperitoneal masses 681
reverse Morton's extension
foot dysfunction 676
RF surgery 424
rhabdomyolysis 588
Rheum 39
rheumatic fever 243, 660
Rheumatic Disease Painful Obstruction (Bi) 406
Rheumatic patters 659
rheumatism 569, 571
rheumatoid 668
factor 243, 244
Rheumatoid and Inflammatory Arthritis 574
rheumatoid arthritis 29, 38, 150, 217, 219, 566, 567, 568, 571, 574, 595, 660, 681
Bi syndromes 660
chronic pain 144
ESR 243
RF 244

vascular or collagen disorders 632
rheumatological disorders 31
rib subluxation
fibromyalgia 627
ribs 55
rickets 244
Righteous-Qi 29, 60, 105, 106, 262, 263, 276, 556
Bi syndroms 660
rigidity 24
Robert's formula 569
Robitussin and fibromyalgia 624
Roland Morris scale and illness behavior questionnaire 159
root 6, 18, 36, 44, 100, 262, 277, 284
palsy 213
rootlet anastomosis 152
rotated leg 479
rotatores 183
rotoscoliosis 217
rough sounds 219
Roussey-Levy syndrome
foot dysfunction 674
rT3 86
rubella 660
ruptured chordae tendineae 222
S
S1 and S2 disc lesions, points 332
sacral
base 187
subluxation 217
torsions 466
sacralization 190
sacroiliac 461, 589
dysfunction and pain, points 330
facet dysfunctions 646
gravitational force 186
joints 183
pelvic girdle 186
sacrospinalis 191
sacrotuberous ligament 183, 186, 187, 189, 197, 505
sacrum 188
S-Adenosylmethionine (SAMe) 139, 569, 572
sadness 36
salicin 569, 575
salicylic acid 569, 575
salivation 135
salix 575
sand-toxin 369
Sarapin 647
sarcoidosis 588, 632
sarcoplasmic reticulum 600
sartorius
pes anserinus bursitis 658
Saturday night palsy 632
saw-tooth 440
scapula 516

scapular & shoulder pain 683
scapular winging 683
scapulothoracic crepitus 220
Scar Tissue 416
interference fields 656
movement 554
treatment 656
scattered needling 294
Schmorl's nod 641
Schwann cell 126
schwannoma 211
sciatic nerve 590
sciatica 76, 332
common points 332
TCM 645
scleroderma 244, 588
sclerotome 152, 207, 280, 600
scoliosis 90, 214
scraping 369
Screening Examination 238
scrofula 39, 40, 41
sea cucumber 569, 571
Sea of Blood 74
Sea of Yin 73
Sea points 54, 165
Secondary Pathogenic Factors 38
summery table 40
second-order neurons 136
segment 278
segmental 276, 288
effects 278
hypermobility 683
innervation figure 150
pain-inhibitory effects 279
segments 308
seizures 76
Selective Tension 224, 280
summary table 223
selenium 575
self-bracing
foot dysfunction 676
self-perpetuating inflammation 553, 595
self-reducing disc disorder 30, 643, 666
semi-conduction 425
semi-placebo 268
sensitive C-reactive protein 245
sensitive thyroid stimulating hormone 243, 244
sensitivity score 205
sensitization 142, 154, 600
sensory 175
neuron 233
tests 232
septic arthritis 25, 30
septic joint 26
septicemia 293
sequelae to S4 disc lesion (cauda equina syndrome) 413
sequestration disc 640

serine 86
serotinergic inhibitory descending system 137
serotonin 37, 137, 138, 139, 145, 169, 271
    fibromyalgia 624
serratia peptidase 574
serum
    calcium 244
    glutamicoxaloacetic transaminase 244
servo systems 49
Sesshoku-Shin techniques 338
sex hormone 245
sexual activity 18, 36, 37, 38
SF-36 questionnaire
    fibromyalgia 625
sham 269, 295
Shao Yang 57, 300, 352
    fibromyalgia 621
    GB and TW 291
Shao-Yin 57
Shao-Yang 103, 161, 167
shear 170, 187, 466
shifting pain 151
short leg 217
Short Leg Syndrome
    assessment 670
short needling 294
Short Upper Arms 672
shortened plantar fascia
    foot dysfunction 675
shortness of breath 40, 93
Shoulder 65, 76, 79, 96, 97, 411
    bursitis 657
    blade 55
    joint
        central line of gravity 213
shrapes fibers 179
side collisions 652
sidebending, spine 185, 191
sideways needling 294
SIgA 86
silken crepitus 220
Sims position 282
Sinew 285
    channels **54**, 218
    channels, activated by 301
    channels, and connecting channels 63
    channels, brain 57
    channels, chronicity 300
    channels, chronology 209
    channels, Defensive Qi 54
    channels, emptiness 303
    channels, Exterior 168
    channels, fullness 302
    channels, points 56
    channels, selective tension 225

channels, six energy zones 57
channels, symptoms & signs 57
channels, treatment 277, 300
channels, well points 284, 299
Sinew and Bone 416
Sinews 63
    Bi 659
    Coldness 166
    damage contemporary classification 546
        stages, summery table 546
    deviation 166
    enlargement 166
    fatigue 166
    flaccidity 166
    Heat 166
    laceration 166
    OM, main topic 165
    rigidity 166
    slippage 166
    turned over 166
    twitching 166
Sinews/Muscles 415
Single Fiber Electromyography (SFEMG) 246
sinusitis 574
six energetic levels 57
six environmental Excesses 23, 39
Six-Divisions 58
Sjogeren's syndrome 244
skin 57
    Bi 659
    impedance 268
    mobility 216
    roll 216
    swelling 63
sleep 588, 589
SMAC 24 243
small emboli 222
Small Hemipelvis 672
Small Intestines 18, 49
small-Fire 81
smoking 38, 184, 555, 683
    disc disorders 641
sodium 84, 138
sodium gate 126
Soft Tissues
    OM classification **165**
    stresses and loads 170
Solid 81, 263, 311
somatic dysfunction 208, **562**, 588
    cross talk 563
    electromyographic 563
    sensitization 563
    summation 564
    windup 563
somatic efferents 175
Somatosensory Evoked Potentials (SSEP) 247, 264

somatovisceral 141, 276, 563
    reflexes 563
sore throat 65
sorrow 34
Source, Entry and Exit points summary 305
source-Fire 42
source-Qi 45
spasm 6, 24, 30, 54, 55, 65, 76, 97, 166, 218, 223, 231, 279, 540, 584, 600, 606
    arthritic joints 589
    bursitis 590
    dislocation 590
    dura mater 590
    early & late 589
    internal derangement 590
    nerve roots 590
    tendon 590
spastic monoplegia
    foot dysfunction 674
spastic paralysis 592
spasticity 594
specificity score 205
Spemann Organizer 53
spermidine 573
spermine 573
spiderweb veins 337
spina bifida
    foot dysfunction 674
spinal
    accessory nerve 683
    ligaments innervation 635
    nerves 133
spinal cord 131, 136
    laminae 131
    segmental innervation figure arms 150
    segmental innervation figure legs 151
    sensitization 132
    sensitized state 132
    suppressed state 132
    ventral horn 132
spinal cord tumors
    foot dysfunction 674
Spinal Movement Characteristics, table 185
Spine
    anterior column 184
    anterior muscles 183
    facet joint 185
    general discussion 181
    intervertebral disc 184
    ligaments 181
    muscles 182
    posterior column 185
    posterior muscles 182
spine 55, 65
spinothalamic tract 131

spinous process 185, 281
    facilitated segment 563
spirit 100
Spirit-Essence 32
Spirit-Essence-Qi 33
spiritless pulse 100
Spleen 33, 39, 45, 49, 60, 87, 288, 556, 558
Spleen Disorders
    and biomedicine 85
        great Connecting (Lou) Channel 299
    Qi-deficiency 86
    Yang-deficiency 86
Spleen/pancreas 18, 34, 39, 51, 220
    fibromyalgia 622, 628
Spleen-Yin 104, 105
spleen and shoulder pain 683
Spondylolisthesis
    hamstring 647
    paresthesia 647
spondylolisthesis 252, 581, 647
Spondylolysis
    imaging 647
    treatment 648
spondylolysis 647
Spondylolysis and Spondylolisthesis **647**
Spondylosis 577, 641
    disc disorders 641
    treatment 577
Sprain Strain 537, 584
    acute stage 539
    alpha 2 macroglobulin 545
    anaesthesia 539
    analgesic 545
    blood letting and acupuncture 541
    chronic phase 542
    complex regional pain 540
    congealed
        Blood (ossification) 545
    contrast therapy 541
    cross
        fiber massage 541
    damage to channels 545
    DMSO 540
    edema 541, 545
    effleurage 541
    electrogalvanic stimulation 541
    elevation 540
    exercise 540, 542
    external herbs summary table 549
    gypsum 543
    heating pad 542
    herbal management 543
    ibuprofen 545
    immobilization 540
    iontophoresis 540
    knee 545
    laceration of bone fragment and OM 545
    laser therapy 541
    ligamentous 540
    massage 541
    minimizing bleeding 539
    mobilization 542
    NSAIDs 545
    OM treatment principles table 548
    oral herbs summary table 547
    osteoarthritis 545
    other natural therapies 545
    periarthritis 545
    proteolytic enzymes 545
    Qi Gong 543
    RSD 540
    salicylate 545
    serratia peptidase 545
    shoulder 545
    silk worm 545
    stabilization and exercise 543
    steroids 540
    subacute stage 541
    surgery collateral knee ligaments 541
    Tai Chi 543
    tendinous 540
    thermacare 542
    thermotherapy 541
    topical herbal soaks 541
    traumatic arthritis 540, 541
    type-3 collagen 540
    ultrasound 540
    zap pac 542
springing techniques 497
Spring-Warm 29, 31, 32
spurs 69, 77
    fibromyalgia 622
stabilization 543
ercises 519
staphylococcal 681
stasis 42
static allodynia 236
Static Blood 38, 40
Static Magnetic Therapy, main topic 443
    acidity 444
    Ah Shi 445
    alertness 444
    alkalinity 444
    athletic performance 444
    bacterial growth 444
    Bi-polar 445
    block magnets 447
    Brain Sand. 446
    bruising 444
    button magnet 447
    button magnets 447
    clinical evidence 445
    depression 444
    dermatomes 447
    diamagnetic 444
    electron 443
    ethmoid 446
    ferromagnetic 443, 444
    fibromyalgia 445
    fluid 444
    fluids 446
    gasses 446
    gauss
        rating 445
    growth hormone 444
    headache 447
    infections 444
    inflammation 444, 446
    ions 444
    magnetic Bars 445
    magnetic Blocks 445
    magnetic buttons 445
    melatonin 444
    MRI 443
    negative magnetic energy 446
    negative polarity 444
    neurons 446
    non-polarized 443
    North 443, 444
    oxygen 444, 446
    paramagnetic 444, 446
    pH 443
    pineal gland 444, 446
    placement 447
    plastiform magnets 447
    polarity of the body 446
    polarized 443
    pole polarity 444
    positive magnetic energy 446
    positive polarity 444
    relax muscle 444
    repetitive strain 447
    sedating 444
    shoulder 447
    side effects and contra-indications 446
    sleep 444
    South 443
    toxins 447
    trigger points 445
    wound healing 445
statin medication
    nerve disorders 637
stellate ganglion 279, 603
stem cell 590
Stenosis **648**
    neurogenic claudication 648
    neurovascular 648
sterilize 298
sternal articulations 194
sternoclavicular 589

sternum 56
steroid treatment 683
stiff neck 24, 44, 94
    Heidi foot
        foot dysfunction 675
stiffness 65, 72, 79
sting nettle 575, 569
Stomach 45, 49, 52, 87, 288, 594
    Qi 100
    Yang-deficiency 220
stomach 389
    back and shoulder pain 211
    disease 211
stone 224
stool 65
straight leg raise 472
Strain 57, 209, 217
    antagonistic 538
    deceleration muscle function 538
    eccentric 538
    grading 538
    hamstring 538
    tendon evulsion 538
    tension 538
strain-counterstrain 487
    fibromyalgia 625
straphylococcus aureus
    bursitis 657
strength 6
stress 145, **149**, 147, 333
    fibromyalgia 621
stretch-and-spray 605
Stretching Techniques 504
stroke 381, 592, 593, 683
strong-Wind 102
strychnine poisoning 632
subarachnoid
    hemorrhage 684
subclavian artery 279
subclavian vein 600
subcoracoid
    bursa 657
subcoracoid bursa 657
subcutaneous tissue 41, 165
subdeltoid
    bursa 657
    bursitis 657
Subluxation 144, **461**, 508, **561**
    nonphysiologic dysfunction 561
suboccipital 65
substance P 139, 571
    fibromyalgia 624, 625
    lamina 131
    main topic 138
    nerve sprouting 141
substantia gelatinosa 136, 138
substantia nigra 138
succinyl dehydrogenase 86
sudden
    halt, passive testing 225
    pain aggravated by deep breath, points 329
sulcus sign 212
sulfonamides 632
sulfur 555, 568
Summer-Heat 23, 26, 28, 32, 39
superficial 277
    collateral vessels 63
    femoral artery 219
    reflexes 233
    skin 220
supportive needling 294
supraclavicular fossa 65
suprarenal (adrenal) glands 84
suprascapular nerve 683
supraspinal descending inhibition of pain 273
supraspinous ligaments 182, 191
supraventricular tachyarrhythmias 600
surface EMG (SEMG) 246
surface needling 294
sweating 44, 92
sweet 37
swelling 218, 220, 289
    Connecting channels 304
    indicate 211
    palpation 212
sympathetic 84, 100, 217, 279, 296, 308
    fibromyalgia 621
    ganglia 134, 333
    ganglion, neck 603
    innervation table 136
        of Organs, Shu, and Mu Points, table 278
    nervous system 134
sympathetically maintained pain 141, 635
symphysis pubis 186, 187
synapses 126
    postsynaptic membrane 126
    presynaptic
        inhibition 127
        membrane 126
    synaptic transmission 126
synarthrosis 187
synovial
    bursitis 657
    culture 243
    gout 244
    joint 475, 560
    membrane 218
synovitis 561
synovium 19, 172, 565
syphilis 244, 595
    foot dysfunction 674
syphilitic 681
systemic inflammation 245
systemic lupus erythematosus 243, 244, 632, 682
systemic sclerosis 682
Systems Science Model 200

T

T3 86
tachycardia 389
Tagament 265
Tai Chi Chuan 148, 172
Tai Yang 57
    UB and SI 291
Tai Yin 57
    LU and Sp 291
Talapi Equino Varus
    foot dysfunction 674
Taping **530**
    lateral epicondylitis 530
    tennis elbow 530
Tarsal Coalition
    foot dysfunction 677
Tarsal Tunnel Syndrome
    foot dysfunction 678
taxation 37
T-cell 86
TCM
    anatomical terminology 7
    degenerative cascade **556**
    terminology 7
tearing 76
tectorial membrane 196
telencephalone 128
temperature 24, 212, 215, 216
temples 95
temporal arteritis 243
temporal lobe 130
tender tendon 218
tenderness 285, 289
tendinitis 211, 280, 571
    chronic treatment 542
    hypermoblile joints 561
    main topic 594
    muscle tension 589
    onset 210
    and tendinosis
        treatment of 596
tendinomuscular 54
tendinosis 265, 373, 596
    eccentric training 596
tendinous 219
    crepitus 220
tendon 57, 165, **179**, 265, 288, 561
    critical zone 595
    insertion 179
    microcurrent 597
    origin 179
    reflex 592
tennis elbow 373, 597
tenoperiosteal junctions 218
tenosynovitis 596
tenovaginitis 596

TENS 262, 269, 277
tensegrity 202
tension 55, 172, 575, 590
    barrier 283
tension myositis syndrome 32
terpenoids 575
Terry's nails 87
testes
    stones 681
tetanus 632
tetany 26
tetracycline
    disc disorders 644
    nerve disorders 637
tetrahedron 267
thalamic
    nuclei 130, 131
thalamocortical projections 130
thalamus 128, 129, 130
The Body Milieu 8
The Electrical Properties of The Body 428
The Placebo Effect 265
theonine 86
thermal allodynia 236
thermal effects 368
thermatomes 278
thermography 562
thick-Phlegm 39
thigh 55, 65, 94
thin Phlegm/Rheum 39
    Yin-Phlegm 39
thirst 44, 65
thoracic 94
    outlet syndrome, vascular disorders 683
    spine 192
Thoracic Inlet and Outlet 193
    fibromyalgia 621, 626
thoracic kyphosis
    forward head posture 679
Thoracic Outlet Syndrome **649**
    electromyography 649
    examination 650
    myofascial pseudo TOS 650
    symptoms 649
    treatment 650
thoracic spine and rib cage 192
    motions in 193
thoracolumbar fascia 182, 186, 191
Thorax muscle
    summary table 191
Three Phases of Joint Degeneration **556**
    bone damage 558
    degenerative
        spondylosis 556
    dysfunction 556
    dysfunction/postural phase and TCM 557

exercise 558
inflammation 558
instability 557
    phase 556
joint dysfunction 558
ligaments
    aging 556
myotomal 556
Pathogenic Factors 558
Qi Gong 559
sclerotome 556
stabilization phase 556, 557
Tai Chi 559
TCM Exterior Pathways 557
TCM Interior Pathways 557
trauma 558
Wind-Cold 557
Wind-Heat 557
threshold 143, 272
throat 76
thrombin time 293
thrombosis 222
thrombotic disorders 87
thromoxane B2 575
through and through acupuncture 287
thymus 52, 134
thyroid 81, 86, 279
    deficiency 243
    function 244
thyroid cancer 682
tibial 278
timidity 78
tingling 6, 34, 389
tinnitus 65, 97, 600
Tissue Congestion and Terminal Lymphatic Drainage **475**
tissue
    biomedical perspective
        joints, connective tissue 169
    lesion-specific 277
    matrix degradation 574
    specific diagnosis 205
    texture 215, 277
T-lymphocyte 305
tobacco 568
toed-out
    foot dysfunction 676
    gait and stance 76
toe-in gait 77
toes and fingers
    cold 220
tomatoes 568
Tong-style acupuncture 277, 288, 289, 350
    analogous areas 350
    bodily reflections 350
toothache 65
total body pain
    fibromyalgia 626

total range of movement 222
toxemia 632
Toxic-Heat 27
toxicity 262
Toxic-Qi 27
toxin and end feel 224
Toxins 15
Toyohari 285, 341
Traction and Distraction **504**
traditional Chinese medicine
    history 1
Tramadol
    fibromyalgia 624
transcutaneous 277
transform 41, 106
Transformative/congested-Fire 34, 39
Transformative/congested-Heat
transformative/congested-Heat 103, 105
    Bi 664
transforming growth factor beta 265
transitory ischemic attack 683
transport needling 294
transverse process 281
transverse processes (TrPrs) 185, 190
trapezius 683
    testing 516
trapped Heat 104
trauma 36, 57, 262, 333
    fibromyalgia 621
    foot dysfunction 674
traumatic 556
    arthritis 25, 209, 218, 542, **576**
        treatment 576
traumatic capsulitis 165
Traumeel
    nerve disorders 637
Treacher-Collins syndrome 344
Treatment of Blood Circulation **375**
Treatment of Painful Obstruction according to TCM Patterns **662**
Treatment Principles 261
    altering tensegrity 266
    abdominal assessment 333
        examination 338
        treatment 338
    Accumulating (Cleft/Xi) points 307
    adverse effects 292
    Alarm (Mu) points 308
    alter neural control 266
    ancillary techniques 368
    ankle points 347
    articulatory techniques 497
    auricular
        examination 345
        therapy 343
        therapy points 344
        therapy treatment 345
    back Shu (transport) points 307

balance and hold 484
balancing
    anterior and posterior 290
    left and right 289
    Qi and Blood 290
    top and bottom 289
    Yin Yang 289
Barrier (Guan) points 312
Blood stagnation 337
blood-letting 371
channel
    activation, downward draining 284
    obstruction 284
    therapies 276
    treatment design 276
Chapman's reflexes 498
cold therapy 371
commonly used Tong-Points, table 354
Connecting channels, network-vessels 299
contractile unit disorders 605
contraindication to manipulations 500
cupping 368
Dampness/Phlegm 338
deactivate trigger points 266
Divergent channels 300
dry needling purpose 265
dynamic functional techniques 484
electrical stimulation 431
electroacupuncture 277
Extra channels 303
facilitated positional release 489
Five Phases
    points 311
    Transporting points 311
four needle technique 314
frequency and number of treatments 291
general Reunion points 312
group Connecting points 311
Heart disorders 336
Hua Tuo Jia Ji points 308
Influential (Meeting) points 307, 309
inhibitory stimulatory techniques 458
integrated neuromuscular inhibition technique 489
ion cord 368
Kidney disorders 336
laser therapy 447
Liver disorders 336
locating points 284
long lever techniques 500
Lower Sea (He) Points 312
Lung disorders 335

Main channels 299
massage/manipulation 453
McKenzie system 526
meridian pulse diagnosis 341
metacarpal bone systems 346
mobilizations without impulse 453
moxibustion 369
muscle energy 489
myofascial-release 496
needling techniques 294
obtaining De-Qi 295
orthopedic integration, channels 277
osteopathic manipulation 460
pain all over 291
point
    gateways 304
    injection fluid acupuncture 296
positioning of patient 283
post treatment care 610
prolotherapy 297
provide blood growth factors 266
Qi circulation 283
rearranging tissue, restoring function 455
regional command points 312
release by countertension-positioning 487
rescue points 314
scraping 369
selecting techniques and points 286
separating adhesions breaking scars 455
serious complications, acupuncture 293
Sinew channels 300
Source points 304
Spleen/pancreas disorders 336
stabilization and exercise 543
status of patient's constitution 333
stimulate
    golgi receptors and muscle spindles 266
strengthen tendons and ligaments 265
subcutaneous fascia 587
tendon insufficiency 597
Tong/Lee-style Acupuncture **350**
    bleeding, cupping, and moxa techniques 356
    points 354
tonification and sedation techniques 295
wrist ankle
    acupuncture 347
    acupuncture selecting points 347
    needling techniques 347

    wrist points 347
Yang
    deficient constitution 334
    Linking (Wei) and Girdle (Dai) 338
    Motility (Qiao) and Governing (GV) 338
Yin
    deficient constitution 335
    Linking (Wei) and Penetrating (Chong) 338
    Motility (Qiao) and Conception (Ren) 338
tremors 6, 24, 77
triamcinolone 573
trigeminal neuralgia 211, 683
trigger points 144, 152, 266, 285, 333, 388, 590, **598**
    active 599
    activated 599
    energy crises 600
    dry needle 265
    examination 603
    false 599
    latent 599
    motor point 606
    primary 599
    referred pain 600
    satellite 599
    secondary 599
triggers 278
trigonum
    bursitis 658
Triple Warmer 18, 29, 39, 68, 81, 89, 585
    and Divergent channels 69
trochanteric
    bursitis 657
trophic factors 18, 174
tropocollagen molecules 169
true-Fire 81
true-Qi 13
    fibromyalgia 621
trusses 183, 201
tryptophan 86, 139
tubercular 681
tuberculi costae 194
tuberculosis 168, 243, 430, 595, 632
Tuina **453**
    commonly used techniques 458
tumors 77, 430
Turner's syndrome 344
twelve Main channels 65
twisted mouth 55
twitching 30, 55
Tylenol
    fibromyalgia 624
type
    I receptor 173

II receptor 127, 173
III receptor 173
IV receptor 173
3 collagen 169
typical cervical spine 194
Typical Pain Quality Descriptions, summery table 155
Typical TCM Intake Form 117
typical vertebrae 194

U

ulcerative colitis 333
ulcers 84, 424
ultrasound 250, 252, 605, 652
    fibromyalgia 624
ultraviolet 430
umbilicus 73
uncovertebral joint 195
unmyelinated 142, 143, 172
unrelated disease processes 106
upper arm 65
upper back 65
upper motor neuron 57, 210, 592
urethritis 74, 95
urgency 389
uric acid
    crystal 244
    level 243, 244
urinalysis 243
Urinary Bladder 18, 214, 305
urinary disorders 65
    infection and stone 681
    retention 72
    symptoms 82
    tract infection 245
urination 135
urine
    strip analysis 243
    tests 245
urogenital 73, 74
urtica dioica 575
uterus 73

V

vacuity of TCM systemic symptoms and signs 104
vacuum 368
vagal complex 134
vagus nerve 135, 279
validity score 205
valine 86
valvular aortic stenosis 222
varicose veins
    fibromyalgia 623
VAS score and fibromyalgia 625
vascular
    claudication 648, 649
    disorders 211, 683
    insufficiencies 219
    somatic dysfunction 562
vasoactive amines 143
vasoconstriction 589, 600
vasodilation 369
vasospasm 683
vasovagal reactions 293
vasulitis 588
vegan diet 569, 575
vegetative 86
veins 475
venenum bufonis 540
venous insufficiency 219
ventral horn 132, 133
ventrobasal thalamus 137
vertebral
    end plates 184
    movements 186
    pedicle 185
Vertebral Dysfunction, 231
    cervical 462
    hypertrophy, points 330
    lumbar 462
    noncapsular pattern 228
    thoracic 462
vertigo 65, 72, 79
Vessels 51
vessels 6
viral infections 681
viral syndrome 31
visceral 588
    afferent nerves 134
    function 282
    imaging 251
    reflex 233
viscerosomatic 141, 153, 563, 634
visible light 423
visual analog scale (VAS) **156**
vital essences 104
Vital Signs 212
vitamin
    B1 555
    B1, B6, B12 681
    B12 389, 553, 575
    B6 632
    C 85, 139, 169, 555, 568, 572, 681
        nerve disorders 637
    D 568, 572
    D excess 244
    d-alpha-tocopheryl acetate 572
    E 572, 568
    folic acid 569, 575, 681
    K deficiency 87
    niacinamide 568, 569
    pantothenic acid 85
volt 426
voltage 126, 268, 429
voluntary muscle guarding 589
vomiting 84, 87, 262, 385, 389
von Recklinghausen's disease 211, 683

W

Waddell signs 148
wandering pains 97
Warmi disease 5, 23, 28, 29, 96, 103
Warm-pestilential-Qi 26
Warm-toxins 29
Wasting Syndromes **593**
Water 48
Water/Fluid 39
Water-type people 336
waves 423
WDR cells 141
weakly ionizing 430
weakness 54, 65, 70, 78, 79, 84, 90, 97
    and tight muscles 599
    and atrophy of muscles, sinews and bones deficiency of Liver and Kidneys 415
    and stroke and acupuncture 593
weather 40
wedge 453
weight 212
weightbearing 188
West Haven-yale multidimensional pain inventory 156
Western Ontario and McMaster Universities osteoarthritis composite index 571
Whiplash 147, 579, **650**
    anterior longitudinal ligament 651, 652
    delay in symptoms 653
    esophagus 651
    headache 653
    longus
        colli 651
    progression of symptoms 653
    treatment of 654
    treatment of chronic-stage . 654
white blood cell 245, 389
wholistic 2
wide dynamic range (WDR) cells 131, 141, 142
willow bark 569, 575
Wilting syndromes 660
Wiltse's evaluation method 156
Wind-Cold-Damp
    Bi 660
Wind-Damp 368
Wind-Damp Obstruction
    Bi 663
Wind-Damp
    Bi 70
Wind-Damp-Cold
    Bi 663
Wind-Damp-Cold—Chronic Disease-Blood-stasis, Qi-stagnation
    Bi 665
Wind-Damp-Cold, Interior Heat
    Bi 664
Wind-Damp-ColdWeakness of Liver, Kidneys, Qi, and Blood

Bi 668
Wind-Damp-Heat Chronic Disease, Blood-stasis
    Bi 668
Wind-Phlegm 39
    paresthesia and numbness 633
Wind-Phlegm-Obstruction—Chronic Disease/ Numbness
    Bi 666
Wind-strike 594
Wind-tetany 26
windup 131, 141
wine 37
winging of the scapula 213
withania somnifera 569, 571
Wolf's Law 171, 180
Wood-type person 336
Worms, Parasites and Insect Bites 38
Wound Healing **553**
    bioelectric battery 553
    cytokines 553
    fibroblasts 554
    gamma-interferon 553
    ground substance 554
    hypothalamic cells 553
    interleukins 1 and 6 553
    tumor necrosis factor 553
Wrist and Ankle Acupuncture 347
wrist extensors 65
wrist flexion 65
Wrist Imaging 257

X
xanthine oxidase 569, 575
xerostomia 262
xiphoid 333
x-ray 39, 184, 205, 250, 378, 423, 430, 576
    collar of the scotty dog 253
    short leg 670
    vacuum sign 253
xylose 85

Y
Yang 39, 63, 283, 289, 429
    arm Sinews channel 301
    constitution 334
    leg Sinews channel 301
    Linking (Wei) channel 70
        accumulating points 307
        use 303
    Ming 57, 220, 221, 291, 350, 593
        LI and St 291
    Motility (Qiao) channel, 70, 214
        accumulating points 307
        balance left right 290
Yin 39, 63, 78, 283, 289, 429, 594
    arm Sinews channel 301
    Blood 26
    deficiency 29, 37, 38, 104, 166
        empty-Heat 220
    Fire 45
    Fluids 39
    leg Sinews channel 301
    Linking (Wei) channel
        accumulating points 307
        musculoskeletal use 303
    Motility (Qiao) channel, 70, 283, 290
        accumulating points 307
        balancing left and right 290
Yin Yang 19
    and biomedicine 21
    and muscles 22
    musculoskeletal medicine 21
Ying 286, 288
yoga 148
    nerve disorders 637
Yoshio Monaka's ion cord treatment of back 332
yucca 568

Z
zinc 571
Zink 86, 585
Zygapophysea Joints **185**
    cervical 195
    joint dysfunctions 561
    spine flexion 191

A note about the author

Alon Marcus received his licensed acupuncturist degree from the American College of Traditional Chinese Medicine in San Francisco, California in 1984, and his Doctor of Oriental Medicine degree from SAMRA University of Oriental Medicine in Los Angeles, California in 1986. He also trained in Japan and China, where he served his internship at the Traditional Chinese Medicine Municipal Hospital in Guangzhou. He studied Orthopaedic and Osteopathic medicines with several physicians through the American Association of Orthopaedic Medicine. Dr. Marcus has published numerous articles in both Eastern and Western medical journals and the books *Acute Abdominal Syndromes Their Diagnosis & Treatment According to Combined Chinese-Western Medicine* (Blue Poppy press 1991) and *Musculoskeletal Disorders: Healing Methods from Chinese Medicine, Orthopaedic Medicine and Osteopathy* (North Atlantic Books 1998). In 1995 he became a diplomate of the American Academy of Pain Management. He has lectured internationally and taught courses in complementary orthopedics for several years. In 1997 he was named Educator of the Year by the American Association of Oriental Medicine. Dr. Marcus is currently in private practice in Oakland, California.